American
Medical
Association

Family
Medical
Guide

Other Books by the American Medical Association

American Medical Association
Complete Medical Encyclopedia

American Medical Association
Diabetes Cookbook

American Medical Association
Healthy Heart Cookbook

American Medical Association
Complete Guide to Men's Health

American Medical Association
Guide to Talking to Your Doctor

American Medical Association
Guide to Home Caregiving

American Medical Association
Complete Guide to Your Children's Health

American Medical Association
Complete Guide to Women's Health

American Medical Association
Handbook of First Aid and Emergency Care

American Medical Association
Family Health Cookbook

American Medical Association
Essential Guide to Asthma

American Medical Association
Essential Guide to Depression

American Medical Association
Essential Guide to Hypertension

American Medical Association
Essential Guide to Menopause

American
Medical
Association

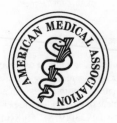

Family
Medical
Guide

Fourth Edition
Completely Revised and Updated

WILEY

John Wiley & Sons, Inc.

Published by John Wiley & Sons, Inc., Hoboken, New Jersey
Published simultaneously in Canada

Design and production by Navta Associates Inc.

Library of Congress Cataloging-in-Publication Data
American Medical Association family medical guide / American Medical
Association.
    p. cm.
 Includes bibliographical references and index.
 ISBN 0-471-26911-5 (cloth)
 1. Medicine, Popular. I. American Medical Association.
 RC81.A543 2004
 613—dc22

2004005764

Printed in the United States of America

10 9 8 7 6 5 4 3 2 1

Foreword

Every day, Americans hear news of the latest medical study or another medical breakthrough. These scientific advances, along with the latest techniques for diagnosing and treating diseases, are helping us live longer and in better health than ever before. With this all-new, completely revised fourth edition of our best-selling *American Medical Association Family Medical Guide,* you have the tools you need to make sense of this abundance of information, enabling you to take charge of your health and health-care needs and make informed medical decisions.

Reviewed by nearly 50 practicing physicians from a cross section of medical specialties and written in clear, easy-to-understand language, this guide provides up-to-date explanations about how specific diseases are diagnosed and treated. The book also explains what you can do to prevent many of the most common chronic diseases and how and why some lifestyle factors (such as diet and exercise—or smoking) can improve your health—or harm it.

We at the AMA believe that good medicine begins with a good patient-doctor relationship. This revised and updated edition of the *American Medical Association Family Medical Guide* will help you and your doctor work closely together to achieve years of good health for you and your family.

Michael D. Maves, MD, MBA
Executive Vice President, CEO
American Medical Association

American Medical Association

	Michael D. Maves, MD, MBA	*Executive Vice President, Chief Executive Officer*
	Robert A. Musacchio, PhD	*Senior Vice President, Publishing and Business Services*
	Anthony J. Frankos	*Vice President, Business Products*
	Mary Lou White	*Chief Operations Officer, AMA Press*
Editorial Staff	Donna Kotulak	*Managing Editor*
	Robin Husayko	*Senior Editor*
	Steve Michaels	*Senior Editor*
	Pam Brick	*Writer*
	Reuben Rios	*Copy Editor*
	Bonnie Chi-Lum, MD, MPH	*Medical Consultant*
	Thomas Houston, MD	*Medical Consultant*
	James J. James, MD	*Medical Consultant*
Illustrations	Mary Ann Albanese	*Art Editor*
	Howard S. Friedman	*Illustrator*
	Kristen Wienandt, CMI	*Illustrator*
Medical Consultants	Kevin P. Bethke, MD	*Surgical Oncology*
	Alan L. Buchman, MD, MSPH	*Gastroenterology/Nutrition*
	Richard Kleven Burt, MD	*Immunotherapy*
	Barbara K. Burton, MD	*Medical Genetics*
	Bruce A. Cohen, MD	*Neurology*
	Suzanne D. Conzen, MD	*Medical Oncology*
	Arthur W. Curtis, MD	*Otolaryngology/Head and Neck Surgery*
	Bruce B. Dan, MD	*Infectious Diseases*
	William J. Frericks, DDS	*General Dentistry*
	Edward R. Garrity, Jr, MD	*Pulmonary/Critical Care*
	David Grinblatt, MD	*Hematology/Oncology*
	Parul Gupta, MD	*Obstetrics and Gynecology*
	Paula J. Harper, LCSW, CADC, CST	*Sex Therapy*
	Philip C. Hoffman, MD	*Hematology/Oncology*
	Cameron Jarrett, MFA	*Fitness Specialist*
	Linda S. Katz, MD	*Obstetrics and Gynecology*
	Rae-Ellen W. Kavey, MD	*Pediatric Cardiology*
	Armen Kelikian, MD	*Orthopedics*
	Karen Koffler, MD	*Internal Medicine/Integrative Medicine*
	Alan R. Leff, MD	*Internal Medicine/Pulmonary Medicine*
	Jerrold Blair Leikin, MD	*Medical Toxicology*
	Gary S. Lissner, MD	*Ophthalmology*
	Fred N. Littooy, MD	*Peripheral Vascular Surgery*
	Magdy Milad, MD, MS	*Reproductive Endocrinology/Infertility*

G. Martin Mullen, MD	*Heart Transplant/Cardiology*
Yu Oyama, MD	*Hematology/Oncology*
Jay Pensler, MD	*Plastic Surgery*
Angela R. Perry, MD	*Internal Medicine*
Louis Philipson, MD	
Endocrinology/Diabetes/Metabolism	
Arthur V. Prancan, PhD	*Pharmacology*
Anthony Thomas Reder, MD	*Neurology*
June K. Robinson, MD	*Dermatology*
Miriam Rodin, MD	*Geriatrics*
Eric Michael Ruderman, MD	*Rheumatology*
Mark J. Schacht, MD	*Urology*
Michael J. Schrift, DO	*Psychiatry*
Irwin M. Siegel, MD	*Orthopedics*
Ramona Slupik, MD	*Gynecology and Obstetrics*
Matthew Sorrentino, MD	*Cardiology*
Kerstin Stenson, MD	*Otolaryngology/Head and Neck*
Surgery	
Wendy Stock, MD	*Hematology/Oncology*
Edward S. Traisman, MD	*Pediatrics*
Ann Traynor, MD	*Hematology/Oncology/Immune*
Therapy	
Linda Van Horn, PhD, RD	*Nutrition*
Cheryl Lynn Walker, MD	*Allergy/Immunology*
Neil Warshawsky, DDS	*Orthodontics*
Dorothy Wawrose, MD	*Infectious Diseases*
Kimberly Ann Workowski, MD	*Infectious Diseases*
Seiko Diane Yamada, MD	*Gynecologic Oncology*
Charles Zugerman, MD	*Dermatology*

Contents

How to Use This Book

A wealth of information on health and disease is at your fingertips in this totally revised and updated fourth edition of the *American Medical Association Family Medical Guide*. To get the most benefit from the book, take some time to familiarize yourself with it—in terms of general information and specific health questions you may have. First, scan the Table of Contents on pages ix through xii for a quick overview of how the book is organized.

When looking up a topic, start with the index. The index contains multiple cross-references to many entries to make it easier for you to find the information you need.

Part One: What You Should Know: Information to Keep You Healthy

Part One is an all-new, full-color section that highlights and illustrates the most important current health issues, including preventive health topics such as nutrition, exercise, weight, and stress reduction, and cutting-edge information about cancer and genetics.

Part Two: Your Healthy Body

Part Two is a completely revised and expanded section that presents up-to-date information on preventive medicine. Families need accurate, easy-to-understand recommendations on topics that are critical to their long-term health. You will learn how and why lifestyle factors—for example, eating a healthy diet, exercising regularly, maintaining a healthy weight, reducing stress, and getting sufficient sleep—have such a profound effect on your health.

Between chapters 7 and 8, you'll find a 32-page full-color section. This section contains an Atlas of the Body, Diagnostic Imaging Techniques, and Visual Aids to Diagnosis. The Atlas is a handy reference for locating bones, muscles, and other parts of the body. Diagnostic Imaging Techniques explains the different types of diagnostic imaging procedures your doctor might recommend, such as ultrasound and magnetic resonance imaging (MRI). This section describes how each diagnostic test is done and which disorders the test might help diagnose. Visual Aids to Diagnosis presents photos of sores, rashes, and other recognizable signs and symptoms, along with brief descriptions of the disorders or conditions to which they might be linked.

Part Three: First Aid and Home Caregiving

Part Three focuses on two important topics—First Aid and Home Caregiving. The First Aid section provides step-by-step advice on how to handle injuries and emergencies including choking, bleeding, burns, and heatstroke. The Home Caregiving section gives practical information to help you take care of a person who is ill or disabled. For example, you will learn how to modify your home to make it easier for you to care for an older family member who has a disabling chronic illness such as Alzheimer's disease.

Part Four: What Are Your Symptoms?

The popular and always-helpful symptoms charts have been completely revised and updated for this edition. Organized like flow charts, the symptoms charts direct you through a series of questions with yes or no answers from a specific symptom to reach a possible diagnosis or recommendation. The charts help you decide when it's important to call your doctor about a problem, when to go to a hospital emergency department immediately, or when to take care of the problem yourself at home.

The symptoms charts contain many cross-references to articles in other parts of the book, especially to Part Five (Health Issues Throughout Life) and Part Six (Diseases, Disorders, and Other Problems). To make the best use of the symptoms charts and to obtain a full explanation of a specific disorder or condition, follow the cross-references to the articles.

Part Five: Health Issues Throughout Life

Part Five is an all-new section that discusses common health concerns that can occur at any time of life. This section has comprehensive chapters on children's health, adolescent health, sexuality, infertility, pregnancy and childbirth, and dying and death. Part Five and Part Six (Diseases, Disorders, and Other Problems), which are both packed with helpful information, are the heart of the book.

Part Six: Diseases, Disorders, and Other Problems

You will probably use Part Six more than any other part of the book because this is where you will find information about hundreds of diseases and disorders. To make it easy for you to find the information you're looking for, the chapters in this part of the book are arranged by body system. The articles in these chapters have an easy-to-follow, straightforward format that usually includes the following headings: Symptoms (describes the most common symptoms and signs of the disorder), Diagnosis (explains how the disorder is diagnosed), Treatment (explores the treatment options for the disorder), and Prevention (tells how the disorder can be prevented, when prevention is possible).

Within the articles on specific diseases, you will also find cross-references to other parts of the book. Use these cross-references, along with the index, to add to your knowledge of or improve your understanding about a particular health problem or concern.

Glossaries

This section contains a general Glossary and a Drug Glossary. The general Glossary defines some common medical terms you might hear or read. The Drug Glossary has two sections—a section on drug classes (the groups into which drugs are categorized) and a section on the top 200 prescription drugs.

American
Medical
Association

Family
Medical
Guide

PART ONE

What You Should Know

Information to Keep You Healthy

Healthy Eating

A wealth of information exists about the fundamental link between diet and health. Although many people think that healthy eating means flavorless, unsatisfying meals, this does not have to be the case. A healthy diet includes plenty of vegetables, fruits, whole grains, legumes, and other high-fiber, high-nutrient foods; supplies the right number of calories; and limits saturated fat and trans fats (such as those found in stick margarine), salt, sugar, and alcohol. The components of a healthy diet translate easily into delicious meals that can appeal to the whole family. For more about a nutritious diet, see pages 35 to 44.

Eat Five a Day for Better Health

We have all heard from experts that eating at least five fruits and vegetables each day is one of the most important things we can do for our health, but only one out of four of us is actually eating this amount. Fruits and vegetables provide a wide assortment of vitamins and minerals, including the antioxidant vitamins—vitamin C, the carotenoids (beta carotene, lycopene, and lutein), and vitamin E—which fight cell damage from free radicals, a major cause of aging and most chronic diseases. Fruits and vegetables also provide fiber, an essential nutrient that promotes healthy bowel function and helps lower the risk of heart disease and some types of cancer. Fruits and vegetables are so good-tasting and so good for you that you should try to consume as many as you can. Five servings a day is the minimum for keeping you healthy (10 a day is better). Here are some tips to help you get your daily dose of fruits and veggies:

- Have one or two servings of fruit at breakfast every day.
- Choose a fruit or vegetable for a snack.
- Have a salad at lunch.
- Stock up on dried, canned, and frozen fruits and vegetables.
- Serve more than one vegetable for dinner.

Eat your colors

Fruits and vegetables come in an array of colors, and the color of a food usually says something about its nutritional value. Each food color confers specific health benefits, so consuming a variety of fruits and vegetables provides the biggest health gains.

BLUES AND PURPLES

Blueberries, blackberries, purple grapes, plums, raisins, and eggplants give you:
- A reduced risk of some cancers
- A healthy urinary tract
- A sharp memory
- A long, healthy life

GREENS

Kiwi, honeydew melons, spinach, broccoli, romaine lettuce, kale, green peas, brussels sprouts, cabbage, and Swiss chard give you:
- Strong bones and teeth
- Good eyesight
- A reduced risk of some cancers

WHITES

Pears, apples, bananas, jicama, mushrooms, cauliflower, onions, and garlic give you:
- A healthy heart
- A good cholesterol profile
- A reduced risk of some cancers

REDS

Watermelon, strawberries, raspberries, cranberries, cherries, tomatoes, and radishes give you:
- A sharp memory
- A healthy heart
- A healthy urinary tract
- A reduced risk of some cancers

YELLOWS AND ORANGES

Oranges, grapefruit, peaches, cantaloupe, mangoes, pineapples, yellow and winter squash, carrots, and corn give you:
- A healthy heart
- A healthy immune system
- Good eyesight
- A reduced risk of some cancers

Reading Food Labels

Nutrition facts panel

The nutrition facts panel is the part of a food package label that lists serving size, the number of servings in the package, the number of calories in a serving, and the percent of daily values (which are the same as the recommended daily allowances) of many important nutrients—fats, carbohydrates, protein, cholesterol, fiber, sugar, sodium, vitamins A and C, and the minerals iron and calcium (no daily values have been set for protein and sugar).

What you can learn from food labels

1 To make it easy to compare different brands of the same food, all serving sizes are required to be the same.

2 This line shows the total calories in one serving and the number of calories from fat contained in the serving.

3 This section displays the amounts of different nutrients in one serving so you can easily compare the nutrient content of similar products and add up the total amounts of a given nutrient that you eat in a day.

4 The percent of daily values are indicated for each nutrient. Percent of daily values are based on a diet of 2,000 calories per day.

5 This area shows the percent of daily values for vitamins A and C and the minerals iron and calcium.

6 This section helps you calculate your daily allowance of various fats, sodium, carbohydrates, and fiber for both a 2,000- and a 2,500-calorie-per-day diet.

7 The number of calories in 1 gram of fat (9), carbohydrate (4), and protein (4) are listed here.

8 The federal government has approved the use of certain health claims on packaged foods. Examples include:

- A diet low in fat and rich in fruits and vegetables may reduce your risk of some cancers.
- A diet rich in fruits, vegetables, and grains may reduce the risk of heart disease.
- A low intake of calcium is one risk factor for osteoporosis.

9 Terms such as "low," "high," and "free" on food labels must meet strict definitions. For example, a food described as "very low sodium" must have no more than 35 milligrams of sodium for every 50 grams of food.

Nutrition Facts

Serving Size 1/2 cup (114 g)
Servings Per Container 4 — 1

Amount Per Serving — 2

Calories 90	Calories from Fat 30

	% Daily Value*
Total Fat 3 g	5%
Saturated Fat 0 g	0%
Cholesterol 0 mg	0%
Sodium 300 mg	13%
Total Carbohydrate 13 g	4%
Dietary Fiber 3 g	12%
Sugars 3 g	
Protein 3 g	

3 ... 4

Vitamin A 80%	■	Vitamin C 60%
Calcium 4%	■	Iron 4%

5

* Percent Daily Values are based on a 2,000 calorie diet. Your daily values may be higher or lower depending on your calorie needs.

	Calories	2,000	2,500
Total Fat	Less than	65 g	80 g
Saturated Fat	Less than	20 g	25 g
Cholesterol	Less than	300 mg	300 mg
Sodium	Less than	2,400 mg	2,400 mg
Total Carbohydrate		300 g	375 g
Dietary Fiber		25 g	30 g

6

Calories per gram: — 7
Fat 9 • Carbohydrate 4 • Protein 4

8 *Many factors affect cancer risk. Eating a diet low in fat and high in fiber may lower risk of this disease.*

9 ☐ GOOD SOURCE OF FIBER
☐ LOW FAT

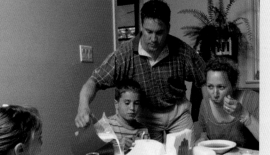

Shared family meals serve up benefits
Eating together as a family improves communication, promotes a strong family bond, and gives children a secure sense of belonging. Shared meals also save money.

Vitamins and Minerals

This table describes the health benefits of the most important vitamins and minerals and some of the foods that contain these nutrients. Vitamins are divided into two categories—fat-soluble and water-soluble. Fat-soluble vitamins are found in fats and oils in foods and are stored in body fat. Water-soluble vitamins dissolve in water and mix easily in the blood. Your body stores only small amounts of water-soluble vitamins (the excess is eliminated in urine). Some vitamins are antioxidants, which protect against damage to cells by free radicals (molecules formed by normal cell processes). Antioxidants can help protect against disease and aging. The best way to get the vitamins and minerals your body needs is to eat a varied diet rich in low-fat, high-fiber vegetables, fruits, legumes, and whole grains; fish; and low-fat dairy products, poultry, and meats.

Vitamin or mineral	Good sources	Health benefits
FAT-SOLUBLE VITAMINS		
Vitamin A	Fortified milk, eggs, cheese, butter, liver, cod and halibut, fish oil	Antioxidant; essential for growth and development; maintains healthy vision, skin, and mucous membranes.
Vitamin D	Salmon, mackerel, fortified milk	Builds bones and teeth; helps the body absorb and use calcium.
Vitamin E	Vegetable oils, whole grains, wheat germ, nuts, green leafy vegetables	Antioxidant; anti-inflammatory; helps form blood cells, muscles, and lung and nerve tissue; boosts the immune system; may help prevent heart disease.
Vitamin K	Dark green leafy vegetables, liver, egg yolks	Essential for blood clotting.
Beta carotene	Orange and deep yellow vegetables and fruits (carrots, sweet potatoes, winter squash, cantaloupe, pumpkins, mangoes); the body converts beta carotene in yellow and orange vegetables and fruits and some dark green leafy vegetables (such as spinach and broccoli) into vitamin A	Antioxidant; used by the body to make vitamin A.
WATER-SOLUBLE VITAMINS		
Vitamin C	Citrus fruits, kiwi, vegetables (tomatoes, bell peppers, cabbage), leafy green vegetables	Antioxidant; keeps bones, teeth, and skin healthy; helps wounds heal.
Thiamin (vitamin B1)	Fortified cereals and breads, whole grains, pork, liver, peas	Helps convert food into energy.
Riboflavin (vitamin B2)	Meats, fish, fortified cereals and breads, whole grains, milk products, dark green vegetables	Helps in energy production and other chemical processes in the body; helps maintain healthy eyes, skin, and nerve function.
Niacin (vitamin B3)	Whole grains, fortified cereals, milk products, pork, poultry, fish, nuts, broccoli, green peas, green beans	Helps convert food into energy; helps maintain brain function.

Vitamin or mineral	Good sources	Health benefits
Vitamin B6	Fortified cereals, whole-wheat products, meat, fish, nuts, green beans, bananas, green leafy vegetables, potatoes	Helps produce essential proteins; helps convert protein into energy.
Vitamin B12	Dairy products, eggs, liver, animal products	Helps convert carbohydrates into energy; helps form red blood cells and maintain the central nervous system; helps make amino acids (the building blocks of proteins).
Folic acid (folate)	Orange juice; dark green leafy vegetables; fruits; dried beans, lentils, and peas; liver	Essential in the first 3 months of pregnancy for preventing birth defects; helps form red blood cells; protects against heart disease by lowering the level of the chemical homocysteine in the blood.
MINERALS		
Calcium	Dairy products, fortified orange juice, fortified cereals and breads, fortified soy milk, legumes, canned fish (with edible bones), dark green leafy vegetables	Builds bones and teeth and maintains bone strength; helps control blood pressure; important in muscle function.
Chromium	Whole grains, bran cereals, green beans, broccoli, spices, processed meats	Enhances the effects of the hormone insulin in converting sugar, protein, and fat into energy.
Copper	Oysters, nuts, legumes, whole grains, vegetables, red meat	Essential for making hemoglobin (oxygen-carrying protein in red blood cells); helps body absorb and use iron; helps in energy production; keeps bones, blood, and nerves healthy.
Iron	Red meat, poultry, fish, dried beans, nuts, dried fruits, whole-grain and enriched grain products	Helps in energy production; helps carry oxygen in the bloodstream and deliver it to muscles.
Magnesium	Leafy green vegetables, nuts, whole grains, dried peas and beans, dairy products, fish, red meat, poultry	Essential for healthy nerve and muscle function and for bone formation; helps prevent irregular heartbeat; helps lower blood pressure.
Phosphorus	Red meat, dairy products, poultry, fish	Essential for building strong bones and teeth; promotes activity of genes and cells; helps produce and store energy.
Potassium	Bananas, oranges, and other fruits; potatoes and other starchy vegetables; nuts; seeds	Essential for maintaining balance of body fluids, transmitting nerve signals, and producing energy; may help lower blood pressure and prevent irregular heartbeat.
Selenium	Fish, red meat, Brazil nuts	Antioxidant; essential for healthy functioning of the heart and the immune system.
Sodium	Table salt, processed foods, canned soups	Essential for maintaining normal blood pressure and the balance of body fluids and for transmitting nerve signals.
Zinc	Fortified cereals and breads, shellfish, red meat, legumes, nuts, eggs, yogurt	Promotes cell reproduction, growth, and development, the immune response, nervous system function, reproduction, and wound healing.

Exercise

Physical activity plays a crucial role in health. Regular exercise protects against the most common disorders—including heart disease, stroke, high blood pressure, obesity, type 2 diabetes, osteoporosis, colon cancer, and depression—and can help you live longer. Still, more than 60 percent of adults in the US fail to get the minimum recommended amount of exercise: half an hour to an hour of moderate activity such as brisk walking on most days of the week. You don't have to do it all at one time: break up the time into 10- or 15-minute sessions scattered throughout the day. The activity you engage in doesn't have to be strenuous to provide health benefits, especially if you have been inactive for some time. Of course, the more vigorous the activity, the more you will get out of it, but what is most important is becoming more active.

The Benefits of Exercise

If exercise were packaged in a pill, it would be the No. 1 prescribed medication in the US—and Americans would be much healthier. Even a small increase in your physical activity can substantially reduce your health risks, especially if you have been inactive. More activity—or activity that is more vigorous—will pay even bigger rewards. In addition, regular exercise provides the following health advantages:

- Lowers your risk of premature death.
- Reduces your risk of heart disease, high blood pressure, diabetes, and some cancers.
- Makes your heart pump more efficiently.
- Fights depression and anxiety.
- Improves strength, flexibility, and balance.
- Helps you maintain a healthy weight.
- Tones your muscles.
- Helps control your appetite.

Fit Exercise Into Your Life

When you look at your busy life, a lot of things seem more important than exercise: your job, chauffeuring your kids to various activities, managing your household, or taking care of aging parents. And a lack of time may not be the only factor. Having too little money or social support—even bad weather—can all conspire against your best intentions to exercise. Here are some tips that might make it easier for you to begin an exercise program and stick with it:

- Choose an exercise you enjoy.
- Schedule time for exercise.
- Find a workout buddy or take an exercise class.
- Vary your activities to avoid boredom.
- Fight inertia by remembering how good exercise makes you feel.

  If you don't want to join a health club or can't make the time for a long workout several times a week, try to incorporate exercise into your daily life in the following ways to accumulate 30 to 60 minutes of exercise every day:

- Climb up and down several flights of stairs at work once or twice a day.
- Take a brisk walk after dinner.
- Walk the dog.
- Pull your children around the neighborhood in a wagon or sled.
- Go to the local mall and walk.
- Park in a parking space farther from the store or office and walk to the building.
- Carry or push a golf bag instead of using a golf cart.
- Wash and wax the car.
- Do yard work.
- Clean the house.
- Jump rope.
- Mow the lawn with a hand mower.
- Lift hand weights, or do lunges, push-ups, and jumping jacks while you watch TV.
- On the weekends, organize a family bike ride, hike, or ball game. Go swimming, ice skating, or in-line skating together. Go dancing.

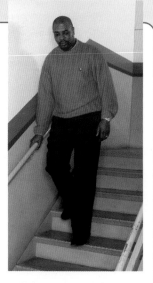

Making time for exercise
It's easier to fit exercise into your busy schedule if you make it part of your daily routine. Try walking up and down several flights of stairs at work every day. It takes only a few minutes and it strengthens your heart, lungs, and bones.

- Keeps your mind sharp.
- Makes you look better.
- Boosts your self-confidence.

Three Types of Exercise

Three different types of exercise—aerobic, flexibility, and strengthening—help you achieve different kinds of physical fitness. Aerobic exercise (such as walking, jogging, and cycling) increases your heart rate to deliver more oxygen to your muscles. Strengthening exercises (such as lifting weights and doing push-ups) build muscle and bone to increase strength. Flexibility exercises (such as stretching or yoga) improve your ability to move your joints through their full range of motion. Including all three types of activity in your exercise regimen will help you reach a high overall level of fitness that can improve your health and reduce your risk of several of the most common chronic diseases, including heart disease and diabetes.

Choosing activities you enjoy will help you stay with your exercise program. Variety is the key, so don't limit yourself to one activity. Jog one day and swim or bike the next. Work out with weights one day and use a stair-climbing machine the next day. Vary your stretching exercises as well. Not only will you maintain your enthusiasm for exercising, you will also be less likely to get injured.

Aerobic exercise

Aerobic exercise includes any activity that uses the large muscles, such as those in the legs, in repetitive motion that can be sustained over a long period. Examples of aerobic activity include walking, jogging, cycling, swimming, skating, cross-country skiing, and stair climbing. Aerobic exercise causes your heart and lungs to work more efficiently as they supply more and more oxygen-rich blood to your working muscles. Aerobic exercise builds endurance and provides a number of other important health benefits, including:

- Improved heart and lung function
- Reduced heart rate
- Lower blood pressure
- Higher blood levels of HDL (good) cholesterol
- Reduced body fat
- Improved weight control
- Increased bone strength
- Improved sleep

Aerobic exercise changes your body composition by lowering your body's percentage of fat and increasing its percentage of muscle, giving you a toned, fitter body. Aerobic exercise also protects against several of the most common chronic health problems, including heart disease, high blood pressure, diabetes, osteoporosis, and some cancers.

If you have been inactive, start your aerobic exercise program with walking. Walking is an excellent aerobic activity that is low impact (and therefore safe for your joints), builds cardiovascular fitness and bone strength, and requires only a pair of sturdy, well-cushioned shoes. At first, try walking 10 to 15 minutes a day on most days of the week. After you build your endurance, add 5 minutes to your daily walking time each week until you can walk up to 30 to 60 minutes a day. You don't have to do all of your walking in one session. Break up the activity into shorter sessions that add up to 30 to 60 total minutes. Walk with a friend or relative so you can encourage each other to stick with the program.

To determine whether you're working out at the right level of intensity, make sure you are exercising at your target heart rate (see page 47), the pulse rate that is best for your age and overall physical condition. Try to do some aerobic exercise on most days of the week. Warm up and cool down before and after you exercise. And remember that the health benefits of aerobic exercise remain only as long as you continue exercising. That is why your goal should be to develop an exercise program that you can stay with for the rest of your life.

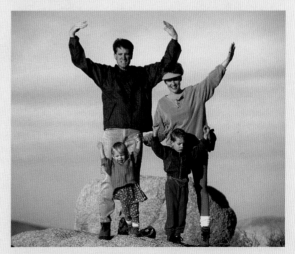

Make exercise a family habit
Exercising together as a family will not only increase your and your children's endurance, build stronger bones, and improve your overall health, it will also help forge a strong family bond. Include physical activities such as hiking in your family vacations.

Flexibility exercises

Flexibility is the ability to move your muscles and joints through their full range of motion. Some people are naturally more flexible than others, but you can always improve your flexibility with exercises that stretch specific muscles. Increased flexibility improves your ability to perform everyday activities, protects your muscles against pulls and tears, and helps relieve arthritis pain. It's important to do stretches gently and slowly—don't bounce. Do each stretch three times for maximum benefit.

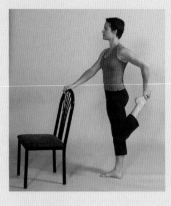

Hip flexor/Quadriceps stretch
While standing, hold on to a sturdy chair back, a counter, or a railing with one hand. Bend one leg and, with the hand on that side, pull your foot up gently behind you, keeping your abdominal muscles pulled in and your knees close together. Maintain the position for at least 30 seconds. Repeat with the other leg.

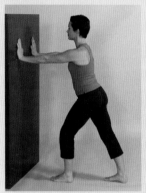
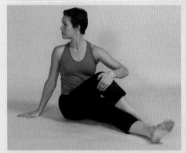

Calf stretch
Stand about 2 to 3 feet from a wall and place your palms on the wall. Step forward with one foot. Keeping both feet flat on the floor and your toes pointing straight ahead, bend the forward leg at the knee and lean forward, keeping your back leg straight (far left). Maintain the position for at least 30 seconds. Repeat with the other leg. Now do a set bending (rather than straightening) the back leg (left); maintain the position for at least 30 seconds.

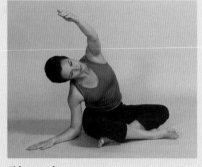

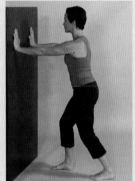

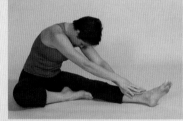

Side stretch
Sit cross-legged on the floor. Inhale and raise one arm to the ceiling and, exhaling, bend from the waist to the opposite side, sliding the other hand along the floor and keeping your buttocks on the floor. Maintain the stretch for at least 30 seconds. Inhale as you return to center, dropping your raised arm and lifting the other arm and repeating the bend to the other side.

Hamstring stretch
Sit with one leg extended in front of you and the other leg bent. Reach forward with both hands along your extended leg as far as it feels comfortable. Bend from your hips, keeping your back straight. Maintain the position for at least 30 seconds. Repeat with the other leg.

Back twist
Sit with your legs out in front of you on the floor. Cross one leg over the other with your knee bent and your foot flat on the floor. Keeping your back straight and your buttocks on the floor, take hold of the bent knee with the opposite hand and gently turn to the bent-knee side, rotating your hips and looking over your shoulder. Maintain the stretch for at least 30 seconds. Repeat on the other side.

Lower back and buttocks stretch
Lie on your back on the floor with one leg stretched out straight and the other leg bent. Pressing your lower back gently to the floor, reach behind the thigh of the bent leg and pull it slowly toward your chest. Maintain the position for at least 30 seconds and release. Repeat with the other leg.

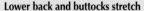
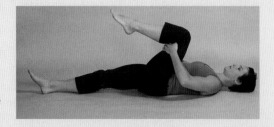

Strengthening exercises

Strength-conditioning exercise is as beneficial for your heart as aerobic exercise, and is essential for keeping you fit and independent as you age. These exercises build muscle by forcing the muscles to work against the weight of your body or an object such as a weight. It's a good idea to alternate strength-building exercises with aerobic exercise. Try to do the following exercises three times a week.

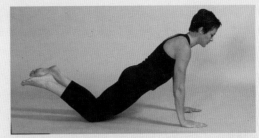

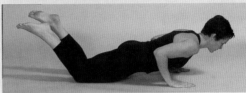

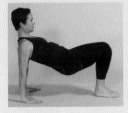 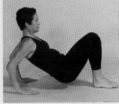

Triceps press
Sit on the floor with your knees bent at a 45-degree angle, your feet flat on the floor, hip-distance apart, and your hands on the floor behind you, fingertips pointing forward. Lift your hips off the floor (left). Bending at the elbows, lower your bottom until it almost touches the floor (right), hold for a count of five, and straighten the arms, returning to hips-up position. Do ten sets.

Modified push-up
Get on your hands and knees on the floor and shift your weight forward, with your hands aligned under your shoulders and your feet raised off the floor (top). Bending your elbows, lower your body from the knees up until your chest almost touches the floor, keeping your hands in the same position on the floor and using your abdominal muscles to keep your back straight (bottom). Still keeping your back straight, push up until your arms are almost straight (but not locked) at the elbows. Repeat as many times as you can without straining. (For an extra challenge, try holding each position for a few seconds.)

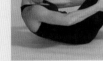

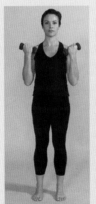 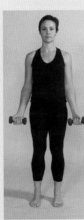

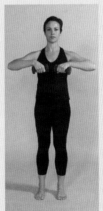 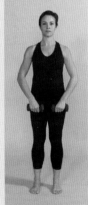

Abdominal curl
Lie on your back with your knees bent and your arms holding the backs of your thighs. Press the small of your back to the floor as you lift your head and upper body until most of your upper back is off the floor. Hold for a count of two. Lower your body to the floor, keeping the small of your back pressed to the floor to work your abdominal muscles and avoid straining your back. As your strength increases, increase the number of repetitions. A more difficult way to do sit-ups is with your arms over your chest and your hands on your shoulders, or with your hands placed lightly behind your neck.

Biceps curl
Standing with your back straight, your knees bent slightly, and your feet slightly apart, hold two hand weights (begin with 1- or 2-pound weights) up to your shoulders, with your elbows bent up at your sides (left). Slowly bring the weights down to your thighs, palms turned out (right). Slowly raise the weights back up to your shoulders, keeping your elbows at your sides. When you can repeat the exercise 12 times, increase the weights by 1 pound.

Pump-up
Standing with your back straight, knees bent slightly and feet slightly apart, hold two hand weights (with ends touching each other) at chest level, elbows bent out to the sides parallel to the floor and shoulders down (left). Lower the weights slowly to thigh level, keeping the ends of the weights together (right). Slowly raise the weights back up to your chest. When you can repeat the exercise 12 times, increase the weights by 1 pound.

Are You at a Healthy Weight?

The percentage of overweight Americans has been steadily increasing over the past several decades. Nearly two out of three adults and about 15 percent of children in the US are overweight. Most alarming, overweight children and adolescents are developing common chronic illnesses—such as heart disease, high blood pressure, and type 2 diabetes—that used to affect only adults.

Body weight results from the complex interaction of inherited, physical, behavioral, socioeconomic, and cultural factors. The major factors contributing to overweight are basic—eating too much and exercising too little. And many Americans tend to eat the wrong kinds of foods: foods that are highly refined, high in salt, and often high in saturated and trans fats and calories and low in fiber.

Health Risks of Being Overweight

Being overweight increases your risk of a number of chronic health problems, including heart disease, high blood pressure, diabetes, and some cancers. The way in which fat is distributed on your body can also increase your health risks. You are at greater risk of health problems if you tend to accumulate fat around your abdomen than if you tend to accumulate fat around your hips and thighs. The risks increase further if your waist is 35 inches or larger (if you're a woman) or 40 inches or larger (if you're a man). To determine if you are overweight, check the BMI chart on the next page. To determine if your child is overweight, have him or her evaluated by the doctor. Your doctor can work with you to develop an effective weight-loss plan.

How to Achieve and Maintain a Healthy Weight

Losing weight and keeping it off is difficult, so it's important to set realistic goals that you can achieve and maintain. If you are overweight, even a moderate reduction in body weight—as little as 10 percent—can significantly improve your health.

The only healthy way to lose weight is to use more calories than you take in. For most people, this means eating less and being more physically active. Losing weight gradually—no more than 1 or 2 pounds per week—improves your chances of keeping it off successfully. Changing your diet and exercise habits gradually will help you to make those changes a permanent part of your life.

Avoid fad diets that promise quick weight loss. Any diet that sounds too good to be true probably is. For more information about losing weight, see page 53.

Be Active

Regular exercise contributes to weight loss, especially when combined with a healthy diet. In addition to weight control, regular exercise helps reduce blood pressure, helps prevent heart disease, helps control cholesterol and blood sugar levels, slows bone loss associated with aging, lowers the risk of some types of cancer, and helps relieve anxiety and depression.

When beginning an exercise program, choose activities you enjoy and can easily fit into your day. Begin exercising slowly, and gradually increase the intensity of your workouts. For example, begin with a 10-minute walk three times a week and work your way up to 30 to 60 minutes of brisk walking five times a week.

If you find it difficult to set aside an entire hour for exercise each day, try scheduling shorter exercise sessions—for example, two or three 20-minute sessions a day. If you miss a day or two, don't be discouraged. Return to your exercise routine as soon as you can. To learn more about what regular exercise can do for you and your family, read the chapter Exercise, Fitness, and Health starting on page 45. Get all members of your family into an active lifestyle:

- Make time for the entire family to participate in regular physical activities that everyone enjoys. Try walking, biking, playing tennis, or in-line skating.
- Plan active family vacations such as hiking, camping, or skiing trips.
- Assign active household chores to every family member, such as vacuuming, mowing the lawn, or washing the car.
- Encourage all family members to enroll in a structured physical activity such as tennis, martial arts, gymnastics, or dancing.
- Limit sedentary activities such as watching TV, playing video games, and surfing the Internet.

Body Mass Index

Body mass index (BMI) is a calculated score that indicates the healthiness of a person's weight. Although the BMI does not directly evaluate body fat percentage, the formula is related to the amount of fat a person carries and is calculated using the person's height and weight. BMI can help determine a person's health risks and is a generally reliable health gauge for people between ages 19 and 70. The index is less reliable, however, for competitive athletes or body builders (who may have a high BMI but whose body is made up mostly of muscle) and for women who are pregnant or breastfeeding.

What's your BMI?

To learn your body mass index (BMI), find your height in the left-hand column in the chart below and read across the row from your height until you reach your weight. Then look at the number at the bottom of your weight column—this is your BMI. In general, the higher your BMI, the higher your health risks.

A healthy BMI is between 18.5 and 24.9. You are considered underweight if your BMI is less than 18.5, overweight if your BMI is between 25 and 29.9, and obese if your BMI is 30 or higher. The risks are even higher in men whose waist is larger than 40 inches and in women whose waist is larger than 35 inches.

Body Mass Index

Height	Body Weight (pounds)													
4'10"	91	96	100	105	110	115	119	124	129	134	138	143	167	191
4'11"	94	99	104	109	114	119	124	128	133	138	143	148	173	198
5'	97	102	107	112	118	123	128	133	138	143	148	153	179	204
5'1"	100	106	111	116	122	127	132	137	143	148	153	158	185	211
5'2"	104	109	115	120	126	131	136	142	147	153	158	164	191	218
5'3"	107	113	118	124	130	135	141	146	152	158	163	169	197	225
5'4"	110	116	122	128	134	140	145	151	157	163	169	174	204	232
5'5"	114	120	126	132	138	144	150	156	162	168	174	180	210	240
5'6"	118	124	130	136	142	148	155	161	167	173	179	186	216	247
5'7"	121	127	134	140	146	153	159	166	172	178	185	191	223	255
5'8"	125	131	138	144	151	158	164	171	177	184	190	197	230	262
5'9"	128	135	142	149	155	162	169	176	182	189	196	203	236	270
5'10"	132	139	146	153	160	167	174	181	188	195	202	209	243	278
5'11"	136	143	150	157	165	172	179	186	193	200	208	215	250	286
6'	140	147	154	162	169	177	184	191	199	206	213	221	258	294
6'1"	144	151	159	166	174	182	189	197	204	212	219	227	265	302
6'2"	148	155	163	171	179	186	194	202	210	218	225	233	272	311
6'3"	152	160	168	176	184	192	200	208	216	224	232	240	279	319
6'4"	156	164	172	180	189	197	205	213	221	230	238	246	287	328
BMI	**19**	**20**	**21**	**22**	**23**	**24**	**25**	**26**	**27**	**28**	**29**	**30**	**35**	**40**

Key: Underweight (less than 18.5)   Healthy weight (18.5 to 24.9)   Overweight (25 to 29.9)   Obese (30 and above)

Stress

Stress affects everybody, but some people react to it more strongly than others. When you experience stress, your body makes two hormones, cortisol and adrenaline, that help you deal with the tense situation. Over the long term, however, too much of these hormones produced for too long can cause anxiety and physical symptoms that can trigger or worsen illnesses such as high blood pressure, asthma, or heart disease. Persistent, prolonged stress can also adversely affect your immune system, making you more susceptible to infections and other illnesses.

A number of natural ways to reduce stress—such as deep breathing, yoga, meditation, biofeedback, exercise, and massage—have been proven to be effective. Try all of them until you find what works best for you. Cognitive-behavioral therapy (see page 710) provided by a mental health professional can also be helpful. If you feel overwhelmed by the stress in your life, talk with your doctor about effective stress-reduction methods (see page 58).

It's Not All in Your Mind

Stress can affect your body in a number of ways. Chronic, long-term stress can be especially harmful. Learning how to manage your response to stress can help you avoid these damaging effects.

Hair
Some forms of baldness, such as alopecia areata, have been linked to stress.

Brain
Stress can trigger headaches and behavioral and emotional problems such as anxiety and depression. A persistent release of the stress hormone cortisol can kill brain cells directly, causing memory and learning problems.

Heart
Heaviness or pain in the chest (angina), rapid heartbeat, and abnormal heart rhythms can occur during or shortly after periods of stress.

Digestive tract
Stress can cause or worsen disorders or diseases of the digestive tract such as indigestion, peptic ulcers, and irritable bowel syndrome. Severe stress can slow digestion.

Abdominal fat
Prolonged or severe stress can cause fat to be deposited at the waist rather than on the hips and buttocks, increasing the risk of heart disease, cancer, type 2 diabetes, and other illnesses.

Bones
High levels of the stress hormone cortisol can cause bone loss.

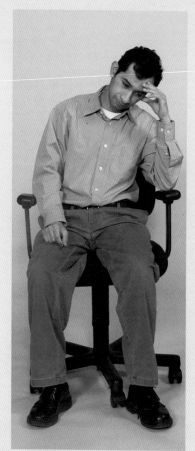

Skin
Some people have outbreaks of skin problems such as eczema and psoriasis when they are under stress. Stress also can increase perspiration.

Mouth
Teeth grinding, mouth ulcers, and dry mouth seem to occur more often during times of stress.

Lungs
People with asthma often find that their condition worsens when they are under stress. Stress can also speed up breathing.

Bladder
Stress can trigger an urgent need to urinate.

Reproductive organs
Severe stress can suppress the reproductive system, causing absence of periods in women and erection problems and premature ejaculation in men.

Muscles
Minor muscular tics become more noticeable, especially on the face and hands, and muscles often become tense when a person is under stress.

Immune system
When a person is under stress, the immune system can become weakened, increasing the risk of infections and other illnesses.

Don't Cheat on Sleep

When it comes to stress, sleep is like medicine, but sometimes you can get caught in a vicious circle. You can't sleep because you feel stressed, and the lack of sleep causes more stress, which affects your sleep. Lacking sufficient sleep for a long period can have harmful effects on your mind and body. Lack of sleep can increase your risk of type 2 diabetes, lower your resistance to illness, and raise your blood pressure—all important reasons to take sleep more seriously.

If you're going through a high-stress period, one way to make sure you get a good night's sleep is to shift your focus away from your daytime worries. When you go to bed at night, try to keep yourself from brooding

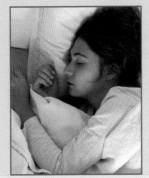

over your daily problems and concerns. Things always seem worse in the middle of the night. Try to look at sleep as an escape from the stresses of the day, not a time for replaying them in your mind.

A midafternoon nap is another way to make up for insufficient sleep at night. Even a short, 20-minute nap will refresh you and improve your mental performance. Just make sure you finish your nap before 3 in the afternoon; napping later can make it harder to fall asleep at bedtime.

Try the tips on pages 57 and 58; they can help you improve your sleep. If you experience sleeplessness for longer than 6 weeks and these suggestions don't seem to help, talk to your doctor. He or she may refer you to a sleep center for treatment.

The Body's Response to Stress

When you are under stress, your body reacts with a cascade of biological responses that begins in a small, grape-sized area of the brain called the hypothalamus. Often referred to as the master gland, the hypothalamus produces many different hormones that tell other glands to jump into action or to quiet down. The hypothalamus communicates to your nervous system to signal the adrenal glands to release adrenaline (epinephrine), a brain messenger that increases alertness and energy and enables you to respond quickly to stress. The hypothalamus also tells a neighboring gland called the pituitary to signal the adrenal glands to release stress hormones (such as cortisol) to enable your body to defend itself. However, over time, if you are under constant stress, these stress-related chemicals (designed to help protect you from harm) can actually turn on your body and be damaging.

Yoga as a Stress Reliever

Yoga is a form of physical activity that helps the body and mind work together to achieve a state of deep relaxation. The practice can lower stress, relieve muscle tension, and increase flexibility. Yoga positions, known as postures, were created thousands of years ago to give the body stability and balance. The deep, controlled breathing that accompanies these postures has a calming effect on the nervous system. The focused attention needed to reach and sustain such postures also helps the mind attain balance. In addition to its physical and mental benefits, yoga has a spiritual aspect that can also increase feelings of well-being.

Western science has shown that yoga produces measurable stress-reducing benefits that can help control conditions such as heart disease, high blood pressure, and asthma. If you are interested in taking a yoga class, contact your local park district, health club, or senior center.

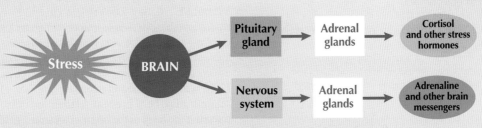

Aging Well

Americans are living longer and healthier, and are more likely to live into their 80s or 90s than ever before. As you grow older, the lifestyle choices you make can either raise or lower your chances of staying healthy and independent well into old age. In fact, your lifestyle choices have twice as much influence as your genes on how well you age and how long you live.

Habits that can increase your longevity and improve your quality of life include eating healthfully, exercising regularly, maintaining social relationships, keeping your weight down, not smoking, drinking alcohol only moderately, and keeping your mind active. No matter what your age, it's never too late to adopt these health-promoting habits and reap their benefits.

Strategies for Successful Aging

The following measures are among the most important things you can do to stay healthy as you age:

- **Eat a nutritious diet.** Consume a varied diet rich in fiber (foods such as vegetables, fruits, whole grains, and legumes) and low in saturated and trans fats, sugar, and salt.
- **Exercise regularly.** Engage in a combination of aerobic, weight-bearing, and stretching exercises for up to an hour most days of the week.
- **Stay connected socially.** Reach out to family and friends, join clubs, volunteer in your community, or start a second career.
- **Maintain a healthy weight.** Keeping your weight down lowers your risk of a number of chronic diseases, including heart disease, diabetes, and some cancers.
- **Don't smoke.** Smoking is the No. 1 cause of preventable premature death in the US.
- **Keep your mind active.** Read books, take a class, do crossword puzzles, help your grandchildren with their homework, learn to play a musical instrument, or go to museums.

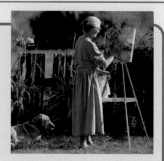

Stay engaged
When it comes to getting older, the more active you are, the healthier you are likely to be, both mentally and physically. Staying active does not mean only physical exercise. It also means staying involved with people and favorite activities.

Memory-Boosting Exercises

Memory loss is not a normal part of aging. It's common to forget where you put your keys—at any age. You don't need to worry about having a memory problem unless you forget what the keys are for. Practicing memory exercises such as the following can help you keep your memory sharp as you age:

- Memorize some poetry.
- Look at a photograph; then look away. Write down all the items in the photo that you remember—for example, how many people, animals, buildings, and other objects—and see how well you did.
- Pick up a paper clip, spool of thread, or other common object. Try to figure out a new use for the object.
- Draw a floor plan of your childhood home, complete with doors, windows, and furniture placement. Tell a story about an event that occurred there.

Preventing Alzheimer's Disease

The following factors seem to have a protective effect against Alzheimer's disease:

- **Education** People who attain a higher level of education tend to have a lower risk of Alzheimer's disease than the general population.
- **Mental activity** Stimulating your mind may protect your brain from Alzheimer's disease by giving you extra connections between cells.
- **Physical exercise** Exercise enlarges blood vessels, supplying more oxygen-rich blood to the brain.
- **Vitamin E** Eating foods rich in vitamin E—such as nuts, vegetable oils, whole grains, and green leafy vegetables—or taking vitamin E supplements may protect against Alzheimer's by reducing the cell-damaging effects of molecules in the brain called free radicals.
- **Folic acid** Consuming adequate amounts of this B vitamin may help prevent Alzheimer's disease by reducing the level in the brain of an amino acid called

homocysteine. Elevated levels of homocysteine can damage cells in the area of the brain involved with learning and memory.

- **Anti-inflammatory drugs**   Over-the-counter anti-inflammatory medications (such as aspirin and ibuprofen) help reduce inflammation in the brain. Inflammation can damage brain cells.
- **Cholesterol-lowering medications**   People who take cholesterol-lowering medications called statins seem to be at significantly lower risk of Alzheimer's disease than other people. The precise effect that elevated cholesterol has on the brain is unknown.

Staying fit as you age

Exercise is the best way to stop or reverse age-related loss of muscle, which can make even simple daily activities such as climbing stairs and getting up from a chair hard to do. Strength-building exercises using handheld weights, elastic exercise bands, or weight machines can help you maintain your independence and lower your risk of falls, even into your 90s. Go for frequent walks; walking regularly can significantly lower your risk of having a heart attack or stroke. At least four times a week, do the following exercises at home (for example, while you watch TV). If you're over 50, talk to your doctor before starting an exercise program.

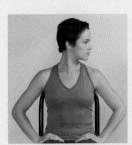

Head turn/Neck stretch
Sit with your back straight, feet flat on the floor, and head in an upright position. Turn your head gently and slowly to one side and hold for a count of 5. Turn your head slowly back to the center and then to the other side and hold for a count of 5. Repeat the sequence 5 to 10 times.

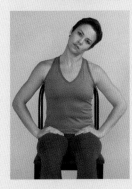

Head roll/Neck stretch
Sit with your back straight, feet flat on the floor, and head in an upright position. Roll your head gently and slowly in a circle from one side to the other, flexing your neck so you are looking up to the point where the wall meets the ceiling at the back of the circle and down at your chest at the front of the circle. Repeat the circle from the other direction. Repeat the sequence 5 to 10 times.

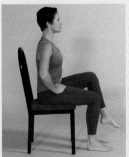
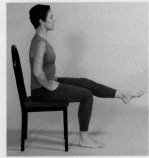

Leg lift/Leg extension
Leg lifts help tone the upper leg muscles. Sitting with your back straight, your knees bent, and both feet flat on the floor, lift one leg off the floor and extend it in front of you, making sure to pull in your abdominal muscles and center your weight over both hips. Bring the leg slowly back to the starting position. Repeat with the other leg. Work up to 10 to 15 repetitions with each leg.

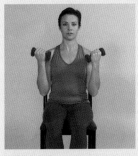
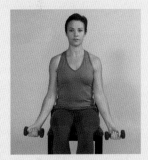

Biceps curl
Sitting with your back straight and feet flat on the floor, hold two small hand weights (begin with 1-pound weights) with your arms bent, the weights up and in toward your shoulders (left). Slowly bring the weights down to the sides of your thighs (right) and then slowly bring them back up to your shoulders. When you can repeat the exercise 12 times, increase the weights by 1 pound.

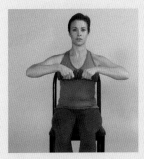
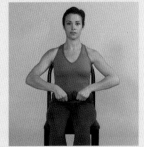

Pump-up
Sit with your back straight and feet flat on the floor, holding the ends of two weights together at chest level, keeping your shoulders down and your elbows out (left). Lower the weights slowly to waist level, keeping the ends of the weights together (right). Raise the weights slowly to chest level again. When you can repeat the exercise 12 times, increase the weights by 1 pound.

Osteoarthritis

Osteoarthritis, also called degenerative joint disease, is the most common type of arthritis, affecting more than 20 million Americans, mostly those over age 45. This form of arthritis is characterized by the breakdown of cartilage, the connective tissue that lines the inside surfaces of joints and that cushions the bones that meet in the joint. When the cartilage wears down, the bones in the joint rub together, causing pain and stiffness.

If you have osteoarthritis, you can still be active and enjoy good health. Learn as much as you can about the disorder and learn how to manage it so you have a sense of control. Your doctor will recommend the best treatment strategies for your condition, including medication, possibly. Your doctor will also recommend modifying lifestyle factors such as regular exercise, sufficient rest, and maintaining a healthy weight.

How Your Joints Work

Your joints are designed to permit free movement between or among two or more bones and to absorb shock when you move. A joint is made up of the following components:

- **Cartilage**   The connective tissue that lines the joint.
- **Joint capsule**   A saclike membrane that holds the bones and other joint parts together.
- **Synovium**   A second, thinner membrane inside the joint capsule.
- **Synovial fluid**   A liquid that lubricates the joint.
- **Ligaments**   Cordlike tissues that connect one bone to another.
- **Tendons**   Fibrous cords that connect muscle to bone.
- **Muscles**   Bundles of cells that contract to produce movement when stimulated by nerves.

How Osteoarthritis Affects Your Joints

Osteoarthritis occurs most often in the joints of the hands, knees, hips, or spine, but it can occur in any joint. The knees, the body's major weight-bearing joints, and the hips are very common sites of osteoarthritis. Osteoarthritis in the knees or hips can limit movement, making everyday tasks difficult. Hip-joint arthritis can produce pain in the groin, inner thighs, buttocks, or knees. Osteoarthritis in the spine can cause weakness or numbness in the arms and legs. Osteoarthritis in the fingers is one form of the disorder that seems to run in families, affecting more women than men, especially after menopause. Small bony knobs appear on the end and middle joints of the fingers, which can become gnarled, sore, and stiff.

A healthy joint
Inside a healthy joint, bones are encased in smooth cartilage. The bones and cartilage lie inside a protective joint capsule lined with a membrane (the synovium) that produces a liquid (synovial fluid) that makes movement easy and painless.

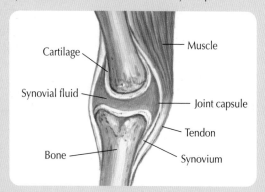

A joint with osteoarthritis
Osteoarthritis causes cartilage to wear away inside the joint. Pieces of bone (spurs) grow out from the edges of the bones that meet in the joint. The bones may begin to rub together, and moving the joint can cause pain and stiffness.

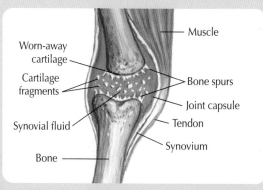

Osteoarthritis affects different people in different ways. In some people, the disease progresses quickly; in others, the process of joint degeneration takes years. The exact cause of osteoarthritis is unknown, but heredity seems to play a role in 25 to 30 percent of cases. A combination of factors—including aging, being overweight, injuring a joint, and stress placed on the joints during work-related or sports activities—probably work together to produce the wearing away of cartilage that is characteristic of the disease.

Exercise and Osteoarthritis

Although exercise may seem like a bad idea when your joints are stiff and painful, regular exercise can actually benefit joints affected by osteoarthritis. Regular exercise lessens pain, improves mobility, strengthens surrounding muscle, and increases flexibility. Exercise also improves your overall fitness and helps control your weight, relieving some of the pressure on overtaxed joints.

To avoid injury, it's important to begin your exercise program slowly. Start with stretching exercises that increase your range of motion and enhance flexibility (see page 8). Then perform strength-conditioning exercises (see page 9).

You don't have to go to a gym to lift weights—buy some hand-held weights to use at home. Add walking, swimming, or bicycling to your routine. Gradually building up your endurance will enable you to exercise longer, and soon you will be stronger and more active and in less pain.

Water exercise is a good choice for people with osteoarthritis because the water supports the body, reducing stress on the hips, knees, and spine. Another good choice is yoga (see page 94), which gently increases joint flexibility as it tones and strengthens the surrounding muscles. Other types of exercise that can benefit people with osteoarthritis include t'ai chi and even jogging. Ask your doctor what exercises are best for you.

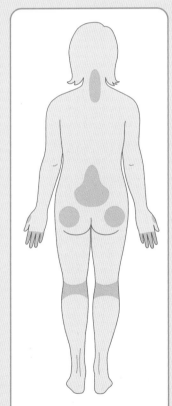

Where does osteoarthritis develop most often?
Osteoarthritis occurs most often in the joints of the fingers, at the base of the thumbs, and in the neck, lower back, knees, and hips.

The Warning Signs of Osteoarthritis

- Steady or intermittent joint pain
- Joint stiffness after getting out of bed or sitting for a long time
- Swelling in a joint
- A crunching sound when bone rubs on bone

Hot, red, or tender joints are usually a sign of another form of arthritis, called rheumatoid arthritis.

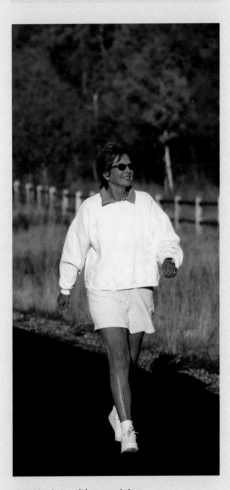

Exercise is good for your joints
Regular physical exercise such as walking is good for people with arthritis. It keeps the joints working as it strengthens the surrounding muscles and ligaments. Exercise can also reduce joint pain, although it can take 4 to 8 weeks of regular exercise before you experience significant pain relief.

Heart Disease

Your heart beats steadily 24 hours a day to pump oxygen-rich blood throughout your body. But if the arteries leading to your heart become clogged with a fatty substance called plaque, they become narrowed, reducing the supply of blood to the heart and causing heart disease. If a plaque ruptures, blood clots can form, blocking the artery and causing a heart attack. Heart disease is the No. 1 killer of both men and women in the US, but many women do not realize they are at risk. The good news is that you can reduce your chances of developing heart disease by adopting the heart-healthy lifestyle described here.

Risk Factors for Heart Disease

Some of the factors that can increase your chances of developing heart disease, such as family history, are not under your control. Many other risk factors, however, can be controlled.

Risk factors you cannot control

- **Age** In men, the risk of heart disease increases after age 45; in women, the risk increases after age 55.
- **Family history** Especially at a young age—a father or brother diagnosed with heart disease before age 55, or a mother or sister diagnosed before age 65.
- **Race** African Americans have a higher risk of heart disease than people of other races.

Risk factors you can control

- **Smoking** Smoking is a major risk factor for heart disease because it raises blood pressure, damages blood vessels, promotes blood clotting, and accelerates plaque formation in artery walls.
- **High blood pressure** High blood pressure (hypertension) puts extra stress on the heart and blood vessels.
- **Undesirable cholesterol profile** A high total cholesterol level, a low HDL (good) cholesterol level, or a high LDL (bad) cholesterol level can promote plaque formation on artery walls.
- **Being overweight** Excess weight increases the heart's workload.
- **Lack of exercise** Regular exercise makes the heart stronger, keeps weight down, improves cholesterol levels, and lowers blood pressure.
- **Diabetes** Over time, diabetes damages blood vessels and boosts the risk of heart attack and stroke.
- **Stress** Unmanaged stress increases heart rate, can cause disturbances in heart rhythm, and can contribute to angina (chest pain from heart disease).

The more of these risk factors you have, the higher your risk of heart disease. Discuss your risk factors with your doctor and ask about steps you can take to avoid heart disease.

Preventing Heart Disease

Doctors have linked many common lifestyle activities to the development of heart disease. By controlling these lifestyle factors, you can prevent heart disease or greatly reduce your chances of getting it—even if you have a family history of the disorder.

What to Do If You're Having a Heart Attack

If you or someone else is having a heart attack, don't delay getting treatment—a heart attack does the most damage to the heart muscle in the first 2 hours. Even if you aren't sure it's really a heart attack because it feels like heartburn or indigestion, call for help anyway. It's better to be wrong than to sustain serious heart damage because you waited too long. Acting quickly can save your life.

- At the first sign of symptoms, sit or lie down.
- If your symptoms last longer than 2 minutes, call 911 or your local emergency number and say you may be having a heart attack.
- If you have nitroglycerin tablets, take one every 5 minutes—up to three pills total.
- If you don't have nitroglycerin, take an aspirin; it can thin the blood and may allow more blood to reach your heart.
- Don't drive yourself to the hospital; wait for the emergency medical team to arrive. They have the special equipment needed to provide emergency care for a heart attack.

- **Don't smoke.**   Cigarette smoking is a major contributor to heart disease. One year after quitting, your risk of heart disease is cut in half; within about 5 years, your risk is equal to that of a person who has never smoked.
- **Eat a healthy diet.**   Consume a diet that is low in saturated fat and trans fats, includes plenty of fruits and vegetables, and incorporates omega-3 fatty acids from fish several times a month. Limiting your intake of saturated fat (found in meat and full-fat dairy products) can lower your blood cholesterol level. Limit your salt intake (salt can raise blood pressure in some people), and drink alcohol in moderation (excessive drinking can raise blood pressure).
- **Exercise regularly.**   Regular physical activity reduces your chances of having a heart attack by at least a third. Regular exercise lowers blood pressure, improves cholesterol levels, and reduces the risk of type 2 diabetes—all major risk factors for heart disease. Exercise also helps control weight.
- **Maintain a healthy weight.**   Being overweight raises blood pressure and cholesterol and can lead to type 2 diabetes. Losing as few as 10 pounds helps lower the risk.
- **Reduce stress.**   Several changes take place in your body when you are under stress. Your heart beats faster, more fat enters your bloodstream, your blood sugar level goes up, and blood clotting increases. All of these factors place an extra load on the heart. Stress also promotes poor health habits such as overeating, smoking, or forgetting to exercise. To counteract the effects of stress, try meditation, yoga, or deep-breathing exercises; have a massage; take a warm bath; exercise; and get plenty of sleep.
- **Avoid smoky environments.**   Secondhand smoke at home or work can cause heart disease and worsen existing heart disease.

What Is a Heart Attack?

Blood reaches the heart through the coronary arteries. Fatty deposits called plaque can build up inside the walls of arteries, making them narrower. This process, called atherosclerosis, or hardening of the arteries, develops gradually over many years. If a plaque ruptures, a blood clot can form, reducing blood flow to the heart even more. If a clot suddenly cuts off most or all of the blood supply to the heart, a heart attack results. Cells in the heart muscle that don't receive enough oxygen-carrying blood begin to die. The more time that passes without treatment to restore blood flow to the heart, the greater the damage to the heart muscle.

Sites of heart attack pain

The symptoms of a heart attack are sometimes hard to identify because a heart attack can feel different to different people. You could feel pain in any of the areas of the body shown here, or you could feel pain in only your arms, jaw, or back. Women's symptoms, especially, can vary considerably from the classic signs of a heart attack. Women are more likely than men to experience dizziness, nausea, sweating, weakness, and faintness along with chest pain.

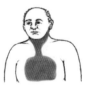

Chest pain that spreads to your neck or jaw

Crushing pain in your chest that radiates to your left shoulder

Deep, dull pain or a tight, heavy, or squeezing sensation under your breastbone

Chest pain that spreads to your back

Pay Attention to Angina

If too little blood reaches the heart because of narrowed arteries, chest pain (called angina) can develop. Angina can feel like erratic pain or heaviness, tightness, burning, or squeezing in the chest. The pain can be mild and intermittent or more pronounced and steady, and can start in the center of the chest and radiate to the left shoulder, arm, jaw, or lower teeth. Angina often occurs during physical exertion or times of stress. Angina is a sign that you have heart disease and are at risk of having a heart attack.

If you think you could have angina, tell your doctor right away. Getting prompt treatment for angina can prevent you from having a heart attack. The most common treatment for angina is a drug called nitroglycerin, which reduces the pain by widening the blood vessels to allow more blood to reach the heart.

Cancer

Cancer is the second leading cause of death in the US (after heart disease), causing more than half a million deaths each year. One out of two men and one out of three women develop some kind of cancer at some time in their life. Most cancers are diagnosed in people over age 55. Early detection and treatment increase your chances for a cure, so be sure to perform routine self-examinations (see page 137), have all the recommended screening tests (see page 143), and report any suspicious symptoms to your doctor.

What Is Cancer?

Cancer is a group of diseases characterized by the uncontrolled multiplication of cells that occurs when genes that control cell division or cell turnover (cell death and replacement) undergo mutations (changes). These genetic mutations are sometimes inherited or present at birth, but usually they result from environmental factors (such as radiation or cigarette smoke) that damage critical regulatory genes.

Cell turnover is a tightly balanced process that keeps the body healthy. In normal tissue, old or damaged cells die naturally before they can become cancerous or cause other problems, and are replaced by healthy new cells—a process called apoptosis. In cancer this balance is upset—when damage occurs to either the genes that tell cells when to stop dividing or to the genes that tell old or damaged cells when to die. The resulting increase in the number of cells creates a growing mass of tissue called a tumor. As more and more dividing cells accumulate, the tumor grows and can disrupt the normal functioning of surrounding tissue.

Cancer can originate anywhere in the body. Common sites include the lungs, breasts, lymph nodes, colon, bladder, and prostate gland. Cancer can spread through the body in two ways: Cancer cells from a tumor can invade neighboring tissues, and cancer cells from a tumor can penetrate blood vessels or lymphatic vessels, circulate through the bloodstream or lymphatic system, and invade healthy tissue in another part of the body.

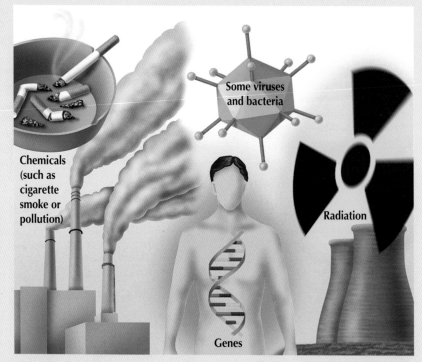

Chemicals (such as cigarette smoke or pollution)

Some viruses and bacteria

Radiation

Genes

What causes cancer?
Some people inherit genes that make them susceptible to developing particular types of cancer. Environmental factors that can trigger the changes in genes that lead to cancer include radiation, some chemicals, and some viruses and bacteria. For example, excessive exposure to radiation from sunlight has been linked to skin cancer. More than 60 different chemicals in cigarette smoke are known to cause cancer. The human papillomavirus, which causes the sexually transmitted disease genital warts, is responsible for most cases of cervical cancer in women, and the bacterium H. pylori causes many cases of stomach cancer.

Preventing Cancer

Many lifestyle factors can either raise or lower your risk of cancer. Although your genes also influence your susceptibility to developing cancer, genes are not necessarily destiny. Even if you have genes that could make you prone to cancer, the following measures can still help you reduce your risk and, at the same time, protect you from other common diseases:

● **Don't smoke or use other tobacco products.** Cigarette smoking is the major cause of lung cancer and contributes to several other cancers, including cancer of the mouth, larynx, esophagus, stomach, pancreas, kidneys, and bladder. Use of smokeless tobacco has been linked to cancers of the mouth and throat.

● **Eat a diet rich in vegetables, fruits, and whole grains.** A number of substances such as antioxidants in plant foods (especially fruits, vegetables, and grains) have been found to interfere with the process that leads to cancer. Consuming foods that are low in fat (especially animal fat) may also help reduce cancer risk.

● **Maintain a healthy weight.** Being overweight increases the risk of some cancers, including cancers of the breast, uterus, and colon.

● **Exercise regularly.** Regular, vigorous exercise may reduce the risk of some cancers. Researchers don't know exactly how physical activity prevents cancer but think that it may enhance the body's immune system.

● **Protect your skin from the sun.** The risk of skin cancer, including melanoma (the most deadly type), can be greatly reduced by avoiding excessive sun exposure, wearing protective clothing in the sun, and using sunscreen.

● **Drink alcohol only in moderation.** Drinking excessive amounts of alcohol increases your risk of cancers of the mouth, throat, and esophagus—especially if you also smoke cigarettes. Together, alcohol and cigarettes make you 40 times more likely than nondrinking nonsmokers to develop these cancers.

● **Engage in safer sex.** The most common known cancer-causing virus in the US is the human papillomavirus (HPV), a sexually transmitted infection that causes cervical cancer in women.

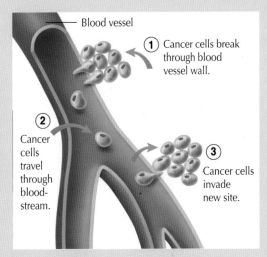

- Blood vessel
1. Cancer cells break through blood vessel wall.
2. Cancer cells travel through bloodstream.
3. Cancer cells invade new site.

When cancer spreads
If cancer cells enter blood vessels, they can be carried through the bloodstream to other parts of the body and invade healthy tissues there. The spread of cancer from one area of the body to another is called metastasis.

● **Have the recommended screening tests.** Having regular cancer screening tests—such as a Pap smear (see page 140) to look for cervical cancer, and a colonoscopy (see page 767) to look for colon cancer—can detect potential problems early, when they are generally easier to treat and the chances for a cure are better.

Most Common Cancers

Although more people have breast cancer or prostate cancer than lung cancer or colon cancer, lung cancer and colon cancer kill more people each year.

Most Common Cancers	Leading Cancer Killers
1 Prostate	1 Lung
2 Breast	2 Colon and rectum
3 Lung	3 Breast
4 Colon and rectum	4 Prostate
5 Bladder	5 Pancreas
6 Non-Hodgkin's lymphoma	6 Non-Hodgkin's lymphoma
7 Melanoma	7 Leukemias
8 Uterus	8 Ovary
9 Leukemias	9 Stomach
10 Kidney	10 Brain and nervous system

Cancer Treatments

When it comes to curing cancer, early detection and treatment are key. Treatment is more likely to be successful if it is done before cancer cells spread from the original tumor to other parts of the body. Cancer is most often treated with surgery, radiation therapy, or chemotherapy, or a combination of all three. Immunotherapy and stem cell transplants are being used increasingly to treat cancer.

Surgery

Conventional surgery is usually the first treatment recommended by doctors to remove a cancerous tumor and any surrounding tissue that may contain cancer cells. Less invasive surgical procedures are continually being developed that try to preserve as much healthy tissue and normal functioning as possible.

Laser surgery

A laser is a highly focused, powerful beam of light that can cut through tissue or vaporize cancers inside the body or on the skin without the need for a large incision. Laser surgery is also sometimes used to relieve symptoms such as breathing or eating problems that can result when large tumors press on the trachea (windpipe) or esophagus.

Cryosurgery

Cryosurgery uses extreme cold (liquid nitrogen spray or a very cold probe) to freeze and destroy abnormal cells. Cryosurgery is most often used to treat external cancers, such as those on the skin, or precancerous conditions, such as those affecting the cervix. However, doctors are using it increasingly to treat tumors inside the body, including tumors in the prostate gland.

Electrosurgery

High-frequency electric current is often used to destroy cancers of the skin and mouth. A procedure called LEEP/LLETZ (loop electrosurgical excision procedure or large-loop excision of the transformation zone) is used to remove abnormal tissue from the cervix.

Mohs surgery

Mohs surgery is a technique to remove cancerous tissue by shaving it off one layer at a time. After each layer is removed, it is examined under a microscope to look for cancer cells. When all the cells in a layer look normal under the microscope, surgery is stopped. This technique is used primarily for skin cancers that have recurred or that have developed around sensitive areas such as the eyelids, nose, or lips. Mohs surgery preserves as much healthy tissue as possible and has a high cure rate.

Experimental forms of cancer surgery

Researchers are investigating other procedures for removing or destroying cancerous tissue using high-intensity focused ultrasound (HIFU), microwaves or radio waves, and magnets.

Immunotherapy

Immunotherapy uses the immune system to fight cancer, either by stimulating a person's immune system (active immunotherapy) or by administering disease-fighting immune system components (such as antibodies) manufactured outside of the body (passive immunotherapy). These techniques, which include cancer vaccines, are currently being studied for treatment of different types of cancer, including melanoma, kidney cancer, blood cancers (such as leukemias, lymphomas, and myelomas), breast cancer, prostate cancer, colon cancer, cervical cancer, and ovarian cancer.

Stem cell transplants and bone marrow transplants

Bone marrow is spongy tissue in the center of bones that makes all the blood cells in the body. Blood cells develop from immature cells called stem cells, which are found in the bone marrow and, in smaller amounts, circulating in the blood. If a cancer destroys bone marrow or if bone marrow is damaged from cancer treatment, doctors may recommend a stem cell transplant or bone marrow transplant (see page 624) to provide healthy new cells. Stem cell transplants are also used to treat cancers that don't respond to normal doses of chemotherapy. After a person receives high doses of chemotherapy, he or she is given an infusion of stem cells to replace those that were destroyed.

Radiation therapy

Radiation therapy uses penetrating beams of high-energy radioactive waves or streams of radioactive particles to treat cancer. This radioactive energy, which is the same as that used in X-rays but in much higher doses, kills the cancer cells or keeps them from dividing. Healthy cells are also affected by radiation but, unlike cancer cells, healthy cells tend to recover from the effects of radiation.

More than half of all people with cancer are treated with some form of radiation. Radiation is often used before surgery to shrink a tumor or after surgery to block the growth of any cancer cells that could remain in the area around the tumor. Radiation therapy is also often combined with chemotherapy (see below).

Radiation therapy can be given either externally or internally. Most people receive the external form, in which a machine directs the high-energy rays at the tumor and a small margin of surrounding tissue. In internal radiation therapy, the radiation is provided by a source placed inside the body, such as an implant, an injection, or a medication.

Side effects from radiation therapy vary from person to person and depend on the dose of radiation and the area of the body being treated. The most common side effects—including fatigue, skin changes, and loss of appetite—usually clear up within a few weeks.

Stereotactic radiation therapy

Some newer radiation techniques are almost as precise as surgery. By aiming radiation at a cancer target from different angles, stereotactic radiation therapy can deliver a large, precise dose of radiation to a small tumor. The procedure is so precise that it is often called stereotactic surgery and the machine that delivers the energy waves is called a gamma knife (even though

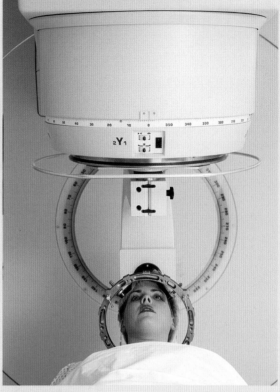

External radiation therapy
The most common type of machine used for external radiation therapy is the linear accelerator, which fires high-energy rays at a tumor to shrink it. In this photograph, the tumor is in the person's head, which is stabilized by a steel frame.

no incision is actually made). Stereotactic radiation therapy has been used mostly to treat tumors in the brain but is being investigated as a way to treat other types of cancer.

Chemotherapy

Chemotherapy is the treatment of cancer with powerful drugs that can destroy cancer cells by preventing them from dividing. Two or more drugs are often given at the same time because they are more effective when combined.

Most people receive chemotherapy on an outpatient basis, usually at home, in a doctor's office, or at a clinic. The drugs can be administered intravenously (through a vein), by mouth, in an injection, or in a skin patch.

During chemotherapy, healthy, normal cells that divide quickly (such as those in hair follicles) can be harmed by the drugs. This damage to healthy cells is the cause of most of the side effects of chemotherapy, including hair loss, fatigue, nausea and vomiting, diarrhea, constipation, pain, anemia, and confusion.

Doctors also treat cancer with drugs that work in other ways. For example, biological therapy uses substances that strengthen the body's immune system to fight the cancer. Other drugs block the effects of specific hormones or other body chemicals that can promote particular types of cancer.

Genetics

Genes play a role in all diseases, including the common cold. Researchers have discovered many of the genes that cause inherited disorders, and they are beginning to find the genes that interact with environmental factors (such as lifestyle) to cause common health problems such as heart disease, cancer, and diabetes. Advances in genetics research will enable us to take steps to modify our habits to avoid many of these disorders. This new knowledge will also spark the development of more effective, more targeted treatments that have fewer adverse effects. The more you know about your genetic makeup, the better able you will be to make informed decisions about your health, your lifestyle, your medical care, and your reproductive options.

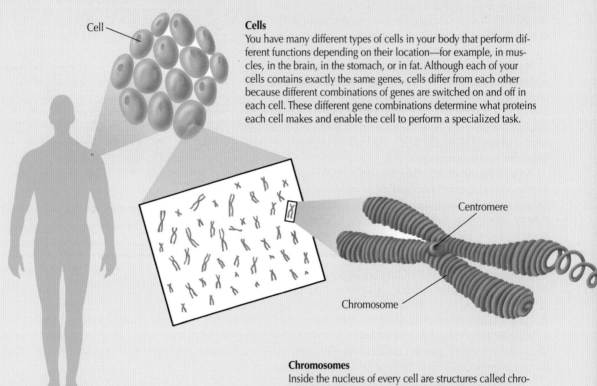

Cell

Cells
You have many different types of cells in your body that perform different functions depending on their location—for example, in muscles, in the brain, in the stomach, or in fat. Although each of your cells contains exactly the same genes, cells differ from each other because different combinations of genes are switched on and off in each cell. These different gene combinations determine what proteins each cell makes and enable the cell to perform a specialized task.

Centromere

Chromosome

DNA: The blueprint of life
Each of us begins life as a single cell containing genetic information from each of our parents. This original cell divides to about 100 trillion specialized cells, each containing a complete set of genes identical to that in the original cell. Your unique set of about 30,000 genes is called your genome. Your genome orchestrates the activity of all the cells in your body, enabling them to work together in harmony to keep your body healthy and functioning normally.

Chromosomes
Inside the nucleus of every cell are structures called chromosomes. Chromosomes are long threads of genetic material made up of strands of deoxyribonucleic acid (DNA). You have 23 pairs of chromosomes; each of your parents contributed one chromosome to every pair. Each chromosome contains from several hundred to several thousand genes. Just before cells divide, the chromosomes make duplicate copies of themselves; the two copies of each chromosome are held together at a narrowed region called a centromere, which gives the chromosome an X shape.

The genetic code

The information carried by a gene is determined by the structure of its DNA. DNA is arranged in the form of a double helix, or ladder, with rungs supported by a twisting ribbon of sugar and phosphates. The two intertwined DNA strands are linked together by varying patterns of substances called nucleotide bases. There are four nucleotide bases—cytosine (C), guanine (G), adenine (A), and thymine (T).

Along each helix, or side of the ladder, the bases are arranged in groups of three, called base triplets, to form words of genetic text. For example, base triplets, such as TAC, CGG, and TCA, carry specific amino acids (the building blocks of proteins) to assembly points in a cell where they are strung together to make functioning proteins. To form the rungs of the DNA ladder, the bases can join in only two ways: C joins only with G, and A joins only with T.

If you think of the nucleotide bases as the letters of the genetic alphabet, then base triplets are the words, genes are the sentences, chromosomes are the chapters, and the genome is each organism's book of life. The human genome contains a total of about 3 billion nucleotide base pairs.

Genes

Genes are the basic physical and functional units of heredity, which provide instructions for making proteins, the building blocks of the body. Scientists believe that genes make up only about 2 percent of the total genome; the rest consists of regions whose functions include keeping the chromosomes intact and regulating where, when, and in what quantity proteins are made.

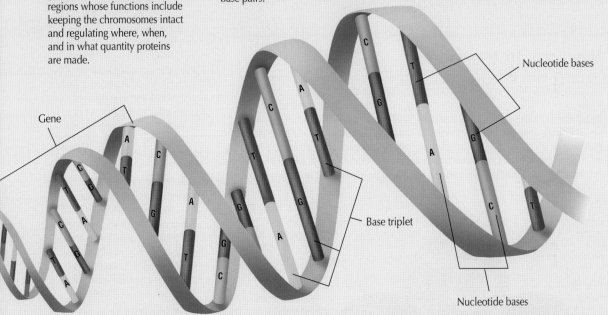

Gene

Nucleotide bases

Base triplet

Nucleotide bases

Proteins: Building Blocks of the Body

Proteins are essential for life. Some proteins make up structures such as muscles and skin; other proteins—including enzymes, antibodies, and many hormones—dissolve in the body's fluids and are carried to wherever they are needed. Genes control the production of proteins inside cells and provide the instructions for making specific proteins in precisely the right number and at precisely the right time. Different proteins have different functions in the body:

- Enzymes regulate the rate of chemical reactions in cells.
- Antibodies, produced by the immune system's white blood cells, destroy invading microorganisms and provide protection against infections.
- Proteins in muscle cells provide mobility, pump blood through the body, and help move food through the digestive tract.
- Hemoglobin carries oxygen in red blood cells and gives the cells their red color.
- Hormones control a variety of biological processes, such as growth, sexual development, and the activities of some organs.

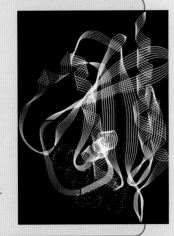

Genetics: The future of medicine

You will one day be able to learn from your unique genome what disorders you are at increased risk of developing, which will enable you to take steps to prevent them. Doctors will be able to prescribe drugs that are more precisely tailored to your individual genome. They would know, for example, what medication or combination of medications for high blood pressure would be most effective for you.

Eventually, scientists hope to find the genes that enable some people to live to 100 or older. Using the information they glean from the genes, they will be able to devise new treatments, drugs, special vitamin formulas, or even combinations of foods that could enhance the activity of the genes and increase healthy life expectancy for everyone—even those of us who were not born with the life-prolonging forms of these genes.

How Genes Are Transmitted

Your genes are continuously being copied inside your cells in a process of cell division called mitosis. Mitosis occurs thousands of times every second to make new cells to replace damaged, dying, or dead cells. Egg and sperm cells are different from other cells in the body and divide in a process called meiosis. Each egg or sperm cell contains half the DNA of body cells, and each is genetically unique. An egg and sperm combine at conception to form a cell with a full set of genes, half from each parent. This random mix of genetic information accounts for the limitless variety of people in the world.

The cycle of life

5 At birth, a child has about 200 billion cells, which will increase to 100 trillion cells in adulthood.

1 Germ cells in females are immature eggs, formed during fetal development, which eventually develop into mature eggs, starting at puberty. In males, germ cells are the cells from which sperm are made.

2 Eggs and sperm are formed in a process called meiosis, in which they each receive half of the genetic makeup of their parent germ cell. Eggs and sperm each have 23 chromosomes instead of the 46 present in all the other cells of the body.

4 A fertilized egg divides many times to form billions of cells with the exact same set of genes to form a fetus.

3 At conception, an egg and a sperm combine their genetic material to produce a fertilized egg containing 46 chromosomes, the full complement of DNA.

Genetic Testing

As you read and hear more and more about genetic testing, you may want to consider being tested for a condition that seems to run in your family. You may want to learn if you carry genes that increase your risk of developing a particular disorder later in life or of transmitting a severe, life-threatening genetic disorder to a child. For many diseases that are inherited through a single gene or pair of genes, tests are available to detect the genes in people who carry them, often from a simple blood test. The odds of passing one of these so-called single-gene disorders to offspring can be calculated relatively easily. However, for other diseases, the risks are more difficult to define, and the best course to follow is not always clear. To be able to make informed decisions, you will need to understand the implications the information has for you personally. For information about genetic counseling, see page 952.

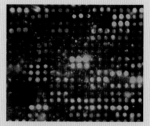

Gene chips
Studying a person's DNA from a small sample of his or her blood or saliva, scientists can detect a wide variety of genes that increase susceptibility to particular disorders. A genetic analysis is made by reading a person's DNA on a gene chip.

The Dangers of Smoking

Cigarette smoking is the major cause of preventable death in the US, causing nearly half a million premature deaths each year. The smoke from a cigarette contains more than 4,000 chemicals—at least 60 of them known to cause cancer. Nicotine, the substance in tobacco that makes smoking highly addictive, raises your heart rate, irritates the lining of your blood vessels, and promotes blood clotting, increasing your risk of heart attack and stroke. The carbon monoxide in cigarette smoke reduces the level of oxygen in your blood.

Smoking causes nearly nine out of ten cases of lung cancer—the No. 1 cancer killer of both men and women—and causes other cancers, including cancer of the mouth, throat, esophagus, bladder, kidneys, cervix, and pancreas. Smoking is also responsible for most cases of emphysema and chronic bronchitis and is a major risk factor for heart disease, the leading cause of death in both men and women. Women over age 35 who both smoke and take birth-control pills increase their risk of having a heart attack or stroke.

Why You're Hooked

Researchers have discovered why smokers have such a hard time quitting. Normally, your brain releases dopamine (a chemical that produces feelings of pleasure) when you perform a rewarding behavior, such as eating when you are hungry. The brain then quickly releases another chemical, called acetylcholine, which stops the release of dopamine.

When you smoke, nicotine triggers the release of dopamine but prevents the brain from turning it off by blocking the release of acetylcholine. As a result, the brain continues pumping out dopamine, making you feel better and better. After nicotine levels in the bloodstream fall, dopamine production declines. The brain, recalling the good feelings, wants more, producing cravings for another cigarette. These processes take place inside a part of your brain that scientists call the reward center.

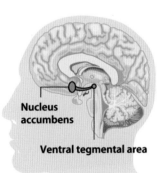

Nucleus accumbens

Ventral tegmental area

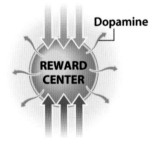

Dopamine

REWARD CENTER

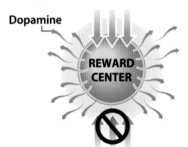

Dopamine

REWARD CENTER

The brain's reward center
Two structures—the nucleus accumbens and the ventral tegmental area—deep in the brain's reward center are responsible for the release of dopamine, which produces feelings of pleasure.

When the brain's reward center works normally

ON: The reward center releases dopamine to reward a good behavior, such as learning a new skill (green arrows).

OFF: Minutes later, another brain chemical, acetylcholine, shuts dopamine production off (red arrows).

When nicotine interferes with the reward center

ON: Nicotine in the bloodstream causes the reward center to release a flood of dopamine (green arrows).

NOT OFF: Nicotine blocks the release of acetylcholine, so the reward center keeps releasing dopamine until blood levels of nicotine fall, producing craving for more nicotine (red arrows).

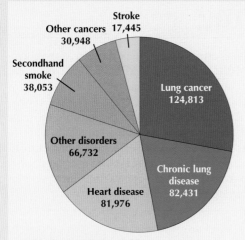

Stroke 17,445

Other cancers 30,948

Secondhand smoke 38,053

Lung cancer 124,813

Other disorders 66,732

Heart disease 81,976

Chronic lung disease 82,431

Deaths from cigarette smoking
This chart uses figures from the Centers for Disease Control and Prevention to show the number and causes of deaths attributed to smoking each year in the US. Of the nearly half a million smoking-related deaths, 7 out of 10 result from lung disease, especially lung cancer and emphysema, and from heart disease and stroke.

How Smoking Affects the Lungs

Smoking is the major cause of lung cancer and emphysema (a chronic lung condition in which damage to the tiny air sacs in the lungs makes breathing difficult). Chronic inflammation of lung tissue from cigarette smoke and tar residue left by the smoke triggers a cascade of changes in cells in the lungs that can lead to cancer, emphysema, or both. In this cross section of a lung with cancer (top), the white area in the upper lobe is cancerous tissue, and the blackened areas are deposits of tar. The lung with emphysema (bottom) has multiple cavities (produced by the destruction of air sacs) that are surrounded by black deposits of tar.

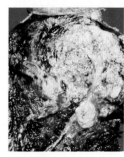

Lung with cancer

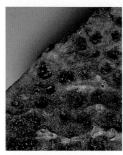

Lung with emphysema

The Benefits of Quitting Smoking

Even if you've been smoking for years, when you quit, your body begins a series of changes to repair the damage caused by smoking and to restore health to affected cells and organs.

Time Since Last Cigarette	Health Benefit
20 minutes	Blood pressure decreases. Pulse rate drops. Circulation improves, making hands and feet feel warmer.
8 hours	Breathing becomes easier because the amount of oxygen-depleting carbon monoxide in the blood decreases, which increases the amount of oxygen in the blood.
24 hours	Risk of heart attack decreases.
48 hours	Senses of smell and taste start to return. Nerve endings begin to grow back.
2 weeks to 3 months	Circulation continues to improve. Walking gets easier. Lung function increases.
1 to 9 months	Symptoms such as coughing, sinus congestion, fatigue, and shortness of breath subside.
1 year	Risk of heart disease is cut in half.
5 to 15 years	Risk of heart disease is reduced to that of a person who has never smoked.
10 years	Risk of lung cancer decreases up to 50 percent. Risk of cancer of the mouth, throat, esophagus, bladder, kidneys, and pancreas drops.
15 years	Risk of stroke decreases to that of a person who has never smoked. Risk of dying of any smoking-related cause is nearly the same as that of a person who has never smoked.

How to quit smoking

Giving up smoking is not easy. But as hard as quitting may be, the results are well worth it. Take some time to think about the many health benefits of being an ex-smoker. This is an important first step in kicking the habit.

Make a Plan

Once you decide to give up smoking, set a target date to quit. Pick a time when you won't be under a lot of stress. On the night before your quit date, throw away all of your cigarettes, matches, lighters, and ashtrays. Plan some special activities to help you get through the next few days without cigarettes. Try these tips:

● **Avoid smoking triggers.**   Familiar activities, such as talking on the phone or drinking alcohol, can bring on the urge to smoke. Make a list of your triggers and avoid as many as you can. Try to avoid being around smokers, especially your smoking friends, until your cravings start to subside.

● **Keep busy.**   Engage in activities that keep your hands busy (such as doing crossword puzzles). When you feel the need to put something in your mouth, chew gum, eat raw vegetables, or suck on a straw.

● **Consider using a nicotine-replacement product.** Nicotine patches, pills, and gum are available over the counter, and other products are available by prescription. These products are safe for most people, but talk to your doctor before using any of them because they can have side effects.

● **Try a stop-smoking program.**   Contact a local hospital or the American Lung Association and ask about smoking cessation programs in your area.

Most people who quit smoking experience unpleasant side effects—including irritability, sleep loss, headaches, fatigue, depression, nervousness, anxiety, and difficulty concentrating—during the first 3 or 4 weeks after quitting. These symptoms result from the body's withdrawal from nicotine and can be severe. Nicotine use causes changes in brain chemistry that make the brain crave higher and higher levels of stimulation and pleasure. Ask your doctor if the prescription medication bupropion could help you through these difficult few weeks.

If You Relapse

If you slip and smoke a cigarette or two after your quit date, don't be hard on yourself. But try to get back on track quickly. Most people relapse several times before they quit for good. If you have a cigarette:

● **Don't be discouraged.** Quitting smoking is difficult—a relapse doesn't mean you can't succeed.

● **Learn from your experience.** Figure out what triggered your urge to light up and try to avoid it.

Secondhand Smoke

Secondhand smoke (also called passive smoking) is a combination of the smoke given off by cigarettes and the smoke exhaled by smokers. Secondhand smoke is classified as a cancer-causing agent and is responsible for about 35,000 deaths from heart disease and 3,000 deaths from lung cancer each year, primarily among nonsmoking spouses of smokers. Every year, nearly 300,000 cases of bronchitis and pneumonia in children under 18 months of age are directly linked to secondhand smoke, which is also responsible for triggering or worsening hundreds of thousands of cases of childhood asthma. Also, children who regularly breathe secondhand smoke are more likely than other children to have frequent ear infections and more dental cavities.

Medical Treatments for Quitting

For smokers who are highly addicted, many doctors recommend nicotine-replacement products. These products—such as nicotine gum, pills, and patches (available over the counter) and inhalers and nasal sprays (available only by prescription)—release small amounts of nicotine into the bloodstream to relieve withdrawal symptoms from nicotine and help reduce cravings for cigarettes. These products provide safer doses of nicotine than cigarettes—the nicotine enters the body less rapidly and in a lower concentration and does not have the thousands of harmful chemicals present in cigarette smoke. Over a period of about 6 to 12 weeks, the dose of nicotine is gradually reduced to slowly lower your craving.

The prescription antidepressant medication buproprion is another proven treatment for helping people quit smoking. Buproprion, taken in pills, acts in the brain, probably by blocking nicotine receptors, preventing them from triggering the release of the feel-good chemical dopamine (which produces the nicotine addiction). Buproprion seems to be most effective for smoking cessation in women and in people who have a history of depression. The drug can be taken along with nicotine replacement products. Together, the two treatments boost the chances of success.

Terrorism

For the average American, the risk of experiencing a terrorist attack firsthand is low. However, despite the low risk, you still may feel worried and frightened during a national security alert. One positive way to cope with your anxiety and fear is to talk about your feelings with family and friends. You will find that most people share your concerns and many will appreciate the opportunity to talk about them. If you continue to feel anxious or depressed or if you are unable to focus on your usual activities, talk to your doctor or a mental health professional. You can also take constructive steps to prepare for a possible terrorist attack (see below), which can help you feel more in control.

The federal government has identified a number of possible terrorist threats and has developed a national emergency response system to coordinate local and state emergency programs throughout the country in the event of terrorist attacks. Types of attacks that could occur involve biological agents (such as bacteria and viruses), chemicals, or radioactive materials.

How to Prepare for a Terrorist Attack

If a terrorist attack occurs, your local emergency response system will activate and local public health authorities will tell you what to do. Listen to news broadcasts to monitor the situation. Follow instructions from your local police and fire departments and from emergency workers on the scene. Although there is no way to predict exactly what might happen during a terrorist attack, there are a number of things you can do to prepare for an attack:

- **Assemble emergency supplies.** Have enough bottled water (1 gallon of water per person per day) and nonperishable foods (such as canned goods, nuts, dried fruit, and boxes of dry cereal) for at least 3 days. Include a first-aid kit, extra eyeglasses and medication, vitamin and mineral supplements, tools, a battery-powered radio, a flashlight, extra batteries, a manual can opener, toilet paper, paper towels, moist towelettes, bleach, soap, and bedding and a change of clothing for each person. If you can, store extra water in containers for washing. If there is a baby in the house, include ready-to-feed formula, baby food, and disposable diapers. Make a list of emergency phone numbers such as the local fire department and police department, a local hospital, and your doctor.
- **Develop an emergency plan.** Plan what your family would do in different emergency situations (for example, if you have to seek shelter at home, if you have to evacuate your house or apartment, or if an attack occurs when you are in a car). Designate a meeting place. Decide how family members will get in touch with one another if you are not together at the time of an attack or if you become separated. It might be helpful for each family member to have a cell phone. Name an out-of-town person for all family members to contact if local phone service is affected.
- **Educate yourself beforehand.** Learn the warning signals used by your community in an emergency. Find out the location of fallout shelters. Take classes in first aid and CPR.

There are also some things you should *not* do when preparing for a terrorist attack. Do not hoard antibiotics—they lose their effectiveness if overused and they don't work against viruses. And don't stock up on gas masks. They are not effective against all gases, they don't protect you from chemicals absorbed through the skin, and (because many gases are odorless and colorless) you probably will not know when to use one. For more information, go to the US Department of Homeland Security Web site (www.ready.gov) or call 1-800-BE-READY.

Biological Attacks

It is unlikely that a bioterrorist attack would be widespread, at least initially, but some biological agents (such as smallpox) can spread from person to person once they enter a population. Biological agents are expensive and difficult to produce, require technical skill and special equipment to handle, and are difficult to deploy. The biological agents on the following page have been identified as those most likely to be used in a bioterrorist attack. If an attack has occurred and you develop symptoms, see a doctor immediately. Rapid detection and treatment are essential for survival.

Anthrax

Possible use as a biological weapon: Envelopes or packages containing anthrax can be sent through the mail, or released as an aerosol in an enclosed space or over a city.

Cause: The bacterium Bacillus anthracis.

Prevention: No vaccine is currently available for routine use for the general public. People exposed to anthrax who have not yet developed symptoms are given antibiotics along with the anthrax vaccine to prevent infection.

Incubation period: Symptoms usually develop within 7 days.

Symptoms:

Cutaneous (skin) anthrax: A small, painless bump that becomes a painless blister; the blister becomes a painless open sore with a black scab in the center.

Inhalation anthrax: Initial symptoms resemble cold or flu symptoms, including sore throat, mild fever, muscle aches, cough, or fatigue. Later symptoms include rapid pulse and severe difficulty breathing. Inhalation anthrax is often fatal.

Treatment: A 60-day course of treatment with antibiotics. The person is kept as comfortable as possible.

Botulinum toxin

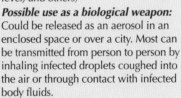

Possible use as a biological weapon: Could be released as an aerosol in an enclosed space or over a city. Most potent known nerve toxin.

Cause: Toxin produced by the bacterium Clostridium botulinum.

Prevention: No vaccine is currently available for the general public.

Incubation period: Symptoms usually develop within 1 to 5 days.

Symptoms: Muscle weakness, double or blurred vision, drooping eyelids, slurred speech, difficulty swallowing, dry mouth, muscle weakness or paralysis, or respiratory failure.

Treatment: Botulism antitoxin stops progression of the disease. The person is kept as comfortable as possible. Breathing may be assisted with a ventilator.

Tularemia

Possible use as a biological weapon: Could be released as an aerosol in an enclosed space or over a city.

Cause: The bacterium Francisella tularensis.

Prevention: No vaccine is currently available for the general public.

Incubation period: Symptoms usually develop within 3 to 5 days (but can take as long as 14 days).

Symptoms: Sudden fever, chills, headache, muscle aches, joint pain, dry cough, weakness, severe difficulty breathing, or pneumonia.

Treatment: A 10- to 14-day course of treatment with antibiotics. The person is kept as comfortable as possible. Breathing may be assisted with a ventilator.

Hemorrhagic fevers

(Ebola, Marburg, Lassa, New World Arenaviridae, Rift Valley, Hantavirus, yellow fever, and others)

Possible use as a biological weapon: Could be released as an aerosol in an enclosed space or over a city. Most can be transmitted from person to person by inhaling infected droplets coughed into the air or through contact with infected body fluids.

Cause: A number of different viruses.

Prevention: Vaccine for yellow fever only. Avoid contact with infected people.

Incubation period: Depending on the virus, symptoms usually develop within 2 to 3 weeks (but can appear as quickly as within a few days or as long as 2 months).

Symptoms: Depending on the virus, initial symptoms usually include fever, fatigue, dizziness, muscle aches, weakness, and exhaustion. Symptoms can also include bleeding under the skin or from body openings, internal bleeding, shock, seizures, or kidney failure.

Treatment: Ribavirin (an antiviral drug) is available for Lassa fever virus, New World Arenaviruses, and Rift Valley fever virus. The person is kept as comfortable as possible. Some hemorrhagic fevers (such as Ebola) are usually fatal.

Plague

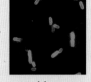

Possible use as a biological weapon: Could be released as an aerosol in an enclosed space or over a city. Can be transmitted from person to person by inhaling infected droplets coughed into the air.

Cause: The bacterium Yersinia pestis.

Prevention: No plague vaccine is currently available. Avoid contact with infected people. Taking antibiotics for 7 days protects those who have had close contact with an infected person.

Incubation period: Symptoms usually develop within 1 to 7 days.

Symptoms: Flulike symptoms including sudden fever, headache, and weakness, followed by shortness of breath, chest pain, cough, bloody or watery phlegm, respiratory failure, or shock.

Treatment: Antibiotics (given within 24 hours after the first symptoms appear). The person is kept as comfortable as possible. Breathing may be assisted with a ventilator. Fatal if not treated.

Smallpox

Possible use as a biological weapon: Could be released as an aerosol in an enclosed space or over a city.

Cause: The variola major virus.

Prevention: Vaccine.

Incubation period: Symptoms usually develop within 7 to 17 days.

Symptoms: High fever, headaches, body aches, and vomiting. A rash appears on the tongue and in the mouth; the rash turns into blisters that break open and spread the virus throughout the mouth and throat. The rash then spreads to the face, arms, legs, hands, feet, and trunk, and turns into pus-filled blisters. Blisters crust over and scab. Scabs begin to fall off, leaving scars.

Treatment: Vaccine (if given within 4 days of exposure). No antiviral treatment is available. The person is kept as comfortable as possible.

Chemical Attacks

A chemical attack is the deliberate release of a toxic gas, liquid (including aerosols), or solid particles (such as dry powders) into the atmosphere. Chemical agents can be released in bombs, sprayed from planes or boats, or discharged from a canister in an enclosed area (such as a building or the subway). A chemical agent can poison people directly or contaminate the environment. Most chemical agents cause symptoms immediately but some can take several hours or even days to have an effect. Symptoms depend on the type of chemical agent used. Chemical agents are classified into the following general categories based on how they affect the body:

- Damage the respiratory system, especially the lungs (phosgene or chlorine)
- Interfere with the body's use of oxygen (cyanide)
- Affect the nervous system (sarin, malathion, soman, tabun, or VX)
- Stun or otherwise cause physical or mental incapacitation (fentanyl)
- Blister the skin (mustard gas)
- Cause irritation (such as chemicals used for crowd control) but usually not permanent or severe damage to health (tear gas, mace, or pepper spray)

Signs of a possible chemical attack:
- A number of people in an area seem to be sick or dying
- Many people have blisters or rashes
- Unusual numbers of birds, fish, insects, or animals are dying
- Vegetation is dead, discolored, or withered
- Strange odors
- An oily film or droplets on outdoor surfaces and water
- Unusual foglike clouds
- Spray devices such as metal canisters or other metal debris that look abandoned

What to do in case of a chemical attack:
- If you think you may have come into contact with a contaminated substance, seek medical help immediately.
- If you are at the scene of a chemical attack, call 911 or your local emergency number.
- If a chemical attack has occurred near your home, stay indoors unless authorities have told you to evacuate the area.
- Do not touch any suspicious substances; report them to the police.
- If the chemical is inside a building you are in, try to get out of the building without passing through the contaminated area.

Radiological Attacks

In a radiological attack, radioactive material could be released into the atmosphere in a number of ways. To contaminate a limited area, a concentrated radioactive material could be placed in a densely populated area and allowed to leak slowly, or a dirty bomb (an ordinary explosive device that contains radioactive material) could be detonated. A 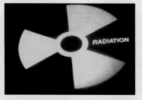 nuclear explosion, caused by detonating a nuclear bomb or by sabotaging a nuclear power plant, could cause widespread destruction and long-term contamination of air, water, and soil.

Experts predict that a radiological attack caused by a radioactive leak or a dirty bomb is far more likely than a nuclear explosion. The radioactive materials used in those types of attacks may be stolen from medical, industrial, or research facilities and are much easier to obtain than the weapons-grade uranium or plutonium required for a nuclear bomb.

If you are in a radiological attack:
- In case of a nuclear explosion, do not look at the flash—it could blind you.
- Try to get to a designated shelter.
- If advised by authorities to stay indoors, try to take cover below ground.
- Stay sheltered until local authorities say it is safe to go outdoors.
- If you are outdoors and can't take cover, try to minimize exposure to the radiation by moving as far away from the explosion as possible as quickly as possible.

After exposure to a radiological substance:
- Remove irradiated clothing, wash the skin, and take other steps to decontaminate.
- Get medical treatment as soon as possible.
- If your doctor recommends it, take a potassium iodide tablet to help protect your thyroid gland (the part of your body that is most susceptible to damage from radiation).
- Have regular medical checkups at least once a year to screen for cancer; exposure to radiation increases the risk of cancer.

Your Healthy Body

Never before have we had such power to control our health. In generations past, the health benefits of regular exercise and the dangers of harmful habits such as smoking were largely unknown. Little was known about the importance of vitamins, antioxidants, fiber, or other nutrients, or the adverse effects of eating too much saturated fat. Today a wealth of information has enabled us to choose health-promoting lifestyle habits that can help us stay fit and live longer.

In this part, you will learn the basics of nutrition and how a healthful diet can help you to lower your risk of heart disease—the No. 1 killer of both men and women in the United States—as well as many of the other common chronic diseases, including type 2 diabetes and some cancers. The critical link between exercise and health, and how to use physical activity to maintain a sensible weight, are also explored. This part also describes ways to reduce stress and avoid harmful behaviors such as smoking and abusing alcohol or other drugs. Information on safety and preventing violence can help you protect your family both at home and when you're away. Other helpful topics discussed here include preventive health care and alternative medicine.

Diet and Health

1

An unhealthy diet is a major factor contributing to the epidemics of obesity, high blood pressure, heart disease, stroke, type 2 diabetes, and some types of cancer. However, diet is one of the most controllable risk factors. You can reduce your risk of developing many chronic diseases by choosing nutritious foods more often and limiting your intake of calories, fat, salt, and sugar. A healthy diet also can help you keep your weight down and your energy levels up. But what constitutes a healthy diet? Nutrition experts agree that you can reduce your risk of many diseases by consuming a diet that contains plenty of fiber-rich vegetables and fruits, an abundance of whole grains, and low-fat sources of dairy, animal, and vegetable protein. This chapter teaches you the basics of good nutrition, explains how nutritional needs change as you get older, and shows you how to improve your diet to prevent disease.

Eating for Good Health

How do you choose nutritious foods to help your family maintain good health? Most doctors agree that the Dietary Guidelines for Americans (see page 37) offer good general guidelines for healthy people. You can tailor these guidelines to meet your individual needs by working with your doctor to identify your personal health risks. As part of a thorough physical examination, your doctor will check your weight, your blood pressure, your cholesterol levels, and your blood glucose (sugar) levels. He or she will ask about your family's health history (see page 131), and calculate your body mass index (BMI; see page 11) and your waist-to-hip ratio to see how fat is distributed on your body. Using this information, you and your doctor can work together to adjust your diet to reduce your risk of disease.

If you have a high cholesterol level and a family history of heart disease, your doctor will probably suggest that you avoid or limit foods high in saturated fat and trans fats (see page 38), exercise regularly, and maintain a healthy weight. If you have a family history of diabetes or are overweight, your doctor will recommend increasing your physical activity and losing weight. If you have a family history of colon cancer or some other cancers, your doctor will recommend reducing your consumption of fat (especially animal fat), increasing your consumption of fiber-rich foods, and increasing your level of physical activity. Depending on your risk factors and your age and gender, the doctor will also tell you what screening tests you need regularly.

The Dietary Guidelines for Americans recommend a diet that is low in fat (especially saturated fat and trans fats) and high in fiber-rich whole grains, vegetables, and fruits. Children under age 2 need breast milk or higher-fat dairy or soy milk or formula to ensure proper brain development. But, after age 2, they should make the transition to low-fat foods. Try to eat at least five half-cup servings of vegetables and fruits and six half-cup servings of grain products and legumes each day. It also is important to eat a wide variety of foods to make sure you are consuming as many essential nutrients as possible. When applying healthy eating principles, consider your diet over several days, but choose wisely meal by meal. Choose low-fat, high-fiber foods more often and use low-fat cooking methods such as broiling and grilling instead of frying.

You don't have to eliminate your favorite high-fat snacks, desserts, or fast foods altogether. If you occasionally indulge in pizza, a burger, or a dish of ice cream, enjoy it. Just try to eat more vegetables, fruits, whole grains, and low-fat foods at your next few meals, a concept known as "fat budgeting." Healthy diets do include certain fats—such as monounsaturated fats—to make you feel full and to provide essential fatty acids.

In fact, some fats are beneficial, improving cholesterol levels and reducing the risk of heart disease. These protective fats come primarily from vegetable oils such as olive, canola, and soy (unsaturated fats); fatty fish such as salmon (omega-3 fatty acids); and some margarines (plant sterols). Other sources of good fats include nuts, seeds, and avocados.

Consume sugar, salt, and alcohol in moderation. Sugar causes tooth decay, and sugar-laden foods such as soft drinks, candy, and pastries contain lots of calories but few nutrients. Many sugary desserts are also high in saturated fat or trans fats. In addition, many fat-free desserts and snacks have replaced fat with sugar and actually have more calories than their full-fat alternatives. You can easily fill up on such foods and exceed your calorie quota, leaving little room for nutritious foods.

Consuming foods that are high in salt (sodium) can elevate blood pressure in salt-sensitive people and also can promote calcium loss from the bones, leading to osteoporosis (see page 989). Although not everyone is salt-sensitive (there is no test to determine if a person is sensitive to salt), your body needs only a very small amount of sodium (fewer than 500 milligrams a day). You can easily exceed the recommended daily allowance for sodium (2,400 milligrams a day), even without adding salt to your food. Processed and commercially packaged foods—including canned soup, pastas, and vegetables; hot dogs; lunch meats; processed cheeses; cereals; flavor packets in rice, dried soup, and noodle packages; crackers; and pretzels—contain high amounts of salt. Check the nutrition labels (see page 3) on packaged foods carefully to determine the sodium content, and look for reduced- or low-sodium versions in the supermarket.

Alcohol, like sugar, provides lots of calories but little or no nutrition. If you choose to drink alcohol, moderation is again the key. Men should have no more than two alcoholic drinks a day and women no more than one. One drink equals one 12-ounce can or bottle of regular or light beer, one 5-ounce glass of wine, or one mixed drink with $1\frac{1}{2}$ ounces of 80-proof liquor. In addition to the many health risks related to excessive drinking, such as liver damage and an increased risk of accidents, excessive alcohol consumption can interfere with your body's ability to absorb nutrients from the food you eat.

A Handful of Nuts Goes a Long Way

Nuts are delicious and, although they are high in fat and calories, they can help you lower your blood cholesterol level and even help you lose weight and keep it off—provided, of course, that you eat them in moderation and maintain an active lifestyle. The portion recommended for the most beneficial effects is 1 ounce a day (about a handful) of nuts or 2 tablespoons of peanut butter. In just a handful of nuts, you get vegetable protein and lots of vitamins—including B vitamins—and minerals—including potassium, magnesium, and phosphorus. Nuts also are packed with heart-healthy nutrients—fiber, vitamin E (an antioxidant that protects blood vessels from the harmful effects of free radicals, which can damage cells), folate (folic acid, which lowers the blood level of homocysteine, a blood chemical linked to heart disease), and copper (which improves cholesterol levels and lowers blood pressure). Just remember that an ounce of nuts also contributes about 200 calories.

The Basics of Nutrition

Carbohydrates, protein, and fat are the main components of a nutritious diet. The goal is to select the best sources in the right proportions every day. Read food labels (see page 3) carefully to find the amounts of these nutrients contained in food products.

USDA Dietary Guidelines for Americans

The Dietary Guidelines for Americans published by the US Department of Agriculture provide reliable, comprehensive nutrition advice. These guidelines show you how to get the nutrients you need to lead a healthier, more active life and to lower your risk for the most common chronic diseases, including heart disease, cancer, high blood pressure, and diabetes. To maintain optimum health:

- Aim for a healthy weight.
- Be physically active every day.
- Eat a variety of grains daily, especially whole grains.
- Eat a variety of fruits and vegetables daily.
- Store food properly.
- Eat a diet low in saturated fat and cholesterol and moderate in total fat.
- Choose beverages and foods that are low in sugar.
- Choose and prepare foods with less salt.
- If you drink alcoholic beverages, do so in moderation.

Carbohydrates

Carbohydrates are the main source of fuel for your body and should make up 45 to 65 percent of your daily calorie intake. Carbohydrates contribute sugar, starches, and fiber from plant foods and come in two forms—simple and complex. Your body absorbs simple carbohydrates—such as those in table sugar, most fruits, and the sugar in milk (lactose)—very quickly. Complex carbohydrates are absorbed more gradually and provide your body with a more constant supply of energy. Complex carbohydrates also help stabilize blood glucose levels, avoiding the up-and-down swings in glucose that can result from eating simple carbohydrates. For these reasons, most of the carbohydrates you eat should be complex carbohydrates from whole grains, vegetables, and whole fruits (including the skins).

Children and adults should consume about 130 grams of carbohydrates every day, which is the minimum amount necessary to get a sufficient amount of glucose to enable the brain to function properly. Most people get much more than this. Sources of added sugars are everywhere in the American food supply and in all food groups. Some obvious sources are candy, soft drinks, fruit drinks, pastries, and other sweets. Some not-so-obvious sources are salad dressings, cereals, ketchup, and breads. People

who eat too many added sugars often take in too many calories and fewer of the essential nutrients than they need. Try to limit your intake of foods and beverages that have added sugars.

Fiber

Fiber, a substance in the cell walls of plants, is an especially important component of complex carbohydrates because it helps lower LDL (bad) cholesterol and reduces your risk of heart disease. Fiber can help you maintain a healthy weight. It also may help lower your risk of colon cancer and other digestive tract disorders such as diverticulosis (see page 772). Dietary fiber occurs in two forms—soluble and insoluble. Neither type is digestible, but they both serve important functions in your diet. Soluble fiber—found naturally in oats, barley, dried

Good Sources of Fiber		
Food	Serving Size	Total Fiber (Grams)
Legumes (Cooked)		
Pinto beans	1 cup	15
Navy beans	1 cup	13
Kidney beans	1 cup	11
Chickpeas	1 cup	9
Vegetables (Cooked)		
Artichoke	1 medium	7
Green peas	1 cup	6
Sweet potato	1 medium	4
Corn	1 medium ear	2.5
Fruits		
Raspberries	1 cup	8
Blueberries	1 cup	6
Apple with skin	1 medium	4
Orange	1 medium	3
Whole Grains		
Packaged wheat-bran cereal	1 cup	8
Whole-grain bread	2 slices	4
Oatmeal (cooked)	1 cup	4
Whole-wheat pasta (cooked)	1 cup	4

beans and peas (legumes), and some fruits—is the type that improves cholesterol. A grass called psyllium, which is added to some cereals and breads and is used in some over-the-counter stool softeners and laxatives, has also been shown to help lower blood cholesterol. Insoluble fiber—contained in whole-wheat bread, wheat bran, and fruit and vegetable skins—provides bulk to stool, helping it pass more easily through the digestive system. For this reason, insoluble fiber, along with plenty of fluid, helps prevent constipation.

The recommended daily intake of fiber for adults up to age 50 is 38 grams for men and 25 grams for women; for adults over 50 (who usually eat less food), the recommendation is 30 grams daily for men and 21 grams for women. Children should have a dietary fiber intake equal to their age plus 5 grams per day. For example, a 6-year-old child needs about 6 plus 5 grams, or 11 grams of fiber per day. Read food labels to determine the fiber content of food products.

Protein

Protein is the major functional and structural component of all the cells in the body, and is essential for building, maintaining, and repairing tissues. Proteins are made up of 21 different amino acids, which can become enzymes, hormones, nucleic acids, or other molecules essential for life. Your body manufactures many of these amino acids, but some must be obtained from the food you eat and are called essential amino acids. Proteins from animal products—such as meat, fish, poultry, eggs, milk, and cheese—are known as complete proteins because they supply all of the essential amino acids.

If you want to limit your intake of animal products, however, eat more plant protein sources, including grains, legumes, nuts, and vegetables. Because none of these foods alone provides all of the amino acids, they are all considered incomplete protein sources. You can, however, get complete proteins by combining plant proteins, such as rice with beans, bread with peanut butter, corn tortillas with beans, and chili with corn bread. Also, you can combine any incomplete protein with dairy protein to further extend or enhance the incomplete protein. For example, macaroni and cheese, beans and cheese, or even whole-grain bread and milk provide good-quality protein.

How Much Protein Do You Need?

The amount of protein you need to fulfill your body's requirements is surprisingly small. Most American adults consume more protein than they need. The recommended daily intake of protein is 63 grams for men and 50 grams for women. Growing children and women who are pregnant or breastfeeding require even more protein.

The more individualized recommendation for adults is 0.8 gram of protein per kilogram (2.2 pounds) of body weight. You can calculate your daily protein need using the following formula. For example, if you weigh 140 pounds:

- To get your weight in kilograms, divide your weight in pounds by 2.2 (140 ÷ 2.2 = 64 kilograms).
- To find out how many grams of protein you need each day, multiply your weight in kilograms by 0.8 gram (64 × 0.8 = 51 grams of protein).

There are 4 calories in each gram of protein. To find out how many calories of protein you should consume each day, multiply your daily gram allowance of protein by 4 calories (51 × 4 = 204 calories of protein). Based on your weight, you should get about 51 grams, or 204 calories, of protein each day. You can easily reach this target if you eat one 3-ounce serving of meat, poultry, or fish; consume a cup of yogurt; drink an 8-ounce glass of low-fat milk; and enjoy a handful of nuts each day. A 3-ounce serving of meat, fish, or poultry is about the size of your palm.

Fat

Your body uses the fat that naturally occurs in food to store energy and carry certain vitamins through the bloodstream. The structural units of fat, called fatty acids, are also used to make hormones. Fat makes you feel full, adds flavor to foods, and makes foods feel smooth in the mouth. It's what makes ice cream taste creamy on your tongue, and it makes cakes and other baked goods soft.

Each type of dietary fat or oil is comprised of a combination of fatty acids, including smaller or larger amounts of saturated and unsaturated fatty acids. Some fats—especially monounsaturated fats (found in foods such as olive oil, canola oil,

Comparing Protein Sources

Food	Serving Size	Total Protein (Grams)
Meat, Poultry, and Fish		
Chicken breast (skinless)	3 ounces	27
Beef (lean)	3 ounces	26
Pork (lean)	3 ounces	26
Turkey (roasted, light meat)	3 ounces	25
Lamb (lean)	3 ounces	24
Salmon (baked or broiled)	3 ounces	23
Tuna (canned in water)	3 ounces	22
Sardines with bones (canned in oil)	3 ounces	21
Shrimp	6 large	10
Dairy Products and Eggs		
Cottage cheese (low-fat)	1 cup	28
Yogurt (nonfat, plain)	1 cup	13
Yogurt (low-fat, with fruit)	1 cup	10
Milk (whole, 1%, skim)	1 cup	8
Cheddar cheese	1 ounce	7
Mozzarella cheese (part skim)	1 ounce	6
American (pasteurized, processed)	1 ounce	6
Egg	1 large	6
Grains, Legumes, and Nuts		
Lentils (cooked)	1 cup	18
Kidney beans (red)	1 cup	13
Tofu, firm	4 ounces	13
Chickpeas (canned)	1 cup	12
Peanut butter (smooth)	2 tablespoons	8
Oatmeal, plain	1 cup	6
Cashews	1 ounce	5
Peanuts (dry-roasted, unsalted)	1 ounce	5
Bread, whole wheat	1 slice	3
Bread, white	1 slice	2
Vegetables		
Peas (boiled from frozen)	1 cup	8
Broccoli, chopped (boiled from raw)	1 cup	5
Potato, baked with skin	1	5
Corn, kernels (cooked from frozen)	1 cup	5

avocados, and nuts) and plant sterols (found in some soft margarines)—are good for you. However, some fats are harmful. Saturated fats (found in meat and full-fat dairy products) and trans fats (found in stick margarines and some commercially baked goods) produce the buildup of fatty deposits in blood vessels that can lead to heart disease. Try to avoid or limit these fats; replace them with healthy, plant-based fats.

Try to consume less than 20 to 30 percent of your total calories from fat. (Infants and young children need a larger proportion of fat—25 to 40 percent of total daily calories.) Also, choose your fats wisely. As few of your calories as possible (less than 5 to 10 percent of total calories) should come from saturated fat and trans fats. Trans fats are found in partially hydrogenated vegetable oils, which are used in many margarines and shortenings to make liquid oils hard at room temperature. Trans fats may be even more harmful to the heart than saturated fats.

Trans fats are often used in packaged baked goods such as cakes, cookies, crackers, and pie crusts; in snacks such as potato chips; and in some dairy products, meats, restaurant fried foods, and fast foods. Consume as little of these fats as possible. Read food labels to find the amounts of trans fats in foods. Take the following steps to limit your consumption of these harmful fats:

• When buying processed foods, read the ingredient list and avoid those that list trans fats or hydrogenated or partially hydrogenated oils. Look for foods that contain unhydrogenated oils.

• Use naturally occurring unhydrogenated oils such as canola or olive oil.

• Choose the soft or liquid margarines sold in tubs or squeeze bottles instead of stick margarines or butter. Look for soft margarines with vegetable oil listed as the first ingredient and that contain no more than 2 grams of saturated fat per tablespoon. Tub margarines that contain plant substances called sterols or phytosterols or stanols have highly beneficial effects on blood cholesterol levels, primarily by lowering the level of harmful LDL. Eating 1 to 2 tablespoons of these margarines with your food each day can reduce total blood cholesterol by as much as 15 to 20 percent.

• Avoid fatty fried foods such as French fries and doughnuts, and snacks such as cookies, crackers, and chips.

Dietary Fat

Different dietary fats can have either beneficial or harmful effects on your blood cholesterol profile. Your blood contains lipo (fat) proteins that influence your risk of heart disease. One lipoprotein, called HDL cholesterol, is good for the heart. Another lipoprotein, called LDL cholesterol, can be harmful to the heart and can increase your risk of heart attack.

Blood cholesterol is a gummy substance your liver makes to help manufacture hormones and bile (a fluid that aids digestion). The liver makes most of the cholesterol from saturated fats that you consume in foods such as meats, baked goods, and full-fat dairy products. A smaller amount of cholesterol is absorbed into the bloodstream directly from cholesterol-containing foods such as egg yolks. The amount of cholesterol in your blood is determined not only by your diet, but also by hereditary factors. Some people inherit a susceptibility to elevated blood cholesterol.

Comparing Types of Fat

Types of Fat	Major Food Sources	Effects on Blood Cholesterol
Monounsaturated fats	Olive oil, canola oil, peanut oil, nuts, avocados	Lower LDL (bad) and total cholesterol and raise HDL (good) cholesterol
Polyunsaturated fats	Corn oil, sunflower oil, safflower oil, flaxseed oil, soybean oil, cottonseed oil, fish	Lower total cholesterol and can lower HDL (good) cholesterol
Omega-3 fatty acids	Fatty, cold-water fish such as salmon, mackerel, and tuna	Lower total cholesterol, lower LDL (bad) cholesterol, and raise HDL (good) cholesterol
Plant sterols	Some tub margarines and salad dressings	Lower total cholesterol and lower LDL (bad) cholesterol
Saturated fats	Fatty red meat, dark meat of poultry, whole and 2% dairy products, butter, chocolate, coconut oil, palm oil	Increase total cholesterol and increase LDL (bad) cholesterol
Trans fats	Most stick margarines, vegetable shortening, partially hydrogenated vegetable oil, deep-fried chips, many fast foods, most commercial baked goods	Increase total cholesterol and LDL (bad) cholesterol and may lower HDL (good) cholesterol
Dietary cholesterol	Egg yolks, shrimp, liver, full-fat dairy products	Raises total cholesterol (but not as much as saturated fats and trans fats do)

Vitamins and Minerals

Vitamins are chemicals in food that your body needs to function normally. Minerals are elements absorbed by plant foods that are essential for your body in very small amounts. With the exception of vitamin D, your body cannot make vitamins or minerals, so you need to get them from the foods you eat. Some people can get sufficient amounts of vitamins and minerals from their diet, but many of us need to take a multivitamin/mineral supplement to ensure that we get all of the essential nutrients. Although food is the best source of nutrients, most doctors now recommend that most people take a daily multivitamin/mineral supplement.

While taking a daily multivitamin can be beneficial, it should not take the place of a healthy diet. Foods supply many nutrients—such as fiber, essential fatty acids, and antioxidants and phytochemicals—that are not present in supplements. Avoid taking massive doses of specific vitamins or minerals, which can be harmful and can increase or reduce your body's absorption of other vitamins

Some Foods That Pack Lots of Nutrients

Nutrition experts recommend consuming a varied diet to make sure you meet all of your nutritional needs. The following foods seem to be especially dense in benefi- cial nutrients. Including them in your diet can go a long way toward ensuring good health and preventing disease.

Food	Nutrient
Cooked tomatoes (tomato sauce or soup, stewed tomatoes, tomato juice), which seem especially potent when cooked in oil	*Lycopene,* a powerful antioxidant that may help prevent certain types of cancer (including prostate cancer) and heart disease; *vitamin C,* an antioxidant that keeps bones, teeth, and skin healthy, helps wounds heal, and fights certain types of cancer; *potassium,* a mineral that helps maintain the body's fluid balance, transmit nerve signals, and produce energy, and may help lower blood pressure and prevent an irregular heartbeat (arrhythmia).
Dark green, leafy vegetables such as spinach, kale, and other greens	*Folate (folic acid),* which prevents birth defects and can lower the risk of heart disease; *calcium,* which builds strong bones and teeth, enhances muscle function, and helps control blood pressure; *lutein,* an antioxidant that helps prevent macular degeneration (a common cause of blindness); *iron,* which prevents anemia; *potassium* (see above); and *vitamin C* (see above).
Cruciferous vegetables such as broccoli, bok choy, brussels sprouts, and cabbage	The antioxidant *beta-carotene,* which fights certain types of cancer; *vitamin C* (see above); *fiber,* which helps reduce the risk of heart disease; and *potassium* (see above).
Unsalted nuts	*Monounsaturated fats, protein, fiber, vitamin E, folate,* and *copper* and *other minerals,* which help protect against heart disease, cancer, and cataracts.
Blueberries, blackberries, raspberries, strawberries	*Antioxidants,* which reduce the risk of cancer and slow the aging process and may aid memory by protecting brain cells.
Fresh (not pickled or smoked) fish, including salmon, herring, mackerel, tuna, and other oily cold-water fish	*Omega-3 fatty acids,* which help protect the heart, improve cholesterol levels, and reduce joint pain and inflammation.
Oats and other whole grains	*Soluble fiber,* which improves cholesterol levels; *B vita- mins,* which help convert proteins to energy and main- tain healthy eyes, skin, and nerve function; and the antioxidant *vitamin E* (see above).
Fat-free dairy foods	*Calcium* (see above); *protein,* which is essential for building, maintaining, and repairing tissues; *vitamin A,* an antioxidant that is essential for growth and develop- ment and for maintaining healthy vision, skin, and mucous membranes; *vitamin D,* which is essential for building bones and teeth and for helping the body absorb and use calcium.

and minerals. For example, fat-soluble vitamins such as A and D (which are not eliminated in urine, as are the water-soluble vitamins) can cause serious health problems. Unless you are a menstruating woman or you have been diagnosed with iron deficiency anemia (see page 610), take a multivitamin that does not contain iron or that has no more than 15 milligrams of iron. Excess levels of iron are linked to an increased risk of heart disease.

Nutrition experts have acclaimed the antioxidant vitamins—vitamin C, the carotenoids (including beta-carotene, lycopene, and lutein) and vitamin E—for their ability to protect cells from damage caused by free radicals, harmful by-products of the body's normal chemical processes. Damage from free radicals is linked to all the common chronic diseases, including heart disease, type 2 diabetes, cancer, and Alzheimer's disease. Damage from free radicals also is responsible for aging. Free radical damage to cells occurs when free radicals outnumber antioxidants in the body. The key is to give antioxidants the upper hand by consuming lots of antioxidant-rich foods—through a diet rich in vegetables, fruits, and whole grains.

Minerals play a significant role in good nutrition. Some minerals, such as chromium, selenium, and zinc, are needed in such tiny amounts that they are called trace minerals. Your body needs other minerals in higher amounts. Magnesium, found in grains, vegetables, and meats, regulates your heartbeat and stimulates the activity of many enzymes (proteins that trigger chemical reactions). Iron, contained in red meat, spinach, and fortified cereals,

helps carry oxygen from your lungs to every other part of your body.

Some people need more of certain vitamins and minerals and other nutrients than other people do. For example, children, teenagers, and adults over age 50 have an especially high requirement for calcium to build bones and to keep bones strong. To ensure proper brain development and to meet their rapid growth requirements, infants and toddlers need to consume more fat than older children and adults. Girls and women who are menstruating need adequate amounts of iron to replace that lost during menstruation. Women of childbearing age should make sure they get enough of the B vitamin folic acid (400 micrograms a day) to prevent birth defects.

Water

Water is an important but often overlooked nutrient. It does not provide energy or calories but, like fiber, it plays a critical role in the body's ability to function normally. Water helps your body distribute nutrients to cells, regulate body temperature, and eliminate waste. Drink six to eight glasses of water each day—more if you consume drinks that contain caffeine or alcohol, both of which increase water loss from the body. Vigorous exercise and hot, humid weather can rapidly use up your body's supply of fluid and increase your need for water, but they are not the only dehydrating factors. Living in a dry climate and dry, indoor heating in the winter can also increase the risk of dehydration and boost your water requirements.

Fluoridated water helps prevent tooth decay. Some parts of the United States have water supplies with naturally occurring fluoride; in others, municipalities add the mineral to the water supply. Many people drink bottled water because they think it's safer. However, most bottled waters do not contain fluoride or naturally occurring minerals. Some supplemented bottled waters contain various nutrients, but they can be expensive and may not be as healthy as water from the tap.

The US government regulates the safety of American drinking water through established standards for water purity. Most public water supplies meet these standards. However, if water treatment systems break down, bacteria and other contaminants can reach unsafe levels. In these situations, local officials usually advise residents to boil their tap water before drinking it or using it for cooking. Lead that

Calcium: Essential at All Ages

Calcium, found in dairy products and calcium-fortified orange juice and other foods, is essential for strong bones and teeth and helps regulate the heartbeat and lower blood pressure. To build strong bones and teeth, children from birth to 6 months should get 400 milligrams of calcium a day, 600 milligrams a day from 7 to 12 months of age, and 800 milligrams a day from 1 to 10 years. Older children, adolescents, and young adults (ages 11 to 24, when the bones reach their peak density) should take in between 1,200 and 1,500 milligrams a day. Adult women and men need about 1,200 milligrams a day. Postmenopausal women need to consume 1,500 milligrams a day (1,000 milligrams daily if they are taking a bone-building medication); men should consume 1,200 milligrams a day after age 50.

leaches from plumbing pipes, solder, or well pumps also can contaminate tap water, especially in older homes. To minimize the level of lead in the tap water in your home, run the cold water for 3 or 4 minutes the first time you use it each day. Always cook with cold tap water instead of hot tap water because hot water pulls lead out of pipes more easily.

Vegetarian Diets

With improved understanding about the role of nutrition in health, vegetarian diets are more popular than ever and are very healthy, as long as they supply adequate amounts of protein, vitamin B12, calcium, vitamin D, iron, and other essential vitamins and minerals that are more abundant in animal-based foods. Vegetarians are less likely than meat eaters to develop heart disease, high blood pressure, and some cancers, or to be overweight. But vegetarians can risk developing iron deficiency anemia (see page 610) or being malnourished if they are not knowledgeable about appropriate food choices.

There are three types of vegetarian diets—ovo-lactovegetarian, lactovegetarian, and vegan. Ovolactovegetarians consume eggs and dairy products along with plant foods. Lactovegetarians eat dairy products but not eggs. Vegans eat only plant foods and, for this reason, are most at risk for vitamin and mineral deficiencies; however, a vegan diet can be very healthy when plant-based foods are combined. A vegetarian diet for children and pregnant women must be planned very carefully to ensure that they consume sufficient calories, calcium, protein, and essential nutrients to meet all their vitamin, mineral, and amino acid (protein) needs.

If you're not ready to be a full-time vegetarian, at least try eating a few vegetarian meals every week. Occasionally having pasta with a meatless sauce, bean or avocado burritos, or mushroom barley soup for lunch or dinner along with salads and fruits will vary your menu, save money, and provide huge health benefits.

Nutritional Needs Change Throughout Life

To a large extent, your age determines your nutritional needs. Newborns and infants have special nutritional needs that are best met by breastfeeding (see page 539). Doctors recommend that mothers breastfeed their babies for the first 12 months of

Food Sensitivities

A food sensitivity is a reaction to an additive or ingredient in a food, but the reaction is not related to the immune system. Sulfites, substances that occur naturally in the fermentation of wine and are used as preservatives on fresh fruits and vegetables, are common additives that cause food sensitivity. Sulfites can trigger severe asthmalike symptoms such as shortness of breath and chest tightness. In the United States, foods and wine that contain sulfites must indicate it on their label. Flavor enhancers (such as monosodium glutamate) and food coloring (mainly yellow dye No. 5) can cause adverse reactions such as headaches. Sometimes a naturally occurring substance called histamine can cause a reaction known as histamine toxicity, which mimics an allergic reaction. Cheese, some wines, and tuna and mackerel sometimes contain large amounts of histamine.

Different people can have different reactions to the same foods. If you think you could be having problems with a particular food, see your doctor; he or she can help you identify the foods that trigger a reaction so you can avoid them.

life. Breast milk supplies better nutrition than commercial formula, promotes healthy brain development, and provides infection-fighting antibodies from the mother. Also, infants should not be given cow's milk until they are 1 year old because it can cause an allergic reaction and is too concentrated for an infant's digestive system.

Toddlers and preschoolers sometimes become picky eaters as their newfound independence propels them into a multitude of activities that seem much more interesting than eating. Start to teach good nutrition habits at this age. Offer your child a variety of foods without forcing him or her to eat any particular food. When deciding how much food to give your child, use this convenient rule of thumb: about 1 tablespoon of each food per meal for every year of age. For example, a typical dinner for a 5-year-old might be 5 tablespoons of chicken along with 5 tablespoons of a vegetable and 5 tablespoons of brown rice.

As your child enters school, he or she will still need lots of calories to fuel growth. However, the number of children in America who are overweight or obese is skyrocketing. Being overweight as a child can lead to health problems such as heart disease and diabetes—and Americans are developing these diseases at younger and younger ages. Limit your child's intake of high-calorie, high-fat snacks, and encourage him or her to be physically active. In general, being physically active is a better solution for an overweight child than a diet that drastically cuts calories because of the risk of developing an eating disorder (see page 725) or of getting insufficient amounts of essential nutrients.

The accelerated body changes that occur during adolescence are sustained by good nutrition. During the rapid growth spurt between ages 15 and 19, athletic teenage boys can require 2,500 to 4,000 calories each day. By contrast, girls usually stop growing at 15 and can easily become overweight if they consume more than 2,000 calories a day. Many teenagers get most of their calories from fast food and junk food. Do what you can to influence your teenager's food choices. Make nutritious food available at home. Offer healthy snacks, such as cut-up vegetables, fresh fruit, whole-grain cereals—or even last night's leftovers. Resist the temptation to buy high-fat, high-calorie, sugar-laden snacks. Remind your teenager to have breakfast every day.

Once a person reaches about 25 years of age, nutritional needs stabilize and stay about the same until middle age and older. Eating a diet that is low in saturated fat and trans fats and high in fiber-rich whole grains, vegetables, fruits, and legumes remains the most sensible path. The average man needs about 2,500 calories each day; the average woman needs about 2,200 daily calories. Consume fewer calories if you are sedentary and more if you are very active.

Avoid weight gain as you age. Excess weight or a body mass index (BMI; see page 11) above the recommended range is always unhealthy and can increase your risk for the most common chronic health problems, including heart disease, high blood pressure, diabetes, and some types of cancer. Although metabolism (the chemical processes that take place in the body) slows down and calorie needs drop with age, your body still needs the same amount of vitamins and minerals. Stay as active as possible; exercise and physical activity can help you maintain muscle strength, boost your metabolism, and fight depression.

The ability to eat nutritiously can be compromised by age-related physical problems resulting from chronic conditions such as arthritis, deteriorating eyesight, and gum disease, or from taking some medications (which can affect your appetite). To make sure you continue to get all the nutrients you need as you age, take advantage of senior citizen programs in your community. Talk to your doctor or to a social worker at your local hospital to find out about available programs. Check with your local senior center to see if it offers inexpensive meals. Home-delivered meals, church-sponsored meal programs, and government-sponsored programs such as food stamps are other options to explore.

If You Are an Athlete

If you are very athletic, your calorie requirements are higher than those for people who are less active. If you train for endurance events such as a marathon or a triathlon, you may need to double your calorie intake each day. Some endurance athletes can develop anemia (see page 610) because vigorous exercise reduces the concentration of iron in the blood. Eating a balanced diet containing iron-rich foods such as fortified cereals and breads, lean beef, pork, the dark meat of poultry, and dried beans is usually enough to prevent sports anemia. Athletes may need slightly more protein than other people, about 1 gram (rather than 0.8 gram) per kilogram (2.2 pounds) of body weight. Protein supplements are unnecessary for athletes because most Americans already consume more protein than they need. However, athletes may need more calcium, potassium, magnesium, and other electrolytes (fluid-balancing minerals) because these minerals are lost in perspiration. Many runners eat lots of carbohydrates just before an event, but this practice is usually not beneficial unless the event is extremely physically demanding, like a marathon.

The most important thing to remember when you are exercising or competing in an athletic event is to drink enough fluids. Water loss from breathing and perspiration can quickly dehydrate you, especially in hot or humid weather. Drink liquids before exercising, every 15 minutes during your workout, and for about 2 hours afterward. Water is the best thirst-quenching liquid, although sports drinks can replace the electrolytes lost during vigorous exercise. But be aware that many sports drinks contain a lot of sugar.

Exercise, Fitness, and Health

2

If doctors could prescribe only one treatment to ensure a long, healthy life, it would be exercise. Regular exercise provides many health benefits, including a reduced risk of heart disease, high blood pressure, diabetes, some cancers, and most of the other common chronic diseases that can affect us as we age. The sedentary lifestyle of increasing numbers of Americans is a serious public health problem in this country. Even if you have been sedentary for years, it's never too late to gain health benefits from exercise.

The Health Benefits of Physical Activity

The human body is designed for movement. We inherited the same efficient mechanisms our primitive ancestors needed for hunting food, traveling long distances on foot, and building shelter. Today, however, most of us drive our cars to the grocery store and sit in offices or classrooms for a large part of the day. Our lack of exercise triggers the processes that lead to common chronic diseases, including osteoporosis, heart disease, high blood pressure, type 2 diabetes, and cancer. Physical activity can help prevent these debilitating chronic diseases and keep you healthy in the following ways:

- Increases the efficiency of your heart and lungs.
- Raises the level of helpful HDL cholesterol and lowers the level of harmful LDL cholesterol in your blood.
- Helps you control your weight.
- Improves sleep.
- Reduces stress, improves your mood, and lowers your risk of depression.
- Boosts the strength and tone of your muscles.

- Builds strong bones.
- Increases the flexibility of your joints.
- Improves your self-image.
- Increases your energy level and endurance.
- Improves your posture.
- Slows the aging process.
- Improves your quality of life as you age.

Exercise also has beneficial effects on the brain. Physical exercise seems to stimulate the growth of brain cells, especially in an area of the brain called the hippocampus, which plays an important role in memory and learning. Physical activity also may improve the brain's defenses against infection.

The Institute of Medicine has established exercise guidelines that set a goal of 1 hour a day of activity, including both low-intensity activities of daily life (such as walking or housecleaning) and more vigorous exercise (such as jogging, swimming, or cycling). If your job is sedentary, you can achieve this goal by, for example, walking at a pace of 4 miles per hour for a total of 60 minutes every day, or by engaging in a high-intensity activity such as jogging for 20 to 30 minutes 4 to 7 days a week. These guidelines are recommended for all children over age 6 and for all adults.

If you have been largely sedentary and start on a moderate exercise program, you can cut your risk of premature death in half. Spread short exercise sessions throughout your day, as long as the total adds up to about 60 minutes. For example, walk your dog briskly for 20 minutes in the morning and 10 minutes more at night. Add a 20-minute walk and a 10-minute stair-climbing session during your lunch hour and you've met your goal.

All types of physical activity are good for you and will lower your risk of heart disease and other illnesses as long as you do them regularly. Of course, the more exercise you do, and the more vigorous, the greater the health benefits. Increase your activity level gradually by adding more vigorous exercises, such as jogging or swimming, to your walking regimen.

People tend to become less active as they get older, but the need for physical activity does not diminish with age. In fact, you will see positive results even if you don't start exercising until you are older. Previously sedentary people who begin exercising in their 50s, 60s, or older can significantly reduce their risk of dying of a heart attack, even if they already have a heart condition. Exercise also increases the flexibility of your joints and the strength of your muscles, reducing your risk of fractures and enabling you to stay active and independent as you age.

Incorporate more physical activity into your daily routine. Get off the bus a stop or two early and walk the rest of the way to work. Use the stairs instead of the elevator whenever you can. Go for bike rides with your children, and take family walks after dinner. Do your own yard work and gardening. In bad weather, walk around the local shopping mall a few times. On weekends, plan active outings such as hiking, skiing, or ice-skating instead of going to the movies. Ride a stationary bike or use hand weights while you watch TV. Take the family on a hiking or biking vacation.

Most physical activities do not demand any particular athletic skills. In fact, many people who dislike participating in sports are surprised to find that exercises such as brisk walking are enjoyable. If you have been inactive for a long time, start exercising gradually to build up your endurance. Stretch before and after your workouts (see page 8), and warm up before each session and cool down afterward by walking at a moderate pace. If you are healthy, you probably don't need to see your doctor before beginning an exercise program as long as you increase your exercise gradually. But you should talk to your doctor before you significantly increase your physical activity if:

- You have a heart condition and your doctor has recommended only medically supervised exercise.
- You have had chest pain within the past month.
- You get dizzy when you exercise.
- You get extremely breathless after only mild exertion.
- You take medication for a heart condition or for high blood pressure.
- You have bone or joint problems that could be worsened by exercise.
- You have diabetes that requires you to take insulin injections.
- You are middle-aged or older, have not been physically active, and plan to start exercising vigorously.

If you feel any pain in your joints or experience any other symptoms when exercising, stop exercising and see your doctor right away.

WARNING!

When to Stop Exercising

Although exercise provides numerous health benefits, it is important to know when to stop. Regular exercise can reduce your risk of a heart attack and early death from heart disease, but overexercising can cause a heart attack, especially if you have been sedentary and you have one or more risk factors for heart disease (such as high blood pressure or angina). If you feel any unusual symptoms or if you have difficulty breathing; feel dizzy; feel pain or pressure on the left side or middle of your chest, or on the left side of your neck, shoulder, or arm; or have an irregular heartbeat, stop exercising immediately. Call 911 or your local emergency number, or have someone take you to the nearest hospital emergency department.

Three Kinds of Exercise

Doctors classify exercise into three types: aerobic, strength conditioning, and flexibility. Each type of exercise has a different effect on the body, and you should try to include all three in your fitness regimen.

Aerobic Exercise

Aerobic exercise refers to any activity that uses oxygen to fuel your muscles. When you do aerobic exercise, your moving muscles and joints send messages to your brain that stimulate your heart to beat faster and your lungs to breathe heavier to take in more oxygen. Aerobic exercise makes your heart work harder, increasing its efficiency even when you are at rest. Any repetitive activity that uses the large muscles of your arms and legs for a sustained period of time is aerobic. Examples of aerobic exercise include brisk walking, running, step and aerobic classes, jumping rope, bicycling, climbing stairs, swimming, rowing, skating, and cross-country skiing.

Aerobic exercise is a good way to reduce the relative amount of fat on your body and boost the amount of muscle. It also burns excess calories, which helps you control your weight. People who maintain a healthy weight have a reduced risk of heart disease, diabetes, some cancers, and other health problems that have been linked to being overweight or obese.

Aerobic exercise also improves your mood. People who do aerobic exercise regularly say that they feel better emotionally and mentally. When you engage in aerobic activity, your body produces chemicals called endorphins, which alter brain chemistry to brighten your mood and reduce pain. If you are like most people, you will feel relaxed after aerobic exercise and you will sleep better.

Doctors recommend engaging in aerobic exercise for 30 to 60 minutes every day. Try to reach a heart rate (beats per minute) that is 50 to 80 percent of the maximum rate for your age. This rate is called your target heart rate (see below). If your heart rate does not reach this range, adjust the intensity of your activity until it does.

Remember to warm up for 5 minutes before every exercise session and to cool down afterward. Begin by stretching the muscles and joints in your spine, arms, and legs and then walk, jog, or bike slowly to raise your heart rate slightly and prepare it for the more intense activity to come. Warm-up and cool-down exercises can increase your flexibility and help prevent injury to your muscles and joints.

Finding Your Target Heart Rate

It's easy to calculate your target heart rate. Let's say that you're 40 years old. First, subtract your age from 220 (220 − 40 = 180). The resulting number (180 beats per minute) is your maximum target heart rate. To find your target heart rate range, multiply that number by 50 percent to find the low end and 80 percent to find the high end (180 × 0.50 = 90 and 180 × 0.80 = 144). Your target heart rate range is 90 to 144 beats per minute.

The easiest way to check your heart rate is to count your heartbeats for 6 seconds right after an exercise session and multiply that number by 10 to find the number of heart beats in a minute. To count your heartbeats, place the tips of your middle and index fingers (don't use your thumb) on your throat to one side of your Adam's apple or on the inside of your wrist. As soon as you feel your pulse, start counting the beats for 6 seconds. Multiply the number of beats by 10. If your rate is below or above your target heart rate range, adjust your exercise by making it more or less strenuous.

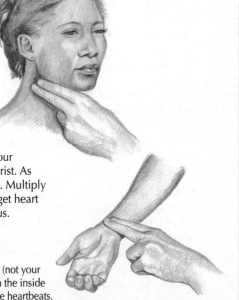

Taking your pulse
To take your pulse, place the tips of your middle and index fingers (not your thumb) on your throat to one side of your Adam's apple (top) or on the inside of your wrist (bottom). When you feel your pulse, start counting the heartbeats.

Staying Strong as You Age

Muscle-building exercises continue to be essential to good health as you age. As you get older, you lose up to half a pound of muscle every year, and the muscle is replaced by fat. This process translates into a 1 to 2 percent loss of strength each year. Over time, the loss in strength can reduce your ability to move, ultimately resulting in a loss of physical independence in old age. Performing strengthening exercises regularly two or three times a week does the following:

- Improves your balance, reducing falls.
- Strengthens your bones, reducing your risk of osteoporosis and fractures.
- Boosts your metabolism (the chemical processes that take place in your body), increasing the rate at which you burn calories.
- Relieves pain from arthritis.
- Improves your state of mind.
- Strengthens your heart.
- Helps you sleep better.
- Improves the quality of your life.

Even if you don't start until your 80s or 90s, strength conditioning will help you perform daily tasks—such as lifting grocery bags or getting up from a chair—that can get more difficult as you get older. A small change in muscle size can make a big difference in strength, which can help you remain independent.

as resistance exercises because they force your muscles to work against, or resist, an object such as a 10-pound weight or the weight of your body.

You don't have to buy any special equipment to build muscle. Lift soup cans or books. Of course, you can buy inexpensive hand and ankle weights or a resistance band at your local sporting-goods store to use at home. Joining a health club will give you access to a variety of weight machines that can condition all of your muscle groups.

If you work out with weights or a weight machine, start with the heaviest weight you can manage to perform 8 to 15 repetitions without stopping. You may have to begin with weights as light as 1 or 2 pounds. Starting with weights that are too heavy can injure your muscles. Exhale as you lift or push the weight, and inhale as you relax. Never hold your breath during strengthening exercises because doing so can affect your blood pressure. Stop if you feel any pain while exercising. Gradually work your way up to heavier weights. (Lighter weights will increase your endurance but not your strength.) Keep using the weights until you can perform a set of 8 to 15 lifts two or three times without stopping between repetitions. Rest between the sets.

For best results, exercise all of your major muscle groups at least twice a week. Don't work on

Keep in mind that if you stop doing aerobic exercise for more than 2 weeks or so, you will start to lose some of the health benefits you have gained. To stay at your more fit level, stick with your aerobic exercise program. Vary your workouts so you won't get bored. Jog or walk briskly a few times each week, swim for a couple of days, and then use a stationary bike or rowing machine for the remaining days of the week. Do an aerobics routine with a video. Think of ways to modify your routine to keep you motivated.

Strength-Conditioning Exercise

Strength-conditioning exercises make you fit by building muscle strength and can be as beneficial for your heart as aerobic exercise. Weight training (using free weights or weight machines) is an efficient way to strengthen your muscles. However, doing sit-ups, push-ups, pull-ups, lunges, and leg lifts can accomplish the same goal. Strength-conditioning exercises are sometimes referred to

Overtraining

Some people—especially those who are training for long-distance endurance events such as a marathon or triathlon—exercise too much without resting between workouts. Up to 60 percent of people who train for such events may exercise to the point of exhaustion, or overtrain. Overtraining can produce changes in the balance of hormones in your body and can suppress your immune system. Common symptoms of overtraining include fatigue, reduced athletic performance, sleep problems, muscle soreness, increased susceptibility to infection, or depression. Women who overtrain can experience potentially serious complications, including absence of periods (see page 846) and osteoporosis (see page 989).

Rest is the usual treatment for overtraining. Your doctor may recommend that you stop exercising for up to 2 weeks to allow your body to repair itself.

the same muscle group 2 days in a row; give your muscles time to rest between workouts. Muscle soreness is natural for a day or two after doing muscle-building exercises.

Flexibility Exercise

As you age, you become less able to move your muscles and joints through their full range of motion. Eventually, decreasing flexibility in your joints can reduce your ability to perform everyday tasks. Exercises such as stretching can help keep your muscles and joints flexible and easier to move. Stretching also protects your muscles from injury as you exercise or perform your daily routine.

You can increase your overall flexibility by making stretching a regular part of your warm-up and cool-down routines (see page 8). Stretching also can prevent or relieve muscle pain or cramps that can occur after vigorous exercise, especially in people who have just begun exercising after a period of inactivity.

The most important muscles to stretch are the hamstring (in the back of the thigh), lower back, and shoulder muscles. When you are stretching, keep the following tips in mind:

- Don't stretch so far that you feel discomfort or pain; pain is a sign that you have stretched too far.
- Stretch slowly and smoothly; avoid bouncing or jerking.
- Hold the stretch. When you have reached a full stretch, hold the position for 30 seconds so your muscles and joints get the full benefit of the stretch.

Exercise-Related Problems

Weight-bearing exercises such as walking or jogging can put a lot of stress on your joints and muscles. Although everyone is at risk when starting an exercise program or when increasing the level of intensity or duration of an activity, overweight people are especially vulnerable to discomfort, pain, or injury from exercise. The most common preventable exercise-related injuries are sprains, strains, inflammation, and pain. If you have a serious injury, such as a broken bone, call 911 or your local emergency number or have someone take you to the nearest hospital emergency department.

Yoga and pilates are excellent forms of exercise for stretching and toning muscles because they put the joints through their full range of motion. These forms of exercise can also improve circulation, relieve tension, and reduce stress. You can probably find a yoga or pilates class at your local health club or community center; many businesses provide exercise classes for their employees. You can also learn the basic yoga postures and pilates exercises from videotapes and books.

Physical Activity and Children's Health

Exercise is as good for children as it is for adults, and the habit of exercising regularly in childhood can lead to an active life in adulthood. Children who engage in regular physical activity gain a number of health benefits, including strong bones, muscles, and joints; lower blood pressure and improved cholesterol levels; weight control; improved self-image; and improved ability to handle stress. Many of these health benefits extend into adulthood. For example, exercising regularly before puberty may reduce the risk of bone fractures and heart disease later in life.

Encourage your children to stay physically active without pressuring them. Give your child a say in the kinds of activities he or she wants to engage in. Make sure the activities are appropriate to the child's physical, mental, emotional, and social maturity. When helping him or her decide, consider the following guidelines:

- **Ages 2 to 5**   Children learn how to run, jump, throw, and catch. Encourage games that use these skills, but keep them simple and don't encourage competition with other children.
- **6 to 9 years**   Children use the skills learned earlier to participate in simplified versions of games and sports. Continue to discourage competition in the early elementary grades. Instead, make sure every child participates.
- **10 to 12 years**   Motor skills and mental abilities are better developed at this age. Children can learn strategy and play organized team sports.

When your child exercises or participates in sports, make sure that he or she wears the proper clothing and uses the right equipment for the activity, including shoes that give good support and traction. Make sure your child has a sturdy bicycle and a helmet that fits properly, and make sure he or she wears it. Mouth guards are essential for protecting the teeth during contact sports such as football and soccer. Because of the way their bones and muscles grow, children and adolescents are prone to muscle tightness, especially in the hamstrings and quadriceps. For this reason, teach your child to stretch before exercising to prevent muscle and joint injury.

Because of their smaller size, children are more susceptible to dehydration than adults. Offer your child plenty of water—even before he or she feels thirsty—especially in hot, humid weather, and send a sports drink along to summer athletic games. Make sure your children wear sunscreen while exercising or participating in any activity outdoors, especially during the summer months.

3

A Healthy Weight

In the United States, two out of three adults and nearly 15 percent of children are overweight. Being overweight increases your risk of developing a number of common chronic illnesses, including heart disease, high blood pressure, type 2 diabetes, and some types of cancer. Overweight children are developing these disorders at younger and younger ages.

Obesity is a complicated chronic disorder caused by a combination of inherited, physical, behavioral, socioeconomic, and cultural factors. People seem to inherit a preset weight range below which it is difficult to stay. While it is possible to keep your weight down near the lower end of your inherited weight range, it would be difficult to stay below it permanently.

Are You Overweight?

Determining if you are at a healthy weight involves the number of pounds you weigh and the percentage of your body that is made up of fat. The way in which fat is distributed on your body—around your waist or around your hips—can also influence your health risks. Women naturally have more body fat than men, especially around the hips and thighs. There is no easy way to measure the amount of fat on your body, but in general, the more active you are, the less your percentage of body fat is likely to be. To find your healthy weight, check the body mass index (BMI) chart on page 11.

The Risks of Being Overweight

Being overweight is a major risk factor for a number of chronic disorders. Where on your body you carry excess weight can also influence your risk of health problems. People who tend to accumulate fat around their waistline are at greater risk of disorders such as high blood pressure, high cholesterol, type 2 diabetes, heart disease, and stroke than are people who tend to accumulate fat around their hips and thighs. Women are at increased risk of health problems if their waistline is larger than 35 inches; men if their waistline is larger than 40 inches. Your risk of health problems increases if your BMI (see page 11) is 25 or greater.

If you already have a health problem associated with being overweight, losing weight will probably help you control it. Even a 10 percent reduction in body weight has health benefits. For some disorders, such as type 2 diabetes and high blood pressure, weight loss can help reduce or even eliminate the need for medication. Even if you are overweight, if you exercise regularly, you can still gain benefits from physical activity, such as a reduced risk of heart disease.

Heart Disease

Being overweight is a major risk factor for heart disease. Although not all the mechanisms involved are known, several factors link obesity to heart disease:

- Being overweight increases the level of total cholesterol and other fats called triglycerides in the blood, which can cause fatty deposits to build up in artery walls.
- Being overweight lowers the blood level of HDL (good) cholesterol, which keeps blood vessels healthy.
- Being overweight increases the risk of diabetes, which increases the risk of having a heart attack.

High Blood Pressure

Being overweight is the No. 1 factor contributing to high blood pressure. In a large percentage of people who have high blood pressure, losing even a modest amount of weight—just 10 pounds—can often bring blood pressure down to a healthy level. Blood pressure readings go down within the first 2 or 3 weeks of weight loss. The percentage of a person's weight that is made up of fat seems to affect blood pressure more than does total body weight. For this reason, strengthening exercises (see page 9) such as weight lifting, push-ups, and leg lifts, which build muscle and reduce body fat, can help keep blood pressure down.

Type 2 Diabetes

More than 16 million Americans have type 2 diabetes, and about a third of them don't know it because the disorder causes no symptoms in the early stages. Type 2 diabetes tends to run in families, but being overweight is a stronger risk factor than heredity. This means that even if you have a family history of diabetes, you can prevent it or delay it by keeping your weight within a healthy range and getting plenty of exercise. Long-term effects of diabetes include blindness, kidney disease, and poor circulation (which frequently results in amputation of lower limbs). People with diabetes also have an increased risk of heart disease, stroke, and high blood pressure.

Cancer

Being overweight appears to increase a person's chances of developing some types of cancer, including cancer of the gallbladder, colon, prostate, uterus, kidney, ovary, and breast. Obesity has also been linked to cancers of the liver, pancreas, rectum, and esophagus. Doctors don't know exactly how obesity increases the risk of cancer because the mechanisms vary for different types of cancer and because obesity results from a complex interaction of inherited and lifestyle factors, any of which could influence the risk of cancer.

For example, kidney cancer is more likely to develop in people who have high blood pressure, which is common in people who are obese. Obesity's role in esophageal cancer appears to be the link between obesity and gastrointestinal reflux disease (GERD; see page 750), which causes inflammation in tissues in the esophagus; chronic inflammation can cause precancerous changes in cells. Some cancers, such as colon cancer, breast cancer, and prostate cancer, seem to result from the interaction of a combination of factors such as diet, weight, and physical activity.

If you have a family history of any type of cancer, especially in a relative who developed cancer before age 60, you should be especially diligent about maintaining a healthy weight. Your doctor also will recommend regular screening tests such as a colonoscopy (see page 767) for colon cancer and a mammogram (see page 141) for breast cancer, usually beginning at about age 40.

Joint Problems

Joint problems frequently develop in people who are overweight. Excess weight increases pressure on the joints in the knees, hips, and lower back, causing the cartilage (the tissue that cushions and protects the joints) to gradually wear away, leading to a type of arthritis called osteoarthritis (see page 996). Over time, the joint damage can become so severe and painful that the joint may have to be surgically replaced (see page 1000). Inflammation of the tendons (tendinitis; see page 984) is also common in overweight people. The tendons can become sore and inflamed from such routine activities as walking. Losing weight reduces wear and tear on joints and tendons and can often help relieve the pain of osteoarthritis.

Sleep Apnea

Sleep apnea (see page 636) is a potentially life-threatening condition that is closely linked to being overweight. The disorder can cause breathing to stop for brief periods of 20 seconds or more several times a night during sleep. Sleep apnea can lead to congestive heart failure (see page 570) because the condition forces the heart to work harder to supply oxygen to the tissues. Weight loss often diminishes or eliminates sleep apnea.

Gallbladder Disease

The risk of developing gallstones (small, hardened masses of cholesterol, calcium salts, and bile pigments) rises as a person's weight increases. Although doctors don't fully understand why this occurs, they think that being overweight causes the liver to produce more cholesterol than usual, and excess cholesterol can form gallstones. People who are overweight also may have an enlarged gallbladder that does not empty normally or completely, which increases their risk of developing gallstones. People who carry excess body fat around the abdomen seem to be at greater risk of having gallstones than people who have excess fat around their hips and thighs.

Yet, although it may seem to be a contradiction, rapid weight loss also increases a person's risk of developing gallstones. Doctors think that losing weight too quickly changes the balance of bile salts and cholesterol in the gallbladder, which increases the risk of gallstones. Also, following a very-low-fat diet or skipping meals can decrease contractions of the gallbladder, preventing it from emptying bile often enough, which can promote gallstone formation. The risk is higher when weight loss exceeds 3 pounds a week—a good reason to lose no more than 1 to 2 pounds a week.

People who lose and regain weight repeatedly also seem to increase their risk of developing gallstones, especially when the losses and gains exceed 10 pounds—the more weight lost and regained during a cycle, the greater the risk of gallstones. The reasons for this are unclear, but doctors think that a rise in cholesterol during the weight-loss phase of the cycle may be responsible.

Losing Weight Sensibly

Many people have tried dieting and exercising to lose weight with only modest success. Losing weight is difficult, and going off of a diet is common, especially during holidays and on other special occasions. Successful weight loss depends on setting realistic goals. For example, losing 10 percent of your total body weight within 6 months is a sensible goal that you can probably reach and, most important, maintain. The sense of accomplishment you get from reaching your goal will encourage you to keep the weight off and possibly lose more.

Fad diets that promise quick and easy results usually deliver nothing but disappointment. Such diets can even harm your health. For example, diets that eliminate entire food groups such as carbohydrates can cause you to become deficient in essential nutrients such as amino acids. High-protein diets are often high in saturated fat, which can raise cholesterol levels. The surest way to lose weight and keep it off is by eating

---

Metabolic Syndrome

Metabolic syndrome is a set of symptoms that refers to a group of factors that, together, indicate a very high risk of developing diabetes and heart disease. Metabolic syndrome is extremely common, affecting about one in every three people between ages 40 and 60. The syndrome increases the likelihood of early death not only from heart disease, but from all causes. A diagnosis of metabolic syndrome is made when a person has at least three of the following five symptoms:

- A waist measurement of at least 40 inches for men and 35 inches for women
- A blood level of triglycerides (a type of fat) of 150 milligrams per deciliter (mg/dL) or higher
- A blood level of HDL (high-density lipoprotein), the good cholesterol, below 40 mg/dL in men and below 50 mg/dL in women
- Blood pressure equal to or higher than 130/85 millimeters of mercury (mm Hg)
- A fasting blood glucose level of 110 mg/dL or higher

Doctors think that lifestyle factors, especially being overweight, play a major role in the development of metabolic syndrome. The two major underlying causes of the syndrome seem to be eating a high-calorie, high-fat diet and not getting enough exercise. You can reduce your risk of having metabolic syndrome by consuming a low-fat, high-fiber diet that includes plenty of fresh vegetables and fruits, legumes, and whole grains, and by making 1 hour of physical activity part of your daily routine.

fewer calories and being more physically active. Follow the healthy eating advice in the Dietary Guidelines for Americans (see page 37).

Doctors recommend losing about 1 to 2 pounds per week. To lose 1 pound per week, you need to burn 3,500 calories more in a week than you take in. You can achieve this by reducing the number of calories you eat by 500 to 1,000 per day or by boosting the number of calories your body burns by the same amount, through increased physical activity. You can lose weight even faster by both reducing calories and exercising more. For example, an inactive 200-pound person who continues to take in the same number of calories but begins walking briskly 1½ miles each day will lose about 14 pounds in a year. By decreasing his or her calorie intake at the same time, he or she will lose substantially more.

About three fourths of the calories you burn every day are used to meet your body's basic needs—sleeping, digesting food, and breathing. Any additional physical activity will burn extra calories. You use only a small number of calories when you sit quietly, but you can burn many more when you walk, ride a bike, jog, swim, lift weights, or play tennis. Engaged in the same activity, a heavier person burns more calories per minute than a lighter person does. For example, a person who weighs 150 pounds burns one third more calories than does a person who weighs 100 pounds. Working harder or faster at a given activity only slightly increases the number of calories you burn.

WARNING!

Over-the-Counter Weight-Loss Drugs

Many over-the-counter weight-loss drugs contain phenyl-propanolamine (PPA), which is also found in some over-the-counter nasal decongestants. (In 2004, the FDA banned the use of ephedra, also called ma huang, in over-the-counter products.) PPA can increase the risk of stroke from bleeding in the brain. Read all package labels carefully, and do not buy any over-the-counter drugs that contain PPA.

Increasing the amount of time you spend on the activity is a better way to burn more calories.

If you plan to start a weight-loss program to lose more than 20 pounds, it's a good idea to talk to your doctor first, especially if you have a health problem, are significantly overweight, or have been inactive for a long time. In the meantime, here are a few helpful suggestions for successful weight loss:

- Get support from friends and family.
- Focus on the many positive health benefits you will get from losing weight.
- Eat smaller, more frequent meals.
- Don't skip meals, especially breakfast.
- Set reasonable goals.
- Make gradual changes in your diet and level of physical activity.
- Exercise for at least 1 hour each day.

If You Are Underweight

Some people are underweight because of an eating disorder (see page 725) or because they have a condition, such as cancer, that causes weight loss. Because they need to maintain their weight or even add pounds, they have to take in more calories each day than they burn.

If you are underweight, you can do a number of things to gain additional pounds. Choose high-calorie foods, but make sure that they are rich in nutrients; good examples are peanut butter, cheese, and milk shakes. Eat high-calorie fruits such as bananas, dried fruit, and canned fruit in syrup. Eat high-calorie vegetables such as olives, avocados, and corn. Eat two or three snacks between the three main meals of your day, but leave plenty of time between your meals and snacks so that you don't feel stuffed.

Add extra calories to your meals by using milk instead of water in soups and sauces. Put a slice of cheese over a baked potato or on your sandwich. Mix wheat germ or powdered milk into casseroles. Make high-calorie shakes with fruit juice, yogurt, and bananas, or buy liquid nutritional supplements.

Reducing Stress

4

The stress response is how the body reacts to threatening, overwhelming, or challenging circumstances. People can experience stress in many different types of situations, positive or negative. Some types of stress—the kind you experience when training for an athletic event, practicing for a piano recital, or meeting a deadline at work—can be useful because you learn or benefit from the experience. Other types of stress—losing a job or being unable to pay your bills—can be emotionally devastating and can affect your health.

The length of time stress lasts is the major factor in how harmful it can be to your health. Acute stress can be severe, but it doesn't last very long. You may have a tight deadline at work, but as soon as it's over, your body recovers from the pressure. In fact, in a situation such as this, the stress response is helpful—it prepares you to meet the challenge. Your nervous system stimulates the production of two stress hormones—cortisol and adrenaline—and increases your heart rate and blood pressure to keep you alert and energized to get the job done.

The most harmful kind of stress is chronic stress—uncontrollable stress that continues with no end in sight. Having a demanding job, caring for a loved one with Alzheimer's disease, or living in extreme poverty are common sources of chronic stress. Long-term situations that are unpredictable, such as living with an abusive spouse, can also produce chronic stress. Traumatic events such as rape, a natural disaster, or military combat can cause a severe psychological disturbance called post-traumatic stress disorder (see page 720).

Chronic stress generates feelings of helplessness and hopelessness that can lead to major depression (see page 709). Constant stress can cause many other health problems, including irritable bowel syndrome (see page 765), high blood pressure, heart disease, and infertility (see page 493). Learning how to handle the stress in your life can help keep your mind and body healthy.

How Your Body Responds to Stress

The human body is designed to cope with sudden, short-term threats. Early humans had to fight for food and shelter and deal with attacks from predators to survive. Their bodies responded to an immediate threat by energizing them and sharpening their attention so they could either stand and fight or escape the danger (called the fight-or-flight response). Today your body responds in the same way—not only to a threat, but also to other pressures such as demands from your employer, children, and family.

When you face a potential threat, your emotions and senses alert a small center in your brain called the hypothalamus. The hypothalamus signals the pituitary gland in the brain and the adrenal glands (two small glands that sit on top of the kidneys) to release a number of different hormones. These hormones work together with your autonomic nervous system, the part of the nervous system that controls involuntary activities of your body such as breathing and heart rate, to prepare your body to respond to the threat.

Cortisol is one of the most important hormones the body releases in response to stress. Cortisol performs a number of functions in the body, but during stress it pumps glucose (sugar) into the bloodstream to fuel the body for action. It also temporarily suppresses some systems of the body that are not critical to the fight-or-flight response, such as the immune system. (See page 13 to learn how the actions of cortisol during chronic stress can adversely affect your health.)

At the same time, your body releases the hormone adrenaline (epinephrine), causing heart rate and breathing to increase, the airways and the blood vessels in the muscles to widen, and the pupils in the eyes to dilate (widen). Blood flows to the brain and muscles, where energy is needed most. Body processes that are not required for the threat response—such as digestion, growth, reproduction, and the immune response—shut down temporarily. Now your body is ready to face or retreat from the challenge.

Once the stressful event is over, your body returns to normal. Your pupils contract, your heart rate and breathing slow, and digestion proceeds as usual. Because the stress response was designed primarily as a survival mechanism, it activates easily but takes a long time to shut down, and you may need to make a conscious effort to bring your body back into equilibrium. Your nervous system triggers the relaxation response. Harnessing this power consciously can help you better handle the stress in your life (see page 59).

Each person's response to stress differs, influenced by a combination of such factors as heredity; childhood experiences; personality; diet, exercise, and sleep habits; having or not having close personal relationships; and income level and social status. Some people seem less able to cope with life's pressures, especially people who experienced severe stress during childhood.

One person may overreact to a relatively minor source of stress (such as missing a bus), activating a cascade of stress hormones that elevates his or her blood pressure and heart rate, while another person might shrug off the situation. Genes, personality, and reactions learned during childhood explain the differences between people's responses to stress. A person may have inherited an overly sensitive stress response or may have learned to respond in this way from one or both parents. The answer probably lies somewhere between the two—an interaction of genetic makeup and experiences.

How Stress Can Make You Sick

The human body is not able to handle the constant release of powerful hormones triggered by chronic stress. The brain can easily become overloaded with the constant release of the stress hormone cortisol, which can kill brain cells directly, impairing a person's ability to remember and learn. The constant release of cortisol makes us feel fatigued but we can't sleep; then we get anxious and depressed.

Most people are aware of the psychological effects of stress, such as an inability to think clearly, make sound judgments, and remember. But stress also can produce angry outbursts, hostility, impatience, and reduced self-esteem, and can lead to depression and a wide range of physical problems, including headaches, indigestion, stomachaches (especially in children), and backaches. Stress can also cause dizziness, a rapid heartbeat, ringing in the ears, and muscle tightness.

Even more serious, stress can contribute to the development of heart disease by damaging the arteries. The increase in blood pressure that occurs during a stress response exerts so much force on the linings of the arteries that it injures them, triggering an immune system response and making the artery walls susceptible to the buildup of plaque—deposits of fat, cholesterol, calcium, and other substances. As these deposits build up, they make the arteries narrower and less able to carry blood to the heart.

The constant release of cortisol during chronic stress also causes high blood sugar (glucose) levels, triggering the release of the hormone insulin, which regulates the body's use of glucose for energy. The excessive, long-term release of insulin can eventually make the body resistant to the effects of the hormone, a condition that causes glucose to build up in the blood. This buildup of glucose in the blood can lead to type 2 diabetes (see page 894).

Are You Under Too Much Stress?

If you are trying to cope with a stressful situation, you may be at increased risk of stress-related illness. Keep in mind that positive changes (such as getting married or having a baby) can produce stress just as easily as negative changes. Here are some examples of common stressful situations:

- Someone close to you died.
- You recently were divorced or separated.
- You or a family member has been hospitalized recently.
- You got married recently.
- You lost your job or retired.
- You are having sex problems.
- You just had a baby.
- Your finances recently became a lot better or worse.
- You changed jobs.
- A child has left home recently or come back home.
- You got a promotion at work.
- You moved, or are remodeling your house.
- Your job is at risk.
- You have taken on substantial debt, such as a mortgage.

Take steps to manage your stress before it overwhelms you or makes you sick. See the next page for the best ways to handle the stress in your life.

Stress and Sleep

Doctors have known for many years that lack of sleep can cause foggy thinking and poor concentration. But lack of sleep also can lead to potentially serious health problems. For example, chronic lack of sleep can place you at risk of developing type 2 diabetes (see page 894). Cortisol, a stress hormone that regulates the blood sugar glucose, seems to be to blame. Prolonged sleeplessness causes the body to continuously release cortisol into the bloodstream. This, in turn, causes a rise in glucose in the blood that prompts the body to release more and more insulin in an attempt to lower the glucose level. Over time, the increased production of insulin leads to insulin resistance, a condition in which the cells no longer respond to the effects of insulin; insulin resistance usually leads to type 2 diabetes. An excess of insulin in the blood also encourages the body to store fat, boosting the risk of obesity.

The chronic release of stress hormones caused by sleep deprivation affects your immune system, making you more susceptible to colds and infections. Also, because your immune system helps your body fight cancer, reduced immune system function from insufficient sleep can put you at increased risk of developing cancer.

Chronic lack of sleep can also accelerate the aging process. When you don't get enough sleep, your brain doesn't make the normal amounts of hormones, producing hormone levels similar to those of a much older person. However, subsequently getting a full night's sleep reverses this aging effect, returning hormone levels to normal.

To get a full night's sleep, try going to bed earlier than you usually do. Use some of the time you might spend relaxing in front of the TV for needed sleep. Keep your bedroom cool (but not cold); most people find it difficult to sleep in a room that is too hot.

If you have trouble getting a good night's sleep, the following strategies may be helpful:

- Go to bed and get up at the same time every day—even on weekends—so you can program a sleep schedule into your body's biological clock.
- Allow enough time each day for at least 8 hours of sleep.
- Engage in relaxing activities before bed. Read a book, listen to soft music, or do relaxation exercises (see page 59).

- Use your bed only for sleep and sex so your mind associates your bed with sleeping and relaxation.
- Drink a glass of fat-free milk before bed. The amino acid tryptophan in the milk will help make you feel sleepy.
- Don't take work-related reading material to bed with you.
- Don't watch an exciting TV show or read a book that is stimulating, frightening, or violent right before bed.
- Don't exercise late in the day. Exercise increases alertness.
- Don't drink alcohol late in the evening. Alcohol disrupts the sleep cycle.
- Don't drink anything containing caffeine and don't smoke for a few hours before bed. Caffeine and nicotine both stimulate the central nervous system.
- Don't go to bed hungry or on a full stomach. Being hungry stimulates you, while being full can make you uncomfortable and restless.

If you continue having difficulty sleeping and it affects your daily routine, talk to your doctor. Insomnia may signal an emotional problem such as anxiety (see page 718) or depression (see page 709). For other possible causes of sleep problems, see the symptom chart on page 212.

How to Handle Stress

No one can avoid stress, but you can deal with it in effective ways that can help prevent health problems. You can learn coping mechanisms to help you manage your time better and change your response to situations that tend to cause you stress. You also can learn how to relieve stress and tension by counteracting the stress response with the relaxation response.

Manage Your Time

You will feel that you have more control over things if you manage your time better. Set goals and break large projects down into smaller, more manageable tasks so you feel that you're accomplishing something. Organize your closet, your desk, your kitchen, and any other storage area so you can find things right away. Plan what you're going to wear the next day the night before so you don't have to rush in the morning. Do tedious tasks first to get them out of the way and limit procrastination. Establish a routine and follow it. If you can, delegate tasks to others. All these techniques can save time and minimize stress.

Exercise Regularly

Regular, vigorous exercise defuses stress by boosting the brain's output of chemicals that counteract the effects of stress hormones. Exercise also gives you a sense of accomplishment, which increases your self-esteem. Improved muscle strength and fitness and the potential for weight loss also can make you feel better about yourself. Exercise fights depression and makes you more alert.

What kind of exercise is best? A combination of aerobic exercise—such as brisk walking, jogging, or swimming—and strengthening exercises such as weight training provide the most health benefits. For more information about exercise and how to incorporate it into your daily routine, see page 6.

Get More Sleep

Getting more sleep will help improve your judgment and make you feel better during the day. A good night's sleep will also keep down the levels of stress hormones. Try to get at least 8 hours of sleep most nights.

Try not to think about your problems late at night. You will probably sleep better if you can relax for a few hours before going to bed. For many people, worries and concerns can seem overwhelming in the middle of the night. For additional suggestions on how to deal with sleep problems, see the previous page.

Eat a Healthy Diet

Eat a low-fat, high-fiber diet that contains plenty of fruits, vegetables, legumes, and whole grains. Avoid high-sugar, high-fat snack foods, which usually are also high in calories. That doughnut may give you a short-term boost but will soon make you feel weak and irritable as your blood sugar level plunges a few hours later. Limit your consumption of foods or drinks that contain caffeine; avoid them completely in the late afternoon and evening. Drink alcohol only moderately (one drink a day for women and two drinks a day for men) because it can disrupt your sleep. Also, because alcohol is a depressant, it can trigger depression in susceptible people.

Maintain a Positive Outlook

A negative attitude can make every task seem daunting. Although it can be difficult if you're feeling low, try to replace negative thoughts with positive ones. For example, look at obstacles as challenges, and defeats as opportunities to try harder. Avoid negative people because it's easy to be drawn into their pessimistic way of thinking. Seeing the humor in a situation can help lighten your mood.

Be Assertive

To get what you need, be assertive—but not aggressive. Aggressive behavior can be unhealthy for your relationships as well as for your health. Learn to ask for what you want. Don't be afraid to say no to additional work you can't possibly handle or to the person who always wants to chat during the workday and keeps you from doing your work. Keep in mind that being assertive doesn't mean being angry or rude, taking advantage of someone, or hurting someone's feelings.

Make Time for Leisure Activities

Plan some time each day for yourself, even if it's just a few minutes to read a book or magazine or take a long bath. On your days off, do something fun with your family or a friend. Take a vacation every year or at least try to get away for a long weekend. If you can't leave town, take time off work to relax at home, finish projects, or enjoy hobbies or other activities.

Concentrate on the Present

Don't brood about things that happened in the past. Holding on to regrets, anger, or old grudges is especially harmful because it can keep you from enjoying life. Don't worry about the future. Think about the future in terms of changes you can make. Try not to worry about circumstances you cannot control.

Take Action

Once you have decided what to do about a problem, act quickly and decisively. Being proactive can give you a sense of accomplishment and can often immediately eliminate a source of stress. However, don't act impulsively—especially if you are angry. Wait until you have calmed down and worked out a sensible plan before you take action.

Don't Play the Blame Game

Avoid blaming other people for your problems. Even if you have been treated badly, holding on to feelings of anger, frustration, or hostility can be harmful to your health. Also, blaming other people prevents you from making positive, constructive changes that can help you avoid similar problems in the future.

Get Help

If you feel that you can no longer cope, get help. Talk to your doctor, contact your hospital social services department, or go to a community mental health agency for a referral to a mental health professional. You also may benefit from joining a support group for people who have similar problems. Your doctor may recommend counseling to help you learn more positive ways to deal with stress or may prescribe medication such as an antidepressant. Medication can sometimes be effective for treating stress, but it is most effective when used in conjunction with one-on-one counseling or therapy.

The Relaxation Response

Developed by Herbert Benson, MD, at Harvard Medical School in the early 1970s, the relaxation response is a simple technique that draws on the meditative practices of Eastern philosophies. The relaxation response has been shown to reverse the effects of stress on the body. It is a simple technique that you can complete in about 20 minutes.

If you are experiencing stress, try to do this exercise twice a day (but wait until at least 2 hours after your last meal):

1. Sit quietly in a relaxed position.
2. Close your eyes.
3. Starting at your feet, consciously relax your muscles. Work your way up your body, relaxing your legs, pelvic region, back, chest, arms, neck, and face.
4. Breathe naturally with your mouth closed. Be conscious of your breathing. Say the word "one" silently to yourself every time you exhale.
5. If distracting thoughts enter your mind, ignore them and concentrate on your breathing. Let the thoughts pass.

6. Stay relaxed and concentrate on your breathing. Keep repeating "one" to yourself for 10 to 20 minutes.
7. When you are finished, don't get up right away. Stay seated for a few minutes, first with your eyes closed and then with your eyes open, to gradually refocus on your surroundings.
8. Don't worry about whether you have done the exercise correctly. Just allow the relaxation to occur at its own pace.

If you don't have time to do the relaxation response exercise twice a day, or if you find yourself in an especially stressful situation, try to do the following exercise. This shorter exercise is especially helpful when you feel overwhelmed by events in your life and need a quick calming fix. You can do it anywhere—waiting in line, stopped at a red light, or on hold on the telephone.

1. Relax and focus on your breathing. Count slowly to yourself backward from 10 to zero, one number per breath.
2. When you reach zero, pause for a moment before resuming your activities.
3. If you don't feel relaxed, repeat the exercise.

5

Staying Safe

Where you live, what you do for a living, and how you spend your leisure time are some of the factors that affect your health and safety. You can take a number of practical steps to help ensure that you and your family are safe at home and on the road. Many of these measures are simple—such as using seat belts each and every time you drive. Others—such as developing a home fire evacuation plan—require preparation and vigilance over time. If you use a commonsense approach to safety and supervise your young children, you can be assured that your family will remain relatively safe.

Keeping Your Children Safe

Young children rely on adults to protect them from accidents and injury because they lack the judgment and experience to protect themselves. A child's natural curiosity and exuberance make him or her more prone to potential danger. Supervise your young child at all times while, at the same time, teaching him or her safe behavior—for example, by explaining why something, such as touching an electrical outlet, is dangerous. You can reduce your child's chances of serious injury by making his or her environment as safe as possible. In addition, make sure that your child knows his or her address and telephone number by age 3 or 4 and how to dial 911 in an emergency.

Preventing Choking and Suffocation

A child can choke on any small object. Small toys, batteries, the tops of pens, safety pins, coins, push-pins, and earrings are just a few of the items that can cause choking. Keep all items that could cause choking out of the reach of young children. Also, children under 4 should not play with any toy that is less than 2¼ inches long.

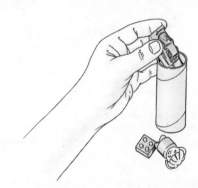

Preventing children from choking on small objects
Young children, especially children under age 4 (who tend to put things into their mouth), have the highest risk of choking on small parts of toys or small toys. A device is available that tests small objects or toys to see if they pose a choking hazard. Or use the cardboard tube inside a roll of toilet paper. Place the toy or part in the tube or tester; if the toy or part fits, a child can choke on it.

Infants and children can easily suffocate if their mouth and nose become blocked. Keep plastic bags away from your children. Don't put pillows or stuffed toys in your young child's bed, and don't put him or her to sleep on a water bed. Always put an infant to sleep on his or her back.

Children under age 2 can easily choke on food. A child's chewing skills are not fully developed until about age 4. Teach your children early on to take small bites of food and to chew food thoroughly. For very young children, cut food into bite-size pieces and watch them while they eat. Don't allow children of any age to talk, walk, or run if they have food in their mouth. Do not allow children to eat in a moving vehicle. If you must eat while traveling, pull over to the side of the road. Encourage children to sit down at the table to eat.

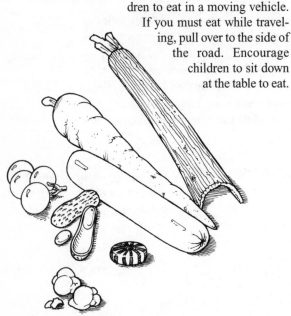

Foods that can cause choking
Never give hard foods such as nuts, hard candy, seeds, popcorn, or raw carrots or celery to children younger than 4 because they usually cannot chew them properly. Other foods young children can choke on include cookies, raisins, and pieces of raw vegetables or fruit. Cut up softer foods such as grapes or hot dogs and other meats into small pieces, or don't give them to your child at all.

Uninflated or broken latex balloons are the No. 1 cause of choking in children. Young children are attracted to colorful, uninflated, or broken balloons and may put them in their mouth. The rubber can become lodged in a child's windpipe, where it obstructs breathing. Never let your children—especially those under age 4—play with latex balloons. To prevent choking, purchase polyester film balloons for children's parties because they don't burst as easily and tend not to break into small parts.

Keeping Your Child Safe Around Pets

Choose pets carefully if you have children. Dogs and cats that are calm and like to be petted are usually good with children. Animals that seem nervous, unfriendly, or afraid can be unpredictable around children and don't make good pets. Pets that become aggressive toward a child (for example, growling or attempting to bite the child) may be capable of causing serious injury. Supervise infants and children under 5 at all times around pets because pets can be jealous and because young children do not always know how to act around animals. Half of all dog bites to children are caused by the family dog. Get obedience training for your dog, and train it to obey commands from all family members. Keep a cat's nails trimmed or get it declawed.

Tell your child to always ask for the owner's permission before approaching an unfamiliar animal. Because dogs can get aggressive when they are defending their territory or themselves, tell children never to put their hands in a place where a dog is confined (such as a pen, car, or yard).

Demonstrate to your child how to safely approach and pet an animal. Keep your arms straight down at your sides, with your hands visible. Speak softly to the animal while lifting your arm slowly and letting the animal sniff your hand. If the animal seems receptive to more contact, gently and slowly touch the side of the animal's head and start petting by scratching the animal behind the ears. Never put your hand on top of an animal's head immediately. Stop right away and slowly back away if the animal shows any signs of aggression.

To be safe around animals, teach your children the following precautions:

- Walk slowly and keep quiet when around strange animals. Never scream or run.
- Avoid staring directly at or teasing an animal.
- Recognize the signs of a disturbed, angry, or frightened animal. For example, avoid dogs that are barking, growling, or showing their teeth; cats that are hissing; and cats or dogs that have their tails up or straight and their ears back.

- Never disturb an animal while it is eating—for example, don't put your hand near a food bowl while the animal is eating.
- Don't attempt to take a toy or bone out of a dog's mouth.
- Don't disturb an animal while it is sleeping.
- Never tease, hit, poke, or throw things at an animal or pull an animal's tail or ears.
- Don't touch or pick up strange animals. Stay away from baby animals because adult animals are protective of their young.
- Get an adult's help if you see animals fighting. Don't try to break up a fight between animals.
- After playing with animals (including turtles and other reptiles), keep your hands away from your mouth, and wash your hands immediately. Try to avoid letting an animal lick your face.

Childproofing Your Home

Hazards in the home injure or kill 2.5 million children nationwide every year. You can prevent injury to your children by childproofing your home before they learn to walk. Use the following guidelines to tackle this project, but keep in mind that no safety device is completely childproof. You still need to closely watch your young children to keep them safe.

- Buy safety latches and locks for cabinets and drawers in the kitchen and bathroom to prevent poisoning and other injuries. These inexpensive devices can stop your child from gaining access to household cleaners and other chemicals, medicines, and sharp objects such as knives. Make sure the latches and locks are sturdy enough to withstand pulling by small hands.
- Put up safety gates to keep children away from stairs and other dangerous areas in the home. At the top of the stairs, anchor the gate to the wall with screws so it can't be dislodged. Check the gate to ensure that it has no openings large enough for a child's head to fit through.
- In the kitchen, turn all stovetop pot handles inward when cooking so your child cannot reach up and pull down a pot.
- Set your water heater temperature no higher than 120°F to prevent scalding, or buy an antiscalding device for your faucets.
- Install spring-loaded electrical outlet covers to prevent electric shock and electrocution.
- Cut your window blind and drapery cords to prevent a child from strangling in the cord loops. You can also install cord cleats or tension devices to keep cords out of reach. Check at your local hardware store. You can get free replacement tassels, cord stops, and tie-down devices from the Window Covering Safety Council (1-800-506-4636).
- Put safety bumpers on the corners and edges of furniture and fireplace hearths to prevent injury should your child fall on them. Remove any furniture that has sharp corners and edges.
- Minimize your child's exposure to lead (see page 425).
- Have your garage door professionally inspected to make sure that it is pinch-resistant and has properly working photo eyes and reversing mechanism. Teach children never to play with the garage door or its control panel or remote controls.
- Don't keep a gun in the house (see page 72).

Crib and High-Chair Safety Standards

New cribs and high chairs must pass rigorous government safety standards before they can be sold, but many parents buy or borrow used cribs and high chairs or use cherished family heirlooms. Before you accept an older crib or high chair, check it to make sure it meets the following standards:

Cribs

- Slats are no more than $2\frac{1}{2}$ inches apart.
- Surfaces contain no lead-based paint.
- End panels have no cutout patterns.
- Corner posts are flush with end panels.
- Mattress fits snugly and extends to all sides of the crib.
- Drop side has a locking latch that does not release accidentally.
- Mattress can be lowered as child gets older so he or she cannot climb out or fall out.

High chairs

- Waist- and crotch-restraining straps are present and do not connect to the tray.
- Tray locks firmly.
- Legs are wide apart, and the base is stable.
- All parts are securely attached.
- Chair locks so it cannot collapse with the child inside.
- Edges are rounded.

Protecting Children From Falls

Active, curious children are prone to falls. Hazards that are clear to adults may not be obvious to children. Supervision is still the best way to prevent injury. Give children extra guidance, especially when they are learning to walk. Make your home a safer place for children by following this simple advice:

- Never leave infants alone on beds or changing tables. Strap infants and toddlers securely into high chairs and strollers. Put guardrails on the beds of young children.
- Don't use infant walkers. Not only can they roll down stairs, but they can also delay a child's development of motor skills and may encourage a child to walk on his or her toes.
- Bolt safety gates to the wall at the top of stairs.
- Do not let children play on balconies or fire escapes.
- Install window locks or guards on all windows, or keep windows closed and locked when children are present.
- Supervise your children closely at all times while grocery shopping. Don't let children of any age play with, push, climb in and out of, or ride on the outside of a grocery cart. Always strap babies and toddlers into a grocery cart; switch to another cart if the belt is broken or missing. Never let a child stand up or lean over while sitting in a cart. Children who weigh more than 35 pounds should not ride in the baby seat of grocery carts (even when the child is strapped in, his or her weight can make the cart top-heavy and tip it over).

Toy Safety

Toys can help a child have fun and learn. However, some toys pose a hazard to young children because they have small parts or can cause a fall. More than 100,000 children are treated at hospital emergency departments every year for injuries caused by toys. Sixty percent of these children are under age 4. Injuries often occur when a young child misuses or plays with a toy designed for older children. Boys are more susceptible than girls to injury from a toy. Most toy-related injuries occur to the head and face. Latex (rubber) balloons (see page 62), which cause choking, are by far the most dangerous toy. Riding toys such as toy cars, scooters, and bicycles account for a large proportion of toy-related injuries and deaths. Most injuries occur when a child falls from the riding toy, but they also occur when the child rides the toy into traffic or into a body of water.

Here are some tips to help you choose toys that are both fun and safe for your child:

- Look for toys that are designed for your child's age group.

Falls From Windows

Unsupervised young children can easily fall from an open window. In the United States, 15,000 children are injured every year and 15 to 20 die after falling from a window. Five times more children who live in apartment buildings—especially those without air conditioning—fall from windows than children who live in single-family homes. A child can be injured or killed falling from a window of any height, even from a first-floor window onto a soft surface.

To keep your child from falling out of an open window, install window guards or window stops. The metal bars of most window guards are spaced no more than 4 inches apart. The guards screw into the side of a window frame, come in different sizes to fit various window types, and can be adjusted for width. Some window guards are designed to be opened easily by an adult (allowing escape from a fire) but are difficult for a young child to open. Window stops are metal locks installed on the sash of a window that can be positioned to allow windows to open no more than 4 inches.

Take these steps now to prevent your child from falling out of an open window:

- Teach your child not to lean on or play near windows.
- Don't leave young children unsupervised in a room with an open window, even if the window is covered by a screen. Screens are designed only to keep insects out, and are not strong enough to keep a child from falling out of a window.
- Move furniture away from windows to discourage children from climbing up to them.
- If you must open a window, do so from the top instead of the bottom.
- Install (or ask your landlord to install) window guards or window stops that allow windows to open only a few inches.

Injuries From Trampolines

Trampolines have become a significant source of injury in children and adolescents. Visits to hospital emergency departments for injuries sustained on home trampolines nearly tripled from 1991 to 1999. Most injuries (including sprains, fractures, cuts, and scrapes) involve the arms, legs, and face, but a few cases of paralysis and death also have occurred. These injuries usually occur when children collide with another person on the trampoline, land improperly, fall or jump off the trampoline, or fall on the springs or frame. Most doctors believe that trampolines of any kind—outdoor or indoor—are unsafe, and doctors often discourage parents from buying them or allowing their children to play on them.

- Don't let your child play with an inflated, uninflated, or broken latex balloon.
- Avoid toys with sharp edges or points, that shoot objects, or that are made of brittle plastic that could break into small pieces or leave jagged edges.
- Throw away plastic bags and wrappings immediately; a child can put these over his or her head and suffocate.
- Use a toy box with a lid that stays open in any position so it cannot fall on your child's head.
- Check your child's toys from time to time for broken parts and potential hazards. Repair or throw away damaged or dangerous toys.
- Instruct older children to keep their toys away from younger siblings and friends.
- Teach your child to put toys away when finished playing with them so no one trips or falls on them.
- Make sure your child wears a helmet every time he or she rides a bicycle, skateboard, or scooter.
- Check with the US Consumer Product Safety Commission (www.cpsc.gov) for toy recalls.

Bicycle Safety

To make each bike ride safe and fun, buy your child a bike that is the right size—not one that he or she needs to grow into. Adjust the seat and handlebars to fit your child properly. Your child should be able to put the balls of both feet on the ground while sitting on the seat. Check to make sure that all of the bike's parts—including the brakes—are secure and in working order. If the bike you buy is used or if your child is using an older bike, have it tuned up and adjusted at a bicycle shop.

Never let your child ride a bike without a helmet, or with a helmet that does not comply with government product safety standards. Bicycle helmets can lower the risk of serious head injury by 85 percent. Choose a helmet that fits snugly and sits flat on the child's head. If necessary, use the extra padding that comes with the helmet to ensure a proper fit. You can remove the padding as your child grows.

Most children are not ready to ride a bike without training wheels until they are 5 or 6 years old. Don't purchase a bike with hand brakes for your child until he or she is older and a more experienced rider.

Children under age 9 should not be allowed to ride in the street. Children between ages 9 and 12 should ride in the street only when accompanied by an older adolescent or an adult. More than 70 percent of all motor vehicle collisions involving bicycles occur near driveways or at street or alley intersections, so tell your child to be especially vigilant at all intersections. Children under age 12 should walk, not ride, a bike through an intersection. They should stop at the intersection; look left, right, and then left again; and then walk their bike across the street before beginning to ride.

If you allow your older child to ride in the street, encourage him or her to wear brightly colored or

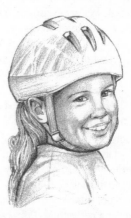

The correct way to wear a bicycle helmet
Bicycle helmets are meant to be worn flat on top of the head, not tilted back at an angle. Make sure that the helmet fits securely and does not block your child's field of vision. The chin strap should be snug, and the buckle should stay fastened throughout the ride. You can adjust the helmet's fit with padded inserts and by loosening or tightening the chin strap.

reflective clothing or reflective tape on his or her ankles, wrists, back, and helmet and to avoid riding at night. Make sure that his or her bike has front and rear reflectors, and install bright lights on the front and back of the bike. No child should ever wear headphones while riding because they block out the sound of traffic.

Bike riders must obey the same traffic laws as drivers of motor vehicles. Teach your child how to signal for turns and to follow other rules of the road. Stress that he or she should always ride in the direction of traffic. Riding against traffic may cause motorists to drive across your child's path or pull into him or her. When riding with your child in the street, observe all traffic laws, not just for safety's sake, but also to set a good example.

A child in a bike passenger seat should not weigh more than 40 pounds or be taller than 3 feet 4 inches. When taking a child for a ride on a bike, use a rear-mounted seat that is firmly fastened over the back wheel. The seat should come with spoke guards that prevent the child's feet and hands from getting caught in the wheel. Make sure that your child wears a bike helmet. Infants under 1 are too young to ride in a rear-mounted seat. Don't carry an infant in a frontpack or backpack carrier that you wear because it will make you top-heavy as you ride, increasing your chances of toppling over with the baby.

If you tow your child in a buggy behind your bike, always strap him or her into the buggy and put a bike helmet on his or her head. Attach a flag on a long pole to the back of the buggy so that other riders and drivers can see you. Always ride on a bike path or street that has little traffic.

Scooter, In-Line Skate, and Skateboard Safety

Scooters, in-line skates, and skateboards account for a large proportion of childhood injuries. Children may be tempted to try difficult stunts while lacking the balance and body control needed to execute them safely. They also can collide with another rider or a pedestrian. Protective gear and common sense go a long way toward avoiding injury during these activities.

Scooters

Lightweight, foot-propelled or motorized scooters can cause injuries requiring a visit to the hospital emergency department. Eighty-five percent of scooter injuries occur in children under age 15. Falls resulting in bone fractures and dislocations, especially in the arms and hands, cause most of the injuries.

To prevent serious injury from a scooter-related fall, instruct your child to wear protective gear when riding a scooter, including a helmet that complies with government safety standards and knee and elbow pads. Check to see that the handlebars and foldable steering column are locked in place and that all nuts and bolts are secure. Encourage your child to ride his or her scooter on smooth, paved surfaces away from traffic (never in the street), avoiding water, gravel, or sand that could cause skidding and falls.

In-line skates

More than 100,000 people go to hospital emergency departments every year seeking treatment for injuries sustained while in-line skating. Skating safely on in-line skates depends on two factors—wearing protective gear and learning how to stop correctly. To prevent injury when in-line skating, your child should always wear a helmet that complies with government safety standards, knee and elbow pads, wrist guards, and gloves. Teach him or her to stop properly by using the brake pads, which are on the heels of most in-line skates: Put one foot in front of the other, raise the toes of the front foot, and push down on the brake with the heel.

Give your child the following tips: Always skate on smoothly paved surfaces, away from traffic. To avoid falls, don't skate on water or gravel. Never skate at night when visibility is poor because you can't see obstacles in your path, and drivers can't see you.

Skateboards

Tens of thousands of people, mostly boys under age 15, are treated in hospital emergency departments for skateboard-related injuries every year. A third of the injuries occur in children who have been skateboarding for less than a week. Common skateboard injuries include sprains, fractures, bruises, and cuts and scrapes from falls. Riding on irregular surfaces, performing risky stunts, and lack of experience, balance, and body control (which is common in children under 15) are factors that contribute to injuries. Falls and collisions with objects or vehicles such as cars can be fatal.

To lower your child's risk of being injured while

riding a skateboard, teach him or her to follow these safety guidelines:

- Check your skateboard after each use. Make sure it doesn't have any broken or loose parts, sharp edges, or cracked wheels. If it does, don't use it again until it has been fixed by a qualified repairperson.
- Wear protective clothing such as a helmet; slip-resistant, closed-toe shoes; elbow and knee pads; wrist guards; gloves; and a padded jacket and shorts. Protective gear is not required to conform to government safety guidelines, so be careful when making a selection. Choose gear that fits properly and does not obstruct your hearing or vision.
- Stay away from irregular surfaces. More than half of all skateboard injuries occur from riding on holes, bumps, rocks, or debris. Check the area where you intend to ride. Better yet, use a designated skateboard park.
- Don't show off. Difficult stunts take careful practice in an area designed for skateboards. Never hitch a ride from a bicycle, car, or other moving vehicle.
- Learn how to fall. If you lose your balance, crouch down low (to shorten the distance you fall), avoid stiffening your body, and roll with the fall. Try to land on the fleshy parts of your body (such as the thighs or buttocks) instead of trying to break the fall with your arms or hands.

Playground Safety

Playgrounds are exciting areas for children to explore and develop motor and social skills. But no national regulations exist for the manufacture or installation of playground equipment, although the federal government has established voluntary guidelines for equipment and ground surfaces. When taking your children to a public playground, it's up to you to check the equipment to make sure it is safe. Look for the following playground safety features:

- Surfaces around the playground equipment should have at least 12 inches of wood chips, mulch, sand, or pea gravel, or be made of safety-tested rubber material.
- The protective surface should extend at least 6 feet from play equipment in all directions. Surfaces around swings should extend to twice the height of the suspending bar both in front and in back.

- Play structures that are more than 30 inches high should be spaced at least 9 feet apart and have guardrails to prevent falls.
- Openings in guardrails or between ladder rungs should be less than $3\frac{1}{2}$ inches or more than 9 inches.
- Sharp points or edges on hardware such as bolt ends should not protrude from the equipment.
- Tripping hazards such as tree roots or stumps or exposed concrete footings should be eliminated.

Don't let young children climb higher than 4 feet (5 feet for older children) because, at greater heights, even recommended surfaces cannot adequately absorb a child's fall. Check your neighborhood playgrounds regularly to make sure the equipment and surfaces are in good condition. Always keep an eye on your children at the playground because supervision is the best way to prevent injuries.

Child Safety Seats

In the United States, motor vehicle collisions are the No. 1 cause of death among children. The best way to protect your child from the risk of injury and death on the road is by using a child safety seat. When purchasing a child safety seat, select one that is right for your child's age and weight, and make sure it fits in your car. Before buying a car seat, try it out in your car to make sure it can be installed properly. Nearly four out of five child safety seats are used improperly because the methods of attachment in different types of motor vehicles vary widely. The three most common mistakes people make when installing car seats are failing to belt the seat into the vehicle tightly enough, keeping the harness straps too loose, and not placing the harness retainer clip at the level of the child's armpit.

All child safety seats manufactured after September 2002 have been standardized. Every new vehicle sold in the United States includes an installation system that uses upper tethers and lower anchors to secure child safety seats. The system, called LATCH (which stands for "lower anchors and tethers for children"), makes it unnecessary to use seat belts to install car safety seats. However, owners of vehicles manufactured before September 2002 must still use the seat-belt method of installation. And parents still have to use seat belts to fasten booster seats for children who weigh 40 to 60 pounds.

Types of Child Safety Seats		
Weight (Age)	**Type of Seat**	**Positioning**
Up to 20 pounds (birth to 1 year)	Infant-only seat or convertible infant-toddler seat	Child and seat face backward. Harness straps are at or below shoulder level.
20 to 40 pounds (over 1 year)	Convertible infant-toddler seat or nonconvertible seat	Child and seat face forward. Harness straps are at or above shoulder level.
Over 40 pounds (about 4 to 8 years), or under 4' 9"	Belt-positioning booster seat or shield booster seat	Child and seat face forward. For the belt-positioning booster seat, use both the lap and shoulder belts, and make sure that the lap belt fits low and tight across the upper thigh (not across the abdomen) and that the shoulder belt fits across the chest and shoulder (not across the neck).

Infant-only seats and convertible infant-toddler seats

Child safety seats for infants under 20 pounds come in two types—infant-only seats and convertible infant-toddler seats. Infant-only seats are more portable and may be more comfortable, but babies outgrow them in the first year, so you will need to buy another safety seat. You can use a convertible infant-toddler safety seat in a rear-facing position until your infant weighs 20 pounds. Then you can use it facing forward when your child weighs 20 to 40 pounds. No matter what type of seat you choose, infants always must face the rear of the vehicle to protect their head, neck, and back in a collision.

Booster seats

Booster seats are designed for children who are too big for a child safety seat but too lightweight and short to use just the vehicle's seat belts. Children need a booster seat if they weigh 40 to 60 pounds or are shorter than 4 feet 9 inches. Riding buckled up in a vehicle without a booster seat forces the shoulder belt to fall across the child's neck. To avoid this discomfort, many children place the shoulder belt under their arms, which can cause serious injury in a collision. Booster seats raise the child up so the shoulder belt falls across the chest and shoulder. The seats come in two types—high-backed, belt-positioning booster seats, and shield booster seats. For either type, make sure the child uses both the lap belt and the shoulder belt, not just the lap belt, for proper protection.

School Bus Safety

A school bus is a relatively safe mode of transportation for children. Even when a school bus is involved in a collision, its occupants are unlikely to sustain serious or fatal injury. But your child can be at risk of being hit by a school bus if he or she does not follow school bus safety procedures. Teach your child the following guidelines to make the ride a safe experience every day:

- While waiting for the bus, stay out of the street and alleys and keep at least 3 feet away from the curb.
- Stay away from the curb and wait to board until the bus has stopped completely and the driver opens the door.
- Use the handrail when getting on the bus.
- Make sure your scarf, book bag, and coat don't get caught in the door of the bus.
- Find a seat right away, sit down and rest your back against the back of the seat, and buckle your seat belt.
- Keep your personal belongings out of the aisle.
- Don't put your arms, hands, or head out the window.
- Wait for the bus to stop completely before unbuckling your seat belt and getting out of your seat.
- If you have to cross the street in front of the bus, walk along the side of the street until you can see the bus driver before walking across the road. Wait until he or she signals that it is OK to cross.

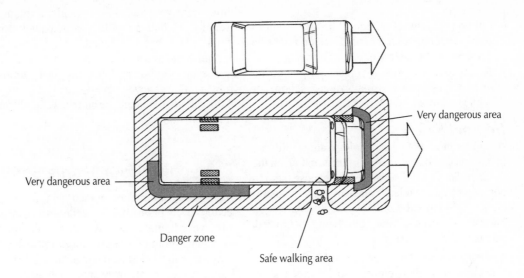

School bus danger zones
A school bus that is stopped on the side of a street creates several danger zones in which it is impossible for the bus driver—and passing drivers—to see pedestrians. Unless they are getting on or off the bus, children should stay at least 10 feet away from the bus on all sides (diagonal lines). Children are the least able to be seen by the bus driver when they are next to the front of the bus and on the right side along the back (shaded area).

Look both ways when you reach the center line of the road.

- Always stay away from the rear wheels of the bus.

Stranger Danger

Tens of thousands of children are reported missing each year. Teach your children not to talk to or get into a car with someone they don't know. Talk to your young children about being observant and cautious around strangers, even seemingly friendly ones (but be careful not to scare them). Adolescents also are vulnerable, so talk to your teenagers about personal safety. Share the following guidelines with your children:

- Always tell your parents where you are going and when you will return. If your plans change, call your parents to tell them where you will be.
- Avoid talking to people you don't know or don't know well. Some strangers pretend they need directions, or help with something. Don't feel guilty about not answering a stranger—adults should ask other adults (not children) for help. Strangers may tell you that your parents are in

trouble and that they will take you to your parents. Don't be tricked into going anywhere with anyone you don't know.

- Never, ever get into a car with a stranger.
- Don't take anything from a stranger.
- Don't accept a message from your parents through another person unless he or she uses a code word that you and your parents have decided on ahead of time.
- Always travel with at least one friend, whether you are walking or riding your bike.
- Never give anyone you don't know well your name, phone number, or address—in person or over the telephone.
- Don't take shortcuts through woods, empty lots, empty buildings, or dark alleys.
- If you are home alone, keep the door locked and don't let anyone in—even someone you know—unless your parents have told you it's OK to do so.
- If you feel that you are in danger, run to a nearby house, restaurant, or store to ask for help.
- If a stranger grabs you, fight back and yell, "I don't know you!" or "You're not my mom (dad)!"

Keep fighting and yelling. Make as much noise as you can.

- Tell your parents if an adult has asked you to keep something a secret—that person might be threatening your safety or that of a friend.
- Tell an adult you trust if you see anyone acting suspiciously around a playground, school, or public rest room.

Internet Safety

Advances in computer technology allow children to have access to new sources of information on the Internet. These same advances can expose them to pornography and violence and leave them vulnerable to exploitation by online sexual predators. To lower the chances of your child being victimized, take the following steps:

- Keep the computer in the den or family room—not in your child's bedroom—so the screen is visible to all family members.
- Use blocking software and other parental control devices provided by your service provider.
- Explain the possibility of online sexual exploitation, especially in chat rooms, to your child.
- Ask your child to show you his or her favorite Web sites and discuss his or her choices.
- Check your child's e-mail messages from time to time, and tell your child why you are doing so.
- Find out if computer safeguards are used by your child's school, the library, and the parents of your child's friends.
- Teach your children never to arrange a face-to-face meeting with strangers they chat with online, never post photographs of themselves on the Internet, and never give out identifying information such as a telephone number.

Here are some signs that your child might be engaging in potentially risky behavior on the Internet:

- Your child turns the computer screen off or changes it when you come into the room.
- Your child spends long periods of time online, especially at night.
- You find pornography on your child's computer.
- Your child gets or makes phone calls to numbers you don't recognize, especially long distance.
- Your child gets mail or gifts from someone you don't know.
- Your child uses an online account belonging to someone else.

If you notice any of these signs, talk to your child about your suspicions openly. Explain that even if your child is a willing participant, he or she is not at fault because the adult always bears full responsibility for such exploitation. If your child ever receives child or adult pornography online or in the mail or if anyone ever sexually solicits your child, call your local police and the Federal Bureau of Investigation.

Keeping Your Home Safe

Many people are injured in their own homes. This section covers basic safety guidelines you can use to make your home as safe as possible. Go through your home room by room to check for safety hazards, especially those that might not be easily visible. Taking a few simple measures, such as installing carbon monoxide detectors and keeping stairs free of clutter, can eliminate many potential dangers.

Preventing Falls in the Home

Falls are the leading cause of accidental death and one of the major causes of injury and death among people older than 65. Most fatal falls occur within the home, mainly on stairs and steps, or from beds and ladders. People over 65 are at increased risk of falling because of reduced vision, slower reaction times, and medical conditions and medications that can affect balance.

You can lower the chances of falls in your home by taking a few simple precautions to fallproof your home. Take steps now to reduce clutter and eliminate slippery surfaces. For ways to protect children from falls, see page 64. Here are some examples of things you can do to make your home safer:

- **Outside** Repair any damaged steps or broken pieces of concrete on sidewalks. Rake or sweep away slippery, wet leaves from sidewalks, stairs, and porches. Eliminate ice from these areas during the winter.
- **All rooms** Keep electrical and telephone cords away from where people walk. Pick up toys, clothes, newspapers, books, and any other items that don't belong on the floor. Pack away and store extra furniture. Keep your floors clean and dry, and don't wax them. Make sure lighting is adequate. Teach pets not to jump on you or weave between your legs. Arrange your furniture to provide open walkways. Eliminate

glass tables, which can shatter during a fall, and furniture that has unprotected sharp edges. If you use area rugs, make sure they have a nonskid backing.

- **Kitchen and bathroom** Clean up spills and wipe away standing water immediately. Don't climb onto the counter to reach items on a high shelf; use a sturdy step stool. Place a night-light in the bathroom and in the hallway that leads to it. Place a rubber mat or nonskid stickers in the tub.
- **Stairways** Pick up clutter and toys on the stairs. Install handrails on both sides. Put a night-light on the stairway. Consider installing a carpet runner if the wooden steps are slippery.

Protecting older people from falls

As people get older, they can become more susceptible to falls because of increased use of medications, disorders that affect the joints (such as arthritis) or nervous system (such as Parkinson's disease), and age-related changes such as decreased vision and hearing. Add such factors as reduced muscle strength and poorly designed living spaces, and the chances of falling rise significantly. Falls can result in serious injuries, such as hip fractures, that can make the difference between a person's being able to live independently and losing his or her independence. To reduce the risk of falling, changes may have to be made to an older person's home. The nature and extent of the changes will depend on his or her physical condition and needs. These changes could be as uncomplicated as moving furniture or as extensive as adding a room. The most important changes to consider are providing adequate lighting, removing clutter, and altering or eliminating slippery surfaces.

Older people need more light than younger people to see properly. Place high-watt bulbs in lamps, and install night-lights in hallways and bathrooms and on stairs. Spatial perception also declines with age, so it's a good idea to have noticeable color contrast between the floors and walls (preferably light carpeting or flooring and dark walls) to prevent bumping into walls. Mark the edge of each stair tread with a contrasting color, and paint or carpet the first and last step with a different color as a cue that steps are beginning or ending. Make sure there is enough contrast between the threshold and the adjoining floor to minimize tripping. Install handrails on both sides of all stairways, including those outside the front and back doors of the home.

Try to minimize changes in the surfaces of floors. Shag carpeting is especially dangerous because it can get caught on toes, canes, and walkers. Avoid using area rugs that can slip or that can trip a person when the edges turn up.

In the bathroom, install two grab bars in the tub or shower area, one positioned for support when getting in and one inside for exiting. They should be parallel to the floor, and their height should be determined by the height of the person most likely to use them. Be sure to attach the grab bars to an underlying stud so they do not pull away from the wall when in use. Put another grab bar next to the toilet in a position that is best for the user. Make sure the bathroom floor has rough, slip-resistant tile because an older person may not be able to wipe up spills and splashes right away. Place a rubber mat or slip-resistant stickers inside the tub.

Older people who use a wheelchair or walker will benefit from wider doors. If possible, increase the door widths to 30 inches, especially in the bathroom. Install a ramp up to the front door for wheelchair access.

Using Medications Safely

When you take different medicines, it can be difficult to remember what each drug is for, how to take it, and when. Expired medications have a way of accumulating, and may lose their potency or undergo a potentially dangerous change in their chemical makeup. You and your family should learn about the medicines you take—both prescription and over the counter—to make sure that you are using them correctly. Here are some tips to help you avoid costly or life-threatening mistakes:

- Make a checklist of all the medicines you take every day, including the name, amount, and times you take them. Put one copy with your medications and another in your wallet.
- Check the label on the container before you take a drug to make sure it is the right one. Never take medications in the dark.
- Take the medication exactly as your doctor prescribed it.
- Don't take medications that are past their expiration date. Check the dates and throw away any medications that have expired.
- Never take medication that has been prescribed for someone else.

- Don't stop taking a drug unless your doctor says it is OK to do so—even if you feel better.
- Don't mix alcohol and medications.
- List all the drugs you are currently taking, and ask your doctor or pharmacist if they can interact when taken together. (Try to use just one pharmacy.)
- Tell your doctor right away about any unwanted side effects.
- Keep medications in a cool, dry place (preferably not in the bathroom medicine cabinet).
- Keep medicines in their original container. (Prescription bottles reduce the amount of light, which can affect some medications.) If you're using a pill organizer, ask your doctor if it's OK to mix the drugs inside the compartments. (When mixed together, some pills interact chemically.)
- Tightly close lids, use child-resistant caps if children live in or visit the home, and keep medications away from children.

Carbon Monoxide Poisoning

Carbon monoxide, a colorless, odorless gas, is the most common cause of death from poisoning in the United States, killing almost 300 people each year. Carbon monoxide is produced when a fuel burns incompletely, and it can easily escape from a defective or improperly vented home heating system. Inhaling carbon monoxide can cause flulike symptoms such as headache, dizziness, nausea, and light-headedness. These early symptoms can quickly progress to seizures, unconsciousness, and death. Entire families have died during the night from carbon monoxide poisoning caused by faulty heating systems.

The following measures can help prevent carbon monoxide poisoning in your home:

- Have new furnaces and gas appliances (such as water heaters) installed professionally.
- Have your furnace inspected and cleaned every year.
- Install a carbon monoxide detector on each floor of your home, including the basement.
- Check the carbon monoxide detector once a month, and replace the batteries at least once a year.
- Make sure all space heaters are properly vented.
- Never use gas or charcoal grills or kerosene lamps indoors.
- Camping equipment (such as portable heaters, lanterns, and stoves) can also emit carbon monoxide. Never use them indoors or while sleeping in a tent or camper.
- Don't run your car in a closed garage, because vehicle exhaust contains carbon monoxide.

If your carbon monoxide detector alarm goes off, call the fire department immediately (even if you think it may only be a low battery) and evacuate your family from your home until the fire department gives you permission to go back inside.

Gun Safety

Half of all homes in the United States contain a firearm. But the risk to the people in the home, especially to children, far outweighs any security benefits—most shooting victims are family members or friends, not intruders. A person living in a home with a gun is 18 times more likely to be killed by the gun than is a stranger. The risk is higher if the home environment includes a person who is violent or verbally abusive, abuses alcohol or drugs, or is depressed. Each year, nearly 6,000 Americans under age 20 die of gun-related injuries, including unintentional injury, homicide, or suicide. For each child killed by a gun, four others are wounded, many so badly that they become permanently disabled.

To protect your family from gun-related injury, don't keep a gun in your home. If you are concerned about protection, take other steps to protect your home and family—buy a home security system, put reinforced bars on your windows and dead-bolt locks on your doors, add outdoor lighting, and start a neighborhood watch program.

Many unintentional injuries occur because a curious child or adolescent plays with or handles an improperly stored gun. If you feel the need to keep a gun in your home for security purposes, or if you keep one or more for hunting, lower your family's risk of injury and death by storing it unloaded (with a gun lock in place) in a locked cabinet or drawer. Make the key available only to responsible adults. Don't tell your child where the gun is stored, because he or she may be tempted to show it off to friends. Keep the ammunition in a separate locked cabinet.

Teach your children never to touch a gun, and tell them to call you or another adult if they ever find one, even if they think it may be a toy. When your children are invited to another child's house to play or if they are going to the home of a babysitter, ask if there is a gun in the home and if it is properly stored. If the gun is not properly stored, invite the other child or the baby-sitter to your home.

Fire Safety

More than 4,000 people in the United States die in fires each year, and an additional 25,000 are injured. Bedrooms are common sites for fires to start—especially electrical fires—and most home fires occur at night when people are asleep. Many fires occur when extension cords are overloaded or portable space heaters are placed too close to bed-clothes or draperies. Other common causes of fires are children playing with matches and smokers falling asleep with a lit cigarette.

Preventing home fires

Fire is a major cause of injury and death and can rob you of your home and your most treasured possessions. Take steps now to protect your family and home from fire:

- Keep matches and lighters locked away from children.
- Keep bedding, clothes, curtains, and other combustible items at least 3 feet away from space heaters.
- Make sure electrical cords are not frayed, especially cords on electric blankets.
- Don't overload wall outlets.
- Never smoke in bed.
- Replace any mattress made before 1973. (Federal mattress flammability standards were raised in 1973.)
- Install smoke detectors (see below) on every floor of your house. Have one close to the bedrooms.
- Avoid planting trees or shrubs that can catch or spread fire easily. Consider planting fire-resistant plants around your home.

- Have your home heating system checked by a professional every year.
- Place a fire screen in front of your fireplace.
- Get your chimney cleaned and inspected each year.
- Consider installing residential fire sprinklers.

The best way to protect your family's safety in a fire is to have an escape plan that you practice every month. Plan at least two ways out of every room. If your secondary exit must be through a window, make sure you'll be able to get to the ground safely. If necessary, buy a collapsible ladder that you can quickly and easily hook on the windowsill and hang out the window. If you have security bars or window guards on your windows, make sure they are the kind that have a quick-release device so they can be opened quickly in an emergency. Check all of your windows to make sure they are not painted shut or otherwise stuck in a closed position.

When you practice your escape plan, rehearse feeling your way out of the house in the dark or with your eyes closed. Practice feeling the doors (not only to be able to find them if you're blinded by smoke, but also to feel if they are hot before exiting through them). Practice crawling low to the ground. Designate a meeting place outside of your house (such as at the end of the driveway or near a certain tree) where family members can meet after everyone has gotten out safely.

What to do in a fire

In a home fire, every second counts. A small fire can go out of control and become a major fire in less than 30 seconds. In only a minute, your house can fill with smoke and become engulfed in flames. The thick, black smoke produced by a fire produces total darkness, making escape more difficult. Room temperatures in a fire can quickly soar to 600°F at eye level, and inhaling superheated air can scorch your lungs. To safely escape a home fire, remember the following tips:

- Leave immediately. Don't try to save your valuables.
- Stay low and keep your mouth covered. Crawl on the floor, under the smoke (which contains toxic gases that can disorient or overcome you).
- Feel closed doors for heat. Use the back of your hand to feel the top of the door, the doorknob, and the door frame. If they feel hot, use another escape route.

Smoke Detectors Save Lives

Smoke detectors—small, battery-powered devices that sound an alarm when exposed to smoke or fire—dramatically increase your chances of survival in a fire. Install a smoke detector on every floor of your home, and make sure one is installed near the bedrooms. Test the smoke detector every month by pressing the test button on the front of the alarm. Change the batteries once a year. Smoke detectors need to be replaced about every 10 years, or according to the manufacturer's guidelines.

- Stop, drop, and roll. If your clothing catches fire, stop running, drop to the ground, and roll over and over until the fire goes out.
- Stay out. Once you are out of the fire, don't go back in for anything.
- Call 911 from a neighbor's house.

Home fire extinguishers

Fire extinguishers can put out a small fire in your home or contain it until firefighters arrive. Put a fire extinguisher on each floor of your home where the risk of fire is the greatest, such as in the kitchen and near the fireplace and furnace. Place it out of the reach of children and near an escape route. Read the manufacturer's instructions so you will know how to use it if you have to.

Fire extinguishers come in different types, or classes. Each type puts out particular kinds of fires. Older fire extinguishers use colored geometric shapes with letter designations and two-word descriptions to differentiate the types of extinguishers. Class A extinguishers are identified by the capital letter A, a green triangle, and the words "ordinary combustibles" and can extinguish fires involving items such as cloth, paper, or wood. Class B extinguishers are identified by a capital B, a red square, and the words "flammable liquids" (such as grease, oil, gasoline, or oil-based paint). Class C extinguishers—identified by a capital C, a blue circle, and the words "electrical equipment"—put out fires involving electrical wiring, appliances, fuse boxes, and circuit breakers. Class D extinguishers are identified by a capital D, a yellow star, and the words "combustible metals."

Many fire extinguishers can put out more than one type of fire and are labeled accordingly. Newer fire extinguishers use self-explanatory pictures and two-word designations to identify the types of fires they fight. The labels may also show a diagonal red line through a picture of a type of fire the extinguisher is not suitable for; for example, a diagonal red line through an illustration of an electrical plug and electrical outlet on fire means that the extinguisher should not be used to put out electrical fires. Some extinguishers can put out all types of fires.

High-rise fires

If you live or work in a high-rise building, become familiar with the special fire-safety and prevention measures required for these structures. Take part in fire drills, and practice escaping from your building

on your own. The following simple fire-safety steps can help prevent loss of life in a high-rise fire:

- Learn your building evacuation plan and practice it.
- Recognize the sound of your building's fire alarm and know the emergency number to call in your area. Don't assume that someone else has already called for help.
- Never lock or prop open fire doors in halls or stairways.
- Install smoke alarms in your apartment or condominium.

If a fire occurs in a high-rise building in which you live or work, try to stay calm and follow these procedures:

- If you are in an apartment or office, feel all doors you use to escape to see if they are warm. If a door feels warm, don't open it. Stay in the room and stuff cloths or tape in the cracks around the door, and cover vents to keep smoke out. Call the fire department and tell them where you are trapped; then wait to be rescued.
- If the door is not warm, stay low while opening it a bit to see if there is smoke or fire in the hallway.
- If you don't see smoke or fire, follow your building's evacuation plan to escape.
- Take the stairs down to the ground floor; never take an elevator.
- If you don't hear the building's fire alarm, pull the nearest fire alarm.
- If smoke or flames block your way out, go to a site far from the source.

Safety With Fireworks

Every year, thousands of people are treated in hospital emergency departments for fireworks-related injuries, and some die. Most of the injured are boys between ages 5 and 14 who play with fireworks such as bottle rockets and sparklers, which are sold legally in many states. Burns to the eyes, hands, and face are the most common injuries. Children lack the physical coordination to handle fireworks safely. The safest way to prevent injury from fireworks is not to buy them and to keep them out of your home and away from children. Enjoy fireworks displays at a local show put on by professionals who are trained to use them safely.

- Once you are out of the building, stay out. Don't go back for anything until the fire department says it is OK to do so.
- Tell the firefighters if you know of anyone who is trapped in the building.

Motor Vehicle Safety

Driving defensively may not be enough to keep you safe on the road. Collisions and breakdowns can make you vulnerable to injury from passing vehicles. Alcohol is a factor in more than 40 percent of all fatal motor vehicle crashes, and nearly 300,000 people are injured in alcohol-related collisions each year. The best defense is to wear your seat belt each and every time you drive. Don't forget to buckle up your children in an age-appropriate safety seat (see page 67), and never let a child age 12 or under ride in the front seat because of the risk of injury and death from a passenger-side air bag (see right).

Seat Belts Save Lives

Seat belts save thousands of lives each year. If you are not wearing a seat belt and you hit something or slam on your brakes, your vehicle will stop but you will keep moving until you hit the windshield, the dashboard, or the back of a front seat. Wearing a seat belt prevents your body from being thrown around inside or out of the vehicle and can help the driver maintain control of the vehicle in a collision. Buckle up on every trip, no matter how short, and teach your children how to buckle up correctly. Here's the right way to wear a seat belt:

- Adjust the lap belt to fit low and tight across your hips and pelvis, not across your abdomen.
- Place the shoulder belt snugly across your chest, away from your neck.
- Never put the shoulder belt behind your back or under your arm.

After a Collision

Each year, about one in every eight drivers has a motor vehicle collision. Many are minor rear-end collisions. If your vehicle is rear-ended and you don't feel safe or are uncomfortable getting out of your vehicle in traffic, signal to the other driver to follow you and then drive to the nearest police station, convenience store, or gas station to look at the

WARNING!

Air Bag Safety for Children

Air bags can save lives in a collision, but they inflate with a force powerful enough to kill or severely injure a child or small adult riding or driving in the front seat. Air bags can inflate after only a slight impact. Also, so-called smart air bags—which are designed to adjust their inflation force according to the size of the passenger or driver (or switch off entirely if the passenger is a young child)—are not 100 percent reliable. Any number of circumstances (such as humidity, shifting body weight on or off seats, the added weight of a child seat, extra tension in safety belts, and reclined seats) can cause air bags to deploy when they shouldn't, or not to inflate when they should. All children age 12 or under (including infants) should ride in the backseat to prevent serious injury or death from inflation of the vehicle's air bag.

damage and exchange insurance information. Some states require vehicles involved in a collision to remain at the site.

The following tips can help keep you safe when you are involved in a more serious collision:

- Stop your vehicle if it is safe to do so, and then carefully move it out of traffic if you can.
- Turn off the ignition of all vehicles involved in the collision.
- Check all the people in each of the vehicles to see if they need medical help.
- Call the police and, if necessary, call emergency medical assistance.

If Your Vehicle Breaks Down

If your vehicle breaks down along a busy road or highway, your greatest danger is getting hit by a passing vehicle. The problem is worsened by the elimination of roadside shoulders, which were designed as a place for disabled vehicles to stop but, in many places, are now being replaced with additional driving lanes. The following steps can minimize the danger if your car breaks down on the highway:

- Pull off the road as far as possible.
- Turn on your hazard lights and the interior dome light.
- Put a white handkerchief or cloth on the antenna, and raise your hood.

- Don't stand next to or behind your car, and don't walk along the highway. If you can, wait on the other side of the guardrail, well away from the highway. Or wait for help inside your vehicle with the doors locked. If you have a flare, place it behind your stalled car.
- If you have a cell phone, call your auto club, a towing service, or the police.
- If someone offers help, don't get in his or her car. Ask the person to call the police.

Driving in Bad Weather

To lower the chances of having your car break down during bad weather, winterize your vehicle according to the suggested maintenance schedule in your owner's manual before winter begins. Regularly check your windshield wipers, lights, and fluid levels (including your windshield-washer solvent). Put snow tires on your car, if needed. Make sure the vehicle's brakes and transmission are functioning properly. Lubricate the door locks and trunk lock to prevent them from freezing.

Prepare an emergency survival kit containing the following items, and keep it in the backseat or trunk of your car:

- Windshield scraper and brush, and snow shovel (in case of snow showers)
- Booster cables
- Flashlight and extra batteries
- Blankets or sleeping bags
- High-calorie, nonperishable food (such as dried fruit)
- First-aid kit
- Knife
- Extra clothing (in case yours gets wet)
- Small metal container and waterproof matches to melt snow for drinking water
- Bag of sand or cat litter for tire traction
- Tool kit
- Tow rope
- Compass and road maps

If a severe storm is forecast, ask yourself if the driving trip is really necessary. If you must drive a long distance and your trip cannot be delayed, listen to weather forecasts (both before you leave and on your car radio as you drive) to find out about current road conditions, or call your state's weather hot line for current information.

Use these guidelines to increase your chances of reaching your destination safely:

- Tell your family or a neighbor where you are going, the route you plan to take, and when you expect to arrive. When you get to your destination, call the person and tell him or her that you have arrived safely.
- Fill your gas tank before you leave to prevent ice from blocking the fuel lines, which could keep the car from starting.
- Ask someone to go along so you don't have to drive alone.
- Clear your windows of snow and ice. Don't start out until your windshield is defrosted.
- Be ready to turn back if weather conditions become threatening.
- In fog, drive with your headlights set on dim, or use fog lights. (Bright lights reflect off the fog, which can decrease visibility.) If the fog gets too dense, pull off the road and wait for the fog to lift. Don't drive at very slow speeds in fog because you can get rear-ended.
- In snow or icy conditions, slow down and keep more distance than usual between your vehicle and the one in front of you.
- Watch for slick spots on bridges and overpasses and in shaded spots.
- If the pavement is slick, start slowly from a stop and brake gently and early. If you have antilock brakes, do not pump your brakes. If your car begins to slide, keep your foot off the gas pedal and brake. Steer into the direction of the skid until you feel the tires' traction; then straighten out the vehicle.
- If a snowplow is coming toward you, stay to the right to allow room for the center line to be cleared. If the snowplow is in front of you, stay back to avoid being sprayed with salt or sand. Pass with care and only when you can see the road ahead of the plow; blowing snow can hide an oncoming vehicle.

Water Safety

Water is an inviting place for family fun, whether at the beach, at a pool, or on a lake or river. But drownings and water-related injuries can occur quickly. The most important step you can take to keep your family safe in and around water is to make sure that every member of your family knows how to swim.

To stay safe whenever you are swimming, boating, or engaging in other water sports, follow these water-safety tips:

- Learn to swim.
- Swim only in supervised areas.
- Obey all posted rules and signs.
- Don't drink alcohol.
- Check the weather conditions; stop swimming in bad weather.
- Know what to do in an emergency.
- Don't swim too far from safety.
- Make sure a pool is deep enough for diving or jumping by easing yourself into the water first.
- Wear a life jacket when boating or rafting.
- Protect yourself from the sun.

Water Safety for Kids

In the United States, drowning is the leading cause of accidental death in children under age 4. A young child can drown in a few seconds in 1 inch of water left in a bucket or wading pool. Even older children are at risk—drowning is a common cause of death in children under age 15. Follow these simple measures to protect children from water accidents:

- Always supervise children closely when they are around water, and make sure they wear a US Coast Guard–approved life preserver or life jacket whenever they are in a boat or near a body of water. Don't rely on inflatable toys or water wings to keep a child afloat.
- Never leave young children alone in the tub, even for a few seconds. Bathtub seats are not safety devices and can tip over, trapping a child underwater.
- Empty the bathtub and all buckets immediately after use.
- Install a toilet lid lock to prevent children from falling into the toilet.
- Sign children up for swimming lessons at about age 5. Children younger than 5 are not yet ready to learn how to swim and may take risks around water.
- Teach children never to swim alone.
- Warn children about the dangers of walking or skating on frozen lakes or rivers.

Home Swimming Pools

Nationwide, hundreds of drownings occur in home swimming pools each year. Most of the casualties are children under age 5. Young children are unpredictable and need to be supervised constantly around water. It takes only a second for a child to become submerged—with no time to scream for help. Some simple measures can lower the chances of having an accident in your home pool:

- Never leave a child in a pool unattended.
- Keep a phone by the pool so you can call for help quickly.
- Learn cardiopulmonary resuscitation (CPR), and insist that all your baby-sitters learn it too.
- Don't get a home swimming pool until your youngest child is 5 years old.
- Encircle your pool with a self-locking fence that is at least 48 inches tall and has vertical bars spaced no more than 4 inches apart. The fence should completely separate the pool from the house. Don't leave furniture or toys near the fence that a child could climb on to reach the pool.
- Keep a pole, rope, and personal flotation device near the pool for rescue purposes.
- Make sure that no standing water has collected in the pool cover; drownings can occur in inches of water.
- Prevent electric shock by keeping electrical appliances away from the pool.

At the Beach

The beach is a great place to take your family for recreation. To make each trip to the beach as safe as possible, follow these beach-safety measures:

- Stay inside the designated swimming area, preferably in sight of a lifeguard.
- Don't swim alone.
- Check beach conditions for bad weather or other potential hazards.
- Don't swim near piers, rafts, docks, pilings, or diving platforms—you could injure your head, neck, or spine, or someone could dive into you. Also, rip currents (seaward-moving water currents, which are difficult to swim against) tend to intensify around fixed objects such as piers.
- If caught in a rip current, swim parallel to shore until you are out of the current. Don't try to swim against the current.
- Be alert for dangerous aquatic life such as jellyfish.
- Stay close to the shore so you have enough energy to swim back.

6

Preventing Violence

Violence is a major public health problem in the United States. The homicide rate is at least two to three times higher in the United States than in any other industrialized nation, and the homicide rate among Americans under age 24 is nearly eight times higher.

This chapter focuses on violence in the home. Family violence includes spouse abuse, child abuse, and elder abuse, but it also extends to violence in the media, which has been shown to increase aggressive behavior in children. You will learn how to prevent violence within your family, what to do if someone you know becomes a victim of violence, and how to protect yourself from sexual assault. You also will find tips on teaching your children to solve problems without resorting to violence.

Family Violence

In the United States, most violence is committed in the home by family members—men against their partners, parents against their children, or adult children against their elderly parents. Spouse abuse, also called domestic violence or battering, is the most common form of family violence and the most common cause of injuries to women. Each year, millions of children and as many as half a million elderly Americans become victims of abuse.

Spouse Abuse

Spouse abuse is recurring coercive behavior intended to intimidate a partner through physical battering (including slapping, punching, kicking, or choking), emotional abuse, sexual assault, or enforced social isolation. Restricted access to or deprivation of food, money, transportation, or employment also is considered spouse abuse. The abuse usually escalates in frequency and severity.

In most cases of spouse abuse, women are abused by their male partner. Women who are at the highest risk of being battered are those who are single, separated, or divorced; who are between ages 17 and 28; who abuse alcohol or other drugs; who are pregnant; or who have excessively jealous or possessive partners.

Spouse abuse occurs in all racial, ethnic, and socioeconomic groups. One out of four American women is abused by a partner at some time in her life. Spouses are not the only victims of domestic violence. Child abuse (see next page) also occurs in up to half of all homes in which a spouse is abused.

Many people who are victims of battering hesitate to seek help or leave their situation. They feel ashamed and humiliated and fear that seeking help will jeopardize their safety or their children's safety by making their partner angry and triggering more violence. Others are prevented from getting help because they are not allowed out of the house or because they lack the money or transportation to leave. Some battered spouses, because they witnessed spouse abuse in their homes during childhood, fail to recognize that their own relationship is abusive. Cultural, ethnic, and religious factors may make it difficult for a spouse to leave an abusive relationship.

Many abusers grew up in families in which they witnessed spouse abuse or experienced child abuse. Use of alcohol and illegal drugs also contribute to violence because mind-altering substances can severely impair judgment and lower inhibitions.

If your partner ever uses violence against you— even once—take it seriously. You are not to blame for being abused. If you are a victim of domestic violence, talk to your doctor. He or she can treat any injuries and can give you the phone numbers of local organizations that can provide help. Don't allow shame or embarrassment to keep you from getting the help you need. Call your local spouse abuse center or battered women's shelter and ask what you should do. If you feel that your life is threatened, call the police. You also can call the National Coalition for Domestic Violence hot line at 1-800-799-7233.

Child Abuse

Because they are young and dependent on adults for care and guidance, children are vulnerable to abuse. Child protective services agencies across the United States receive nearly 3 million reports of child abuse every year, but because many more cases go unreported, the actual incidence of child abuse is thought to be much higher. About three American children die each day from abuse or neglect. Child abuse or neglect is the No. 1 cause of death in children under age 5.

The abuser usually is a child's parent or caregiver, and the problem occurs in all racial, ethnic, and socioeconomic groups. Child abuse is a repeated pattern of any of the following types of abusive behavior:

- **Physical neglect** Failure to meet a child's physical needs, including lack of supervision; inadequate food, shelter, or clothing; abandonment; denial of medical care; or poor hygiene. Physical neglect is the most common form of child abuse.
- **Emotional neglect** Failure to give a child affection and the guidance needed to develop

emotionally by ignoring him or her, withholding affection or attention, or withholding praise.
- **Educational neglect** Failure to enroll a child in school, or overlooking or encouraging truancy.
- **Emotional abuse** Impairing a child's emotional development by screaming, name-calling, shaming, belittling, or telling the child that he or she is bad or worthless.
- **Sexual abuse** Sexual exploitation of a child, including sexual contact between an adult and a child, child pornography, child prostitution, or on-line solicitation of a child for sexual purposes.
- **Physical abuse** Slapping, punching, shaking, burning, biting, choking, throwing, whipping, or paddling a child, whether or not an injury results. Any intentional injury to a child.

The incidence of all types of child abuse is roughly equal among boys and girls, with the exception of sexual abuse, which occurs more frequently to girls than to boys.

Various factors contribute to child abuse, including parental use of alcohol or other drugs, poverty, inadequate parenting skills, and violence within the family. (Some experts also consider witnessing violence in the home to be a form of child abuse.) Children with special needs are especially vulnerable to abuse because their caregivers may be unprepared to provide adequate care or consider them less valuable than other children.

Corporal punishment (such as spanking) has the same effect on children as child abuse. Younger children, especially, cannot distinguish between being spanked as punishment and being spanked in anger. Although spanking a child may make him or her obey immediately, it will not affect a child's behavior over the long term, teach him or her right from wrong, or prevent future misbehavior. Being disciplined with violence teaches children to resolve problems with violence. For these reasons, you should never use corporal punishment to discipline a child. Instead, give your child a time-out or take away a privilege. Some states allow corporal punishment in schools; if your child's school allows corporal punishment, protect him or her by working with the school to eliminate this practice.

Child abuse can have serious, long-lasting consequences for a child and can lead to a psychological disorder called posttraumatic stress disorder (see page 720). Girls who are sexually abused are at especially high risk of smoking, abusing drugs, dropping out of school, stealing, engaging in sexual activity at a young age, or having multiple sexual partners. Many children who were abused have difficulty forming and maintaining healthy relationships in adulthood.

If you know a child who you think may be a victim of abuse or if you think you may be at risk of abusing a child yourself, get help. Call your local child protective services agency or the national child abuse hot line at 1-800-4-A-CHILD (1-800-422-4453).

Teaching Your Child Nonviolent Problem-Solving

Young children often express their needs and emotions without thinking about how they affect other people. Teach your child to be assertive enough to have his or her needs met, without being aggressive. The following steps can help your child become a person who is thoughtful and considerate of other people:

- Give your child plenty of love, respect, and attention. He or she will feel secure and will imitate your behavior when interacting with others.
- When your child says or does something hurtful to another person, ask him or her to think about how the other person must be feeling and to apologize.
- Teach your child to use positive problem-solving skills such as talking instead of yelling or hitting.
- Teach your child to treat everyone with respect.
- Don't use corporal punishment to discipline your children. Violence doesn't change behavior in the long run and teaches children to resolve problems with violence.
- Don't let your child watch violent TV shows, movies, DVDs, or videotapes or play violent interactive video or computer games. Frequent exposure to media violence increases aggressive behavior in children.
- Never allow your child to carry a weapon for self-defense. Knives or guns can easily be stolen or cause unintentional injury.

Media Violence

More than half of all current television programming contains some type of violence. Two thirds of programming targeted to children contains violence. Exposure to violence on television can have a long-term negative impact on children. In addition to

desensitizing children to violence, viewing violence on television may increase aggression, as children try to imitate the violence they see. They may learn to accept violence as a legitimate way of solving problems. Seeing violent images on TV also can make a child afraid. Movies, music videos, interactive video games, and computer games are additional sources of violent images.

The two most important things you can do to protect your children from media violence are to prohibit them from watching TV programs and playing video games with violent content. Here are some additional tips:

- Never put a TV or video game player in your child's bedroom.
- Watch what your children are watching so you can monitor their viewing and talk about the programs.
- Teach your children the difference between real life and the fantasy portrayed on TV. Tell them about the real-life consequences of the violent acts they see in the media. Talk about nonviolent ways the characters could have solved their problems.
- Don't buy violent video games or computer games for your children.
- Don't take your children to movies or let them watch rented movies that are not recommended for children.
- Write letters to TV station program managers to request better programming for children.

Gang Violence

A street gang is a group of young people who engage in antisocial, destructive, or violent behavior, often involving criminal activity. A street gang typically claims a particular city block or street corner as its turf and vigorously defends it. Gang problems occur primarily in large cities, but gang activity is occurring increasingly in the suburbs and in rural communities. Although the majority of gang members are boys, girls organize and are involved in their own gangs in many areas.

Much violence occurs between gangs and inside the gang itself. For example, gangs often initiate new members through vicious beatings and may expect new members to commit violent crimes such as armed robbery, rape, drive-by shootings, or even murder to gain acceptance by the group.

Sometimes innocent bystanders become victims of gang violence.

You can make a difference by volunteering to work with young people, serving as a mentor, or providing opportunities for young people to engage in productive neighborhood projects and activities. Be vigilant about potential gang activity by always removing graffiti on your property and asking the police to discourage young people from loitering. Organize a neighborhood watch program and always report gang activity to the police. Find out what the local gang colors and styles of dress are, and discourage your children from wearing them so they won't be mistaken for a gang member.

Elder Abuse

Experts estimate that more than 450,000 older Americans living at home are abused or neglected every year. People age 80 or older experience abuse and neglect two to three times more often than younger people, and older women are abused more often than older men. Two thirds of all abusers of the elderly are their adult children or spouses. The most common forms of elder abuse include:

- **Neglect** Failure to provide or pay for care, shelter, or other necessities for an older person.
- **Emotional abuse** The use of insults, threats, humiliation, social isolation, or verbal assaults to inflict emotional pain.
- **Physical abuse** The use of physical force to inflict pain, injury, or impairment.
- **Abandonment** Desertion of an older person at a hospital, nursing home, shopping center, or other public location by a caregiver.
- **Financial exploitation** Personal use of an older person's financial resources by a caregiver.
- **Sexual abuse** Any kind of nonconsensual sexual contact with an older person, as well as taking sexually explicit photographs.

Signs of elder abuse can vary widely, ranging from bruises or broken bones and untreated bedsores to sudden changes to a will or bank account. Older people and their caregivers share a complex relationship in which the caregiver has power over the person's basic needs. This power can easily deteriorate into control or coercion, especially when family members are not equipped to handle the role of caregiver, are under extreme stress, or have personal problems such as substance abuse or emotional disorders.

If you provide care for an older person and you feel that you cannot handle your caregiving responsibilities, talk to the person's doctor or to a social worker at your local hospital. They can refer you to community resources, such as respite care, that can provide needed help. If you suspect an older person might be a victim of neglect or abuse, call your local police department, your local public health department, or your state or local area agency on aging.

Sexual Assault

Sexual assault is any type of forced or nonconsensual sexual contact, including rape and forced touching or fondling. Rape is a crime of violence and aggression during which an offender (usually a man) forces a victim (usually a woman) to have sexual intercourse as a way of expressing dominance and control. Women are more likely to be raped by someone they know—a friend, a boyfriend, a date, or a neighbor—than by a stranger.

Do what you can to help people who have been victims of sexual assault. Work with others to prevent future sexual assaults. For example, ask your neighborhood group, school, employer, church, or library to sponsor a talk on rape prevention. Volunteer your time at a rape crisis center.

Protecting Yourself From Sexual Assault

To protect yourself from sexual assault—by someone you know or by a stranger—take the following precautions:

- Take self-defense classes.
- Set clear limits in your romantic relationships.
- Understand that sexually provocative actions and dress could invite unwanted attention.
- Don't let alcohol or other drugs impair your judgment.
- If a situation makes you feel uncomfortable, leave.
- When walking, be aware of your surroundings.
- At home, keep doors and windows locked, especially at night. Install a peephole in your front door. Never open the door to strangers.
- Check the identification of all service people

before allowing them into your home. Don't admit anyone with whom you have not made an appointment in advance.

- Be vigilant in isolated areas such as apartment building laundry rooms, parking lots and garages, and your workplace after hours.
- Don't walk or jog alone in deserted areas or at night.
- Have your key ready as you approach your door or car.
- Park in well-lighted areas and check the backseat of your car before getting in.
- Never pick up a hitchhiker or offer a ride to a casual acquaintance.

What to Do If You Are Sexually Assaulted

Most experts say that fighting back and trying to run away are the best defenses against rape. A rapist is motivated by the need to overpower and control you; he wants you to be compliant. Fight back, scream, and try to run away if you are attacked.

Take the following steps if you have been raped:

- Report the rape immediately to the police or to a rape crisis center to increase the chances that the rapist will be caught. Most sexual offenders repeat their crime until they are caught.
- Preserve the physical evidence. Don't shower or bathe, change clothes, brush your teeth, or wash or throw away any of your clothing until the police tell you that it's OK to do so.
- Immediately go to a hospital emergency department, a rape crisis center, or your doctor's office for medical treatment.
- Seek professional help to cope with your feelings.
- Don't blame yourself.

Complementary and Alternative Medicine

7

Complementary and alternative medicine refers to healing approaches or philosophies that are generally not offered by conventional medical institutions or Western medical schools. People use these treatments in a variety of ways—alone or in combination with other alternative therapies, instead of conventional treatments, or, most often, in addition to conventional treatments.

If you are using an alternative therapy or are considering trying one, tell your medical doctor. Using an alternative therapy as a substitute for conventional therapy without receiving an accurate diagnosis from a doctor can be harmful to your health. In addition, combining some treatments can be dangerous. For example, some herbs can interact with prescription or over-the-counter medications. Although results from an increasing number of studies on alternative therapies are being published in mainstream medical literature, there remains a general lack of understanding about how conventional and alternative therapies function together. Ask your doctor for scientific information about the safety and effectiveness of a particular treatment you are considering, or consult a reliable source, such as the National Center for Complementary and Alternative Medicine at the National Institutes of Health, for guidance.

The complementary and alternative approaches discussed here are a few examples of the more popular treatments people are trying. These discussions are not endorsements by the American Medical Association of any treatments or therapies. The most widely used alternative treatments include herbal therapies and dietary supplements, acupuncture, mind-body therapies such as meditation, and manipulative therapies such as massage and chiropractic.

Alternative Medical Systems

Alternative medical systems are complete systems of medical theory and practice that have developed outside of conventional medicine. Some systems, such as homeopathy and naturopathy, evolved inside Western culture. Others, such as Chinese medicine and Ayurveda, developed in Eastern cultures. Other traditional medical systems exist in Native American, African, Middle Eastern, and South American and other cultures. Fragments of these medical systems still exist in the folk medicine practices of many of the people in these cultures, as well as those of many immigrants to the United States.

Homeopathy

Developed in Germany in the 1790s by a physician, homeopathy is based on the theory that "like cures like." According to this theory, natural ingredients that produce certain symptoms in a healthy person can cure the same symptoms in a sick person when the substances are highly diluted and given in small doses. Homeopathic doctors believe that the more highly diluted the substance, the stronger the medicine. They consider medicines produced in this way to be safer, producing fewer side effects than conventional medicines. The homeopath takes into account the person's personality and mental and emotional states before prescribing a remedy. Homeopathy is used to treat a wide variety of illnesses. Its theoretical base has not been proven by medical science. A variety of published studies on homeopathy have had mixed results.

Naturopathy

Naturopathy is an alternative medical system in which practitioners use natural healing forces in the body to help the body cure itself. Typical therapies include changes in diet, massage, water therapy, light therapy, soft tissue manipulation, and exercise as well as interventions such as acupuncture (see below) and minor surgery. Naturopathy views disease as an alteration in the process by which the body stays healthy and emphasizes the reestablishment of health over the treatment of disease. The effectiveness of naturopathy has not been proven scientifically.

Chinese Medicine

Traditional Chinese medicine is an ancient system of health care that is based on the concept of chi, or qi (pronounced "chee"), the vital energy that flows throughout the body in specific pathways called meridians. According to this theory, disease occurs when the balance of chi is disrupted in the body. Chinese medicine uses a constellation of herbal remedies, nutritional therapy, physical exercises such as t'ai chi, meditation, acupuncture, acupressure, and massage to bring chi back into balance, a process that is thought to cure disease.

Acupuncture

Acupuncture is a Chinese medical technique in which a practitioner punctures the person's skin with very fine needles at points along the meridians through which chi travels to relieve the blockage of the body's vital energy. Sometimes the needles are twirled, warmed, or stimulated electronically. The needles have tapered tips and usually do not draw blood or cause bruising when placed into the skin. In the United States, acupuncture is used primarily for pain disorders, including back pain and migraines, and is sometimes used as an anesthetic. In China the technique is used widely to treat many medical problems and as an anesthetic during surgery.

Moxibustion and cupping are two treatment methods that are closely related to acupuncture. Both use the meridian system central to acupuncture theory and are often performed at the same time as acupuncture. In moxibustion, practitioners burn a herb called mugwort over the skin or on the acupuncture needles to intensify their effects. In cupping, a substance is burned under a glass or bamboo cup, which is then placed over an acupuncture site. The process causes suction that draws blood to the surface of the skin.

In Western medicine, there is no equivalent to the concept of chi, and researchers are looking for a scientific explanation for acupuncture's effectiveness. The meridians along which the needles are placed do not correspond to the nervous system or any other major body system. However, acupuncture treatments for pain have been shown by imaging techniques such as magnetic resonance angiography (MRA) to produce changes in the body that seem to be associated with pain relief.

Acupressure

Another component of ancient Chinese medical practice, acupressure is the application of sustained fingertip pressure on specific points of the body (meridians) to prevent or alleviate disease by balancing the flow of the body's vital energy (chi). The fingertips may be rotated slightly to activate the flow of energy. Acupressure, which is based on the same concept of meridians as acupuncture, is used to treat headaches, pain in the lower back, and a number of other problems.

A Japanese offshoot of acupressure called shiatsu also uses finger pressure on the meridians of the body, but applies different techniques to stimulate the flow of energy. Shiatsu was developed in Japan centuries ago.

Ayurveda

Ayurveda, which means "knowledge of life," is an ancient medical system dating back to 3000 BC and is still practiced in India today. Ayurveda attempts to restore the innate harmony of a person by treating the body, mind, and spirit equally. As in Chinese medicine, health is believed to be determined by the balanced flow of the life force, called prana in India. Traditional Ayurvedic treatments include diet (which recommends some foods and restricts others), fasting, exercise, meditation, herbal remedies, massage, sun exposure, and controlled breathing exercises. Yoga (see page 94) is an important practice of Ayurvedic medicine. If illness cannot be cured using such methods, stronger treatment is given, including purges, emetics (drugs that induce vomiting), and enemas.

Folk Medicine

Folk medicine is the treatment of illness according to the traditional practices of the people of a given culture. Virtually every culture has its own traditional folk medicine practices. Folk remedies typically use herbs and other natural substances. Treatment may be given in the person's home or at the home of a local healer. Many folk remedies have been used for thousands of years and may have health benefits that are poorly understood by medical science. Others may be useless or harmful.

While folk medicine may be appropriate in its traditional setting, it can be dangerous when taken out of its cultural context and practiced by someone outside of the culture. Always talk to your doctor before trying any folk medicine practice.

Herbal Remedies and Dietary Supplements

Plants have been used for centuries to prevent and cure diseases and disorders and to relieve pain. Many drugs in use today are derived from plants, but the Food and Drug Administration (FDA) also has approved more than 200 plant products for sale as dietary supplements. In the United States, dietary supplements are regulated as foods, not drugs. This means that the FDA does not require dietary supplements to undergo the same rigorous approval process required of prescription and over-the-counter medications before they appear on the market. In addition, manufacturers are not required to provide the FDA with evidence that their dietary supplements are safe or effective before marketing them. However, the FDA can remove a supplement from the market if it determines that the product is unsafe.

As with pharmaceutical drugs, the effects of herbs can vary greatly from one person to another, influenced by factors such as weight, sex, age, and general physical condition. In addition, the effects of herbs can be more subdued than those of pharmaceutical drugs, and herbs tend to have less noticeable side effects. But unlike most standard medications, herbal remedies can contain potentially harmful substances because of the lack of regulations for production. A manufacturer's growing conditions, storage, handling, and preparation also can affect potency.

Always let your doctor know about any herbal remedies or dietary supplements you are taking. Don't self-medicate with herbs or supplements without talking to your doctor first and getting a diagnosis. Some of these products can have harmful interactions with prescription and over-the-counter medications. For example, ginkgo biloba can cause excessive bleeding when taken with anticlotting medications such as aspirin or warfarin.

Some doctors recommend that people stop using supplements for at least 3 weeks before having elective surgery. Although adverse effects are rare, taking some herbs or dietary supplements before undergoing surgery can be harmful. Some supplements can speed or slow heart rate, intensify the effects of anesthesia, inhibit blood clotting, or cause the body to reject a transplanted organ.

The herbs and supplements discussed here are among the most common in the United States. Research has supported the use of some of these substances. For others, however, there is no scientific proof of effectiveness.

Aloe Vera

The gel of the aloe vera plant is used to treat burns and heal skin infections. Companies that make skin-care and cosmetic products incorporate aloe into many of their preparations, including hand lotions and shaving creams. The dried outer leaf of the aloe plant is ingested as a powder or dissolved in liquids to aid digestion and relieve constipation. Aloe may cause intestinal cramping, so you should not consume it if you have an inflammatory intestinal disorder (see page 764) such as Crohn's disease or ulcerative colitis or if you have an intestinal obstruction. Do not take aloe during pregnancy because it can trigger contractions of the uterus. Children younger than age 12 should not consume aloe because of its laxative effect.

Black Cohosh

Also known as black snakeroot or bugbane, black cohosh is a traditional Native American remedy for snakebites and gynecologic disorders. Derived from a plant from the buttercup family, black cohosh is used as a dietary supplement to treat hot flashes and other symptoms of menopause, such as mood swings, insomnia, and vaginal dryness. It also is taken for the relief of premenstrual syndrome (PMS; see page 850).

Several scientific studies have shown that black cohosh improves menopausal symptoms. However, most of these studies have been short-term, and little is known about the long-term effects of the supplement. For this reason, you should not take black cohosh for more than 6 months, and must not take it if you are pregnant or breastfeeding. Side effects can include stomach discomfort, headaches, and possible weight gain.

Cayenne

Also called capsicum, capsaicin, or red hot pepper, cayenne is an antioxidant that when eaten stimulates blood flow and metabolic rate and strengthens the heartbeat. It may also reduce blood cholesterol and triglyceride levels. Cayenne tastes hot, but it actually lowers body temperature by stimulating the cooling center of the hypothalamus in the brain. When applied to the skin, cayenne first stimulates and then blocks pain receptors. It is used as an active ingredient in creams and lotions to decrease pain associated with conditions such as arthritis (see page 996), fibromyalgia (see page 985), and shingles (see page 936). Although eating foods seasoned with hot pepper (such as cayenne) does not cause ulcers, people who have ulcers sometimes have discomfort after eating spicy foods.

Chamomile

When taken internally, usually in the form of tea, chamomile is a digestive aid and mild sedative. It contains a compound called coumarin, which

---

Alternative Therapies for Menopause

Deciding whether to use alternative therapies after menopause is a decision that many women face as they get older. Hormone therapy (see page 853) with estrogen is very effective in relieving symptoms of menopause—such as hot flashes and vaginal dryness—but some forms of hormone therapy carry small but known health risks, especially with long-term use. Many women are considering alternatives to hormone therapy in hopes of alleviating their symptoms and possibly reducing the risks of heart disease and osteoporosis.

Options that postmenopausal women have explored include natural or plant estrogens, acupuncture, and herbal supplements such as black cohosh, red clover, hops, dong quai, and ginseng. Of the herbal supplements, black cohosh seems to be the most effective in reducing symptoms of menopause, but not enough evidence exists to determine whether any of these therapies are safe over the long term. Limited studies have shown that plant estrogens—such as those present in soy products, wild yams, and flaxseed—may benefit some women who have hot flashes. With so many women seeking effective alternatives to estrogen, researchers are studying many of these plant substances to understand their effects on women's health. The best course is to talk to your doctor about your personal risks and the possible benefits and risks of using hormone therapy or alternative therapies to reduce your menopausal symptoms.

Vitamin Megadoses

Taking large doses of some vitamins—especially antioxidants (nutrients that destroy cell-damaging substances called free radicals)—is a popular way to try to prevent disease, maintain health, and slow aging. Theoretically, antioxidants such as selenium and vitamins C and E can prevent disease and slow aging by blocking damage to cells. However, there is little scientific evidence to support these theories.

Fat-soluble vitamins—such as vitamins A, D, E, and K—are stored in the body's fat cells. If you take too much of a fat-soluble vitamin, it can build up in your body and cause harm. Most vitamins work together with other nutrients to finely balance the complex chemical processes in your body. Taking too much of one vitamin or mineral without a similar increase in the other nutrients can upset this delicate balance. It is best to get most of your vitamins and minerals from a varied diet that contains plenty of fruits and vegetables, supplemented by a daily multivitamin that contains the recommended doses of vitamins and minerals.

relieves muscle spasms, including spasms of the intestine. Allergic reactions to chamomile are common, especially in people who are allergic to ragweed. Externally, chamomile extract is used in cosmetics to treat inflammation of the skin and mucous membranes. But avoid using chamomile around the eyes because it can cause irritation.

Coenzyme Q-10

Coenzyme Q-10, also known as ubiquinone, is a compound made naturally by the body. It helps cells produce energy and acts as an antioxidant, protecting cells from damaging free radicals (harmful by-products of the body's normal chemical processes). Naturally made quantities of coenzyme Q-10 in the body decrease as people age. Coenzyme Q-10 is marketed in the United States as a dietary supplement in pill form that protects the heart and stimulates the immune system. Coenzyme Q-10 may also be beneficial as an addition to conventional treatments for cancer and congestive heart failure. No serious side effects have been reported from the use of coenzyme Q-10; it does, however, lower the effectiveness of the anticlotting drug warfarin, so you should not take coenzyme Q-10 if you are taking warfarin.

Melatonin

Melatonin is a hormone produced by the pineal gland in the brain at night, when it is dark, to help regulate the sleep-wake cycle. The level of the hormone falls in the morning, when it is light.

Some people take melatonin supplements to help ease the symptoms of jet lag (brought on by a change in time zone that disrupts the sleep-wake cycle) or as a temporary sleep aid. However, there are no definitive studies proving melatonin's effectiveness for either jet lag or insomnia, and doctors caution that taking it could reduce the body's own production of the hormone. Also, because melatonin can interact with other hormones, it should not be taken by women who are pregnant or breastfeeding, or by children. In people with asthma, the supplement may increase asthma symptoms during the night. Possible side effects associated with melatonin include headache, diminished sex drive and fertility, and excessive sleepiness.

If you are thinking about taking melatonin, talk to your doctor. Melatonin may interact with some medications, and the long-term effects of taking melatonin supplements are not known. Also, like all supplements, its manufacture is not regulated by the FDA, and dosages have not been standardized.

Echinacea

Also called purple coneflower, echinacea was initially applied to the skin as a folk remedy to heal wounds. Today it is taken internally to boost the immune system and to treat upper respiratory infections such as colds and the flu. Studies testing its effectiveness in reducing cold symptoms have had mixed results. Echinacea can cause allergic reactions in some people or interfere with immune-suppressing drugs (such as those prescribed to prevent rejection after an organ or tissue transplant).

Ephedra

Also called ma huang, ephedra is a herbal Chinese medicine used for treating asthma and hay fever. Ephedra contains chemicals that have powerful stimulating effects on the nervous system and heart. Because ephedra suppresses appetite and burns fat, it was frequently used as a weight-loss supplement. The supplement was implicated in several deaths, and, for this reason, the FDA banned its use in products in 2004.

Green Tea

Green tea is a drink made from the steamed and dried leaves of the Camellia sinesis plant, a shrub that is native to Asia. The Chinese have been drinking green tea for thousands of years to promote health. Green tea is used to relieve stomach problems (including vomiting and diarrhea), to prevent tooth decay, and to reduce blood pressure and cholesterol levels. Because green tea contains cancer-fighting antioxidants, some researchers think it may protect against some cancers. Research is ongoing to understand the effects of green tea against cancer. In some people, green tea can cause allergic reactions. Because green tea contains caffeine, you should not drink more than 2 cups a day if you have an irregular heartbeat or panic attacks.

Evening Primrose Oil

Evening primrose oil, extracted from the seeds of the primrose plant (a tiny wildflower), is sometimes used for breast pain and the skin conditions allergic dermatitis and eczema. It is also used to reduce the symptoms of premenstrual syndrome (PMS) and menopause, rheumatoid arthritis, nerve damage from diabetes, asthma, and headaches. There is no scientific evidence showing that the supplement is beneficial. Do not use evening primrose oil with an antiseizure medication because it can lower the medication's effectiveness.

Feverfew

The herb feverfew is a folk remedy used to help regulate the menstrual cycle. Some people take it to treat migraine headaches and the symptoms of rheumatoid arthritis. Do not use feverfew with nonsteroidal anti-inflammatory drugs or with anticlotting medications such as warfarin or aspirin because it can increase bleeding. Because feverfew can induce menstruation, it should not be used during pregnancy.

Garlic

The cloves of the garlic plant are thought to have antibacterial, antiviral, and antifungal effects. These immune-boosting effects may also help prevent some cancers. People use garlic to treat a variety of conditions including colds and other upper respiratory infections. Garlic contains an ingredient that has been shown to lower cholesterol and triglyceride levels, help prevent blood clots, and possibly help lower blood pressure.

The only known side effects of garlic are allergic reactions in some people, stomach upset, and bad breath. You should not use garlic with anticlotting medications such as warfarin or aspirin (because it can increase bleeding) or if you are breastfeeding (because it can alter the taste of breast milk and possibly cause colic in your infant).

Ginger

Ginger ingested as a powder or in liquids is taken to prevent motion sickness and to relieve nausea and vomiting, including that caused by chemotherapy, pregnancy, or anesthesia. It is considered a natural anti-inflammatory and can be helpful for inflammatory conditions such as rheumatoid arthritis. Ginger can cause mild stomach upset or allergic reactions in some people. Do not use ginger with anticlotting medications such as warfarin or aspirin because it can increase bleeding.

Ginkgo Biloba

The dried leaf of the ginkgo tree taken internally as a powder or dissolved in liquids is an antioxidant that may help improve blood circulation. Scientific studies have shown that ginkgo biloba may be helpful for people who have mild to moderate dementia, but it appears to be ineffective in enhancing memory in healthy older people. Do not use ginkgo biloba with anticlotting medications such as warfarin or aspirin because it can increase bleeding.

Ginseng

Ginseng is taken internally to increase stamina, lower blood cholesterol, stimulate immune function, and lower blood glucose. Ginseng may also heighten the effects of the female hormone estrogen or corticosteroids (which relieve inflammation). Do not take ginseng if you have diabetes (unless your doctor says it's OK to do so), if you have high blood pressure (because it can raise blood pressure), or if you are taking anticlotting medications such as warfarin or aspirin (because it can increase bleeding). When used with the antidepressant phenelzine sulfate, ginseng can cause headaches and possibly manic episodes.

Goldenseal

Goldenseal is taken to treat colds, flu, sore throat, and other upper respiratory or sinus infections and to relieve digestive problems such as peptic ulcers or colitis. It is also used as a topical antiseptic. Do not ingest goldenseal during pregnancy (because it stimulates the involuntary muscles of the uterus) or while breastfeeding (because it can cause jaundice in nursing infants). In large doses, goldenseal can cause upset stomach, high blood pressure, and seizures.

Kava

Kava, a plant found throughout the islands of the South Pacific, where it is considered a relaxing intoxicant, is used in the United States to relieve muscle tension and reduce anxiety. Long-term use of the herb in high doses has been associated with a skin condition called kava dermopathy (characterized by scaly sores on the skin). In some European countries, kava has been linked to liver damage, and kava-containing products have been removed from the market. For this reason, you should not use products containing kava if you have liver disease or liver problems or if you are taking drugs that can affect the liver (including some drugs used for chemotherapy). The FDA is investigating the relationship between the use of kava and liver damage.

Saw Palmetto

Saw palmetto is used primarily for treating conditions that involve the male reproductive system, usually benign prostatic hyperplasia (see page 832) or prostatitis (see page 831). The herb seems to work by blocking the conversion of the male hormone testosterone into a form of the hormone that is thought to enlarge the prostate. The herb also is being marketed to treat male pattern baldness. Use of the herb can be traced back centuries to Native Americans of Florida, who used the berries of the plant as a food staple.

Saw palmetto can cause stomach problems or headaches, and the tannic acid contained in it can inhibit the body's absorption of iron.

Shark Cartilage

Cartilage tissue taken from sharks is a controversial alternative cancer treatment that gained popularity in the 1980s after a study showed that a substance in shark cartilage could block the growth of blood vessels that nourish cancerous tumors. However, shark cartilage has not been proven scientifically to be of benefit to people with cancer. Treatment with shark cartilage is undergoing clinical trials (testing on people) to determine definitively if claims about its benefits have any merit. Because shark cartilage has few side effects, cancer patients do not harm themselves by trying this approach, as long as it doesn't replace a conventional cancer treatment.

St John's Wort

St John's wort is used for treating mild to moderate depression, inflammation, and anxiety. However, studies conducted in the United States by the National Institutes of Health (NIH) have found it to be ineffective for relieving depression. Applied to the skin, St John's wort is used to treat mild burns and other superficial wounds.

In high doses, the herb can cause extreme sensitivity to sunlight. The tannic acid in St John's wort can inhibit the body's absorption of iron. Do not use St John's wort with antidepressants, birth-control pills, digoxin (a heart disease drug), anti-retroviral medications (such as AIDS drugs), or cyclosporine (an immune-suppressing drug) because it can interfere with the effects of these medications.

Aromatherapy

Aromatherapy is the practice of using essential oils from plants to promote health and well-being. While the practice dates back thousands of years, the modern form of aromatherapy was developed in France in the 1920s by a physician and a chemist. Today many French doctors incorporate essential oils in their treatment plans for patients. Essential oils are extracted and distilled from the leaves, flowers, twigs, and roots of plants such as eucalyptus, geranium, rose, and lavender. The oils are then used in massages, baths, compresses, or salves. They may also be applied to the skin in creams, inhaled in steam, or dispersed into the air using an air pump, candle, or water spray.

Odors can affect the limbic system of the brain (which governs emotions), and it is thought that aromatherapy exerts its effects in this way. Therapeutic claims for aromatherapy include improvement in mood, skin conditions, fatigue, joint problems, and pain. Such claims have not been studied or verified by medical research. Aromatherapy is not meant to be used as a substitute for medical care, but as a way to promote relaxation and relieve stress.

Valerian

Valerian is a herb that is widely used in Europe as a sleeping aid. It seems to have few side effects but in rare cases can cause headaches, heart palpitations, and insomnia. Valerian should not be used with barbiturates because it intensifies their sedative effects.

Manipulative Therapies

Manipulative therapies attempt to treat illness by manipulating or moving parts of the body. Manipulative therapies include chiropractic, massage therapy, and reflexology. Osteopathic medicine is included in this section, even though it is part of mainstream medical practice, because of its emphasis on the study and treatment of the musculoskeletal system through manipulation. Chiropractic focuses on the relationship between the structure of the body (primarily the spine) and how the body works. It is based on the belief that health can be restored through manipulation of the spine. Massage therapists manipulate the soft tissues of the body to relieve so-called restrictions (tightenings) and return the tissues to normal function.

Manipulative therapies have had varying degrees of success at treating chronic diseases, but are generally recognized as being effective for the treatment of lower back problems and pain.

Chiropractic

Chiropractic is a system of therapy based on the theory that disease results from a lack of normal nerve function. Treatment focuses on the physical adjustment and manipulation of the muscle, tissue, and joints of the spinal column instead of using medication or surgery. To diagnose a medical problem, chiropractors usually take a health history, order X-rays of the spine, and perform a physical examination of the back. Once a diagnosis is made, the chiropractor then manually adjusts the vertebrae of the spine suspected of causing the problem. The number of treatments needed and the length of visits vary.

Chiropractic seeks to bring the skeletal structure into balance to restore or increase the range of motion of the spinal column. It can be effective in treating lower back problems, but claims that it can also treat such medical problems as high blood pressure, heart disease, or diabetes have not been proven scientifically.

Osteopathic Medicine

Osteopathic medicine is similar to conventional medical practice, with an emphasis on the study of the musculoskeletal system (bones, muscles, tendons, tissues, nerves, and the spinal column). Osteopathic medicine takes a holistic approach to health care, teaching that the human body is a unified system and that the musculoskeletal system plays a central role in a person's overall health.

A doctor of osteopathy (DO) is a fully trained and licensed physician who has attended a 4-year osteopathic medical school and served a 1-year internship and a 2- to 6-year residency in a specialty area, as medical doctors (MDs) do. An osteopath can prescribe drugs and is qualified to practice all branches of medicine and surgery. Osteopaths use manipulation techniques such as stretching and thrusting in addition to conventional drugs and therapies to treat illness.

Craniosacral therapy

Craniosacral therapy is a form of osteopathic manipulation that involves gentle manual manipulation of the cranial (skull) bones to relieve tightening of the tissues that surround the brain and spinal cord. Osteopaths think that relieving this tightening (which they call restriction) allows the cerebrospinal fluid that bathes these structures to flow smoothly, thereby correcting the neurologic dysfunction. Studies have demonstrated the effectiveness of craniosacral therapy in treating cerebral palsy, seizure disorders, attention deficit disorders, headaches, and other neurologic disorders. The therapy is also effective in treating ear infections in children.

Massage Therapy

In massage therapy, the practitioner manipulates the soft tissues of the body to improve health and well-being. Massage is believed to enable the body to heal itself by increasing the circulation of blood and lymph (a body fluid that plays an important role in the immune system) and by normalizing the tissues of the nervous system and the musculoskeletal system. Massage can also help relax tightened muscles and eliminate the lactic acid that can accumulate in muscles after vigorous exercise. As a form of relaxation therapy, massage provides important psychological benefits.

There are three main types of massage: Swedish massage, pressure point therapy, and sports massage. Swedish massage is a traditional, gentle, whole-body massage that uses large, gliding strokes. In pressure point therapy—including deep tissue massage, neuromuscular therapy, acupressure, and shiatsu—concentrated finger pressure is applied to parts of the body that are in pain or have been injured. Sports massage concentrates on muscle groups that have been used excessively for a particular sport and is especially useful for improving athletic performance, relieving injuries, and promoting recovery.

A massage therapy session usually lasts 1 hour. You probably will be asked to remove as much clothing as you are comfortable removing and then lie down on a padded massage table. The therapist will then drape a cloth across your body, exposing one area at a time to be massaged. A lotion or oil may be applied to your skin to facilitate the motion of the therapist's hands.

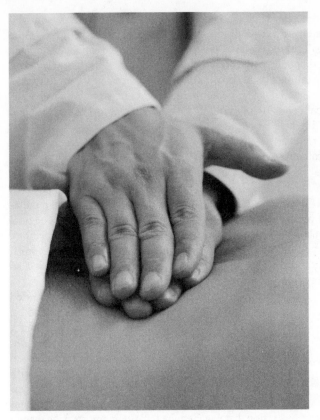

Massage therapy
Massage manipulates the muscles to increase blood flow and reverse the buildup of lactic acid in the muscles that accumulates after vigorous exercise.

study human function, eventually developing the theory that physical dysfunction results when a faulty learned movement is repeated over and over throughout a person's life. These faulty movements can be corrected, the theory goes, when a person becomes more aware of them and learns specific small movements that, with practice, eventually become larger, more complex, more efficient movements that replace the previous damaging ones. Conditions that have benefited by the Feldenkrais approach include back pain, cerebral palsy, chronic fatigue syndrome, head and neck pain, irritable bowel syndrome, and stroke.

Mind-Body Therapies

Mind-body therapies use a number of techniques that are believed to increase the mind's ability to heal the body. The most common forms of alternative mind-body therapies are guided imagery, meditation, prayer, yoga, and art and music therapy. Relaxation therapy, another popular mind-body technique, is discussed on page 59. Hypnosis and biofeedback are not included in this section because they are now generally accepted by the medical profession. Another mind-body technique that has become an accepted part of mainstream medical practice is cognitive-behavioral therapy (see page 710).

Mind-body therapies have been shown to provide many health benefits, including relieving stress, understanding illness, and restoring a person's sense of control.

Reflexology

Reflexology is an ancient form of therapy based on the theory that certain areas of the feet correspond to certain glands, organs, and systems of the body. Stimulation of these areas through finger and hand pressure is believed to have beneficial effects on the corresponding body part. Proponents of reflexology claim that it can improve a wide variety of health conditions, but it is primarily used as a stress-reduction technique. The effectiveness of reflexology has not been proven scientifically.

Feldenkrais

Feldenkrais is a method of movement therapy named after an Israeli scientist who, after injuring his knee, faced surgery that posed the risk of his not being able to regain movement in the joint. He considered the odds unacceptable and began to

Guided Imagery

Guided imagery refers to the use of the imagination to produce positive images that may bring about healing changes in the body. The process is often guided by the voice of a practitioner or by a voice recording that leads the person to visualize a suggested relaxing or healing scenario (such as being on a beach) in which healing can begin. The theory behind guided imagery is that the body will react as if the positive image is real, and undergo healthful changes. Guided imagery is used in hospitals and other health care settings for its proven benefit in managing pain, reducing anxiety, and strengthening the immune system.

Meditation

Meditation is a technique in which a person rests or sits quietly, usually with his or her eyes closed, and performs mental exercises that help focus attention, achieve relaxation, and increase mental awareness. The person often reaches this state by silently focusing on his or her breathing or on a word or an object. The stillness of mind and deep relaxation achieved during meditation help relieve stress and can have a beneficial effect on many medical conditions, including high blood pressure and heart disease. Meditation is also used to help relieve chronic pain, headaches, and respiratory problems such as asthma.

Prayer

Several scientific studies have shown that prayer may have an objective and positive effect on health outcomes. In these studies, the health of people who were prayed for improved substantially more than that of people who were not prayed for. This outcome occurred whether or not the person who was ill knew about the praying or believed in the power of prayer. Medical science cannot explain the connection between prayer and healing. However, many doctors encourage it because it can strengthen an ill person's emotional and psychological well-being and give encouragement to caregivers and loved ones.

Yoga

Yoga is a discipline developed in India over thousands of years that teaches a series of body postures and movements, breathing techniques, and meditation to calm the mind and relax the body. The goal of practitioners is to reach a state of harmony between the mind and the body that leads to spiritual enlightenment. This state of harmony is also believed to produce optimal health.

The physical benefits of yoga include increased flexibility, better balance, and stronger muscles. Yoga has been shown to reduce blood pressure, breathing rate, and anxiety. Yoga is also helpful for fighting insomnia, increasing range of motion in the joints, and decreasing pain in people with osteoarthritis (see page 996) or carpal tunnel syndrome (see page 699). The sustained focus of attention that yoga requires may help improve the mental abilities of older people.

Yoga postures should be learned from a practitioner and then practiced at home. If you are pregnant or have a chronic disorder such as high blood pressure, you may have to modify or avoid certain postures.

Art Therapy, Music Therapy, and Dance Therapy

Sometimes doctors use art, music, and dance to treat emotional and physical problems in a way that complements more conventional drug and therapy treatments. Art, music, and dance therapies attempt to release the healing potential of the creative arts. These therapies are frequently used in hospitals, nursing homes, psychiatric facilities, and hospices to ease pain, promote relaxation, and treat depression. Therapists are trained in the creative arts as well as in human development, psychological theory, and physical therapy.

Art therapy increases a person's self-awareness and may help him or her cope better with symptoms. Music therapy uses the emotional response

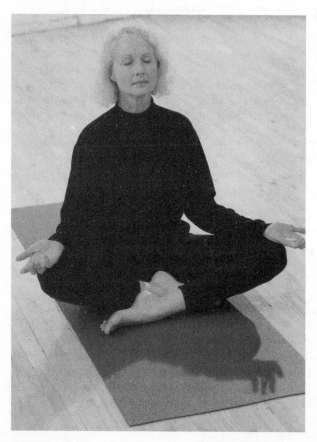

Yoga
Yoga is a good way to increase your joint flexibility and muscle tone while learning to relax and counteract stress.

generated by music to achieve these results. Also, listening to or playing music can reduce heart rate and blood pressure and can lower the levels of stress hormones released by the body. Dance therapy uses movement to express emotions and promote well-being.

Energy Therapies

Energy therapies seek to restore health by affecting energy fields originating in and extending out from the body. The existence of such energy fields has not been proven scientifically. Some types of energy therapy—including Reiki and therapeutic touch—attempt to manipulate the energy fields by placing the hands in or through these fields. Electronic field therapies, on the other hand, use magnetic fields or electric current fields to treat illness or manage pain. Research exploring these phenomena is ongoing.

Reiki

Reiki, which means universal life force energy, is a method of natural healing that attempts to direct the flow of chi, or qi (pronounced "chee"), believed to be the vital energy that circulates throughout the body, to promote physical and spiritual well-being. Developed in Japan in the late 19th century, Reiki principles probably originated from a branch of Tibetan Buddhism. The healing abilities they bring are believed to be transmitted from teacher to pupil, not taught.

During a Reiki healing, the practitioner places his or her hands on the sick person and "wills" Reiki energy to flow. The energy is supposed to flow naturally and "know" where to go in the sick person's body to promote healing. The practitioner believes that he or she is only the facilitator of the energy and does not consciously intervene in the healing process. Although no large-scale studies have proven the effectiveness of Reiki, the National Institutes of Health is studying the practice to determine if it can help relieve pain and increase exercise tolerance in people who have diabetes and improve the quality of life in people who have AIDS.

Therapeutic Touch

An outgrowth of the ancient healing therapy called the "laying on of hands," therapeutic touch is the manipulation of a person's energy field to induce healing by passing the hands a few inches above the person's body. Developed in the 1970s by a nurse and a natural healer, therapeutic touch is practiced primarily in the nursing community, but is gaining growing acceptance in the medical community. The therapy is based on the theory that the human body, the mind, and the emotions form a harmonious and ordered energy field that is balanced during times of health but that falls out of balance during illness. By passing the hands over a person's energy field, the practitioner directs and rebalances this energy.

During the process, the ill person sits or lies down comfortably while the practitioner runs his or her hands up and down the person's body a few inches above the skin to identify energy imbalances. Therapeutic touch has not been scientifically proven to bring about healing, although anecdotal reports from people who have undergone the procedure have been positive. Some studies suggest that therapeutic touch may help relax people who have dementia and may help substance abusers remain drug-free.

Electromagnetic Field Therapy

Electromagnetic field therapy uses magnets or magnetic fields and more unconventional methods, such as pulsed fields and alternating or direct electrical current fields, to treat illness. Practitioners of electromagnetic field therapy believe that they can use such fields to alter the behavior of cells in the body to induce positive health changes. For example, pulses of electromagnetic fields may be used to prevent bone loss or to restore bone mass. Electromagnetic fields also have been used to treat asthma, cancer, and migraine headaches, and to manage pain. Because electromagnetic field therapies have not been studied by medical science, their effectiveness is not known.

Atlas of the body

This atlas illustrates the anatomy of the major organs and systems of the body and provides brief descriptions of each. For more information about a specific body system or to learn about the symptoms, diagnosis, and treatment of a specific health problem, consult the index at the back of the book.

Torso

The upper part of the torso is the chest, which contains the heart and lungs. The chest is separated from the lower part of the torso—the abdomen—by the diaphragm, a dome-shaped sheet of muscle. The edge of the diaphragm is attached to the bottom of the rib cage.

Inside the abdomen are the organs of the digestive system and the urinary system. The digestive system is composed of the digestive tract—the tube running from the mouth to the anus that processes the food you eat—plus two other organs, the liver and the pancreas, which aid digestion by manufacturing digestive fluids. The urinary system includes the kidneys, ureters, bladder, and urethra. The lower part of the abdomen, cradled within the hipbone, is called the pelvis. See also Organs of the Lower Abdomen, page 107.

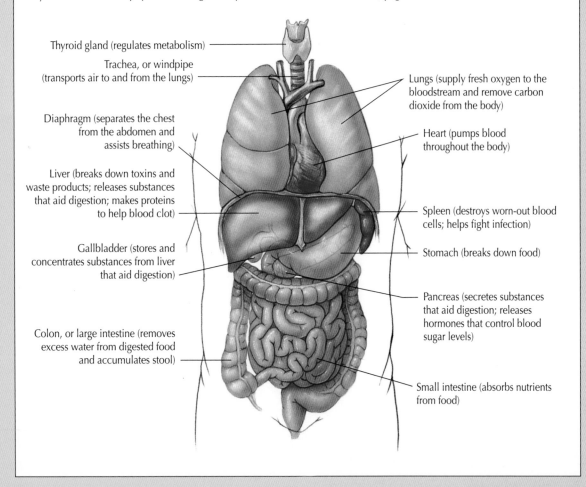

Thyroid gland (regulates metabolism)

Trachea, or windpipe (transports air to and from the lungs)

Diaphragm (separates the chest from the abdomen and assists breathing)

Liver (breaks down toxins and waste products; releases substances that aid digestion; makes proteins to help blood clot)

Gallbladder (stores and concentrates substances from liver that aid digestion)

Colon, or large intestine (removes excess water from digested food and accumulates stool)

Lungs (supply fresh oxygen to the bloodstream and remove carbon dioxide from the body)

Heart (pumps blood throughout the body)

Spleen (destroys worn-out blood cells; helps fight infection)

Stomach (breaks down food)

Pancreas (secretes substances that aid digestion; releases hormones that control blood sugar levels)

Small intestine (absorbs nutrients from food)

Muscles

The more than 600 muscles in your body are composed of bundles of interlocking fibers that have the ability to contract (shorten) and relax (lengthen). The skeletal muscles are attached (directly or with a tendon) to two or more bones; when these muscles contract, the bones move. A group of muscles can often work together—one contracts, another relaxes, and nearby muscles provide stability.

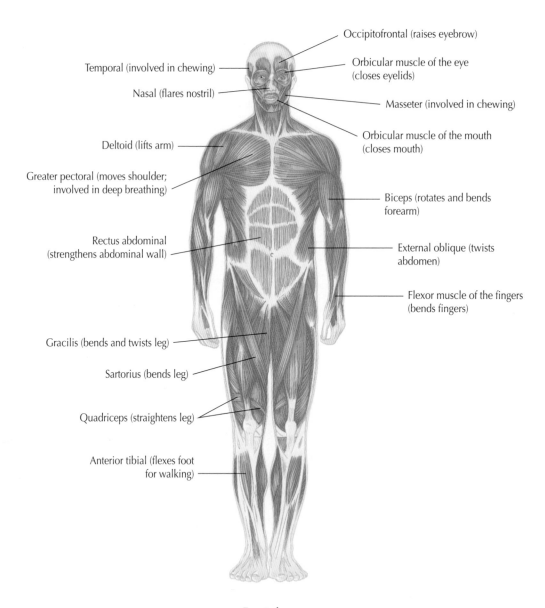

Occipitofrontal (raises eyebrow)

Orbicular muscle of the eye (closes eyelids)

Temporal (involved in chewing)

Nasal (flares nostril)

Masseter (involved in chewing)

Orbicular muscle of the mouth (closes mouth)

Deltoid (lifts arm)

Greater pectoral (moves shoulder; involved in deep breathing)

Biceps (rotates and bends forearm)

Rectus abdominal (strengthens abdominal wall)

External oblique (twists abdomen)

Flexor muscle of the fingers (bends fingers)

Gracilis (bends and twists leg)

Sartorius (bends leg)

Quadriceps (straightens leg)

Anterior tibial (flexes foot for walking)

Front view

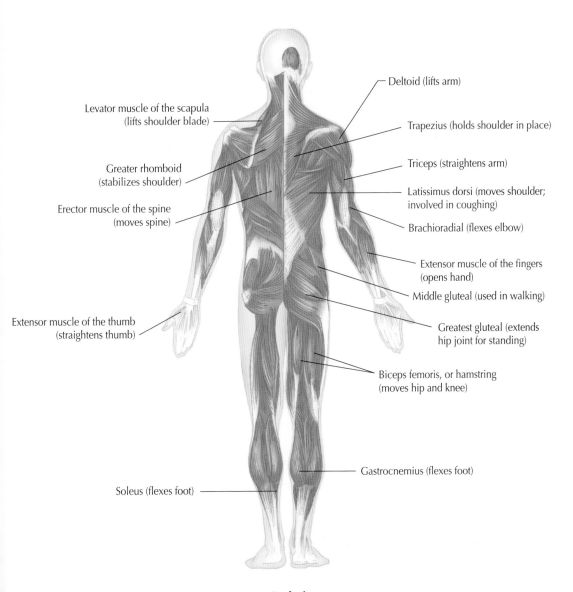

Levator muscle of the scapula
(lifts shoulder blade)

Greater rhomboid
(stabilizes shoulder)

Erector muscle of the spine
(moves spine)

Extensor muscle of the thumb
(straightens thumb)

Soleus (flexes foot)

Deltoid (lifts arm)

Trapezius (holds shoulder in place)

Triceps (straightens arm)

Latissimus dorsi (moves shoulder;
involved in coughing)

Brachioradial (flexes elbow)

Extensor muscle of the fingers
(opens hand)

Middle gluteal (used in walking)

Greatest gluteal (extends
hip joint for standing)

Biceps femoris, or hamstring
(moves hip and knee)

Gastrocnemius (flexes foot)

Back view

Immune System

Your immune system provides your body with a wide variety of mechanisms—both internal and external—that protect you from disease-causing microorganisms such as viruses and illnesses such as cancer. The immune system is a complex, tightly orchestrated network of proteins, cells, organs, and the lymphatic vessels, all of which work together to keep you healthy.

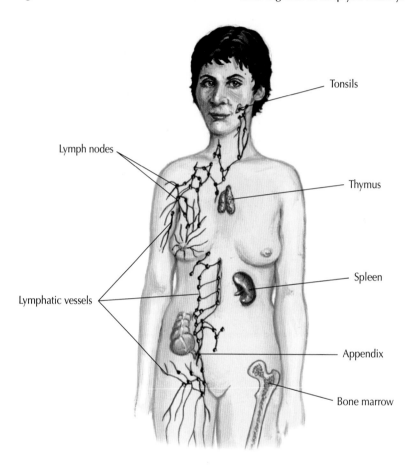

Lymphatic system

The major organs of the immune system are called lymph nodes. Lymph nodes—clustered in your neck, armpits, and groin—contain white blood cells called lymphocytes that mount the response against potentially harmful invading microorganisms such as viruses or bacteria. Like all blood cells, white blood cells are produced in the soft marrow inside bones. White blood cells leave the bone marrow and are carried in the blood to the lymph nodes.

A system of fluid-filled ducts (called lymphatic vessels) channels white blood cells from the lymph nodes back into the bloodstream. White blood cells patrol the entire body—circulating in the blood, lymph nodes, and lymphatic vessels—to watch for harmful microorganisms and to remove damaged cells.

The thymus, an organ that lies behind the breastbone, is where a group of lymphocytes called T cells grows to maturity. The spleen, a fist-sized organ in the upper left corner of the abdomen, contains large numbers of white blood cells, including many lymphocytes. The tonsils and nearby adenoids (not shown) and the appendix are clumps of lymphoid tissue that provide lines of defense at sites in the body where potentially harmful microorganisms are likely to enter or multiply.

Bones

Your bones and muscles work together to support your body and enable you to move. The average human skeleton has 206 bones—32 bones in each arm, 31 in each leg, 29 in the skull, 26 in the spine, and 25 in the chest. In some people, the number of bones varies slightly from the norm—for example, about 5 percent of us have an extra pair of ribs, and some of us may have a few extra bones in our hands or feet or may be missing one or more bones.

Bones meet at joints, of which there are several types. Fixed joints, such as those in the skull, hold the bones firmly together. Partly movable joints, such as those between the bones of the spine, allow limited flexibility. Freely movable joints, such as in the jaw, hip, knee, or shoulder, provide variable flexibility in several planes of movement.

The skeletons of men and women differ very little. Men's bones are generally slightly larger and heavier than women's bones. The cavity in the female pelvis, surrounded by the hipbones and sacrum, is wider than the cavity in the male pelvis, to accommodate the passage of a baby during delivery.

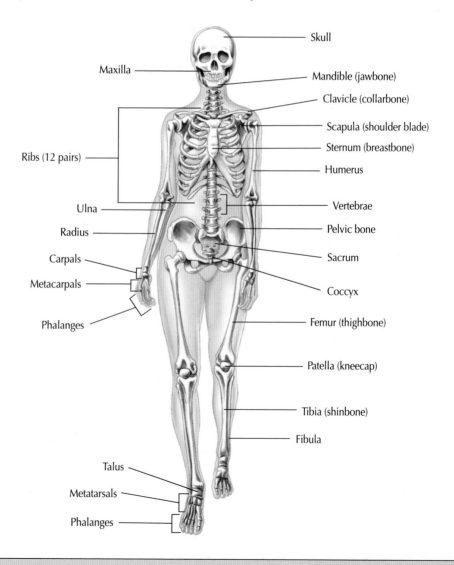

Skull

Maxilla

Mandible (jawbone)

Clavicle (collarbone)

Scapula (shoulder blade)

Sternum (breastbone)

Ribs (12 pairs)

Humerus

Ulna

Vertebrae

Radius

Pelvic bone

Carpals

Sacrum

Metacarpals

Coccyx

Phalanges

Femur (thighbone)

Patella (kneecap)

Tibia (shinbone)

Fibula

Talus

Metatarsals

Phalanges

Heart and Blood Vessels

Blood delivers life-sustaining oxygen and other vital nutrients to cells throughout the body and carries away wastes produced by the cells. The pumping action of the heart keeps the blood in constant circulation, sending it to the lungs to pick up a fresh supply of oxygen and then pushing it back out to the organs and tissues. Every minute, the heart pumps about 5 quarts of blood through the entire circulatory system.

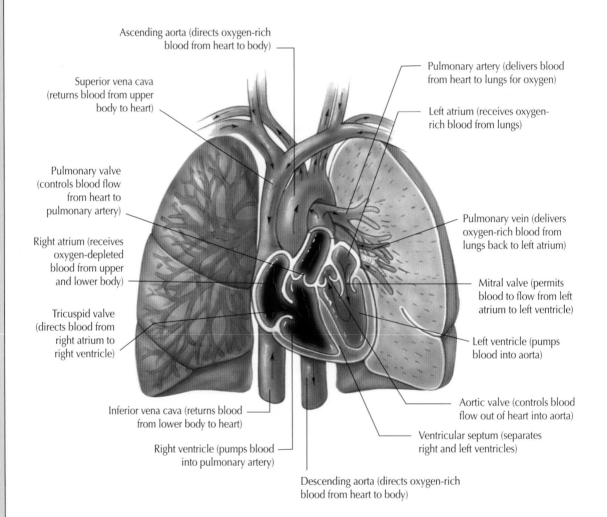

Ascending aorta (directs oxygen-rich blood from heart to body)

Superior vena cava (returns blood from upper body to heart)

Pulmonary valve (controls blood flow from heart to pulmonary artery)

Right atrium (receives oxygen-depleted blood from upper and lower body)

Tricuspid valve (directs blood from right atrium to right ventricle)

Inferior vena cava (returns blood from lower body to heart)

Right ventricle (pumps blood into pulmonary artery)

Pulmonary artery (delivers blood from heart to lungs for oxygen)

Left atrium (receives oxygen-rich blood from lungs)

Pulmonary vein (delivers oxygen-rich blood from lungs back to left atrium)

Mitral valve (permits blood to flow from left atrium to left ventricle)

Left ventricle (pumps blood into aorta)

Aortic valve (controls blood flow out of heart into aorta)

Ventricular septum (separates right and left ventricles)

Descending aorta (directs oxygen-rich blood from heart to body)

Heart

The heart is a muscular organ about the size and shape of a fist, consisting of two side-by-side pumps. The right side sends blood from the veins into the lungs, where the blood receives fresh oxygen. The oxygen-rich blood then enters the left side of the heart, which pumps it through the aorta and out to the entire body.

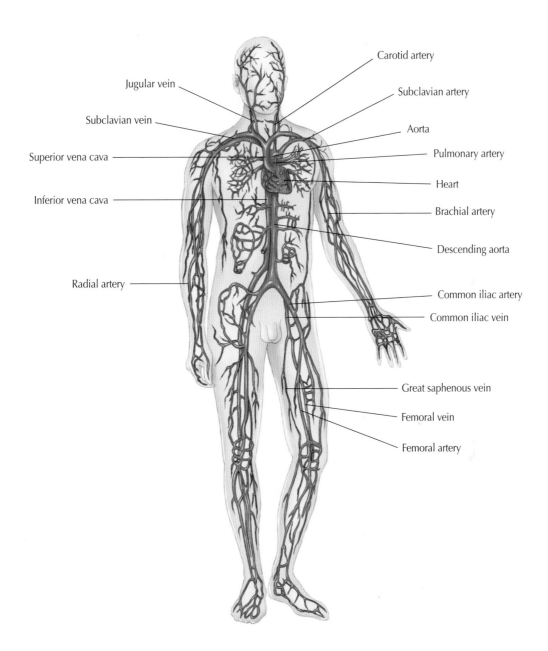

Carotid artery

Jugular vein

Subclavian artery

Subclavian vein

Aorta

Superior vena cava

Pulmonary artery

Heart

Inferior vena cava

Brachial artery

Descending aorta

Radial artery

Common iliac artery

Common iliac vein

Great saphenous vein

Femoral vein

Femoral artery

Circulatory system

The circulatory system consists of the heart, lungs, and blood vessels. Your veins (blue in illustration) carry used, oxygen-depleted blood to the right side of your heart, which pumps it to the lungs for a fresh supply of oxygen. The newly oxygenated blood returns to the left side of the heart and is pumped through the aorta, a large blood vessel that directs blood to a system of arteries (red in illustration) that deliver the blood to tissues throughout the body. The veins return the used blood to the heart and the process starts again, about 10,000 times every day.

Brain and Nervous System

The nervous system has two major parts—the central nervous system and the peripheral nervous system. The brain and spinal cord make up the central nervous system, which coordinates all the body's interactions with the environment. The brain, which is the most complex organ of the body, regulates most of your body's functions. Each area of the brain is responsible for different functions, such as language, vision, movement, or emotions. The peripheral nervous system consists of nerves that radiate from the brain and spinal cord to all parts of the body. The peripheral nerves transmit information from different parts of the body to the brain and carry messages back to those parts of the body from the brain. The brain is always working, even during sleep.

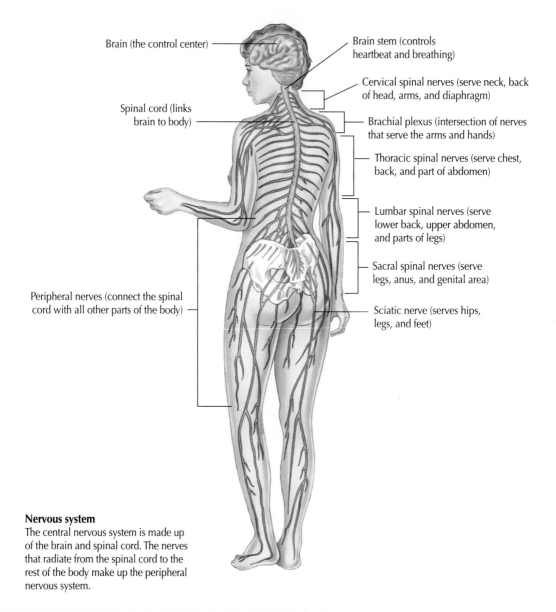

Brain (the control center)

Brain stem (controls heartbeat and breathing)

Cervical spinal nerves (serve neck, back of head, arms, and diaphragm)

Spinal cord (links brain to body)

Brachial plexus (intersection of nerves that serve the arms and hands)

Thoracic spinal nerves (serve chest, back, and part of abdomen)

Lumbar spinal nerves (serve lower back, upper abdomen, and parts of legs)

Sacral spinal nerves (serve legs, anus, and genital area)

Peripheral nerves (connect the spinal cord with all other parts of the body)

Sciatic nerve (serves hips, legs, and feet)

Nervous system
The central nervous system is made up of the brain and spinal cord. The nerves that radiate from the spinal cord to the rest of the body make up the peripheral nervous system.

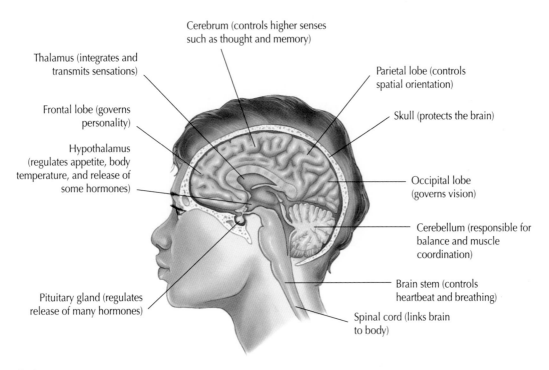

Cerebrum (controls higher senses such as thought and memory)

Thalamus (integrates and transmits sensations)

Frontal lobe (governs personality)

Hypothalamus (regulates appetite, body temperature, and release of some hormones)

Parietal lobe (controls spatial orientation)

Skull (protects the brain)

Occipital lobe (governs vision)

Cerebellum (responsible for balance and muscle coordination)

Brain stem (controls heartbeat and breathing)

Pituitary gland (regulates release of many hormones)

Spinal cord (links brain to body)

Brain

The brain lies inside a rigid, bony container called the skull. The two cerebral hemispheres, the cerebellum, and the brain stem are the major components of the brain. The cerebral hemispheres make up nearly 90 percent of brain tissue. Each hemisphere is about 6 inches from front to back, and together they measure about 4½ inches across. The hemispheres consist of intricate folds of nerve tissue that have a total surface area equal to that of a large newspaper spread.

The cerebellum, which lies beneath the back of the cerebral hemispheres, is concerned with muscle coordination. Like the cerebral hemispheres, the cerebellum consists of nerve cells and is divided into two hemispheres.

The brain stem contains tracts of nerve fibers that connect the brain to the rest of the body by way of the spinal cord. The brain stem also controls breathing and heart rate.

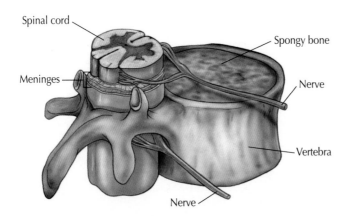

Spinal cord

Meninges

Spongy bone

Nerve

Vertebra

Nerve

Spinal cord

The spinal cord is covered by three layers of protective membranes called the meninges. The spinal cord has a central canal that contains cerebrospinal fluid. Spinal nerves send and receive messages about body sensation and move to and from the brain by way of the spinal cord. A column of bones called vertebrae surrounds and protects the spinal cord. The vertebral column enables you to stand upright and maintain your balance.

Urinary Tract

The urinary tract filters waste products and excess fluid from the bloodstream and eliminates them from the body in urine. The kidneys filter out excess water, salts, and waste products from the blood, and the remaining substances are reabsorbed into the blood in the exact amounts the body needs. The kidneys then expel the excess water, salts, and waste products as urine (through tubes called ureters) into the bladder, where it is stored until you feel the urge to urinate. Urine is expelled from the body through a narrow tube called the urethra.

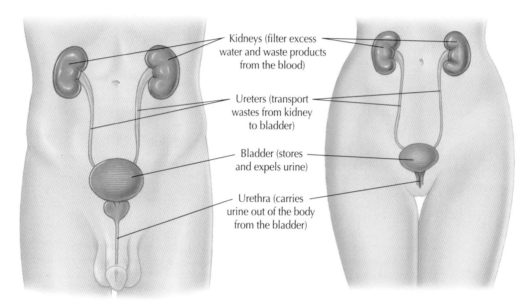

Kidneys (filter excess water and waste products from the blood)

Ureters (transport wastes from kidney to bladder)

Bladder (stores and expels urine)

Urethra (carries urine out of the body from the bladder)

Male urinary tract   Female urinary tract

Male and female urinary tracts
The urinary tracts differ somewhat in males and females. A male's urethra is much longer than a female's, and the male bladder sits higher in the pelvis.

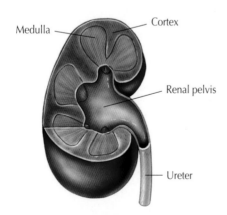

Medulla   Cortex

Renal pelvis

Ureter

How the kidneys work
The kidneys play a role in regulating blood pressure, producing red blood cells, and filtering waste from the body. Blood first passes through the tiny blood vessels in the cortex, which remove waste products from the blood. The filtered blood flows into small tubes (in the medulla) that reabsorb the nutrients and water that the body needs. The filtered and replenished blood returns to the circulation, and the leftover waste by-product (urine) collects in the renal pelvis. Urine drains through the ureter into the bladder, where it is stored until it is eliminated from the body.

Organs of the Lower Abdomen

The organs of the lower abdomen are involved primarily with reproduction and with removing wastes from the body (in urine and stool). The lower abdominal organs are sometimes called the pelvic organs. Except for the reproductive organs, these organs function the same way in both males and females.

The bladder, a muscular sac that is about 3 inches in diameter when full, stores urine until it is eliminated from the body through a tube called the urethra. The urethra is much longer in males than in females. Digested food passes from the stomach through the intestines and out of the body via the rectum and anus.

Male reproductive organs
In addition to the visible male genitals—the penis and testicles—a system of glands and ducts is located inside the abdomen. The internal male reproductive organs, which produce, store, and transport sperm, are the prostate gland, two seminal vesicles, and two tubes called the vas deferens.

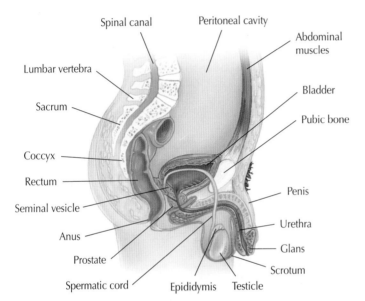

Lower abdomen in males

Female reproductive organs
The female reproductive organs are located inside the pelvis. The ovaries, which contain a female's eggs, are connected to the uterus on either side by a fallopian tube. During each menstrual cycle, a mature egg travels from an ovary through a fallopian tube into the uterus (ovulation).

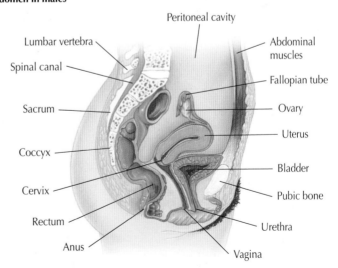

Lower abdomen in females

Diagnostic imaging techniques

Diagnostic imaging is a branch of medicine that helps doctors diagnose medical disorders and is often used in addition to a physical examination and laboratory tests. For example, after taking a health history and performing a physical examination on a person who has a chronic cough, a doctor may recommend a chest X-ray to determine the cause of the cough. For a person who may have had a stroke, a doctor might recommend computed tomography (CT) or magnetic resonance imaging (MRI) to examine the brain. These procedures can often find the cause of symptoms or narrow down the possible causes. In many imaging techniques (such as angiography), contrast mediums (dyes) or contrast agents (such as air or water) are used to make specific parts of the body easier to see.

X-rays, discovered in 1895, were the first imaging technique used for diagnosing medical problems. Ultrasound, which was developed in 1952 to evaluate fetuses and monitor pregnancies, uses sound waves to create an image. Diagnostic imaging advanced significantly in the 1960s with SPECT (single photon emission computed tomography), in the 1970s with the introduction of conventional CT scans, in the 1980s with MRI and PET (positron emission tomography), and in the 1990s with functional MRI (fMRI). New imaging techniques continue to be developed.

Using viewing devices called endoscopes, which are inserted directly into the body, doctors can see inside the body to evaluate tissues and organs and to perform procedures.

Imaging the Brain

With computerized imaging techniques such as MRIs and PET scans, doctors can look inside the living, thinking brain. These newer imaging techniques have improved the ability of doctors to diagnose and locate the site of brain disorders. The techniques have also enabled them to understand the relationship between different areas of the brain, to learn about the functions of specific areas of the brain, and to develop new treatments for brain disorders.

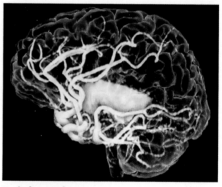

Brain hemorrhage
This three-dimensional angiogram shows a brain after a type of stroke caused by a hemorrhage, or bleeding inside the brain. The white areas are major arteries. The large yellow area in the center is the hemorrhage.

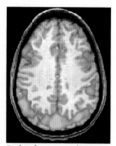 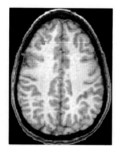

Brain of an aggressive teen   Brain of a nonaggressive teen

Brains of aggressive and nonaggressive teens
For these images, a technique called functional MRI (fMRI) shows brain activity (orange areas at top of images) in teens who have disruptive behavior disorder (which makes them aggressive) and in healthy, nonaggressive teens as they play a violent video game. The images show less activity in the frontal lobe of a teen with the behavior disorder (left) than in the frontal lobe of the healthy teen (right), indicating that the teen with the disorder is less able to inhibit the violent emotions triggered by the video game.

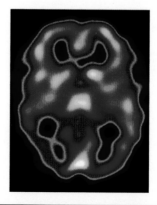

Brain during a migraine
This single photon emission computed tomography (SPECT) scan of a brain was taken during a migraine headache. Areas of high brain activity are yellow or red. Areas of low activity are gray or blue. Migraines usually affect one side of the brain. The grayish area at the lower left is an area of reduced blood flow (and low brain activity) from the migraine.

X-Rays

X-rays are high-energy electromagnetic waves that have a shorter wavelength than visible light or radio waves. When a beam of X-rays is passed through the body, some parts of the body absorb more radiation than other parts, producing a darker, shadowy image on the X-ray film, or radiograph. X-ray images can also be viewed on a fluorescent screen, or monitor. Dense structures (such as bone) allow few X-rays to pass through, so these structures appear lighter, or white, on the film. Fat and other soft tissues absorb less radiation, and so they look somewhat gray. Hollow structures (such as the lungs) allow even more radiation to pass through, making them appear darker, or black, on film.

Structures that are hollow (such as the intestines and blood vessels) can show up more clearly on X-rays if they are filled with a contrast medium (dye) such as barium sulfate, which blocks the X-rays. For example, for an X-ray examination of the upper digestive tract, a person fasts for several hours and then drinks a barium sulfate liquid. As the barium moves through the digestive tract, it highlights the outlines of the esophagus, stomach, and upper intestine on the X-ray film. For an X-ray examination of the lower intestine, barium is introduced into the intestine through the rectum (called a barium enema). Iodine is used as a contrast medium to examine the thyroid gland, blood vessels, and urinary tract.

THE PROCEDURE

Before an X-ray examination, you may be asked to remove some of your clothing to help produce a better X-ray image. The part of your body to be examined will be positioned between the X-ray machine and the film, usually touching or very close to the machine. The technician will position you or immobilize the body part to obtain the best possible view. Several images may be taken from various angles. The X-rays themselves cause no discomfort because you cannot feel X-rays pass through your body.

The parts of your body not being examined may be shielded from the X-rays in some way (such as with a lead apron) to protect them from exposure to radiation. Your exposure to the radiation lasts only a fraction of a second. Because of a small risk of tissue damage from exposure to radiation, X-rays are performed only when necessary, and never during pregnancy.

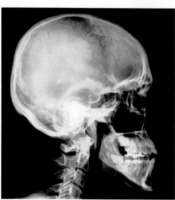

Skull
This X-ray shows the dense bone of a healthy human skull, which encloses and protects the brain. Because X-rays provide little information about the brain itself, they are used primarily to diagnose and evaluate skull fractures.

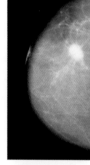

Mammogram
Mammography uses low doses of X-rays to produce images of the soft tissues of the breast to detect abnormal growths such as tumors. This mammogram shows a cancerous tumor (bright white spot) in its early stages.

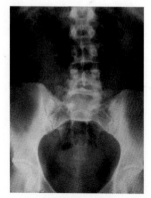

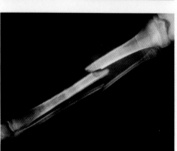

Broken arm
This X-ray shows severe fractures of both bones in the lower arm—the radius and the ulna.

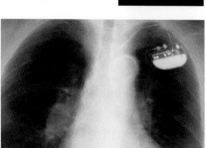

Pacemaker in chest cavity
In this X-ray of the chest, the hollow lungs are the two large dark areas, and the heart is barely visible between the lungs. A pacemaker, which is implanted just beneath the skin, is attached to the heart with wires to regulate the heartbeat.

Lower spine and pelvis
The vertebrae of the spine and the thick hip bones are easy to see on this X-ray. The tailbone of the spine can be seen faintly in the hollow between the hip bones.

Angiography

Angiography is an imaging procedure used to examine blood vessels, particularly arteries (arteriography). Angiograms can help doctors diagnose blood vessel disorders and are frequently performed before surgery on a blood vessel to locate the sites of blockages or other problems. Before an angiogram, a contrast medium (dye) containing iodine (which shows up on X-rays) is injected through a thin, flexible tube (catheter) inserted through a small incision into the femoral artery in the groin, the brachial artery in the elbow, or one of the carotid arteries in the neck. A rapid series of X-ray pictures is then taken of the arteries. Any abnormalities in the arteries will show up on the X-rays.

Magnetic resonance angiography (MRA) uses MRI (page 113) with angiography. In MRA, specific radio-pulse sequences are used (usually without using X-rays and usually without injecting a contrast medium) to create and enhance images.

THE PROCEDURE

If you are having an angiogram, you will be asked to lie very still on an examining table. The area in which the catheter is inserted will be numbed with an anesthetic. A needle is inserted through the skin into the artery, and a long, thin wire with a soft tip is inserted through the needle. The needle is then removed and the catheter threaded over the wire into the blood vessel. When the contrast medium is injected, you will feel a sensation of warmth for a few seconds. The procedure lasts from a few minutes to a few hours. After the examination, you may be asked to lie still for a few hours. Angiography poses a slight risk of damage to blood vessels (at the site of the injection or anywhere along the blood vessel during passage of the catheter) and a risk of an allergic reaction to the contrast medium.

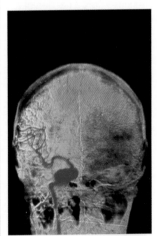

Aneurysm in a carotid artery

This angiogram reveals an aneurysm, an abnormal ballooning of a weakened area in the wall of an artery (red area on left), as viewed from the back of the head. This aneurysm is in a carotid artery (one of two main arteries that supply blood to the head and neck). If an aneurysm in the brain ruptures, it can cause a stroke.

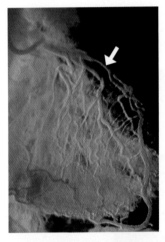

Narrowed coronary artery

An angiogram of the arteries of the heart (called a cardiac arteriogram) is used to diagnose heart disease. In this image, the contrast medium reveals a narrowed section in the left coronary artery (arrow) that has reduced blood flow to that part of the heart muscle. A total blockage can cause a heart attack. The long, pink, unbroken areas in the image are healthy blood vessels.

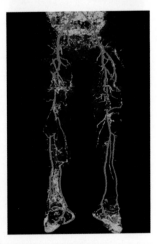

Inflamed arteries in legs

This angiogram (taken with MRA) shows diseased arteries (dark pink areas) in the legs of a person with arteritis (inflammation in the walls of the arteries). The arteries in the legs originate in the iliac arteries of the groin (the groin is the brownish, circular area at top center).

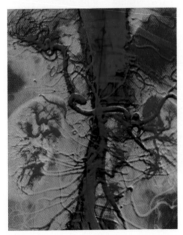

Arteries to the kidneys

The arteries that supply blood to the kidneys (the renal arteries) are red in this angiogram. The kidneys appear yellow. The renal arteries branch off the abdominal aorta (the large red blood vessel running vertically down the center of the image). The vertebrae of the spine and several ribs are barely visible.

Ultrasound

Ultrasound is an imaging procedure that uses high-frequency sound waves to produce an image. Although ultrasound was initially used to view fetuses, it is now used to examine every organ of the body, including the heart (an echocardiogram). Because ultrasound does not pose a risk of exposure to radiation, it is increasingly taking the place of conventional X-rays (see page 109) for diagnosing many different conditions. In ultrasound, sound waves are directed into the body through a wandlike device called a transducer, which is moved around the skin over the area to be examined. Ultrasound produces clear images of soft tissues and fluid-filled organs (such as the ovaries) but is less useful for examining organs filled with gas or air (such as the lungs). Also, ultrasound waves do not penetrate bone. The ultrasound images are displayed on a computer screen. Ultrasound is often used to guide the positioning of a needle during a biopsy (removal of a small piece of tissue for microscopic examination).

Doppler ultrasound is an ultrasound technique that can evaluate movement such as blood flow through the beating heart of a fetus or through arteries and veins.

Because flowing blood cells in a blood vessel reflect sound waves, the speed and direction of blood flow through the vessels can be measured and analyzed with ultrasound. This information is displayed on a screen as a graph. Doppler ultrasound is often used along with or, in some cases, instead of angiography (see previous page).

THE PROCEDURE

If you are having an ultrasound of the abdominal area, you will be asked to fast for at least 12 hours before the procedure. If the scan involves the pelvic area (such as to examine pelvic organs or to view a fetus), you will be asked to drink three or four glasses of water about 20 to 30 minutes before the examination to fill your bladder (so it will reflect sound waves). The technician will spread a gel on your skin over the area to be examined; the gel provides good contact for the transducer and allows it to move easily and smoothly over the skin. The room is darkened slightly to make the images on the computer screen clearly visible to the technician. Most ultrasounds take about 15 to 30 minutes. The procedure is very safe and has no known side effects or risks.

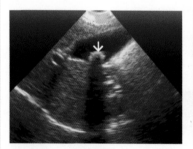

Gallstone in gallbladder
This ultrasound scan of the gallbladder (the dark oval area at the top of the image) shows a gallstone (arrow) inside the gallbladder. Gallstones form when bile (which is stored in the gallbladder) hardens. The major component of most gallstones is cholesterol.

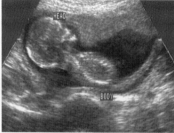

Four-month-old fetus
During pregnancy, ultrasound is a safe method for determining the approximate age, rate of growth, and position of a fetus. This ultrasound image is of a healthy 4-month-old fetus (the head of the fetus is at the left, facing up).

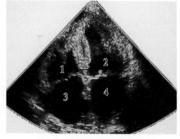

Heart
An ultrasound of the heart (called an echocardiogram) can help diagnose heart abnormalities. This echocardiogram shows a healthy heart. The four chambers of the heart are numbered, and appear as dark spaces surrounded by the walls of the chambers: 1 indicates the right ventricle; 2, the left ventricle; 3, the right atrium; and 4, the left atrium.

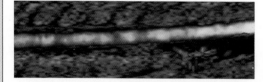

Vein in leg
This Doppler ultrasound shows blood flow (orange) through the longest vein in the body—the vein in the leg from the foot to the groin that drains blood back to the heart.

CT scanning

Computed tomography (CT) uses a combination of X-rays (see page 109) and a computer to create images. A CT scanner uses X-rays in a different way than a conventional X-ray machine does. Instead of taking an X-ray photograph, a CT scanner sends large numbers of X-ray beams from many directions through the part of the body being examined, records the amount of radiation that has been absorbed, and uses an internal computer to construct an image. In CT, the computer produces a series of horizontal or vertical (or even three-dimensional) cross-sectional slice images of the body. These images offer clear pictures of all the organs in the part of the body being studied. CT scanning is able to create more fully defined pictures of the head and body than conventional X-rays and has reduced the need for uncomfortable, invasive, and risky diagnostic procedures such as exploratory surgery.

A newer type of CT—called electron beam tomography (EBT)—is ten times faster than any other scanning technique. EBT is also called spiral, or helical, tomography. The EBT X-ray tube revolves around the body, allowing a continuous flow of images. The data are collected on a computer, and can be enhanced to provide clearer and more detailed images than those produced with conventional CT. Three-dimensional images can be created by combining many cross-sectional slice images. Because of its speed, EBT reduces the amount of time a person is exposed to radiation. Full-body scanning with EBT is being used to diagnose heart disease, lung disorders, and tumors at early stages, before they cause symptoms.

THE PROCEDURE

Before you have a CT scan, a technician may inject a contrast medium (dye), such as iodine, into a vein in your arm to help get a better image of the blood vessels and any tumors. If your abdomen and pelvis are being scanned, you will be asked to drink a weak solution of barium sulfate (another contrast medium) to expand your intestines and improve the image. The technician will also position you (or the scanner) to get the best image possible. You will be asked to lie very still on a table while you are inside the scanner. CT scanning is painless. However, the procedure may take an hour or more, depending on the number of angles and exposures required.

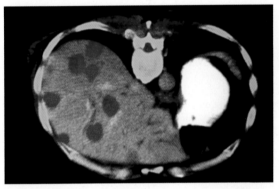

Liver cancer
The large brownish mass at left is a liver to which cancerous tumors (red spots) have spread from the colon. The spine (at the top) and the ribs (surrounding the internal organs) are yellow.

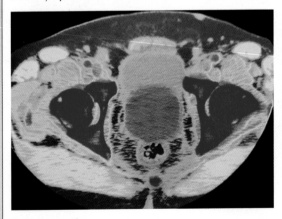

Prostate cancer
This is a view of a male pelvis showing an enlarged, cancerous prostate gland (green). The bones of the pelvis are the red areas on either side of the prostate. The rectum is the circular blue area below the prostate. The bladder is the yellow oval (slightly indented by the enlarged prostate) directly above the prostate.

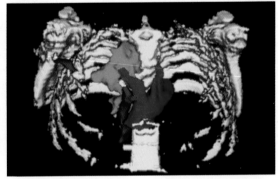

Pancreatic cancer
CT scans are useful for revealing small pancreatic tumors or swelling of the pancreas caused by inflammation. Here, a cancerous tumor of the pancreas (green) is evident. Also seen are the ribs and spine (white); the aorta (red), which is the major artery that carries blood away from the heart; and a vena cava (blue), one of the two major veins that drain blood from the body into the right side of the heart.

MRI

Magnetic resonance imaging (MRI) makes cross-sectional images by measuring changes in the body's natural magnetic field as parts of the body are exposed to strong magnets and various radio frequencies. Using these techniques, a doctor can examine the structure and appearance of internal organs. Like computed tomography (CT) scanning (see previous page), MRI uses a computer to construct images from information recorded by the scanner. In MRI, however, the information is not provided by X-rays. Instead, the person being examined is placed inside a powerful magnet, which arranges the nuclei of some of the hydrogen atoms in the body in a precise pattern (like iron shavings around a magnet). A pulse of radio waves is then passed through the person's body, moving the nuclei of the aligned hydrogen atoms briefly out of alignment. The nuclei then return to their original pattern, emitting radio signals as they do so. Different tissues such as tumors emit a more or less intense signal. These signals are detected by the machine and analyzed by the computer. The information is then used by the computer to construct an image. MRI can sometimes produce more detailed three-dimensional images than CT.

MRI technology includes magnetic resonance angiography (MRA) and magnetic resonance spectroscopy (MRS). MRA, like other types of angiography (see page 110), is used to evaluate blood flow but does not use dyes or radioactive tracers. MRS is different from conventional MRI in that MRS uses a continuous band of radio waves to excite hydrogen atoms in a variety of chemical compounds other than water. The compounds absorb and emit radio energy at certain frequencies (or spectra) that can be used to identify them. A color image is created by assigning a color to each distinct spectral emission. MRS is used to produce color images of brain function and to identify the chemical composition of diseased tissue.

Functional magnetic resonance imaging (fMRI)—also called brain mapping—uses the same MRI scanner hardware to provide noninvasive images of the brain's activity, and to detect changes resulting from biological function. Functional MRI tracks blood flow in the brain. The more active an area of the brain is, the more blood flows to it. Functional MRI enables doctors to take a series of images in quick succession and to analyze the differences between them. It also allows doctors to identify the parts of the brain that "light up" (are active) when a person is asked to perform specific tasks or is exposed to certain stimuli.

THE PROCEDURE

Because the MRI scanner creates a very strong magnetic field, you cannot carry or wear any metal objects (such as jewelry, eyeglasses, or hair clips) during the examination. Make sure you let your doctor know if you have any metal implants (such as artificial joints, plates, screws, or clips), metal attachments (such as dental braces), or electrical devices (such as a hearing aid), which could be affected by the magnet. It is especially important to tell your doctor if you have a pacemaker

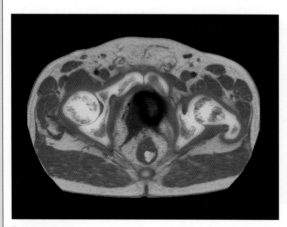

Prostate cancer
This MRI scan of a male pelvis shows an enlarged prostate gland (dark brown) with a cancerous tumor (black kidney-shaped area). The bones of the pelvis (on either side of the prostate) are yellow. The rectum (blue) is below the prostate. The reddish brown areas are muscle.

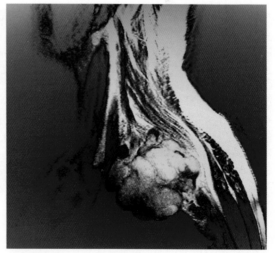

Lung cancer
This side view of a lung shows a cancerous tumor (yellow area) that is extending into the neck.

MRI *(continued)*

because the magnet can make the pacemaker stop working. Although MRI is not known to pose any health risks to a fetus, tell your doctor before having the procedure if you are (or could be) pregnant.

For an MRI, you lie on your back on a narrow padded table with a cushion under your knees. You are given a signal button to alert the technician if you begin to feel uncomfortable during the test. (If you don't like confined spaces, ask your doctor for a sedative before the test.) Because the scanner is very noisy, you are given earplugs or headphones to help block the noise. You may be given a contrast medium through a needle inserted into a vein. You must lie still during the MRI, and you may be asked to hold your breath occasionally. In closed MRI, the table slides into a narrow tunnel inside the scanner. In open MRI, the scanner is quieter and less confining. MRI is painless, and the test can last from 20 to 90 minutes or longer.

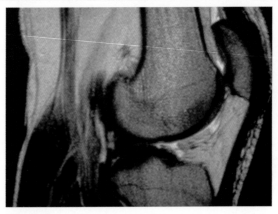

Knee joint
MRI can provide clear images of the structures in a joint. This is a side view of the knee joint; the gray areas are the two long bones that meet in the joint (the femur and tibia) and the kneecap (at right on the image).

Nuclear Medicine Imaging

Nuclear medicine imaging (also called radionuclide scanning) shows not only what organs or other structures of the body look like but also evaluates how they function. In nuclear medicine imaging, a small amount of a radioactive substance (called a radionuclide or radioisotope—or tracer) is either swallowed or injected into a blood vessel. The doctor chooses a tracer that confines itself to the organ being examined (for example, iodine concentrates in the thyroid gland). After entering the bloodstream, the tracer travels to the target organ, emitting very small amounts of gamma rays (similar to X-rays). The gamma rays are detected by an instrument called a gamma camera. Depending on the type of tissue, an abnormality may absorb more or less radiation than healthy tissue. For example, a cancerous tumor may absorb more radiation, while dead heart tissue will absorb less. The information is then analyzed by computer and constructed into an image of the organ called

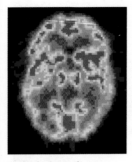

Brain during a dream
In this image, PET scanning has produced a slice image of the brain during a dream. In the REM (rapid eye movement) sleep phase (when dreaming occurs), the brain is active (red areas). The blue areas indicate low brain activity.

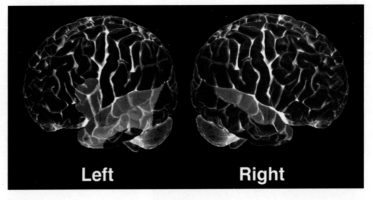

Brain
In this image, PET data (brightly colored areas) are combined with three-dimensional MRI scans of the left and right sides of the brain to show the activity in the brain when a person hears a language he or she knows well. The front of the brain is at the far left and far right of the two images. Red and green areas indicate the auditory (hearing) areas of the brain; yellow, the language or word areas; and pink, the area of the brain responsible for speech (Broca's area).

Nuclear Medicine Imaging *(continued)*

a gamma scan (also called a scintiscan or scintigram).

Radionuclide scanning can also be used with a computer to help form images with techniques such as single photon emission computed tomography (SPECT). In SPECT, cross-sectional images of the body (usually the brain) are created using a gamma camera that rotates around the person. PET (positron emission tomography) scans combine nuclear scanning with chemical analysis to show blood flow and chemical processes in action. In SPECT/PET, chemicals such as the sugar glucose (the brain's energy source) and key neurotransmitters (brain cell messengers) are made slightly radioactive and injected into the person. As they work in the brain, the chemicals emit photons (particles of light) that can be picked up like X-rays. SPECT and PET are often used to study the working brain.

THE PROCEDURE

Because the radioactive chemicals used during nuclear imaging can affect a fetus, tell your doctor before the procedure if you are (or could be) pregnant. After the radioactive tracer is swallowed or injected, you may need to wait for it to travel through your bloodstream and collect in the target organ before you are examined by the gamma camera. Because this may take several hours, you may be allowed to leave the facility and return later to take the scan. While you are having the scan, you lie or sit on the examination table, and the gamma camera is moved close to the area being examined. You must stay very still during the scan, but you may be asked to change positions; the technician will reposition you and the camera if necessary. The amount of time the procedure takes varies from about 1 to 5 hours. In some cases, a second or third scan is required. Radionuclide scanning is painless (except for the injection of the tracer). The tracer quickly breaks down into harmless substances and is eliminated from the body.

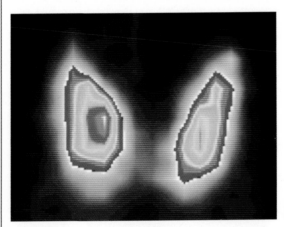

Thyroid gland
This is a gamma scan (front view) of the two lobes of a healthy thyroid gland (located at the base of the neck). The radioactive tracer has highlighted areas of activity in the gland. Areas of high activity are green or red; areas of low activity are blue.

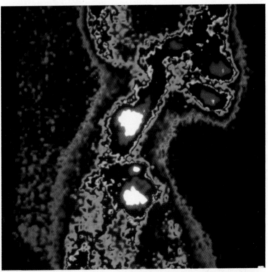

Bone cancer
This gamma scan shows a side view of the head, neck, and upper chest of a person who has cancer that has spread to the vertebrae in the neck (white area). Cancerous bone appears as bright "hot spots" on the image because the radionuclide tracer concentrates in cancerous bone more strongly than it does in normal bone.

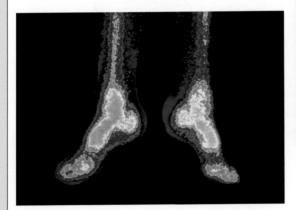

Lower legs and feet
This image is a gamma scan of the bones in the lower legs and feet. Bone shows up on the image in blue or yellow.

Endoscopy

An endoscope is a thin (usually flexible) viewing tube that enables a doctor to examine the inside of the body directly. Endoscopes have a light source, flexible bundles of glass or plastic fibers (called fiberoptic bundles) that transmit light, an eyepiece at one end, and lenses or a video computer chip at the other. Endoscopes also have a suction channel and a channel or tube through which instruments can be passed and manipulated.

Endoscopes are used to view the upper airways and lungs (bronchoscope); the esophagus, stomach, and first part of the small intestine (gastroscope); the abdominal cavity (laparoscope); the entire large intestine (colonoscope); the lower part of the large intestine and rectum (sigmoidoscope); the bladder (cystoscope); the cervix and uterus (hysteroscope); and the joints, particularly the knee (arthroscope).

THE PROCEDURE

If the endoscopic examination is of some part of the digestive tract, you may be asked to fast for a certain amount of time (usually overnight) before undergoing the procedure. Depending on the type of examination (usually the more invasive the procedure, the more uncomfortable it may be), you may be given a mild sedative, either intravenously or by mouth, or a local or general anesthetic. The doctor will then insert the endoscope directly through a natural opening in the body (such as the mouth or anus) or insert it through a small incision and guide it to the area being examined. The procedure usually takes about 30 to 60 minutes.

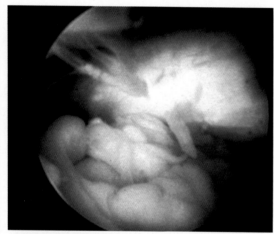

Calcium deposits in knee
A thin, rigid type of endoscope (called an arthroscope) is used to see directly inside a joint. This arthroscopic image shows calcium deposits inside a knee joint.

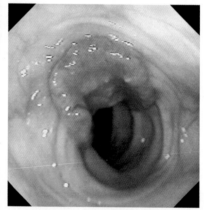

Colon cancer
Doctors can use two types of endoscopes to see the inside of the colon (large intestine) directly—a colonoscope to view the entire large intestine, and a sigmoidoscope to see just the lower third. This image is of a cancerous growth (the dark pink area in the upper part of the image) on the inside wall of the large intestine.

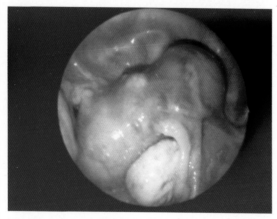

Uterus
This image is the inside of a uterus as seen through a special endoscope called a hysteroscope. The hysteroscope is guided into the uterus through the vagina and cervix.

Visual aids to diagnosis

The purpose of this section is to help you identify visual signs of illness. The color photographs on the following pages show some skin, eye, and nail disorders or problems. As a backup to the photographs, review the appropriate symptoms chart (see pages 201 to 369). If you are concerned about any symptom, talk to your doctor.

While you are looking at these photographs, keep in mind that many skin, eye, and nail problems look similar to one another. Symptoms can vary from person to person, and your symptoms may not resemble those shown here. But doctors are familiar with the full range of a disorder's visual signs and can usually make an accurate diagnosis based on these signs.

Birthmarks

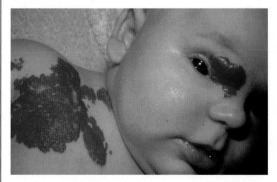

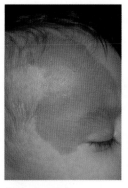

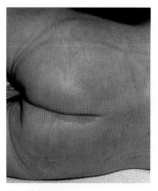

Strawberry hemangioma
A strawberry hemangioma (see page 1058) is a raised bright-red patch of skin that grows in the first few months of life and may bleed easily. After 6 to 10 months, the mark begins to shrink and fade. Most disappear by the time a child is 5 years old.

Port wine stain
A port wine stain (see page 1058) is a flat or pebbled patch of purplish red skin that usually occurs on the face and may cover a large area. A port wine stain usually remains the same throughout life but may fade over time.

Mongolian spot
Mongolian spots (see page 1058) are bluish patches on a baby's buttocks or lower back. The spots affect mostly babies of African or Asian descent, but they can also occur in white babies, usually in those of Hispanic or Mediterranean descent. They usually disappear by the time a child is 5 years old.

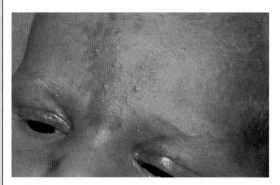

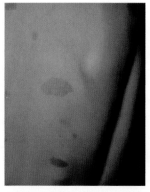

Café au lait spots
Café au lait spots are flat pigmented patches of skin that usually join and appear as a single patch. They are present from birth and remain unchanged throughout life. The presence of several café au lait spots may be a symptom of a genetic disorder called neurofibromatosis (see page 968).

Stork bites
Stork bites, which are common, are flat, salmon-colored skin patches made up of blood vessels. They most often appear on the forehead, eyelids, upper nose, and the back of the neck in newborns. They may become darker when the baby is crying and turn white when pressed. Stork bites usually disappear by the time a baby is 18 months old.

Abnormal Coloration

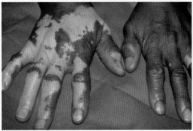
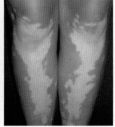
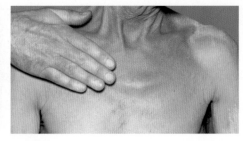

Vitiligo
In vitiligo (see page 1072), irregularly shaped patches of skin lose all of their normal color and become much paler than the surrounding skin, although the texture of the skin remains the same. The unpigmented skin patches are often symmetrical mirror images on each side of the body. Vitiligo seems to result from an abnormal immune response. In most cases, the loss of pigment is permanent.

Jaundice
Jaundice (see page 785) is yellowing of the skin (as on the chest here) and the whites of the eyes, usually caused by liver disorders. Jaundice results from a buildup in the blood of bilirubin, a yellowish brown pigment that is normally removed from the bloodstream by the liver and excreted in bile.

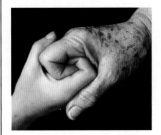
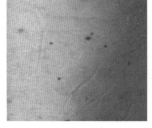
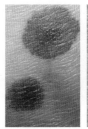
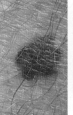
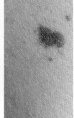

Age spots
Age spots (see page 1059), also called liver spots or solar lentigos, are flat, tan to dark brown or black patches of skin caused by long-term sun exposure. They usually develop by middle age in areas of skin (such as the hands, face, and chest) that have been repeatedly exposed to the sun.

Cherry angiomas
Cherry angiomas (see page 1059) are flat or dome-shaped small red spots on the skin that are caused by leaks in blood vessels. Although they can first appear in early adulthood, cherry angiomas usually result from a loss of elasticity in the skin that occurs as people age.

Dysplastic nevi
Dysplastic nevi are large, round moles that have not been present from birth. They usually appear around puberty but can occur at any age. Dysplastic nevi usually have irregular borders with indistinct margins and may be slightly asymmetrical. They can be varying shades of tan or brown and darker in the center. Dysplastic nevi should be examined regularly by a doctor because they can become cancerous (malignant melanoma; see page 1069).

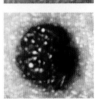
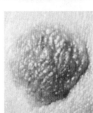

Normal moles
Moles are round or oval spots on the skin that are pigmented with melanin, the substance that gives skin, hair, and eyes their color. Moles are very common. They can be flat (top left and right) or evenly raised (bottom left and right) and are usually clearly outlined against surrounding skin. Large moles may have coarse hairs growing out of them. Some people have many moles all over their body (dysplastic nevi; above right). Some moles can become cancerous (malignant melanoma; see page 1069).

Skin Cancer

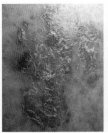 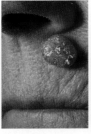 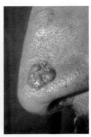

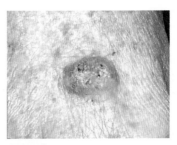

Basal cell carcinoma

Basal cell carcinoma (see page 1068) is a common form of skin cancer usually caused by overexposure to the sun. Basal cell carcinomas grow slowly, rarely spread, and are seldom life-threatening. They vary in appearance but usually start as small, flat nodules that gradually turn into ulcers (open sores) with raised edges. A close-up of one type of basal cell carcinoma is shown here (left). Basal cell tumors frequently appear on the face, usually around the eyes, near the nose (center) or on the nose (right) and on other sun-exposed areas (including the back, chest, arms, and legs).

Squamous cell carcinoma

Squamous cell carcinoma (see page 1069) is a common skin cancer that is rarely life-threatening. Squamous cell tumors start as small, firm, usually painless lumps or patches and can resemble warts or ulcers (open sores). They are associated with sun exposure and can occur anywhere on the body but are common on the backs of the hands (as shown here) or on the lips. In rare cases, squamous cell tumors can spread to other parts of the body and can be fatal, especially if they develop in a scar from a burn or vaccination.

MALIGNANT MELANOMA

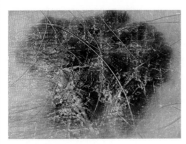

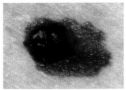

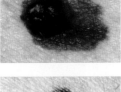

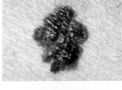

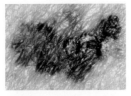

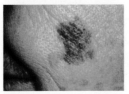

Malignant melanoma

Malignant melanoma (see page 1069) is the most deadly form of skin cancer. It is sometimes associated with exposure to the sun but can occur anywhere on the body, including parts of the body that are normally not exposed to the sun. Malignant melanomas most often appear on the face, upper trunk, or legs, and usually grow from existing moles, although they can also develop on seemingly normal skin. Malignant moles may bleed and can resemble sores that don't heal.

Asymmetry
Cancerous moles are often asymmetrical—one half of the mole looks different from the other half if you draw an imaginary line horizontally or vertically through the center of it.

Border
The outline of a cancerous mole can be uneven or have poorly defined edges and may change over time. Normal moles have clean borders.

Color
Melanomas can be very dark and can contain shades of tan, brown, white, red, or blue. They can also change color.

Diameter
Moles or colored areas of skin that grow larger than $\frac{1}{2}$ inch across (about the width of a pencil eraser) may be a sign of malignant melanoma, although smaller moles can also indicate malignant melanoma.

Dermatitis

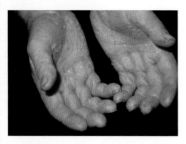

Irritant dermatitis

Irritant dermatitis (see page 1062) is a nonallergic form of contact dermatitis caused by exposure to any substance (including soap and water) that damages the skin or strips it of its protective oils. Symptoms include dry, itchy, irritated skin. Irritant dermatitis is common in adults with sensitive skin.

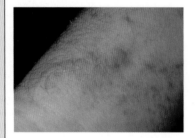

Poison ivy

Touching plants such as poison ivy, poison oak, and poison sumac (see page 169) can cause a severe case of allergic contact dermatitis in most people, although sensitivity declines with age. Symptoms develop within 24 to 48 hours of exposure and include patches of red bumpy skin or blisters that itch intensely and eventually break open and release a watery discharge. The oil from the plant that causes the initial rash can spread from the area of contact to other parts of the body.

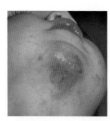

Infantile eczema

Infantile eczema (see page 1062) is a form of atopic dermatitis that causes skin inflammation in infants and small children. It produces an itchy rash or small red pimples, and can be accompanied by oozing blisters that crust over. Infantile eczema can occur anywhere on the body but usually develops on the cheeks or chin, behind the knees, or on the insides of the elbows.

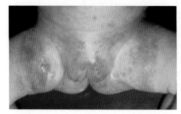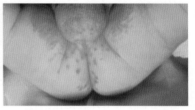

Diaper rash

Diaper rash (see page 386) is slight redness to severe inflammation of the skin around the thighs, genitals, and buttocks in babies (left). It can sometimes be accompanied by a yeast infection that causes tender sores and oozing pimples (right). Skin contact with urine and stool, along with moisture and chafing from the diaper itself, can cause diaper rash.

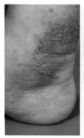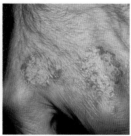

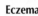

Eczema

Eczema (see page 1062) appears as red, itchy lumps or blisters on the skin that sometimes join to form patches. When eczema is persistent, the skin in the affected area may become dry and lighter or darker than the surrounding skin, and may look like leather. In nummular eczema, the patches of skin are round, raised, and flaky. The legs (left) and hands (right) are commonly affected sites.

Seborrheic dermatitis

Seborrheic dermatitis (see page 1063) is chronic skin inflammation that makes the skin red, flaky, and itchy. In adults, it usually affects the scalp, face, and neck, but it can occur anywhere on the body. Dandruff is a form of seborrheic dermatitis.

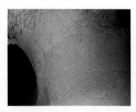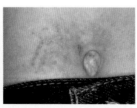

Allergic contact dermatitis

Allergic contact dermatitis (see page 1062) is an allergic reaction to a substance such as hair dye, metal, or wool (as on neck in the image at far left). The itchy, flaky skin of allergic contact dermatitis is limited to the area of contact. A metal button made of nickel caused the rash in the illustration at right.

Lumps and Bumps on or Under the Skin

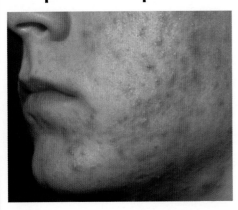

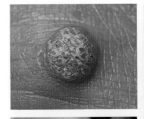

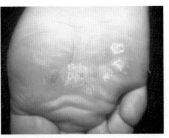

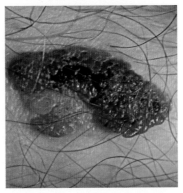

Acne

Acne (see page 1065) is a chronic skin condition in which various types of blemishes recur persistently on the upper part of the body, mostly on the face. Acne blemishes include small dark plugs imbedded in the skin (blackheads), small red lumps, tiny raised white spots (whiteheads), and small to large firm swellings (nodules and cysts). Acne is common in adolescents but can occur at any age.

Warts

Warts (see page 1060) are small areas of persistent viral infection in the upper layer of skin. The typical common wart is a hard lump with a rough, cauliflowerlike surface (top left). Warts on the bottom of the feet are called plantar warts (top right). Tiny black flecks may be visible in the body of the wart. Flat-topped, flesh-colored warts occur mainly on the wrists, the backs of the hands, and the face (left). Flat warts can itch.

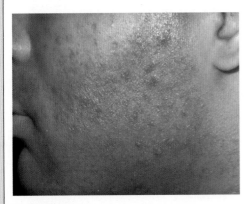

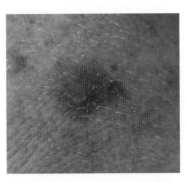

Shaving bumps

Shaving bumps (known medically as pseudo-folliculitis) are ingrown hairs (see page 1075) that can develop when the sharp ends of shaved hair grow back into the skin and become trapped under the skin. The small, hard bumps that appear around hair follicles cause slight inflammation and are common in men with curly hair. If the hair follicles become infected, the condition is called folliculitis (see page 1076).

Seborrheic keratoses

Seborrheic keratoses (see page 1063) are dark, sometimes rough-surfaced lumps that often appear on the skin in large numbers later in life. They are harmless but can resemble malignant melanoma (see page 1069), a life-threatening form of skin cancer. Seborrheic keratoses are sometimes called seborrheic warts.

Actinic keratoses

Actinic keratoses (see page 1069) are small wartlike growths that develop on sun-exposed areas of the body. They are not actually skin cancer but must always be removed because they can become cancerous.

Lumps and Bumps on or Under the Skin *(continued)*

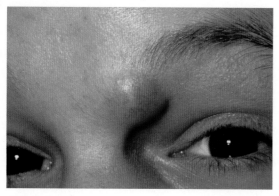

Epidermal cysts

Epidermal cysts (see page 1070), also called sebaceous cysts, usually appear as soft, smooth, sometimes yellowish lumps just beneath the surface of the skin. Sometimes a small dark dot can be seen in the skin over the center of the cyst. Epidermal cysts usually occur on the scalp, face, neck, or ears. They are harmless but can grow large and can become infected.

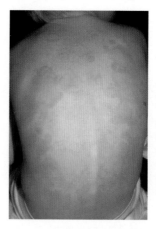

Hives

Hives (see page 1066) usually take the form of one or more raised, red, itchy patches of skin called wheals that have clearly defined edges. They are caused by allergic reactions to food, medication, cosmetics, or heat or cold. Hives usually disappear after a few hours but can recur.

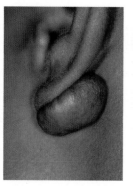 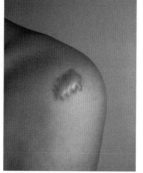

Keloids

When skin is injured, the damage is repaired by scar tissue. Keloids (see page 1071) are raised, hard, itchy scars caused by an abnormality in the healing process. Keloids are more common in dark-skinned people.

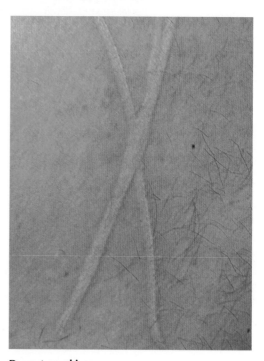

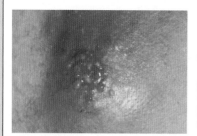

Boils

Boils are infected hair follicles that start as red lumps under the skin and gradually become bigger and more painful as they swell with pus.

Dermatographism

Dermatographism is an allergic reaction that is activated when the skin is scratched or otherwise touched with a finger or object. The resulting marks are hives that follow exactly where the skin has been touched. The red, raised, itchy patches (wheals) from these types of hives may not appear immediately and can develop up to several hours after the skin was touched.

Infections and Inflammatory Conditions

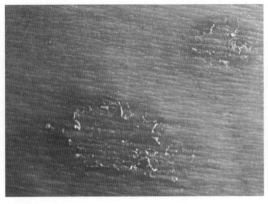

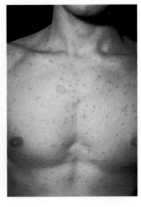

Pityriasis rosea

Pityriasis rosea (see page 1071) usually starts as one or two oval patches (left) called herald patches on the chest (right) or back. Over a few weeks, similar (usually smaller) patches appear and may spread to the upper arms and the thighs. The rash is sometimes itchy and may have a slightly scaly surface and appear orangish red in people with light skin and dark brown in people with dark skin.

Ringworm

Ringworm is a tinea (a fungus) infection (see page 1073) that is marked by red, itchy, ring-shaped rashes. The characteristic rings form when the fungus spreads uniformly outward, leaving normal skin in the center.

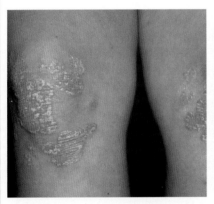

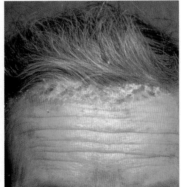

Psoriasis

Psoriasis (see page 1064) consists of patches of thick, raised skin that are pink or red and covered with silverish white scales. Small patches may join to form larger patches. In rare cases, the affected area can be slightly itchy or sore. Common sites for psoriasis are the knees (left), elbows, and scalp (right). When psoriasis affects the head, lumps can appear on the scalp and temporary hair loss can occur. Psoriasis can also affect the nails.

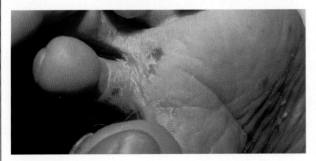

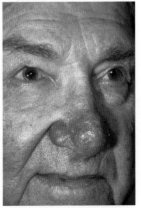

Rosacea

In rosacea (see page 1066), the face (usually the skin on the cheeks and nose) becomes abnormally red and flushed, and pus-filled pimples develop on the affected areas. In some cases, the nose becomes large and bulbous and the eyes become red.

Athlete's foot

Athlete's foot is a tinea (a fungus) infection (see page 1073) that causes itchy, cracked skin on the feet, usually between and under the toes. The skin may peel away and occasionally blister.

Infections and Inflammatory Conditions (continued)

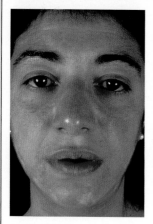

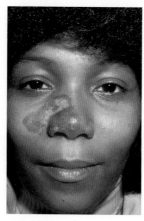

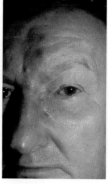
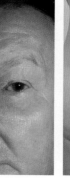

Systemic lupus
Systemic lupus erythematosus (see page 920) is a chronic disease that causes inflammation of connective tissues such as tendons and cartilage. Systemic lupus causes a red, itchy, butterfly-shaped rash over the cheeks and the bridge of the nose.

Discoid lupus
Discoid lupus erythematosus, the more common form of lupus (see page 1072), affects exposed areas of skin. In discoid lupus, the rash starts as red, circular areas of thick skin, usually on the face, behind the ears, and on the scalp. The affected area may eventually scar.

Shingles
Shingles (see page 936), caused by the herpes zoster virus, usually appears as a rash around an eye (left) or in a narrow strip on one side of the body such as around the waist, on a shoulder, or down the hip (right). Before the rash appears, a person will feel burning or stinging in the affected area. The rash is made up of many small blisters that usually dry up and scab over within a week. A shingles rash that occurs near an eye can cause severe pain, redness, and tearing.

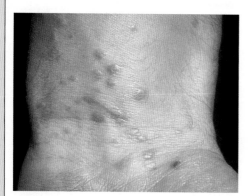

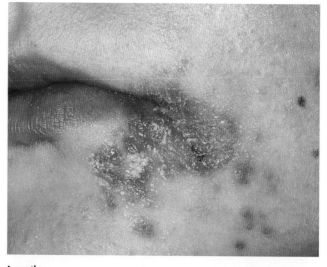

Lichen planus
Lichen planus (see page 1071) usually occurs as a rash of tiny, purplish red lumps on the inside of the wrist. The cause is unknown.

Impetigo
Impetigo (see page 1067) is a highly contagious bacterial infection that usually appears as small blisters around the mouth and nose, although the blisters can appear anywhere on the body. The infection spreads quickly. The blisters eventually break open and form a yellowish brown crust.

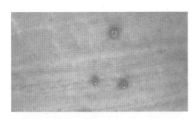

Molluscum contagiosum

Molluscum contagiosum (see page 1061) is a harmless, highly contagious viral infection characterized by small, shiny, circular, pearly lumps. The lumps have a tiny depression in the center that produces a white, waxy substance when squeezed. The infection is most common in children but can also be transmitted sexually.

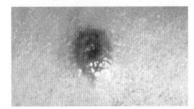

Anthrax lesion

Cutaneous anthrax (see page 1074) usually begins as an itchy, swollen sore that resembles an insect bite on exposed skin areas such as the head, neck, or hands. The sore forms a blister, which develops into an ulcer that eventually turns into a scab.

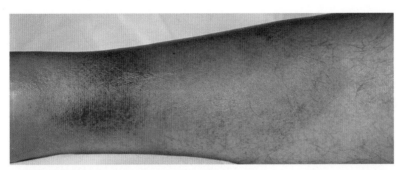

Cellulitis

Cellulitis (see page 1067) is a skin and tissue infection caused by bacteria that usually enter the skin through a wound or other break in the skin. The affected area is often hot, red, and tender, and red lines may run from the infected area to nearby lymph glands. The face, neck, and legs are the areas affected most frequently.

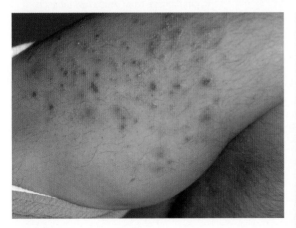

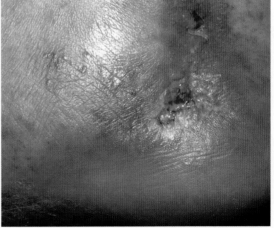

Folliculitis

Folliculitis (see page 1076) is inflammation of hair follicles resulting from a bacterial infection. It can occur almost anywhere on the skin but frequently occurs on the neck, thighs, buttocks, or armpits, causing boils (see page 1060). In men, a severe form of folliculitis can produce pus-filled blisters on the face in the beard area.

Varicose ulcers

Varicose ulcers are open, infected sores caused by twisted, swollen veins in the legs (varicose veins; see page 602) that result from insufficient circulation to the legs. Varicose ulcers usually appear around or on the ankle.

Bites and Infestations

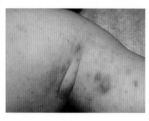

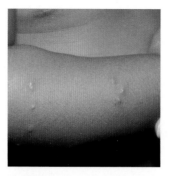

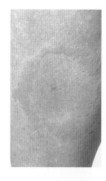

Lyme disease
Lyme disease (see page 942) is caused by a bacterium that is transmitted by the bites of infected ticks. A red dot may appear at the site of the bite. The dot gradually gets larger and forms a circular red rash. Other symptoms include fever, headache, and muscle and joint aches.

Scabies
Scabies (see page 938) is an itchy skin condition caused by the bites of scabies mites that burrow under the skin and lay eggs. The bites cause small red bumps; the burrows look like thin white lines. The bites usually occur in warm, moist areas of the skin such as on the genitals, buttocks, wrists, and around the waist and between the fingers.

Flea bites
Flea bites produce small, inflamed, itchy spots on the skin. Fleas usually bite around the ankles or lower part of the legs, although the bites can occur anywhere on the body. The area may also be swollen and turn white when pressed.

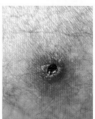

Tick bite
To feed on blood, ticks use their hooked mouthparts to pierce and attach themselves to the skin. After they finish feeding, they drop off, leaving a small wound and an area of inflammation.

Mouth and Lip Disorders

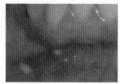

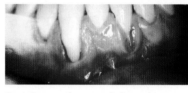

Canker sores
Canker sores (see page 743) are small, round, painful ulcers (open sores) that usually occur inside the mouth, on the tongue, or around the lips. Canker sores can be white, gray, or yellow and are surrounded by red, inflamed tissue.

Gum damage from smokeless tobacco
Smokeless tobacco can cause changes in the mouth and gums such as discolored teeth, tooth abrasion, receding gums (exposing the roots of the teeth), and loss of supporting bone and gum tissue. The damage may be permanent. Using smokeless tobacco can also lead to other mouth conditions, such as leukoplakia (see page 744) or oral cancer (see page 747).

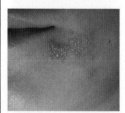

Cold sores
Cold sores (see page 744) are small blisters caused by a herpes virus. They frequently occur on or around the lips but can occur anywhere. The blisters, which are usually preceded by a tingling sensation, are small at first but eventually grow larger and break open and crust over within a few days. An area of inflamed, red skin surrounds the blisters.

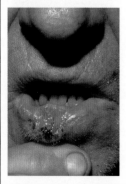

Oral cancer
Oral cancer (see page 747) is usually caused by smoking cigarettes or cigars or by using smokeless tobacco. Cancer on the lips or just inside the mouth (left, squamous cell carcinoma) can also be caused by sun exposure. Signs include a painless or painful discolored area or lump anywhere in the mouth, including on the tongue, that does not heal within a couple of weeks.

Leukoplakia
Leukoplakia (see page 744) is a disorder of the mucous membranes of the mouth in which raised, white patches develop in the mouth or on the tongue. The condition results from chronic irritation caused

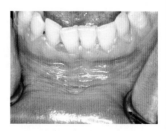

by smoking, using smokeless tobacco, poor dental hygiene, poorly fitting dental appliances, or a jagged tooth. If left untreated, leukoplakia can lead to oral cancer (see page 747).

Nail and Scalp Disorders

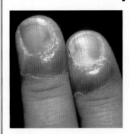

Paronychia

In paronychia (see page 1077), the cuticles and nail fold become swollen, inflamed, and painful as a result of a bacterial or fungal infection. Abscesses called whitlows make the base of the nail swell. In some cases, the nails are also thick and powdery.

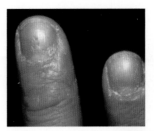

Psoriasis of the nails

Some skin disorders can also affect the nails. When psoriasis (see page 1064) affects the nails, they become pitted, rough, and abnormally thick.

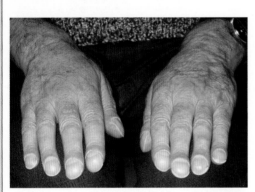

Clubbed nails

Clubbed, or spoon-shaped, fingernails often occur in people with lung or heart disease and occasionally in people with inflammatory bowel disease (see page 1078). The tips of the fingers are bulbous and rounded. (Fingernails and fingertips that have been rounded since birth usually do not result from an underlying disorder.)

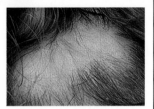

Bald patches on the scalp

Hair loss that occurs in round patches on the scalp may result from a condition called alopecia areata (see page 1076), which can be triggered by stress.

Eye Disorders

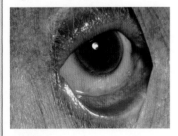

Jaundice

Jaundice (see page 785), a condition resulting from too much of a pigment called bilirubin in the blood, causes the skin and the whites of the eyes (above) to turn yellow. Jaundice usually results from liver disorders.

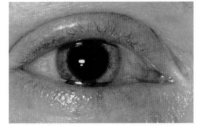

Corneal ulcer

A corneal ulcer (see page 1037) is a break or open sore in the outer layer of the cornea (the clear, protective covering at the front of the eye). An ulcer on the cornea may make the white of the eye turn pink or red. In some cases, an ulcer can appear as a whitish patch that may impair vision.

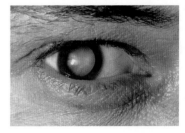

Cataract

A cataract (see page 1041) is a clouding of the normally clear lens of the eye. An advanced, or mature, cataract resembles a gray or misty-looking circle within the normally black pupil. Cataracts can reduce vision.

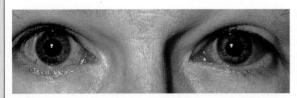

Conjunctivitis

In conjunctivitis (see page 1038), a membrane called the conjunctiva (the membrane that lines the eye) becomes painful, red, and inflamed. The eye may feel gritty and itchy and have a sticky discharge. In some cases, the eye may be sensitive to light.

Eye Disorders *(continued)*

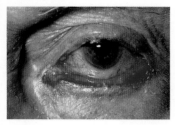

Ectropion
In ectropion (see page 1035), the lower eyelid hangs away from the eyeball, giving the appearance that the eyelashes are turned outward. The inner surface of the eyelid is exposed and the lining and the eyeball become sore and dry. A person with ectropion has excess tearing because the tears cannot drain properly.

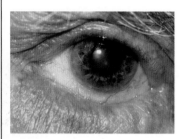

Entropion
In entropion (see page 1035), either the upper or the lower eyelid turns inward. The eyelashes rub on the surface of the eyeball, causing pain and irritating the eyeball. Entropion can cause extreme discomfort and lead to eye inflammation.

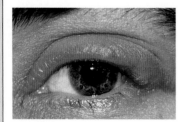

Stye
A stye (see page 1034) is an infected eyelash follicle. A follicle in the eyelid becomes red, inflamed, and painful as it fills with pus.

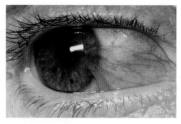

Pterygium
A pterygium is a thickening of the conjunctiva (the membrane that lines the eye), causing it to grow and cover part of the cornea (the clear, protective covering at the front of the eye), usually in a winglike or fanlike pattern. Pterygiums usually appear on the inner corner of the eye and may grow large enough to interfere with sight. In some cases, pterygiums become red and irritated.

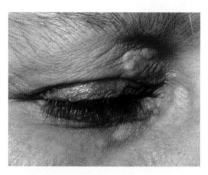

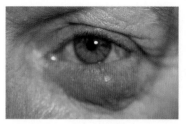

Chalazion
A chalazion (see page 1034) is a painless swelling (cyst) on the upper or lower eyelid that can grow to the size of a pea (although most are much smaller). If the cyst becomes infected, the eyelid can become red, painful, and more swollen. Chalazions are caused by blockage of the glands that lubricate the edges of the eyelids.

Xanthelasma
Xanthelasma (see page 1035) is a condition in which small, yellowish deposits of fatty material grow in the skin around the eyes, usually near the nose. The fatty deposits are harmless but, in rare cases, can be a sign of an abnormally high level of cholesterol in the blood.

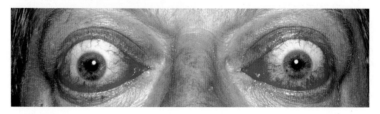

Exophthalmos
Exophthalmos (see page 1054) is the medical term for eyes that appear to stare or to protrude from their sockets, exposing more of the whites of the eyes than usual. Exophthalmos can make closing the eyes difficult. Protruding eyes are a symptom of a number of disorders but are usually a symptom of hyperthyroidism (see page 901). The bulging is caused by a buildup of tissue behind the eyeballs that pushes them forward in their sockets.

8

Preventive Health Care

One of the most important things you can do is to take responsibility for keeping yourself healthy. Although genes play a role in all diseases, lifestyle factors—such as exercise habits and diet—are even more important influences on your health risks. Your doctor can help you evaluate your health risks and recommend steps to take to reduce them. See your doctor regularly to make sure you have all the recommended checkups, screening tests, and vaccinations. In general, the earlier a disorder is diagnosed and treated, the better the outcome.

Routine Health Care

You may need to choose a new doctor for a number of reasons: a move to another community, your doctor's retirement or relocation, new health insurance requirements, the need for a specialist, a problem with your current doctor, or to get a second opinion. Try to explore your options while you are well so that you don't have to rush into a decision during a crisis. Get a copy of your medical records from your former doctor or ask his or her office to send them to your new doctor. Everyone wants his or her doctor to be well trained, competent, and accessible. Compassion and high ethical standards are also important qualities in a doctor and are basic to good health care.

How to Choose a Doctor

If you are in a health insurance plan, or if you need a doctor who will accept Medicare, the range of doctors you can choose from may be restricted. With this in mind, ask friends and relatives if they have had good experiences with their doctors. What do they like about their doctors? (Remember, however, that what they like about their doctors may not be the same qualities you are looking for.) Ask your current doctor or other health care professionals for recommendations. Find out from local medical societies which doctors are currently accepting new patients. Locate a medical center that specializes in a particular area of health you're interested in, and ask your doctor for a referral to the center or call the center yourself and find out how to get an appointment.

Many organizations (such as hospitals) have no-fee physician-referral services. You can also get information from doctor-selection services online or over the telephone. Most of these services organize their information according to type of practice and location. Others also provide information about a doctor's background, education, training, and professional achievements.

Doctor Finder

You can locate doctors in your area by specialty through a physician-referral service called Doctor Finder, or AMA Physician Select, from the American Medical Association Web site (www.ama-assn.org/aps/amahg.htm). This service provides basic professional information about virtually every licensed physician in the United States, including more than 690,000 doctors of medicine (MDs) and doctors of osteopathic medicine (DOs). All credential data have been verified for accuracy and authenticated by accrediting agencies, medical schools, residency training programs, and licensing boards.

Talking to Your Doctor

When you see a new doctor for a routine physical examination, he or she will ask you a series of questions to find out what diseases or disorders you and your closest family members have had. Your answers to these questions make up your health history. This is valuable information your doctor needs to evaluate your current health status, determine what screening tests you might need, diagnose and treat any disease or disorder you might have, and recommend steps you can take to prevent future health problems.

Also be ready to provide your doctor with information about previous medical care, dates of immunizations, and your lifestyle. Have this information in writing—don't rely on your memory.

To help determine if any diseases or disorders run in your family, try to learn as much as possible about the health history of your close relatives. Ask them about health problems they have now or may have had in the past. To learn about the health problems of a family member who has died, ask another family member or contact the person's local health department to obtain a death certificate, which lists the cause of death.

After you have interviewed all of your relatives, use the information you have gathered to construct a family health history tree like the one on the next page. You and your doctor can then review the information in the finished tree to identify any patterns in the health of your family and evaluate your health risks.

Here are some other things to consider when choosing a doctor:

- What kind of doctor do you need?
- Do you have a personal preference concerning culture, gender, or age? For example, do you want a doctor who comes from a similar background or speaks the same language as you do? Would you prefer a doctor who is the same sex as you or close in age?
- Do you need a doctor who is skilled in performing a particular procedure or in treating a particular illness?
- Is the doctor's office easily accessible? Are his or her office hours and days of operation convenient? How far in advance would you have to make an appointment?
- Does your doctor have a good reputation among other doctors?
- Does he or she have privileges at a good hospital?
- How many years of residency training or fellowship has he or she completed?
- Is he or she certified by a medical specialty board?

Your Health History

Create your own written personal health history so you can monitor your medications and any changes in your health. Fill out the personal health history form on pages 132 to 134. Take your written personal health history with you each time you have an appointment with a new doctor or other health care professional. The information can help your doctors become familiar with you, your health, and your health care needs. The more completely you fill out the form, the better able your doctor will be to determine your health care needs.

What Does It Mean to Be Board-Certified?

To become board-certified, a doctor must complete at least 7 years of medical training (4 years of medical school plus 3 years or more of residency) and pass a comprehensive examination in his or her chosen specialty, such as surgery or internal medicine. Only when the doctor passes the examination is he or she board-certified. To find out if a doctor is board-certified, call the American Board of Medical Specialties (ABMS) at 866-275-2267, or visit the ABMS Web site (www.abms.org).

Family Health History Tree

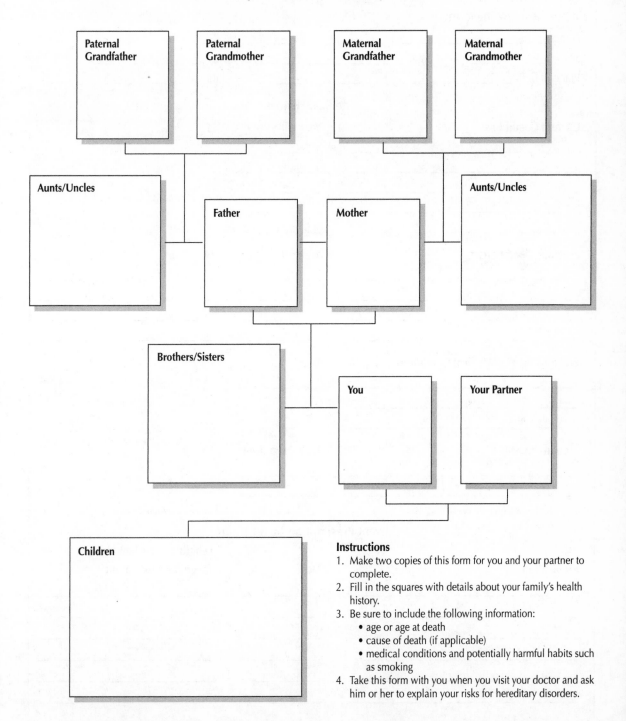

Paternal Grandfather

Paternal Grandmother

Maternal Grandfather

Maternal Grandmother

Aunts/Uncles

Father

Mother

Aunts/Uncles

Brothers/Sisters

You

Your Partner

Children

Instructions

1. Make two copies of this form for you and your partner to complete.
2. Fill in the squares with details about your family's health history.
3. Be sure to include the following information:
   - age or age at death
   - cause of death (if applicable)
   - medical conditions and potentially harmful habits such as smoking
4. Take this form with you when you visit your doctor and ask him or her to explain your risks for hereditary disorders.

Personal Health History

Fill out the following form:

Name _____

Sex _____   Birth date _____   Age _____

Place of birth _____   Ethnicity _____

Medical History

Current Conditions	Year Diagnosed
_____	_____
_____	_____
_____	_____
_____	_____
_____	_____

Previous Operations	Year	Hospital
_____	_____	_____
_____	_____	_____
_____	_____	_____
_____	_____	_____

Previous Injuries/Medical Conditions	Year
_____	_____
_____	_____
_____	_____

Mental Illnesses	Year Diagnosed
_____	_____
_____	_____

Current Prescription Medications

Medication	Dose	Length of Time You Have Taken the Medication
_____	_____	_____
_____	_____	_____
_____	_____	_____
_____	_____	_____
_____	_____	_____
_____	_____	_____
_____	_____	_____

Current Nonprescription Medications

Medication	Dose	Length of Time You Have Taken the Medication
_____	_____	_____
_____	_____	_____
_____	_____	_____
_____	_____	_____

Drug Allergies

Medication	Reaction
_____	_____
_____	_____

Social History

Marital status: Married or single   No. of children _____

Sexual history:

   No. of sex partners in your lifetime _____

   Sex of sex partners: Male, female, or both

   Practice safer sex? Yes or No

Lifestyle

Tobacco

Have you ever used tobacco products? Yes or No
No. of cigarettes smoked per day _____
No. of cigars smoked per day _____
No. of years you smoked _____
Amount of chewing tobacco or snuff used per day _____
No. of years you used chewing tobacco or snuff _____
Have you ever quit? Yes or No

Alcohol

No. of drinks per week _____
Have you ever quit? Yes or No
Have you abused alcohol? Yes or No

Illicit drugs

Have you ever used illicit drugs? Yes or No
Which drug(s) have you used? _____
When was your last use? _____

Exercise

Do you regularly exercise? Yes or No
If yes, what type of exercise? _____
How often do you exercise per week? _____
Length of exercise sessions _____

Vaccinations

Vaccination	Year of Last Vaccination	Vaccination	Year of Last Vaccination
Tetanus/diphtheria	_____	Varicella (chickenpox)	_____
Pneumococcal vaccine	_____	Hepatitis A	_____
Flu vaccine	_____	Hepatitis B	_____
Measles, mumps, rubella	_____	Meningitis	_____
Polio	_____		

Family Health History

Relative	Living (yes/no)	Age at Death	Medical Conditions and/or Cause of Death
Father	_____	_____	_____
Mother	_____	_____	_____
Partner	_____	_____	_____
Brothers	_____	_____	_____
	_____	_____	_____
Sisters	_____	_____	_____
	_____	_____	_____
Grandparents			
Paternal grandfather	_____	_____	_____
Paternal grandmother	_____	_____	_____
Maternal grandfather	_____	_____	_____
Maternal grandmother	_____	_____	_____
Uncles and aunts	_____	_____	_____
	_____	_____	_____

Doctors

Current Doctor(s)— Medical Specialty	Address	Phone No.
Primary doctor _____	_____	_____
_____	_____	_____
_____	_____	

Past Doctor(s)— Medical Specialty	Address	Phone No.
Primary doctor _____	_____	_____
_____	_____	_____
_____	_____	

Health Insurance

Health insurance company _____

Your identification no. _____

Phone no. of insurance company _____

Make the Most of a Doctor Visit

Time is valuable—for both you and your doctor—so make the most of your doctor visit. Be on time for your appointment, and make your questions clear and brief. Listen carefully to the answers; take notes if you have to. Try not to get off the subject. Deal only with present health concerns; your doctor will ask you about past health concerns if they are related to your current health. Identify and describe your symptoms clearly. Answer questions completely and truthfully. Ask questions, especially if your doctor uses words or medical terms you don't understand. Go over the list of medications you are currently taking—make sure you include all vitamins and other nutritional supplements. Also, discuss any alternative therapies or self-treatments you are using.

Your doctor makes his or her diagnosis based on your symptoms, a physical examination, and, often, test results. After he or she identifies your health problem, make sure you understand the diagnosis—and don't leave until you do.

After the doctor's visit, think about what you have learned. Call your doctor or his or her assistant or nurse if you still have questions or if you are not sure what you heard. Try to learn as much as you can about your disorder and about any recommended tests or treatment options by reading books or pamphlets and researching on the Internet. Make sure the information is from a reliable source, such as the federal government, a reputable national health organization such as the American Medical Association, or an organization that provides information about your specific disorder. Talk to other people who have the disorder.

Follow your doctor's instructions completely and carefully. Take responsibility for improving your health by improving your lifestyle. You may be able to monitor some conditions at home between appointments. For example, you can use a blood pressure monitor at home to check your blood pressure or test your blood regularly for glucose if you have diabetes. Don't hesitate to call your doctor if you have any problems with your treatment or any other aspects of your care.

How to Manage Medications

When your doctor prescribes medication, he or she will tell you how, when, and how often to take it. Find out all you can about your medication. Don't hesitate to ask your doctor or pharmacist questions about each medication you are taking.

Your doctor will examine you regularly and ask questions to determine if your medication is working. He or she will make any necessary adjustments, such as changing the dosage or prescribing a different medication, based on the results of the examination and the information you provide.

The following general guidelines will help you manage your medications safely:

- Have all of your prescriptions filled at the same pharmacy so that all of your medication records are in one place. Your pharmacist will be able to advise you about all of your medications and help you avoid potentially serious problems such as drug interactions.

- Take your medication exactly as directed. Follow your doctor's instructions carefully. If you miss a dose, take the next dose at the scheduled time; do not take a double dose. If you are not sure what to do, talk to your doctor or pharmacist.

- If you are having difficulty swallowing your medication, talk to your doctor. Do not split or crush pills or tablets or open capsules unless he or she tells you to do so.

- Don't drink alcohol if your doctor or pharmacist has told you it can interact with your medication

When to Get a Second Opinion

Your health insurance company may insist that you get a second opinion before you have surgery or some other procedure. If your insurance plan requires a second opinion, the insurance company may help you find a doctor and will pay for the cost of the doctor's appointment. In many cases Medicare will pay for the cost of a second opinion.

If you are the one who wants a second opinion, you may have to pay for it yourself. But don't let cost be the deciding factor. You have a right to get a second opinion. Try to choose a doctor for a second opinion who is not affiliated or associated with your primary doctor, and make sure that the second doctor receives a copy of your medical records so you don't have to repeat any diagnostic tests or procedures.

or make it ineffective. (Some cold and cough remedies and mouthwashes contain alcohol.)

• Because one medication can interact with another or with other substances, your doctor needs to know about all the medications you are taking, especially if another health care provider prescribed them. Make a list of everything you are taking—including prescription and over-the counter drugs; vitamins, minerals, and other nutritional supplements; and herbal remedies—and bring it with you when you visit your doctor.

• Tell your doctor if you have ever had an allergic reaction to a medication. Some allergic reactions can lead to anaphylactic shock, a life-threatening condition.

• Tell your doctor if you have diabetes, kidney disease, or liver disease. These conditions can influence how your body handles medication.

• Tell your doctor if you are pregnant or breast-feeding. Medication can be passed to a fetus through the placenta or the bloodstream and to an infant through breast milk.

• Tell your doctor if you smoke or chew tobacco. Some medications may not work if you use tobacco.

• Don't stop taking your medication because you are feeling better—unless your doctor has told you to do so. For example, if you stop taking an antibiotic too soon, your symptoms may return, or treatment could be ineffective. It is essential to continue taking medication to control a long-term condition such as high blood pressure.

• Don't stop taking your medication because it is causing side effects. Instead, contact your doctor, who will adjust the dosage or prescribe a different medication. Continue taking your medication until your doctor tells you to stop.

• Store all medications properly, preferably in their original containers. Never store more than one drug in a single container. Keep your medication out of direct sunlight and away from heat and moisture, which could alter the effectiveness of the drug. Never store medication in a bathroom medicine cabinet or kitchen cupboard. Instead, store it in a cool, dry place. If your medication needs to be refrigerated, store it on the top shelf of the refrigerator, which is usually the coldest, but make sure it doesn't freeze.

• If you have children in your home, request child-proof caps on all your prescriptions and store all medications (including over-the-counter drugs and vitamins) in a locked cabinet or drawer.

• Always check the label carefully before taking a medication to ensure that you are taking the correct drug. To avoid mistakes, never take medication in the dark.

• Never share prescription medication with others, and never take medication that was prescribed for someone else.

• Keep your prescriptions up-to-date. To avoid interrupting your treatment, check labels from time to time, and tell your doctor as soon as possible when a prescription is about to expire.

• Dispose of all expired medications, including over-the-counter drugs that are past their expiration date. Keep the medication in its original container with a child-resistant cap, put it in a sealable plastic bag, and throw it in the trash.

• Keep the phone number of your local poison-control center next to the telephone. Call the number if you take an overdose.

• If you have any questions about your medication, contact your doctor or pharmacist.

Managing Medication for Older People

Many older people are treated for more than one condition or by more than one doctor. They may need to take several different prescription and non-prescription medications every day, and can easily become confused about what medication to take at what time. Some older people may accidentally skip doses or take extra doses, while others may have trouble swallowing their medication. All of these problems can present serious health risks.

The following tips can help an older person or his or her caregiver manage medications safely:

• Make a list of the medications (both prescription and over-the-counter) the person is taking, and keep it up-to-date. Bring the list (or the containers) along to each office visit. This information helps the doctor prescribe and properly monitor the person's medications.

• Tell the doctor promptly about any side effects or changes in the way the drug affects the person.

• If the person has trouble remembering to take medication, try associating doses with specific times of the day—such as first thing in the morning, at bedtime, or with meals.

- Keep a medication schedule on a calendar, and check off each dose as the person takes it.
- Use a divided container to sort the person's doses of medication for the week. Plastic containers designed for this purpose are available at drugstores. Make sure that the container is labeled correctly.
- Have the person take his or her medications exactly as prescribed. Never change the dosage or stop any prescribed medication unless the doctor tells you to do so.
- Ask the doctor to prescribe medication in the form that is easiest for the person to take. For example, if the person has problems swallowing pills, the medication may be available in liquid form.
- Encourage the person to take medication when sitting or standing rather than when lying down.
- If the person has trouble opening containers, ask the pharmacist to use containers with easy-to-open lids. Always keep the containers out of the reach of children.
- Make sure that the instructions on the labels can be read and understood. Request that medication labels be printed in large type.
- Avoid keeping medications on a bedside table. This helps to prevent the person from taking the wrong drug or overdosing when he or she is not fully awake.
- Keep the person's prescriptions up-to-date. If the doctor wants the person to continue taking a medication that is nearing its expiration date, be sure to inform the doctor as soon as possible so that he or she can call the pharmacist to renew the prescription or write a new one.
- Dispose of all unused and expired prescription medications and over-the-counter medications. Throw them away.
- Make sure that the person never takes any medication that was prescribed for someone else, and never gives his or her medication to anyone else.

Self-Examinations

In addition to the screening tests recommended by your doctor, you should do some self-examinations regularly at home that can help identify early signs of cancer. When you are familiar with your body, you are more likely to notice any abnormal changes. Regular self-examinations—especially of the breasts, skin, and testicles—provide the best chance of detecting a tumor at an early stage, when it is small, easier to treat, and usually has a better chance for a cure.

Breast Self-Examination

Early detection of breast cancer improves the chances for a cure. Many breast lumps are found by women themselves during regular breast self-examinations. All women should start examining their breasts for changes each month at age 18 and continue performing regular exams throughout their life. Any changes in the shape or feel of your breasts or changes in the skin or nipples can be early signs of breast cancer. Look for hard or soft lumps, changes in skin texture (such as scaling) or color (such as redness), puckering or depression (such as dimpling) in part of the breast, a newly inverted nipple, or a discharge of any kind from a nipple. Each woman's breasts are unique, so it's important to get to know your breasts to be able to tell what's normal for you.

Perform a breast self-examination every month at the same time in your menstrual cycle. The best time to do a self-exam is right after your menstrual period ends (about 7 to 10 days after your period starts), when your breasts are less tender or swollen. If you take oral contraceptives, do the self-exam when you start a new pill pack each month. If you are on hormone therapy (see page 853), ask your doctor about the best time to perform a breast self-examination. After menopause, choose a specific day of the month and perform the exam on that day each month.

If you detect anything unusual in a breast, let your doctor know right away. Although most breast lumps and other changes are not cancerous, they all should be evaluated by a doctor.

- Repeat the examination by raising both arms straight over your head and looking again for changes in your breasts, and then clasp your hands behind your head and pull your arms forward as you look for changes.
- Put your hands on your hips, push your elbows forward, and look for skin or nipple changes.

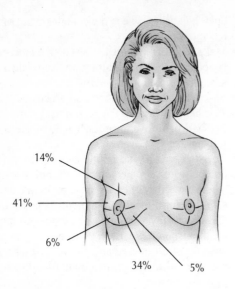

14%

41%

6%

34%   5%

Percentage of cancerous tumors
Breast cancer is more likely to occur in some parts of the breast than in others. Most breast tumors occur in the upper, outer part of the breast (toward the armpit) or behind the nipple. Examine all parts of your breasts, but pay special attention to these areas. The percentage of cancerous tumors that are found in each part of the breast are shown here.

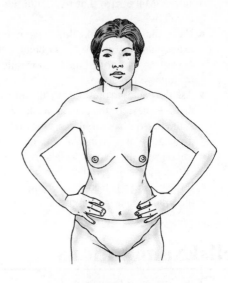

Place your hands on your hips and flex your chest muscles

How to Perform a Breast Self-Examination

Positioning yourself correctly can make a difference in how easily you can feel lumps in your breasts. To perform a breast self-examination:

- Stand in front of a mirror with your arms at your sides and look carefully for lumps or other changes in each breast.

- Squeeze both nipples between your thumb and forefinger and check for discharge.
- Lie on a flat surface (such as a firm bed or the floor) and put a pillow under the shoulder on the side of the breast you will be examining first. Raise the arm on that side and rest it over your head on the bed or floor. If you have large breasts, adjust your position until the tissue of the breast you are examining is evenly distributed.

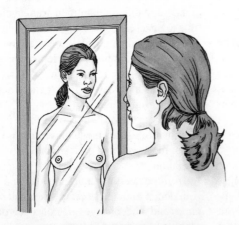

Use a mirror to examine your breasts

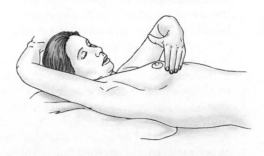

Lie down with a pillow under your shoulder

- Using the pads, not the tips, of the middle three fingers of the hand opposite the breast, start examining your breast at the armpit. Use small, circular motions—about the size of a dime. Move your fingers around your breast in decreasing concentric circles, or up and down your breast in rows. Whichever technique you use, don't take your fingers off your breast until you have covered every part of the breast. (Some women use body oil, lotion, or powder to make their fingers glide more easily over the breast.)
- Use lighter pressure to feel the skin. Increase the pressure slightly to feel for changes just below the skin surface. Use deep pressure to feel for changes closer to the ribs.
- Be sure to feel all the way from the middle of your armpit over to your breastbone (which runs down the center of your chest), and from your collarbone down to the crease under your breast.
- Repeat the entire examination on the other breast.
- Call your doctor right away if you think you feel a lump or detect any changes.

Testicle Self-Examination

All males who have reached puberty or are over age 15 should perform a testicle examination at least once a month (once a week is better) to check for any change that may be an early sign of cancer of the testicle (see page 824). In addition to any lump found in a testicle, any enlargement or shrinking of one of the testicles, buildup of fluid, feeling of heaviness, or ache, pain, or other discomfort in the testicles, scrotum, groin, or abdomen can be a sign of cancer and should be reported immediately to a doctor. Another sign of testicle cancer is enlargement or tenderness of the breasts.

Examining your testicles will help you become familiar with their normal feel and appearance. If you find a lump or swelling (painful or not), see a doctor right away. Although it is possible for cancerous lumps to occur on the front of a testicle, they develop more often on the sides.

How to Perform a Testicle Self-Examination

The best time to examine your testicles is after a warm bath or during a shower. Heat relaxes the muscles of the scrotum, making it easier to detect an abnormality.

To perform a testicle examination:

- Stand in front of a full-length mirror. Check your testicles and scrotum for any swelling or to see if one testicle seems noticeably larger than the other. (It is normal for one testicle to be slightly larger than the other.)
- Find the epididymis (the soft, tubelike structure on top of and behind each testicle that collects and carries sperm) to become familiar with the way it feels so you won't mistake it for a cancerous lump.
- Examine each testicle with both hands. Place your thumbs on top and your index and middle fingers under the testicle you are examining.
- Using both hands, roll the testicle gently between your fingers and thumb. Spend about 30 to 60 seconds examining each testicle.

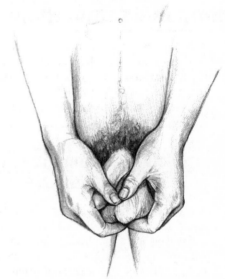

Roll the testicle between your fingers and thumb

- Feel the surface of the testicle to search for any lump or swelling, no matter how small.
- Repeat the examination on the other testicle.

Skin Cancer Check

All adults over age 20 (especially people who have had frequent, prolonged exposure to the sun) should examine their skin regularly (at least once a month) for any skin changes. Become familiar with your own pattern of birthmarks, freckles, moles, and blemishes. Changes such as a new mole or newly pigmented spot or patch of skin, a change in an existing mole, or an area that continuously grows, bleeds, itches, or fails to heal may indicate skin cancer (see page 119).

How to Perform a Skin Cancer Check

While examining your skin, pay special attention to skin areas that get direct or frequent sun exposure. Make sure you do the skin check in good light. To perform a skin self-examination:

- Stand in front of a full-length mirror. Do a superficial check of your entire body, front and back.
- Closely examine your face (especially your chin, nose, and cheeks), the front of your ears and neck, chest (women should look under their breasts), and abdomen. Check your shoulders. Raise your arms and look at your right and left sides.
- Bend your elbows and look carefully at your forearms, the backs of your upper arms, and the backs and palms of your hands (including your fingernails).
- Use a hand mirror along with the full-length mirror. Lift and part your hair all over your head to see all parts of your scalp. Check the back of your neck and the top and back of each ear.
- Examine your back (upper and lower), buttocks, and the backs of your legs.
- Sit down. Look at your genitals, the front of your thighs and shins, the tops and bottoms of your feet, and the spaces between your toes.

Common Examinations and Tests

One of the most important things you can do to stay healthy is to have all the medical checkups and screening tests your doctor recommends. Some screening tests, such as the fecal occult blood test, are recommended for everybody after a certain age, while other tests are recommended for women or men specifically. For example, the Pap smear is recommended for women (to detect cervical cancer) and the PSA test is recommended for men (to detect prostate cancer).

Pelvic Examination and Pap Smear

A pelvic examination is often performed as part of a routine gynecologic checkup. During the examination, you lie on your back on an examining table with your feet in stirrups and your knees apart and bent. The doctor will insert an instrument called a speculum into your vagina to hold it open while he or she checks for any abnormalities in the walls of your vagina and cervix (the opening into the uterus).

In a procedure called a Pap smear, the doctor swabs a few cells from the cervix to send to a laboratory, where they are examined for abnormal changes that could become cancerous. After taking the sample cells, the doctor will remove the speculum and insert one or two gloved fingers into your vagina to check for abnormalities in the uterus, ovaries, or fallopian tubes. Your doctor may examine your rectum as well at this time and take a sample of stool for laboratory testing.

The results of your Pap test usually come back in a few weeks. The test result is negative if the cells

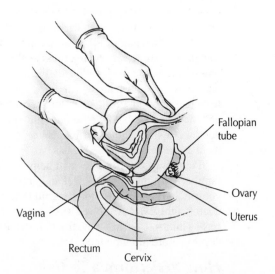

The pelvic examination
During a pelvic examination, a doctor examines the pelvic organs by hand to feel for any abnormalities of the uterus, ovaries, and fallopian tubes.

are normal; the result is positive if the cells are pre-cancerous or cancerous. If the results indicate cancerous or precancerous cells, your doctor will arrange for further tests and treatment. If the results are inconclusive—referred to as ASCUS (for atypical squamous cells of undetermined significance)—the test may have to be repeated every 3 months until definite results come back or until the doctor performs a colposcopy (see page 874) to examine the cervix directly.

Many laboratories perform genetic tests on Pap smears to identify specific strains of the human papillomavirus (HPV) that are known to increase a woman's risk of cervical cancer. If the results of your Pap smear show that you have been exposed to a cancer-causing strain of HPV, your doctor may recommend that you have more frequent Pap smears or a colposcopy.

You should have your first Pap smear when you are planning to become sexually active or by age 18. To help prevent cervical cancer, see your doctor regularly—every year or as often as your doctor recommends—for a Pap smear, which makes early detection of cervical dysplasia (see page 874) possible. A Pap smear can help prevent cancer by detecting highly treatable precancerous changes in the cervical cells, which can then be destroyed at an early stage.

Mammograms

A mammogram is a low-intensity X-ray that provides a picture of the internal structure of the breast. Digital mammography records the X-rays in computer code rather than on X-ray film. Mammograms are used as a screening test for breast cancer in women over 40 to detect cancers at an early stage, when they are generally easier to treat and more likely to be cured. Diagnostic mammograms are used to evaluate breast changes such as lumps, pain, or nipple discharge and to look more closely at abnormalities found on a screening mammogram. Although lung cancer kills more women each year, breast cancer is the most common cancer in American women, especially those between ages 50 and 69.

Most doctors recommend that women have a baseline screening mammogram at about age 40 and then have mammograms every 1 to 2 years. For women who are at increased risk of breast cancer (see page 857)—such as those who have a family

history of breast cancer (especially in a mother or sister)—a doctor may recommend starting regular mammograms at a younger age. You can obtain a high-quality mammogram at a breast clinic, the radiology department of a hospital, a private radiology office, or at a doctor's office.

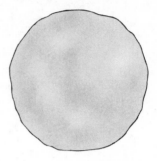

Found by chance (1½ inches)

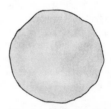

Found on self-examinations done infrequently (1 inch)

Found on regular self-examinations (½ inch)

Found with regular mammograms (⅛ inch)

Detecting breast tumors early
In general, the earlier breast cancer is detected and treated, the higher the chances for a cure. The average size of cancerous tumors found by chance is significantly larger than the average size of tumors found on a regular mammogram or with regular or infrequent breast self-examinations.

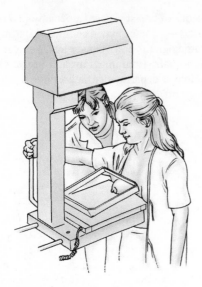

Having a mammogram
For a mammogram, each breast is compressed between two plastic plates on the mammogram machine. The technician will position your breast to flatten it as much as possible between the plates to get a good image and to spot abnormalities more easily. Once the breast is compressed, a low-intensity X-ray is taken. Screening mammograms usually take two images of each breast—one from the top and one from the side. The procedure takes about 10 to 15 minutes.

All mammography facilities in the United States must meet stringent standards established by the Mammography Quality Standards Act (MQSA), be accredited by the Food and Drug Administration (FDA), and have annual inspections to ensure their safety and reliability. Before making an appointment for a mammogram, ask if the facility has an up-to-date MQSA certificate. You can call the National Cancer Institute at 1-800-4-CANCER (1-800-422-6237) to find a qualified facility in your area. If you are menstruating, schedule your mammogram during the week after your period (about 7 to 10 days after the first day of your period), when your breasts are less likely to be swollen and tender.

Fecal Occult Blood Test

Blood in the stool can be an early sign of cancer of the colon or rectum but also of less serious conditions such as hemorrhoids. A screening test for colon cancer, called the fecal occult blood test, detects the presence of hidden blood in the stool. Because small tumors in early stages may bleed infrequently and in tiny amounts, the blood is impossible to see with the naked eye and can be detected only with a chemical test. Most fecal occult blood tests are performed at home, but doctors also often take a stool sample with a gloved finger during a routine pelvic examination or rectal examination. Doctors recommend that everyone have a fecal occult blood test every year starting at age 50. People who have risk factors for colon cancer, such as a family history of colon cancer or having previous colon polyps, should start having annual tests at age 40.

Your doctor may give you a testing kit to use at home. For this test (called the guaiac smear test), you take small samples of stool from three different bowel movements and place them on a special card. You mail the card to your doctor's office or to a laboratory, where the samples are tested for the presence of blood.

You can get a flushable reagent stool blood test from a pharmacy without a prescription. For this test, you place a chemically treated tissue in the toilet after a bowel movement. You look for a change of color in the tissue and note it on the card provided with the kit. You repeat the procedure for two or more bowel movements and then mail the results to your doctor.

With either kit, follow the instructions carefully. Before taking the test, you will be asked to make some changes in your diet and to avoid some medications that could affect the test results. For example, you will be asked not to take aspirin and other nonsteroidal anti-inflammatory drugs for 7 days before the test. (It is OK to take acetaminophen because it doesn't increase bleeding.) For 3 days before the test, don't consume more than 250 milligrams a day of vitamin C (in food or supplements) or eat red meat or raw broccoli, cauliflower, horseradish, parsnips, radishes, turnips, or melons. Don't perform the test during or for 3 days after your menstrual period, if you have hemorrhoids that are bleeding, or if you have blood in your urine. Avoid using toilet bowl cleaners for several days before the test because they can affect test results. Protect the card on which you put the stool samples from heat, light, and chemicals (such as iodine, bleach, and household cleaners).

Recommended Screening Tests

The following table lists frequently performed screening tests, how often people of average risk should have the tests, and at what age the tests should be performed. These are general guidelines. Depending on your health, your health risks, your family health history, and your health history, your doctor may recommend that you have some of these tests more frequently or less frequently.

Age Group	Test	When to Have the Test
Adults younger than 30	Physical examination (including blood pressure measurement)	Every 1 or 2 years, or as often as your doctor recommends.
	Dental examination	Every 6 months.
	Eye examination	Once between ages 20 and 29.
	Pelvic examination	Once a year, starting at age 18.
	Pap smear	Once a year for sexually active women, or as often as your doctor recommends; every 6 months if you have more than one sex partner.
	Cholesterol test	Not needed unless you are at increased risk of heart disease because of smoking, obesity, high blood pressure, diabetes, or a family history of heart disease; if you're at increased risk, have a baseline test at age 20 and every 5 years if last test result was normal.
Ages 30 to 39	Physical examination (including blood pressure measurement)	Every 1 or 2 years, or as often as your doctor recommends.
	Dental examination	Every 6 months.
	Eye examination	Once between ages 30 and 39.
	Pelvic examination	Once a year.
	Pap smear	Once a year for sexually active women, or as often as your doctor recommends; every 6 months if you have more than one sex partner.
	Cholesterol test	Every 5 years if last test result was normal.
Ages 40 to 49	Physical examination (including blood pressure measurement)	Every 1 or 2 years, or as often as your doctor recommends.
	Dental examination	Every 6 months.
	Eye examination	Every 2 to 4 years.
	Pelvic examination	Once a year.
	Pap smear	Once a year for sexually active women or as often as your doctor recommends; every 6 months if you have more than one sex partner.
	Cholesterol test	Every 5 years if last test result was normal.
	Mammogram	Baseline at age 40 and then once a year or every 2 years.
	Prostate examination	At age 45 for all black men and for white men who have a family history of prostate cancer.
	Bone density test	All women approaching menopause; women or men who are at risk of osteoporosis; whenever doctor recommends.

(continued)

Recommended Screening Tests *(continued)*

Age Group	Test	When to Have the Test
Ages 50 and older	Physical examination (including blood pressure measurement)	Every 1 or 2 years, or as often as your doctor recommends.
	Dental examination	Every 6 months.
	Eye examination	Every 2 to 4 years; every 1 to 2 years after age 65.
	Pelvic examination	Once a year.
	Pap smear	Once a year for sexually active women, or as often as your doctor recommends; not needed after age 70 in women who have had three normal Pap smears or no abnormal results in 10 years.
	Blood cholesterol test	Every 5 years if last test result was normal.
	Mammogram	Once a year.
	Colon and rectum examination	Rectal examination and fecal occult blood test once a year; sigmoidoscopy every 5 years; colonoscopy every 10 years or as often as your doctor recommends.
	Prostate examination	Once a year.
	Bone density test	All women approaching or at menopause; all women over age 65; men who are at risk of osteoporosis; whenever doctor recommends.

If a fecal occult blood test shows that you have blood in your stool, your doctor may recommend repeating the test or having additional tests such as a colonoscopy (see page 767), barium enema, or sigmoidoscopy (see right) to examine your colon and rectum.

Digital Rectal Examination

A digital rectal examination checks for abnormalities in the pelvis and lower abdomen. During a digital rectal examination, a doctor inserts a lubricated, gloved finger into the rectum and may use the other hand to press on the lower abdomen or pelvic area. A digital rectal exam is frequently done as part of a routine physical examination in men and a routine pelvic examination in women, or to find the cause of symptoms such as pelvic pain or rectal bleeding. During the exam, the doctor usually takes a sample of stool from the rectum to test it for blood, which can be an early sign of colon cancer. In men, a doctor can feel the prostate during a digital rectal examination; in women, the doctor can feel the uterus and ovaries to check for abnormalities. Other organs, such as the bladder, can sometimes also be felt during a digital rectal examination.

Sigmoidoscopy

Flexible sigmoidoscopy is used as a screening test for cancer in the lower part of the large intestine (the sigmoid or descending colon), which runs from the rectum through the last section of the colon. Sigmoidoscopy is also used to find the cause of diarrhea, abdominal pain, and constipation, or to diagnose and monitor conditions such as ulcerative colitis or Crohn's disease. For the procedure, a doctor inserts a short, flexible, lighted viewing tube (sigmoidoscope) into the rectum and slowly guides it into the lower colon. As the doctor withdraws the tube, he or she looks through it, carefully examining the rectum and colon.

If the doctor finds anything unusual, such as an abnormal growth (polyp) or inflamed tissue, he or she will remove a small sample of tissue (biopsy), using instruments inserted through the scope. The tissue sample is sent to a laboratory for examination under a microscope. If you have polyps, which can sometimes become cancerous, your doctor will recommend that you have a colonoscopy (see page 767), which allows the doctor to examine the entire colon.

Before having a sigmoidoscopy, you will be given instructions about emptying your intestine. For example, your doctor may recommend that you have one or two enemas before the procedure, and you may be asked to use a laxative or to modify your diet in some way. For the procedure, you lie on your side on an examining table while the doctor inserts the flexible tube (about the thickness of a finger) into your anus and rectum and slowly directs it up through the lower colon. You may feel some discomfort, such as pressure and slight cramping in your lower abdomen. The procedure takes about 5 to 10 minutes.

Blood Tests

Doctors order blood tests for a number of reasons. By taking a sample of blood and having it evaluated in a laboratory, a doctor can learn if you are susceptible to developing a particular disorder or can determine the cause of an existing disorder and how to treat it. Many factors, such as taking prescription or nonprescription medications, drinking alcohol, or eating before the test, can affect the test results. You will be given instructions on how to prepare for a blood test.

Complete Blood Cell Count
A doctor takes a complete blood cell (CBC) count to check the quantity and quality of red blood cells, white blood cells, and platelets—three major types of cells in the blood. A CBC count consists of six different tests.

Red blood cell count
The red blood cell (RBC) count is used to determine if the level of red cells (which transport oxygen to tissues) in the blood is too high or too low. Extremely high levels of red blood cells may be a sign of a blood disorder such as polycythemia; extremely low levels may be a sign of anemia.

Routine Vaccinations for Adults

In addition to periodic health checkups and screening tests, your doctor will probably recommend that you have vaccinations against some potentially dangerous infectious diseases. The vaccinations you should have will depend on your risk factors. Talk to your doctor about having the following vaccinations.

Vaccination	Who Should Have It?	When?
Tetanus booster	All adults.	Every 10 years.
Diphtheria booster	All adults.	Every 10 years.
Chickenpox	Adults who have never had chickenpox or the vaccination.	Any time.
Pneumococcal pneumonia vaccine	Adults over age 60 or who have a chronic disease, live in a long-term care facility, are health care workers, or have an impaired immune system.	Every 5 to 10 years.
Influenza vaccine	All adults.	Every fall (at the beginning of the flu season).
Measles, mumps, and rubella	Everyone who was born after 1956 and has not had these infections or a vaccination.	Any time.
Hepatitis B	Health care workers and anyone who has a chronic disease or multiple sex partners.	Any time.
Meningitis	College students or travelers to areas where meningitis is prevalent.	Any time; for travelers, at least 1 week before departure.

Hematocrit

The hematocrit test, like the RBC count, is used to look for extremely high or low levels of red blood cells. In the hematocrit test, the doctor pricks a person's finger, and puts a drop of the person's blood into a glass tube. The tube is then spun in a machine at high speed, causing the red blood cells to sink to the bottom and leaving the liquid part of the blood at the top.

White blood cell count

The white blood cell (WBC) count is used to determine if the level of white blood cells (which fight infection) is too high or too low. High or low levels of white blood cells may be a sign that you have an infection or are at increased risk of an infection. High levels of white blood cells can also indicate a blood cancer such as leukemia.

Differential blood cell count

A differential blood cell count measures the amounts of the five different types of white blood cells—neutrophils, lymphocytes, monocytes, eosinophils, and basophils. High or low levels of any of the different types of cells may be a sign of infection or allergies or of more serious disorders such as cancer, leukemia, heart attack, or AIDS.

Hemoglobin

The hemoglobin test measures the amount of hemoglobin (the oxygen-carrying pigment that gives blood its red color). The hemoglobin test is also used to determine if levels of red blood cells are normal. A low level of hemoglobin indicates iron deficiency anemia.

Platelet count

The platelet count measures the amount of platelets (cell fragments that enable blood to clot) in the blood. It is important to know the number of platelets if you are going to have surgery. Low platelet counts can result from leukemia and other cancers or from treatment for cancer. High platelet counts can result from bone marrow diseases or iron deficiency anemia. Very low platelet counts can be a sign of internal bleeding.

Blood Chemistry Tests

A blood chemistry profile consists of a number of tests that measure the levels of certain chemical substances in blood serum (the liquid part of the blood). Abnormal blood chemistry test results may, but not always, indicate a health problem, and normal test results can occur in people who have a medical disorder. If you have an abnormal test result, your doctor will order another blood test to see if the results are consistent before recommending further medical tests. The ranges given for

Measuring Cholesterol Levels

Beginning at age 20, you should have a cholesterol test at least every 5 years, and more frequently if you have a family history of heart disease. The numbers provided on your cholesterol profile can help your doctor evaluate your risk of developing heart disease. Your risk of heart disease is low if your total cholesterol level is less than 200 milligrams per deciliter (mg/dL), your LDL (bad) cholesterol level is below 100 mg/dL, your HDL (good) cholesterol level is 60 mg/dL or higher, and your triglyceride level is less than 150 mg/dL. The measurement is most reliable when performed after you have fasted for 12 hours.

Total Cholesterol	Level of Risk for Heart Disease
Less than 200 mg/dL	Low
200–239 mg/dL	Borderline high
240 mg/dL and above	High
LDL Cholesterol	
Less than 100 mg/dL	Low
100–129 mg/dL	Moderately low
130–159 mg/dL	Borderline high
160–189 mg/dL	High
190 mg/dL and above	Very high
HDL Cholesterol	
60 mg/dL and above	Low
50–59 mg/dL	Moderately low
40–49 mg/dL	Borderline high
39 mg/dL or less	High
Triglycerides	
Less than 150 mg/dL	Low
151–199 mg/dL	Borderline high
200–499 mg/dL	High
500 mg/dL and above	Very high

normal results can vary slightly from laboratory to laboratory.

Cholesterol and lipids

A cholesterol and lipids test measures the levels of various fats in the blood, including triglycerides; HDL (high-density lipoprotein), the good cholesterol; and LDL (low-density lipoprotein), the bad cholesterol. Increased levels of triglycerides or LDL cholesterol and decreased levels of HDL cholesterol can indicate an increased risk of cardiovascular disease, including heart disease, atherosclerosis, and stroke. Doctors use the cholesterol test to evaluate heart disease risk. Drugs such as corticosteroids, thiazide diuretics, and oral contraceptives can affect cholesterol levels. Excess alcohol intake, kidney and liver diseases, obesity, menopause, diabetes, and hypothyroidism (an underactive thyroid gland) also can affect cholesterol and lipid levels.

Glucose

Glucose is a sugar that the body uses for energy. The hormone insulin, which is produced by the pancreas, regulates the level of glucose in the blood. Increased levels of glucose can be a sign of diabetes. Decreased levels of glucose can be a sign of adrenal insufficiency (underfunctioning of the adrenal glands). Conditions such as a stroke or heart attack can temporarily increase glucose levels. Medications such as corticosteroids, diuretics, and tricyclic antidepressants also can increase glucose levels. In general, low blood glucose is a rare condition in people who are otherwise healthy. The normal glucose range is 65 to 109 milligrams per deciliter (mg/dL).

Albumin

The albumin test measures the amount in the blood of the protein albumin, which keeps water inside blood vessels and is the most plentiful protein in the body. The albumin level is a good indicator of a person's general nutritional status. Disorders such as hepatitis, cirrhosis, and malnutrition can cause a decrease in the level of albumin. The level of albumin is also decreased during pregnancy. The albumin test can help diagnose liver disease, kidney disease, and intestinal disorders such as Crohn's disease that can reduce the absorption of nutrients. People who have cancer or chronic diseases such as autoimmune disorders or AIDS often have a low albumin level. The normal albumin range is 3.7 to 5.2 grams per deciliter (g/dL).

Alkaline phosphatase

Alkaline phosphatase (ALP) is an enzyme that is present in all tissues of the body. High concentrations of ALP are normally found in the liver, in bile ducts, in bones, and, in pregnant women, in the placenta. Extremely high levels of ALP can be a sign of several abnormal conditions, including bone disease, leukemia, and liver disease. The enzyme can also be elevated in normal conditions such as healthy bone growth or can result from an abnormal response to a medication. The normal ALP range is 40 to 157 international units per liter (IU/L).

Alanine aminotransferase

Alanine aminotransferase (ALT) is an enzyme found in many tissues, but is present in high levels in the liver. Doctors use the ALT test to detect liver damage, which can cause ALT to be released into the blood. Extremely high levels of ALT can be a sign of liver diseases such as hepatitis and cirrhosis. The normal ALT range is 5 to 35 international units per liter (IU/L).

Aspartate aminotransferase

Aspartate aminotransferase (AST) is an enzyme found mostly in the heart muscle, skeletal muscle cells, and liver cells. Conditions such as liver disease, infectious mononucleosis, and muscle disease can increase the level of AST in the blood. Recent surgery, exercise, and pregnancy can also raise levels of AST. Doctors use the AST test mainly to diagnose or monitor liver disease and, occasionally, to monitor people who have had a heart attack. The normal AST range is 10 to 34 international units per liter (IU/L).

Blood urea nitrogen

Blood urea nitrogen (BUN) is a by-product of the breakdown of proteins in the liver. An elevated BUN level can be a sign of kidney disease or, occasionally, severe gastrointestinal bleeding. Medications such as antibiotics and diuretics can also affect BUN levels. Doctors use the BUN test to evaluate kidney function and to diagnose conditions such as gastrointestinal bleeding. The normal BUN range is 8 to 23 milligrams per deciliter (mg/dL).

Calcium

The serum calcium test measures the amount of calcium in blood serum. Increased levels of calcium can be a sign of cancer that has spread to the bones from another part of the body, multiple myeloma, hyperthyroidism (an overactive thyroid gland), or hyperparathyroidism (overactive parathyroid glands). Medications such as lithium, thiazide diuretics, and antacids can also increase the levels of calcium in the blood. Doctors use the serum calcium test to diagnose or monitor conditions such as bone disease, kidney disease, endocrine disorders, and cancer. A low calcium level can result from severe, acute pancreatitis. The normal total calcium range is 8.4 to 10.3 milligrams per deciliter (mg/dL).

Carbon dioxide

Carbon dioxide is a waste product of normal metabolism. The lungs eliminate carbon dioxide from the blood through breathing. Increased levels of carbon dioxide can indicate disorders that affect the lungs, such as emphysema or other obstructive lung diseases, or loss of stomach acid from vomiting. Drugs such as corticosteroids and excessive use of antacids can also increase the blood levels of carbon dioxide. Decreased levels of carbon dioxide can result from severe, uncontrolled diabetes, kidney failure, or severe diarrhea. The normal carbon dioxide range is 21.3 to 30.3 milliequivalents per liter (mEq/L).

Creatinine

Creatinine is a muscle enzyme that is present in the blood at various levels based on a person's size and muscle mass and that is filtered out by the kidneys and excreted in urine. Doctors measure the levels of creatinine to diagnose kidney disease. The normal creatinine range is 0.6 to 1.1 milligrams per deciliter (mg/dL).

Total bilirubin

Bilirubin is an orange-yellow pigment in bile, a liquid secreted by the liver to remove waste products and break down fats during digestion. Doctors use the total bilirubin test to diagnose liver disease, jaundice (yellowing of the skin and the whites of the eyes), and obstruction of the bile duct (the tube that carries bile from the liver). The normal total bilirubin range is 0.2 to 1.1 milligrams per deciliter (mg/dL).

Direct bilirubin

The direct bilirubin test measures the blood level of a form of bilirubin called conjugated bilirubin. The blood usually contains very small amounts of conjugated bilirubin. However, damage to the liver can increase the amount of bilirubin in the blood. The normal direct bilirubin range is 0.04 to 0.20 milligram per deciliter (mg/dL).

Indirect bilirubin

An elevated level of indirect (unconjugated) bilirubin can be a sign of hemolytic anemia, pernicious anemia, or neonatal jaundice. The normal indirect bilirubin range is 0.2 to 0.7 milligram per deciliter (mg/dL).

Gamma glutamyltransferase

Gamma glutamyltransferase (GGT) is an enzyme that is usually found at high levels in the kidneys, liver, and bile ducts. Doctors use the GGT test to help diagnose disorders of the liver, bile ducts, and gallbladder, which can increase the levels of GGT in the blood. Use of some drugs such as phenobarbital and excessive intake of alcohol can increase GGT levels. The normal GGT range is 0 to 51 international units per liter (IU/L).

Lactate dehydrogenase

Lactate dehydrogenase (LDH) is an enzyme found in many tissues, especially the brain, heart, liver, kidneys, lungs, blood cells, and skeletal muscles. Doctors use the LDH test to detect tissue damage. Increased levels of LDH may be a sign of a heart attack, liver disease, lung problems, or advanced cancer. Drugs such as aspirin and some anesthetics and narcotics can also increase LDH levels. The normal LDH range is 105 to 333 international units per liter (IU/L).

Phosphorus

Phosphorus is a substance that the body uses, along with calcium, for bone development and growth. Increased levels of phosphorus in the blood can be a sign of kidney failure or hypoparathyroidism (underactive parathyroid glands). The normal serum phosphorus range is 2.4 to 4.4 milligrams per deciliter (mg/dL).

Potassium

Potassium is a mineral that is essential for maintaining nerve impulses, water balance in the body, normal heart rhythm, and muscle function. Increased levels of potassium in the blood can be a sign of kidney failure and can occur when a person is undergoing hemodialysis (a treatment for kidney failure in which a machine temporarily performs the functions of the kidneys). Decreased levels of potassium can result from fluid loss such as from excessive sweating, vomiting, or diarrhea. Medications such as angiotensin-converting enzyme (ACE) inhibitors can increase the level of potassium in the blood. Medications such as laxatives, insulin, or salicylates can decrease the amount of potassium in the blood. The normal potassium range is 3.5 to 5.3 milliequivalents per liter (mEq/L).

Sodium
Sodium is a chemical that plays an important part in maintaining the balance of water and salt in the body. Some hormones can cause a loss of sodium. Increased levels of sodium can indicate excessive loss of water (dehydration). Eating too many salty foods and not drinking enough water can also increase sodium levels. Decreased levels of sodium can be a sign of kidney disease, severe brain disease, or lung disease. Medications such as diuretics and some medications used for treating diabetes can also decrease sodium levels. The normal sodium range is 133 to 145 milliequivalents per liter (mEq/L).

Total protein
Doctors measure the level of protein in the blood to detect a variety of diseases including liver disease, kidney disease, and a blood cancer called multiple myeloma. Medications such as corticosteroids, insulin, and growth hormone can increase protein levels in the blood. Medications such as the hormone estrogen can decrease protein levels. The normal total protein range is 6 to 8 grams per deciliter (g/dL).

Uric acid
Uric acid is a by-product of metabolism that normally is excreted by the kidneys in urine. An increase in the amount of uric acid can be a sign of gout, kidney failure, or lead poisoning. Drugs such as alcohol, diuretics, and caffeine can increase the amount of uric acid in the blood. The normal uric acid range is 2.6 to 7.8 milligrams per deciliter (mg/dL).

Blood Culture
In a blood culture, blood is drawn from a vein on the inside of an elbow or from the back of the hand and examined over several days. A blood culture is used to check for the growth of bacteria and other microorganisms in the blood. The presence of bacteria in the blood indicates a life-threatening infection called bacteremia.

PSA Test
The PSA (prostate-specific antigen) test measures the level in the blood of a protein called PSA, which is produced by cells in the prostate gland. The level can be increased when a man has prostate cancer or a noncancerous condition such as inflammation of the prostate or enlargement of the prostate. The test is often used along with a digital rectal examination to screen for and diagnose prostate cancer in men age 50 or older. Because blacks are at higher risk than whites of developing prostate cancer, black men (and all men who have a family history of prostate cancer) should start having the PSA test at about age 45. The test is also used, with other tests, to detect a recurrence of prostate cancer in men who have undergone treatment for prostate cancer.

A PSA level of fewer than 4 nanograms per milliliter (ng/mL) is considered normal. If your PSA level is elevated, your doctor will recommend further testing, including imaging tests or a biopsy (taking a small tissue sample from the prostate for examination under a microscope). Most men who have an elevated PSA level, especially those over age 50, are found not to have prostate cancer on further testing. Talk to your doctor about the pros and cons of having an annual PSA test and possible follow-up procedures if the level is elevated.

CA-125 Test
In the CA-125 test, a sample of a woman's blood is examined for the presence of a chemical marker (antigen) called CA-125 on the surface of cells to help diagnose ovarian cancer. Most women who have ovarian cancer have an elevated level of CA-125 in their blood. However, this test is not used as a screening test for ovarian cancer or to make a definite diagnosis of ovarian cancer because levels of CA-125 also can be elevated in noncancerous conditions such as inflammation in the abdomen, pelvic infections, uterine fibroids, ovarian cysts, endometriosis, and liver diseases such as hepatitis and cirrhosis. The CA-125 test is often used, usually along with other tests, to monitor the effectiveness of treatment of ovarian cancer in women who are undergoing chemotherapy.

A CA-125 level below 35 units per milliliter (U/mL) is considered normal. If your level of CA-125 is higher than normal, your doctor will recommend further tests, such as a vaginal ultrasound (see page 510), to make a diagnosis.

Thyroid Hormones

The thyroid gland produces two thyroid hormones, called thyroxine (T4) and triiodothyronine (T3), which can be measured in the blood to help doctors evaluate thyroid function. The thyroid's hormone production is triggered by secretion of a hormone called thyroid-stimulating hormone (TSH) by the pituitary gland in the brain. Doctors usually use a combination of two or more tests to diagnose thyroid disorders. For example, a high level of TSH and a low level of T4 can indicate an underactive thyroid gland (hypothyroidism). An abnormally low level of TSH and high level of T4 can indicate an overactive thyroid gland (hyperthyroidism). The normal range for total T4 is 4.6 to 12 micrograms per deciliter (mcg/dL). The normal range for total T3 is 80 to 180 nanograms per deciliter (ng/dL). The normal range for TSH is 0.5 to 6 microunits per milliliter (mcU/mL).

Urine Tests

Doctors use urine tests to evaluate urine for signs of infection in the kidneys or bladder, or for the presence of blood or other substances. A person may have a urine test for a number of reasons, including as part of an annual physical examination, before surgery, to diagnose a urinary tract infection, and to confirm and monitor a pregnancy. A urine sample can be taken at the doctor's office or at home (and brought to the doctor's office).

It is essential for urine samples to be taken under clean conditions. Before having a urine test, you will be asked to wash your genital area to make sure that the urine is not contaminated by bacteria that normally live on the skin. You will be given a clean container in which to urinate. To get a midstream or clean-catch urine sample, you will be asked to urinate into the toilet for a few seconds before urinating into the container.

Urinalysis

A doctor performs a urinalysis to diagnose or monitor conditions that affect the kidneys, such as kidney disease or diabetes. The doctor will use a test strip to check for specific suspected abnormalities, such as the presence of bacteria. The sample is also examined more closely under a microscope to look for bacteria or other microorganisms and for specific substances, such as mucus, red blood cells, or white blood cells that can be signs of health problems.

Urine Culture

Doctors perform urine cultures to diagnose urinary tract infections. After the urine is collected, a sample is put on a slide in the laboratory and placed in an incubator for 24 hours. If bacteria, yeast, or other microorganisms grow on the sample, the test result is considered positive. The sample is then tested with various drugs to determine what medication to use to treat the infection.

First Aid and
Home Caregiving

First Aid

The main goal of first aid is to help an injured (or, in some cases, ill) person recover or to prevent an injury from getting worse. The person giving first aid should also provide reassurance and make the person as comfortable as possible until professional help arrives. For many minor injuries, first aid may be all that is needed. More serious injuries may require medical attention and further treatment.

The more knowledge you have before an injury or emergency occurs, the more helpful you can be. Review this section and familiarize yourself with first-aid techniques and procedures. Some topics such as allergic reactions (see page 912), asthma attacks (see page 640), seizures (see page 686), and diabetic coma (see page 897) are covered in other sections of the book. Sports injuries and the standard treatment for most athletic injuries are covered on pages 978 to 982.

Make a practice run to the nearest hospital emergency department so you know the best route in case you have to drive an injured person there yourself. Information is no substitute for hands-on experience; take first-aid classes to prepare yourself for an emergency. Because cardiopulmonary resuscitation (CPR) should be used only by a person trained in the procedure, this book does not include instructions for CPR.

Priority Checklist for Emergencies

Rapid and accurate assessment of what needs to be done is crucial. Follow these steps in an emergency:

1. **Call or have someone else call 911** or your local emergency number, or send someone for help.
2. **Check breathing.** If the person is choking, perform the Heimlich maneuver (see page 155). If breathing has stopped, immediately start mouth-to-mouth resuscitation (see page 156).
3. **Check heartbeat.** If the person's heart has stopped, perform cardiopulmonary resuscitation (CPR) if you have had CPR training.
4. **Control any bleeding** (see page 160).
5. **Treat any burns** (see page 163) or **broken bones** (see page 167).
6. **Prevent shock** (see page 162).

Index to First-Aid Procedures

Allergic reactions (see pages 170 and 916)
Artificial respiration (see page 156)
Asthma attacks (see page 641)
Bites
  • animal (see page 173)
  • insect (see page 170)
  • snake (see page 172)
  • spider (see page 171)
  • tick (see page 171)
Bleeding
  • minor (see page 173)
  • from nose (see page 177)

Absence of Breathing

The simplest and most effective method of restoring breathing in a person who is not breathing is to exhale your breath into the person's lungs. If a person's breathing has stopped, mouth-to-mouth resuscitation (also called artificial respiration) is needed immediately because if the brain is deprived of oxygen for more than 4 or 5 minutes, permanent brain damage or death can occur. Call or have someone call 911 or your local emergency number, or send someone for help.

When someone has stopped breathing, his or her chest or abdomen does not rise and fall, his or her face may turn blue or gray, and you will not be able to feel any air coming out of his or her mouth or nose.

If, for some reason (such as a mouth injury), you can't give the person mouth-to-mouth resuscitation, try to resuscitate him or her by putting your mouth around his or her nose. For an infant or small child, put your mouth over the child's mouth and nose.

Choking

A person who is choking will involuntarily grasp his or her neck. Complete obstruction of an airway is an emergency that requires immediate attention. If the person can speak, cough, or breathe and his or her skin color is good (he or she does not look bluish or gray), the airway may be only partly blocked. Do not interfere with his or her efforts to cough up the food or object.

The Heimlich Maneuver

The Heimlich maneuver is an effective first-aid measure for dislodging food or another foreign object in a choking person.

*If the choking person is
conscious or standing:*

1. Stand behind the person and place your fist (with your thumb folded in your fist) slightly above the person's navel and below the ribs and breastbone. Do not touch the breastbone.
2. Place your other hand under the first and give several quick, forceful, upward thrusts. Squeeze only the person's abdomen; do not squeeze the ribs. Repeat until the person coughs up the object.

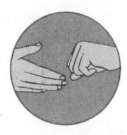
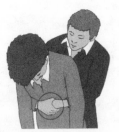

3. If the object is dislodged but the person stops breathing, start mouth-to-mouth resuscitation immediately (see next page).

If the choking person is unconscious or lying down:

1. Turn the person on his or her back and straddle him or her.
2. Place the heel of one hand on the person's stomach, slightly above the navel and below the ribs (dotted line). Put your other hand on top of the first hand. Keeping your elbows straight, give several quick, forceful, downward and forward thrusts (toward the person's head). Do not press on the person's ribs; press on the abdomen only. Repeat until the person coughs up the object.
3. If the object is dislodged but the person stops breathing, start mouth-to-mouth resuscitation immediately (see next page).

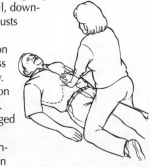

**Straddle the person and give
several forward thrusts**

Mouth-to-Mouth Resuscitation

To provide mouth-to-mouth resuscitation, follow these steps:

1. Lay the person down on his or her back on a firm, rigid surface.

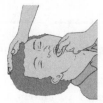

2. Turn the person's head to the side and clear the mouth of any visible foreign material (such as food or loose dentures) by sweeping a finger inside the person's mouth.

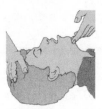

Clear the mouth of foreign material

3. If the person's neck does not appear to be injured, tilt his or her head back by lifting the chin up while gently holding down the forehead with the palm of your other hand. This will open the airway by lifting the tongue from the back of the throat. (Don't tip a small child's head back too far.)

Tilt the head back by lifting the chin

4. Pinch the person's nostrils closed with the fingers of the hand that is holding down the person's forehead (below). (For a person with a facial injury or for a small child, don't pinch the nostrils.) Open your mouth wide, take a deep breath, and blow two full breaths into the person's mouth.

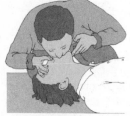

5. If the person has a mouth injury, blow into his or her nose (below left). For an infant or small child, don't pinch the nose; blow into both the mouth and nose (below right).

Blow into the mouth

6. Continue breathing into the person's mouth. Remove your mouth after each breath and turn your head so that your ear is over the person's mouth to listen for air coming out of his or her lungs. You may also be able to feel the exhaled air. Inhale deeply before blowing into the person's mouth again. Give one breath about every 5 seconds (one breath every 3 seconds for small children).

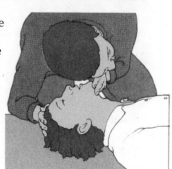

Listen and feel for exhaled breath

7. Watch the person's chest. If the chest does not rise with each breath, the airway is not clear or is not open enough. Recheck the person's airway; clear it of any foreign material and adjust the person's chin to try to open the airway.

8. Continue breathing into the person's mouth until he or she is breathing on his or her own or until medical help arrives.

9. Check the person's neck (or wrist) artery for a pulse. If there is no pulse, begin chest compressions if you have been trained in CPR. Either way, continue doing mouth-to-mouth resuscitation until the person is breathing on his or her own or until medical help arrives.

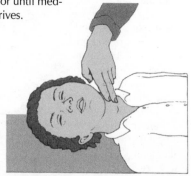

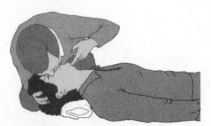

Blow into the nose for a facial injury

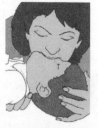

Blow into a small child's mouth and nose

Check the neck artery for a pulse

To Revive a Choking Infant or Baby

1. Sit down and lay the child facedown across your knee (an infant can be held facedown along your arm with your hand supporting his or her jaw).
2. Give the child several thumps between the shoulder blades with the heel of your hand. The back blows should be strong but not forceful enough to hurt the child.

3. If this does not expel the food or object, turn the child onto his or her back (keeping the head lower than the trunk). Place two fingers slightly below and centered between the child's nipples. Give five quick thrusts to the child's chest with your fingers. The thrusts should be strong but not forceful enough to hurt the child.

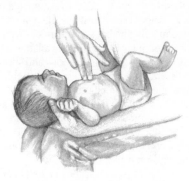

Turn the child on his or her back and give five thrusts with your fingers

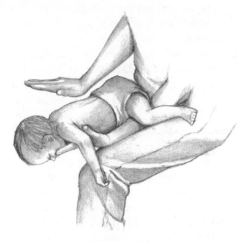

Thump the child between the shoulder blades

4. Repeat both procedures (facedown and faceup) until the child coughs up the food or object.

If the person can't speak and is having difficulty breathing, have someone call 911 or your local emergency number or get help while you start the Heimlich maneuver. The Heimlich maneuver works by putting pressure on the abdomen. Putting pressure on the abdomen, in turn, pushes up the diaphragm, which increases air pressure in the lungs and forces the object out of the windpipe.

Drowning

Call or have someone call 911 or your local emergency number, or send someone for help. Do not move the person if you think he or she may have a neck injury (see page 167). If you must move the person, always keep his or her head, neck, and body in alignment (see page 169).

If the person is breathing, place the person on his or her side, preferably with the head slightly backward (to open the airway) and lower than the body (to drain fluids). Do not give the person anything to eat or drink. Keep the person warm, but do not massage the skin because massaging can worsen any muscle damage.

If the person is not breathing, start mouth-to-mouth resuscitation immediately (see previous page). The air you breathe into the person's lungs will pass through any water in the lungs. Continue mouth-to-mouth resuscitation until medical help arrives or until the person is breathing on his or her own. If the person's heart has stopped beating, perform CPR if you have had CPR training.

Heart Attack

A heart attack (see page 567) is a life-threatening emergency that results from a lack of blood and oxygen to a portion of the heart muscle, usually caused by a narrowing or obstruction of one of the coronary arteries that supply the heart muscle. If a part of the heart muscle is deprived of blood and oxygen for too long, it will die. A person's chances of surviving a heart attack decrease 10 percent for every minute that elapses without treatment.

Automated External Defibrillators

A lifesaving device called an automated external defibrillator (AED) can shock the heart from an abnormal rhythm back to a normal rhythm. AEDs are increasingly being made available in public places such as airports, schools, and shopping malls. They are intended for use by nonmedical personnel and can be used by anyone without prior training (although AED classes are available in most communities). The devices come with written and audio instructions. An AED is easier to use and more effective than cardiopulmonary resuscitation (CPR).

The AED first checks the person's heart rhythm to determine if a shock is needed. The AED will not administer a shock unless the person needs it. In addition, the AED will work even if the pads aren't placed in the exact position. Always ask if an AED is available if you think someone may be having or may have had a heart attack.

Symptoms of a heart attack include constant pain (which may last several minutes) or a sensation of tightness or pressure in the center of the chest; chest pain or discomfort that moves from the chest to an arm or shoulder or to the neck, jaw, back, or abdomen; profuse sweating; nausea or vomiting; anxiety; pale skin or bluish nails or lips; weakness; dizziness; and difficulty breathing.

If you think someone may be having a heart attack:

1. Call or have someone call 911 or your local emergency number, or send someone for help. Tell emergency personnel that the person may be having a heart attack.
2. Find out if there is an automated external defibrillator (AED) available where you are. Take the person immediately to the nearest hospital emergency department after following steps 3, 4, or 5 below.
3. *If the person is conscious,* help the person into a comfortable sitting position (lying down may make breathing difficult) and (if the person is not allergic to aspirin) give him or her an aspirin. Chewable aspirin is best, but you can have him or her chew a regular aspirin. Don't give him or her anything else to eat or drink. Loosen any tight clothing and keep the person calm, comfortable, and warm.
4. *If the person is unconscious and not breathing and an AED is not available,* start CPR if you have had CPR training. Start mouth-to-mouth resuscitation immediately (see page 156) until breathing has been restored or until medical help arrives.
5. *If the person is unconscious and not breathing and an AED is available,* open the person's clothing and place the electrode pads on the person's chest as directed on the machine—one pad on the person's upper right side (between the nipple and collarbone) and the other pad on the person's lower left side (just below the armpit). Make sure no one (including the person administering the defibrillator) is touching the person. Press the "analyze" button on the machine, which checks to see if a shock should be administered. If the defibrillator says to give the person a shock, again make sure no one is touching the person, and press the "shock" button. Repeat this sequence (of pressing the analyze and shock buttons) up to three times if necessary. If there is still no pulse, start CPR if you have had CPR training.

Unconsciousness

When a person is unconscious, the body's normal reflexes are not functioning. The person will not respond to attempts to rouse him or her. The main danger when a person is unconscious is obstruction of the airway, which can result when the tongue or some other object such as food or vomit blocks the airway. Some causes of unconsciousness include heart attack (see previous page), stroke (see page 669), head injury (see page 167), severe bleeding (see next page), severe burn (see page 163, diabetic coma (hypoglycemia; see page 897), broken bones (see page 167), poisoning (see page 169), drug overdose, heatstroke (see page 166), choking (see page 155), a severe allergic reaction to food or to an insect bite or sting (see page 170), snakebite (see page 172), and an electric shock or lightning strike (see page 163).

Call or have someone call 911 or your local emergency number, or send someone for help. If you can't call or send for help, take the person immediately to the nearest hospital emergency department. Do not leave an unconscious person alone.

How to Treat a Person Who Is Unconscious

If the person is not breathing:

1. Start mouth-to-mouth resuscitation immediately (see page 156). If the person has no heartbeat, perform CPR if you have had CPR training.

If the person is breathing:

1. Don't move the person, especially if you think he or she may have a neck or back injury.
2. If you are sure that the person does not have a neck or back injury, place him or her on his or her side (to prevent choking), with the head tilted back slightly (to open the airway) and lower than the rest of the body (to drain fluids).
3. Loosen any tight clothing, particularly around the person's neck, and keep him or her comfortable and warm.
4. Do not give the person anything to eat or drink.

Severe Bleeding

Blood flow from a vein usually flows more slowly and steadily than blood flow from an artery, which usually spurts from a wound. Large quantities of blood can be lost very rapidly from a severed or torn artery. In a severe wound, blood may flow so freely that there is no chance for a clot to form. Severe blood loss can lead to shock and unconsciousness and, if the bleeding is not stopped, can be fatal. Blood loss is considered severe if an adult loses more than $1\frac{1}{2}$ pints of blood or if a child loses $\frac{1}{2}$ pint of blood.

The body normally seals a wound by contracting the muscles in the wall of a damaged artery and

forming a blood clot. If the blood does not clot for any reason, such as because the person has hemophilia (see page 618) or is taking anticlotting medications (see page 563), bleeding will be more difficult to control. The goal of first aid is to stop the flow of blood as quickly as possible (see next page). Call or have someone call 911 or your local emergency number, or send someone for help. If you can't call or send for help, take the person immediately to the nearest hospital emergency department.

Severed Arm, Leg, Finger, or Toe

If a person has severed a limb, finger, or toe, the first concern is saving the person's life. Call or have someone call 911 or your local emergency number, or send someone for help. If you have the severed body part, tell hospital personnel. Get the person and the severed part to a hospital emergency department immediately.

A person who has severed a body part is usually bleeding profusely. To treat severe bleeding, see next page.

The longer the severed part goes without a blood supply, the less the chance that it can be successfully rejoined. **Follow these steps to try to save the severed part** (after you have treated the wound):

1. Clean the severed body part by rinsing it with water or a saline solution, but do not scrub it or use soap on it.
2. Place the body part in a clean, dry, sealable plastic bag.
3. Keep the severed body part as cool as possible by placing the bag containing it in ice water (but don't freeze the severed part or let it come in direct contact with ice because extreme cold can cause tissue damage).

Chest Wounds

Various types of chest wounds may require different methods of first aid. For example, if an object penetrates the chest wall, air can enter the chest cavity, displacing and collapsing a lung and reducing the amount of air entering the lungs. This is called a sucking chest wound. You will be able to hear the air being sucked in as the person inhales

To Stop Severe Bleeding

1. Raise the injured part of the body. Lifting the bleeding body part higher than the person's heart will reduce the flow of blood from the wound.

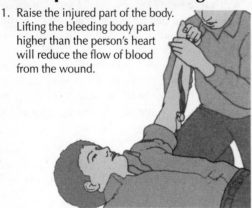

Raise the injured body part

2. Pick out any visible and easily removable objects (such as glass or metal), but do not probe the wound for deeply embedded objects.

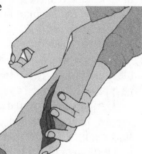

Pick out visible objects

3. Use something that is as clean as possible (such as a clean cloth or piece of clothing, but use your hand if you have to) and press hard, directly on the wound. Avoid pressing on objects in the wound that you cannot easily remove. Keep pressure on the wound for 5 to 10 minutes until all visible bleeding stops. If the edges of the wound are gaping, hold them together firmly.

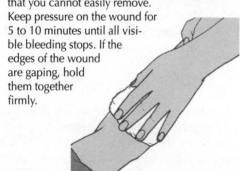

Press hard on the wound

4. Bind the entire wound tightly (with any clean material such as an item of clothing) to maintain pressure, but do not tie the bandage so tightly that blood circulation is completely cut off, and do not use a tourniquet.

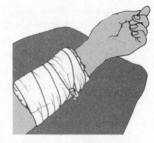

Bind the wound tightly

5. Check to make sure that there is blood circulation below the bandage by checking for a pulse along an artery that is farther away from the heart than the bandage.

6. If the bandage becomes bloody, do not remove it. Instead, put more gauze or fabric over the bloody bandage and wrap it or tape it again tightly while continuing to apply direct pressure.

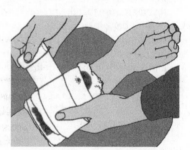

Place additional padding over the previous bandage

7. If direct pressure fails to slow or stop the bleeding, press on an arterial pressure point (see next page) in addition to applying direct pressure to the wound and keeping it elevated above the heart.

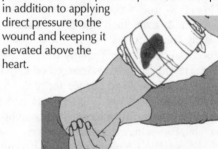

If bleeding continues, apply pressure to a pressure point

Arterial Pressure Points

Sometimes applying direct pressure to a wound does not stop the bleeding or the wound is too extensive to be able to put pressure on the entire area. Pressing firmly on an artery that supplies blood to the wound can help. Apply pressure at a point between the wound and the heart where the artery can be compressed against a bone. Apply pressure only until the bleeding stops

The circled areas on the arteries show the places to apply pressure to control bleeding.

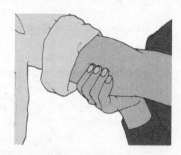

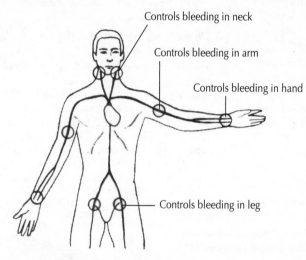

- Controls bleeding in neck
- Controls bleeding in arm
- Controls bleeding in hand
- Controls bleeding in leg

Pressure points on the body

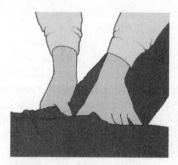

Bleeding from the arm

An artery runs along the inner side of the upper arm. To stop bleeding in an arm, press the artery against the arm bone with your fingertips at a point between the armpit and elbow, in line with the muscle.

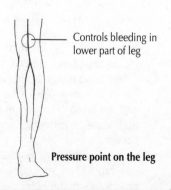

Bleeding from the leg

An artery runs across the groin and down the leg. To stop bleeding in the leg, hold the person's upper thigh with both hands and press hard in the center of the groin with both thumbs, one on top of the other.

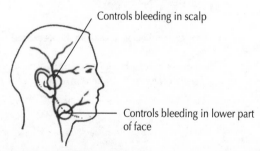

- Controls bleeding in scalp
- Controls bleeding in lower part of face

Pressure points on the head

Scalp injuries usually bleed profusely because the scalp has a rich supply of blood. If you are treating a superficial head wound, apply steady pressure. Don't apply pressure to the wound if a fracture, broken skull fragments, or other foreign material is visible (or if you suspect a fracture) because you could press the fragments or other material into the brain. If the head wound is very severe, press carefully around the edges of the wound and tie a bandage loosely around it.

If a clear, watery fluid (which is cerebrospinal fluid) comes out of the injured person's ear or nose, the base of the skull may be fractured. Place a clean pad over the ear or nose but don't try to stop the fluid from draining.

- Controls bleeding in lower part of leg

Pressure point on the leg

and see blood-stained bubbles around the wound as the person exhales. If you are not sure if the object has penetrated the chest wall completely, treat the wound as a sucking chest wound.

Call or have someone call 911 or your local emergency number, or send someone for help. **Take the following steps to treat the chest wound:**

1. Do not remove any object that is embedded in the wound.
2. Using the palm of your hand, press firmly over the site of the wound, using a clean pad or piece of clothing.
3. If the wound is not a sucking wound (see page 159), cover the entire wound and about 2 inches around it with a petroleum gauze dressing, large cloth, sheet of foil, or plastic wrap. Try to make the dressing airtight using tape or another adhesive. If you don't have tape, place a hand on each side of the wound and firmly push the skin together to close the wound.
4. If the wound seems to be sucking in air, seal the wound after the person has exhaled, but leave one corner untaped, which will prevent air from being trapped in the chest cavity and pressing on the collapsed lung.
5. Lay the person down with the head and shoulders raised and the body leaning slightly toward the injured side.
6. Don't give the person anything to eat or drink.

Shock

Shock is a life-threatening reduction in the flow of blood to body tissues. Shock usually results from a serious illness or injury, such as a heart attack (see page 157), spinal injury (see page 167), severe bleeding (see page 159), severe burn (see next page), poisoning (see page 169), or a severe allergic reaction (see page 916).

A person who is in shock looks pale and sweaty; has cool, moist skin and a weak, rapid pulse; and acts confused. The person may say that he or she feels faint or drowsy. Eventually the person will become unconscious. A person who is in shock requires immediate treatment. Call or have someone call 911 or your local emergency number, or send someone for help.

To Treat Shock

After calling or having someone call 911 or your local emergency number, or sending someone for help, take the following measures to treat shock:

If the person is not breathing:

1. Start mouth-to-mouth resuscitation immediately (see page 156). If the person has no heartbeat, perform CPR if you have had CPR training.

If the person is breathing:

1. Do not move a person who may have head, neck, or back injuries.
2. Treat any severe injuries or illness (see those listed under "Shock" below left).
3. If the person is vomiting or unconscious, lay the person down on his or her side with his or her head tilted back slightly (with the mouth open) to prevent choking on fluids or vomit.
4. If the person is not vomiting, is conscious, and does not have back, spine, neck, head, or chest injuries, raise his or her legs about a foot to allow blood to flow to the upper body.

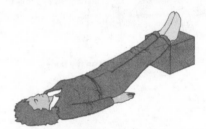

Lay the person down with the feet raised

5. Loosen any tight clothing, and keep the person comfortable and warm.

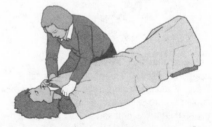

Keep the person warm

6. Don't give the person anything to eat or drink.

Electric Shock or Lightning Shock

Exposure to ordinary household current in the United States seldom causes serious problems, but an electric shock from a high-voltage wire can be fatal. Being struck by lightning can also be fatal. The shock of an electric current entering and leaving the body can disrupt the electrical activity in the brain that controls breathing and can make the heart stop beating. It can also knock a person down and cause unconsciousness, internal injuries, and broken bones (from muscle contractions). There may be only small marks where the current entered and left the body.

To treat a person for electric shock:

1. Call or have someone call 911 or your local emergency number, or send someone for help. Get medical attention no matter how minor the burn or shock seems to be.
2. Turn off the current if possible, or safely separate the person from the source of the current using a material that doesn't conduct electricity, such as a wooden chair, broom handle, or dry rope. A person who has been struck by lightning can be safely touched immediately.

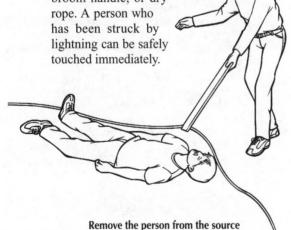

Remove the person from the source of the electric current

3. If the person is not breathing, start mouth-to-mouth resuscitation immediately (see page 156). If there is no heartbeat, perform CPR if you have had CPR training.
4. Treat any burns (see right).
5. Treat any broken bones (see page 167).

Burns

Burns can be caused by dry heat (such as a fire), moist heat (such as steam or hot liquids), electricity, friction, corrosive chemicals, or the sun.

Get medical help immediately for burns to the eyes (such as from hot ashes or cinders). Do not let the person rub his or her eyes, and gently cover both eyes (which helps minimize eye movement and therefore pain) with a sterile compress and bandage. For chemical burns to the eyes, see page 176.

Burns are divided into three categories—first degree, second degree, and third degree—depending on the depth of skin damage. All burns require medical attention. A first-degree burn damages only the outer layer of skin and causes slight redness, pain, and swelling. The skin is not broken, blisters do not form, and the burn usually heals within 5 days. A mild sunburn is a first-degree burn. A second-degree burn causes injury to the layers of skin beneath the surface and severe pain and red, blotchy, swollen, moist skin that usually blisters. A burn that destroys all the layers of skin (a third-degree burn) may cause little pain because the nerve endings have been destroyed. The skin may look white and charred.

To treat a burn:

1. If the burn is severe or covers an extensive skin area, call or have someone call 911 or your local emergency number or send someone for help.
2. If the person has stopped breathing (which is common with burns or smoke inhalation), start mouth-to-mouth resuscitation immediately (see page 156).
3. Do not remove clothing that is stuck to the burn, but do carefully try to remove clothing that has been in contact with a corrosive chemical. Try to remove shoes, jewelry, or anything constricting from the burned area because of possible swelling.
4. Decrease the temperature of the burned skin as quickly as possible to help limit tissue damage. Put cool (not cold) water or another cool liquid such as milk or beer on the burn. (Do not put ice or very cold water on the burned area because it can further damage the skin and, if the burn is severe, cause shock.) Depending on the size, site, and severity of the

burn, pour cool water on the burn, immerse the entire burned area in cool water, or apply cool-water compresses using a nonfluffy material (which will not stick to the burn).

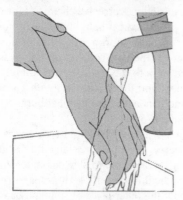

Pour cool, running water on the burn

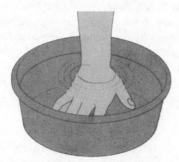

Immerse the burn in cool water

5. Don't apply any lotions, creams, ointments, sprays, antiseptics, or home remedies of any kind. You can apply calamine lotion to skin that has been mildly sunburned. Don't prick any blisters.
6. Lightly cover the burn with a clean, dry, non-fluffy material.

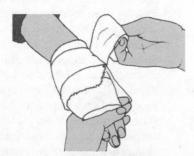

Cover the burn

7. A burned arm or leg should be elevated to reduce swelling. Protect it inside a clean plastic bag if possible.

Elevate a burned arm, leg, hand, or foot

8. If the burn is very minor, give the person an over-the-counter pain reliever.
9. If the burn is more severe or extensive (for example, it covers the entire chest), don't put anything cold on it (you could lower the person's body temperature to a dangerous level). Instead, cover the person with a clean blanket.
10. Do not give the person anything to eat or drink. However, if the burn is relatively minor (and the person is conscious and not vomiting), give him or her frequent sips of cool water to prevent fluid loss.
11. Treat for shock (see page 162) if necessary.

WARNING!

Unusual Burns

You should suspect that someone (especially a child or an incapacitated or older person) has been a victim of abuse if he or she has any of the following signs:
- A burn with a distinctive or recognizable shape or the pattern of an object such as an iron
- Multiple circular burns (as from a cigarette)
- A burn with a clear-cut edge (as if the affected area were immersed in scalding water)
- Multiple burns in various stages of healing

Blisters

Blisters on the skin are usually caused by skin damage from friction (such as from shoes or repetitive use of tools or equipment) or burns (including chemical burns). New skin forms under a blister, and the fluid inside the blister is gradually absorbed; eventually the outer skin layer comes off. First aid is needed only if the blister breaks or if the raw skin area is likely to be damaged by friction, which can lead to pain and infection.

To treat a blister:

1. Gently wash the blister and surrounding area with soap and water. Do not prick the blister or try to remove it.
2. Cover the blister with a sterile gauze pad and tape the pad in place.
3. If the blister was caused by a chemical, is larger than 2 inches across, or occurs on the hands, face (especially around the mouth and nose), or genitals, see your doctor.

Hypothermia

Hypothermia is a drop in internal body temperature below 95°F. Hypothermia usually occurs from prolonged exposure to extreme cold or after submersion in cold water, although it can occur in relatively warm water if the water temperature is lower than body temperature and exposure is long enough. During prolonged exposure to extreme cold, more body heat is lost than can be replaced, and body temperature drops. In young, healthy people, hypothermia occurs only after extreme, prolonged exposure. In older people and very young children, hypothermia occurs faster and more easily.

The drop in body temperature may not be noticeable at first but can cause clumsiness, irritability, slurred speech, confusion, and drowsiness as a person's physical and mental abilities slow. Breathing and heartbeat become weaker and slower, and the person may eventually go into a coma and die.

To treat hypothermia:

1. Call or have someone call 911 or your local emergency number, or send someone for help.
2. If the person's breathing has stopped, start mouth-to-mouth resuscitation immediately (see page 156). If there is no heartbeat, perform CPR if you have had CPR training.
3. Have the person lie down, and keep him or her as still as possible, which reduces the risk of a dangerous drop in blood pressure or heart rhythm abnormalities that can occur when cold blood returns to the heart from the extremities.
4. If outside, shelter the person from the cold and wind in any way you can. Insulate him or her from the ground to prevent further heat loss. Cover him or her with warm, dry clothing and blankets, and make sure his or her head is covered. Use your own body to provide additional warmth.

5. If you can, bring the person into a warm room. Remove any wet clothing. Do not overheat the person too quickly by placing him or her in front of a heater. Rewarming the body too quickly can cause a rush of blood to the body's surface and a drop in internal body temperature when cold blood from the arms and legs returns to the heart and brain.
6. If the person is conscious, give him or her a warm (not hot) beverage such as broth or warm water with lemon or honey or gelatin dissolved in it. Do not give the person alcohol, beverages that contain caffeine (such as tea, coffee, or hot chocolate), or cigarettes. Alcohol can restrict blood flow to the extremities and inhibit the shivering mechanism, which helps warm the body. Caffeine accelerates the symptoms of hypothermia and can cause the heart to beat faster, possibly causing heart-rhythm abnormalities. Tobacco directs warm blood away from the surface of the skin. Alcohol, caffeine, and tobacco are also diuretics (which increase the output of water in urine) and can cause dehydration.
7. Don't rub or massage the skin, which can cause skin damage. Check and treat for frostbite (below) if necessary.

Frostbite

Frostbite is damage to skin and other tissues resulting from exposure to extremely low temperatures. Most cases of frostbite occur at temperatures below 44°F after 7 to 10 hours of exposure. Frostbite occurs when the fluid that is normally inside skin and tissue cells freezes and crystallizes, blocking blood flow to an area and causing tissue damage. Frostbite usually affects the ears, hands and fingers, feet and toes, and nose.

In the early stages, symptoms of frostbite include red skin that stings or burns or feels cold. Later, the skin may look white, grayish yellow, or waxy, and may throb and swell or become numb. If only the skin and underlying tissues are affected, recovery is usually complete. If blood vessels are affected, damage is usually permanent and the frostbitten part may have to be amputated.

To treat frostbite:

1. If the frostbite seems severe or extensive, call or have someone call 911 or your local emergency number, or send someone for help.

2. Until you get the person to a warm place, cover the frozen part with extra clothing or blankets. Tuck frostbitten hands and fingers under the person's armpits, or cup a frostbitten ear or nose with a hand. Do not massage or rub the frostbitten part.

3. Once inside a warm place, remove any wet, cold, or constricting clothing.

4. Rewarm the frostbitten body part rapidly, which can cause some pain. Put the frostbitten part in warm (not hot) water (104°F to 107°F) for 15 to 30 minutes. Do not place the frozen body part too close to a direct heat source (such as a heat lamp, heating pad, radiator, or hot stove); burns can occur because the frostbitten area is numb.

5. Keep the frostbitten parts elevated if possible to prevent swelling, which can cause more tissue damage.

6. Give the person warm, nonalcoholic beverages (alcohol restricts blood flow). Do not let the person smoke, because smoking constricts the arteries and directs warm blood away from the surface of the skin.

7. Give the person an over-the-counter pain reliever (such as ibuprofen) if necessary. Ibuprofen is most helpful at an adult dose of 400 milligrams every 12 hours.

8. As frostbitten parts warm up, have the person move them gently, but don't let a person who has frostbite of the feet walk. The weight of the body can damage frostbitten toes.

9. Stop the warming process when the skin returns to its normal color and feeling returns to the frostbitten area. Do not break any blisters. To aid healing, apply aloe vera to frostbitten skin every 6 hours.

Heat Exhaustion

Heat exhaustion occurs when someone is exposed for prolonged periods to high (especially humid) temperatures or exercises excessively in hot weather without taking in enough salt and water to replace salt and fluids lost through excessive sweating.

The person may feel generally ill and dizzy and may faint; may look pale; and may have cool, clammy skin. He or she will sweat profusely, and his or her pulse rate and breathing may become rapid. Usually the person's temperature is normal or only slightly elevated (100°F). The person may also have a headache and muscle cramps and may vomit. He or she may faint. Heat exhaustion may lead to heatstroke (see below), which is more serious.

To treat heat exhaustion:

1. If the symptoms are severe or become worse, call or have someone call 911 or your local emergency number or send someone for help.

2. Lay the person down in a cool, shady place, and elevate the person's feet. Move the person to an air-conditioned room if possible.

3. Loosen any tight clothing.

4. Cool the person in any way you can. Fan the person by hand, with a blow dryer set on cool, or with an electric fan. Sponge him or her with cool water; spray him or her with water from a hose or spray bottle; place cool, wet cloths on his or her forehead; or place ice packs on his or her neck, groin, and armpits. Cool him or her in a tub or shower using cool (not cold) water but do not immerse the entire body.

5. If the person is conscious and is not vomiting, give him or her cool water, a rehydration solution (¼ to ½ teaspoon of salt or salt tablets dissolved in a quart of water), clear juice, or a sports drink with a concentration of less than 6 percent glucose. Do not give undissolved salt tablets.

Heatstroke

Heatstroke usually occurs because of prolonged exposure to very hot conditions. Heatstroke caused by direct exposure to the sun is called sunstroke. The mechanism in the brain that normally regulates body temperature stops functioning, and the person's temperature rises higher than 103°F. The person may be confused and lose consciousness and is flushed, with hot, dry skin and a strong, rapid pulse. He or she may vomit and may have seizures. Heatstroke is a medical emergency.

To treat heatstroke:

1. Call or have someone call 911 or your local emergency number, or send someone for help.

2. Cool the person down as soon as possible by having him or her lie down in a cool, shady place. Move the person to an air-conditioned room if possible.

3. Remove excess or tight clothing such as vapor-impermeable clothing or sports uniforms.

4. Cool the person in any way you can. Fan the person by hand, with a blow dryer set on cool, or

with an electric fan. Sponge him or her with cool water; spray him or her with water from a hose or spray bottle; place cool, wet cloths on his or her forehead; or place ice packs on his or her neck, groin, and armpits. Cool him or her in a tub or shower using cool (not cold) water but do not immerse the entire body.

Broken or Dislocated Bones

Without an X-ray, it is usually impossible to tell for sure if a bone is broken (fractured), although sometimes the broken bone may stick out through the skin in what is called an open break. An open break is usually more serious than a closed break (in which the skin is intact) because of bleeding and the possibility of infection. Suspect a broken bone if someone heard the bone snap. A broken bone may also produce a grating sensation as the bone ends rub together.

A broken or dislocated bone will be tender or painful when touched or moved, and the person may have difficulty moving the injured part. The site of the break may look deformed or swollen, may move abnormally, and may be bruised. Mishandling broken bones or dislocations can cause extensive damage to nerves and blood vessels. Any movement can cause further tissue damage.

To treat a suspected broken or dislocated bone:

1. If the injured area is severely deformed or if the skin is broken, call or have someone call 911 or your local emergency number.
2. If the injury does not seem too serious, take the person to the nearest hospital emergency department.
3. Treat any severe bleeding (see page 160). If the wound is open, do not wash it or apply any medication. Gently apply pressure with a large sterile or clean pad to stop the bleeding. Cover the

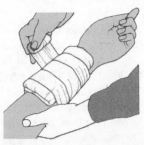

Cover the bone with a bandage

entire wound, including the protruding bone, with a bandage.
4. Do not try to put a dislocated or broken bone back in place.
5. If the person must be moved, immobilize the injured part with a splint (see next page).
6. Keep the person comfortable and warm.

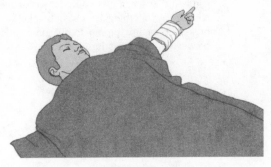

Keep the person warm

7. Do not give the person anything to eat or drink.
8. Watch for signs of shock, and treat for shock (see page 162) if necessary.

WARNING!

Unusual Patterns of Broken Bones or Dislocations

You should suspect that someone (especially a child or an incapacitated or older person) has been a victim of abuse if he or she has any of the following signs:
- Repeated broken bones or recurring dislocations in the same part of the body
- Fractures in the breastbone, back, skull, end of the collarbone, or ribs in the back

Head, Back, or Spinal Injury

Any person who is found unconscious must be assumed to have a head injury. Anyone with a head injury may also have a neck injury. If a person has been injured and has severe pain in the neck or spine, any tingling or loss of feeling or control in his or her arms or legs, or any loss of bladder or bowel control, the spinal column may be fractured or dislocated.

To treat a head, back, or spinal injury:

1. Call or have someone call 911 or your local emergency number, or send someone for help.

Applying a Splint

Splinting prevents a fracture from moving, which reduces pain and keeps the break from getting worse. A splint should be rigid and long enough to immobilize the joints above and below the fracture. Splints can be made with pieces of wood, cardboard, magazines, or newspapers padded with pillows, clothing, towels, or blankets. For a broken upper arm, be sure to put some padding between the arm and the torso.

Splints can be tied in place with neckties, torn strips of cloth, belts, string, or rope. But make sure you do not tie the splint so tightly that it interferes with blood circulation. Loosen splint ties if you notice swelling, numbness or tingling, or discoloration not caused by the injury; if the person cannot feel his or her fingers or toes; or if you cannot feel a pulse in the area of the splint. These are signs of lack of blood to the area.

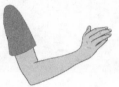 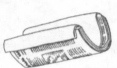 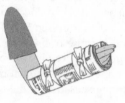 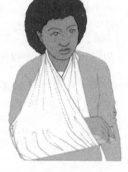

Place arm at a right angle   **Make a padded splint**   **Tie splint in place above and below the break**

Support arm with a wide sling

Splinting a broken lower arm

Place the person's lower arm at a right angle across the person's chest, with his or her palm facing the chest and his or her thumb pointing upward. Put a padded splint around the lower arm. The splint should reach from the elbow to beyond the wrist.

Tie the splint in place above and below the break. Support the lower arm (the fingers should be slightly higher than the elbow) with a wide sling tied around the neck.

Splinting an injured leg

Gently straighten the knee of the injured leg. Place some padding between the person's legs. Tie the injured leg to the other leg in several places, but don't tie directly over the break. If you are using a board as a splint, it should run the entire length of the leg.

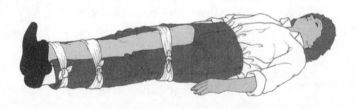

2. Do not move the person unless he or she is in immediate danger or is choking or vomiting.
3. If the person must be moved, immobilize the head, back, neck, and spine. Do not let the neck or back bend or twist. Place pads or other material on each side of the injured person's head, neck, and trunk to keep them from moving from side to side. Do not lift the person without a back support such as a board. If the person must be dragged, do not drag him or her sideways. Grasp the person by the armpits or legs and pull in the direction of the length of the body. Always keep the head in line with the rest of the body.
4. If the person is not breathing, start mouth-to-mouth resuscitation immediately (see page 156), moving the head and neck as little as possible.
5. Do not give the person anything to eat or drink.

WARNING!

Immobilize the Head of a Person With a Neck Injury

Any movement of the head of a person with a neck injury (either forward, backward, or from side to side) can result in paralysis or death. Do not remove a helmet from a person who has a possible neck injury. If necessary, try to remove the face guard from a helmet with a screwdriver.

If you must remove a helmet (to give mouth-to-mouth resuscitation because the person has stopped

breathing or to treat a severe head injury), keep the person's head completely immobile until the helmet is removed. Have someone else hold the injured person's head by applying pressure to the jaw with the thumb and fingers of one hand while firmly holding the base of the skull with the other hand while you stretch out the sides of the helmet as you carefully remove it.

Swallowed Poisons

Call 911 or your local emergency number or the national poison center (1-800-222-1222) for instructions before doing anything for a person who has swallowed a poison (see list of common poisons at right). Be ready to provide the following information:

- The person's age
- Name of the poison
- How much poison was swallowed
- When the poison was swallowed
- If the person has vomited
- How much time it may take to get the person to the nearest hospital emergency department
- The phone number where you can be reached immediately

Follow the instructions you are given exactly. Usually milk or water is given to dilute the poison, but you will need to be told which fluid to use, depending on the poison. Do not give fruit juice or vinegar; they might not be effective and they could be harmful. Do not induce vomiting or give syrup of ipecac or activated charcoal unless you have been told to do so by a doctor or by the poison center.

To treat poisoning:

1. If the person is not breathing, start mouth-to-mouth resuscitation immediately (see page 156).
2. If the person is vomiting, turn the person's head to the side or facedown, with the head lower than the rest of the body to prevent choking on vomit. Place a child facedown across your knees.
3. Collect any vomited material in a container to take to the emergency department.
4. Bring the poison container with the person to the emergency department.

Common Household Poisons

The following poisonous substances are found in most homes. They are extremely harmful, and possibly fatal, if swallowed. Keep them in correctly labeled childproof containers, and store them out of the reach of children.

- Antifreeze
- Cigarettes and other forms of tobacco
- Cosmetics, colognes, or perfumes
- Drugs of any kind
- Gardening products such as fertilizer, fungicide, or weed killer
- Household cleaners such as bleach, dishwasher and dishwashing detergent, drain cleaner, furniture polish, glass cleaner, grease remover, laundry detergent, oven cleaner, scouring powder, or toilet bowl cleaner
- Insecticides
- Liquor
- Nail polish and removers
- Paint and paint thinner
- Certain plants (such as dieffenbachia, philodendrons, and spider plants)

Poisonous Plants

Some plants can cause an allergic reaction or direct chemical reaction on the skin, such as a burn or a blister. Poison ivy, poison oak, and poison sumac are three of the most common plants that cause this reaction in susceptible people. When a person touches a poisonous plant (or touches clothing or a pet that has been in contact with the plant), an oily substance on the leaves gets on the skin and can cause an itchy, oozing rash (see color illustration on page 120). The rash can be easily spread to other parts of the body. The smoke from burning poison ivy, oak, or sumac can cause skin irritation and, if inhaled, can cause severe wheezing or difficulty breathing.

An over-the-counter lotion containing bentoquatam (which blocks the irritating oil that causes the allergic reaction) can be applied before a potential exposure to prevent or reduce an allergic skin reaction. It should be applied at least 15 minutes before the possible exposure (and every 4 hours after), and the skin should be washed after exposure even if the lotion was applied. The medication will not stop or prevent a reaction if applied after exposure.

To treat poison ivy, oak, or sumac:

1. Wear gloves if you are helping someone who has been exposed to a poisonous plant remove his or her clothing.
2. Wash the skin and clean the fingernails immediately (within 15 minutes) with mild soap and water to remove the oily plant substance.
3. Apply cool packs to the affected areas.
4. Tell the person not to scratch or rub the affected areas; scratching can worsen or spread the rash.
5. Take frequent warm (not hot) showers or oatmeal baths, apply calamine lotion or topical corticosteroids to the affected areas, and take oral antihistamines or over-the-counter pain relievers to help relieve itching.
6. Wash clothing thoroughly, using warm water and a laundry detergent that can remove oil.
7. If the reaction is severe or if the rash is on the person's face (especially around the eyes or mouth) or genitals, get medical attention right away.

Insect Stings

Insect stings cause more deaths per year than snakebites, but most insect stings cause only mild reactions, such as redness and swelling. Some stings can be life-threatening and cause anaphylactic shock (see page 916) if a person is allergic to the insect's venom. The most common stinging insects are honeybees, hornets, wasps, yellow jackets, bumblebees, and fire ants. Only honeybees leave a stinger in the skin.

Some symptoms of insect stings are pain, swelling, redness, itching, and burning. Multiple insect stings can cause rapid swelling, headache, muscle cramps, fever, and drowsiness. Severe allergic reactions to insect stings include severe swelling and itching (including in areas of the body away from the sting), hives, coughing or wheezing, difficulty breathing, stomach cramps, nausea and vomiting, weakness, dizziness, bluish skin color, and unconsciousness.

To treat a severe allergic reaction to an insect sting:

1. If the person seems to be having a severe allergic reaction, call or have someone call 911 or your local emergency number, or send someone for help. If the person has an anaphylaxis kit, help him or her administer a shot of epinephrine (adrenaline); if he or she is unable to administer the injection, give it to him or her yourself by following the instructions on the kit.
2. Give the person an oral antihistamine to help stop the allergic reaction and relieve the symptoms.

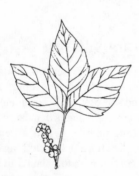

Poison ivy
Poison ivy has three shiny leaflets on a stem and may grow as a plant, bush, or vine.

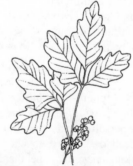

Poison oak
Like poison ivy, poison oak has three leaflets on a stem and may grow as a plant, bush, or vine. The three leaflets resemble oak leaves.

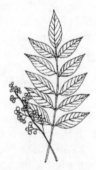

Poison sumac
Poison sumac has two rows of leaflets opposite each other and a leaflet at the tip. It grows as a bush or a tree.

3. If the person stops breathing, start mouth-to-mouth resuscitation immediately (see page 156). If the person's heart stops beating, perform CPR if you have had CPR training.

To treat an insect sting:

1. If the stinger is embedded in the skin, carefully remove the stinger by gently scraping the skin with a dull knife blade, fingernail, or piece of cardboard. Do not squeeze the stinger with tweezers, which can push the venom into the body.
2. Wash the area gently with soap and water, being careful not to break any blisters.
3. Put ice (wrapped in a cloth) or cold compresses on the sting to decrease absorption and spread of the venom.
4. If the area is swollen or itchy, have the person take an oral antihistamine to stop the reaction and relieve the symptoms.

Poisonous Spider Bites and Scorpion Stings

Bites from poisonous spiders and the stings of some scorpions are especially dangerous for young children, older people, and people who are ill. Two kinds of poisonous spiders are found in the United States—the black widow and the brown recluse (also known as the fiddleback spider). Scorpions are found in the southwestern United States.

Black widow spiders are shiny and black and are about an inch long, including their legs. They have a red hourglass marking on the underside of their body. Brown recluse spiders are dark brown and are about ¾ to 1½ inches long, including their legs. They have a violin-shaped marking on the top of their body, toward the head. Scorpions look like 2-inch-long lobsters or crabs and have a set of pincers. Their tail arches over their back and has a stinger at the tip.

Symptoms of a black widow spider bite include slight redness and swelling and sharp pain around the bite, sweating, nausea and vomiting, stomach cramps, a hard abdomen, muscle cramps, weakness, facial swelling, and tightness in the chest and difficulty breathing.

Symptoms of a brown recluse spider bite include a stinging sensation at the time of the bite, redness at the site of the bite (which turns into a blister), pain at the site that becomes more severe with time, fever with chills, nausea and vomiting, joint pain, and a rash. The person may have blood in his or her urine within a day of the bite. An open ulcer will form around the bite that can persist for months.

Symptoms of a scorpion sting include severe burning pain at the site of the sting, nausea and vomiting, stomach pain, numbness and tingling in the affected area, difficulty opening the mouth, fast heart rate, blurred vision, muscle spasms, seizures, and unconsciousness.

To treat a bite by a poisonous spider or a scorpion sting:

1. If a person has been bitten by a poisonous spider or stung by a scorpion, call or have someone call 911 or your local emergency number or the national poison center (1-800-222-1222), or send someone for help.
2. If the person is not breathing, start mouth-to-mouth resuscitation (see page 156) immediately. If the person's heart has stopped beating, perform CPR if you have had CPR training.
3. Keep the bitten area lower than the person's heart.
4. Place ice wrapped in a cloth or cold compresses on the bite.
5. Keep the person calm and comfortable.
6. If you can catch the spider or scorpion safely, take it with you to the emergency department.

Tick Bites

Ticks can be found anywhere but thrive in wooded and grassy areas. They can transmit diseases such as Lyme disease (see page 942) and Rocky Mountain spotted fever (see page 942). Initial symptoms of a tick bite include irritation, pain, bruising, and a

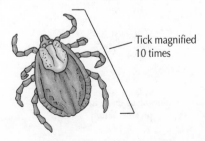

Tick magnified 10 times

Tick
Ticks are about ⅛ inch long. When a tick becomes engorged with blood, it can expand to up to seven times its normal size.

round, red rash or blotch (see color illustration on page 126) that may not appear at the site of the bite. If you think you have been bitten by a tick, see your doctor right away. The doctor will perform a blood test to determine if the tick has caused an infection; if the infection is in an early stage, he or she will prescribe antibiotics. To remove a tick, see page 943.

Snakebites

Poisonous snakes include the rattlesnake, cottonmouth (water moccasin), and copperhead (all three are pit vipers), and the coral snake. Rattlesnakes are responsible for two out of three poisonous snakebites and are found all over the United States. Cottonmouth and copperhead snakes are found primarily in the Southeast and South Central United States. Coral snakes are found in the Southeast.

It is important to know whether a snake is poisonous. Poisonous, or venomous, snakes have a triangular-shaped head, while nonvenomous snakes have a more rounded head. Pit vipers such as the rattlesnake, copperhead, and cottonmouth have pits (which look like another set of nostrils) between their nostrils and their slitlike eyes. Rattlesnakes have a rattle at the end of their tail. Cottonmouths have a white lining in their mouth. Copperheads have a copper-colored head and a pinkish gray body with a brown hourglass shape on the skin.

The symptoms of a pit viper bite include severe pain, rapid swelling, discoloration, and redness at the site of the bite. The person may also experience weakness, nausea and vomiting, blurred vision, seizures, numbness in the arms and legs, and difficulty breathing.

Coral snakes are not pit vipers, but they are venomous. They have round eyes and a black nose and alternating rings of red, yellow, and black (the narrow yellow rings always separate the red rings from the black). All poisonous snakes have long fangs.

Symptoms of a coral snake bite include slight pain and swelling at the site of the bite, blurred vision, drooping eyelids, difficulty speaking or swallowing, drooling, drowsiness, sweating, nausea and vomiting, confusion, weakness, dizziness, joint pain, paralysis, and difficulty breathing.

If there is no swelling within 4 hours (for a pit viper bite) and 6 hours (for a coral snake bite), the snake was probably not poisonous.

If someone has been bitten by a poisonous snake:

1. Call 911 or your local emergency number or the national poison center (1-800-222-1222). Do not try to suck out the venom (you could poison yourself).
2. If the person is not breathing, start mouth-to-mouth resuscitation immediately (see page 156). If the person's heart has stopped, perform CPR if you have had CPR training.
3. If a snakebite kit is available, immediately use the suction cups from the kit to draw out body fluids containing the venom.
4. Keep the person calm, which will slow circulation and help stop the spread of the venom.
5. Remove any jewelry.
6. Immobilize the bitten arm or leg, and keep it below the level of the heart. Keep the person calm, and do not let him or her walk.
7. Wash the bite area thoroughly. Do not apply ice

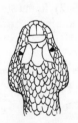

Poisonous snake in the pit viper family

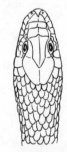

Nonpoisonous snake

Top view of a pit viper
Pit vipers such as rattlesnakes, cottonmouths, and copperheads have a triangular head when viewed from above (left). Nonpoisonous snakes have a more rounded head (right).

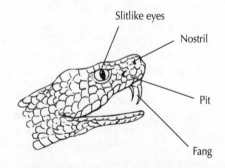

Identifying pit vipers
Poisonous snakes such as pit vipers have long fangs, slitlike eyes, and pits that contain sacs of poison between their eyes and their nostrils.

or very cold water; it could damage the skin. Cover the bite with a sterile dressing.

8. If the person is not nauseated or vomiting, is not having seizures, and is conscious, give him or her small sips of water. Do not give alcoholic beverages.

9. If you can safely capture and kill the snake (preferably without damaging its head), take it with you to the emergency department. Do not handle the head. The severed head of a snake can inject poison for up to an hour after the snake has died. If you cannot bring the snake with you to the doctor, try to describe the snake.

Animal Bites

Bites from a domesticated animal (such as a dog or cat) or a wild animal (such as a squirrel or raccoon) can result in serious infection and tissue damage. The animal must be caught and tested for rabies. Call the police or health department to catch and confine or kill the animal so it can be tested for rabies. The person may need to get a tetanus shot and, in rare cases, a series of rabies shots.

To treat an animal bite:

1. Call or have someone call 911 or your local emergency number, or send someone for help if the bite is deep or extensive. If the bite is not too severe, take the person to the emergency department yourself.

2. Clean the wound with soap and running water for at least 5 minutes to wash out contaminating organisms. After cleaning the bite with soap and water, irrigate it for 5 minutes with a povidone-iodine solution or a 1 percent to 2 percent quaternary ammonium solution. Do not put any other medications or home remedies on the wound because they can cause infections or tissue damage.

3. Treat any bleeding (see page 160).

Human Bites

Human bites that break the skin can lead to serious infection from bacteria or viruses that can contaminate the wound. All human bites need immediate medical treatment. Treat a human bite as you would an animal bite, and get medical attention immediately.

4. Put a sterile bandage or a clean, dry cloth over the wound.

5. If a body part or skin has been bitten off, try to bring it with you to the emergency department.

Foreign Object in the Ear or Nose

Children often put small objects in their ears or nose. If your child puts an object in his or her ear or nose, do not try to remove it yourself. Take your child to the doctor to have the object removed safely.

To kill a live insect in the ear before it can be removed:

1. Have the person tilt his or her head with the affected ear up. Pull the earlobe gently backward and upward to straighten the ear canal.

2. If you think the eardrum has not been damaged, slowly pour a small amount of warmed mineral, olive, vegetable, or baby oil into the ear. The oil will smother the insect.

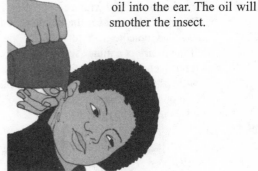

Slowly pour a small amount of warm oil into the ear

3. If the insect floats to the top and you can easily remove it, take it out of the ear with tweezers. If removal seems difficult, have a doctor remove the insect.

Minor Cuts and Scrapes

Slight bleeding from a minor cut or scrape usually stops on its own within a few minutes. If blood spurts from a wound or cannot be stopped after applying pressure for a few minutes, the bleeding is severe and requires immediate medical attention (see page 160). If a cut is on the face, or is deep (you can see yellow fatty tissue), irregular, or gapes so badly that you cannot bring the edges together, get the person to an emergency department immediately. Such cuts probably need stitches to aid healing and reduce scarring. A doctor should clean a cut or scrape caused by an obviously dirty object, that has visible dirt or foreign material embedded in it, or that was caused by an animal or human bite. A doctor should evaluate any cut or scrape that becomes infected or has red streaks leading from it (which is a sign that the infection is spreading in the bloodstream).

To treat a minor cut or scrape:

1. Wash your hands before treating the cut or scrape.
2. Use a clean gauze or cotton pad to gently wash the wound with soap and water. Remove all bits of dirt if you can do so without further damaging the skin. For a scrape that has foreign material or dirt in it, gentle scrubbing may be necessary. Rinse thoroughly under running water for at least 5 minutes.
3. Pat the wound dry with a clean or sterile cloth. Do not apply any over-the-counter medications or home remedies.
4. If the injury is a minor scrape or scratch, leave it uncovered and exposed to the air. Cover a cut with a sterile dressing, and tape it in place. Use one or two strips of surgical tape to hold the edges of a slightly gaping cut closed.

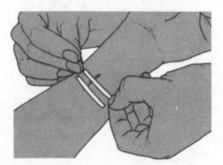

Hold the edges of a cut closed with surgical tape

Puncture Wound

A deep wound caused by a long, narrow object (such as a nail or a tooth) that does not produce much bleeding is more likely than other wounds to become infected because dirt and bacteria are carried deep into the tissues and are not washed out by blood. All puncture wounds should be examined and treated by a doctor, especially if they become infected, if red streaks radiate from them (which is a sign that the infection is spreading in the bloodstream), or if they were caused by an animal bite. Numbness, tingling, or weakness in an arm or leg after a puncture wound may indicate that nerves or tendons are damaged. Antibiotics and a tetanus shot may be necessary after a deep wound to prevent infection.

To treat a puncture wound:

1. Wash your hands before treating the wound.
2. Do not poke around in the wound or put any medication in it.
3. Do not try to remove an object that is deeply embedded in the wound because the object may break off in the wound or because removing it could cause severe bleeding. If the piercing object is small and goes no deeper than the skin, remove it with tweezers that have been sterilized with rubbing alcohol or placed over an open flame or in boiling water and cooled.
4. Encourage bleeding (to wash out germs) by gently pressing on the edges of the wound. Don't press too hard because you could cause additional tissue damage.
5. Using a clean gauze or cotton pad, wash the wound with soap and water. Rinse thoroughly under running water for at least 5 minutes.
6. Pat the wound dry with a clean cloth. Do not apply any medications or home remedies.
7. Cover the wound with a sterile dressing, and tape it in place.

Bruises

Bruises occur when an injury breaks small blood vessels under the skin but the skin is not broken. The discoloration and swelling in the skin are caused by blood seeping into the tissues. The skin will usually turn colors—from reddish blue, to green and yellow, to brown—before fading. Bruises usually disappear without treatment after 10 to 14 days.

Bruises on the head or shin or around the eye (a black eye) may swell significantly because bone is just beneath the skin and there is little fatty tissue to cushion the blow. If a bruise does not fade or disappear completely or if it becomes painful and swollen, or if bruises continue to appear for no reason, see your doctor. You may have a broken bone or other injury or a blood-clotting disorder.

To treat a bruise:

1. Gently apply an ice pack or a cold, wet cloth to the bruise to reduce bleeding, pain, and swelling. Don't apply too much pressure.
2. If the bruise is on an arm or leg, elevate it above the level of the heart to decrease blood flow to the area.
3. After 24 hours, apply a warm washcloth or a heating pad to aid healing.

WARNING!

Unusual Bruises

You should suspect that someone (especially a child or an incapacitated or older person) has been a victim of abuse if he or she has any of the following signs:

- Bruises on fleshy areas such as the face, back, abdomen, thighs, or buttocks
- Bruises in generally protected areas such as the neck (possibly from choking), chest, or genitals
- Bruises with distinctive and recognizable shapes of objects such as clothes hangers or belt buckles
- Multiple bruises in various stages of healing

Splinters

A small splinter usually can be removed easily with tweezers. A splinter in the eye should be removed only by a doctor. If a splinter breaks off in the skin, is deeply lodged, or cannot be removed, see your doctor as soon as possible. You should also see a doctor if the wound becomes infected or if red streaks radiate from the wound (which is a sign that the infection is spreading in the bloodstream).

To remove a splinter from the skin:

1. Wash your hands and the skin around the splinter with soap and water.
2. Sterilize tweezers (and any other instrument you may need, such as a needle or razor blade) with rubbing alcohol or by placing them over an open flame or in boiling water and letting them cool. If the splinter is sticking out of the skin, place the open tweezers directly on the skin on either side of the splinter (pushing on the skin slightly), and gently pull on the splinter in the direction in which it entered the skin.
3. If the splinter is embedded just under the skin, gently loosen the skin around the splinter with a sterilized needle or the tip of a sterilized razor blade. Lift the end of the splinter with the end of the needle or tip of the razor blade. Carefully

remove all of the splinter with the sterilized tweezers.
4. Squeeze the wound gently to promote slight bleeding, which will force out some of the germs.
5. Wash the area with soap and water, and apply a bandage.

Foreign Object in the Eye

Never try to remove anything that is stuck in the eye or is on the pupil of the eye. If a person has something embedded in his or her eye, do not let the person rub it. Gently cover both eyes with a sterile compress and lightly bandage it in place. Covering both eyes helps stop eye movement, which can help minimize eye damage and pain. Call 911 or your local emergency number, or get the person to a hospital emergency department immediately.

If an object such as a piece of dirt or an eyelash is floating on the white or inside corner of the eye or on the inside of the eyelid, you can try to remove it. Symptoms of something in the eye include pain, a burning sensation, tearing, redness, or sensitivity to light.

To remove a foreign object that is not embedded in the eye:

1. Wash your hands with soap and water.
2. If the person is wearing contact lenses, remove (or have the person remove) the lenses if they can be removed easily.
3. Gently pull the upper eyelid out and down over the lower eyelid, and hold the upper lid down for a few seconds. This should cause tears to flow, which may wash out the particle. The upper lid sliding over the lower lid also may dislodge the particle.

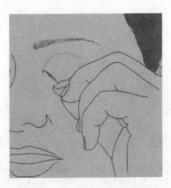

Pull the upper eyelid over the lower eyelid

4. If the person still can feel the particle, gently cover the eye with a clean cloth and get medical help immediately.

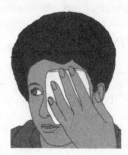

Cover the eye with a clean cloth

Chemicals in the Eye

Chemicals that come in contact with the eye must be washed out right away to avoid permanent injury or blindness. Damage to the eye can occur immediately. Do not let the person rub the eye.

To treat a chemical burn to the eye:

1. Call or have someone call 911 or your local emergency number, or send someone for help.
2. If the person is wearing contact lenses, remove (or have the person remove) the lenses if they can be removed easily.
3. Hold the person's head under a faucet (or a hose or pitcher of water) and allow cool water to run gently from the inside corner of the eye (next to the nose) outward, flowing over the entire eye, for at least 30 minutes. If running water is not available, use bottled water or milk. Hold the eyelids open. Make sure that none of the chemical runs into the unaffected eye. (If both eyes are affected, let the water flow over both eyes or quickly alternate between one eye and the other.) You can also put the top of the person's face in a bowl or sink filled with water, with his or her eyes immersed in the water. Tell the person to blink a few times under the water. If the person is lying down and can't stand up, pour large quantities of water into the inside corner of the eye and let it flow outward, keeping the eyelids open; continue this for up to 30 minutes.
4. Cover the injured eye or eyes with a sterile pad or a clean cloth, and tape it in place with the eyelids closed.
5. Take the person to the nearest hospital emergency department immediately.

Sprains and Strains

A tear in a muscle or tendon is called a strain; a tear in a ligament or joint capsule is called a sprain. Both sprains and strains result from overstretching the tissues, and the symptoms for both injuries are the same: pain, swelling, and bruising.

Applying a Figure-Eight Bandage

1. Anchor the bandage by making one or two turns around the foot.

2. Bring the bandage diagonally across the top of the foot and around the ankle. Continue to bring the bandage down across the top of the foot and under the arch of the foot.

3. Continue figure-eight turns. Make each turn overlap the last one by about three fourths of the width of the bandage.

4. Bandage until the foot (but not the toes), ankle, and lower leg are covered. Secure the bandage with tape or clips.

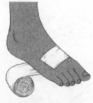

Make one or two turns around the foot with the bandage

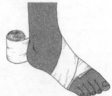

Bring the bandage across the top of the foot and around the ankle

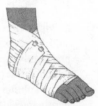

Overlap the last turn of the bandage by three fourths of the bandage width

Bandage until the entire foot (but not the toes) is covered

A severe sprain can feel the same as a fracture, so you should get medical attention to rule out a broken bone.

To treat either a sprain or a strain:

1. Place cold packs or a small bag of ice wrapped in cloth on the affected area (20 minutes on, 20 minutes off) for the first 24 to 48 hours to decrease swelling.
2. Keep weight off the injury by supporting it in a splint (if it's a wrist, elbow, or shoulder injury) or by not walking on it (if it's an ankle, foot, or knee injury). If the sprain is in the foot or ankle, support the injured joint or muscle with an elastic bandage wrapped in a figure-eight pattern (see box on previous page).
3. Apply heat to a sprain or strain after the first 24 hours to promote healing.

Nosebleeds

Nosebleeds can result from an injury, a scratch in the lining of the nose, repeatedly blowing the nose, or an infection. Usually the bleeding comes from only one nostril. Nosebleeds are seldom a cause for concern and usually stop in a few minutes. Nosebleeds that occur repeatedly (especially in older people) may have an underlying medical cause and should be evaluated by a doctor. Get medical attention if your nose could be broken, if the bleeding doesn't stop, or if you feel light-headed, are pale, or have a rapid heart rate.

To stop a nosebleed:

1. Sit down and lean forward, keeping your mouth open to prevent blood from blocking the airway.
2. Breathe through your mouth and pinch together both sides of your nose below the bridge for

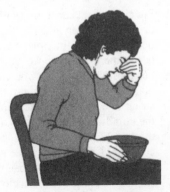

Sit and lean forward

about 10 minutes. (This is usually enough time for a blood clot to form and seal the damaged vessels.)
3. Slowly release your fingers from your nose. Do not blow your nose or even touch it.

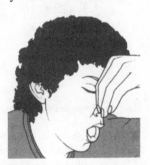

Pinch the fleshy part of the nose

4. If the bleeding continues, pinch your nose again for another 10 minutes.
5. Place a cold, wet cloth or a cloth filled with ice over the bridge of your nose and face to help constrict the blood vessels.
6. Avoid blowing, moving, or touching your nose for at least 12 hours after the bleeding has stopped.

Fainting

Fainting is a brief loss of consciousness caused by a reduced blood supply to the brain. A person may feel faint because of a temporary drop in blood pressure caused by blood pressure medication, getting up from a sitting or lying position too quickly, exercising too strenuously, heat exhaustion (see page 166), or low blood sugar (hypoglycemia; see page 897). People usually recover from a fainting spell after a few minutes.

If a person feels faint or has fainted:

1. Lay the person down with his or her legs elevated 8 to 12 inches. If the person is conscious, have him or her sit down and slowly bend forward so the head is between the knees.

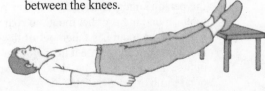

Lay the person down with the legs elevated

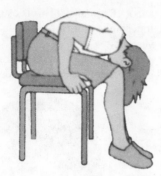

Have the person sit down and slowly bend forward

2. If a person remains unconscious for longer than a few minutes, call or have someone call 911 or your local emergency number, or send someone for help. See page 155 if the person is not breathing.
3. Loosen any tight clothing, especially around the neck.
4. Bathe the person's face with cool water (but don't pour or throw water on the face).
5. Do not give the person anything to eat or drink until he or she is fully conscious. If you think the fainting may have been caused by dehydration, give the person cool water if he or she is conscious and not vomiting.
6. If the person is vomiting, turn the person on his or her side with the head tilted back slightly (to open the airway and prevent choking on vomit).

Knocked-Out Tooth

A whole tooth that has been knocked out and is not cracked or otherwise damaged can usually be successfully reimplanted by a dentist within 30 minutes. Touch only the crown (or top part) of the tooth; never hold the tooth by the root. Do not try to reimplant a baby tooth. Get the person to a dentist as quickly as possible.

To save a permanent tooth:

1. If the person is conscious and the tooth is still in the person's mouth, have him or her roll the tooth around in his or her mouth to coat it with saliva. If the tooth has fallen out of the mouth and is dirty, quickly rinse it in cool water (without touching the root), but don't use soap, and don't scrub or dry the tooth.
2. Holding it by the crown with a clean cloth or piece of gauze, immediately place the tooth

firmly back in the socket. Have the person hold the tooth in place with his or her tongue or fingers or by gently biting down on it until you can get the person to a dentist.
3. If the tooth cannot be replaced in the socket immediately, place the tooth in the salt solution found in most first-aid kits, which is specifically designed for transporting teeth that have been knocked out. If you don't have the salt solution, place the tooth in a container of the person's saliva or of cold whole-fat milk (not skim milk), which should keep the tooth alive until you can get to the dentist. Use regular saline solution or tap water with a little salt in it to preserve the tooth only if you can't use the person's saliva or whole-fat milk. Do not transport the tooth in cloth or gauze or let the tooth dry out.

Emergency Childbirth

Sometimes childbirth occurs suddenly and unexpectedly or labor proceeds too fast to get to a hospital in time for delivery. If the woman's contractions are about 2 minutes apart, if she feels like pushing, or if the baby's head is visible in the vaginal opening, birth will usually occur very soon.

Childbirth is a natural process, and most deliveries do not have complications. However, delivery is bloody. Call or have someone call 911 or your local emergency number, or send someone for help. Try to get the woman to the nearest hospital emergency department if possible. If not, a doctor may be able to give you instructions over the phone. Do not try to delay or prevent the birth by crossing the woman's legs or pushing on the baby's head, which can seriously harm the baby.

To help deliver a baby:

1. Put clean sheets on a bed (with a rubber sheet or shower curtain underneath if possible). If a bed is not available, place clean clothing or newspapers under the woman or at least under her hips and thighs. If you can, gather clean blankets or towels (to wrap the baby); clean string, shoelaces, cord, or strips of cloth (to tie the umbilical cord); scissors or a knife (to cut the umbilical cord); a large plastic bag or other container (in which to place the afterbirth, or placenta, so a doctor can examine it later); and sanitary napkins or a clean cloth (to place over the woman's vagina after the birth).

2. Make the woman as comfortable as possible.

3. Wash your hands with soap and water. Sterilize the scissors or knife with rubbing alcohol, or place them in boiling water for at least 5 minutes or over an open flame for 30 seconds and cool them before using them.

4. Have the woman lie on her back with her knees bent, feet flat, and knees and thighs wide apart.

5. Do not place your hands or any objects in the vagina, interfere with the delivery in any way, or touch the baby until the head is completely out of the vagina. Once the baby's head is visible, support the baby's head but don't pull. If the baby's head is inside a fluid-filled bag (the placenta), carefully puncture the bag with the sterile scissors or your finger and remove the membranes from the baby's face.

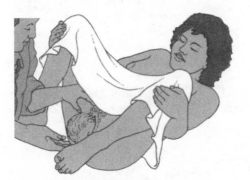

Support the baby's head as it emerges

6. Once the head has emerged, if you can feel or see that the umbilical cord is around the baby's neck, quickly but gently slip the cord over the baby's head. If the cord is wrapped around the neck too tightly, cut the cord immediately and tie off the ends (see step 14). If the cord is not wrapped around the neck, do not cut it at this time.

7. Continue to support the head as the shoulders emerge, but don't pull the baby out (even by the armpits). Carefully hold the baby as the rest of his or her body comes out.

8. After delivery, if you can, note the time.

9. Support the baby's head and body with one hand while grasping the baby's legs and ankles with the other (get a firm grip because the baby will be very slippery). Position the baby so that his or her head is lower than the feet to allow any membranes or fluid to drain from the baby's lungs, mouth, and nose. Do not hold the baby completely upside down by the ankles or slap or hit him or her.

10. Gently wipe any fluid or membranes out of the baby's mouth and nose (preferably with a sterile gauze or clean cloth).

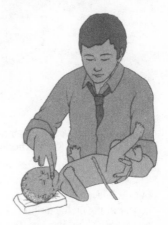

Wipe fluid or membranes from the mouth and nose

11. If the baby has not cried or is not breathing, gently rub his or her chest, or tap the bottoms of the feet. If the baby still is not breathing, perform artificial respiration (see page 156).

12. Once the baby has started breathing, wrap him or her up snugly (including the top of the head). Do not clean the cheesy white coating from the baby's skin, eyes, or ears (it is a protective covering).

13. If the woman can be taken to a hospital immediately after the delivery of the placenta (which occurs about 5 to 20 minutes after delivery), the baby can be left attached to the cord and placenta.

14. If you must cut the umbilical cord, do not cut or tie it until it has stopped pulsating. Using a string, shoelace, cord, or cloth, tie a tight knot in the umbilical cord at least 4 inches from the baby's navel and then tie another knot 6 to 8 inches away from the baby. Cut the cord between the two knots with the sterile scissors or knife. (At the hospital, a doctor will clamp the umbilical cord at the baby's abdomen in the usual way.)

15. Within 20 minutes, the placenta (which is attached to the umbilical cord) will emerge.

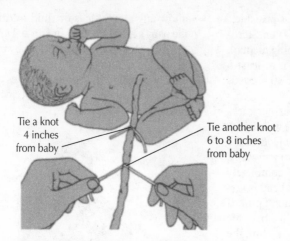

Tie a knot
4 inches
from baby

Tie another knot
6 to 8 inches
from baby

Tie a knot in the umbilical cord 4 inches away from the baby and another one 6 to 8 inches away from the baby

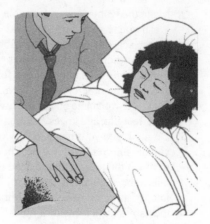

Massage the woman's lower abdomen

The woman's contractions will eventually push out the placenta. Do not pull on the umbilical cord. Pulling on the umbilical cord may pull off a section of the placenta from the wall of the uterus and cause severe or continuous bleeding. Gently but firmly massage the woman's lower abdomen in a circular motion to help the uterus contract and reduce heavy bleeding.

16. After delivery of the placenta, place it in a plastic bag or other container to take to the hospital with the woman and baby for examination. Continue to massage the woman's abdomen after delivery of the placenta.

17. Place sanitary napkins or a clean cloth over the woman's vagina to absorb blood. Keep the woman warm and comfortable, and give her something nonalcoholic to drink to replace lost fluids.

2

Home Caregiving

At one time or another, most families need to provide home care for a family member who is ill, aging, disabled, or recovering from surgery. Caring for a person at home can improve his or her sense of well-being, which can lead to a quicker, more complete recovery.

Preparing for Home Care

Home caregiving requires a well-thought-out care plan, which must be flexible enough to meet the continually changing needs of the person who is being cared for. Discussing expectations and potential problems in advance with all members of the caregiving team—such as doctors, nurses, therapists, social workers, and family members—will help you to develop a support network and the best care plan possible. The members of the caregiving team will consider the following factors when developing the care plan:

- How long the illness is expected to last

- How the person's condition might improve or worsen
- Whether it is possible for the person to fully recover
- Whether rehabilitation therapies—such as physical, occupational, or speech therapy—will be needed to promote recovery, and who will provide these services
- The specific medical emergencies that might occur and how these emergencies should be handled
- Caregiving adjustments you will need to make

Setting Priorities and Goals

The best time to begin planning the transition from hospital care to home care is shortly after a person has been admitted to the hospital. A hospital social worker, primary care nurse, or case manager can guide you through this transition and help you plan successful home care strategies so you can concentrate on providing the best possible care for a person, once he or she leaves the hospital. Consider the following questions when developing your care plan:

- What types of care are needed, and what is the best way to provide them? Can you provide this care at home?
- Will the person require 24-hour care?
- If you need to monitor health indicators such as blood pressure or blood glucose levels, or administer and adjust medications, who will train you to perform these tasks? Who can you call for advice and help?
- Who will be part of your caregiving team, and what roles will they play? You may need the services of a variety of people, such as doctors,

181

specialists, visiting nurses, therapists, and home health aides.

- What type of care is available, and from which agencies? Is the care effective and dependable, and what are the costs?
- Will you need any special equipment, such as that used to provide oxygen or intravenous feeding? Who will train you to operate it, what type of maintenance does it require, and who will provide the maintenance?
- Will physical changes have to be made to the person's home to enhance his or her mobility and safety? For example, you may need to have ramps, railings, or electric stair lifts installed on stairways, or grab bars and handrails installed in bathrooms to help make it safer to use the toilet or bathtub.
- Will the person need specialized equipment to help him or her perform daily tasks? Various useful devices, such as a handheld device called a grabber that can help a person grasp objects that otherwise would be out of reach, are available from drugstores and medical supply companies.
- Will pets in the home create any problems? Some pet-related routines and behaviors may need to be adjusted to prevent accidents. For example, you might install a child safety gate to keep a dog from getting in the way of a person who is learning to use a walker.
- What are the person's likely transportation needs? You may be able to use your own car or van, or you may need to use a specially equipped van. Transportation services are available at reasonable cost in many communities; ask a hospital social worker for recommendations, or check your phone book.

In most families, a spouse, parents, siblings, or children provide most of the routine care, with assistance from various health care professionals and under the supervision of a doctor. To provide quality care, learn as much as you can about the person's illness or condition:

- Talk with designated contact members of the health care team about the person's condition. Write down questions and take notes or tape record sessions with care instructors. If you feel your questions are not being addressed in these meetings, schedule a separate meeting to resolve them.
- Consult a private clinical social worker, gerontologist (aging specialist), or other appropriate care provider. These people are trained to evaluate your family's needs and can help you find a qualified physical therapist or household helper, as well as supplies you may need such as a hospital bed. They also can help you find a nursing home in your community that meets your loved one's needs.
- Use the services offered by local and national support groups and organizations, community outreach programs at nearby hospitals, and help hot lines. Consult your local public library, bookstores, and the Internet for additional information and resources.

Caregiving Skills

Once the person is home, your daily routine will focus on meeting his or her needs. In some cases, the person needs the expertise and training of a registered nurse or other professional caregiver. But with proper training and guidance, you will learn to perform the required tasks on your own. Always call on the experience of professionals whenever you need to.

Giving Medications

Learn all you can about the person's medications, starting with the names of the drugs. If he or she is taking several medications, keep a list of their names and a written schedule of the daily doses of each so that you can check off each dose as you give it. Get the instructions about each prescribed medication from your doctor or pharmacist, and make sure you understand them. Read the package insert that comes with each medication. You may want to ask the doctor or pharmacist the following questions:

- When should the medication be taken (with meals, first thing in the morning, at bedtime, or two or more times a day)?

- How long should the medication be taken? Will refills be necessary?
- What are the possible side effects? What should be done about them?
- Does the medication interact with any other drugs that the person is taking?
- Should the person avoid certain foods?
- Does the medication have lasting effects?
- Does the medication have any warnings?
- Does the medication come in various forms? For example, if the person has problems swallowing pills, ask if the medication is available as a liquid.

Remember that all medications must be taken exactly as prescribed by the doctor. Never stop giving medication without the doctor's permission.

WARNING!

Allergic Reactions and Unpleasant Side Effects

Some medications can cause an allergic reaction (producing symptoms such as hives, itching, a rash, or wheezing) or side effects (such as nausea or dizziness). If the person develops any of these symptoms, call the doctor immediately to find out if you should stop giving the medication. The doctor may need to adjust the dosage or change medications.

Providing a Healthy Diet

Healthy eating is essential for maintaining the person's health and well-being and also can promote successful recovery. If the doctor has not prescribed a special diet for the person, you can provide the foods that he or she normally eats.

Adequate fluid intake also is an important part of a healthy diet. Most people should drink at least eight glasses of fluid every day, including water, milk, juice, broth, or caffeine-free coffee, tea, or soft drinks. If the doctor limits the person's daily fluid intake, follow the doctor's instructions.

The following tips can make it easier for the person to consume a healthful diet. Adapt them to the person's needs:

- Slice, dice, chop, mash, or purée foods to make them easier to chew and swallow.
- Look for ways to add calories and nutrients to the diet of a person who is at risk for weight loss. For example, fortified milk shakes can be tasty and nutritious. Ask your doctor if the person you are caring for could benefit from nutritional supplements that provide added nutrients and calories.
- People with decreased appetites may consume more calories by eating five or six smaller meals throughout the day rather than three large meals.
- Ask the person what foods he or she likes or dislikes.
- Make meals look attractive.
- Eat meals together whenever possible. Mealtime rituals can be comforting and can help restore a sense of normalcy to a person's life.
- If a stroke has paralyzed one side of a person's body, food may tend to collect in the paralyzed cheek. If this occurs, gently knead the cheek with your finger while the person is chewing, to help move the food along.
- If the person is able to exercise, encourage and help him or her to do so. Regular exercise stimulates the appetite and helps prevent constipation. Ask the doctor which exercises are best.

Assisting With Eating

If the person cannot feed himself or herself, you must feed him or her. Cut food into small, bite-size pieces, or purée it to make it easy to chew and swallow. Before feeding the person, be sure he or she is sitting upright in a comfortable position. Tuck a napkin or hand towel under the chin to catch any spills. Taste the food to be sure it is not too hot. Because feeding someone can be a lengthy process, keep the food warm in a warming dish.

If the person cannot chew or swallow—because of oral radiation treatments, jaw injury, or stroke, for example—you may need to provide nutrition through a feeding tube or intravenously (directly into a vein). The doctor or nurse will teach you how to do this correctly and safely. Watch closely for any signs of infection: pain, redness, or swelling at the insertion site of the intravenous needle or feeding tube, or fever.

Good oral hygiene is essential for maintaining a healthy diet. Make sure that the person practices good oral hygiene (daily brushing and flossing) and that he or she sees the dentist regularly.

Special Diets

If the person needs to follow a special diet, your doctor can recommend a nurse or registered dietitian who can teach you how to prepare the food. A registered dietitian can assess the person's dietary needs, provide guidance, and answer any questions you may have. Common special diets include low-sodium, low-protein, and liquid diets.

Low-sodium diet

You can easily reduce the amount of sodium in a person's diet by not adding salt to food when you cook or serve it. Avoid serving foods—such as cured or tenderized meat (including ham, bacon, and cold cuts), smoked fish or meat, cheese, pickles, canned foods other than fruit, processed and prepared foods, and salted butter or margarine—that are high in sodium. Always check package labels for the sodium content of canned, prepared, and processed foods. Buy canned foods labeled "no salt added."

If you need to further restrict the person's salt intake, your doctor can tell you how to cut down on or eliminate foods that contain even small amounts of sodium. To add flavor to foods without adding salt, season them with spices, herbs, or lemon juice. Ask your doctor if it is all right to use a salt substitute. Most people find that after several salt-free weeks, they do not miss the salt.

Low-protein diet

To reduce the amount of protein in the person's diet, cut down on protein-rich foods such as eggs, meat, fish, and dairy products. Because protein supplies much of the body's energy requirements, you will need to compensate by adding extra carbohydrates to the diet. If your loved one needs to cut back on protein, ask the doctor or dietitian for guidance.

Liquid diet

Sometimes doctors prescribe a liquid diet, in which the person cannot eat any solid food. In this case, ask the doctor to recommend a dietitian who can plan an appropriately balanced diet. You also may want to ask the doctor about giving the person liquid nutritional supplements, which are widely available in single-serving cans.

When giving liquids, always elevate the person's head slightly to help prevent choking and spilling. The best way to do this is to hold the cup or glass while the person drinks through a flexible drinking straw. Keep the person's head elevated for at least 20 minutes after eating to help prevent choking or regurgitation.

Meal Services

Special meal services such as Meals-On-Wheels provide home delivery of nutritionally balanced hot and cold meals for older or disabled people who are not able to prepare their own meals. Fees for this service are based on a person's ability to pay. Because the demand for such services is high in some communities, preference may be given to people with limited income. In other communities, anyone who can pay the full fee is eligible. Special diets require a written order from a doctor.

Preventing Pressure Sores

A person who is confined to bed is at risk of developing pressure sores, especially if his or her movement is restricted or sensation impaired. Pressure sores develop on the parts of the body that bear weight or rub against bedding. They are the result of continuous pressure that interferes with blood circulation to the tissue in the surrounding area. Poor nutrition and incontinence also can contribute to the development of pressure sores.

A pressure sore begins as a patch of tender, reddened, inflamed skin. Gradually the skin turns purple, breaks down, and forms an open sore. The sore gradually grows larger and deeper, and can become

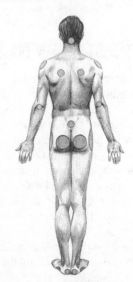

Pressure sores
The most common sites for pressure sores are the base of the skull, shoulders, shoulder blades, elbows, lower back, hips, buttocks, sides of the knees, ankles, sides of the feet, and heels.

infected. Pressure sores are usually very slow to heal. They will not heal at all unless pressure on the affected area is greatly reduced or eliminated.

The best way to prevent pressure sores is to change the person's position every 2 hours during waking hours. Gently move the person from one side onto his or her back, then to the other side; rotate positions throughout the day. Never drag the person from one position to another in bed—you could damage the skin, increasing the risk of developing pressure sores.

About once every hour, have the person stimulate circulation and prevent joint stiffening by wiggling his or her toes, rotating the ankles, flexing the arms and legs, tightening and relaxing the muscles, and stretching the entire body. If the person is immobile or very weak, you can perform passive exercises by gently bending and straightening his or her joints several times a day.

Help the person out of bed as often as possible (see page 191). Moving around also will help prevent fluid from collecting in his or her lungs, a major risk factor for pneumonia. If the person cannot get out of bed, encourage him or her to move around in bed frequently.

Place cushions and pillows between the person's knees and under his or her shoulders to help relieve pressure. Alternating pressure mattresses, synthetic sheepskin mattress pads, and heel protectors allows air to circulate around the person's skin and helps reduce pressure and friction against the bedding. A bed or foot cradle (a tentlike device placed at the foot of the bed) helps to keep the weight of blankets and other coverings off the person's feet. You can rent or purchase these items from drugstores and medical supply companies. Remember that, even when you use them, you still need to turn the person frequently to prevent pressure sores.

Keep the person's skin clean and dry, especially in areas most vulnerable to pressure sores. Bathe the person frequently (see right). Ask the doctor or nurse to recommend an alcohol-free skin cream. Apply the cream using a circular motion. Check the person's skin each day for signs of pressure sores such as reddening. If you see any changes in the skin, tell the doctor; a pressure sore may be forming.

Remove soiled underwear (including disposable briefs) promptly. Be sure to keep sheets pulled tight to prevent wrinkles, and keep them clean, dry, and free of crumbs.

Provide a healthy diet (see page 183) and plenty of fluids to help keep the person's skin healthy. Eating high-protein foods (such as lean meat, fish, dried peas and beans, and whole grains) and taking nutritional supplements also can help prevent and treat pressure sores.

Bathing

Unless a person is extremely ill, he or she usually can bathe independently with minimal help. Place a large towel under the person to protect the bedding before bringing him or her a basin of warm water, mild soap, and a washcloth. Be sure that the room is warm, and provide another large towel to drape over the person for warmth and privacy. The person should give himself or herself a sponge bath once a day.

If the person you are caring for is unable to bathe without help, you can give him or her a bath in bed. Although giving a bed bath presents its own challenges, it is not a difficult task to perform once you have mastered the routine. Make sure that the room is warm before undressing the person, taking care to provide as much privacy as possible. Cover him or her with a large towel and place another towel underneath to protect the bedding. Before you begin, check the water to make sure it is at a comfortable temperature. When you use soap, make sure it is a mild soap that will not dry out or irritate the person's skin.

As you bathe the person, look carefully for sores, rashes, or other skin problems. If the person is recovering from surgery, be sure to examine the incision carefully to make sure it is healing properly. Some indications of possible infection include fever; redness, pain, and swelling around the incision; and pus. It is important to report any of these signs to the doctor or nurse immediately.

When giving a bed bath, wash and dry one area of the person's body at a time, uncovering only the part of the body you are washing. This helps keep the person warm and maintains a sense of privacy. Follow these steps:

1. Use plain water to bathe the person, starting at the head. Use soap only in sweaty areas (such as the armpits, groin, and buttocks); wash between skin folds. Be thorough but gentle. Change the water as needed.

2. Gently pat the person dry with a fresh, soft towel; don't rub.

3. Roll the person onto one side to wash and dry his or her back.
4. Let the person dip his or her hands into a basin of fresh water. This is more refreshing than having the hands wiped with a washcloth.
5. Before helping the person dress, make sure that every area of his or her body is thoroughly dry. Provide or apply deodorant, lotion, or body powder as needed.

Helping With Toileting Needs

Bladder and bowel movements can be difficult for people who cannot use the toilet. A person who is confined to bed will need to use a bedpan or commode; a man may be able to use a handheld urinal. If a person cannot use these devices, he or she may need to wear absorbent disposable briefs. Always give the person complete privacy.

If the person cannot wipe after urinating or having a bowel movement, you will need to do it for him or her. Keeping the genital and anal areas clean helps prevent the skin from breaking down. Always wipe a woman or girl gently from front to back (from the vagina to the anus) to ensure that bacteria do not enter the vagina or urinary tract and cause infection.

Some caregivers need to give an enema (by injecting a liquid into the rectum) to relieve constipation (see page 769) or an accumulation of hardened feces in the rectum (fecal impaction). If the person has an indwelling catheter (a plastic tube inserted directly into the bladder) that drains urine into a bag, you will need to empty and clean the bag regularly. (A doctor or other health care professional will change the catheter periodically.) Learn to perform these tasks correctly from a trained health care professional. Ask for clear, precise instructions.

Using a Commode

If the person is able to get out of bed for brief periods, using a bedside commode may be easiest. Assist the person out of bed and onto the commode. If necessary, help the person wipe himself or herself, and then help him or her back into bed. Empty the removable pan into the toilet. Rinse the pan out, clean it thoroughly with a household disinfectant diluted with water, and return it to the commode.

Using a Bedpan

A person who is confined to bed will need to use a bedpan, which can be awkward. In addition to giving the person privacy, be sure to give him or her plenty of time. A person who is embarrassed about using a bedpan or who feels pressured while using one may be reluctant to ask for it when he or she needs it. Resisting the urge to have a bowel movement can lead to constipation and fecal impaction. Remember to ask the person frequently if he or she needs to use the bedpan—and keep it within easy reach and in the same place so it can be found quickly when needed.

Before giving the person a bedpan, sprinkle a small amount of body powder on the rim of the bedpan to make it easier to slip under the buttocks. The open end of the bedpan should always be toward the person's feet. Keep toilet paper and moist towelettes within easy reach and help the person with cleanup if necessary. After use, empty the contents of the bedpan into a toilet and rinse and wash the bedpan with a household disinfectant diluted with water.

A person who cannot lift himself or herself up may be able to use a bedpan with assistance. If possible, have someone help you. Lift the person's hips while the other caregiver places the bedpan beneath the person's buttocks. If another caregiver is not available, roll the immobile person away from you onto his or her side. Gently position the bedpan against his or her buttocks and press the bedpan firmly into the mattress while rolling the person back on top of it. To remove the bedpan without spilling its contents, hold it firmly in place and gently roll the person away from you, and off the bedpan. Thoroughly clean and dry the genital and anal areas.

Using a Handheld Urinal

Always keep a handheld urinal in the same place and within the man's easy reach. Have him put the urinal in a large bowl or bucket to prevent and contain spills until you can empty it. Empty the urinal into a toilet after each use, rinse the urinal, and wash it thoroughly with a household disinfectant diluted with water.

Monitoring Symptoms

As a person's main caregiver, you are in the best position to observe any changes in his or her condition that may indicate an improvement or decline in health. What you need to watch for depends on the person's illness or injury. In general, it is important to closely watch his or her alertness, memory, mobility, vision, hearing, emotions, sleep patterns, eating habits, personal interactions, and sensory responses such as touch. Even small, seemingly insignificant changes can indicate a serious underlying health problem and should be reported to the doctor or nurse as soon as possible. Common signs to watch for include:

- Changes in breathing patterns, including shallow breathing, hyperventilation (abnormally deep, rapid, or prolonged breathing), raspy breathing, gurgling noises in the throat, temporary cessation of breathing (including during sleep), difficulty breathing, or wheezing
- Changes in mobility such as limping, problems maintaining balance, restricted use of arms or legs, or paralysis
- Tremors, shaking, facial tics, twitching, drooping eyelids or mouth, or facial paralysis
- Unusual sneezing or coughing
- Discharge, such as through a bandage; a bloody nose or leaking eye; or pus oozing from an open sore
- Fever, chills, or sweating
- Insomnia (difficulty falling asleep or staying asleep) or fatigue
- Constipation, diarrhea, loss of bladder or bowel control, or vomiting
- Changes in urination or bowel movements, including frequency, smell, appearance, and quantity, and pain or difficulty urinating or moving the bowels
- Changes in skin appearance, including rashes, sores, tenderness, dryness, moistness, itchiness, pallor (paleness), jaundice (yellowing of the skin and whites of the eyes), or swelling
- Unexplained weight loss or gain
- Changes in appetite

Incontinence

Incontinence, the inability to control the passage of urine (urinary incontinence) or stool (fecal incontinence), usually is caused by an underlying disease or condition. Urinary and fecal incontinence can occur separately or together. Do not accept incontinence as a normal part of aging. An older person who is experiencing problems with incontinence should be examined by a doctor as soon as possible.

Incontinence can be a major problem when caring for a person at home. One way to deal with incontinence is to establish a toilet routine: encourage the person to go to the bathroom at frequent, regular intervals (for example, every 2 to 3 hours). Provide help promptly to prevent accidents. Make sure that the toilet facilities are readily accessible and easy to use. If the person is confined to bed, make sure that a commode, bedpan, or handheld urinal is within easy reach.

A number of incontinence aids, such as absorbent incontinence pads, disposable briefs, and condom catheters are available from drugstores and medical supply companies. Ask your doctor about them.

If a person has both urinary and fecal incontinence, loss of bladder control usually occurs before loss of bowel control. His or her doctor will examine the person to find the underlying cause.

Depression

A person who is ill or disabled is at high risk for depression. In older people, early detection and treatment of depression are extremely important because of the high risk of suicide. If you notice that the person you are caring for has any of the following signs or symptoms for more than a few days, talk to his or her doctor immediately:

- Changes in appetite (decrease or increase)
- Weight loss or weight gain
- Changes in mood or emotions
- Lack of responsiveness or attentiveness
- Loss of interest in favorite activities
- Feelings of hopelessness or helplessness

Some people incorrectly assume that symptoms of depression are a normal part of aging or mistake symptoms of depression for Alzheimer's disease (see page 688), dementia (see page 689), or another illness. If the diagnosis is depression, it can be successfully treated with medication, psychotherapy, or a combination of both, at any age.

Fever

Although a fever is not usually dangerous, notify the person's doctor if the person you are caring for has a fever. Always check with the person's doctor before giving aspirin or an aspirin substitute. The doctor may prescribe a medication to reduce the fever. If the person's temperature continues to rise after he or she has been given medication to reduce it, call his or her doctor immediately. Never try to raise the temperature of a person who has a fever (such as by turning up the heat or putting extra blankets or other coverings on him or her). Raising a person's temperature abnormally high can cause seizures or loss of consciousness.

To help reduce the person's temperature, sponge his or her face, neck, trunk, arms, and legs with lukewarm water and let it evaporate on the skin. Evaporation brings down the temperature of the skin. Encourage the person to drink plenty of water, a sports drink, fruit juice, or broth to replace the fluids that will be lost through the excessive perspiration that accompanies a fever.

Vomiting

Medications and treatments such as radiation therapy can cause nausea and vomiting. However, because vomiting can also be a sign of an illness or underlying health problem, tell the doctor if the person you are caring for is vomiting, especially if he or she is vomiting repeatedly. The doctor may tell you to watch for signs of dehydration such as thirst, dry lips and mouth, dizziness, headache, confusion, muscle weakness, shakiness, and a reduced output of urine. Dehydration is a potentially dangerous condition that can lead to coma and death.

If the person is confined to bed or cannot get to a bathroom quickly, leave a container (such as a bowl or dishpan) at the bedside for him or her to vomit into. Some people want to be left alone when vomiting, while others find it comforting to have someone with them. If the person finds it reassuring, hold his or her forehead while he or she is vomiting. After the person has vomited, offer some water to rinse out his or her mouth and a bowl to spit into. Then gently wipe off his or her face using cool or lukewarm water.

As soon as the nausea ends, give sips of water, tea, ginger ale, broth, or fruit drinks to replace lost body fluids. Unless told to do so by the doctor, do not give the person solid food for several hours after he or she has stopped vomiting, and then give something that won't upset his or her stomach (such as gelatin).

Memory Problems

People of all ages can forget to call a relative on his or her birthday or leave some of the ingredients out of a favorite recipe. These types of memory problems are normal and do not interfere with the ability to function. More serious memory problems sometimes accompany aging. When an older person realizes that his or her memory is not as good as it once was, he or she may begin to feel apprehensive, fearful, and anxious. Forgetfulness may cause an older person to assume that he or she is developing dementia (see page 689) or Alzheimer's disease (see page 688). Reassure the person, and try the following strategies to help him or her remember better:

- Make signs to remind the person to do things such as take medication, turn off the stove, or lock the doors. Place the signs in a visible location. Put signs along the way to the bathroom, with a sign that reads "BATHROOM" attached to the bathroom door.
- Give the person a large calendar with large numbers to help him or her keep track of dates and events by checking off each day of the week.
- Circle dates on the calendar as a reminder of important appointments and dates.
- Provide clocks with large, easy-to-read numbers to help the person stay time-oriented.
- Follow a regular mealtime schedule; people with memory problems often forget to eat.
- Post a daily checklist on the refrigerator door to remind the person of the things he or she needs to do.
- Place items to bring upstairs near the foot of the stairs (but never on the stairs).
- Place items to be taken along on outings near the front door.
- Label boxes with their contents so the person will know at a glance what is inside.
- Store items such as keys, eyeglasses, and medications in the same place (and be sure to always return them to their proper place) so they are easy to find when needed.
- If the person is disoriented, have him or her wear an identification bracelet at all times. It should list the person's name, address, and telephone number. This identification will be helpful if he or she wanders away or becomes lost.

If the person's memory problems begin to interfere with day-to-day living, he or she should be examined by a doctor who has experience diagnosing and treating people with Alzheimer's disease and other forms of dementia.

Reducing the Risks of Immobility

Many people who are confined to bed develop health problems from immobility. Because of the potential risk of problems with circulation, breathing, and muscle stiffness, a person who can get out of bed needs to do so regularly.

Increasing Circulation

Immobility decreases a person's heart output, or circulation, increasing his or her chances of developing blood clots. A person's heart rate, or pulse, is a good indicator of how well his or her cardiovascular system can handle being out of bed.

If the person's heart rate is between 50 and 100 beats per minute when out of bed and sitting in a chair, it may be OK for him or her to stay up. If the person's heart rate is higher than 100 beats per minute when sitting in a chair, sitting up may be too strenuous; ask his or her doctor if the person should stay in bed.

The person's doctor may suggest that the person start exercising in bed to increase his or her strength and endurance enough to get out of bed. Always check with the person's doctor first before starting an exercise program. These simple exercises may include range-of-motion exercises (see next page), turning from side to side in bed, and sitting on the edge of the bed for short periods of time. If the person's heart rate goes below 50 beats per minute or above 110 beats per minute, call his or her doctor right away. A heart rate below 50 beats per minute could indicate problems such as dehydration, anemia (see page 610), or heart failure (see page 570). A heart rate above 110 beats per minute could indicate problems such as an arrhythmia (see page 580) or high blood pressure (see page 574).

Maintaining Lung Function

Being immobile reduces lung function and increases the risk of pneumonia, so it is important to maintain lung function in a person who is confined to bed. If the person's doctor has recommended it, encourage the person to cough and do deep breathing exercises every hour while awake to expand his or her lungs. Encourage the person to breathe through his or her nose as deeply as possible and then breathe out through the mouth slowly but forcibly.

If possible, obtain a device called a spirometer (which is used to measure air expulsion) from a respiratory therapist and have him or her show you how to help the person use it.

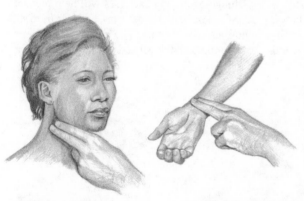

In the carotid artery   In the radial artery

Checking a pulse
To check a person's heart rate, place your index and middle fingers on the artery inside his or her wrist or along the artery at the side of the neck. (Do not use one of your thumbs to take a person's pulse because you could mistake your own pulse in an artery in your thumb for the person's pulse.) You should be able to feel blood pulsing in the person's artery as his or her heart beats. Count the number of beats that occur in exactly 20 seconds and multiply this number by 3. The resulting number is the person's heart rate.

> ### WARNING!
> ### Difficulty Breathing
> Call the person's doctor immediately if the person you are caring for has difficulty breathing or coughs up green, gray, yellow, or brown phlegm. He or she may have pneumonia.

Preventing Deep Vein Thrombosis

Blood clots are another potential complication of immobility. They usually develop in the veins of the legs. If the person cannot bear his or her own weight or walk, ask the doctor if the person should move his or her legs while in bed to prevent blood clots. Also, ask the doctor about using special elastic stockings that can help prevent blood clots from forming in the legs. Don't massage the person's legs unless told to do so by the doctor.

Pulmonary Embolism

Never massage the legs of a person who is confined to bed. Massaging an immobile person's legs (especially the calves) can dislodge a blood clot, which can then travel through the bloodstream to the lungs, causing a life-threatening blockage of an artery (pulmonary embolism; see page 606). Symptoms of pulmonary embolism include difficulty breathing, pain in the chest, rapid pulse, sweating, slight fever, and a cough that produces blood-tinged phlegm. If these symptoms occur, call 911 or your local emergency number, or take the person to the nearest hospital emergency department right away.

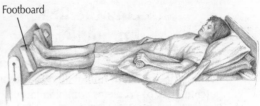

Footboard

Supporting the feet with a footboard

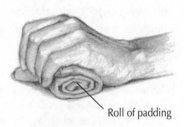

Roll of padding

Supporting the hand with foam-rubber padding

Keeping the Arms and Legs Strong

A person begins to lose muscle strength after being confined to bed for just 1 day; after 1 week in bed, he or she may be too weak to stand up. A period of bed rest often is required after surgery or a major illness. A person who is confined to bed for any reason must be encouraged to change positions frequently to prevent joint stiffness, loss of muscle tone, and contraction of the limbs from prolonged inactivity.

To help prevent joint stiffness, carefully place the person's arms and legs in comfortable, natural, strain-free positions and support them on pillows, cushions, or pads. Rest the person's elbows on pillows, and keep his or her legs from turning outward with foam-rubber cushions or pillows. Support the person's feet with a footboard to prevent footdrop (a condition in which the foot hangs limply from the ankle). Place the person's hands around small rolls of foam-rubber padding.

Range-of-motion exercises will help prevent a bedridden person's hands, arms, and legs from stiffening and contracting. The person should move each limb up and down and away from and toward

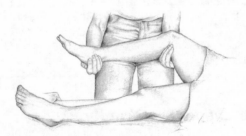

Exercising the leg

Range-of-motion exercises
If the person you are caring for is immobile or has difficulty moving, help him or her to perform range-of-motion exercises to prevent the hands and limbs from contracting. Gently bend and straighten each elbow and wrist, and the fingers and thumb of each hand. Raise each leg, bending and straightening the hip, knee, and ankle.

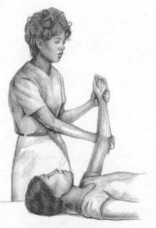

Straightening the elbow and wrist

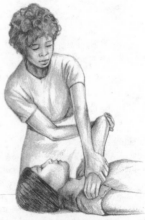

Bending the elbow and wrist

the middle of the body. This process is called active range of motion. If the person cannot move a limb, the caregiver should perform passive range-of-motion exercises. Gently hold the person's limb at each joint and move the limb in all the directions in which it can move normally. These exercises also help stimulate blood circulation and help prevent blood clots from forming in the legs. A visiting nurse can teach you how to correctly perform range-of-motion exercises.

Encourage the person to move each joint through its entire range of motion several times a day. To prevent injury, do not try to move any joint that resists motion. Never move any limb beyond the point at which it causes discomfort or pain. If resistance or pain occurs, tell the doctor as soon as possible.

Helping the Person Get Out of Bed

A person who has been confined to bed for a long time is likely to feel weak and dizzy when getting out of bed for the first time. To prevent a fall, have the person sit up slowly and rest on the edge of the bed for a few minutes before trying to stand up. Place a sturdy chair beside the bed. When the person feels steady, stand directly in front of him or her so he or she can lean on you for support. Hold the person under the arms. Then help the person turn slowly, and gently and carefully lower him or her into the chair. As the person begins to feel stronger, have him or her try to take a few steps, using your arms for support.

Positioning an Immobile Person in Bed

A person who is confined to bed often tends to slide toward the foot of the bed. To move an immobile person toward the head of the bed, you first need to help him or her to a sitting position.

An immobile person's body should always be properly positioned to help prevent deformities. Proper positioning can be achieved using pillows and bolsters. For example, when a person is lying on his or her side, instead of elevating the head of

Moving a Person in Bed

1. To help the person sit up in bed, first arrange the pillows so that his or her shoulders are elevated. Cross the person's arms at his or her waist. Place your hands over the person's shoulders and place your knee on the bed, next to his or her hip. Place your other foot firmly on the floor next to the bed, slightly ahead of your knee and even with the person's waist.

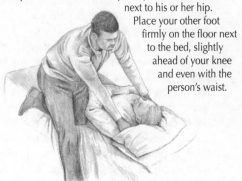

2. Firmly grasp the person's shoulders, keeping your arms straight, and slowly move back, using your weight to pull him or her up toward you.

3. If you want to move the person toward the head of the bed, keep your hand on the shoulder closer to you and get in position behind him or her. Place your knee on the bed behind the person and place your other foot firmly on the floor. Cross the person's forearms in front of his or her waist and hold them firmly from behind. Slowly move back, using your weight to pull the person toward you.

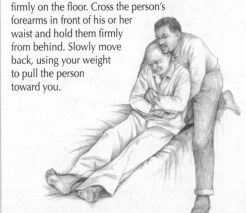

the bed, place a pillow under the upper leg and arm. And place a pillow or bolster behind the person's back to prevent him or her from rolling backward. A person who has little fat on the hips should not be positioned fully on his or her side. Instead, position him or her in a 30-degree side-lying position to help prevent the development of pressure sores in the hip area.

An immobile person who is confined to bed should not remain in the same position for longer than 2 hours while the caregiver is awake. Move the person from his or her side, onto his or her back, and onto the other side every 2 hours. When the immobile person is on his or her back, position a pillow under each arm and on the side of each thigh to prevent outward hip rotation. Also, place a small pillow under the knees and a footboard at the foot of the bed to keep the person's feet positioned at a right angle to the mattress. This positioning will prevent the development of footdrop (a condition in which the foot hangs limply from the ankle) and keep the person from sliding down the bed.

Do not tuck sheets and blankets tightly around the person's feet and legs; keep blankets and other coverings elevated with a bed or foot cradle (a tentlike device placed at the foot of the bed). Keep bottom sheets taut to prevent them from wrinkling or gathering under the person's body, which could cause pressure sores.

When feeding a person in bed, elevate the head of the bed at least 30 degrees to prevent choking, and keep the bed raised for at least an hour after eating. This positioning helps prevent the person from regurgitating food, which can cause him or her to accidentally breathe food into the lungs and choke. Breathing foreign particles into the lungs can lead to pneumonia.

Moving an Immobile Person

When moving an immobile person to a chair, wheelchair, or commode, wear sturdy shoes with nonskid soles, and make sure that the person you are moving is also wearing sturdy, nonskid shoes or slippers. To prevent falls, do not attempt to move a person who is barefoot or wearing only socks. You may need to use a transfer belt, a specially designed belt that is placed around the person's waist. The belt provides leverage and makes it easier to firmly grip the person when you help him or her to a standing or sitting position. Your doctor, nurse, or home health aide can teach you how to use a transfer belt properly. You can purchase one from a medical supply company.

WARNING!

Transfer Belts

Never use a regular belt as a transfer belt when moving an immobile person or you could cause serious injury to the person.

Before you move the person:

- Talk about each step with the person.
- If you are moving the person from a hospital bed, lock the bed's brakes.
- If you are moving the person to a wheelchair, lock the wheelchair's brakes.
- If needed, put a transfer belt on the person.

To move an immobile person:

1. Carefully help the person to a sitting position on the side of the bed, with his or her feet on the floor. If the person has been confined to bed for a long time, allow him or her to rest on the edge of the bed until he or she feels secure. Stand directly in front of the person, and brace his or her knees with your knees. Carefully slide the person's hips toward you.
2. Help the person to a standing position, using the transfer belt if necessary, to firmly hold him or her around the waist.
3. Slowly pivot the person around until his or her back is directly in front of the chair, wheelchair, or commode; have the person feel the seat of the chair or commode with the back of his or her legs before attempting to sit.
4. Slowly lower the person to a sitting position. Once he or she is securely seated, remove the transfer belt.

To help the person back into bed, perform the steps described above in reverse order. Be sure to lock the brakes on the bed and wheelchair before you begin, and use the transfer belt. If you are using a hospital bed, don't forget to raise the bed rails after the person is back in bed.

Modifying the Home Environment

A safe environment is often the most immediate concern when an older or disabled person lives alone. Take a careful look around the home and take the following steps to make the home safe:

- Modify the home as needed to help prevent falls (see below right).
- Install smoke alarms (especially near bedrooms and the kitchen) and a carbon monoxide detector. Check the batteries frequently and replace them on the same day every year, whether they need it or not.
- Plan an escape route in case of fire. Have regular fire drills.
- Keep a clear path to all doors that lead outside.

- Set the temperature of the water heater below 110°F to prevent burns.
- Keep a fire extinguisher in the kitchen, and learn how to use and maintain it properly.
- Repair or replace any electrical appliances that have frayed wires or damaged plugs.
- Do not overload electrical outlets.
- Remove electrical cords from under rugs or carpets.
- Install deadbolt locks on outside doors, sturdy locks on all windows, and motion-detector lights on the grounds of the home.
- Have the furnace and thermostat inspected by a qualified professional.

Organizing the Room

When organizing the person's room, think about his or her needs. Consider how ill he or she is and how long you are likely to be caring for him or her. Arrange the room to make it as comfortable and convenient as possible for the person who is being cared for and the caregivers. Here are some helpful tips:

- In a two-story house, it is better for the person to stay on the first floor. He or she will feel less isolated, you will eliminate a lot of trips up and down the stairs, and you can prevent falls.
- Provide a single bed, positioned so it is accessible from both sides. If you need a hospital bed, you can rent one from a medical supply company.
- Provide a bedside table stocked with medications, water, tissues, a whistle or bell (to call for help), and any other important items.
- If the person can get out of bed but cannot get to the bathroom easily, you will need to get a commode (a portable chair that contains a removable bedpan). You can rent or buy one from a drugstore or medical supply company or, in some communities, borrow one from a local health agency or volunteer organization. If the person is confined to bed, keep a bedpan (and a handheld urinal for a man or boy) near the bed at all times.
- Keep the temperature in the room comfortable

and the air circulation adequate, but keep the room free of drafts.

Preventing Falls

Carefully and thoroughly inspect the house or apartment of the person you are caring for and make all necessary changes to help prevent falls. Here are some things you can do:

- Make sure that light switches are within easy reach of doorways so the person does not have to cross a dark room to turn on a light. Lighting that is too dim can make it difficult to see. Use high-watt bulbs but make sure they are frosted to reduce glare.
- Place a lamp within reach of the person's bed. Put night-lights along the pathways between the bedrooms and the bathroom and a night-light in the bathroom.
- Remove loose rugs, mats, and runners. Make sure that all other carpets and rugs have slip-resistant backing or that they are tacked down to prevent trips and slips.
- Arrange furniture so the person has a clear, unobstructed path from one place to another. Keep hallways and stairs clear and uncluttered. Take special care with placement of furniture that has sharp or pointed corners or that is easy to bump into or fall over such as ottomans and coffee tables. Remove any furniture that is not being used. Provide a remote control for the television.

- Keep telephone and electrical cords out of pathways.
- Provide sturdy handrails on both sides of all stairways, 30 inches above the steps. Use nonskid treads on all bare steps. If a stairway is carpeted, make sure that the carpeting is tacked down securely on every step. Do not put loose rugs at the top or bottom of stairways. All stairways should be well lit. Do not keep toys or other items on stairs. Have an electric stair lift installed if the person can no longer climb the stairs. If there is a bathroom on the first floor, move the person's bedroom there.
- Make sure chairs and tables are sturdy, stable, and balanced in case the person leans on them for support.
- Set the thermostat at a warm temperature (at least 72°F) to help keep an older person's joints from stiffening. Stiff joints can lead to falls.
- Place guardrails on the bed or a sturdy chair bedside to help the person get in and out of bed. Place a telephone with volume control and a lighted dial next to the bed.
- Place a nonslip rubber mat on the floor in front of the sink. Clean up spills on the floor and countertops immediately. Keep frequently used items within easy reach to avoid having to bend or climb up on a chair or stepladder to reach them. Be sure that the person wears low-heeled, slip-resistant shoes that fit properly.
- Put a nonslip rubber mat or nonslip adhesive strips on the floor of the tub or shower. Install handrails and grab bars that are attached to underlying studs on the walls around the toilet and along the bathtub. Tell the person you are caring for never to use towel bars for support—they are not strong enough. Place a nonslip bath mat on the floor outside the tub or shower. Some people find an elevated toilet seat easier to use.
- Do not lock the bathroom door. It may be necessary to remove locks to prevent the person from accidentally locking himself or herself in the bathroom.
- Have all medications reviewed by the person's doctor to be sure that they are necessary, especially drugs with possible side effects such as drowsiness, dizziness, or fainting.
- When going outdoors, have the person wear comfortable, sturdy walking shoes with soles that grip the pavement. If he or she uses a cane or walker, make sure it is sturdy and in good condition.

Encourage the person to stay indoors, if possible, when the weather is bad, especially when the pavement is wet or icy. During the winter, keep porches, steps, sidewalks, and driveways clear of snow and ice. Always spread sand or salt on icy surfaces.

- A person who has difficulty walking may benefit from working with a physical therapist, either as an outpatient or through a home health care agency. If walking is a problem, talk to your doctor about having a gait evaluation and starting an exercise program to improve the person's ability to walk and increase his or her strength.

In spite of the best preventive measures, falls still may occur. If the person you are caring for falls, don't move him or her; try to determine the nature and extent of any injuries, and call for emergency medical assistance immediately.

Regulating Home Temperature

As you age, your body becomes less able to regulate temperature. A life-threatening drop in body temperature (hypothermia; see page 165) can develop quickly in an older person if the room temperature is lower than 65°F. Make sure that the heating system in your loved one's home is in proper working order and that there is enough heat throughout the day, especially if the person lives in an apartment building, where tenants usually do not have control over the heat. It also is vital to have the furnace checked regularly for carbon monoxide leaks.

Older people also are vulnerable to the effects of high temperatures, which can lead to life-threatening conditions such as heat exhaustion and heatstroke (see page 166). Experts strongly recommend that room temperature be maintained at a constant 72°F, if possible. In the summer, fans may be helpful, but in many parts of the United States, air-conditioning is the only way to keep the temperature at a comfortable level. However, many older people do not own an air conditioner or cannot afford to pay high electric bills. Watch the person carefully for signs of heat exhaustion and heatstroke. In some communities, social service agencies provide air conditioners free to older people on limited incomes. Check with your local area agency on aging for more information.

Personal Emergency Response Systems

Personal emergency response systems (PERS) provide an easy way for a disabled person to call for help in an emergency. The system includes an electronic monitor (about the size of a small radio or answering machine) that can be placed on a bedside table. The monitor is plugged into an electrical outlet and connected to the person's telephone line. Most systems require the person to push a help button to activate the system. There is a button on the monitor and also on a wristband or pendant that the person wears at all times. Some systems also may be voice-activated or use motion detectors.

When the system is activated, the signal goes to a monitoring center, where a response is set into motion. First, the center attempts to contact the person. Depending on the situation (or if the person does not respond), the center then attempts to contact a designated person or people (such as a relative, friend, or neighbor), or calls for emergency assistance (from emergency medical services, the fire department, or the police).

Personal emergency response systems are available by subscription in many communities, usually with a one-time installation charge and a monthly fee. In some communities, local hospitals, fire departments, and various community organizations provide this service. If the person has limited income and assets, the service may have a reduced fee or be free. In any case, you should not have to purchase any equipment or sign a long-term contract. Ask your doctor or contact your local hospital for information about these systems.

Telephone Check-in and Reassurance

Telephone check-in and reassurance services provide a way of monitoring the health and safety of an older person who lives alone. Paid staff or trained volunteers call the person at home at prearranged times throughout the day. If there is a problem or if the person does not answer the phone, the caller will follow specific procedures such as contacting a doctor or a designated family member, or calling for emergency assistance. These services also can provide older people with companionship and a sense of security. Contact your doctor, nurse, social worker, or local hospital for information about the availability of telephone check-in and reassurance services in your area.

Care for the Caregiver

Taking good care of yourself is an essential part of good caregiving. Because successful caregiving requires an enormous amount of time and energy, it is vital that you remain physically and emotionally healthy. Don't be shy about asking for and accepting help from others.

Taking Care of Yourself

Keeping yourself healthy physically, mentally, and emotionally will enable you to provide the best care possible to a person who is ill. Here are some guidelines that will help you cope with the demands of caregiving:

• Set realistic goals and limits. Educate yourself about your loved one's condition so that you know what to expect, now and in the future. Knowing what to expect will help you to adjust your care plan as time passes. Decide under what conditions you will no longer be able to care for your loved one at home, and begin planning for that possibility well in advance. For example, if your loved one has a terminal illness, find out about hospice programs.

• Learn all you can about caregiving. There are many sources of useful information, including libraries, hospitals, agencies, and associations. Ask your doctor, a nurse, or a hospital social worker for information sources.

• Do not confuse doing with caring. Let your loved one remain as independent as possible for as long as possible. Resist the urge to do everything, and encourage your loved one to participate in his or her daily care routine.

• Get plenty of rest every day. Every caregiver needs some uninterrupted sleep during the day, every day. Most people need about 8 hours of sleep each day. If possible, sleep at the same time your loved one is sleeping, or try to get some sleep while another caregiver takes over for you.

• Be sure to keep all of your own medical and dental appointments. It is important that you stay as healthy as possible. Arrange to have a dependable family member, friend, or neighbor stay with your loved one while you visit your doctor or dentist.

• Maintain a healthy diet so you have enough energy to get through all of the day's activities. Eat lots of fruits, vegetables, and whole grains, and be sure you are getting a sufficient amount of calcium every day. Consider taking a daily multivitamin/mineral supplement.

• Try to exercise every day. Choose a type of exercise you enjoy. For example, 30 minutes of brisk walking each day will tone your muscles and stimulate your circulation. It also will get you out of the house.

• Do not neglect your personal life. Regularly take time away from caregiving to enjoy yourself and take care of personal business. Continue to participate in the activities you have always enjoyed. Having fun is a good way to relieve stress and take your mind off of caregiving.

• Take advantage of respite care when you need a break. A responsible family member or friend may be able to take over your caregiving responsibilities for several hours each week. Adult day care programs are often available at senior citizen centers and community service organizations, either free or for a modest fee. Some hospitals and nursing facilities provide respite care services for longer periods (from several days to several weeks) for a fee. Your doctor can recommend appropriate respite care services in your area.

• Keep a diary throughout the caregiving process. Writing things down at the end of the day can help you organize your thoughts, express your feelings, and find solutions to problems.

• Try to stay in touch with your feelings and find positive ways to deal with them. It is common for caregivers to experience feelings of guilt, anger, resentment, or depression. When these feelings are not addressed, they can interfere with the caregiving process and have adverse effects on your health. Discussing your feelings with family, friends, and other members of the caregiving team may be helpful. Joining a support group for caregivers can reduce your sense of isolation, help you find ways to cope with your feelings, and solve caregiving-related problems. Watch for symptoms of depression (see page 187); if you are depressed, get professional help as soon as possible.

Asking for and Accepting Help From Others

Share your caregiving responsibilities with others whenever possible to ensure the health and well-being of the person being cared for, and your own health and well-being. Get in the habit of asking for help as soon as you need it. Do not wait until a situation becomes unmanageable. Every member of the household should participate or contribute in some way—doing chores, running errands, preparing meals, making telephone calls, or providing company.

Be ready to ask for help by keeping a list handy of all the things that need to be done. For example, ask friends or family to come over and stay with the person so you can go out. To get time on your own at home, ask them to go shopping for you or to accompany the person to the doctor's office. And do not hesitate to accept help when it's offered.

If you cannot rely on friends, neighbors, or family members, ask your doctor for a referral to a visiting nurse association, which can send a nurse to evaluate the situation and provide some needed help. Consider hiring a household helper, home health aide, or companion to help you with day-to-day tasks. If family members cannot give their time, perhaps they can offer financial support for help you need. Some hospitals and nursing homes have respite facilities where you can bring your loved one for a short period while you go away on a trip, make up the needed sleep you might have lost, or just stay home and enjoy the solitude. Inquire about the governmental services the person may be entitled to that could help you with required tasks—meal delivery service, homemaker service, respite care, shopping service, case management, transportation service, or taxi service. You may want to attend a support group in your community. Ask your doctor to recommend one.

Caregiver Self-Assessment Questionnaire

Caregivers often are so concerned with caring for another person's needs that they lose sight of their own well-being. If you are a caregiver, answer the following questions and then do the self-evaluation to determine your level of stress.

During the past week or so, I:

1.	Had trouble keeping my mind on what I was doing	____ Yes	____ No
2.	Felt that I couldn't leave my relative alone	____ Yes	____ No
3.	Had difficulty making decisions	____ Yes	____ No
4.	Felt completely overwhelmed	____ Yes	____ No
5.	Felt useful and needed	____ Yes	____ No
6.	Felt lonely	____ Yes	____ No
7.	Was upset that my relative has changed so much from his or her former self	____ Yes	____ No
8.	Felt a loss of privacy or personal time	____ Yes	____ No
9.	Was edgy or irritable	____ Yes	____ No
10.	Had my sleep disturbed to care for my relative	____ Yes	____ No
11.	Had a crying spell	____ Yes	____ No
12.	Felt strained between work and family responsibilities	____ Yes	____ No
13.	Had back pain	____ Yes	____ No
14.	Felt ill (headaches, stomach problems, or a cold)	____ Yes	____ No
15.	Felt satisfied with the support my family has given me	____ Yes	____ No
16.	Found my relative's living situation inconvenient or a barrier to care	____ Yes	____ No
17.	On a scale of 1 to 10, with 1 being not stressful and 10 being extremely stressful, rate your current level of stress.	____	
18.	On a scale of 1 to 10, with 1 being very healthy and 10 being very ill, rate your current health compared to what it was this time last year.	____	

Self-Evaluation

To determine your score:

1. For questions 5 and 15, count a No response as a Yes, and a Yes response as a No.
2. Total the number of Yes responses.

Interpreting Your Score

Chances are that you are experiencing a high degree of stress if:

- You answered Yes to question 4 or 11; or
- Your score on question 17 is 6 or higher; or
- Your score on question 18 is 6 or higher; or
- Your total score is 10 or higher

What Should You Do Now?

If you are experiencing a high degree of stress:

- Consider seeing your doctor for a checkup.
- Consider having some relief from caregiving. Ask the doctor or a social worker about caregiving resources in your community. Contact the National Family Caregivers Association (800-896-3650) and Eldercare Locator (800-677-1116), which can also direct you to caregiving resources in your area.
- Consider joining a support group in which you can learn from and share experiences with other caregivers.

Stress Relief for Caregivers

Caring for a loved one at home can be a major cause of stress for the entire household, but it is especially stressful for the caregiver. The person you are caring for may be confused, angry, or depressed. He or she may be demanding or difficult to please, making you feel inadequate, frustrated, angry, and trapped. You may feel guilty for having negative feelings. Such feelings are understandable, but you need to cope with them so you can go on. Take steps early in your caregiving to arrange for respite care.

Preventing Burnout

Caregiver burnout is physical or emotional exhaustion resulting from the prolonged stress of caregiving. The condition usually occurs gradually; the first signs and symptoms may not appear until long after you have settled into a daily caregiving routine. Burnout affects your ability to provide good quality care. Because different people have different coping abilities, burnout levels vary from person to person. Common signs and symptoms of caregiver burnout include:

- Anger or irritability
- Feeling frustrated or overwhelmed
- Lack of energy; tiring easily
- Feeling isolated
- Crying regularly
- Difficulty handling minor problems or making minor decisions
- Frequent headaches or colds
- Change in appetite
- Sleeping problems
- Skin problems such as acne or rashes
- Inability to concentrate
- Feeling anxious, depressed, or resentful
- Nervous habits (such as nail-biting, chain smoking, or overeating)

To help prevent burnout, have a dependable support system consisting of people you can talk to or visit regularly to express your feelings and discuss concerns. Many caregivers are relieved just to have someone to talk to. If nothing is done to relieve it, burnout can quickly lead to depression. If you have any symptoms of caregiver burnout, seek help from a social worker, doctor, nurse, psychologist, or professional counselor as soon as possible. A visit with your clergyperson also may help.

Relieving Stress

If you are a caregiver, respite can take a variety of forms. It may be something simple, such as enjoying a hot bath at the end of the day or watching a favorite TV show. It can be an organized program, such as adult day care, or a respite care program in which the person you are caring for goes to a health care facility for care or treatment. Or it may take the form of a respite worker or volunteer who comes to stay with the person at home. Either way, you can get away or spend some time at home alone.

Maintain your activities and relationships outside the home as much as possible. If you are employed outside the home, for example, try to keep your job if at all possible. Continue to participate in the leisure activities you enjoyed before your loved one became ill. Accept offers of help

What You Can Do to Help a Caregiver

As a friend or relative of a caregiver, you can do many things to help make the person's job easier. Although the following actions are relatively simple, they can have a profound, positive impact on a caregiver's day.

- Keep in touch. Call or visit the caregiver as often as you can. Caregivers often feel isolated, and it can be a great relief to talk with friends or relatives.

- Offer to help. Ask the caregiver what he or she would like you to do. Because many caregivers are reluctant to ask others for help, you may need to be persistent.
- Be a good listener. It is important for caregivers to discuss their feelings and concerns, and doing so can often help relieve stress and anxiety. Let the caregiver know that you are available if he or she needs to talk.

from others, including family members, friends, respite workers, and volunteers.

Many people find comfort in sharing their experiences with others in support groups. In such groups, people share their concerns about caregiving or about a specific illness such as diabetes, cancer, or Alzheimer's disease. Consult your local hospital for information about groups in your area. Your doctor or other members of your health care team also may be able to recommend a support group. The Internet also is a good place to look for a support group that will meet your needs. If you cannot find a support group in your area, consider starting your own.

PART FOUR

What Are Your Symptoms?

How to Use the Self-Diagnosis Symptoms Charts

The charts in this section are designed to help you find the possible cause (or causes) of a symptom you have. Through a series of questions and answers, you are led to a possible diagnosis or to other charts or articles in this book. You also may be advised to see a doctor or to go immediately to a hospital emergency department.

To use the charts:

- Find the symptoms chart you want by consulting the Chart-Finder Index on the next page.
- Turn to the chart and read the description of

the symptom under the chart title to be sure it's the chart you need.

- Always start each chart with the beginning question.
- Follow the YES and NO answer paths all the way through to the diagnosis or other instructions.
- Except in emergencies, make sure that you read all the cross-references to get as much information as possible.
- **For a definite diagnosis and for treatment, always see a doctor.**

Chart Title
The chart title is a short term that describes the symptom.

Description
A simple description of the symptom (or more information about the symptom) is given here.

Sex and Age Group
The section at the upper left of each chart indicates the people the chart is designed to help.

Questions
Each question is phrased to require either a YES or a NO answer. Follow the path to the next question (or recommendation).

Answers
Possible reasons for your symptom or a possible diagnosis appear here. You may be referred to another symptoms chart or section of the book, or given other instructions. For an emergency, you will be told to get medical help immediately.

Information in Boxes
Some charts contain additional important information such as self-help advice or warnings about possible symptoms of life-threatening conditions that require immediate medical attention.

Visual Aids to Diagnosis
To help you find the possible cause of a skin or eye disorder, a number of disorders are illustrated in full color in the Visual Aids to Diagnosis section starting on p. 117.

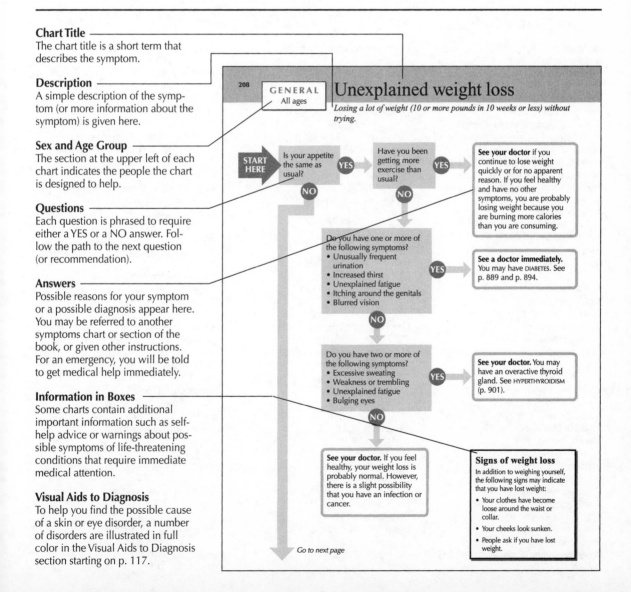

How to Find the Chart You Need

The index below directs you to the page number of the chart that deals with your symptom. To find the chart you want, follow these steps:

1. Single out your major symptom. If you have two or more symptoms (such as a high fever, a cough, and a runny nose), determine which one bothers you the most.
2. Look for the symptom in the Chart-Finder Index below and on the next page. The charts are listed in the index by key words. For example, difficulty sleeping is listed under both "Difficulty sleeping" and "Sleeping difficulty."
3. If you can't find your main symptom in the index, look for a chart that deals with another symptom you have.
4. When you find the correct chart in the index, go to the page indicated and answer the questions on the chart to find the cause of your symptoms. A detailed explanation of how to use the charts is on the previous page.

Chart-Finder Index

Feeling generally ill

A vague sense of not being well.

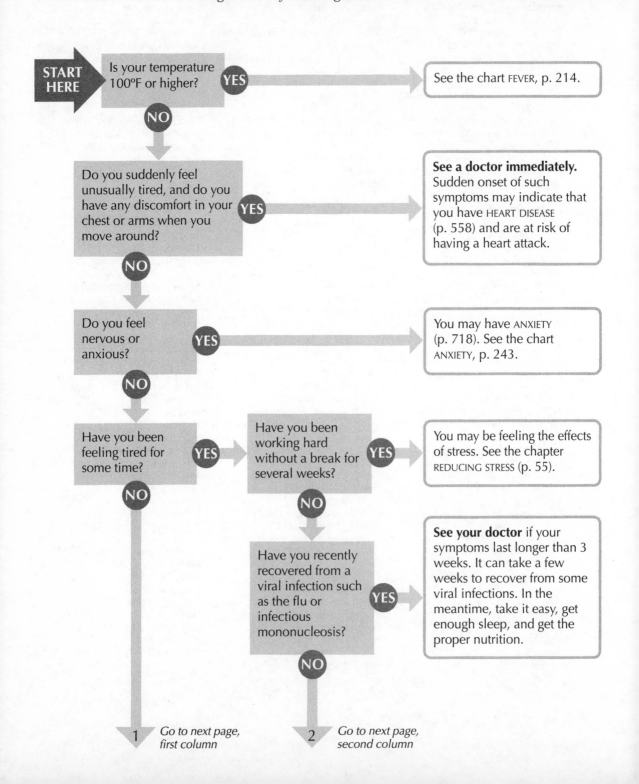

START HERE

Is your temperature 100°F or higher? — **YES** → See the chart FEVER, p. 214.

NO ↓

Do you suddenly feel unusually tired, and do you have any discomfort in your chest or arms when you move around? — **YES** → **See a doctor immediately.** Sudden onset of such symptoms may indicate that you have HEART DISEASE (p. 558) and are at risk of having a heart attack.

NO ↓

Do you feel nervous or anxious? — **YES** → You may have ANXIETY (p. 718). See the chart ANXIETY, p. 243.

NO ↓

Have you been feeling tired for some time? — **YES** → Have you been working hard without a break for several weeks? — **YES** → You may be feeling the effects of stress. See the chapter REDUCING STRESS (p. 55).

NO ↓ (from "working hard")

Have you recently recovered from a viral infection such as the flu or infectious mononucleosis? — **YES** → **See your doctor** if your symptoms last longer than 3 weeks. It can take a few weeks to recover from some viral infections. In the meantime, take it easy, get enough sleep, and get the proper nutrition.

NO ↓ (from "feeling tired for some time")

1 *Go to next page, first column*

NO ↓ (from "viral infection")

2 *Go to next page, second column*

1 *Continued from previous page, first column*

2 *Continued from previous page, second column*

Do you have one or more of the following symptoms?
- Difficulty sleeping
- Inability to concentrate or make decisions
- Lack of interest in sex
- Recurring headaches
- Frequently feeling sad

YES → **See your doctor.** You may have DEPRESSION (p. 709). See the chart DEPRESSION, p. 242. Or you may have IRON DEFICIENCY ANEMIA (p. 610), HYPOTHYROIDISM (p. 903), or CHRONIC FATIGUE SYNDROME (p. 931).

NO ↓

Are you overweight according to the body mass index chart on p. 11?

YES → **See your doctor.** Being overweight puts a strain on your body. Losing weight may help you feel better. See THE RISKS OF BEING OVERWEIGHT (p. 51) and LOSING WEIGHT SENSIBLY (p. 53).

NO ↓

Do you exercise regularly?

NO → Regular exercise keeps you fit both physically and mentally. See THE HEALTH BENEFITS OF PHYSICAL ACTIVITY (p. 45).

YES ↓

Are you taking any medication?

YES → **Talk to your doctor.** Some drugs can make you feel tired or sick.

NO ↓

Have you lost a lot of weight (10 or more pounds in 10 weeks or less) without trying?

YES → See the chart UNEXPLAINED WEIGHT LOSS, next page.

NO ↓

See your doctor if you are unable to make a diagnosis from this chart.

GENERAL
All ages

Unexplained weight loss

Losing a lot of weight (10 or more pounds in 10 weeks or less) without trying.

START HERE

Is your appetite the same as usual?

 YES

Have you been getting more exercise than usual?

YES

See your doctor if you continue to lose weight quickly or for no apparent reason. If you feel healthy and have no other symptoms, you are probably losing weight because you are burning more calories than you are consuming.

NO

NO

Do you have one or more of the following symptoms?
• Unusually frequent urination
• Increased thirst
• Unexplained fatigue
• Itching around the genitals
• Blurred vision

 YES

See a doctor immediately. You may have DIABETES. See p. 889 and p. 894.

NO

Do you have two or more of the following symptoms?
• Excessive sweating
• Weakness or trembling
• Unexplained fatigue
• Bulging eyes

 YES

See your doctor. You may have an overactive thyroid gland. See HYPERTHYROIDISM (p. 901).

 NO

See your doctor. If you feel healthy, your weight loss is probably normal. However, there is a slight possibility that you have an infection or cancer.

Signs of weight loss

In addition to weighing yourself, the following signs may indicate that you have lost weight:

• Your clothes have become loose around the waist or collar.

• Your cheeks look sunken.

• People ask if you have lost weight.

Go to next page

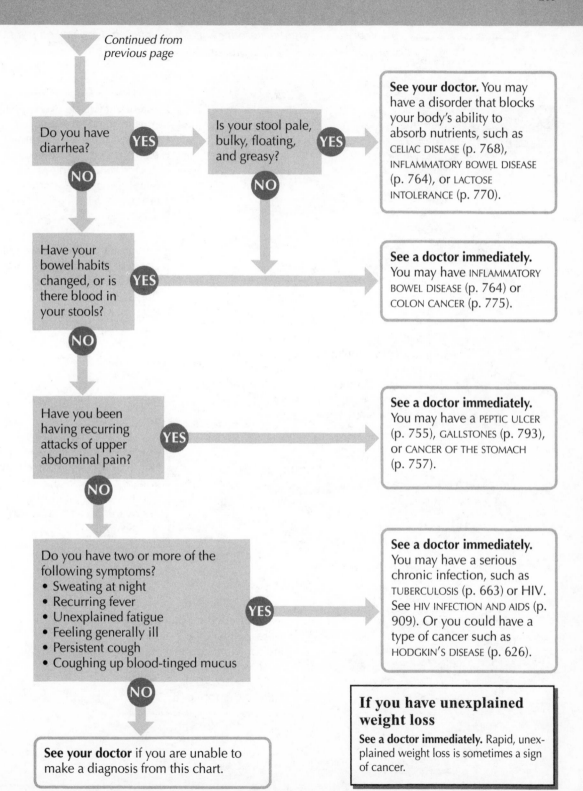

Continued from previous page

Do you have diarrhea?

YES → **Is your stool pale, bulky, floating, and greasy?**

YES → **See your doctor.** You may have a disorder that blocks your body's ability to absorb nutrients, such as CELIAC DISEASE (p. 768), INFLAMMATORY BOWEL DISEASE (p. 764), or LACTOSE INTOLERANCE (p. 770).

NO

NO

Have your bowel habits changed, or is there blood in your stools?

YES → **See a doctor immediately.** You may have INFLAMMATORY BOWEL DISEASE (p. 764) or COLON CANCER (p. 775).

NO

Have you been having recurring attacks of upper abdominal pain?

YES → **See a doctor immediately.** You may have a PEPTIC ULCER (p. 755), GALLSTONES (p. 793), or CANCER OF THE STOMACH (p. 757).

NO

Do you have two or more of the following symptoms?
- Sweating at night
- Recurring fever
- Unexplained fatigue
- Feeling generally ill
- Persistent cough
- Coughing up blood-tinged mucus

YES → **See a doctor immediately.** You may have a serious chronic infection, such as TUBERCULOSIS (p. 663) or HIV. See HIV INFECTION AND AIDS (p. 909). Or you could have a type of cancer such as HODGKIN'S DISEASE (p. 626).

NO

See your doctor if you are unable to make a diagnosis from this chart.

If you have unexplained weight loss

See a doctor immediately. Rapid, unexplained weight loss is sometimes a sign of cancer.

Overweight

If you are overweight according to the body mass index chart on p. 11, you may be putting your health at risk.

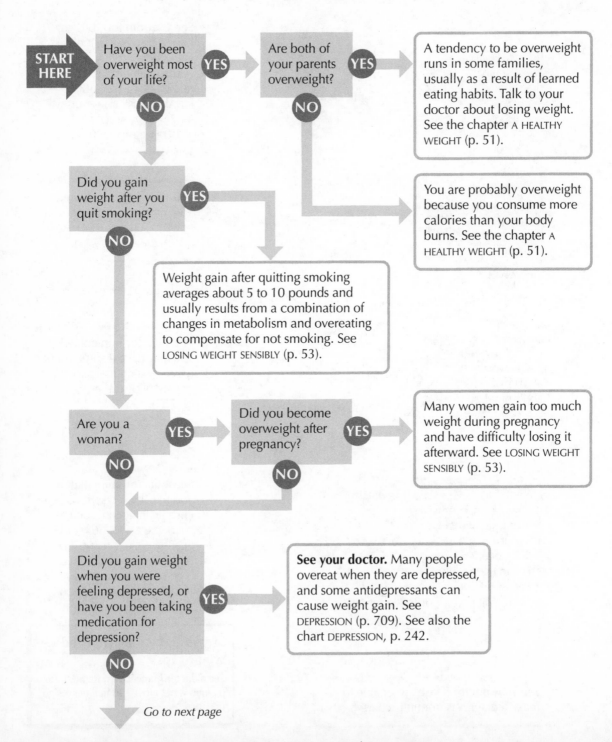

START HERE

Have you been overweight most of your life? **YES** → Are both of your parents overweight? **YES** → A tendency to be overweight runs in some families, usually as a result of learned eating habits. Talk to your doctor about losing weight. See the chapter A HEALTHY WEIGHT (p. 51).

NO ↓

Did you gain weight after you quit smoking? **YES** →

NO ↓

NO (from parents) → You are probably overweight because you consume more calories than your body burns. See the chapter A HEALTHY WEIGHT (p. 51).

Weight gain after quitting smoking averages about 5 to 10 pounds and usually results from a combination of changes in metabolism and overeating to compensate for not smoking. See LOSING WEIGHT SENSIBLY (p. 53).

Are you a woman? **YES** → Did you become overweight after pregnancy? **YES** → Many women gain too much weight during pregnancy and have difficulty losing it afterward. See LOSING WEIGHT SENSIBLY (p. 53).

NO ↓

NO ↓

Did you gain weight when you were feeling depressed, or have you been taking medication for depression? **YES** → **See your doctor.** Many people overeat when they are depressed, and some antidepressants can cause weight gain. See DEPRESSION (p. 709). See also the chart DEPRESSION, p. 242.

NO ↓

Go to next page

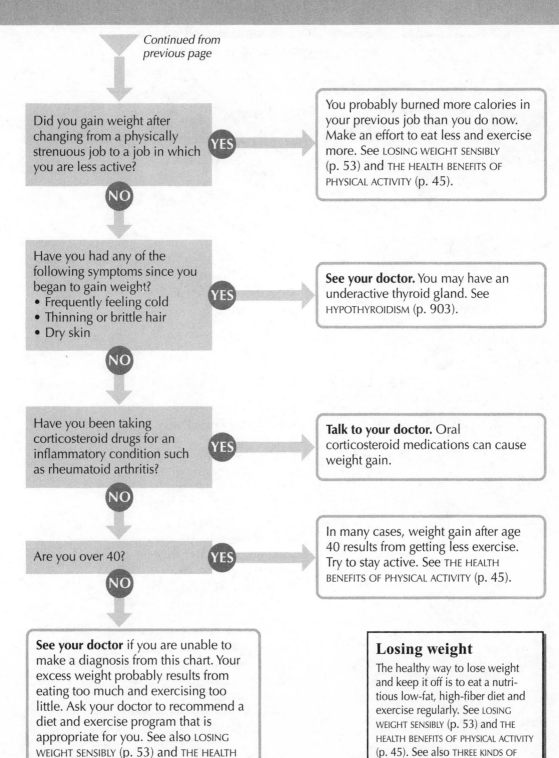

Continued from previous page

Did you gain weight after changing from a physically strenuous job to a job in which you are less active?

YES → You probably burned more calories in your previous job than you do now. Make an effort to eat less and exercise more. See LOSING WEIGHT SENSIBLY (p. 53) and THE HEALTH BENEFITS OF PHYSICAL ACTIVITY (p. 45).

NO

Have you had any of the following symptoms since you began to gain weight?
• Frequently feeling cold
• Thinning or brittle hair
• Dry skin

YES → **See your doctor.** You may have an underactive thyroid gland. See HYPOTHYROIDISM (p. 903).

NO

Have you been taking corticosteroid drugs for an inflammatory condition such as rheumatoid arthritis?

YES → **Talk to your doctor.** Oral corticosteroid medications can cause weight gain.

NO

Are you over 40?

YES → In many cases, weight gain after age 40 results from getting less exercise. Try to stay active. See THE HEALTH BENEFITS OF PHYSICAL ACTIVITY (p. 45).

NO

See your doctor if you are unable to make a diagnosis from this chart. Your excess weight probably results from eating too much and exercising too little. Ask your doctor to recommend a diet and exercise program that is appropriate for you. See also LOSING WEIGHT SENSIBLY (p. 53) and THE HEALTH BENEFITS OF PHYSICAL ACTIVITY (p. 45).

Losing weight

The healthy way to lose weight and keep it off is to eat a nutritious low-fat, high-fiber diet and exercise regularly. See LOSING WEIGHT SENSIBLY (p. 53) and THE HEALTH BENEFITS OF PHYSICAL ACTIVITY (p. 45). See also THREE KINDS OF EXERCISE (p. 46).

GENERAL
All ages

Difficulty sleeping

Frequent problems falling asleep or staying asleep. For children under 5 years, see the chart WAKING AT NIGHT IN CHILDREN, p. 342.

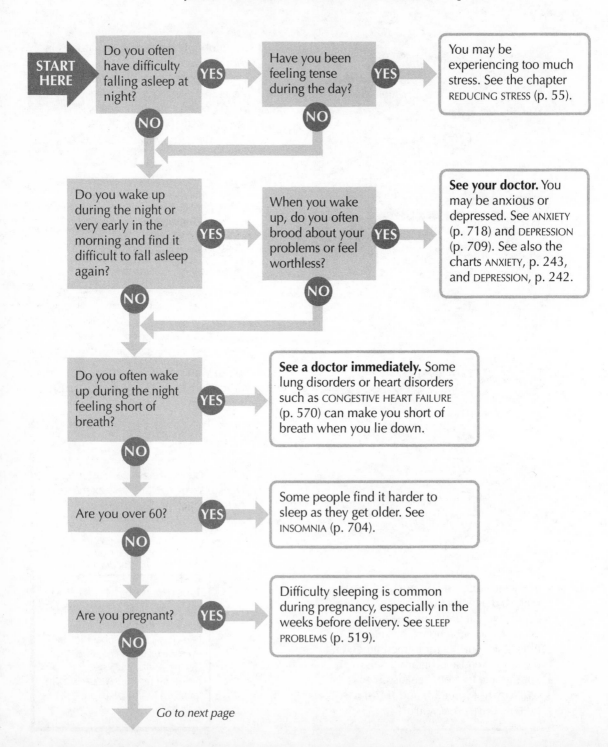

START HERE

Do you often have difficulty falling asleep at night?

YES → Have you been feeling tense during the day? **YES** → You may be experiencing too much stress. See the chapter REDUCING STRESS (p. 55).

NO

NO

Do you wake up during the night or very early in the morning and find it difficult to fall asleep again?

YES → When you wake up, do you often brood about your problems or feel worthless? **YES** → **See your doctor.** You may be anxious or depressed. See ANXIETY (p. 718) and DEPRESSION (p. 709). See also the charts ANXIETY, p. 243, and DEPRESSION, p. 242.

NO

NO

Do you often wake up during the night feeling short of breath?

YES → **See a doctor immediately.** Some lung disorders or heart disorders such as CONGESTIVE HEART FAILURE (p. 570) can make you short of breath when you lie down.

NO

Are you over 60?

YES → Some people find it harder to sleep as they get older. See INSOMNIA (p. 704).

NO

Are you pregnant?

YES → Difficulty sleeping is common during pregnancy, especially in the weeks before delivery. See SLEEP PROBLEMS (p. 519).

NO

Go to next page

Continued from previous page

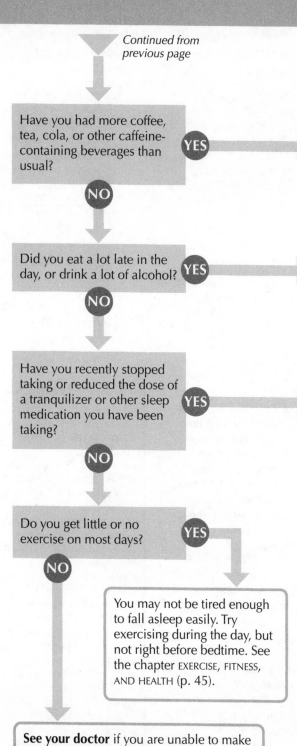

Have you had more coffee, tea, cola, or other caffeine-containing beverages than usual?

YES → Caffeine is a stimulant that can cause sleeplessness. Avoid or reduce your intake of caffeine, especially in the late afternoon and evening.

NO ↓

Did you eat a lot late in the day, or drink a lot of alcohol?

YES → Try eating a lighter meal earlier in the evening or reduce your alcohol intake to a moderate level. See ALCOHOL ABUSE AND ALCOHOL DEPENDENCE (p. 733).

NO ↓

Have you recently stopped taking or reduced the dose of a tranquilizer or other sleep medication you have been taking?

YES → **Talk to your doctor.** If you have been using tranquilizers or sleep medication, suddenly stopping or reducing the dose can interfere with sleep and cause other problems. Your doctor can help you gradually and safely reduce the dose.

NO ↓

Do you get little or no exercise on most days?

YES → You may not be tired enough to fall asleep easily. Try exercising during the day, but not right before bedtime. See the chapter EXERCISE, FITNESS, AND HEALTH (p. 45).

NO ↓

See your doctor if you are unable to make a diagnosis from this chart and the self-help measures at right do not work.

Improving your sleep

If you have difficulty sleeping for any reason, try the following self-help measures:

- Cut back on caffeinated beverages and alcohol or eliminate them completely.

- Avoid eating heavy meals just before going to bed.

- Drink a glass of warm milk before going to bed. Milk contains an essential amino acid called tryptophan, which acts as a natural sleep inducer.

- Take a warm bath to help you relax.

- Do not use your bed for any activities other than sleeping and sex.

- Make sure the bedroom is not too warm and that your mattress is comfortable.

See also STRESS AND SLEEP (p. 57).

GENERAL
Over 12 years

Fever

A temperature of 100°F or higher. For children under 2 years, see the chart FEVER IN YOUNG CHILDREN, *p. 354. For children 2 to 12 years, see the chart* FEVER IN CHILDREN, *p. 356.*

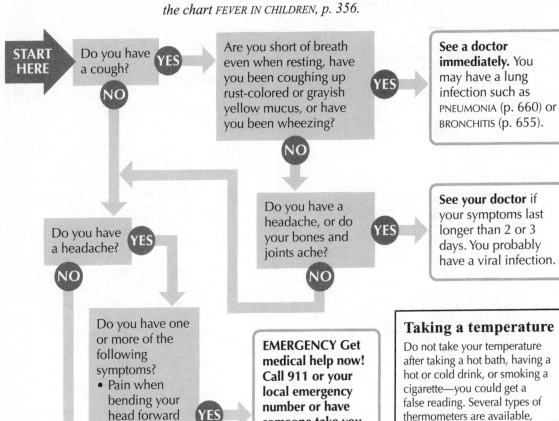

START HERE

Do you have a cough? → **YES** → Are you short of breath even when resting, have you been coughing up rust-colored or grayish yellow mucus, or have you been wheezing? → **YES** → **See a doctor immediately.** You may have a lung infection such as PNEUMONIA (p. 660) or BRONCHITIS (p. 655).

NO

NO

Do you have a headache, or do your bones and joints ache? → **YES** → **See your doctor** if your symptoms last longer than 2 or 3 days. You probably have a viral infection.

NO

Do you have a headache? → **YES**

NO

Do you have one or more of the following symptoms?
• Pain when bending your head forward
• Nausea or vomiting
• Sensitivity of eyes to bright light
• Drowsiness or confusion

→ **YES** → **EMERGENCY Get medical help now! Call 911 or your local emergency number or have someone take you to the nearest hospital emergency department.** You may have MENINGITIS (p. 692), a potentially life-threatening infection of the brain.

Have you vomited or had diarrhea? → **YES** → **See your doctor.** You may have an infection of the digestive tract. See GASTROENTERITIS (p. 781).

NO

Go to next page

Taking a temperature

Do not take your temperature after taking a hot bath, having a hot or cold drink, or smoking a cigarette—you could get a false reading. Several types of thermometers are available, including mercury and digital thermometers and temperature strips. Concerns about possible exposure to mercury have led doctors to recommend digital thermometers, which are safe and accurate (but slightly more expensive than glass thermometers). Temperature strips (which can be placed on the forehead) measure temperature quickly but are less accurate than digital or glass thermometers.

Normal body temperature is about 98.6°F but can be different for everyone and vary by 1 or 2 degrees during the day. Body temperature is usually lowest in the early morning.

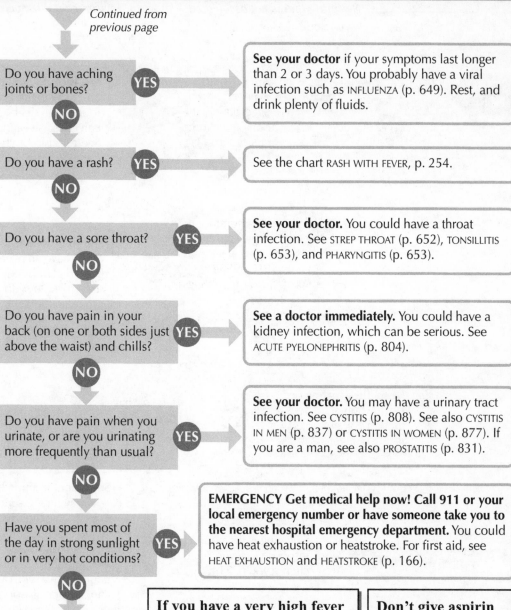

Continued from previous page

Do you have aching joints or bones? — **YES** → **See your doctor** if your symptoms last longer than 2 or 3 days. You probably have a viral infection such as INFLUENZA (p. 649). Rest, and drink plenty of fluids.

NO ↓

Do you have a rash? — **YES** → See the chart RASH WITH FEVER, p. 254.

NO ↓

Do you have a sore throat? — **YES** → **See your doctor.** You could have a throat infection. See STREP THROAT (p. 652), TONSILLITIS (p. 653), and PHARYNGITIS (p. 653).

NO ↓

Do you have pain in your back (on one or both sides just above the waist) and chills? — **YES** → **See a doctor immediately.** You could have a kidney infection, which can be serious. See ACUTE PYELONEPHRITIS (p. 804).

NO ↓

Do you have pain when you urinate, or are you urinating more frequently than usual? — **YES** → **See your doctor.** You may have a urinary tract infection. See CYSTITIS (p. 808). See also CYSTITIS IN MEN (p. 837) or CYSTITIS IN WOMEN (p. 877). If you are a man, see also PROSTATITIS (p. 831).

NO ↓

Have you spent most of the day in strong sunlight or in very hot conditions? — **YES** → **EMERGENCY Get medical help now! Call 911 or your local emergency number or have someone take you to the nearest hospital emergency department.** You could have heat exhaustion or heatstroke. For first aid, see HEAT EXHAUSTION and HEATSTROKE (p. 166).

NO ↓

See your doctor if you are unable to make a diagnosis from this chart, if your temperature has not returned to normal within 24 hours, or if it is very high or rises again.

If you have a very high fever

Call your doctor immediately. A temperature of 104°F or higher is potentially dangerous. Wiping your head and body with lukewarm (not cold) water may give you some relief. Replace lost fluids by drinking lots of fluids, particularly water and a rehydration solution or sports drink. Talk to your doctor before taking aspirin or an aspirin substitute to help bring down a fever.

Don't give aspirin to children or adolescents

Do not give aspirin to children or adolescents who have a fever; taking aspirin has been linked with REYE'S SYNDROME (p. 411)—a rare but potentially fatal childhood disorder.

GENERAL
All ages

Excessive sweating

Sweating that is not associated with warm environmental temperatures or exercise.

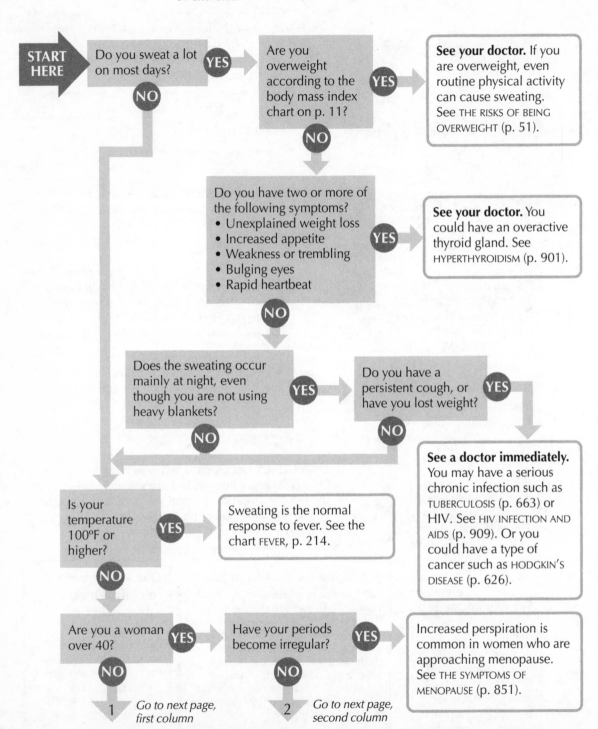

START HERE

Do you sweat a lot on most days? — **NO** / **YES**

Are you overweight according to the body mass index chart on p. 11? — **NO** / **YES**

See your doctor. If you are overweight, even routine physical activity can cause sweating. See THE RISKS OF BEING OVERWEIGHT (p. 51).

Do you have two or more of the following symptoms?
• Unexplained weight loss
• Increased appetite
• Weakness or trembling
• Bulging eyes
• Rapid heartbeat — **NO** / **YES**

See your doctor. You could have an overactive thyroid gland. See HYPERTHYROIDISM (p. 901).

Does the sweating occur mainly at night, even though you are not using heavy blankets? — **NO** / **YES**

Do you have a persistent cough, or have you lost weight? — **NO** / **YES**

See a doctor immediately. You may have a serious chronic infection such as TUBERCULOSIS (p. 663) or HIV. See HIV INFECTION AND AIDS (p. 909). Or you could have a type of cancer such as HODGKIN'S DISEASE (p. 626).

Is your temperature 100°F or higher? — **NO** / **YES**

Sweating is the normal response to fever. See the chart FEVER, p. 214.

Are you a woman over 40? — **NO** / **YES**

Have your periods become irregular? — **NO** / **YES**

Increased perspiration is common in women who are approaching menopause. See THE SYMPTOMS OF MENOPAUSE (p. 851).

1 *Go to next page, first column*

2 *Go to next page, second column*

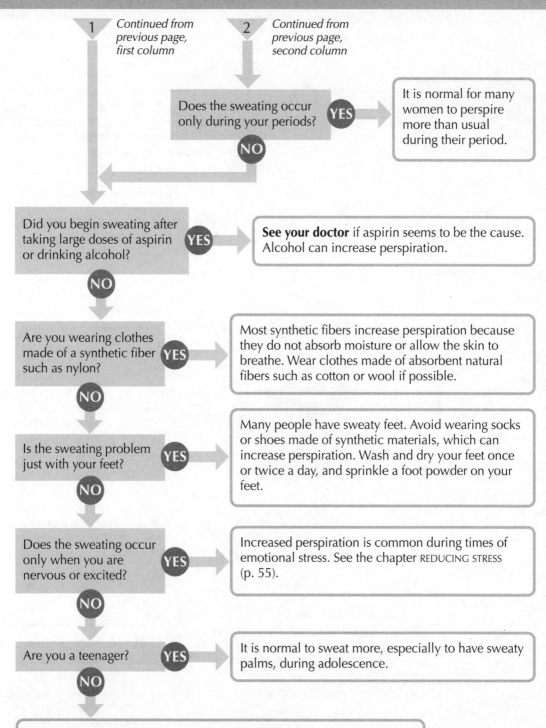

1 *Continued from previous page, first column*

2 *Continued from previous page, second column*

Does the sweating occur only during your periods? — **YES** → It is normal for many women to perspire more than usual during their period.

NO

Did you begin sweating after taking large doses of aspirin or drinking alcohol? — **YES** → **See your doctor** if aspirin seems to be the cause. Alcohol can increase perspiration.

NO

Are you wearing clothes made of a synthetic fiber such as nylon? — **YES** → Most synthetic fibers increase perspiration because they do not absorb moisture or allow the skin to breathe. Wear clothes made of absorbent natural fibers such as cotton or wool if possible.

NO

Is the sweating problem just with your feet? — **YES** → Many people have sweaty feet. Avoid wearing socks or shoes made of synthetic materials, which can increase perspiration. Wash and dry your feet once or twice a day, and sprinkle a foot powder on your feet.

NO

Does the sweating occur only when you are nervous or excited? — **YES** → Increased perspiration is common during times of emotional stress. See the chapter REDUCING STRESS (p. 55).

NO

Are you a teenager? — **YES** → It is normal to sweat more, especially to have sweaty palms, during adolescence.

NO

See your doctor if you are unable to make a diagnosis from this chart or if you are concerned about the excessive sweating.

GENERAL
Over 12 years

Swellings under the skin

A new lump or swelling under the skin that you can see or feel. For children up to 12 years, see the chart SWELLINGS IN CHILDREN, p. 362.

START HERE

Is the lump or swelling painful, red, and warm? **YES**

See your doctor. You may have a skin infection such as a BOIL (p. 1060). If you recently injured the area, you could have a hematoma, an accumulation of blood caused by bleeding from an injured blood vessel.

NO

Do you have any lumps or swellings in any of the lymph nodes in your neck, armpit, or groin? **YES**

 Is your temperature 100°F or higher? **YES**

See your doctor. You could have an infection such as INFECTIOUS MONONUCLEOSIS (p. 935).

NO

Do you smoke? **YES**

See your doctor. A lump in the neck can be a sign of throat cancer. See TUMORS OF THE LARYNX (p. 637).

NO

Did you have a vaccination (such as a typhoid shot) within the past few days? **YES**

Talk to your doctor. Vaccinations can sometimes cause swollen glands.

NO

Are you currently taking any medication? **YES**

Talk to your doctor. Some drugs, especially those used to treat epilepsy and some thyroid disorders, can cause swollen glands.

NO

See a doctor immediately. You may have an infection, but there is also a slight possibility that you have cancer of the lymphatic system. See HODGKIN'S DISEASE (p. 626) and NON-HODGKIN'S LYMPHOMA (p. 625).

NO

If you have a new, unexplained lump

See a doctor immediately to have the lump evaluated. Any lump under or on the skin may be a sign of cancer. For example, a lump in the neck can indicate throat or thyroid cancer.

Go to next page

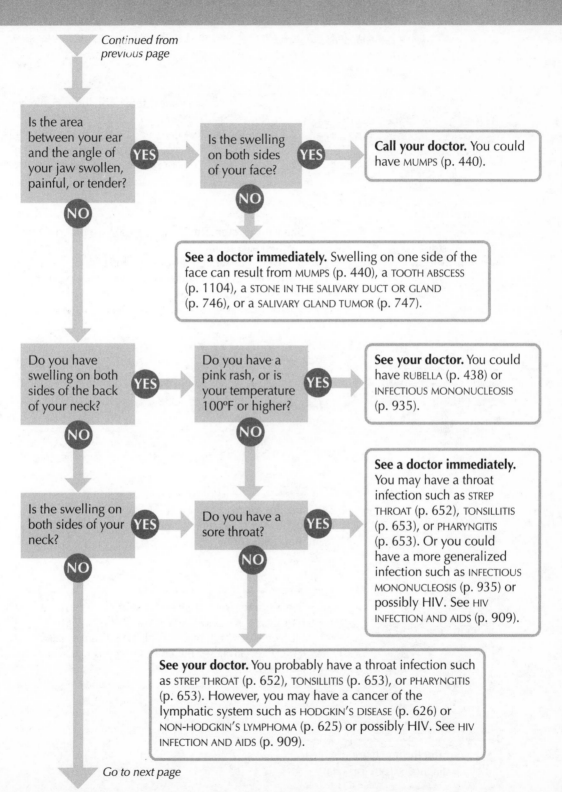

Continued from previous page

Is the area between your ear and the angle of your jaw swollen, painful, or tender? — **YES** → **Is the swelling on both sides of your face?** — **YES** → **Call your doctor.** You could have MUMPS (p. 440).

NO (from "Is the swelling on both sides of your face?") →

See a doctor immediately. Swelling on one side of the face can result from MUMPS (p. 440), a TOOTH ABSCESS (p. 1104), a STONE IN THE SALIVARY DUCT OR GLAND (p. 746), or a SALIVARY GLAND TUMOR (p. 747).

NO (from "Is the area between your ear...") ↓

Do you have swelling on both sides of the back of your neck? — **YES** → **Do you have a pink rash, or is your temperature 100°F or higher?** — **YES** → **See your doctor.** You could have RUBELLA (p. 438) or INFECTIOUS MONONUCLEOSIS (p. 935).

NO (from "Do you have a pink rash...") ↓

Do you have a sore throat? — **YES** → **See a doctor immediately.** You may have a throat infection such as STREP THROAT (p. 652), TONSILLITIS (p. 653), or PHARYNGITIS (p. 653). Or you could have a more generalized infection such as INFECTIOUS MONONUCLEOSIS (p. 935) or possibly HIV. See HIV INFECTION AND AIDS (p. 909).

NO (from "Do you have swelling on both sides of the back of your neck?") ↓

Is the swelling on both sides of your neck? — **YES** → **Do you have a sore throat?**

NO (from "Do you have a sore throat?") ↓

See your doctor. You probably have a throat infection such as STREP THROAT (p. 652), TONSILLITIS (p. 653), or PHARYNGITIS (p. 653). However, you may have a cancer of the lymphatic system such as HODGKIN'S DISEASE (p. 626) or NON-HODGKIN'S LYMPHOMA (p. 625) or possibly HIV. See HIV INFECTION AND AIDS (p. 909).

NO (from "Is the swelling on both sides of your neck?") ↓

Go to next page

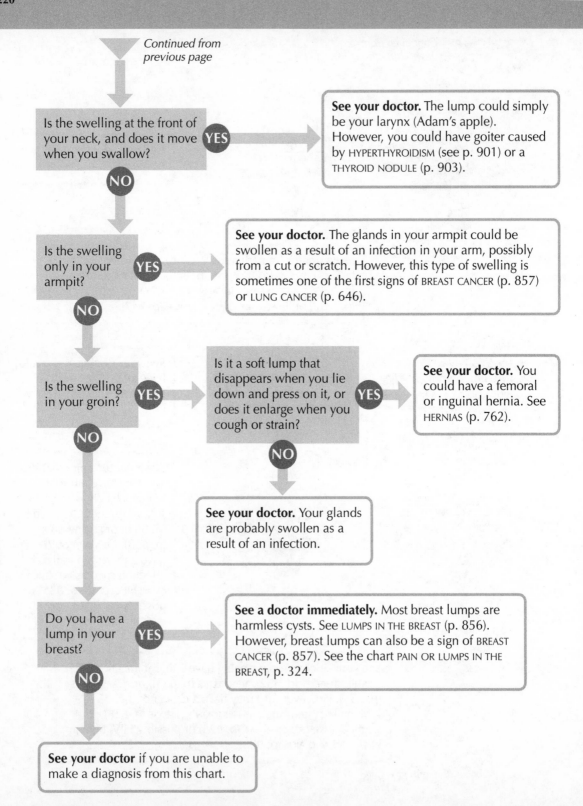

Continued from previous page

Is the swelling at the front of your neck, and does it move when you swallow? YES → **See your doctor.** The lump could simply be your larynx (Adam's apple). However, you could have goiter caused by HYPERTHYROIDISM (see p. 901) or a THYROID NODULE (p. 903).

NO ↓

Is the swelling only in your armpit? YES → **See your doctor.** The glands in your armpit could be swollen as a result of an infection in your arm, possibly from a cut or scratch. However, this type of swelling is sometimes one of the first signs of BREAST CANCER (p. 857) or LUNG CANCER (p. 646).

NO ↓

Is the swelling in your groin? YES → **Is it a soft lump that disappears when you lie down and press on it, or does it enlarge when you cough or strain?** YES → **See your doctor.** You could have a femoral or inguinal hernia. See HERNIAS (p. 762).

NO ↓

See your doctor. Your glands are probably swollen as a result of an infection.

NO ↓

Do you have a lump in your breast? YES → **See a doctor immediately.** Most breast lumps are harmless cysts. See LUMPS IN THE BREAST (p. 856). However, breast lumps can also be a sign of BREAST CANCER (p. 857). See the chart PAIN OR LUMPS IN THE BREAST, p. 324.

NO ↓

See your doctor if you are unable to make a diagnosis from this chart.

Itching without a rash

The skin itches but there is no change in its appearance. For children 2 to 12 years, see the chart ITCHING IN CHILDREN, p. 359.

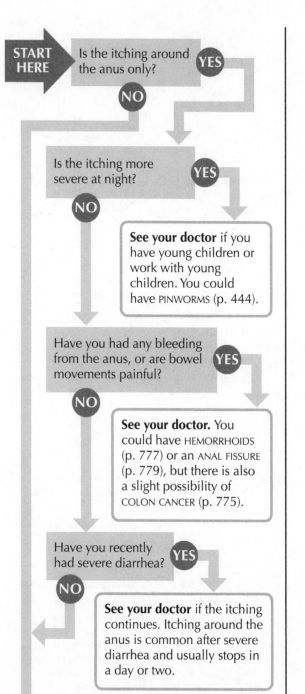

START HERE

Is the itching around the anus only? **YES**

NO

Is the itching more severe at night? **YES**

NO

See your doctor if you have young children or work with young children. You could have PINWORMS (p. 444).

Have you had any bleeding from the anus, or are bowel movements painful? **YES**

NO

See your doctor. You could have HEMORRHOIDS (p. 777) or an ANAL FISSURE (p. 779), but there is also a slight possibility of COLON CANCER (p. 775).

Have you recently had severe diarrhea? **YES**

NO

See your doctor if the itching continues. Itching around the anus is common after severe diarrhea and usually stops in a day or two.

Go to next column

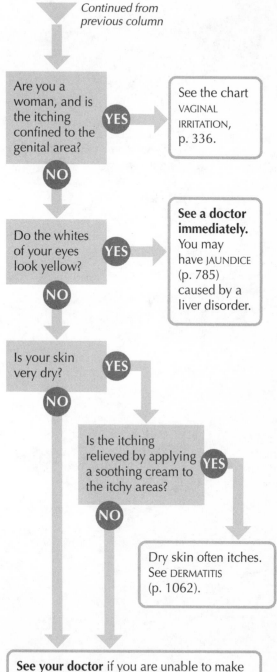

Continued from previous column

Are you a woman, and is the itching confined to the genital area? **YES**

NO

See the chart VAGINAL IRRITATION, p. 336.

Do the whites of your eyes look yellow? **YES**

NO

See a doctor immediately. You may have JAUNDICE (p. 785) caused by a liver disorder.

Is your skin very dry? **YES**

NO

Is the itching relieved by applying a soothing cream to the itchy areas? **YES**

NO

Dry skin often itches. See DERMATITIS (p. 1062).

See your doctor if you are unable to make a diagnosis from this chart.

Feeling faint and fainting

A sudden feeling of weakness and unsteadiness that may result in brief loss of consciousness.

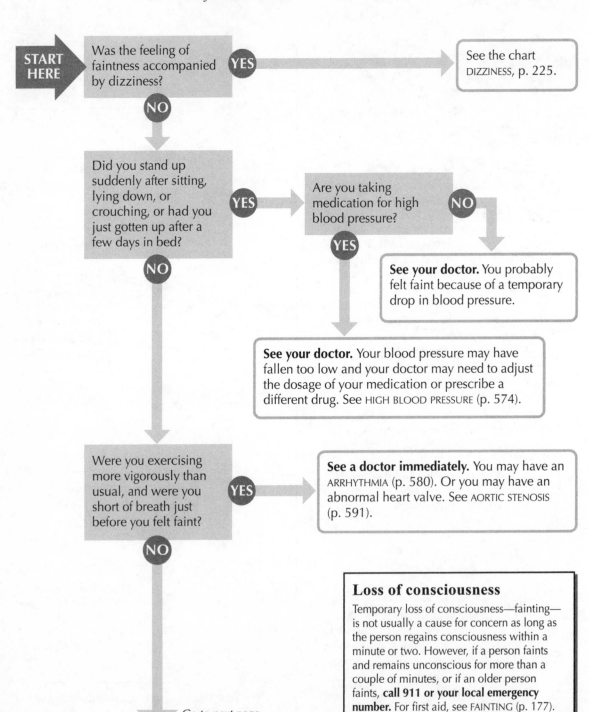

START HERE

Was the feeling of faintness accompanied by dizziness?

YES → See the chart DIZZINESS, p. 225.

NO ↓

Did you stand up suddenly after sitting, lying down, or crouching, or had you just gotten up after a few days in bed?

YES → Are you taking medication for high blood pressure?

NO → **See your doctor.** You probably felt faint because of a temporary drop in blood pressure.

YES → **See your doctor.** Your blood pressure may have fallen too low and your doctor may need to adjust the dosage of your medication or prescribe a different drug. See HIGH BLOOD PRESSURE (p. 574).

NO ↓

Were you exercising more vigorously than usual, and were you short of breath just before you felt faint?

YES → **See a doctor immediately.** You may have an ARRHYTHMIA (p. 580). Or you may have an abnormal heart valve. See AORTIC STENOSIS (p. 591).

NO ↓

Go to next page

Loss of consciousness

Temporary loss of consciousness—fainting— is not usually a cause for concern as long as the person regains consciousness within a minute or two. However, if a person faints and remains unconscious for more than a couple of minutes, or if an older person faints, **call 911 or your local emergency number.** For first aid, see FAINTING (p. 177).

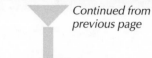

Continued from previous page

Have you not eaten for some time, or do you have diabetes?

 YES → **See your doctor** if you have diabetes so you can discuss ways to control your blood sugar better. Low blood sugar may be causing you to feel faint. Drinking something sweet or eating something sugary or starchy will probably make you feel better. See HYPOGLYCEMIA (p. 897).

NO

If you feel faint

If you feel faint, lie down with your legs raised. If this is not possible, sit bent forward with your head between your knees until you feel better. For first aid, see FAINTING (p. 177).

Did you spend several hours in strong sunlight or in very hot or stuffy conditions?

 YES → **EMERGENCY Get medical help now! Call 911 or your local emergency number or have someone take you to the nearest hospital emergency department.** You could have heat exhaustion, which can lead to heatstroke, a life-threatening condition. For first aid, see HEAT EXHAUSTION and HEATSTROKE (p. 166).

NO

Have you had one or more of the following symptoms?
- Numbness or tingling in any part of your body
- Blurred vision
- Confusion
- Difficulty speaking
- Loss of movement in your arms or legs

 YES → **EMERGENCY Get medical help now! Call 911 or your local emergency number or have someone take you to the nearest hospital emergency department.** You may have had a STROKE (p. 669) or a TRANSIENT ISCHEMIC ATTACK (p. 675).

NO

Do you have heart disease, or did your heartbeat speed up or slow down just before you felt faint?

 YES → Did you lose consciousness?

 YES → **See a doctor immediately.** Your loss of consciousness may have been caused by a serious abnormal heart rhythm. See HEART BLOCK (p. 583).

NO

→ **See your doctor.** You may have a disorder of heart rate and rhythm, such as an ARRHYTHMIA (p. 580).

NO

Go to next page

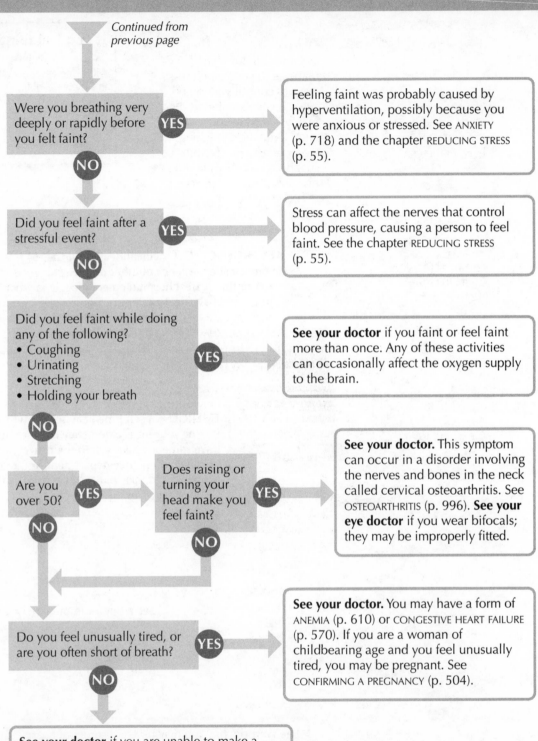

Continued from previous page

Were you breathing very deeply or rapidly before you felt faint?

YES → Feeling faint was probably caused by hyperventilation, possibly because you were anxious or stressed. See ANXIETY (p. 718) and the chapter REDUCING STRESS (p. 55).

NO ↓

Did you feel faint after a stressful event?

YES → Stress can affect the nerves that control blood pressure, causing a person to feel faint. See the chapter REDUCING STRESS (p. 55).

NO ↓

Did you feel faint while doing any of the following?
- Coughing
- Urinating
- Stretching
- Holding your breath

YES → **See your doctor** if you faint or feel faint more than once. Any of these activities can occasionally affect the oxygen supply to the brain.

NO ↓

Are you over 50?

YES → **Does raising or turning your head make you feel faint?**

YES → **See your doctor.** This symptom can occur in a disorder involving the nerves and bones in the neck called cervical osteoarthritis. See OSTEOARTHRITIS (p. 996). **See your eye doctor** if you wear bifocals; they may be improperly fitted.

NO ↓

Do you feel unusually tired, or are you often short of breath?

YES → **See your doctor.** You may have a form of ANEMIA (p. 610) or CONGESTIVE HEART FAILURE (p. 570). If you are a woman of childbearing age and you feel unusually tired, you may be pregnant. See CONFIRMING A PREGNANCY (p. 504).

NO ↓

See your doctor if you are unable to make a diagnosis from this chart.

Dizziness

A spinning sensation accompanied by light-headedness and unsteadiness.

START HERE

Do you feel as though the room is spinning around you?

YES → **Have you noticed one or more of the following symptoms?**
- Weakness in your arms or legs
- Numbness or tingling in any part of your body
- Blurred vision
- Difficulty speaking

YES →

NO ↓

See the chart FEELING FAINT AND FAINTING, p. 222.

NO →

EMERGENCY Get medical help now! Call 911 or your local emergency number or have someone take you to the nearest hospital emergency department. You may have had a STROKE (p. 669) or a TRANSIENT ISCHEMIC ATTACK (p. 675).

Do you have any hearing loss, or do you hear noises in your ear when there is no external source of noise?

YES → **See your doctor.** You could have an inner ear disorder such as LABYRINTHITIS (p. 1014) or MÉNIÈRE'S DISEASE (p. 1013).

NO ↓

Are you over 50?

YES → **Does raising your head bring on dizziness?**

YES → **See your doctor.** This symptom can occur in a disorder involving the nerves and bones in the neck called cervical osteoarthritis. See OSTEOARTHRITIS (p. 996). **See your eye doctor** if you wear bifocals; they may be improperly fitted.

NO ↓

NO →

Do you have recurring severe headaches in the mornings, accompanied by nausea or vomiting?

YES → **Did you injure your head recently?**

YES → **EMERGENCY Get medical help now! Call 911 or your local emergency number or have someone take you to the nearest hospital emergency department.** You could have a SUBDURAL HEMORRHAGE AND HEMATOMA (p. 678).

NO ↓

NO ↓

EMERGENCY Get medical help now! Call 911 or your local emergency number or have someone take you to the nearest hospital emergency department. You could have increased fluid pressure inside your brain, which is life-threatening. However, you may be having MIGRAINE HEADACHES (p. 684).

See your doctor if you are unable to make a diagnosis from this chart.

If you have severe, recurring headaches

See a doctor immediately. Episodes of dizziness or unsteadiness, particularly in the morning, can be signs of a brain tumor, especially if accompanied by symptoms such as recurring headaches and sudden, unexpected vomiting (without initial nausea).

GENERAL
All ages

Headache

Mild to severe pain in the head.

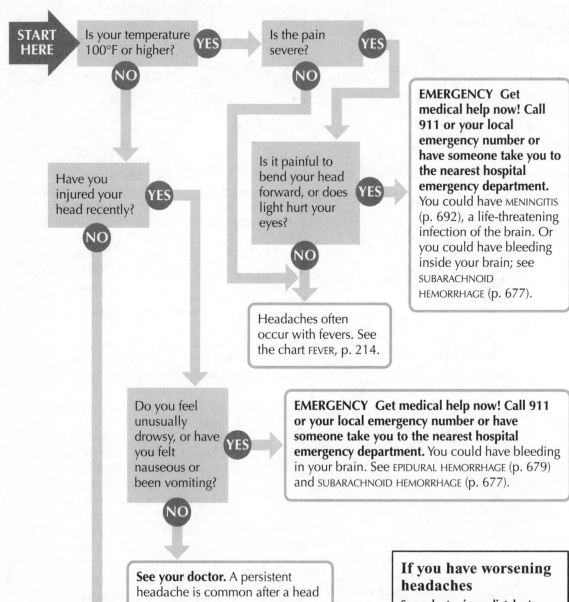

START HERE → Is your temperature 100°F or higher? — **YES** → Is the pain severe? — **YES** →

EMERGENCY Get medical help now! Call 911 or your local emergency number or have someone take you to the nearest hospital emergency department. You could have MENINGITIS (p. 692), a life-threatening infection of the brain. Or you could have bleeding inside your brain; see SUBARACHNOID HEMORRHAGE (p. 677).

Is your temperature 100°F or higher? — **NO** →

Is the pain severe? — **NO** → Is it painful to bend your head forward, or does light hurt your eyes? — **YES** → *(to EMERGENCY box above)*

Is it painful to bend your head forward, or does light hurt your eyes? — **NO** →

Headaches often occur with fevers. See the chart FEVER, p. 214.

Have you injured your head recently? — **YES** → Do you feel unusually drowsy, or have you felt nauseous or been vomiting? — **YES** →

EMERGENCY Get medical help now! Call 911 or your local emergency number or have someone take you to the nearest hospital emergency department. You could have bleeding in your brain. See EPIDURAL HEMORRHAGE (p. 679) and SUBARACHNOID HEMORRHAGE (p. 677).

Do you feel unusually drowsy, or have you felt nauseous or been vomiting? — **NO** →

See your doctor. A persistent headache is common after a head injury. See BRAIN INJURY (p. 680).

Have you injured your head recently? — **NO** →

Go to next page

If you have worsening headaches

See a doctor immediately. A headache that is present when you wake in the morning and worsens progressively throughout the day may be a sign of a brain tumor, particularly if you also have vomiting without nausea.

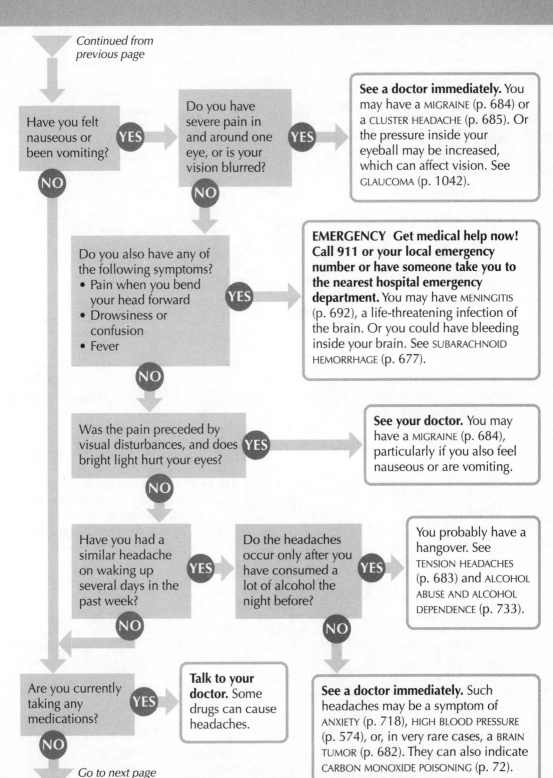

Continued from previous page

Have you felt nauseous or been vomiting? — **YES** → Do you have severe pain in and around one eye, or is your vision blurred? — **YES** → **See a doctor immediately.** You may have a MIGRAINE (p. 684) or a CLUSTER HEADACHE (p. 685). Or the pressure inside your eyeball may be increased, which can affect vision. See GLAUCOMA (p. 1042).

NO ↓   **NO** ↓

Do you also have any of the following symptoms?
• Pain when you bend your head forward
• Drowsiness or confusion
• Fever
— **YES** → **EMERGENCY Get medical help now! Call 911 or your local emergency number or have someone take you to the nearest hospital emergency department.** You may have MENINGITIS (p. 692), a life-threatening infection of the brain. Or you could have bleeding inside your brain. See SUBARACHNOID HEMORRHAGE (p. 677).

NO ↓

Was the pain preceded by visual disturbances, and does bright light hurt your eyes? — **YES** → **See your doctor.** You may have a MIGRAINE (p. 684), particularly if you also feel nauseous or are vomiting.

NO ↓

Have you had a similar headache on waking up several days in the past week? — **YES** → Do the headaches occur only after you have consumed a lot of alcohol the night before? — **YES** → You probably have a hangover. See TENSION HEADACHES (p. 683) and ALCOHOL ABUSE AND ALCOHOL DEPENDENCE (p. 733).

NO ↓   **NO** ↓

Are you currently taking any medications? — **YES** → **Talk to your doctor.** Some drugs can cause headaches.

See a doctor immediately. Such headaches may be a symptom of ANXIETY (p. 718), HIGH BLOOD PRESSURE (p. 574), or, in very rare cases, a BRAIN TUMOR (p. 682). They can also indicate CARBON MONOXIDE POISONING (p. 72).

NO ↓

Go to next page

Continued from previous page

Do you or did you recently have a stuffy or runny nose? 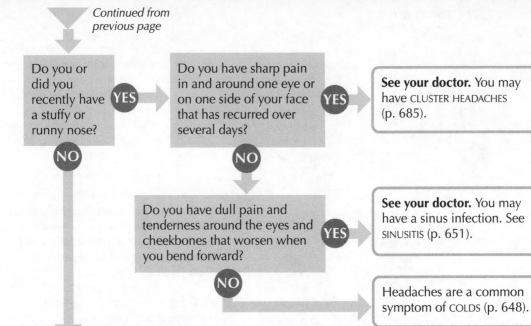 **YES** → Do you have sharp pain in and around one eye or on one side of your face that has recurred over several days? **YES** → **See your doctor.** You may have CLUSTER HEADACHES (p. 685).

NO ↓ (from first box)

NO ↓ (from second box)

Do you have dull pain and tenderness around the eyes and cheekbones that worsen when you bend forward? **YES** → **See your doctor.** You may have a sinus infection. See SINUSITIS (p. 651).

NO ↓

Headaches are a common symptom of COLDS (p. 648).

Are you feeling anxious or under stress, or are you having difficulty sleeping? **YES** → **See your doctor.** Anxiety, stress, and lack of sleep often cause headaches. See the chapter REDUCING STRESS (p. 55). See also the chart ANXIETY, p. 243.

NO ↓

Did the headache occur after you had been reading or doing close-up work such as sewing? **YES** → **Talk to your doctor.** Strain on your neck muscles may have caused a TENSION HEADACHE (p. 683). **See your eye doctor** if you wear glasses; you may need a new prescription.

NO ↓

Did any of the following occur within the 12 hours before your headache started?
• You were exposed to strong sunlight.
• You were in stuffy, smoky, or noisy surroundings.
• You drank more alcohol than usual.
• You missed a meal.
YES → These factors often bring on headaches. See TENSION HEADACHES (p. 683) or MIGRAINES (p. 684).

NO ↓

See your doctor if you are unable to make a diagnosis from this chart and your headache persists overnight or if you develop other symptoms.

Numbness or tingling

Loss of feeling or a prickly sensation in any part of the body.

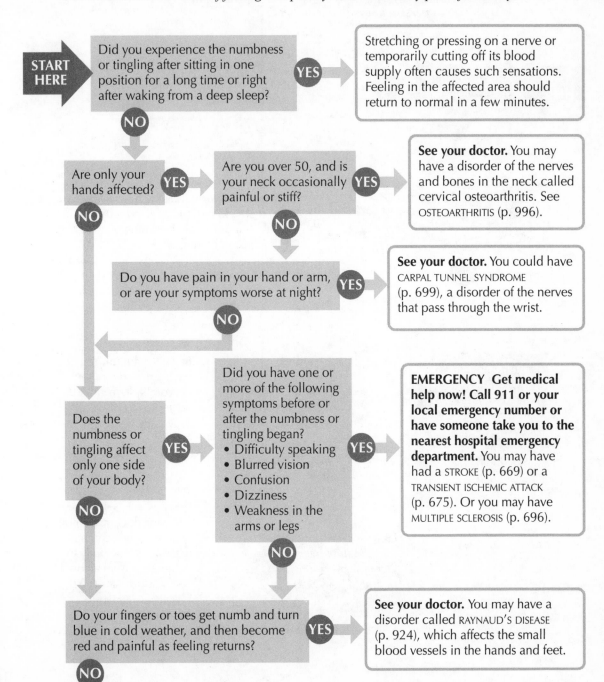

START HERE

Did you experience the numbness or tingling after sitting in one position for a long time or right after waking from a deep sleep?

YES → Stretching or pressing on a nerve or temporarily cutting off its blood supply often causes such sensations. Feeling in the affected area should return to normal in a few minutes.

NO

Are only your hands affected? **YES** → Are you over 50, and is your neck occasionally painful or stiff? **YES** → **See your doctor.** You may have a disorder of the nerves and bones in the neck called cervical osteoarthritis. See OSTEOARTHRITIS (p. 996).

NO

NO

Do you have pain in your hand or arm, or are your symptoms worse at night? **YES** → **See your doctor.** You could have CARPAL TUNNEL SYNDROME (p. 699), a disorder of the nerves that pass through the wrist.

NO

Does the numbness or tingling affect only one side of your body? **YES** → Did you have one or more of the following symptoms before or after the numbness or tingling began?
• Difficulty speaking
• Blurred vision
• Confusion
• Dizziness
• Weakness in the arms or legs
YES → **EMERGENCY Get medical help now! Call 911 or your local emergency number or have someone take you to the nearest hospital emergency department.** You may have had a STROKE (p. 669) or a TRANSIENT ISCHEMIC ATTACK (p. 675). Or you may have MULTIPLE SCLEROSIS (p. 696).

NO

NO

Do your fingers or toes get numb and turn blue in cold weather, and then become red and painful as feeling returns? **YES** → **See your doctor.** You may have a disorder called RAYNAUD'S DISEASE (p. 924), which affects the small blood vessels in the hands and feet.

NO

See your doctor if you are unable to make a diagnosis from this chart.

Twitching and trembling

Involuntary muscle movements including sudden, brief twitching and persistent trembling or shaking.

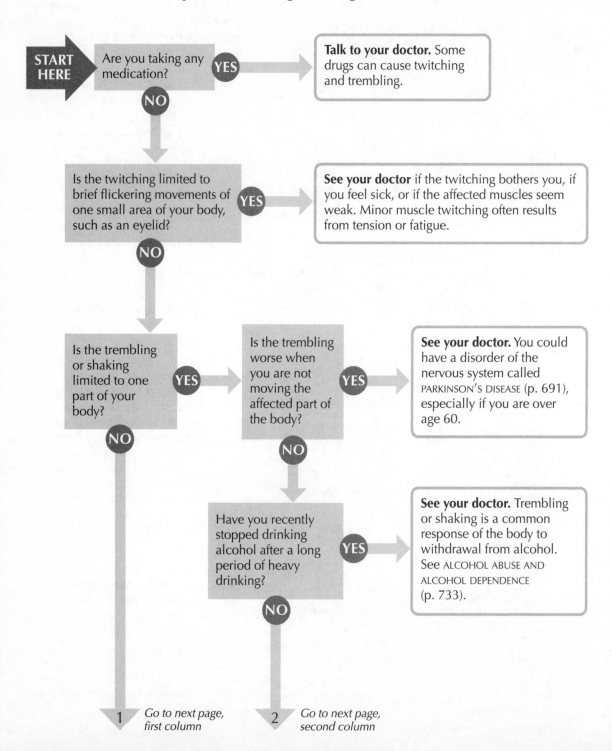

START HERE → Are you taking any medication?

YES → **Talk to your doctor.** Some drugs can cause twitching and trembling.

NO ↓

Is the twitching limited to brief flickering movements of one small area of your body, such as an eyelid?

YES → **See your doctor** if the twitching bothers you, if you feel sick, or if the affected muscles seem weak. Minor muscle twitching often results from tension or fatigue.

NO ↓

Is the trembling or shaking limited to one part of your body?

YES → Is the trembling worse when you are not moving the affected part of the body?

YES → **See your doctor.** You could have a disorder of the nervous system called PARKINSON'S DISEASE (p. 691), especially if you are over age 60.

NO ↓

Have you recently stopped drinking alcohol after a long period of heavy drinking?

YES → **See your doctor.** Trembling or shaking is a common response of the body to withdrawal from alcohol. See ALCOHOL ABUSE AND ALCOHOL DEPENDENCE (p. 733).

NO ↓

1 *Go to next page, first column*

2 *Go to next page, second column*

1 *Continued from previous page, first column*

2 *Continued from previous page, second column*

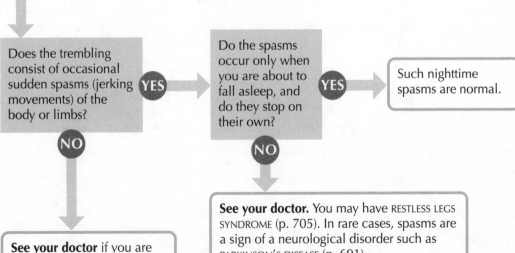

Have you been drinking a lot more caffeine-containing beverages (such as coffee or cola) than usual?

YES → Caffeine is a stimulant and can make you jittery. The trembling should stop when you stop consuming caffeine.

NO ↓

Do you have two or more of the following symptoms?
- Excessive sweating
- Unexplained fatigue
- Bulging eyes
- Unexplained weight loss

YES → **See your doctor.** You may have an overactive thyroid gland. See HYPERTHYROIDISM (p. 901).

NO ↓

Call your doctor. A tendency to tremble or shake can run in families and is often brought on by ANXIETY (p. 718) or stress. See the chapter REDUCING STRESS (p. 55).

Does the trembling consist of occasional sudden spasms (jerking movements) of the body or limbs?

YES → Do the spasms occur only when you are about to fall asleep, and do they stop on their own?

YES → Such nighttime spasms are normal.

NO ↓

See your doctor if you are unable to make a diagnosis from this chart.

NO ↓

See your doctor. You may have RESTLESS LEGS SYNDROME (p. 705). In rare cases, spasms are a sign of a neurological disorder such as PARKINSON'S DISEASE (p. 691).

Pain in the face

Pain in one or both sides of the face or forehead.

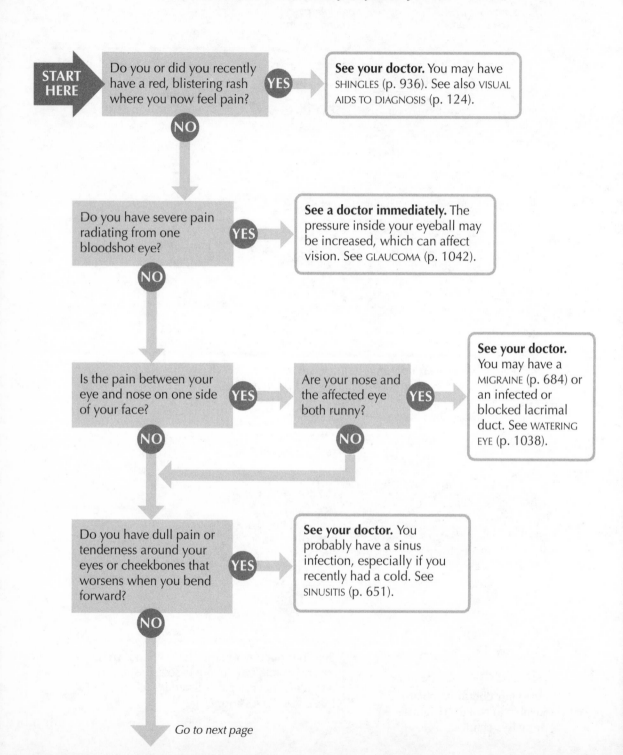

START HERE

Do you or did you recently have a red, blistering rash where you now feel pain?

YES → **See your doctor.** You may have SHINGLES (p. 936). See also VISUAL AIDS TO DIAGNOSIS (p. 124).

NO ↓

Do you have severe pain radiating from one bloodshot eye?

YES → **See a doctor immediately.** The pressure inside your eyeball may be increased, which can affect vision. See GLAUCOMA (p. 1042).

NO ↓

Is the pain between your eye and nose on one side of your face?

YES → Are your nose and the affected eye both runny?

YES → **See your doctor.** You may have a MIGRAINE (p. 684) or an infected or blocked lacrimal duct. See WATERING EYE (p. 1038).

NO ←

NO ↓

Do you have dull pain or tenderness around your eyes or cheekbones that worsens when you bend forward?

YES → **See your doctor.** You probably have a sinus infection, especially if you recently had a cold. See SINUSITIS (p. 651).

NO ↓

Go to next page

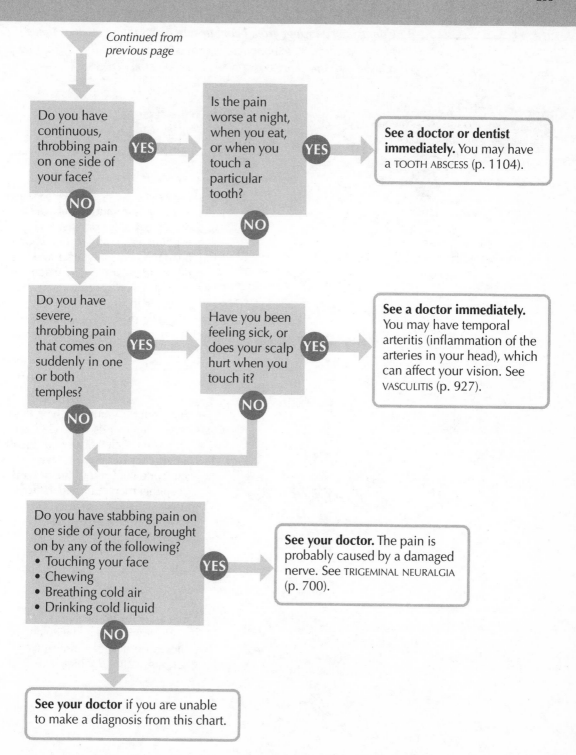

Continued from previous page

Do you have continuous, throbbing pain on one side of your face?

YES → Is the pain worse at night, when you eat, or when you touch a particular tooth?

YES → **See a doctor or dentist immediately.** You may have a TOOTH ABSCESS (p. 1104).

NO

NO

Do you have severe, throbbing pain that comes on suddenly in one or both temples?

YES → Have you been feeling sick, or does your scalp hurt when you touch it?

YES → **See a doctor immediately.** You may have temporal arteritis (inflammation of the arteries in your head), which can affect your vision. See VASCULITIS (p. 927).

NO

NO

Do you have stabbing pain on one side of your face, brought on by any of the following?
• Touching your face
• Chewing
• Breathing cold air
• Drinking cold liquid

YES → **See your doctor.** The pain is probably caused by a damaged nerve. See TRIGEMINAL NEURALGIA (p. 700).

NO

See your doctor if you are unable to make a diagnosis from this chart.

Confusion

Confusion can range from being unsure about things such as times, places, and events to complete loss of contact with reality. If you are over 65, see also the chart CONFUSION IN OLDER PEOPLE, p. 368.

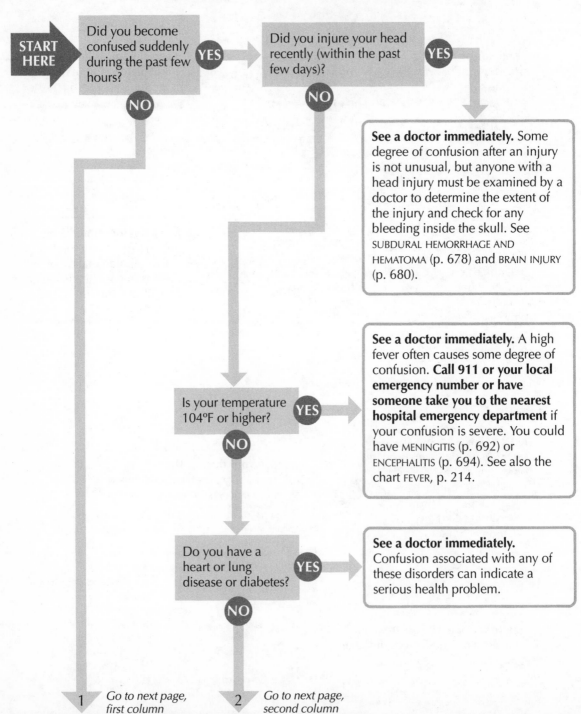

START HERE

Did you become confused suddenly during the past few hours? **YES** → Did you injure your head recently (within the past few days)? **YES** →

See a doctor immediately. Some degree of confusion after an injury is not unusual, but anyone with a head injury must be examined by a doctor to determine the extent of the injury and check for any bleeding inside the skull. See SUBDURAL HEMORRHAGE AND HEMATOMA (p. 678) and BRAIN INJURY (p. 680).

NO ↓ (from "Did you injure your head")

Is your temperature 104°F or higher? **YES** →

See a doctor immediately. A high fever often causes some degree of confusion. **Call 911 or your local emergency number or have someone take you to the nearest hospital emergency department** if your confusion is severe. You could have MENINGITIS (p. 692) or ENCEPHALITIS (p. 694). See also the chart FEVER, p. 214.

NO ↓

Do you have a heart or lung disease or diabetes? **YES** →

See a doctor immediately. Confusion associated with any of these disorders can indicate a serious health problem.

NO ↓

1   *Go to next page, first column*

2   *Go to next page, second column*

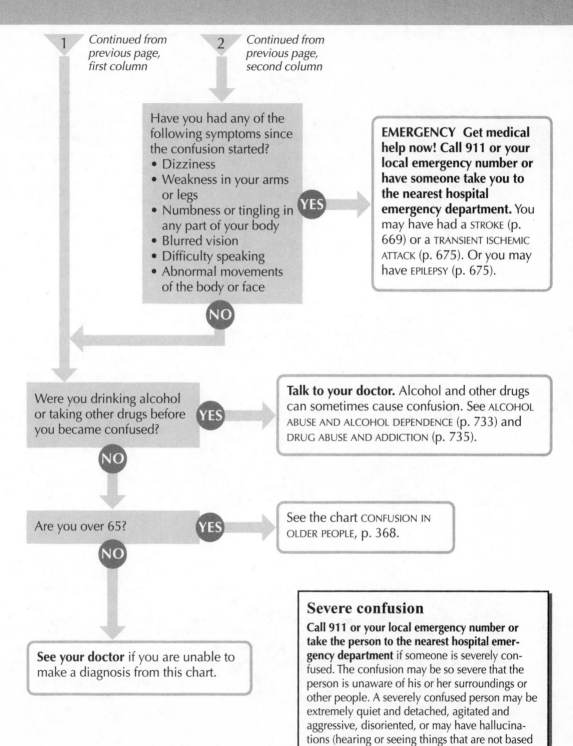

1 Continued from previous page, first column

2 Continued from previous page, second column

Have you had any of the following symptoms since the confusion started?
• Dizziness
• Weakness in your arms or legs
• Numbness or tingling in any part of your body
• Blurred vision
• Difficulty speaking
• Abnormal movements of the body or face

YES

EMERGENCY Get medical help now! Call 911 or your local emergency number or have someone take you to the nearest hospital emergency department. You may have had a STROKE (p. 669) or a TRANSIENT ISCHEMIC ATTACK (p. 675). Or you may have EPILEPSY (p. 675).

NO

Were you drinking alcohol or taking other drugs before you became confused?

YES

Talk to your doctor. Alcohol and other drugs can sometimes cause confusion. See ALCOHOL ABUSE AND ALCOHOL DEPENDENCE (p. 733) and DRUG ABUSE AND ADDICTION (p. 735).

NO

Are you over 65?

YES

See the chart CONFUSION IN OLDER PEOPLE, p. 368.

NO

See your doctor if you are unable to make a diagnosis from this chart.

Severe confusion

Call 911 or your local emergency number or take the person to the nearest hospital emergency department if someone is severely confused. The confusion may be so severe that the person is unaware of his or her surroundings or other people. A severely confused person may be extremely quiet and detached, agitated and aggressive, disoriented, or may have hallucinations (hearing or seeing things that are not based on reality). A severely confused person needs prompt medical attention.

Impaired memory

Difficulty remembering specific facts, events, or periods of time.

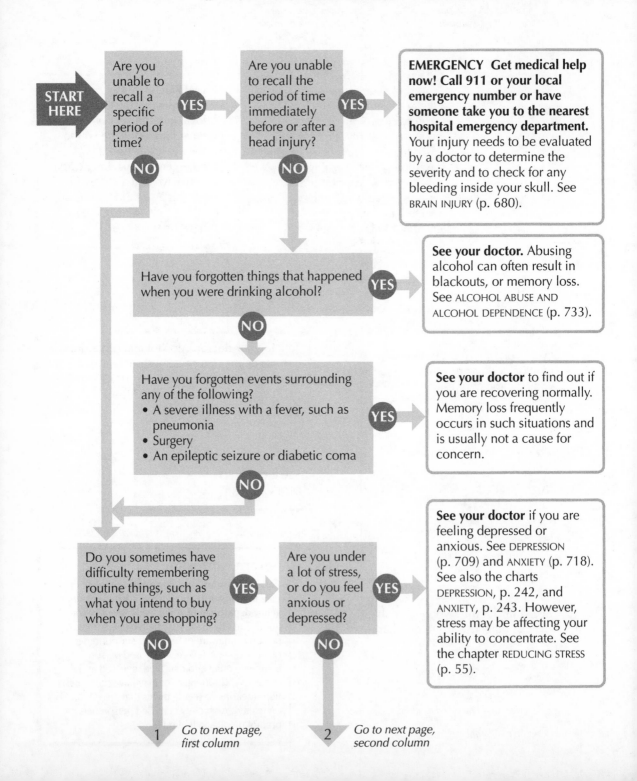

START HERE → Are you unable to recall a specific period of time?

YES → Are you unable to recall the period of time immediately before or after a head injury?

YES → **EMERGENCY Get medical help now! Call 911 or your local emergency number or have someone take you to the nearest hospital emergency department.** Your injury needs to be evaluated by a doctor to determine the severity and to check for any bleeding inside your skull. See BRAIN INJURY (p. 680).

NO ↓

Have you forgotten things that happened when you were drinking alcohol?

YES → **See your doctor.** Abusing alcohol can often result in blackouts, or memory loss. See ALCOHOL ABUSE AND ALCOHOL DEPENDENCE (p. 733).

NO ↓

Have you forgotten events surrounding any of the following?
- A severe illness with a fever, such as pneumonia
- Surgery
- An epileptic seizure or diabetic coma

YES → **See your doctor** to find out if you are recovering normally. Memory loss frequently occurs in such situations and is usually not a cause for concern.

NO ↓

Do you sometimes have difficulty remembering routine things, such as what you intend to buy when you are shopping?

YES → Are you under a lot of stress, or do you feel anxious or depressed?

YES → **See your doctor** if you are feeling depressed or anxious. See DEPRESSION (p. 709) and ANXIETY (p. 718). See also the charts DEPRESSION, p. 242, and ANXIETY, p. 243. However, stress may be affecting your ability to concentrate. See the chapter REDUCING STRESS (p. 55).

NO ↓ 1 — *Go to next page, first column*

NO ↓ 2 — *Go to next page, second column*

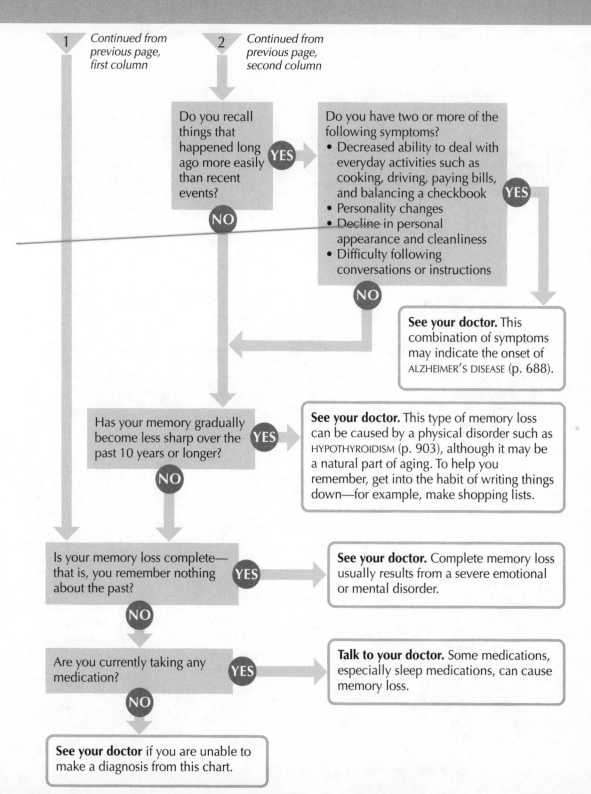

1 *Continued from previous page, first column*

2 *Continued from previous page, second column*

Do you recall things that happened long ago more easily than recent events?

YES →

Do you have two or more of the following symptoms?
• Decreased ability to deal with everyday activities such as cooking, driving, paying bills, and balancing a checkbook
• Personality changes
• Decline in personal appearance and cleanliness
• Difficulty following conversations or instructions

YES →

See your doctor. This combination of symptoms may indicate the onset of ALZHEIMER'S DISEASE (p. 688).

NO

NO

Has your memory gradually become less sharp over the past 10 years or longer?

YES →

See your doctor. This type of memory loss can be caused by a physical disorder such as HYPOTHYROIDISM (p. 903), although it may be a natural part of aging. To help you remember, get into the habit of writing things down—for example, make shopping lists.

NO

Is your memory loss complete—that is, you remember nothing about the past?

YES →

See your doctor. Complete memory loss usually results from a severe emotional or mental disorder.

NO

Are you currently taking any medication?

YES →

Talk to your doctor. Some medications, especially sleep medications, can cause memory loss.

NO

See your doctor if you are unable to make a diagnosis from this chart.

GENERAL
All ages

Difficulty speaking

Difficulty choosing, using, or pronouncing words.

START HERE

Have you had one or more of the following symptoms?
- Dizziness
- Headache
- Weakness in your arms or legs
- Numbness or tingling in any part of your body
- Blurred vision
- Difficulty swallowing

 YES →

EMERGENCY Get medical help now! Call 911 or your local emergency number or have someone take you to the nearest hospital emergency department. You may have had a STROKE (p. 669) or a TRANSIENT ISCHEMIC ATTACK (p. 675).

NO ↓

Do you think that you are pronouncing words correctly but what you say does not seem to make sense to others?

 YES →

Do you have two or more of the following symptoms?
- Decreased ability to deal with everyday activities such as cooking, driving, paying bills, and balancing a checkbook
- Decline in personal appearance or cleanliness
- Difficulty following complex conversations and instructions

YES →

NO ↓

See your doctor. You may have a mental disorder such as SCHIZOPHRENIA (p. 728).

NO ↓

See your doctor. This combination of symptoms may indicate the onset of ALZHEIMER'S DISEASE (p. 688). In rare cases, these symptoms can result from a BRAIN TUMOR (p. 682) or STROKE (p. 669).

Is it difficult to speak because of pain inside your mouth or in your tongue?

 YES →

See the chart SORE MOUTH OR TONGUE, p. 276.

NO ↓

Have you been drinking alcohol?

 YES →

Drinking can make you slur your speech.

 NO ↓

Go to next page

Continued from previous page

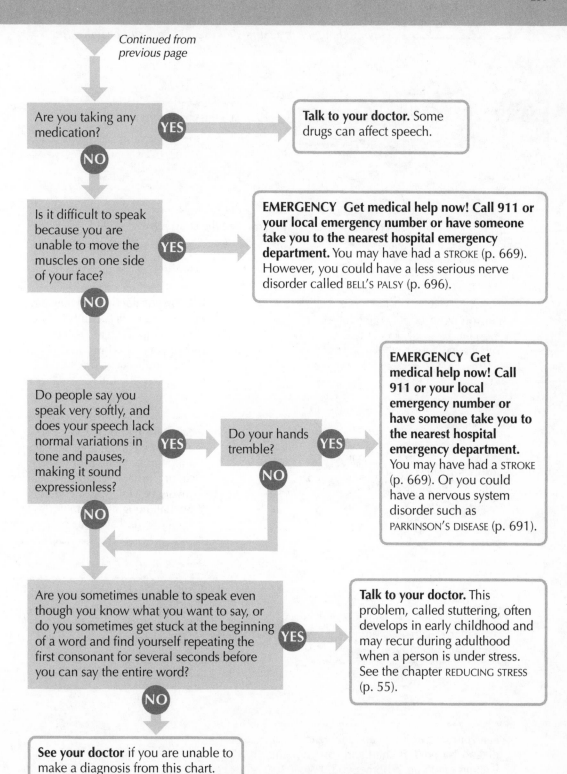

Are you taking any medication?

YES → **Talk to your doctor.** Some drugs can affect speech.

NO ↓

Is it difficult to speak because you are unable to move the muscles on one side of your face?

YES → **EMERGENCY Get medical help now! Call 911 or your local emergency number or have someone take you to the nearest hospital emergency department.** You may have had a STROKE (p. 669). However, you could have a less serious nerve disorder called BELL'S PALSY (p. 696).

NO ↓

Do people say you speak very softly, and does your speech lack normal variations in tone and pauses, making it sound expressionless?

YES → **Do your hands tremble?**

YES → **EMERGENCY Get medical help now! Call 911 or your local emergency number or have someone take you to the nearest hospital emergency department.** You may have had a STROKE (p. 669). Or you could have a nervous system disorder such as PARKINSON'S DISEASE (p. 691).

NO ↓

Are you sometimes unable to speak even though you know what you want to say, or do you sometimes get stuck at the beginning of a word and find yourself repeating the first consonant for several seconds before you can say the entire word?

YES → **Talk to your doctor.** This problem, called stuttering, often develops in early childhood and may recur during adulthood when a person is under stress. See the chapter REDUCING STRESS (p. 55).

NO ↓

See your doctor if you are unable to make a diagnosis from this chart.

Disturbing thoughts or feelings

Having thoughts or feelings that seem abnormal or unhealthy.

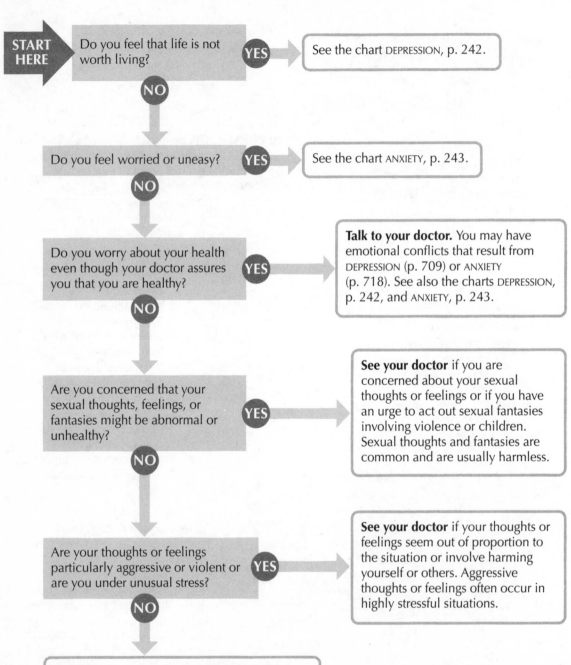

START HERE

Do you feel that life is not worth living? **YES** → See the chart DEPRESSION, p. 242.

NO

Do you feel worried or uneasy? **YES** → See the chart ANXIETY, p. 243.

NO

Do you worry about your health even though your doctor assures you that you are healthy? **YES** → **Talk to your doctor.** You may have emotional conflicts that result from DEPRESSION (p. 709) or ANXIETY (p. 718). See also the charts DEPRESSION, p. 242, and ANXIETY, p. 243.

NO

Are you concerned that your sexual thoughts, feelings, or fantasies might be abnormal or unhealthy? **YES** → **See your doctor** if you are concerned about your sexual thoughts or feelings or if you have an urge to act out sexual fantasies involving violence or children. Sexual thoughts and fantasies are common and are usually harmless.

NO

Are your thoughts or feelings particularly aggressive or violent or are you under unusual stress? **YES** → **See your doctor** if your thoughts or feelings seem out of proportion to the situation or involve harming yourself or others. Aggressive thoughts or feelings often occur in highly stressful situations.

NO

See your doctor if you are unable to make a diagnosis from this chart and your thoughts or feelings continue to bother you.

Unusual behavior

Behavior that is significantly different from a person's usual behavior.

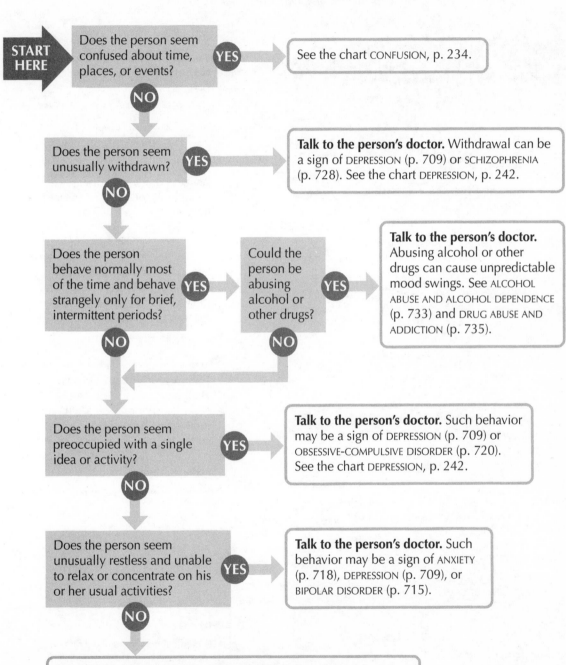

START HERE

Does the person seem confused about time, places, or events?

YES → See the chart CONFUSION, p. 234.

NO ↓

Does the person seem unusually withdrawn?

YES → **Talk to the person's doctor.** Withdrawal can be a sign of DEPRESSION (p. 709) or SCHIZOPHRENIA (p. 728). See the chart DEPRESSION, p. 242.

NO ↓

Does the person behave normally most of the time and behave strangely only for brief, intermittent periods?

YES → Could the person be abusing alcohol or other drugs?

YES → **Talk to the person's doctor.** Abusing alcohol or other drugs can cause unpredictable mood swings. See ALCOHOL ABUSE AND ALCOHOL DEPENDENCE (p. 733) and DRUG ABUSE AND ADDICTION (p. 735).

NO   **NO**

Does the person seem preoccupied with a single idea or activity?

YES → **Talk to the person's doctor.** Such behavior may be a sign of DEPRESSION (p. 709) or OBSESSIVE-COMPULSIVE DISORDER (p. 720). See the chart DEPRESSION, p. 242.

NO ↓

Does the person seem unusually restless and unable to relax or concentrate on his or her usual activities?

YES → **Talk to the person's doctor.** Such behavior may be a sign of ANXIETY (p. 718), DEPRESSION (p. 709), or BIPOLAR DISORDER (p. 715).

NO ↓

Take the person to a doctor immediately if you are unable to make a diagnosis from this chart. There is a chance that a BRAIN TUMOR (p. 682) could be causing the person's unusual behavior.

Depression

A mood disorder characterized by feelings of sadness, hopelessness, and helplessness, usually combined with poor self-esteem, apathy, and withdrawal from social situations.

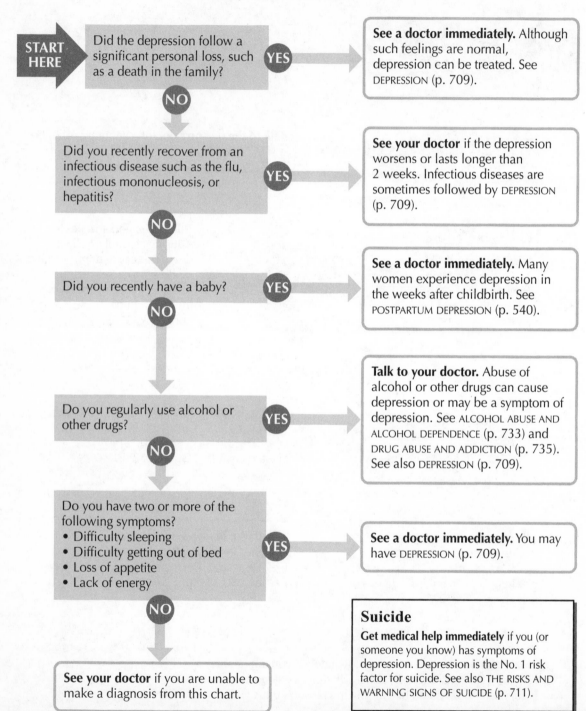

START HERE

Did the depression follow a significant personal loss, such as a death in the family?

YES → **See a doctor immediately.** Although such feelings are normal, depression can be treated. See DEPRESSION (p. 709).

NO ↓

Did you recently recover from an infectious disease such as the flu, infectious mononucleosis, or hepatitis?

YES → **See your doctor** if the depression worsens or lasts longer than 2 weeks. Infectious diseases are sometimes followed by DEPRESSION (p. 709).

NO ↓

Did you recently have a baby?

YES → **See a doctor immediately.** Many women experience depression in the weeks after childbirth. See POSTPARTUM DEPRESSION (p. 540).

NO ↓

Do you regularly use alcohol or other drugs?

YES → **Talk to your doctor.** Abuse of alcohol or other drugs can cause depression or may be a symptom of depression. See ALCOHOL ABUSE AND ALCOHOL DEPENDENCE (p. 733) and DRUG ABUSE AND ADDICTION (p. 735). See also DEPRESSION (p. 709).

NO ↓

Do you have two or more of the following symptoms?
- Difficulty sleeping
- Difficulty getting out of bed
- Loss of appetite
- Lack of energy

YES → **See a doctor immediately.** You may have DEPRESSION (p. 709).

NO ↓

See your doctor if you are unable to make a diagnosis from this chart.

Suicide

Get medical help immediately if you (or someone you know) has symptoms of depression. Depression is the No. 1 risk factor for suicide. See also THE RISKS AND WARNING SIGNS OF SUICIDE (p. 711).

GENERAL
All ages

Anxiety

A feeling of tension, apprehension, or edginess, sometimes accompanied by physical symptoms such as palpitations (heartbeats that you're aware of) or diarrhea.

START HERE

Do you feel anxious most of the time? → **YES** → **Have you been feeling anxious only since giving up cigarettes, alcohol, or drugs such as sleep medications?** → **YES** →

NO ↓ (from first question)

NO ↓ (from second question)

Talk to your doctor. Anxiety often follows the sudden withdrawal of tobacco, alcohol, or other drugs. See HOW TO QUIT SMOKING (p. 29), ALCOHOL ABUSE AND ALCOHOL DEPENDENCE (p. 733), and DRUG ABUSE AND ADDICTION (p. 735).

Have you lost weight, or do your eyes seem to be bulging? **YES** → **See your doctor.** You may have an overactive thyroid gland. See HYPERTHYROIDISM (p. 901).

NO ↓

See your doctor. Your anxiety may be brought on by stress. See ANXIETY (p. 718). See also the chapter REDUCING STRESS (p. 55).

Do you feel anxious only in specific situations—for example, when you are in a confined space or when you are unable to do things a certain way? **YES** → **See your doctor.** Your anxiety may result from a PHOBIA (p. 721) or from OBSESSIVE-COMPULSIVE DISORDER (p. 720).

NO ↓

See your doctor if you are unable to make a diagnosis from this chart.

Panic attacks

In some people, severe anxiety can lead to sudden episodes of overwhelming fear called panic attacks, which produce symptoms such as light-headedness, shortness of breath, chest pain, palpitations, sweating, or numbness or tingling in the hands. Because the symptoms are similar to those of a heart attack, a panic attack is sometimes mistaken for a heart attack. If you have these symptoms (and have never had a panic attack before), suspect a heart attack. **Call 911 or your local emergency number or have someone take you to the nearest hospital emergency department.**

Hallucinations

*Abnormal sensory perceptions that occur without an external stimulus
and are not based on reality.*

START HERE

Do you have one or more of the following symptoms?
- General confusion about time, places, or events
- Agitated behavior
- Signs of physical illness

YES → **See a doctor immediately.** You could be experiencing delirium. See the chart CONFUSION, p. 234.

NO ↓

Do the hallucinations occur only just before you fall asleep or just after you wake up?

YES → It is normal for hallucinations to occur at the point between sleeping and waking.

NO ↓

Do you drink a lot of alcohol, or do you use illegal drugs?

YES → **Talk to your doctor.** Abuse of alcohol or other drugs can cause hallucinations. See ALCOHOL ABUSE AND ALCOHOL DEPENDENCE (p. 733) and DRUG ABUSE AND ADDICTION (p. 735).

NO ↓

Did you think that you saw or heard a close relative or friend who died recently?

YES → **Talk to your doctor,** although this type of hallucination often occurs as part of the grieving process.

NO ↓

Do you hear voices?

YES → **See a doctor immediately.** Hearing voices may be a sign of a mood disorder or a psychotic disorder, especially if the hallucinations are accompanied by feelings of guilt. See DEPRESSION (p. 709), SCHIZOPHRENIA (p. 728), and DELUSIONAL DISORDER (p. 729).

NO ↓

See your doctor if you are unable to make a diagnosis from this chart.

Nightmares

Frightening dreams that may be disturbing enough to wake you.

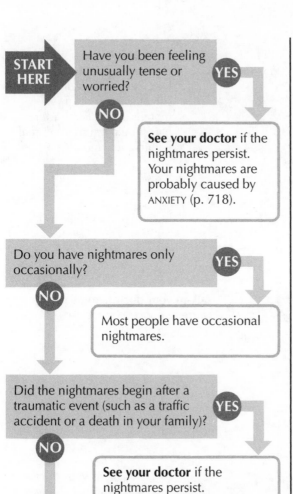

START HERE

Have you been feeling unusually tense or worried?

YES → **See your doctor** if the nightmares persist. Your nightmares are probably caused by ANXIETY (p. 718).

NO ↓

Do you have nightmares only occasionally?

YES → Most people have occasional nightmares.

NO ↓

Did the nightmares begin after a traumatic event (such as a traffic accident or a death in your family)?

YES → **See your doctor** if the nightmares persist. Nightmares often follow such experiences and usually stop within a few weeks.

NO ↓

Do you have a physical illness such as a viral infection?

 YES → Vivid dreams are common during illness, especially when a person has a fever.

NO ↓

Go to next column

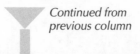 *Continued from previous column*

Have you recently stopped taking sleep medication?

 YES → **See your doctor** about stopping your medication gradually and safely. Stopping sleep medication too quickly is a common cause of nightmares. Your dreams should return to normal in a few days.

NO ↓

Have you recently been drinking more alcohol than usual, or have you recently stopped drinking?

 YES → **See your doctor.** Drinking large quantities of alcohol or suddenly stopping drinking after drinking for a long time can disturb sleep patterns and cause nightmares.

NO ↓

Are you currently taking any medication?

 YES → **Talk to your doctor.** Some drugs can cause nightmares.

NO ↓

See your doctor if you are unable to make a diagnosis from this chart and your nightmares persist.

Hair loss

Thinning of hair or hair loss on all or part of the head.

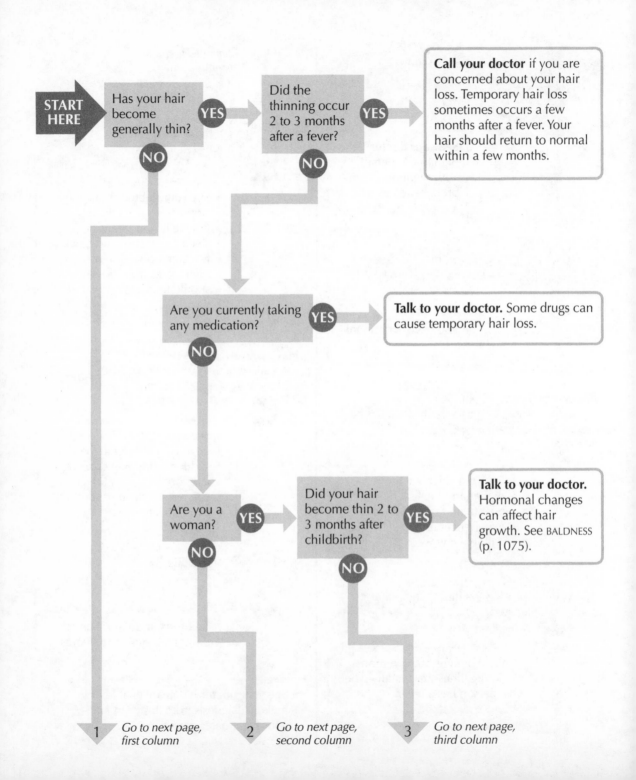

START HERE

Has your hair become generally thin? — YES → **Did the thinning occur 2 to 3 months after a fever?** — YES → **Call your doctor** if you are concerned about your hair loss. Temporary hair loss sometimes occurs a few months after a fever. Your hair should return to normal within a few months.

NO ↓

NO ↓

Are you currently taking any medication? — YES → **Talk to your doctor.** Some drugs can cause temporary hair loss.

NO ↓

Are you a woman? — YES → **Did your hair become thin 2 to 3 months after childbirth?** — YES → **Talk to your doctor.** Hormonal changes can affect hair growth. See BALDNESS (p. 1075).

NO ↓

NO ↓

1 | *Go to next page, first column*

2 | *Go to next page, second column*

3 | *Go to next page, third column*

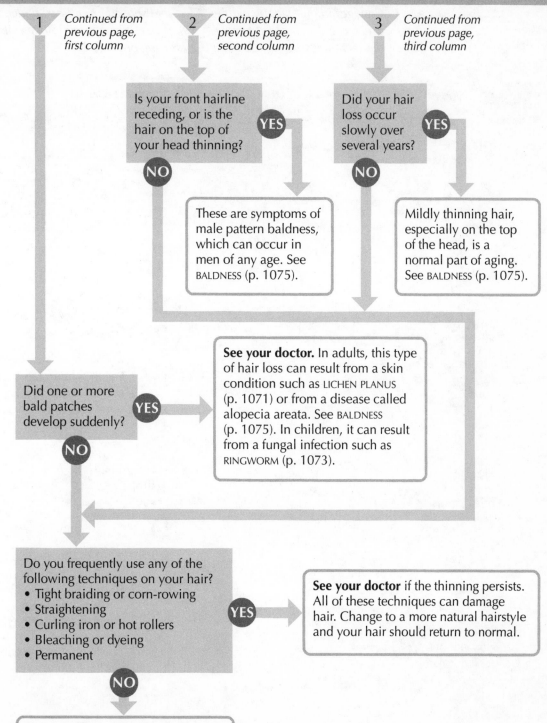

1 *Continued from previous page, first column*

2 *Continued from previous page, second column*

3 *Continued from previous page, third column*

Is your front hairline receding, or is the hair on the top of your head thinning?

YES →

These are symptoms of male pattern baldness, which can occur in men of any age. See BALDNESS (p. 1075).

Did your hair loss occur slowly over several years?

YES →

Mildly thinning hair, especially on the top of the head, is a normal part of aging. See BALDNESS (p. 1075).

NO

NO

Did one or more bald patches develop suddenly?

YES →

See your doctor. In adults, this type of hair loss can result from a skin condition such as LICHEN PLANUS (p. 1071) or from a disease called alopecia areata. See BALDNESS (p. 1075). In children, it can result from a fungal infection such as RINGWORM (p. 1073).

NO

Do you frequently use any of the following techniques on your hair?
• Tight braiding or corn-rowing
• Straightening
• Curling iron or hot rollers
• Bleaching or dyeing
• Permanent

YES →

See your doctor if the thinning persists. All of these techniques can damage hair. Change to a more natural hairstyle and your hair should return to normal.

NO

See your doctor if you are unable to make a diagnosis from this chart.

General skin problems

Changes in the skin, including rashes and spots. For children under 2 years, see the chart SKIN PROBLEMS IN YOUNG CHILDREN, p. 350. See also the section VISUAL AIDS TO DIAGNOSIS starting on page 117.

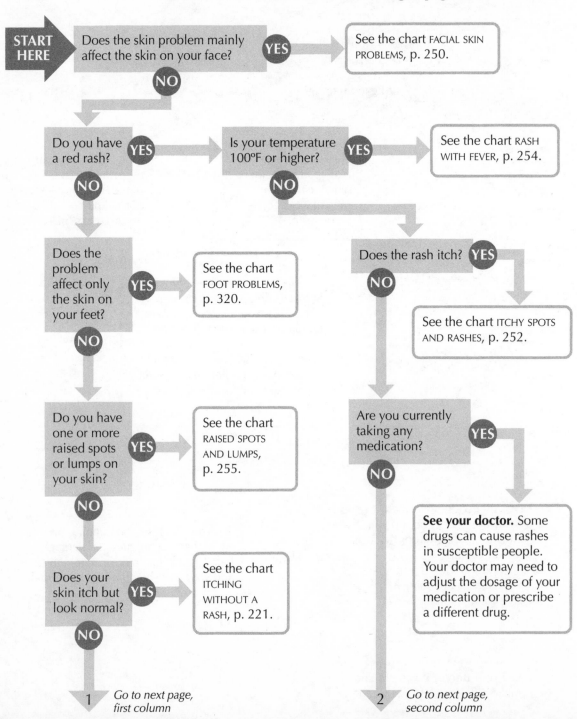

START HERE

Does the skin problem mainly affect the skin on your face?

YES → See the chart FACIAL SKIN PROBLEMS, p. 250.

NO

Do you have a red rash?

YES → Is your temperature 100°F or higher?

YES → See the chart RASH WITH FEVER, p. 254.

NO

Does the problem affect only the skin on your feet?

YES → See the chart FOOT PROBLEMS, p. 320.

NO

Do you have one or more raised spots or lumps on your skin?

YES → See the chart RAISED SPOTS AND LUMPS, p. 255.

NO

Does your skin itch but look normal?

YES → See the chart ITCHING WITHOUT A RASH, p. 221.

NO

Does the rash itch?

YES →

NO

See the chart ITCHY SPOTS AND RASHES, p. 252.

Are you currently taking any medication?

YES →

NO

See your doctor. Some drugs can cause rashes in susceptible people. Your doctor may need to adjust the dosage of your medication or prescribe a different drug.

1 *Go to next page, first column*

2 *Go to next page, second column*

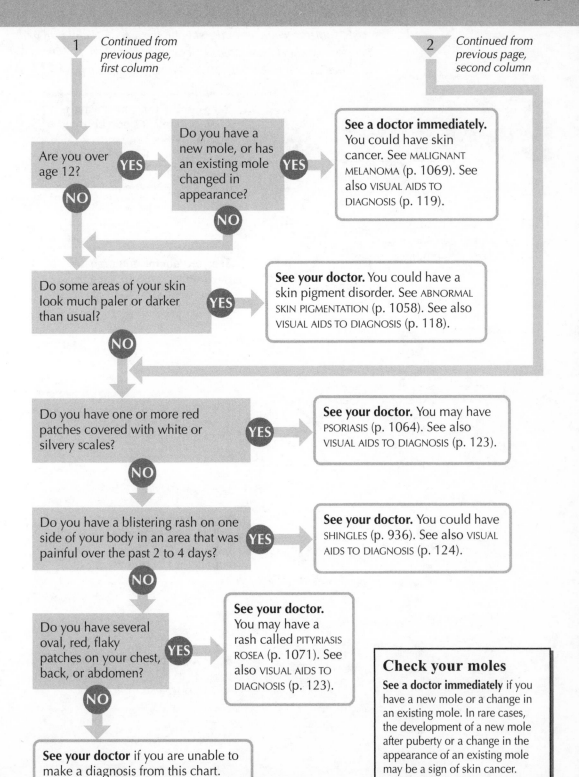

1 *Continued from previous page, first column*

2 *Continued from previous page, second column*

Are you over age 12?

YES → Do you have a new mole, or has an existing mole changed in appearance?

YES → **See a doctor immediately.** You could have skin cancer. See MALIGNANT MELANOMA (p. 1069). See also VISUAL AIDS TO DIAGNOSIS (p. 119).

NO / **NO**

Do some areas of your skin look much paler or darker than usual?

YES → **See your doctor.** You could have a skin pigment disorder. See ABNORMAL SKIN PIGMENTATION (p. 1058). See also VISUAL AIDS TO DIAGNOSIS (p. 118).

NO

Do you have one or more red patches covered with white or silvery scales?

YES → **See your doctor.** You may have PSORIASIS (p. 1064). See also VISUAL AIDS TO DIAGNOSIS (p. 123).

NO

Do you have a blistering rash on one side of your body in an area that was painful over the past 2 to 4 days?

YES → **See your doctor.** You could have SHINGLES (p. 936). See also VISUAL AIDS TO DIAGNOSIS (p. 124).

NO

Do you have several oval, red, flaky patches on your chest, back, or abdomen?

YES → **See your doctor.** You may have a rash called PITYRIASIS ROSEA (p. 1071). See also VISUAL AIDS TO DIAGNOSIS (p. 123).

NO

See your doctor if you are unable to make a diagnosis from this chart.

Check your moles

See a doctor immediately if you have a new mole or a change in an existing mole. In rare cases, the development of a new mole after puberty or a change in the appearance of an existing mole may be a sign of skin cancer.

Facial skin problems

*Any rash, spots, or changes in the skin on the face. For children under
2 years, see the chart SKIN PROBLEMS IN YOUNG CHILDREN, p. 350.
See also the section VISUAL AIDS TO DIAGNOSIS starting on page 117.*

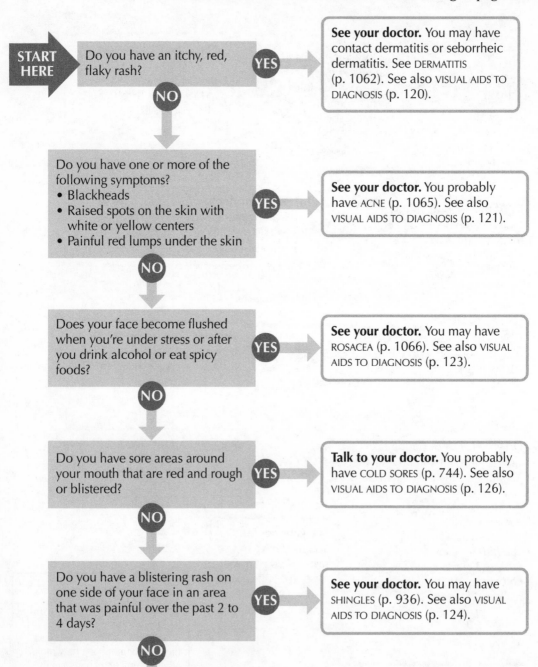

START HERE

Do you have an itchy, red, flaky rash?

YES → **See your doctor.** You may have contact dermatitis or seborrheic dermatitis. See DERMATITIS (p. 1062). See also VISUAL AIDS TO DIAGNOSIS (p. 120).

NO ↓

Do you have one or more of the following symptoms?
• Blackheads
• Raised spots on the skin with white or yellow centers
• Painful red lumps under the skin

YES → **See your doctor.** You probably have ACNE (p. 1065). See also VISUAL AIDS TO DIAGNOSIS (p. 121).

NO ↓

Does your face become flushed when you're under stress or after you drink alcohol or eat spicy foods?

YES → **See your doctor.** You may have ROSACEA (p. 1066). See also VISUAL AIDS TO DIAGNOSIS (p. 123).

NO ↓

Do you have sore areas around your mouth that are red and rough or blistered?

YES → **Talk to your doctor.** You probably have COLD SORES (p. 744). See also VISUAL AIDS TO DIAGNOSIS (p. 126).

NO ↓

Do you have a blistering rash on one side of your face in an area that was painful over the past 2 to 4 days?

YES → **See your doctor.** You may have SHINGLES (p. 936). See also VISUAL AIDS TO DIAGNOSIS (p. 124).

NO ↓

Go to next page

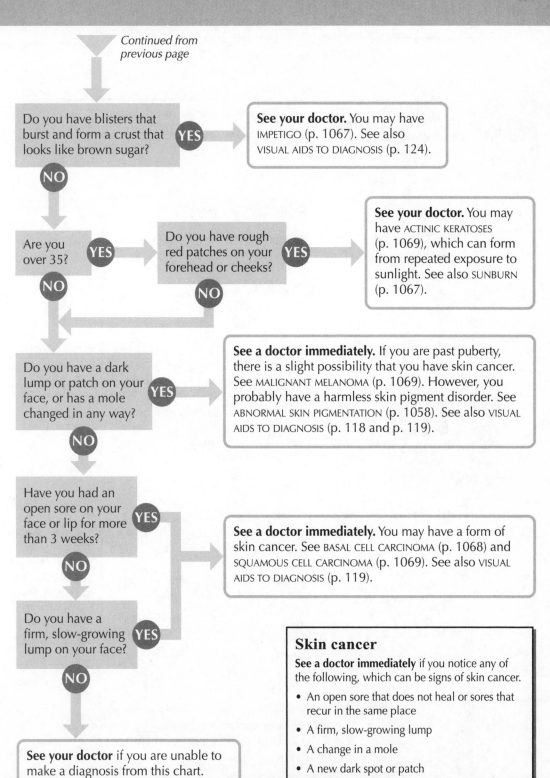

Continued from previous page

Do you have blisters that burst and form a crust that looks like brown sugar?

YES → **See your doctor.** You may have IMPETIGO (p. 1067). See also VISUAL AIDS TO DIAGNOSIS (p. 124).

NO ↓

Are you over 35?

YES → Do you have rough red patches on your forehead or cheeks?

YES → **See your doctor.** You may have ACTINIC KERATOSES (p. 1069), which can form from repeated exposure to sunlight. See also SUNBURN (p. 1067).

NO ↓

NO ↓

Do you have a dark lump or patch on your face, or has a mole changed in any way?

YES → **See a doctor immediately.** If you are past puberty, there is a slight possibility that you have skin cancer. See MALIGNANT MELANOMA (p. 1069). However, you probably have a harmless skin pigment disorder. See ABNORMAL SKIN PIGMENTATION (p. 1058). See also VISUAL AIDS TO DIAGNOSIS (p. 118 and p. 119).

NO ↓

Have you had an open sore on your face or lip for more than 3 weeks?

YES → **See a doctor immediately.** You may have a form of skin cancer. See BASAL CELL CARCINOMA (p. 1068) and SQUAMOUS CELL CARCINOMA (p. 1069). See also VISUAL AIDS TO DIAGNOSIS (p. 119).

NO ↓

Do you have a firm, slow-growing lump on your face?

YES

NO ↓

See your doctor if you are unable to make a diagnosis from this chart.

Skin cancer

See a doctor immediately if you notice any of the following, which can be signs of skin cancer.

- An open sore that does not heal or sores that recur in the same place
- A firm, slow-growing lump
- A change in a mole
- A new dark spot or patch

GENERAL Over 2 years

Itchy spots and rashes

Discolored or raised areas of itchy skin. For children under 2 years, see the chart SKIN PROBLEMS IN YOUNG CHILDREN, p. 350.

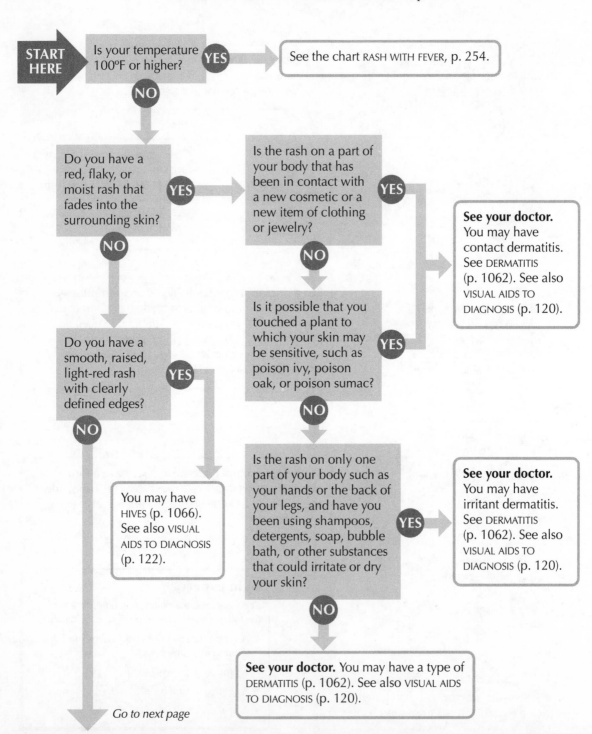

START HERE

Is your temperature 100°F or higher?

YES → See the chart RASH WITH FEVER, p. 254.

NO ↓

Do you have a red, flaky, or moist rash that fades into the surrounding skin?

YES → Is the rash on a part of your body that has been in contact with a new cosmetic or a new item of clothing or jewelry?

YES → **See your doctor.** You may have contact dermatitis. See DERMATITIS (p. 1062). See also VISUAL AIDS TO DIAGNOSIS (p. 120).

NO ↓

Is it possible that you touched a plant to which your skin may be sensitive, such as poison ivy, poison oak, or poison sumac?

YES → (to See your doctor, contact dermatitis)

NO ↓

NO (from red, flaky rash) ↓

Do you have a smooth, raised, light-red rash with clearly defined edges?

YES → You may have HIVES (p. 1066). See also VISUAL AIDS TO DIAGNOSIS (p. 122).

NO ↓

Is the rash on only one part of your body such as your hands or the back of your legs, and have you been using shampoos, detergents, soap, bubble bath, or other substances that could irritate or dry your skin?

YES → **See your doctor.** You may have irritant dermatitis. See DERMATITIS (p. 1062). See also VISUAL AIDS TO DIAGNOSIS (p. 120).

NO ↓

See your doctor. You may have a type of DERMATITIS (p. 1062). See also VISUAL AIDS TO DIAGNOSIS (p. 120).

Go to next page

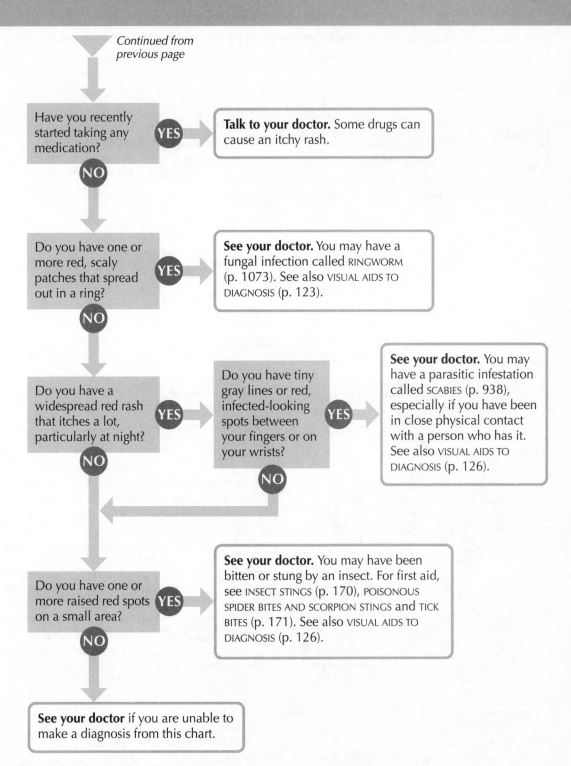

Continued from previous page

Have you recently started taking any medication?

YES → **Talk to your doctor.** Some drugs can cause an itchy rash.

NO ↓

Do you have one or more red, scaly patches that spread out in a ring?

YES → **See your doctor.** You may have a fungal infection called RINGWORM (p. 1073). See also VISUAL AIDS TO DIAGNOSIS (p. 123).

NO ↓

Do you have a widespread red rash that itches a lot, particularly at night?

YES → Do you have tiny gray lines or red, infected-looking spots between your fingers or on your wrists?

YES → **See your doctor.** You may have a parasitic infestation called SCABIES (p. 938), especially if you have been in close physical contact with a person who has it. See also VISUAL AIDS TO DIAGNOSIS (p. 126).

NO ↓

Do you have one or more raised red spots on a small area?

YES → **See your doctor.** You may have been bitten or stung by an insect. For first aid, see INSECT STINGS (p. 170), POISONOUS SPIDER BITES AND SCORPION STINGS and TICK BITES (p. 171). See also VISUAL AIDS TO DIAGNOSIS (p. 126).

NO ↓

See your doctor if you are unable to make a diagnosis from this chart.

Rash with fever

Spots, discolored areas, or blisters on the skin and a temperature of 100°F or higher.

 START HERE

Do you have red spots or blotches on your skin?

YES → Do you have two or more of the following symptoms?
- Runny nose
- Sore, red eyes
- Dry cough

 YES → **See your doctor.** You may have MEASLES (p. 437) or a similar viral infection, especially if the rash is mainly on your face or trunk.

NO ↓

Do you have swelling down the sides of the back of your neck or at the base of your skull?

 YES → **See your doctor.** You may have RUBELLA (p. 438).

NO ↓

NO ↓

Do you have raised, red, itchy spots that turn into blisters? **YES** → **See your doctor.** You may have CHICKENPOX (p. 439).

NO ↓

Do you have one or more reddish brown spots that have become bigger and developed a whitish center? **YES** → **See your doctor.** You may have LYME DISEASE (p. 942), a viral infection that is spread by ticks. For first aid, see TICK BITES (p. 171). See also VISUAL AIDS TO DIAGNOSIS (p. 126).

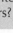 **NO** ↓

Do you have a rash of purple spots? **YES** → Do you have two or more of the following symptoms?
- Vomiting
- Headache
- Sensitivity of eyes to bright light
- Pain when you bend your head forward

YES → **EMERGENCY Get medical help now! Call 911 or your local emergency number or have someone take you to the nearest hospital emergency department.** You could have MENINGITIS (p. 692).

 NO ↓

 NO ↓

 See your doctor if you are unable to make a diagnosis from this chart.

See a doctor immediately. You may have a serious blood disorder called ALLERGIC PURPURA (p. 423).

Raised spots and lumps

Raised areas on the skin that may be inflamed, dark-colored, rough, or hard.

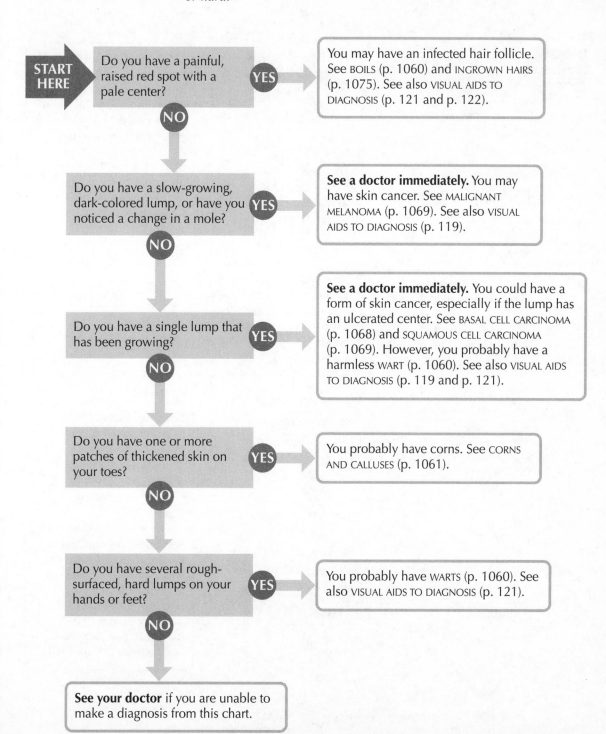

START HERE

Do you have a painful, raised red spot with a pale center?

YES → You may have an infected hair follicle. See BOILS (p. 1060) and INGROWN HAIRS (p. 1075). See also VISUAL AIDS TO DIAGNOSIS (p. 121 and p. 122).

NO ↓

Do you have a slow-growing, dark-colored lump, or have you noticed a change in a mole?

YES → **See a doctor immediately.** You may have skin cancer. See MALIGNANT MELANOMA (p. 1069). See also VISUAL AIDS TO DIAGNOSIS (p. 119).

NO ↓

Do you have a single lump that has been growing?

YES → **See a doctor immediately.** You could have a form of skin cancer, especially if the lump has an ulcerated center. See BASAL CELL CARCINOMA (p. 1068) and SQUAMOUS CELL CARCINOMA (p. 1069). However, you probably have a harmless WART (p. 1060). See also VISUAL AIDS TO DIAGNOSIS (p. 119 and p. 121).

NO ↓

Do you have one or more patches of thickened skin on your toes?

YES → You probably have corns. See CORNS AND CALLUSES (p. 1061).

NO ↓

Do you have several rough-surfaced, hard lumps on your hands or feet?

YES → You probably have WARTS (p. 1060). See also VISUAL AIDS TO DIAGNOSIS (p. 121).

NO ↓

See your doctor if you are unable to make a diagnosis from this chart.

Painful eye

Continuous or intermittent pain in or around the eye.

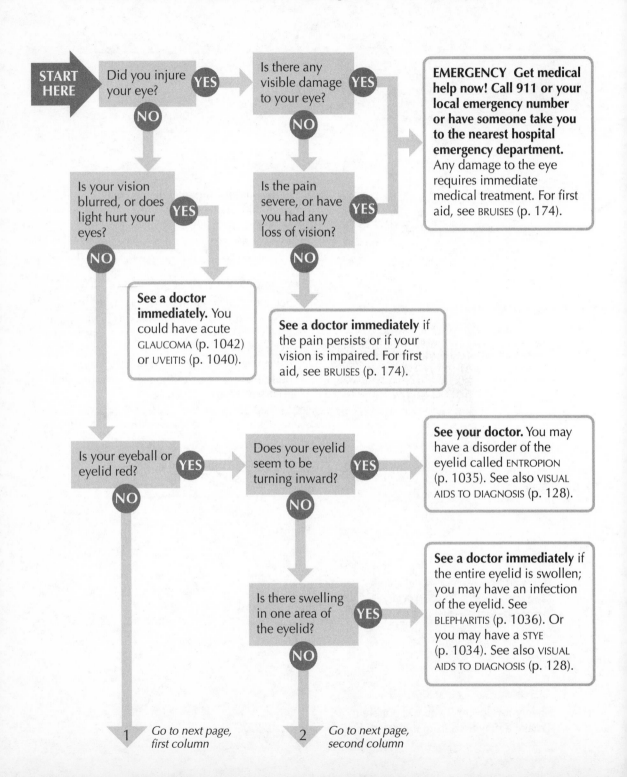

START HERE → Did you injure your eye?

— **YES** → Is there any visible damage to your eye?

— **YES** → **EMERGENCY Get medical help now! Call 911 or your local emergency number or have someone take you to the nearest hospital emergency department.** Any damage to the eye requires immediate medical treatment. For first aid, see BRUISES (p. 174).

— **NO** → Is the pain severe, or have you had any loss of vision?

— **YES** → *(to EMERGENCY box above)*

— **NO** → **See a doctor immediately** if the pain persists or if your vision is impaired. For first aid, see BRUISES (p. 174).

— **NO** → Is your vision blurred, or does light hurt your eyes?

— **YES** → **See a doctor immediately.** You could have acute GLAUCOMA (p. 1042) or UVEITIS (p. 1040).

— **NO** → Is your eyeball or eyelid red?

— **YES** → Does your eyelid seem to be turning inward?

— **YES** → **See your doctor.** You may have a disorder of the eyelid called ENTROPION (p. 1035). See also VISUAL AIDS TO DIAGNOSIS (p. 128).

— **NO** → Is there swelling in one area of the eyelid?

— **YES** → **See a doctor immediately** if the entire eyelid is swollen; you may have an infection of the eyelid. See BLEPHARITIS (p. 1036). Or you may have a STYE (p. 1034). See also VISUAL AIDS TO DIAGNOSIS (p. 128).

— **NO** →

1 *Go to next page, first column*

2 *Go to next page, second column*

1 *Continued from previous page, first column*

2 *Continued from previous page, second column*

Does your eye feel gritty? **YES** → Is your eye sticky? **YES** →

See your doctor. You probably have CONJUNCTIVITIS (p. 1038). See also VISUAL AIDS TO DIAGNOSIS (p. 127).

NO ↓ (gritty)
NO ↓ (sticky)

See your doctor. You may have DRY EYE (p. 1037).

Is your eye watering? **YES** →

You may have a foreign object in your eye. For first aid, see FOREIGN OBJECT IN THE EYE (p. 175). See also WATERING EYE (p. 1038).

NO

Does the pain seem to come from behind your eye? **YES** →

Do you have two or more of the following symptoms?
• Severe headache
• Sensitivity of eyes to bright light
• Pain when you bend your head forward
• Drowsiness or confusion

YES →

EMERGENCY Get medical help now! Call 911 or your local emergency number or have someone take you to the nearest hospital emergency department. You could have MENINGITIS (p. 692) or a SUBARACHNOID HEMORRHAGE (p. 677).

NO ↓

NO ↓

Is there an area of tenderness in the temple above the affected eye? **YES** →

See a doctor immediately. You may have temporal arteritis (inflammation of arteries in the head). See VASCULITIS (p. 927).

NO ↓

Is there an area of tenderness over your nose or in your cheekbones? **YES** →

See a doctor immediately. You may have SINUSITIS (p. 651). Or you may have an infection of the eye socket. See ORBITAL CELLULITIS (p. 1055).

NO ↓

See your doctor if you are unable to make a diagnosis from this chart.

Disturbed or impaired vision

Vision problems, including blurring, double vision, or seeing flashing lights or floating spots.

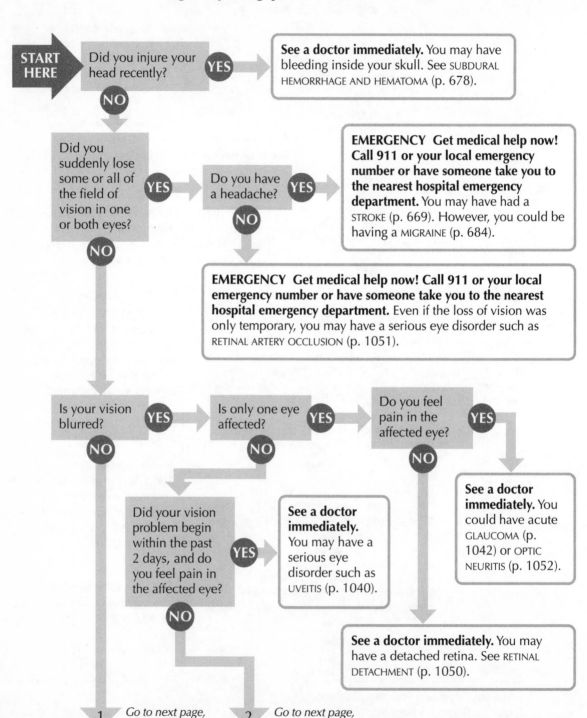

START HERE → Did you injure your head recently? — **YES** → **See a doctor immediately.** You may have bleeding inside your skull. See SUBDURAL HEMORRHAGE AND HEMATOMA (p. 678).

NO ↓

Did you suddenly lose some or all of the field of vision in one or both eyes? — **YES** → Do you have a headache? — **YES** → **EMERGENCY Get medical help now! Call 911 or your local emergency number or have someone take you to the nearest hospital emergency department.** You may have had a STROKE (p. 669). However, you could be having a MIGRAINE (p. 684).

NO ↓ (from headache)

EMERGENCY Get medical help now! Call 911 or your local emergency number or have someone take you to the nearest hospital emergency department. Even if the loss of vision was only temporary, you may have a serious eye disorder such as RETINAL ARTERY OCCLUSION (p. 1051).

NO ↓ (from field of vision)

Is your vision blurred? — **YES** → Is only one eye affected? — **YES** → Do you feel pain in the affected eye? — **YES** → **See a doctor immediately.** You could have acute GLAUCOMA (p. 1042) or OPTIC NEURITIS (p. 1052).

NO ↓ (only one eye affected)

Did your vision problem begin within the past 2 days, and do you feel pain in the affected eye? — **YES** → **See a doctor immediately.** You may have a serious eye disorder such as UVEITIS (p. 1040).

NO ↓ (pain in affected eye)

See a doctor immediately. You may have a detached retina. See RETINAL DETACHMENT (p. 1050).

NO (blurred vision) ↓

1 *Go to next page, first column*

2 *Go to next page, second column*

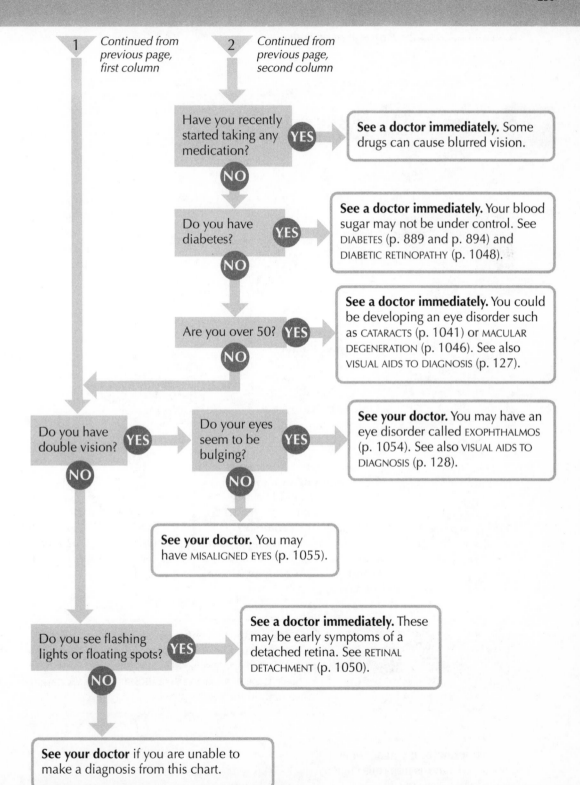

1 Continued from previous page, first column

2 Continued from previous page, second column

Have you recently started taking any medication?
YES → **See a doctor immediately.** Some drugs can cause blurred vision.
NO ↓

Do you have diabetes?
YES → **See a doctor immediately.** Your blood sugar may not be under control. See DIABETES (p. 889 and p. 894) and DIABETIC RETINOPATHY (p. 1048).
NO ↓

Are you over 50?
YES → **See a doctor immediately.** You could be developing an eye disorder such as CATARACTS (p. 1041) or MACULAR DEGENERATION (p. 1046). See also VISUAL AIDS TO DIAGNOSIS (p. 127).
NO ↓

Do you have double vision?
YES → Do your eyes seem to be bulging?
YES → **See your doctor.** You may have an eye disorder called EXOPHTHALMOS (p. 1054). See also VISUAL AIDS TO DIAGNOSIS (p. 128).
NO ↓ (from "Do your eyes seem to be bulging?") → **See your doctor.** You may have MISALIGNED EYES (p. 1055).
NO ↓ (from "Do you have double vision?")

Do you see flashing lights or floating spots?
YES → **See a doctor immediately.** These may be early symptoms of a detached retina. See RETINAL DETACHMENT (p. 1050).
NO ↓

See your doctor if you are unable to make a diagnosis from this chart.

GENERAL
All ages

Earache

Pain in one or both ears.

START HERE

Does the pain get worse when you pull down on your earlobe?

 YES → **See your doctor.** You probably have an INFECTION OF THE EAR CANAL (p. 1025).

NO

Do you have a blocked-up feeling in your ear that cannot be cleared by swallowing?

YES → Did the pain begin after an airplane flight?

 YES → **See a doctor immediately.** Changes in air pressure may have damaged your middle ear. See BAROTRAUMA (p. 1021).

NO

NO

Does the affected ear have a sticky yellow discharge?

 YES → **See your doctor.** You could have an INFECTION OF THE EAR CANAL (p. 1025) or an ACUTE MIDDLE EAR INFECTION (p. 1023).

Has your hearing worsened in the past few weeks or months?

YES → **See your doctor.** You could have an EARWAX BLOCKAGE (p. 1025).

NO

NO

Do you have a cold?

YES → **See your doctor** if the pain is severe; you could have a MIDDLE EAR INFECTION (p. 1023). Earaches are a common symptom of colds that involve the upper respiratory tract, and usually subside when the cold clears up.

See your doctor. You could have an ACUTE MIDDLE EAR INFECTION (p. 1023) or a CHRONIC MIDDLE EAR INFECTION (p. 1023).

NO

Do you also have pain in your teeth, jaw, or neck?

 YES → **See your doctor or dentist.** Tooth and gum problems frequently cause pain in the ear. See TOOTH DECAY (p. 1100) and TEMPOROMANDIBULAR DISORDER (p. 1005). A STRAINED OR TORN MUSCLE (p. 983) in the neck can also cause pain in the ear.

 NO

See your doctor if you are unable to make a diagnosis from this chart.

Noises in the ear

Sounds (such as ringing, buzzing, or hissing) that have no external source and that only you can hear.

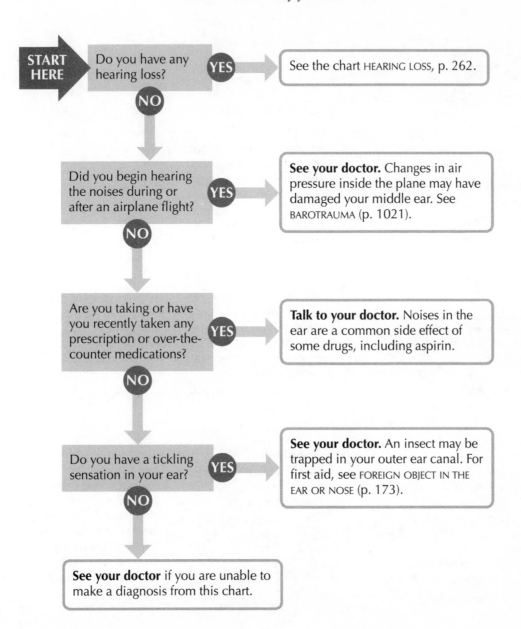

START HERE

Do you have any hearing loss?
YES → See the chart HEARING LOSS, p. 262.

NO ↓

Did you begin hearing the noises during or after an airplane flight?
YES → **See your doctor.** Changes in air pressure inside the plane may have damaged your middle ear. See BAROTRAUMA (p. 1021).

NO ↓

Are you taking or have you recently taken any prescription or over-the-counter medications?
YES → **Talk to your doctor.** Noises in the ear are a common side effect of some drugs, including aspirin.

NO ↓

Do you have a tickling sensation in your ear?
YES → **See your doctor.** An insect may be trapped in your outer ear canal. For first aid, see FOREIGN OBJECT IN THE EAR OR NOSE (p. 173).

NO ↓

See your doctor if you are unable to make a diagnosis from this chart.

Hearing loss

Impaired ability to hear in one or both ears.

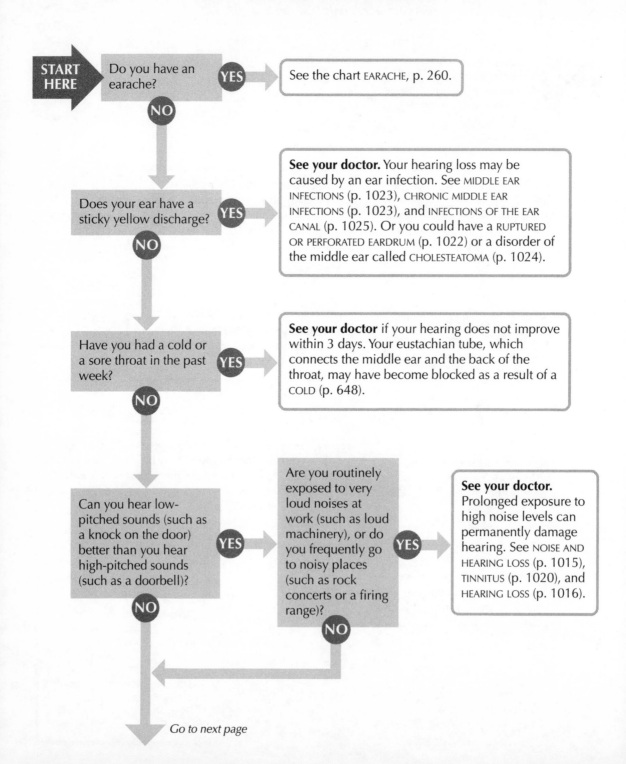

START HERE — Do you have an earache? — **YES** → See the chart EARACHE, p. 260.

NO ↓

Does your ear have a sticky yellow discharge? — **YES** → **See your doctor.** Your hearing loss may be caused by an ear infection. See MIDDLE EAR INFECTIONS (p. 1023), CHRONIC MIDDLE EAR INFECTIONS (p. 1023), and INFECTIONS OF THE EAR CANAL (p. 1025). Or you could have a RUPTURED OR PERFORATED EARDRUM (p. 1022) or a disorder of the middle ear called CHOLESTEATOMA (p. 1024).

NO ↓

Have you had a cold or a sore throat in the past week? — **YES** → **See your doctor** if your hearing does not improve within 3 days. Your eustachian tube, which connects the middle ear and the back of the throat, may have become blocked as a result of a COLD (p. 648).

NO ↓

Can you hear low-pitched sounds (such as a knock on the door) better than you hear high-pitched sounds (such as a doorbell)? — **YES** → Are you routinely exposed to very loud noises at work (such as loud machinery), or do you frequently go to noisy places (such as rock concerts or a firing range)? — **YES** → **See your doctor.** Prolonged exposure to high noise levels can permanently damage hearing. See NOISE AND HEARING LOSS (p. 1015), TINNITUS (p. 1020), and HEARING LOSS (p. 1016).

NO ↓ (from both)

Go to next page

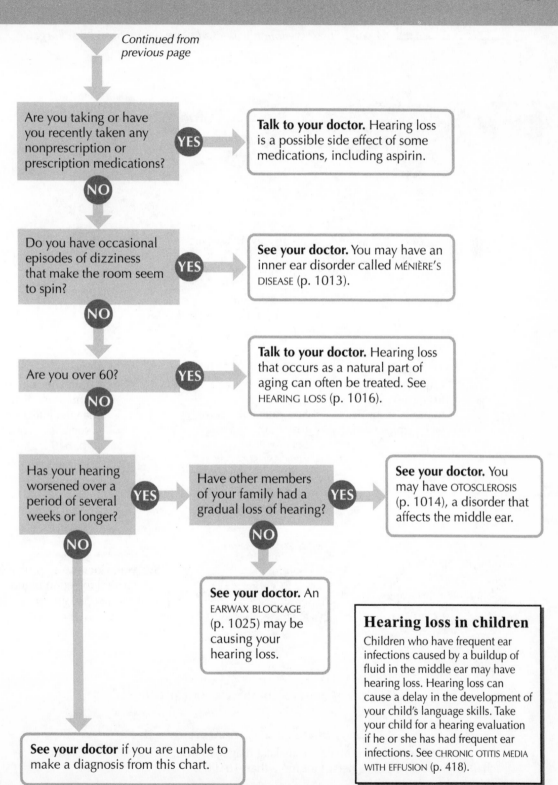

Continued from previous page

Are you taking or have you recently taken any nonprescription or prescription medications?

YES → **Talk to your doctor.** Hearing loss is a possible side effect of some medications, including aspirin.

NO ↓

Do you have occasional episodes of dizziness that make the room seem to spin?

YES → **See your doctor.** You may have an inner ear disorder called MÉNIÈRE'S DISEASE (p. 1013).

NO ↓

Are you over 60?

YES → **Talk to your doctor.** Hearing loss that occurs as a natural part of aging can often be treated. See HEARING LOSS (p. 1016).

NO ↓

Has your hearing worsened over a period of several weeks or longer?

YES → Have other members of your family had a gradual loss of hearing?

YES → **See your doctor.** You may have OTOSCLEROSIS (p. 1014), a disorder that affects the middle ear.

NO ↓

See your doctor. An EARWAX BLOCKAGE (p. 1025) may be causing your hearing loss.

NO ↓

See your doctor if you are unable to make a diagnosis from this chart.

Hearing loss in children

Children who have frequent ear infections caused by a buildup of fluid in the middle ear may have hearing loss. Hearing loss can cause a delay in the development of your child's language skills. Take your child for a hearing evaluation if he or she has had frequent ear infections. See CHRONIC OTITIS MEDIA WITH EFFUSION (p. 418).

Runny nose

A partially or completely blocked nose, with a liquid discharge.

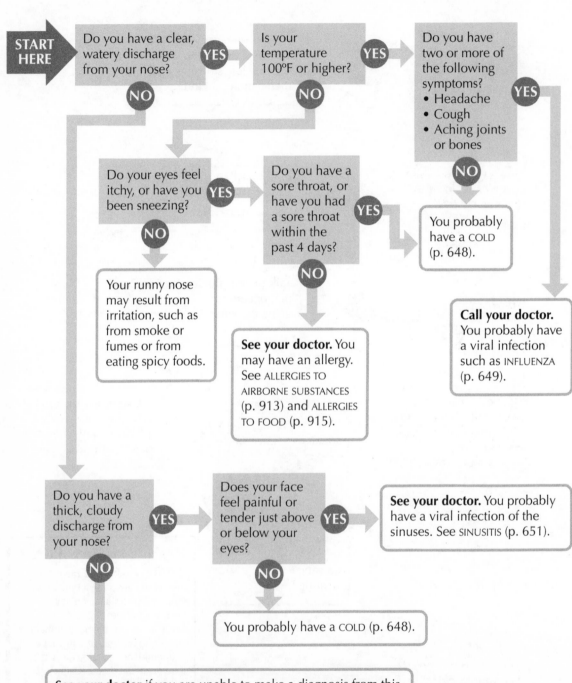

START HERE

Do you have a clear, watery discharge from your nose? — **YES** → **Is your temperature 100°F or higher?** — **YES** → **Do you have two or more of the following symptoms?**
• Headache
• Cough
• Aching joints or bones — **YES** →

NO ↓ (from clear watery discharge)

NO ↓ (from temperature)

NO ↓ (from two or more symptoms)

Do your eyes feel itchy, or have you been sneezing? — **YES** → **Do you have a sore throat, or have you had a sore throat within the past 4 days?** — **YES** → **You probably have a COLD (p. 648).**

NO ↓ (from eyes itchy)

NO ↓ (from sore throat)

Your runny nose may result from irritation, such as from smoke or fumes or from eating spicy foods.

See your doctor. You may have an allergy. See ALLERGIES TO AIRBORNE SUBSTANCES (p. 913) and ALLERGIES TO FOOD (p. 915).

Call your doctor. You probably have a viral infection such as INFLUENZA (p. 649).

Do you have a thick, cloudy discharge from your nose? — **YES** → **Does your face feel painful or tender just above or below your eyes?** — **YES** → **See your doctor.** You probably have a viral infection of the sinuses. See SINUSITIS (p. 651).

NO ↓ (from thick cloudy discharge)

NO ↓ (from face painful)

You probably have a COLD (p. 648).

See your doctor if you are unable to make a diagnosis from this chart and your symptoms persist for more than 10 days.

Sore throat

A rough or raw feeling at the back of the throat that causes discomfort, especially when swallowing.

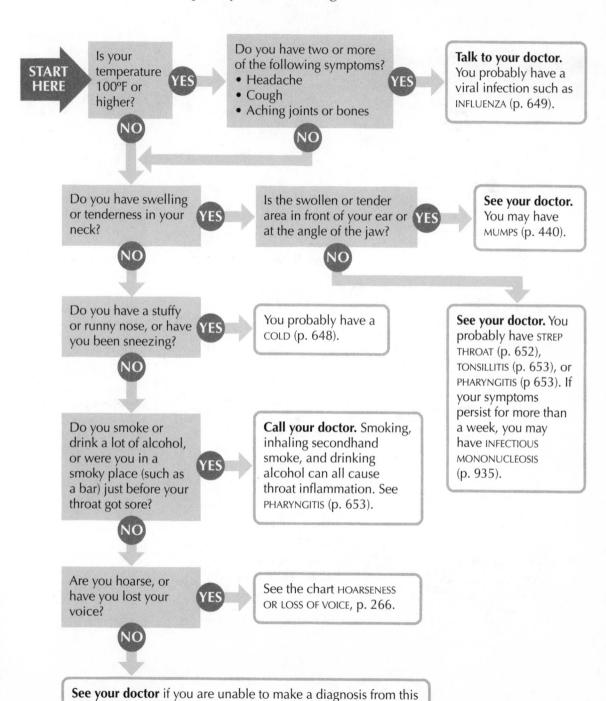

START HERE

Is your temperature 100°F or higher? **YES** → Do you have two or more of the following symptoms?
• Headache
• Cough
• Aching joints or bones **YES** → **Talk to your doctor.** You probably have a viral infection such as INFLUENZA (p. 649).

NO ↓

NO ↓

Do you have swelling or tenderness in your neck? **YES** → Is the swollen or tender area in front of your ear or at the angle of the jaw? **YES** → **See your doctor.** You may have MUMPS (p. 440).

NO ↓

NO →

Do you have a stuffy or runny nose, or have you been sneezing? **YES** → You probably have a COLD (p. 648).

See your doctor. You probably have STREP THROAT (p. 652), TONSILLITIS (p. 653), or PHARYNGITIS (p 653). If your symptoms persist for more than a week, you may have INFECTIOUS MONONUCLEOSIS (p. 935).

NO ↓

Do you smoke or drink a lot of alcohol, or were you in a smoky place (such as a bar) just before your throat got sore? **YES** → **Call your doctor.** Smoking, inhaling secondhand smoke, and drinking alcohol can all cause throat inflammation. See PHARYNGITIS (p. 653).

NO ↓

Are you hoarse, or have you lost your voice? **YES** → See the chart HOARSENESS OR LOSS OF VOICE, p. 266.

NO ↓

See your doctor if you are unable to make a diagnosis from this chart and your sore throat persists for more than 2 days.

Hoarseness or loss of voice

Abnormal huskiness in the voice.

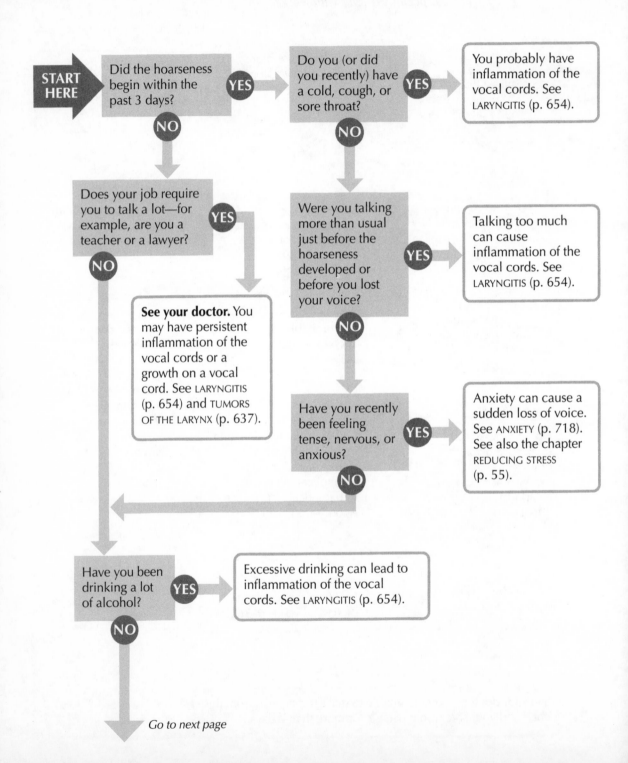

START HERE → Did the hoarseness begin within the past 3 days?

YES → Do you (or did you recently) have a cold, cough, or sore throat?

YES → You probably have inflammation of the vocal cords. See LARYNGITIS (p. 654).

NO ↓ (from "Did the hoarseness begin within the past 3 days?")

Does your job require you to talk a lot—for example, are you a teacher or a lawyer?

YES → **See your doctor.** You may have persistent inflammation of the vocal cords or a growth on a vocal cord. See LARYNGITIS (p. 654) and TUMORS OF THE LARYNX (p. 637).

NO ↓

NO ↓ (from "Do you have a cold, cough, or sore throat?")

Were you talking more than usual just before the hoarseness developed or before you lost your voice?

YES → Talking too much can cause inflammation of the vocal cords. See LARYNGITIS (p. 654).

NO ↓

Have you recently been feeling tense, nervous, or anxious?

YES → Anxiety can cause a sudden loss of voice. See ANXIETY (p. 718). See also the chapter REDUCING STRESS (p. 55).

NO ↓

Have you been drinking a lot of alcohol?

YES → Excessive drinking can lead to inflammation of the vocal cords. See LARYNGITIS (p. 654).

NO ↓

Go to next page

Continued from previous page

Do you smoke, or have you been in a smoky place (such as a bar)?

YES → **See your doctor.** Smoking can lead to inflammation of the vocal cords. See LARYNGITIS (p. 654). However, it can also cause cancer. See TUMORS OF THE LARYNX (p. 637). See also HOW TO QUIT SMOKING (p. 29).

NO

Do you have two or more of the following symptoms?
• Sensitivity to cold weather
• Dry skin or dry hair
• Unexplained weight gain
• Unexplained fatigue

YES → **See your doctor.** You may have an underactive thyroid gland. See HYPOTHYROIDISM (p. 903).

NO

Has the hoarseness or loss of voice lasted longer than a week?

YES →

NO

See a doctor immediately. You could have a polyp on a vocal cord or cancer of the larynx. See TUMORS OF THE LARYNX (p. 637).

Have you had several episodes of hoarseness or voice loss in the past 6 months?

YES →

NO

See your doctor if you are unable to make a diagnosis from this chart and your hoarseness persists for more than a week.

If you have persistent hoarseness

See a doctor immediately.
Chronic hoarseness or loss of voice or an episode of hoarseness that lasts more than a week may be a sign of cancer of the larynx.

GENERAL
Over 12 years

Coughing

A sudden, forceful release of air from the lungs that helps clear material from breathing passages. A cough that clears mucus from the lungs is called a productive cough. A cough that does not produce mucus (usually brought on by minor irritation in the throat) is called a dry cough. For children 2 to 12 years, see the chart COUGHING IN CHILDREN, p. 360.

START HERE

Is the cough dry? **YES** → Are you hoarse, or have you lost your voice? **YES** → See the chart HOARSENESS OR LOSS OF VOICE, p. 266.

 NO

Could you have inhaled a small object or piece of food (such as a peanut)? **YES** → **See your doctor** if coughing fails to clear your lungs or continues for more than an hour.

 NO

Have you inhaled the fumes of an irritating chemical such as a cleaning fluid that contains ammonia? **YES** → **See your doctor.** The fumes have probably irritated your lungs and caused the coughing. See also OCCUPATIONAL LUNG DISEASES (p. 645).

 NO

Do you have a dry cough with no other symptoms?  **YES** → Is your cough deep, raspy, and persistent? **YES** → **See your doctor.** You may have a form of ASTHMA (p. 640).

 NO

 NO

Are you currently taking any medication? **YES** → **Talk to your doctor.** A dry cough is a side effect of some drugs.

 NO

Is your cough often worse when you are lying down or when you wake up in the morning? **YES** → **See a doctor immediately.** You could have GASTROESOPHAGEAL REFLUX DISEASE (p. 750).

NO

See a doctor immediately. A dry cough may be a symptom of a tumor. See LUNG CANCER (p. 646).

Go to next page

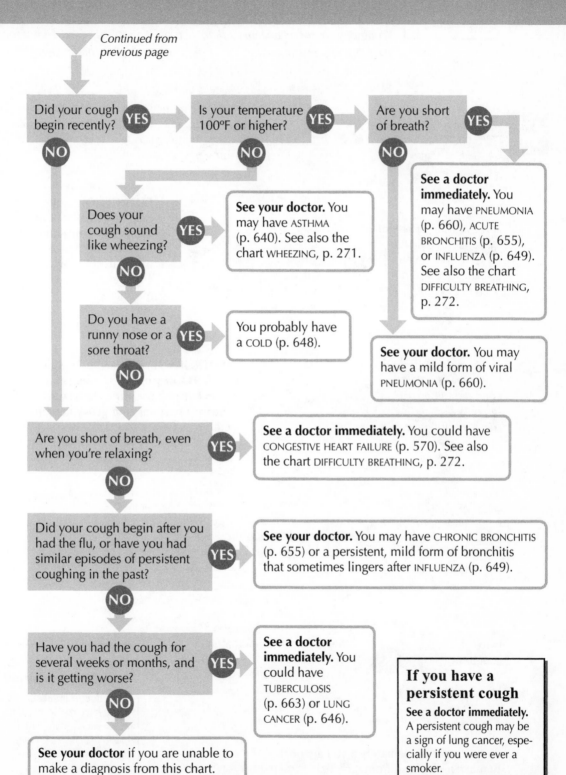

Continued from previous page

Did your cough begin recently? **YES** → Is your temperature 100°F or higher? **YES** → Are you short of breath? **YES** →

NO ↓

NO ↓

NO ↓

Does your cough sound like wheezing? **YES** → **See your doctor.** You may have ASTHMA (p. 640). See also the chart WHEEZING, p. 271.

NO ↓

Do you have a runny nose or a sore throat? **YES** → You probably have a COLD (p. 648).

NO ↓

See a doctor immediately. You may have PNEUMONIA (p. 660), ACUTE BRONCHITIS (p. 655), or INFLUENZA (p. 649). See also the chart DIFFICULTY BREATHING, p. 272.

See your doctor. You may have a mild form of viral PNEUMONIA (p. 660).

Are you short of breath, even when you're relaxing? **YES** → **See a doctor immediately.** You could have CONGESTIVE HEART FAILURE (p. 570). See also the chart DIFFICULTY BREATHING, p. 272.

NO ↓

Did your cough begin after you had the flu, or have you had similar episodes of persistent coughing in the past? **YES** → **See your doctor.** You may have CHRONIC BRONCHITIS (p. 655) or a persistent, mild form of bronchitis that sometimes lingers after INFLUENZA (p. 649).

NO ↓

Have you had the cough for several weeks or months, and is it getting worse? **YES** → **See a doctor immediately.** You could have TUBERCULOSIS (p. 663) or LUNG CANCER (p. 646).

NO ↓

See your doctor if you are unable to make a diagnosis from this chart.

If you have a persistent cough
See a doctor immediately. A persistent cough may be a sign of lung cancer, especially if you were ever a smoker.

Coughing up blood

Coughing up blood or mucus that is colored or streaked bright red or rusty brown, contains dark flecks or spots, or is pink and frothy.

START HERE

Is your temperature 102°F or higher? — **YES** → **See a doctor immediately.** You may have PNEUMONIA (p. 660) or ACUTE BRONCHITIS (p. 655), especially if you are coughing up mucus that is rusty brown or streaked with red.

NO ↓

Are you short of breath and unable to lie flat on your back, even though you have not been exercising? — **YES** → **Are you coughing up mucus that is pink and frothy?** — **YES** → **EMERGENCY Get medical help now!** Call 911 or your local emergency number or have someone take you to the nearest hospital emergency department. You may have CONGESTIVE HEART FAILURE (p. 570).

NO ↓ (from "pink and frothy")

NO ↓

Have you recently had surgery, been confined to bed, or sat for prolonged periods during a trip? — **YES** → **EMERGENCY Get medical help now!** Call 911 or your local emergency number or have someone take you to the nearest hospital emergency department. You may have a blood clot in your lung. See PULMONARY EMBOLISM (p. 606).

NO ↓

Have you had a cold or the flu within the past month that has left you with a persistent cough? — **YES** → **See your doctor.** Coughing may have ruptured a small blood vessel in your airway.

NO ↓

Have you had a cough for many weeks or months? — **YES** → **See a doctor immediately.** You could have LUNG CANCER (p. 646) or TUBERCULOSIS (p. 663).

NO ↓

See a doctor immediately if you are unable to make a diagnosis from this chart.

If you are coughing up blood

See a doctor immediately. If you have had a cough for many weeks, coughing up blood may be a sign of lung cancer, especially if you were ever a smoker.

Wheezing

Noisy, difficult breathing.

START HERE → Did you begin wheezing within the past few hours?

YES → Have you coughed up mucus that is frothy and pink or white?

YES → **EMERGENCY Get medical help now! Call 911 or your local emergency number or have someone take you to the nearest hospital emergency department.** You may have CONGESTIVE HEART FAILURE (p. 570).

NO (from "Did you begin wheezing...") → Is your temperature 100°F or higher?

YES → **See your doctor.** You may have ACUTE BRONCHITIS (p. 655).

NO (from "Have you coughed up mucus...") → Do you have a feeling of tightness in your chest, or do you feel as if you are suffocating?

YES → **EMERGENCY Get medical help now! Call 911 or your local emergency number or have someone take you to the nearest hospital emergency department.** You may be having a severe asthma attack. See ASTHMA (p. 640). Or you may be hyperventilating. See ANXIETY (p. 718).

NO → **See a doctor immediately** if you have not been previously diagnosed with asthma. You are probably having a mild asthma attack. See ASTHMA (p. 640).

NO (from "Is your temperature...") → Do you wheeze on most days?

YES → Do you cough up gray or greenish yellow phlegm on most days?

YES → **See your doctor.** You may have a lung disease such as CHRONIC BRONCHITIS (p. 655) or EMPHYSEMA (p. 656).

NO (from "Do you wheeze on most days?") and **NO** (from "Do you cough up gray...") → **See your doctor** if you are unable to make a diagnosis from this chart.

GENERAL
All ages

Difficulty breathing

Shortness of breath or tightness in your chest that makes you aware of your breathing.

START HERE

Did your breathing difficulty begin within the past few days?

YES → Do you have chest pain?

NO → 1

Do you have chest pain?

YES → Is the pain crushing, or does it radiate from the breastbone or upper abdomen to your jaw, neck, or arms?

NO → Is your temperature 100°F or above, or are you coughing up greenish yellow or rust-colored phlegm?

Is your temperature 100°F or above, or are you coughing up greenish yellow or rust-colored phlegm?

YES → **See a doctor immediately.** You could have PNEUMONIA (p. 660) or ACUTE BRONCHITIS (p. 655).

NO → 2

Is the pain crushing, or does it radiate from the breastbone or upper abdomen to your jaw, neck, or arms?

YES → **EMERGENCY Get medical help now! Call 911 or your local emergency number or have someone take you to the nearest hospital emergency department.** You could be having a HEART ATTACK (p. 567). For first aid, see HEART ATTACK (p. 157).

NO → Is the pain worse when you inhale?

Is the pain worse when you inhale?

YES → **EMERGENCY Get medical help now! Call 911 or your local emergency number or have someone take you to the nearest hospital emergency department.** You may have a blood clot in a lung, a collapsed lung, or pleurisy. See PULMONARY EMBOLISM (p. 606), PNEUMOTHORAX (p. 644), and OTHER LUNG PROBLEMS (p. 639).

NO → **EMERGENCY Get medical help now! Call 911 or your local emergency number or have someone take you to the nearest hospital emergency department.** If the pain persists after you rest for 5 minutes, you could be having a HEART ATTACK (p. 567). For first aid, see HEART ATTACK (p. 157). However, you could also be having an attack of angina, a symptom of HEART DISEASE (p. 558).

1 *Go to next page, first column*

2 *Go to next page, second column*

1 *Continued from previous page, first column*

2 *Continued from previous page, second column*

Have you been wheezing? **YES** → See the chart WHEEZING, p. 271.

NO ↓

Do you feel light-headed, or are your hands and feet numb and tingling? **YES** → **See your doctor.** Your problem is probably hyperventilation resulting from ANXIETY (p. 718). See the chart ANXIETY, p. 243.

NO ↓

If you have severe difficulty breathing
If you have severe difficulty breathing EMERGENCY Get medical help now! Call 911 or your local emergency number or have someone take you to the nearest hospital emergency department, especially if you are also increasingly anxious, fearful, or agitated, or if your skin or lips are blue.

Has your breathing become increasingly difficult in the past weeks or months? **YES** → Do you cough up thick gray or greenish yellow mucus most days? **YES** → Do you work in a dusty atmosphere (such as a mine or quarry)? **YES**

NO

NO ↓

NO

Do your ankles look unusually puffy, or does pressing on them with your fingers leave an indentation? **YES**

NO

You could have a lung disease caused by long-term exposure to dust. See OCCUPATIONAL LUNG DISEASES (p. 645).

See your doctor. You may have CONGESTIVE HEART FAILURE (p. 570).

See your doctor. You probably have a lung disease such as CHRONIC BRONCHITIS (p. 655), EMPHYSEMA (p. 656), or PNEUMONIA (p. 660).

Do you have new pets or new carpeting, has your carpet or upholstery been cleaned recently, or have you been inhaling the fumes of any cleaning agents? **YES**

NO

See your doctor if you are unable to make a diagnosis from this chart.

See your doctor. You may be having an allergic reaction to the new pet or reacting to toxic fumes. See ALLERGIES TO AIRBORNE SUBSTANCES (p. 913).

GENERAL
All ages

Toothache

Pain in the teeth or gums.

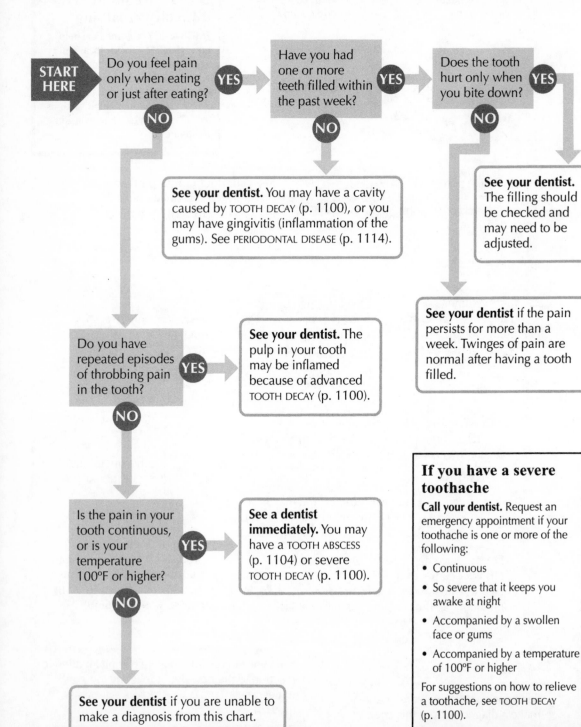

START HERE

Do you feel pain only when eating or just after eating?

YES → Have you had one or more teeth filled within the past week?

YES → Does the tooth hurt only when you bite down?

YES →

See your dentist. The filling should be checked and may need to be adjusted.

NO (from bite down question) →

See your dentist if the pain persists for more than a week. Twinges of pain are normal after having a tooth filled.

NO (from teeth filled question) →

See your dentist. You may have a cavity caused by TOOTH DECAY (p. 1100), or you may have gingivitis (inflammation of the gums). See PERIODONTAL DISEASE (p. 1114).

NO (from eating question) →

Do you have repeated episodes of throbbing pain in the tooth?

YES →

See your dentist. The pulp in your tooth may be inflamed because of advanced TOOTH DECAY (p. 1100).

NO →

Is the pain in your tooth continuous, or is your temperature 100°F or higher?

YES →

See a dentist immediately. You may have a TOOTH ABSCESS (p. 1104) or severe TOOTH DECAY (p. 1100).

NO →

See your dentist if you are unable to make a diagnosis from this chart.

If you have a severe toothache

Call your dentist. Request an emergency appointment if your toothache is one or more of the following:

- Continuous
- So severe that it keeps you awake at night
- Accompanied by a swollen face or gums
- Accompanied by a temperature of 100°F or higher

For suggestions on how to relieve a toothache, see TOOTH DECAY (p. 1100).

Difficulty swallowing

Discomfort or pain when swallowing, or the inability to swallow.

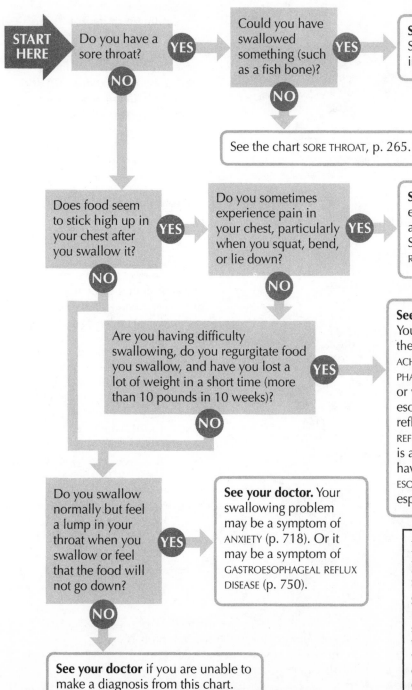

START HERE

Do you have a sore throat?

YES → Could you have swallowed something (such as a fish bone)?

YES → **See a doctor immediately.** Something may be lodged in your throat.

NO (from "Could you have swallowed something") → See the chart SORE THROAT, p. 265.

NO (from "Do you have a sore throat?")

Does food seem to stick high up in your chest after you swallow it?

YES → Do you sometimes experience pain in your chest, particularly when you squat, bend, or lie down?

YES → **See your doctor.** Your esophagus may be scarred as a result of acid reflux. See GASTROESOPHAGEAL REFLUX DISEASE (p. 750).

NO (from "Do you sometimes experience pain...")

Are you having difficulty swallowing, do you regurgitate food you swallow, and have you lost a lot of weight in a short time (more than 10 pounds in 10 weeks)?

YES → **See a doctor immediately.** You may have a disorder of the esophagus such as ACHALASIA (p. 752) or a PHARYNGEAL POUCH (p. 748), or you may have a scarred esophagus from chronic acid reflux. See GASTROESOPHAGEAL REFLUX DISEASE (p. 750). There is also a possibility that you have CANCER OF THE ESOPHAGUS (p. 754), especially if you are over 40.

NO (from "Does food seem to stick...") and **NO** (from "Are you having difficulty...")

Do you swallow normally but feel a lump in your throat when you swallow or feel that the food will not go down?

YES → **See your doctor.** Your swallowing problem may be a symptom of ANXIETY (p. 718). Or it may be a symptom of GASTROESOPHAGEAL REFLUX DISEASE (p. 750).

NO → **See your doctor** if you are unable to make a diagnosis from this chart.

If you have persistent difficulty swallowing

See a doctor immediately. Difficulty swallowing that persists or worsens over time or that is accompanied by rapid weight loss may be a symptom of cancer of the esophagus, especially if you are over 40.

Sore mouth or tongue

Soreness inside the mouth or on or around the tongue or lips.

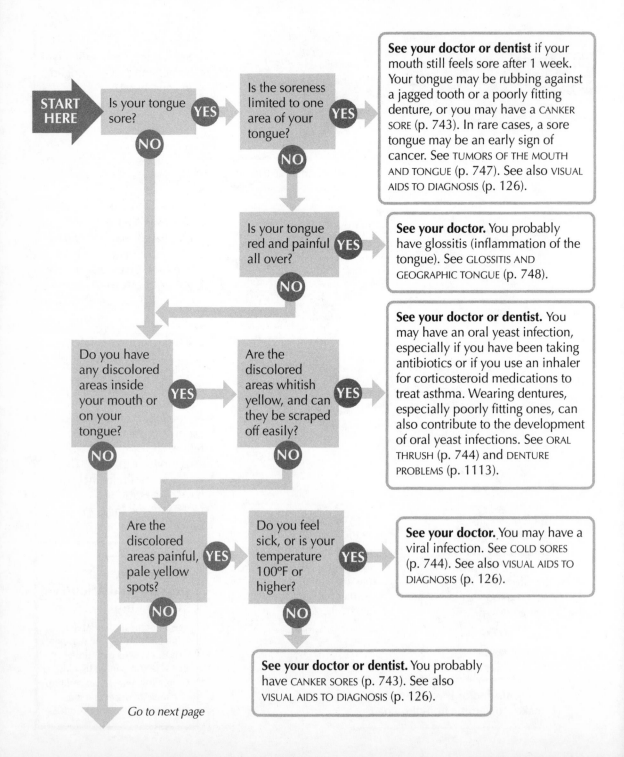

START HERE

Is your tongue sore?

YES → **Is the soreness limited to one area of your tongue?**

YES → **See your doctor or dentist** if your mouth still feels sore after 1 week. Your tongue may be rubbing against a jagged tooth or a poorly fitting denture, or you may have a CANKER SORE (p. 743). In rare cases, a sore tongue may be an early sign of cancer. See TUMORS OF THE MOUTH AND TONGUE (p. 747). See also VISUAL AIDS TO DIAGNOSIS (p. 126).

NO ↓

Is your tongue red and painful all over?

YES → **See your doctor.** You probably have glossitis (inflammation of the tongue). See GLOSSITIS AND GEOGRAPHIC TONGUE (p. 748).

NO ↓

NO (from "Is your tongue sore?")

Do you have any discolored areas inside your mouth or on your tongue?

YES → **Are the discolored areas whitish yellow, and can they be scraped off easily?**

YES → **See your doctor or dentist.** You may have an oral yeast infection, especially if you have been taking antibiotics or if you use an inhaler for corticosteroid medications to treat asthma. Wearing dentures, especially poorly fitting ones, can also contribute to the development of oral yeast infections. See ORAL THRUSH (p. 744) and DENTURE PROBLEMS (p. 1113).

NO ↓

Are the discolored areas painful, pale yellow spots?

YES → **Do you feel sick, or is your temperature 100°F or higher?**

YES → **See your doctor.** You may have a viral infection. See COLD SORES (p. 744). See also VISUAL AIDS TO DIAGNOSIS (p. 126).

NO ↓

See your doctor or dentist. You probably have CANKER SORES (p. 743). See also VISUAL AIDS TO DIAGNOSIS (p. 126).

NO ↓

Go to next page

Continued from previous page

Are your gums painful, red, and swollen? **NO** / **YES**

Do you have bad breath, or do you have a bad taste in your mouth? **NO** / **YES**

See your dentist. You may have severe gingivitis (inflammation of the gums). See PERIODONTAL DISEASE (p. 1114).

See your doctor. You may have a COLD SORE (p. 744). See also VISUAL AIDS TO DIAGNOSIS (p. 126).

Do you have sores on or around your lips? **NO** / **YES**

Are the sores red, rough, or blistered? **NO** / **YES**

See your doctor. You probably have COLD SORES (p. 744). See also VISUAL AIDS TO DIAGNOSIS (p. 126).

Do you have cracks at the corners of your mouth? **NO** / **YES**

See your doctor or dentist. You may have an oral yeast infection, especially if you have been taking antibiotics or if you use an inhaler for corticosteroid medications to treat asthma. Wearing dentures, especially poorly fitting ones, can also increase the risk of oral yeast infections. See ORAL THRUSH (p. 744) and DENTURE PROBLEMS (p. 1113).

Did you recently start using any new cosmetics or lotions on your lips? **NO** / **YES**

The soreness may be an allergic reaction to an ingredient in the cosmetic or lotion. See DERMATITIS (p. 1062). See also VISUAL AIDS TO DIAGNOSIS (p. 120).

See your doctor if you are unable to make a diagnosis from this chart.

If you have sores in your mouth that don't heal

See a doctor or dentist immediately. A sore in the mouth or on the tongue that does not begin to heal within a week and is not healed completely within 2 weeks may be a sign of cancer.

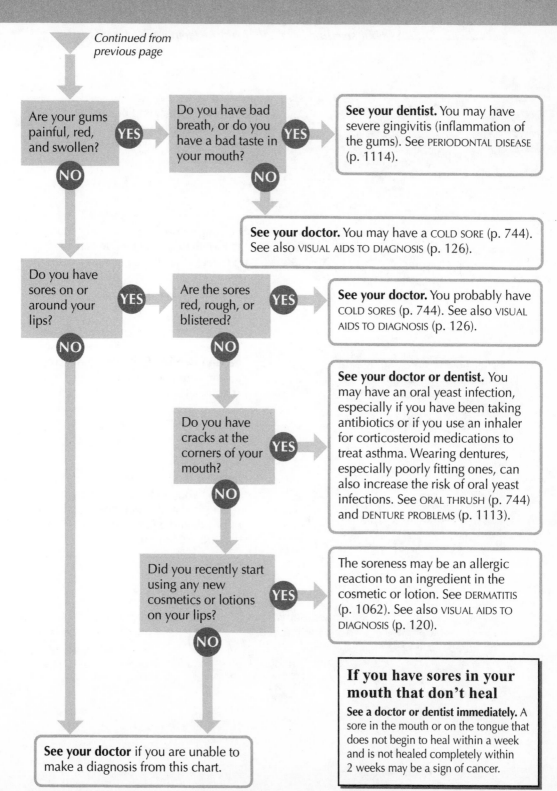

Bad breath

Foul-smelling breath that may be temporary or persistent.

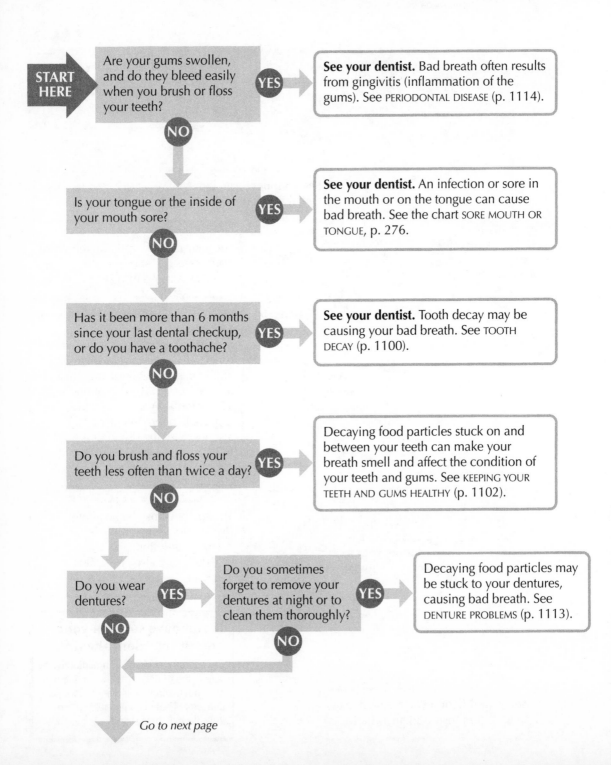

START HERE

Are your gums swollen, and do they bleed easily when you brush or floss your teeth?

YES → **See your dentist.** Bad breath often results from gingivitis (inflammation of the gums). See PERIODONTAL DISEASE (p. 1114).

NO ↓

Is your tongue or the inside of your mouth sore?

YES → **See your dentist.** An infection or sore in the mouth or on the tongue can cause bad breath. See the chart SORE MOUTH OR TONGUE, p. 276.

NO ↓

Has it been more than 6 months since your last dental checkup, or do you have a toothache?

YES → **See your dentist.** Tooth decay may be causing your bad breath. See TOOTH DECAY (p. 1100).

NO ↓

Do you brush and floss your teeth less often than twice a day?

YES → Decaying food particles stuck on and between your teeth can make your breath smell and affect the condition of your teeth and gums. See KEEPING YOUR TEETH AND GUMS HEALTHY (p. 1102).

NO ↓

Do you wear dentures?

YES → **Do you sometimes forget to remove your dentures at night or to clean them thoroughly?**

YES → Decaying food particles may be stuck to your dentures, causing bad breath. See DENTURE PROBLEMS (p. 1113).

NO

Go to next page

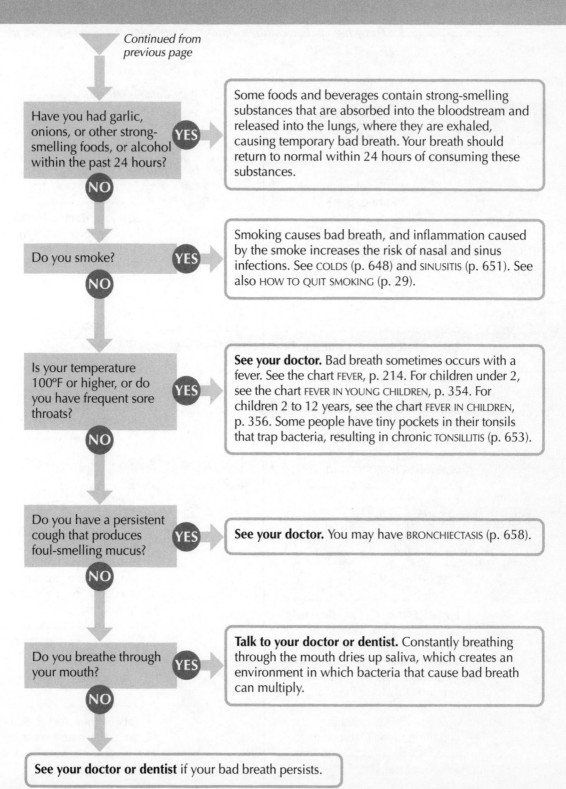

Continued from previous page

Have you had garlic, onions, or other strong-smelling foods, or alcohol within the past 24 hours? **YES** → Some foods and beverages contain strong-smelling substances that are absorbed into the bloodstream and released into the lungs, where they are exhaled, causing temporary bad breath. Your breath should return to normal within 24 hours of consuming these substances.

NO

Do you smoke? **YES** → Smoking causes bad breath, and inflammation caused by the smoke increases the risk of nasal and sinus infections. See COLDS (p. 648) and SINUSITIS (p. 651). See also HOW TO QUIT SMOKING (p. 29).

NO

Is your temperature 100°F or higher, or do you have frequent sore throats? **YES** → **See your doctor.** Bad breath sometimes occurs with a fever. See the chart FEVER, p. 214. For children under 2, see the chart FEVER IN YOUNG CHILDREN, p. 354. For children 2 to 12 years, see the chart FEVER IN CHILDREN, p. 356. Some people have tiny pockets in their tonsils that trap bacteria, resulting in chronic TONSILLITIS (p. 653).

NO

Do you have a persistent cough that produces foul-smelling mucus? **YES** → **See your doctor.** You may have BRONCHIECTASIS (p. 658).

NO

Do you breathe through your mouth? **YES** → **Talk to your doctor or dentist.** Constantly breathing through the mouth dries up saliva, which creates an environment in which bacteria that cause bad breath can multiply.

NO

See your doctor or dentist if your bad breath persists.

Vomiting

Throwing up. For children under 6 months, see the chart VOMITING IN INFANTS, *p. 346.*

 START HERE

Have you been having episodes of vomiting for a week or longer? **YES**

NO

See the chart RECURRING VOMITING, p. 282.

Do you have severe abdominal pain that has lasted at least 1 hour and has not been relieved by vomiting? **YES**

NO

EMERGENCY Get medical help now! Call 911 or your local emergency number or have someone take you to the nearest hospital emergency department. You probably have a serious abdominal condition such as PERITONITIS (p. 759) or an INTESTINAL OBSTRUCTION (p. 759).

Have you vomited blood, or black or dark brown matter that looks like coffee grounds (partially digested blood)? **YES**

NO

EMERGENCY Get medical help now! Call 911 or your local emergency number or have someone take you to the nearest hospital emergency department. You probably have internal bleeding, possibly from a PEPTIC ULCER (p. 755) or another condition in the digestive tract.

 Go to next column

Continued from previous column

Do you have diarrhea? **YES**

NO

See your doctor. You may have an infection of the digestive tract. See GASTROENTERITIS (p. 750).

Did you eat a lot of rich food in the past few hours or drink a lot of alcohol? **YES**

NO

You probably have INDIGESTION (p. 749).

Have you eaten food that may have spoiled? **YES**

NO

See your doctor. You may have FOOD POISONING (p. 783), especially if someone who ate the same food has the same symptoms.

Are you currently taking any medication? **YES**

NO

Talk to your doctor. Some drugs can cause vomiting.

 Go to next page, first column

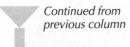

Continued from previous page

Do you have severe pain in or around one eye, and is your vision blurred? **YES**

 NO

> **See an eye doctor immediately.** You could have acute GLAUCOMA (p. 1042).

Do you have a headache? **YES**

 NO

Before vomiting, did you feel so dizzy that the room seemed to be spinning? **YES**

 NO

> **See your doctor.** You may have a disorder of the inner ear such as LABYRINTHITIS (p. 1014) or MÉNIÈRE'S DISEASE (p. 1013).

Do the whites of your eyes and your skin look yellow? **YES**

NO

> **See your doctor.** You may have a disorder of the liver or gallbladder. See HEPATITIS (p. 786) and GALLSTONES (p. 793).

See your doctor if you are unable to make a diagnosis from this chart and your vomiting persists for more than 24 hours.

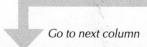 *Go to next column*

Continued from previous column

Did you injure your head within the past 24 hours? **YES**

> **EMERGENCY Get medical help now! Call 911 or your local emergency number or have someone take you to the nearest hospital emergency department.** You may have a BRAIN INJURY (p. 680).

 NO

Do you have one or more of the following symptoms?
- Pain when you bend your head forward
- Sensitivity of eyes to bright light
- Drowsiness or confusion
- Fever

YES

 NO

See the chart HEADACHE, p. 226.

> **EMERGENCY Get medical help now! Call 911 or your local emergency number or have someone take you to the nearest hospital emergency department.** You could have MENINGITIS (p. 692) or a SUBARACHNOID HEMORRHAGE (p. 677).

If you have persistent vomiting

See a doctor immediately. Persistent vomiting can cause dehydration and loss of essential body salts, resulting in a chemical imbalance that if not treated promptly can lead to SHOCK (p. 579). Symptoms of dehydration include light-headedness, a rapid pulse, and decreased urination. For first aid, see p. 162.

If you are vomiting blood

EMERGENCY Get medical help now! Call 911 or your local emergency number or have someone take you to the nearest hospital emergency department. Vomit that contains dark red blood or a black or dark brown substance that looks like coffee grounds (partially digested blood) is a sign of life-threatening gastrointestinal bleeding.

GENERAL
Over 6 months

Recurring vomiting

Vomiting several times within a week. For children under 6 months, see the chart VOMITING IN INFANTS, p. 346.

START HERE

Are you a woman of childbearing age, and do you vomit at about the same time on most days? **YES**

→ **See your doctor.** You may be pregnant; this type of vomiting is common early in pregnancy. See NAUSEA (p. 516).

NO

Do you usually vomit within a few hours after drinking alcohol? **YES**

→ **See your doctor.** Alcohol can cause inflammation of the stomach lining, especially if you drink a lot of alcohol. See INDIGESTION (p. 749). See also ALCOHOL ABUSE AND ALCOHOL DEPENDENCE (p. 733).

NO

Do you have burning pain in your chest or upper abdomen when you bend over or lie down? **YES**

→ **See your doctor.** You may have GASTROESOPHAGEAL REFLUX DISEASE (p. 750).

NO

Do you have abdominal pain or tenderness an hour or two after meals? **YES**

→ **Is the pain or tenderness in the center of your upper abdomen, and is the pain relieved by vomiting?** **YES**

→ **See your doctor.** You may have a PEPTIC ULCER (p. 755).

NO

NO

Have you lost your appetite? **YES**

→ **Do the whites of your eyes and your skin look yellow?** **YES**

→ **See your doctor.** You may have a disorder of the liver or gallbladder. See JAUNDICE (p. 785), HEPATITIS (p. 786), CIRRHOSIS OF THE LIVER (p. 790), and GALLSTONES (p. 793).

NO

NO

If you have recurring vomiting

See a doctor immediately. Recurring vomiting, especially if it is accompanied by a feeling that your stomach fills too easily or too quickly, may be a sign of cancer of the stomach.

If you have blood in your vomit

EMERGENCY Get medical help now! Call 911 or your local emergency number or have someone take you to the nearest hospital emergency department. Vomit that contains dark red blood or a black or dark brown substance that looks like coffee grounds (partially digested blood) is a sign of life-threatening gastrointestinal bleeding.

---

1 *Go to next page, first column*

2 *Go to next page, second column*

3 *Go to next page, third column*

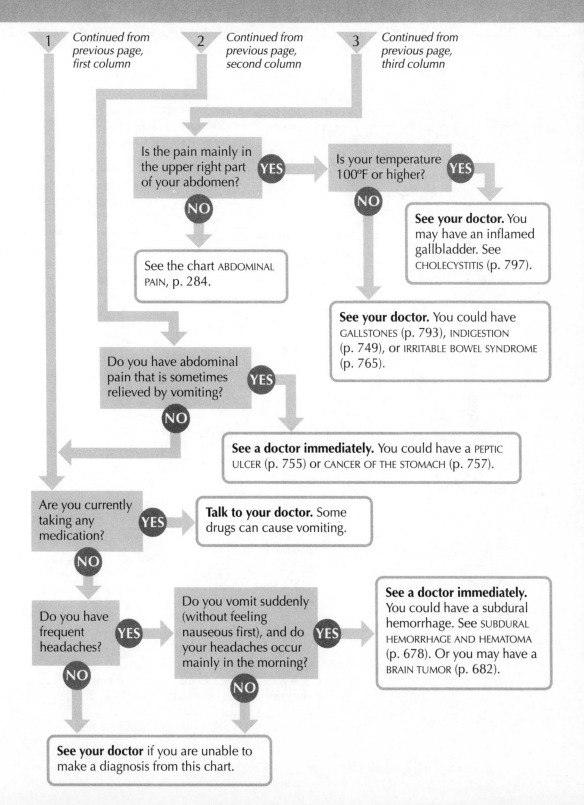

283

1 *Continued from previous page, first column*

2 *Continued from previous page, second column*

3 *Continued from previous page, third column*

Is the pain mainly in the upper right part of your abdomen? **YES** → Is your temperature 100°F or higher? **YES** →

NO ↓

See the chart ABDOMINAL PAIN, p. 284.

See your doctor. You may have an inflamed gallbladder. See CHOLECYSTITIS (p. 797).

NO ↓

See your doctor. You could have GALLSTONES (p. 793), INDIGESTION (p. 749), or IRRITABLE BOWEL SYNDROME (p. 765).

Do you have abdominal pain that is sometimes relieved by vomiting? **YES** →

NO ↓

See a doctor immediately. You could have a PEPTIC ULCER (p. 755) or CANCER OF THE STOMACH (p. 757).

Are you currently taking any medication? **YES** → **Talk to your doctor.** Some drugs can cause vomiting.

NO ↓

Do you have frequent headaches? **YES** → Do you vomit suddenly (without feeling nauseous first), and do your headaches occur mainly in the morning? **YES** →

See a doctor immediately. You could have a subdural hemorrhage. See SUBDURAL HEMORRHAGE AND HEMATOMA (p. 678). Or you may have a BRAIN TUMOR (p. 682).

NO ↓

NO ↓

See your doctor if you are unable to make a diagnosis from this chart.

Abdominal pain

Pain between the bottom of the rib cage and the groin. For children 2 to 12 years, see the chart ABDOMINAL PAIN IN CHILDREN, p. 358.

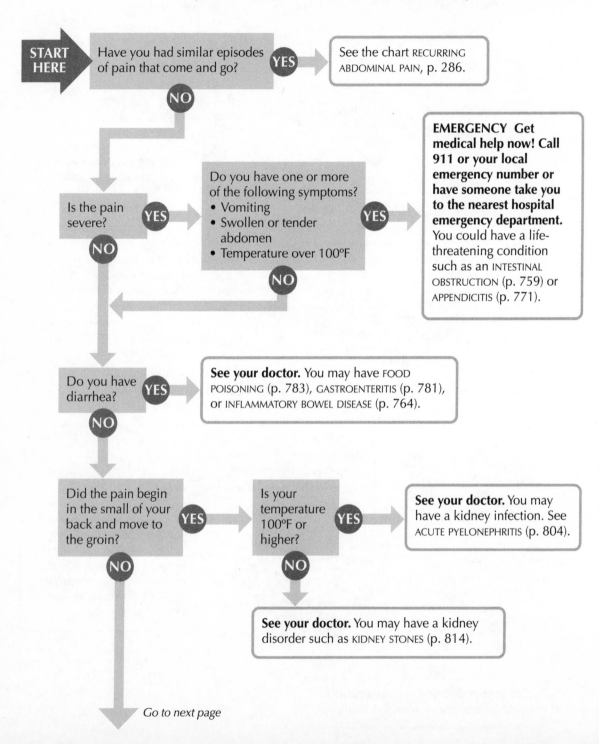

START HERE

Have you had similar episodes of pain that come and go?

YES → See the chart RECURRING ABDOMINAL PAIN, p. 286.

NO

Is the pain severe?

YES → Do you have one or more of the following symptoms?
• Vomiting
• Swollen or tender abdomen
• Temperature over 100°F

YES → **EMERGENCY** Get medical help now! Call 911 or your local emergency number or have someone take you to the nearest hospital emergency department. You could have a life-threatening condition such as an INTESTINAL OBSTRUCTION (p. 759) or APPENDICITIS (p. 771).

NO

NO

Do you have diarrhea?

YES → **See your doctor.** You may have FOOD POISONING (p. 783), GASTROENTERITIS (p. 781), or INFLAMMATORY BOWEL DISEASE (p. 764).

NO

Did the pain begin in the small of your back and move to the groin?

YES → Is your temperature 100°F or higher?

YES → **See your doctor.** You may have a kidney infection. See ACUTE PYELONEPHRITIS (p. 804).

NO

NO → **See your doctor.** You may have a kidney disorder such as KIDNEY STONES (p. 814).

Go to next page

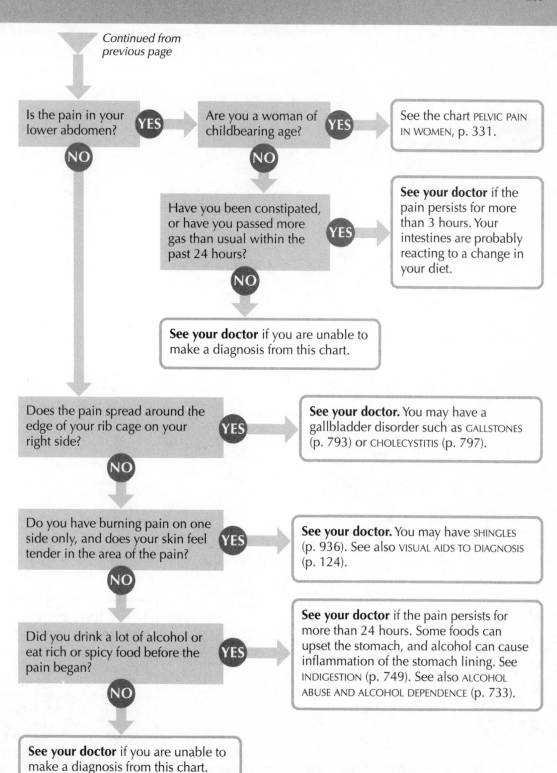

Continued from previous page

Is the pain in your lower abdomen?

NO ↓ **YES** →

Are you a woman of childbearing age?

NO ↓ **YES** →

See the chart PELVIC PAIN IN WOMEN, p. 331.

Have you been constipated, or have you passed more gas than usual within the past 24 hours?

NO ↓ **YES** →

See your doctor if the pain persists for more than 3 hours. Your intestines are probably reacting to a change in your diet.

See your doctor if you are unable to make a diagnosis from this chart.

Does the pain spread around the edge of your rib cage on your right side?

NO ↓ **YES** →

See your doctor. You may have a gallbladder disorder such as GALLSTONES (p. 793) or CHOLECYSTITIS (p. 797).

Do you have burning pain on one side only, and does your skin feel tender in the area of the pain?

NO ↓ **YES** →

See your doctor. You may have SHINGLES (p. 936). See also VISUAL AIDS TO DIAGNOSIS (p. 124).

Did you drink a lot of alcohol or eat rich or spicy food before the pain began?

NO ↓ **YES** →

See your doctor if the pain persists for more than 24 hours. Some foods can upset the stomach, and alcohol can cause inflammation of the stomach lining. See INDIGESTION (p. 749). See also ALCOHOL ABUSE AND ALCOHOL DEPENDENCE (p. 733).

See your doctor if you are unable to make a diagnosis from this chart.

Recurring abdominal pain

Abdominal pain that comes and goes. For children 2 to 12 years, see the chart ABDOMINAL PAIN IN CHILDREN, p. 358.

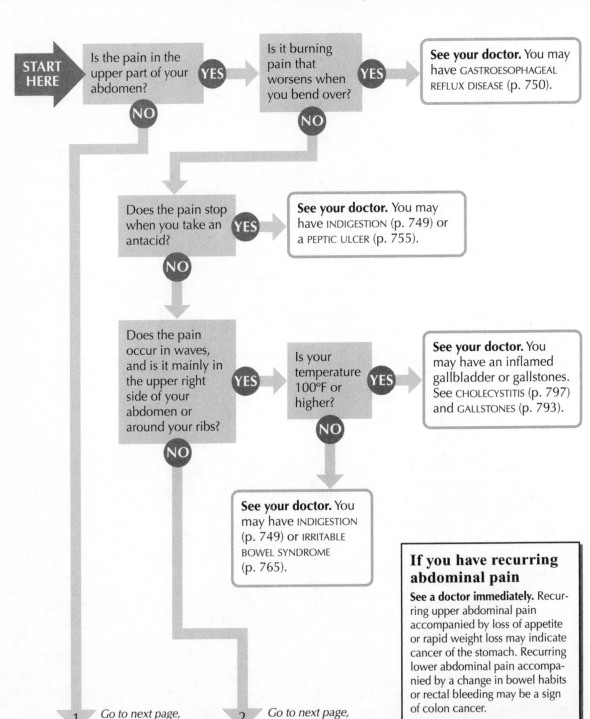

START HERE

Is the pain in the upper part of your abdomen? — **YES** → Is it burning pain that worsens when you bend over? — **YES** → **See your doctor.** You may have GASTROESOPHAGEAL REFLUX DISEASE (p. 750).

NO ↓ (1)

NO ↓

Does the pain stop when you take an antacid? — **YES** → **See your doctor.** You may have INDIGESTION (p. 749) or a PEPTIC ULCER (p. 755).

NO ↓

Does the pain occur in waves, and is it mainly in the upper right side of your abdomen or around your ribs? — **YES** → Is your temperature 100°F or higher? — **YES** → **See your doctor.** You may have an inflamed gallbladder or gallstones. See CHOLECYSTITIS (p. 797) and GALLSTONES (p. 793).

NO ↓ (2)

NO ↓

See your doctor. You may have INDIGESTION (p. 749) or IRRITABLE BOWEL SYNDROME (p. 765).

If you have recurring abdominal pain

See a doctor immediately. Recurring upper abdominal pain accompanied by loss of appetite or rapid weight loss may indicate cancer of the stomach. Recurring lower abdominal pain accompanied by a change in bowel habits or rectal bleeding may be a sign of colon cancer.

1 *Go to next page, first column*

2 *Go to next page, second column*

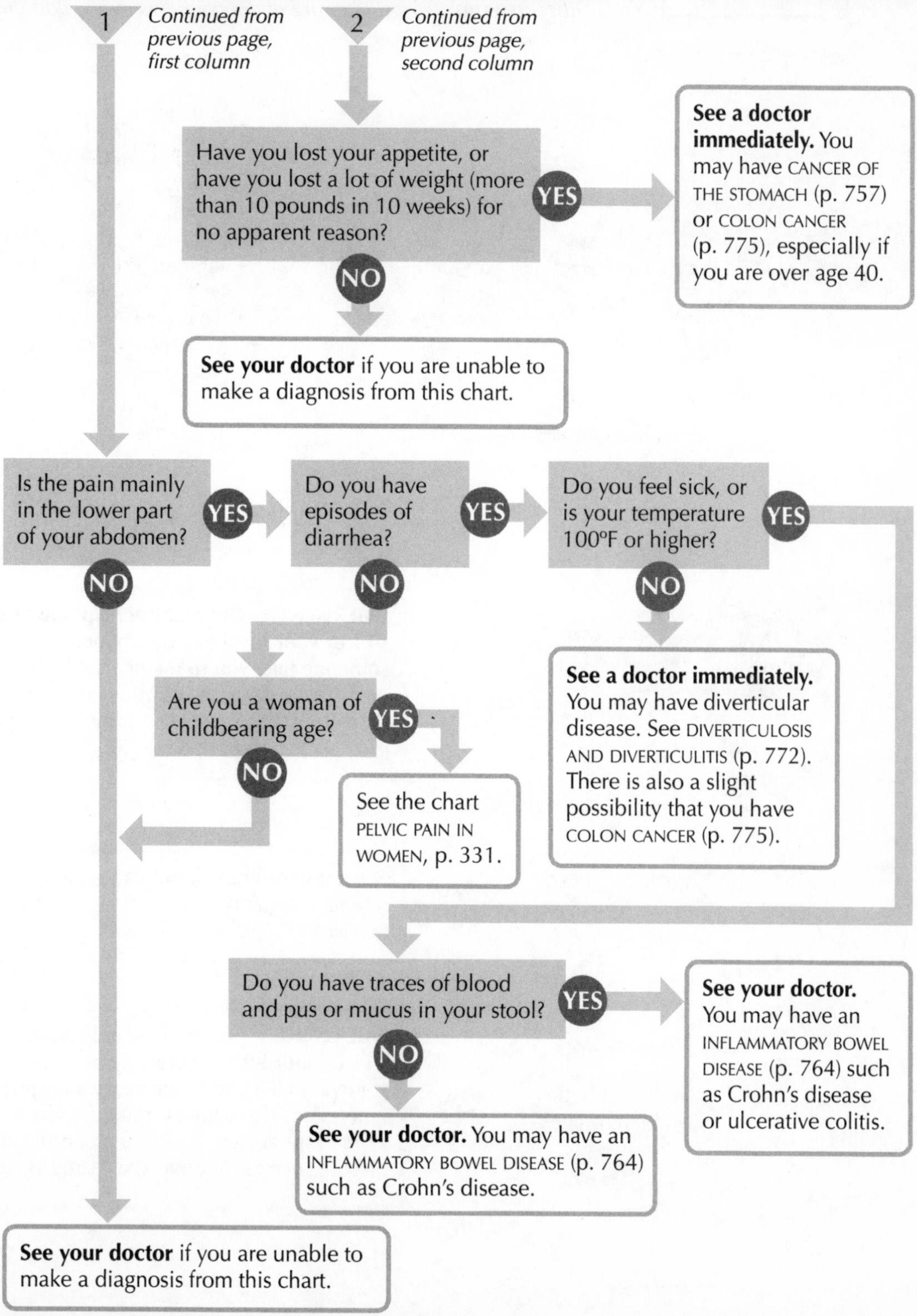

1 *Continued from previous page, first column*

2 *Continued from previous page, second column*

Have you lost your appetite, or have you lost a lot of weight (more than 10 pounds in 10 weeks) for no apparent reason?

YES → **See a doctor immediately.** You may have CANCER OF THE STOMACH (p. 757) or COLON CANCER (p. 775), especially if you are over age 40.

NO ↓

See your doctor if you are unable to make a diagnosis from this chart.

Is the pain mainly in the lower part of your abdomen? **YES** → Do you have episodes of diarrhea? **YES** → Do you feel sick, or is your temperature 100°F or higher? **YES** →

NO (lower part of abdomen)

NO (diarrhea) ↓

NO (temperature) ↓

Are you a woman of childbearing age? **YES** →

NO ←

See the chart PELVIC PAIN IN WOMEN, p. 331.

See a doctor immediately. You may have diverticular disease. See DIVERTICULOSIS AND DIVERTICULITIS (p. 772). There is also a slight possibility that you have COLON CANCER (p. 775).

Do you have traces of blood and pus or mucus in your stool? **YES** → **See your doctor.** You may have an INFLAMMATORY BOWEL DISEASE (p. 764) such as Crohn's disease or ulcerative colitis.

NO ↓

See your doctor. You may have an INFLAMMATORY BOWEL DISEASE (p. 764) such as Crohn's disease.

See your doctor if you are unable to make a diagnosis from this chart.

Swollen abdomen

Generalized swelling over the entire abdomen between the bottom of the rib cage and the groin.

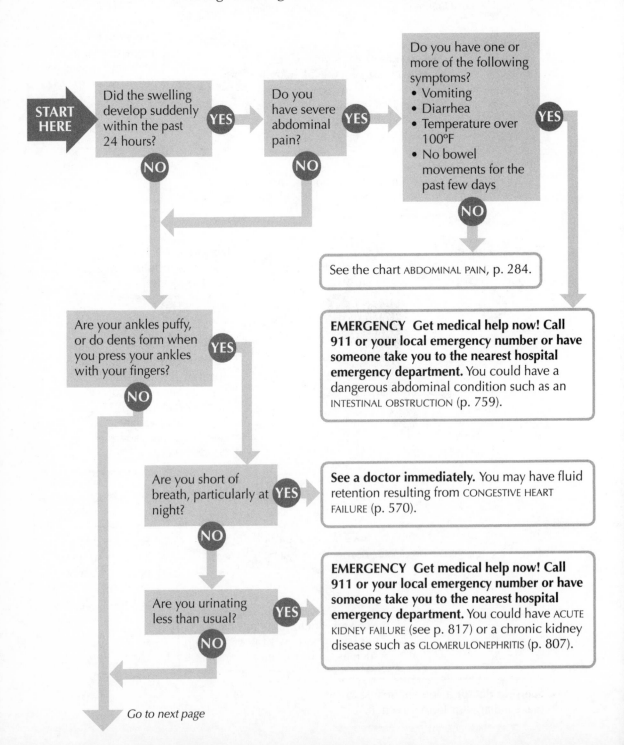

START HERE → Did the swelling develop suddenly within the past 24 hours?

YES → Do you have severe abdominal pain?

YES → Do you have one or more of the following symptoms?
- Vomiting
- Diarrhea
- Temperature over 100°F
- No bowel movements for the past few days

NO → See the chart ABDOMINAL PAIN, p. 284.

YES → **EMERGENCY Get medical help now! Call 911 or your local emergency number or have someone take you to the nearest hospital emergency department.** You could have a dangerous abdominal condition such as an INTESTINAL OBSTRUCTION (p. 759).

Are your ankles puffy, or do dents form when you press your ankles with your fingers?

YES → Are you short of breath, particularly at night?

YES → **See a doctor immediately.** You may have fluid retention resulting from CONGESTIVE HEART FAILURE (p. 570).

NO → Are you urinating less than usual?

YES → **EMERGENCY Get medical help now! Call 911 or your local emergency number or have someone take you to the nearest hospital emergency department.** You could have ACUTE KIDNEY FAILURE (see p. 817) or a chronic kidney disease such as GLOMERULONEPHRITIS (p. 807).

Go to next page

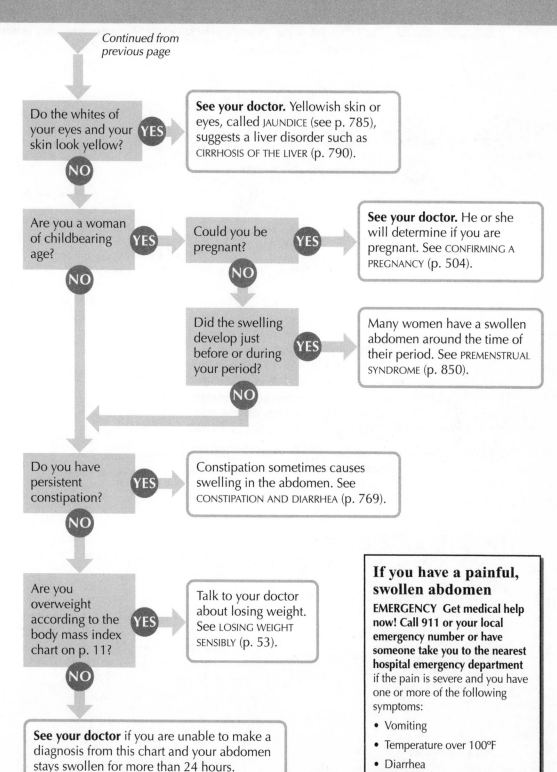

Continued from previous page

Do the whites of your eyes and your skin look yellow? **YES** → **See your doctor.** Yellowish skin or eyes, called JAUNDICE (see p. 785), suggests a liver disorder such as CIRRHOSIS OF THE LIVER (p. 790).

NO ↓

Are you a woman of childbearing age? **YES** → Could you be pregnant? **YES** → **See your doctor.** He or she will determine if you are pregnant. See CONFIRMING A PREGNANCY (p. 504).

NO ↓

Did the swelling develop just before or during your period? **YES** → Many women have a swollen abdomen around the time of their period. See PREMENSTRUAL SYNDROME (p. 850).

NO ↓

Do you have persistent constipation? **YES** → Constipation sometimes causes swelling in the abdomen. See CONSTIPATION AND DIARRHEA (p. 769).

NO ↓

Are you overweight according to the body mass index chart on p. 11? **YES** → Talk to your doctor about losing weight. See LOSING WEIGHT SENSIBLY (p. 53).

NO ↓

See your doctor if you are unable to make a diagnosis from this chart and your abdomen stays swollen for more than 24 hours.

If you have a painful, swollen abdomen

EMERGENCY Get medical help now! Call 911 or your local emergency number or have someone take you to the nearest hospital emergency department if the pain is severe and you have one or more of the following symptoms:

- Vomiting
- Temperature over 100°F
- Diarrhea

GENERAL
All ages

Gas and belching

The expulsion of gas from the digestive tract through the mouth or the anus (also called flatulence).

 START HERE

Is the gas expelled by belching?

YES → **Can you taste a sour or bitter fluid when you belch, especially if you are bending over or lying down?**

YES → **See your doctor.** You may have GASTROESOPHAGEAL REFLUX DISEASE (p. 750).

 NO ↓

Do you often have a bloated, uncomfortable feeling after meals?

YES → You may be unconsciously swallowing air while you eat and then regurgitating it to relieve your discomfort. See INDIGESTION (p. 749).

 NO ↓

See your doctor. You probably swallow large amounts of air without realizing it while eating or chewing gum or as a nervous habit. See RELIEVING AND PREVENTING INDIGESTION (p. 750).

 NO ↓

Have you recently eaten large quantities of high-fiber foods such as beans, bran, or fruit?

YES → Most high-fiber foods cause gas.

 NO ↓

Do you have episodes of lower abdominal pain that are relieved by passing gas or having a bowel movement?

YES → **See your doctor.** You may have IRRITABLE BOWEL SYNDROME (p. 765).

 NO ↓

Are your stools pale, greasy, and foul-smelling?

YES → **See your doctor.** You may have an intestinal disorder such as CELIAC DISEASE (p. 768).

 NO ↓

See your doctor if you are unable to make a diagnosis from this chart.

Diarrhea

Frequent passing of unusually loose stools. For infants up to 6 months, see the chart DIARRHEA IN INFANTS, p. 348.

START HERE

Have you had other episodes of diarrhea in the past few weeks? **YES** →

Do the attacks occur when you are under stress? **YES** →

See your doctor. Stress can often cause diarrhea. See the chapter REDUCING STRESS (p. 55). If you have episodes of cramping abdominal pain with alternating episodes of constipation and diarrhea, you may have IRRITABLE BOWEL SYNDROME (p. 765).

NO ↓

NO ↓

Have you felt ill or have you been vomiting? **YES** →

You may have inflammation of the digestive tract. See GASTROENTERITIS (p. 781).

Do you have pain in the lower part of your abdomen? **YES** →

NO ↓

NO ↓

Have you eaten food that may have spoiled, or do you think you may be allergic to a food you ate recently? **YES** →

Call your doctor if the symptoms last longer than 48 hours. You may have FOOD POISONING (p. 783), especially if other people who ate the same food have the same symptoms. Or you could have an ALLERGY TO FOOD (p. 915).

NO ↓

Is there blood or pus in your stools? **YES** →

See a doctor immediately. Blood or pus in stools could result from an INFLAMMATORY BOWEL DISEASE (p. 764).

See the charts ABDOMINAL PAIN, p. 284, and RECURRING ABDOMINAL PAIN, p. 286.

NO ↓

Have you recently started taking any medication? **YES** →

See your doctor. Sensitivity to some drugs can cause diarrhea.

NO ↓

See your doctor if you are unable to make a diagnosis from this chart and your diarrhea persists for more than 48 hours or recurs.

If you have severe, persistent diarrhea

See a doctor immediately. If your diarrhea is severe, you may lose a dangerous amount of body fluids. Drink lots of water or a rehydration solution or sports drink.

Constipation

Infrequent, difficult passage of hard stools.

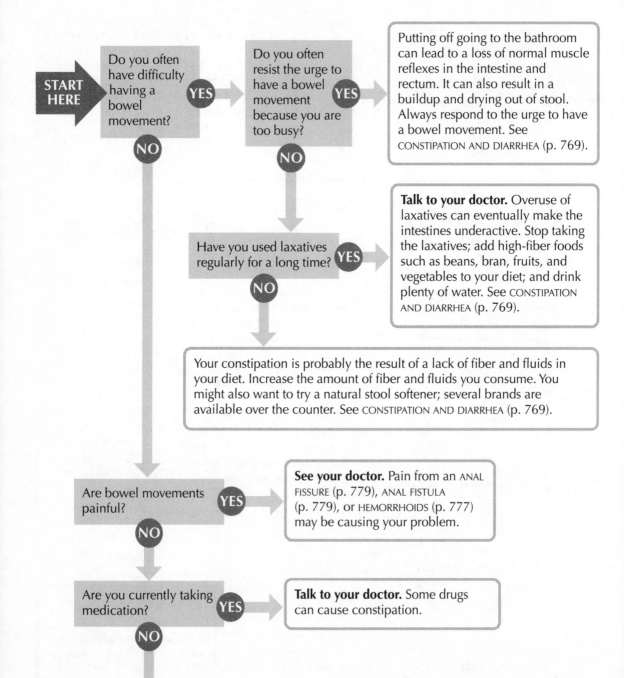

START HERE

Do you often have difficulty having a bowel movement?

YES → Do you often resist the urge to have a bowel movement because you are too busy?

YES → Putting off going to the bathroom can lead to a loss of normal muscle reflexes in the intestine and rectum. It can also result in a buildup and drying out of stool. Always respond to the urge to have a bowel movement. See CONSTIPATION AND DIARRHEA (p. 769).

NO ↓

Have you used laxatives regularly for a long time?

YES → **Talk to your doctor.** Overuse of laxatives can eventually make the intestines underactive. Stop taking the laxatives; add high-fiber foods such as beans, bran, fruits, and vegetables to your diet; and drink plenty of water. See CONSTIPATION AND DIARRHEA (p. 769).

NO ↓

Your constipation is probably the result of a lack of fiber and fluids in your diet. Increase the amount of fiber and fluids you consume. You might also want to try a natural stool softener; several brands are available over the counter. See CONSTIPATION AND DIARRHEA (p. 769).

NO (from first question) ↓

Are bowel movements painful?

YES → **See your doctor.** Pain from an ANAL FISSURE (p. 779), ANAL FISTULA (p. 779), or HEMORRHOIDS (p. 777) may be causing your problem.

NO ↓

Are you currently taking medication?

YES → **Talk to your doctor.** Some drugs can cause constipation.

NO ↓

Go to next page

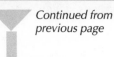 *Continued from previous page*

Are you on a diet, or does your diet lack sufficient amounts of water and high-fiber foods such as fruit, vegetables, whole grains, and legumes? **YES**

 NO

You may not be eating enough or you may not be getting enough water or fiber in your diet to stimulate bowel movements. See the chapter DIET AND HEALTH (p. 35).

If you have any change in bowel movements
See a doctor immediately. Any change in bowel movements (especially in people over 40), including constipation that develops suddenly after years of regularity, may indicate colon cancer.

Are you pregnant? **YES**

 NO

Constipation is common during pregnancy. See CONSTIPATION AND HEMORRHOIDS (p. 518).

Do you have two or more of the following symptoms?
• Frequently feeling cold
• Dry skin or hair
• Unexplained weight gain
• Unexplained fatigue **YES**

 NO

See your doctor. You may have an underactive thyroid gland. See HYPOTHYROIDISM (p. 903).

Do you have lower abdominal pain? **YES**

 NO

Have you had similar episodes of pain and constipation for many years? **YES**

 NO

See your doctor. You probably have IRRITABLE BOWEL SYNDROME (p. 765).

See a doctor immediately. You may have diverticular disease. See DIVERTICULOSIS AND DIVERTICULITIS (p. 772), or you could have COLON CANCER (p. 775).

See your doctor if you are unable to make a diagnosis from this chart and the constipation persists for more than 2 weeks or you do not have any bowel movements for 3 days or more.

Abnormal-looking stools

Stools that are not the usual color or consistency.

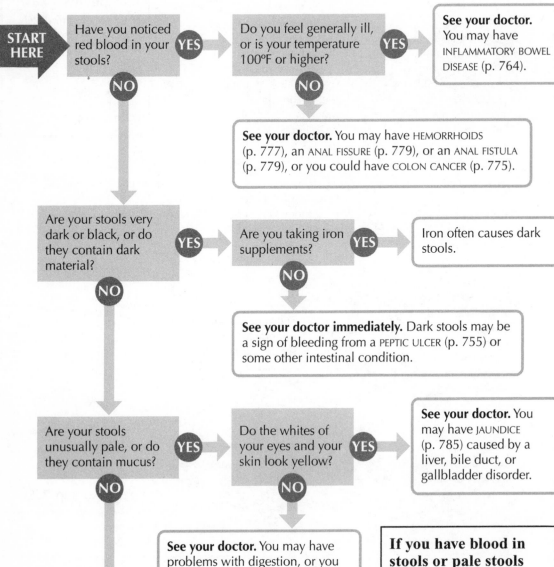

START HERE

Have you noticed red blood in your stools?

YES → Do you feel generally ill, or is your temperature 100°F or higher?

YES → **See your doctor.** You may have INFLAMMATORY BOWEL DISEASE (p. 764).

NO ↓

NO → **See your doctor.** You may have HEMORRHOIDS (p. 777), an ANAL FISSURE (p. 779), or an ANAL FISTULA (p. 779), or you could have COLON CANCER (p. 775).

Are your stools very dark or black, or do they contain dark material?

YES → Are you taking iron supplements?

YES → Iron often causes dark stools.

NO ↓

NO → **See your doctor immediately.** Dark stools may be a sign of bleeding from a PEPTIC ULCER (p. 755) or some other intestinal condition.

Are your stools unusually pale, or do they contain mucus?

YES → Do the whites of your eyes and your skin look yellow?

YES → **See your doctor.** You may have JAUNDICE (p. 785) caused by a liver, bile duct, or gallbladder disorder.

NO ↓

NO → **See your doctor.** You may have problems with digestion, or you may have an intestinal disorder such as CELIAC DISEASE (p. 768) or LACTOSE INTOLERANCE (p. 770).

See your doctor if you are unable to make a diagnosis from this chart.

If you have blood in stools or pale stools

See a doctor immediately. Red blood in stools may indicate hemorrhoids but can also be a sign of colon cancer. Pale stools can result from hepatitis or gallstones but can also be a sign of pancreatic cancer, especially if your skin and eyes are abnormally yellow.

Palpitations

A feeling that your heart is beating irregularly or more strongly or rapidly than usual.

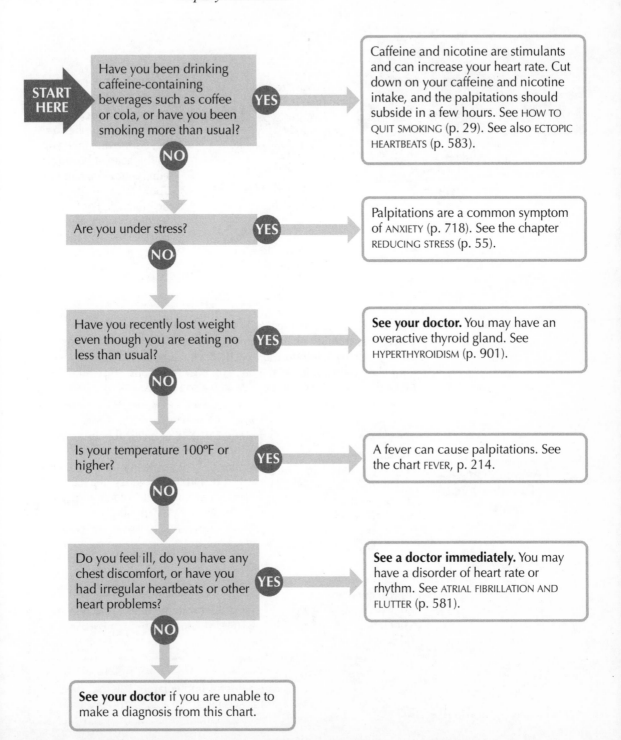

START HERE

Have you been drinking caffeine-containing beverages such as coffee or cola, or have you been smoking more than usual?

YES → Caffeine and nicotine are stimulants and can increase your heart rate. Cut down on your caffeine and nicotine intake, and the palpitations should subside in a few hours. See HOW TO QUIT SMOKING (p. 29). See also ECTOPIC HEARTBEATS (p. 583).

NO ↓

Are you under stress?

YES → Palpitations are a common symptom of ANXIETY (p. 718). See the chapter REDUCING STRESS (p. 55).

NO ↓

Have you recently lost weight even though you are eating no less than usual?

YES → **See your doctor.** You may have an overactive thyroid gland. See HYPERTHYROIDISM (p. 901).

NO ↓

Is your temperature 100°F or higher?

YES → A fever can cause palpitations. See the chart FEVER, p. 214.

NO ↓

Do you feel ill, do you have any chest discomfort, or have you had irregular heartbeats or other heart problems?

YES → **See a doctor immediately.** You may have a disorder of heart rate or rhythm. See ATRIAL FIBRILLATION AND FLUTTER (p. 581).

NO ↓

See your doctor if you are unable to make a diagnosis from this chart.

GENERAL
All ages

Chest pain

Any pain between the neck and the bottom of the rib cage.

START HERE

Is the pain pressing or crushing, or does it radiate out from your chest to other parts of your body (such as your breastbone, the upper part of your abdomen, or your jaw, neck, or arms)?

YES

Is this the first time you have had this type of chest pain?

YES

EMERGENCY Get medical help now! Call 911 or your local emergency number or have someone take you to the nearest hospital emergency department. You may be having a heart attack. For first aid for heart attack, see p. 157. See also HEART ATTACK (p. 567).

NO

Is the pain similar to that of a previous heart attack?

YES

EMERGENCY Get medical help now! Call 911 or your local emergency number or have someone take you to the nearest hospital emergency department. You may be having a heart attack, although your chest pain could be angina caused by HEART DISEASE (p. 558). For first aid, see HEART ATTACK (p. 157). See also HEART ATTACK (p. 567).

NO

NO

Are you short of breath?

YES

Have you recently had surgery, or has an injury or illness kept you in bed?

YES

EMERGENCY Get medical help now! Call 911 or your local emergency number or have someone take you to the nearest hospital emergency department. You may have a blood clot in a lung. See PULMONARY EMBOLISM (p. 606).

NO

NO

Are you coughing, and is your temperature 100°F or higher?

YES

See a doctor immediately. You may have ACUTE BRONCHITIS (p. 655) or PNEUMONIA (p. 660).

NO

See a doctor immediately. You may have a collapsed lung. See PNEUMOTHORAX (p. 644).

Go to next page

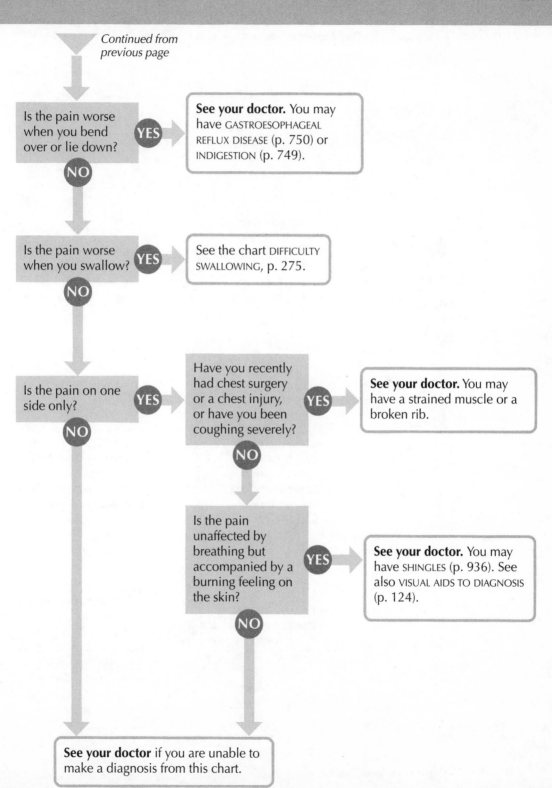

Continued from previous page

Is the pain worse when you bend over or lie down?

YES → **See your doctor.** You may have GASTROESOPHAGEAL REFLUX DISEASE (p. 750) or INDIGESTION (p. 749).

NO ↓

Is the pain worse when you swallow?

YES → See the chart DIFFICULTY SWALLOWING, p. 275.

NO ↓

Is the pain on one side only?

YES → Have you recently had chest surgery or a chest injury, or have you been coughing severely?

YES → **See your doctor.** You may have a strained muscle or a broken rib.

NO ↓

Is the pain unaffected by breathing but accompanied by a burning feeling on the skin?

YES → **See your doctor.** You may have SHINGLES (p. 936). See also VISUAL AIDS TO DIAGNOSIS (p. 124).

NO ↓

NO ↓

See your doctor if you are unable to make a diagnosis from this chart.

Abnormally frequent urination

Feeling the urge to urinate and urinating more often than usual.

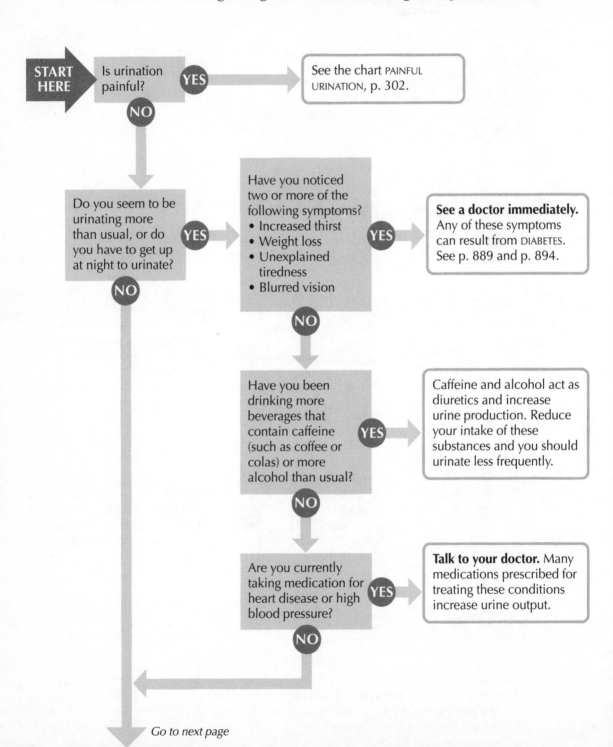

START HERE → Is urination painful? — **YES** → See the chart PAINFUL URINATION, p. 302.

NO ↓

Do you seem to be urinating more than usual, or do you have to get up at night to urinate? — **YES** → Have you noticed two or more of the following symptoms?
• Increased thirst
• Weight loss
• Unexplained tiredness
• Blurred vision
— **YES** → **See a doctor immediately.** Any of these symptoms can result from DIABETES. See p. 889 and p. 894.

NO ↓

Have you been drinking more beverages that contain caffeine (such as coffee or colas) or more alcohol than usual? — **YES** → Caffeine and alcohol act as diuretics and increase urine production. Reduce your intake of these substances and you should urinate less frequently.

NO ↓

Are you currently taking medication for heart disease or high blood pressure? — **YES** → **Talk to your doctor.** Many medications prescribed for treating these conditions increase urine output.

NO ↓

Go to next page

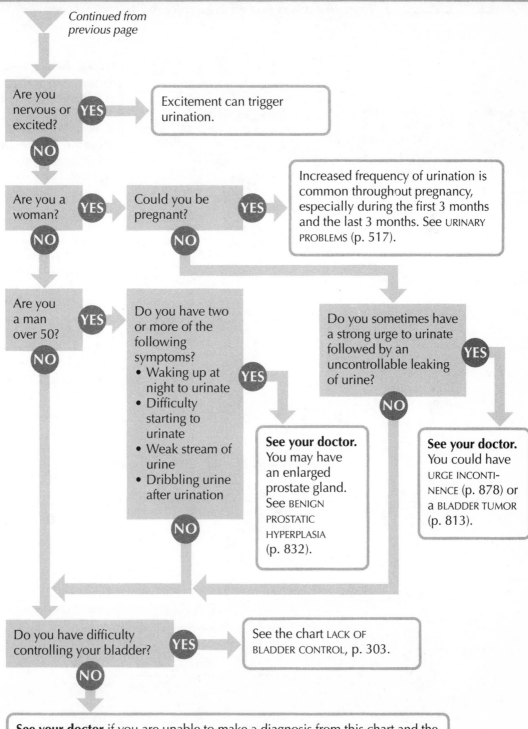

Continued from previous page

Are you nervous or excited? **YES** → Excitement can trigger urination.

NO

Are you a woman? **YES** → Could you be pregnant? **YES** → Increased frequency of urination is common throughout pregnancy, especially during the first 3 months and the last 3 months. See URINARY PROBLEMS (p. 517).

NO **NO**

Are you a man over 50? **YES** → Do you have two or more of the following symptoms?
• Waking up at night to urinate
• Difficulty starting to urinate
• Weak stream of urine
• Dribbling urine after urination

NO **YES** →

Do you sometimes have a strong urge to urinate followed by an uncontrollable leaking of urine? **YES** →

NO

See your doctor. You may have an enlarged prostate gland. See BENIGN PROSTATIC HYPERPLASIA (p. 832).

See your doctor. You could have URGE INCONTINENCE (p. 878) or a BLADDER TUMOR (p. 813).

NO

Do you have difficulty controlling your bladder? **YES** → See the chart LACK OF BLADDER CONTROL, p. 303.

NO

See your doctor if you are unable to make a diagnosis from this chart and the urge to urinate wakes you at night or continues for more than 1 week.

Abnormal-looking urine

Urine that differs from its usual color or that is cloudy or tinged with blood.

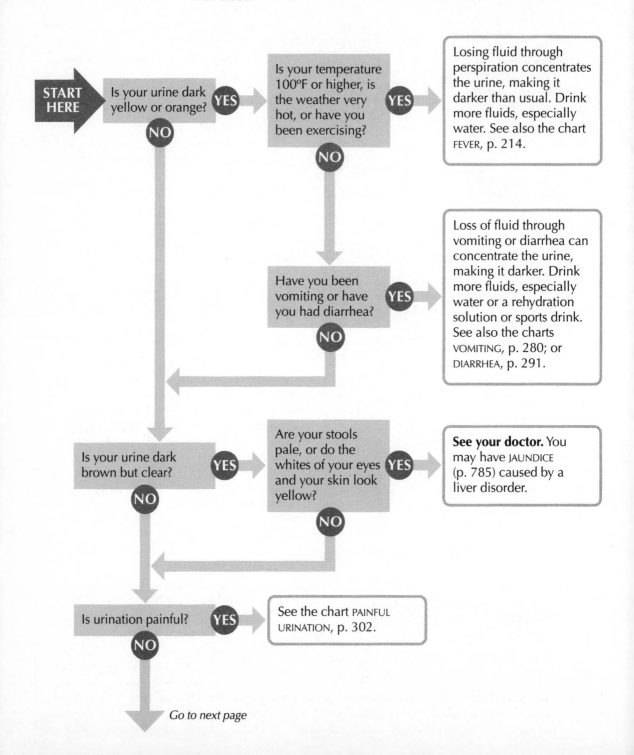

START HERE

Is your urine dark yellow or orange? **YES** → Is your temperature 100°F or higher, is the weather very hot, or have you been exercising? **YES** → Losing fluid through perspiration concentrates the urine, making it darker than usual. Drink more fluids, especially water. See also the chart FEVER, p. 214.

NO ↓ / **NO** ↓

Have you been vomiting or have you had diarrhea? **YES** → Loss of fluid through vomiting or diarrhea can concentrate the urine, making it darker. Drink more fluids, especially water or a rehydration solution or sports drink. See also the charts VOMITING, p. 280; or DIARRHEA, p. 291.

NO

Is your urine dark brown but clear? **YES** → Are your stools pale, or do the whites of your eyes and your skin look yellow? **YES** → **See your doctor.** You may have JAUNDICE (p. 785) caused by a liver disorder.

NO / **NO**

Is urination painful? **YES** → See the chart PAINFUL URINATION, p. 302.

NO

Go to next page

Continued from previous page

Is your urine pink, red, or smoky brown?

YES → Are you taking a laxative that contains senna, or have you started to take any new medications or vitamins within the past 24 hours?

YES → Senna contains substances that can darken the urine temporarily, and some drugs (including some vitamins) can darken urine.

NO ↓

Have you eaten any foods within the past 24 hours that contain red or dark artificial dyes (such as brightly colored candies) or that are dark in color (such as rhubarb, beets, or blackberries)?

YES → Many artificial food dyes and the natural coloring of some foods can discolor urine.

NO ↓

See a doctor immediately. You may have blood in your urine or a urinary tract infection such as CYSTITIS (p. 808). See also CYSTITIS IN MEN (p. 837) and CYSTITIS IN WOMEN (p. 877). There is also a slight chance that you may have a KIDNEY TUMOR (p. 812), BLADDER TUMOR (p. 813), or TUBERCULOSIS (p. 663). If you are a man, you may have an enlarged prostate gland. See BENIGN PROSTATIC HYPERPLASIA (p. 832).

NO (from "Is your urine pink, red, or smoky brown?") ↓

Is your urine green or blue?

YES → Green or blue urine is almost always the result of artificial coloring in food or medication.

NO ↓

See your doctor if you are unable to make a diagnosis from this chart.

If you have pink, red, or smoky brown urine

See a doctor immediately. If you pass pink, red, or smoky brown urine for no obvious reason, you may have blood in your urine, possibly caused by a kidney tumor or a bladder tumor.

Painful urination

Discomfort when urinating, sometimes accompanied by pain in the lower abdomen.

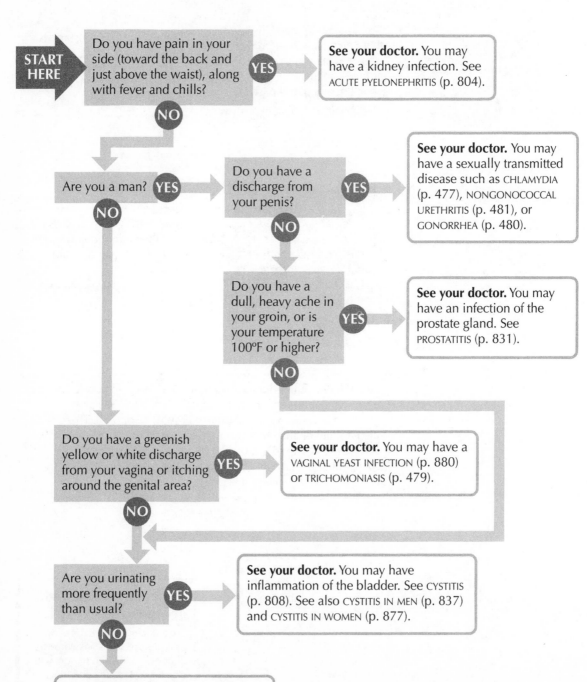

START HERE

Do you have pain in your side (toward the back and just above the waist), along with fever and chills?

YES → **See your doctor.** You may have a kidney infection. See ACUTE PYELONEPHRITIS (p. 804).

NO

Are you a man? **YES** → Do you have a discharge from your penis?

YES → **See your doctor.** You may have a sexually transmitted disease such as CHLAMYDIA (p. 477), NONGONOCOCCAL URETHRITIS (p. 481), or GONORRHEA (p. 480).

NO

Do you have a dull, heavy ache in your groin, or is your temperature 100°F or higher?

YES → **See your doctor.** You may have an infection of the prostate gland. See PROSTATITIS (p. 831).

NO

Do you have a greenish yellow or white discharge from your vagina or itching around the genital area?

YES → **See your doctor.** You may have a VAGINAL YEAST INFECTION (p. 880) or TRICHOMONIASIS (p. 479).

NO

Are you urinating more frequently than usual?

YES → **See your doctor.** You may have inflammation of the bladder. See CYSTITIS (p. 808). See also CYSTITIS IN MEN (p. 837) and CYSTITIS IN WOMEN (p. 877).

NO

See your doctor if you are unable to make a diagnosis from this chart.

Lack of bladder control

Involuntary urination. If you are over 65, see also the chart LACK OF BLADDER CONTROL IN OLDER PEOPLE, p. 366.

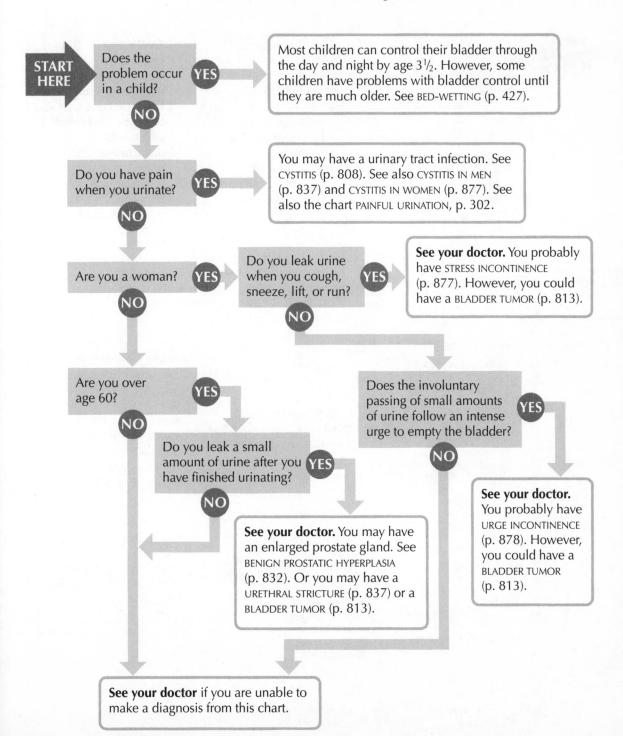

START HERE

Does the problem occur in a child? **YES** → Most children can control their bladder through the day and night by age 3½. However, some children have problems with bladder control until they are much older. See BED-WETTING (p. 427).

NO

Do you have pain when you urinate? **YES** → You may have a urinary tract infection. See CYSTITIS (p. 808). See also CYSTITIS IN MEN (p. 837) and CYSTITIS IN WOMEN (p. 877). See also the chart PAINFUL URINATION, p. 302.

NO

Are you a woman? **YES** → Do you leak urine when you cough, sneeze, lift, or run? **YES** → **See your doctor.** You probably have STRESS INCONTINENCE (p. 877). However, you could have a BLADDER TUMOR (p. 813).

NO

NO

Are you over age 60? **YES** →

Does the involuntary passing of small amounts of urine follow an intense urge to empty the bladder? **YES** →

NO

Do you leak a small amount of urine after you have finished urinating? **YES** →

NO

NO

See your doctor. You may have an enlarged prostate gland. See BENIGN PROSTATIC HYPERPLASIA (p. 832). Or you may have a URETHRAL STRICTURE (p. 837) or a BLADDER TUMOR (p. 813).

See your doctor. You probably have URGE INCONTINENCE (p. 878). However, you could have a BLADDER TUMOR (p. 813).

See your doctor if you are unable to make a diagnosis from this chart.

Backache

Continuous or intermittent pain or stiffness in the back.

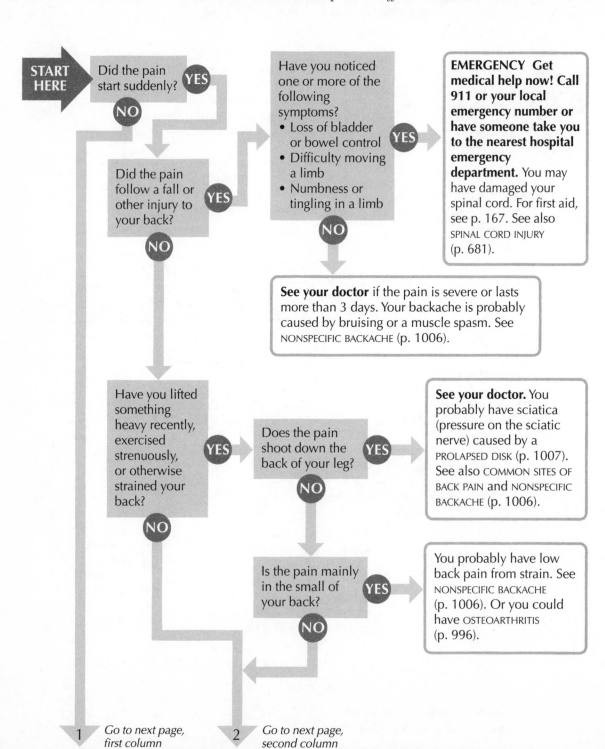

START HERE

Did the pain start suddenly?

YES → Have you noticed one or more of the following symptoms?
- Loss of bladder or bowel control
- Difficulty moving a limb
- Numbness or tingling in a limb

YES → **EMERGENCY Get medical help now! Call 911 or your local emergency number or have someone take you to the nearest hospital emergency department.** You may have damaged your spinal cord. For first aid, see p. 167. See also SPINAL CORD INJURY (p. 681).

NO ↓

Did the pain follow a fall or other injury to your back?

YES ↑

NO ↓ (from symptoms)

See your doctor if the pain is severe or lasts more than 3 days. Your backache is probably caused by bruising or a muscle spasm. See NONSPECIFIC BACKACHE (p. 1006).

NO ↓

Have you lifted something heavy recently, exercised strenuously, or otherwise strained your back?

YES → Does the pain shoot down the back of your leg?

YES → **See your doctor.** You probably have sciatica (pressure on the sciatic nerve) caused by a PROLAPSED DISK (p. 1007). See also COMMON SITES OF BACK PAIN and NONSPECIFIC BACKACHE (p. 1006).

NO ↓

Is the pain mainly in the small of your back?

YES → You probably have low back pain from strain. See NONSPECIFIC BACKACHE (p. 1006). Or you could have OSTEOARTHRITIS (p. 996).

NO ↓

NO ↓

1 *Go to next page, first column*

2 *Go to next page, second column*

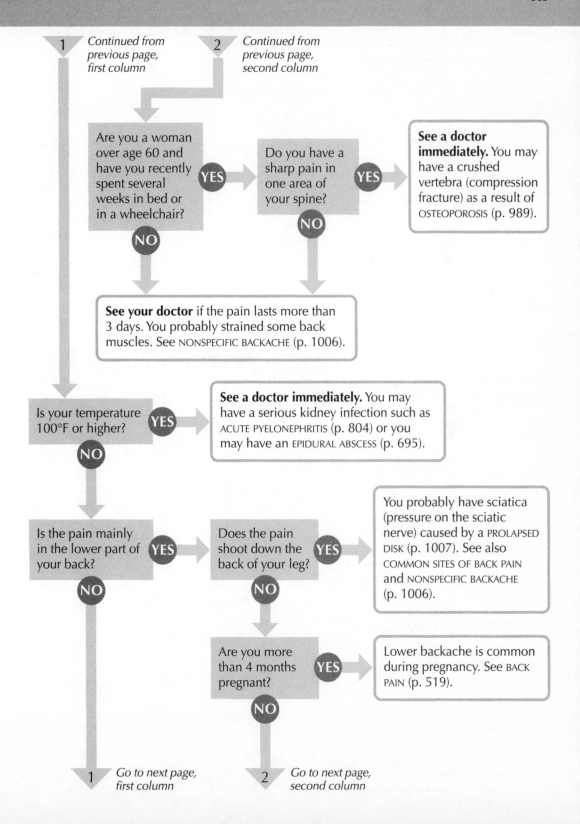

1 *Continued from previous page, first column*

2 *Continued from previous page, second column*

Are you a woman over age 60 and have you recently spent several weeks in bed or in a wheelchair?

YES → **Do you have a sharp pain in one area of your spine?**

YES → **See a doctor immediately.** You may have a crushed vertebra (compression fracture) as a result of OSTEOPOROSIS (p. 989).

NO ↓

NO ↓

See your doctor if the pain lasts more than 3 days. You probably strained some back muscles. See NONSPECIFIC BACKACHE (p. 1006).

Is your temperature 100°F or higher?

YES → **See a doctor immediately.** You may have a serious kidney infection such as ACUTE PYELONEPHRITIS (p. 804) or you may have an EPIDURAL ABSCESS (p. 695).

NO ↓

Is the pain mainly in the lower part of your back?

YES → **Does the pain shoot down the back of your leg?**

YES → You probably have sciatica (pressure on the sciatic nerve) caused by a PROLAPSED DISK (p. 1007). See also COMMON SITES OF BACK PAIN and NONSPECIFIC BACKACHE (p. 1006).

NO ↓

NO ↓

Are you more than 4 months pregnant?

YES → Lower backache is common during pregnancy. See BACK PAIN (p. 519).

NO ↓

1 *Go to next page, first column*

2 *Go to next page, second column*

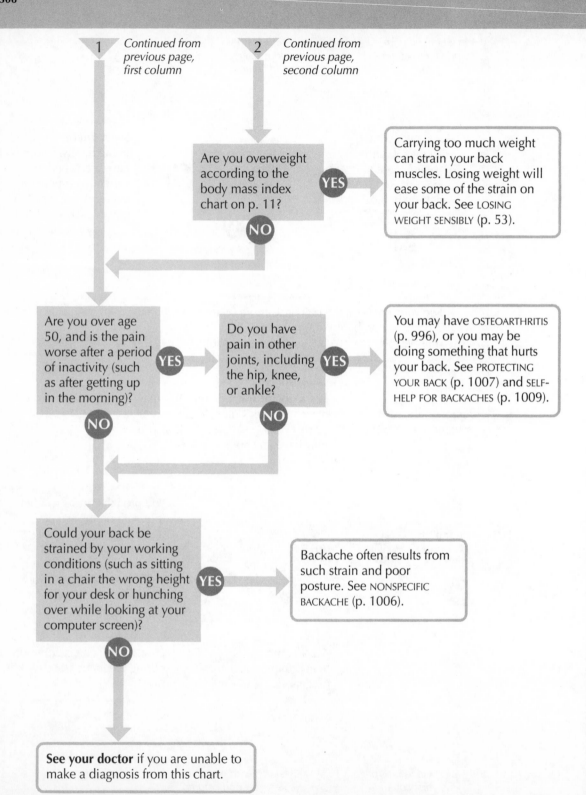

1 *Continued from previous page, first column*

2 *Continued from previous page, second column*

Are you overweight according to the body mass index chart on p. 11?

YES → Carrying too much weight can strain your back muscles. Losing weight will ease some of the strain on your back. See LOSING WEIGHT SENSIBLY (p. 53).

NO

Are you over age 50, and is the pain worse after a period of inactivity (such as after getting up in the morning)?

YES → Do you have pain in other joints, including the hip, knee, or ankle?

YES → You may have OSTEOARTHRITIS (p. 996), or you may be doing something that hurts your back. See PROTECTING YOUR BACK (p. 1007) and SELF-HELP FOR BACKACHES (p. 1009).

NO

NO

Could your back be strained by your working conditions (such as sitting in a chair the wrong height for your desk or hunching over while looking at your computer screen)?

YES → Backache often results from such strain and poor posture. See NONSPECIFIC BACKACHE (p. 1006).

NO

See your doctor if you are unable to make a diagnosis from this chart.

Cramp

Involuntary, painful tightening of muscles other than the abdominal muscles. For abdominal cramps, see the chart ABDOMINAL PAIN, p. 284.

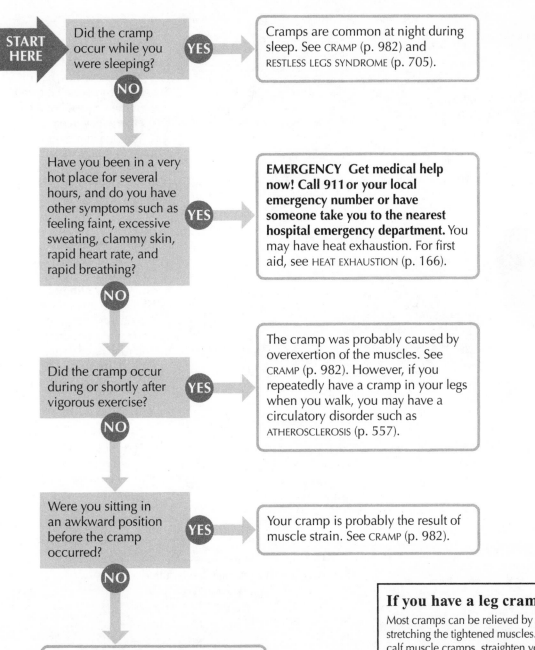

START HERE

Did the cramp occur while you were sleeping?

YES → Cramps are common at night during sleep. See CRAMP (p. 982) and RESTLESS LEGS SYNDROME (p. 705).

NO ↓

Have you been in a very hot place for several hours, and do you have other symptoms such as feeling faint, excessive sweating, clammy skin, rapid heart rate, and rapid breathing?

YES → **EMERGENCY Get medical help now! Call 911 or your local emergency number or have someone take you to the nearest hospital emergency department.** You may have heat exhaustion. For first aid, see HEAT EXHAUSTION (p. 166).

NO ↓

Did the cramp occur during or shortly after vigorous exercise?

YES → The cramp was probably caused by overexertion of the muscles. See CRAMP (p. 982). However, if you repeatedly have a cramp in your legs when you walk, you may have a circulatory disorder such as ATHEROSCLEROSIS (p. 557).

NO ↓

Were you sitting in an awkward position before the cramp occurred?

YES → Your cramp is probably the result of muscle strain. See CRAMP (p. 982).

NO ↓

See your doctor if you are unable to make a diagnosis from this chart and you continue to have cramps.

If you have a leg cramp

Most cramps can be relieved by stretching the tightened muscles. If a calf muscle cramps, straighten your leg and bend the foot upward. Massaging the calf or standing on the leg may also help.

Painful or stiff neck

Pain or discomfort or inability to move the neck.

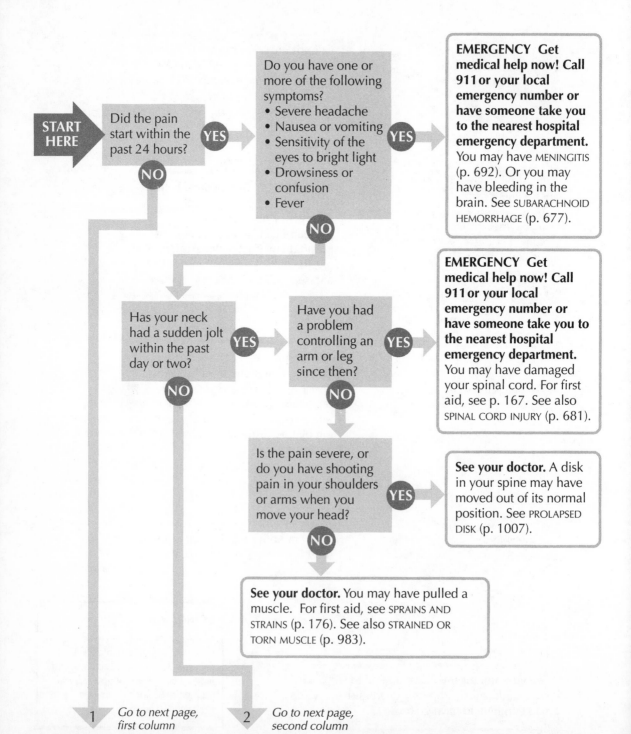

START HERE

Did the pain start within the past 24 hours?

YES →

Do you have one or more of the following symptoms?
- Severe headache
- Nausea or vomiting
- Sensitivity of the eyes to bright light
- Drowsiness or confusion
- Fever

YES →

EMERGENCY Get medical help now! Call 911 or your local emergency number or have someone take you to the nearest hospital emergency department. You may have MENINGITIS (p. 692). Or you may have bleeding in the brain. See SUBARACHNOID HEMORRHAGE (p. 677).

NO (from first question)

NO (from symptoms question)

Has your neck had a sudden jolt within the past day or two?

YES →

Have you had a problem controlling an arm or leg since then?

YES →

EMERGENCY Get medical help now! Call 911 or your local emergency number or have someone take you to the nearest hospital emergency department. You may have damaged your spinal cord. For first aid, see p. 167. See also SPINAL CORD INJURY (p. 681).

NO (from sudden jolt question)

NO (from controlling arm/leg question)

Is the pain severe, or do you have shooting pain in your shoulders or arms when you move your head?

YES →

See your doctor. A disk in your spine may have moved out of its normal position. See PROLAPSED DISK (p. 1007).

NO

See your doctor. You may have pulled a muscle. For first aid, see SPRAINS AND STRAINS (p. 176). See also STRAINED OR TORN MUSCLE (p. 983).

1 *Go to next page, first column*

2 *Go to next page, second column*

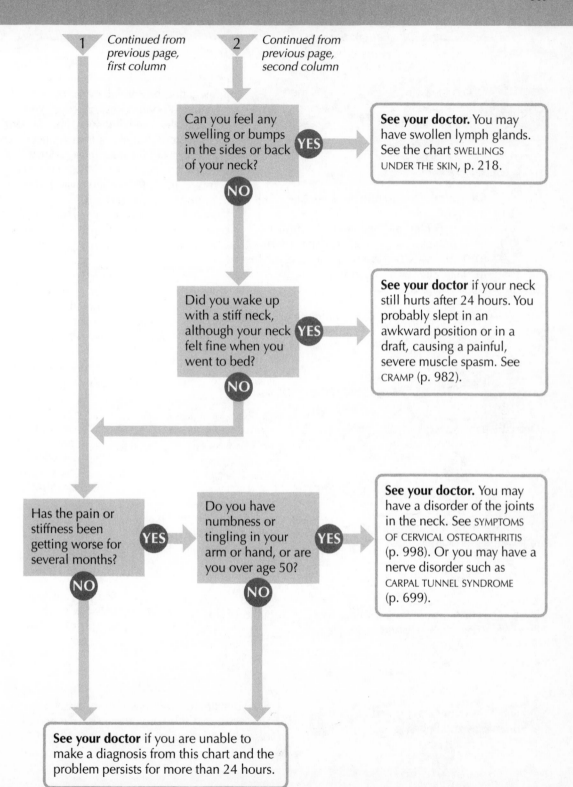

1 *Continued from previous page, first column*

2 *Continued from previous page, second column*

Can you feel any swelling or bumps in the sides or back of your neck?

YES → **See your doctor.** You may have swollen lymph glands. See the chart SWELLINGS UNDER THE SKIN, p. 218.

NO

Did you wake up with a stiff neck, although your neck felt fine when you went to bed?

YES → **See your doctor** if your neck still hurts after 24 hours. You probably slept in an awkward position or in a draft, causing a painful, severe muscle spasm. See CRAMP (p. 982).

NO

Has the pain or stiffness been getting worse for several months?

YES → Do you have numbness or tingling in your arm or hand, or are you over age 50?

YES → **See your doctor.** You may have a disorder of the joints in the neck. See SYMPTOMS OF CERVICAL OSTEOARTHRITIS (p. 998). Or you may have a nerve disorder such as CARPAL TUNNEL SYNDROME (p. 699).

NO

NO

See your doctor if you are unable to make a diagnosis from this chart and the problem persists for more than 24 hours.

GENERAL
All ages

Painful arm or hand

Pain in the arm, elbow, wrist, or hand. For pain in the shoulder, see the chart PAINFUL SHOULDER, p. 316.

START HERE

Did the pain immediately follow an injury? **YES** → Is the pain severe? **YES** →

See a doctor immediately. You may have broken a bone or dislocated a joint (especially if the area looks misshapen) or severely strained or torn a muscle or tendon. For first aid, see BROKEN OR DISLOCATED BONES (p. 167) and SPRAINS AND STRAINS (p. 176). See also FRACTURES (p. 987), DISLOCATED JOINT (p. 1001), STRAINED OR TORN MUSCLE (p. 983), TORN OR SEVERED TENDON (p. 983), BASEBALL FINGER (p. 979), and SKIER'S THUMB (p. 980).

NO ↓   **NO** ↓

See your doctor (to rule out a fracture). You may have pulled a muscle, ligament, or tendon. For first aid, see SPRAINS AND STRAINS (p. 176). See also STRAINED OR TORN MUSCLE (p. 983), SPRAINED LIGAMENT (p. 983), TENDINITIS (p. 984), and ELBOW BURSITIS (p. 979).

Does the pain extend down the upper arm toward the wrist? **YES** → Did the pain begin during exercise and disappear within a few minutes of stopping? **YES** →

See a doctor immediately, especially if you also have chest pain. Your pain could be angina. See HEART DISEASE (p. 558).

NO ↓   **NO** ↓

Does the pain get worse with use and better with rest? **YES** → Do the joints nearest your fingernails look swollen? **YES** →

See your doctor. You may have OSTEOARTHRITIS (p. 996).

NO ↓   **NO** ↓

Does a warm bath or shower relieve the pain somewhat? **YES** →

See your doctor. You may have OSTEOARTHRITIS (p. 996) or RHEUMATOID ARTHRITIS (p. 918).

NO ↓

Do you have stiffness in the morning that lasts longer than an hour? **YES** → Are the joints near your knuckles swollen? **YES** →

See your doctor. You may have RHEUMATOID ARTHRITIS (p. 918).

NO ↓   **NO** ↓

Do you have numbness or tingling in your hands and fingers only? **YES** →

See your doctor. You may have CARPAL TUNNEL SYNDROME (p. 699). Or you may have a nerve disorder related to DIABETES. See p. 889 and p. 894.

NO ↓

Go to next page

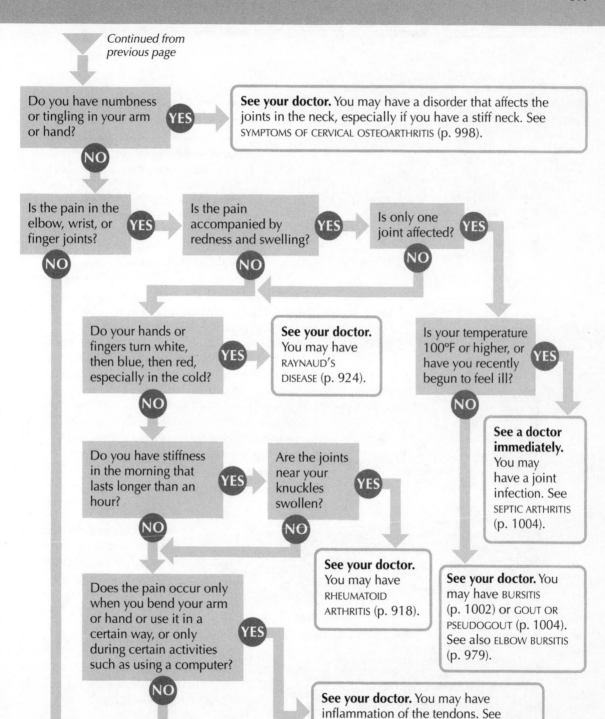

Continued from previous page

Do you have numbness or tingling in your arm or hand? — **YES** → **See your doctor.** You may have a disorder that affects the joints in the neck, especially if you have a stiff neck. See SYMPTOMS OF CERVICAL OSTEOARTHRITIS (p. 998).

NO ↓

Is the pain in the elbow, wrist, or finger joints? — **YES** → **Is the pain accompanied by redness and swelling?** — **YES** → **Is only one joint affected?** — **YES** ↓

NO ↓ (Is the pain in the elbow, wrist, or finger joints?)

NO ↓ (Is the pain accompanied by redness and swelling?)

NO ↓ (Is only one joint affected?)

Do your hands or fingers turn white, then blue, then red, especially in the cold? — **YES** → **See your doctor.** You may have RAYNAUD'S DISEASE (p. 924).

NO ↓

Is your temperature 100°F or higher, or have you recently begun to feel ill? — **YES** ↓

NO ↓

Do you have stiffness in the morning that lasts longer than an hour? — **YES** → **Are the joints near your knuckles swollen?** — **YES** ↓

NO ↓ (Do you have stiffness...)

NO ↓ (Are the joints near your knuckles swollen?)

See a doctor immediately. You may have a joint infection. See SEPTIC ARTHRITIS (p. 1004).

See your doctor. You may have RHEUMATOID ARTHRITIS (p. 918).

See your doctor. You may have BURSITIS (p. 1002) or GOUT OR PSEUDOGOUT (p. 1004). See also ELBOW BURSITIS (p. 979).

Does the pain occur only when you bend your arm or hand or use it in a certain way, or only during certain activities such as using a computer? — **YES** → **See your doctor.** You may have inflammation of the tendons. See TENDINITIS (p. 984). See also GOLFER'S ELBOW AND TENNIS ELBOW (p. 979).

NO ↓

See your doctor if you are unable to make a diagnosis from this chart.

GENERAL
All ages

Painful leg

Intermittent or continuous pain in the thigh or calf.

START HERE

Did the muscles in your leg suddenly tighten painfully for a few minutes and then return to normal? **YES** → See the chart CRAMP, p. 307.

NO

Did the pain immediately follow a fall or other injury? **YES** → Can you walk on the affected leg? **YES** →

See your doctor. You may have pulled a muscle, ligament, or tendon. For first aid, see SPRAINS AND STRAINS (p. 176). See also STRAINED OR TORN MUSCLE (p. 983), SPRAINED LIGAMENT (p. 983), TENDINITIS (p. 984), ACHILLES TENDINITIS (p. 981), and PULLED HAMSTRING MUSCLE and CALF MUSCLE TEAR (p. 980).

NO

NO

See a doctor immediately. You may have broken your leg or severely torn a muscle or tendon. For first aid, see BROKEN OR DISLOCATED BONES (p. 167) and SPRAINS AND STRAINS (p. 176). See also FRACTURES (p. 987), STRAINED OR TORN MUSCLE (p. 983), TORN OR SEVERED TENDON (p. 983), ACHILLES TENDINITIS (p. 981), and PULLED HAMSTRING MUSCLE and CALF MUSCLE TEAR (p. 980).

Does the pain shoot down the back of your leg, especially when you cough or strain? **YES** → **See your doctor.** You probably have sciatica (pressure on the sciatic nerve) caused by a PROLAPSED DISK (p. 1007).

NO

Do you have persistent pain in one area of your leg? **YES** → Is your temperature 100°F or higher, or do you have chills and feel generally ill? **YES** → **See a doctor immediately.** You may have OSTEOMYELITIS (p. 433), a bone infection that is most common in children.

NO **NO**

Do both of your legs ache and do your ankles swell sometimes, particularly after you stand for long periods? **YES** → Are the veins in your legs twisted, swollen, and unusually prominent? **YES** →

NO **NO**

Go to next page

See your doctor. You probably have VARICOSE VEINS (p. 602).

Continued from previous page

Is your hip painful or stiff on the same side as the affected leg? **YES** → **See your doctor.** You may have OSTEOARTHRITIS (p. 996).

NO

Is the pain mainly in your calf? **YES** → Is your calf swollen, and does it hurt when you walk? **YES** → **See a doctor immediately.** You may have a blood clot in your leg. See DEEP VEIN THROMBOSIS (p. 605).

NO

NO

Is just one of your veins red and inflamed? **YES** → **See a doctor immediately.** You may have THROMBOPHLEBITIS (p. 604).

NO

Does your leg hurt when you walk but not when you are resting? **YES** → **See your doctor.** Pain in the calf during exercise that disappears promptly when you stop may be a sign of a circulatory problem such as ATHEROSCLEROSIS (p. 557). It could also be a pulled muscle, ligament, or tendon. For first aid, see SPRAINS AND STRAINS (p. 176). See also STRAINED OR TORN MUSCLE (p. 983), SPRAINED LIGAMENT (p. 983), TENDINITIS (p. 984), ACHILLES TENDINITIS (p. 981), and CALF MUSCLE TEAR (p. 980).

NO

Did your leg become painful following unusually strenuous exercise? **YES** → **See your doctor.** You may have pulled a muscle, ligament, or tendon. For first aid, see SPRAINS AND STRAINS (p. 176). See also STRAINED OR TORN MUSCLE (p. 983), SPRAINED LIGAMENT (p. 983), TENDINITIS (p. 984), ACHILLES TENDINITIS (p. 981), and CALF MUSCLE TEAR (p. 980).

NO

See your doctor if you are unable to make a diagnosis from this chart and the pain persists for more than 48 hours or gets worse.

Painful knee

Pain in or around the knee joint.

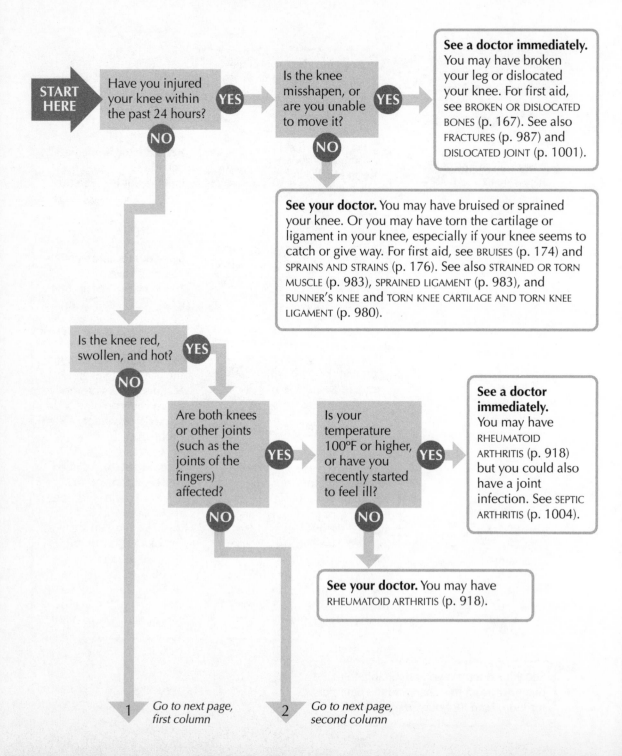

START HERE

Have you injured your knee within the past 24 hours?

YES → Is the knee misshapen, or are you unable to move it?

YES → **See a doctor immediately.** You may have broken your leg or dislocated your knee. For first aid, see BROKEN OR DISLOCATED BONES (p. 167). See also FRACTURES (p. 987) and DISLOCATED JOINT (p. 1001).

NO (from "Is the knee misshapen") → **See your doctor.** You may have bruised or sprained your knee. Or you may have torn the cartilage or ligament in your knee, especially if your knee seems to catch or give way. For first aid, see BRUISES (p. 174) and SPRAINS AND STRAINS (p. 176). See also STRAINED OR TORN MUSCLE (p. 983), SPRAINED LIGAMENT (p. 983), and RUNNER'S KNEE and TORN KNEE CARTILAGE AND TORN KNEE LIGAMENT (p. 980).

NO (from "Have you injured your knee") → Is the knee red, swollen, and hot?

YES → Are both knees or other joints (such as the joints of the fingers) affected?

YES → Is your temperature 100°F or higher, or have you recently started to feel ill?

YES → **See a doctor immediately.** You may have RHEUMATOID ARTHRITIS (p. 918) but you could also have a joint infection. See SEPTIC ARTHRITIS (p. 1004).

NO (from "Is your temperature") → **See your doctor.** You may have RHEUMATOID ARTHRITIS (p. 918).

NO (from "Are both knees") →

NO (from "Is the knee red") →

1 *Go to next page, first column*

2 *Go to next page, second column*

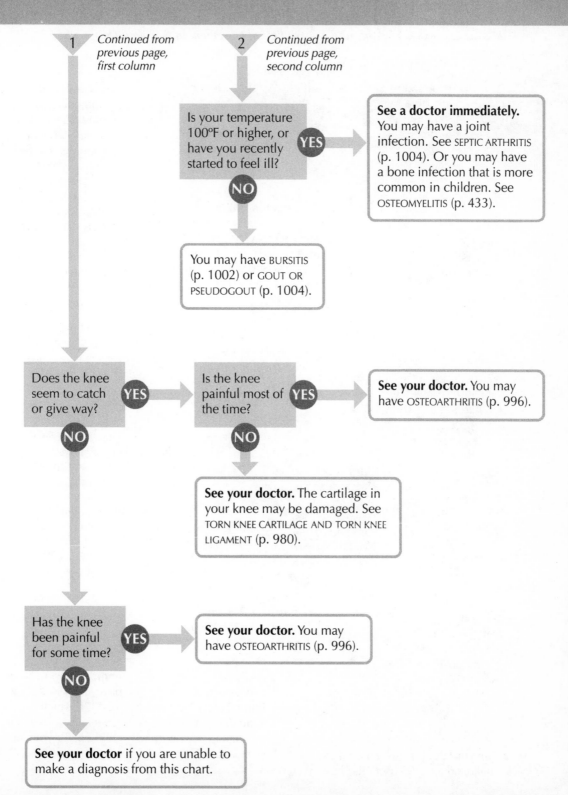

1 *Continued from previous page, first column*

2 *Continued from previous page, second column*

Is your temperature 100°F or higher, or have you recently started to feel ill?

YES →

See a doctor immediately. You may have a joint infection. See SEPTIC ARTHRITIS (p. 1004). Or you may have a bone infection that is more common in children. See OSTEOMYELITIS (p. 433).

NO ↓

You may have BURSITIS (p. 1002) or GOUT OR PSEUDOGOUT (p. 1004).

Does the knee seem to catch or give way?

YES →

Is the knee painful most of the time?

YES →

See your doctor. You may have OSTEOARTHRITIS (p. 996).

NO ↓

See your doctor. The cartilage in your knee may be damaged. See TORN KNEE CARTILAGE AND TORN KNEE LIGAMENT (p. 980).

NO ↓

Has the knee been painful for some time?

YES →

See your doctor. You may have OSTEOARTHRITIS (p. 996).

NO ↓

See your doctor if you are unable to make a diagnosis from this chart.

Painful shoulder

Pain, stiffness, or limited movement in the shoulder.

START HERE

Did you injure your shoulder within the past 24 hours? **YES**

Is it impossible or very painful to move your shoulder, or does your shoulder seem misshapen? **YES**

See a doctor immediately. You may have broken or dislocated your shoulder. For first aid, see BROKEN OR DISLOCATED BONES (p. 167). See also FRACTURES (p. 987), DISLOCATED JOINT (p. 1001), and DISLOCATED SHOULDER AND SEPARATED SHOULDER (p. 979).

NO

NO

See your doctor. You may have pulled or torn a muscle or ligament. For first aid, see SPRAINS AND STRAINS (p. 176). See also STRAINED OR TORN MUSCLE (p. 983), SPRAINED LIGAMENT (p. 983), and SWIMMER'S SHOULDER (p. 979).

Did the pain begin suddenly? **YES**

NO

Do you have pain, swelling, or redness in other joints, such as your finger joints? **YES**

See your doctor. You may have RHEUMATOID ARTHRITIS (p. 918).

Is your temperature 100°F or higher, or have you recently started to feel ill? **YES**

NO

See your doctor. You may have BURSITIS (p. 1002) or TENDINITIS (p. 984).

NO

Does the pain occur only when you move your arm?  **YES**

Has your shoulder become increasingly painful and stiff over several weeks, and are you barely able to move your arm? **YES**

See your doctor. You may have inflammation and thickening of the lining of the joint capsule. See FROZEN SHOULDER (p. 1004).

NO

NO

See your doctor. You may have BURSITIS (p. 1002).

Does the pain occur when you exert yourself or exercise the shoulder, and subside when you stop? **YES**

See a doctor immediately. Your shoulder pain may be angina. See HEART DISEASE (p. 558).

See a doctor immediately. You may have RHEUMATIC FEVER (p. 432), which is especially common in children. Or you could have TENDINITIS (p. 984).

NO

See your doctor if you are unable to make a diagnosis from this chart.

Painful ankles

Pain in or around one or both ankles.

START HERE

Did the pain follow an injury?

YES → **Is it impossible or very painful to move your ankle?**

YES → **See a doctor immediately.** You may have a broken bone. For first aid, see BROKEN OR DISLOCATED BONES (p. 167). See also FRACTURES (p. 987). Or you may have strained a ligament. For first aid, see SPRAINS AND STRAINS (p. 176). See also SPRAINED LIGAMENT (p. 983) and SPRAINED ANKLE (p. 981).

NO ↓ (from injury question)

NO (from move ankle) → **See your doctor.** You have probably strained a ligament. For first aid, see SPRAINS AND STRAINS (p. 176). See also SPRAINED LIGAMENT (p. 983) and SPRAINED ANKLE (p. 981).

Is the pain accompanied by redness and swelling?

YES → **Are both ankles or any other joints (such as your knee or finger joints) affected?**

YES → **Is your temperature 100°F or higher, or have you recently started to feel ill?**

YES → **See your doctor.** You may have RHEUMATOID ARTHRITIS (p. 918).

NO (from redness and swelling) ↓

NO (from both ankles affected) → **Is your temperature 100°F or higher, or have you recently started to feel ill?**

YES → **See a doctor immediately.** You may have RHEUMATOID ARTHRITIS (p. 918), or you could have a joint infection. See SEPTIC ARTHRITIS (p. 1004).

NO (from temperature) ↓

See your doctor. You may have GOUT OR PSEUDOGOUT (p. 1004).

Are you over age 50?

YES → **See your doctor.** You may have OSTEOARTHRITIS (p. 996) or GOUT OR PSEUDOGOUT (p. 1004).

NO ↓

See your doctor if you are unable to make a diagnosis from this chart.

Swollen ankles

Swelling or puffiness in one or both ankles.

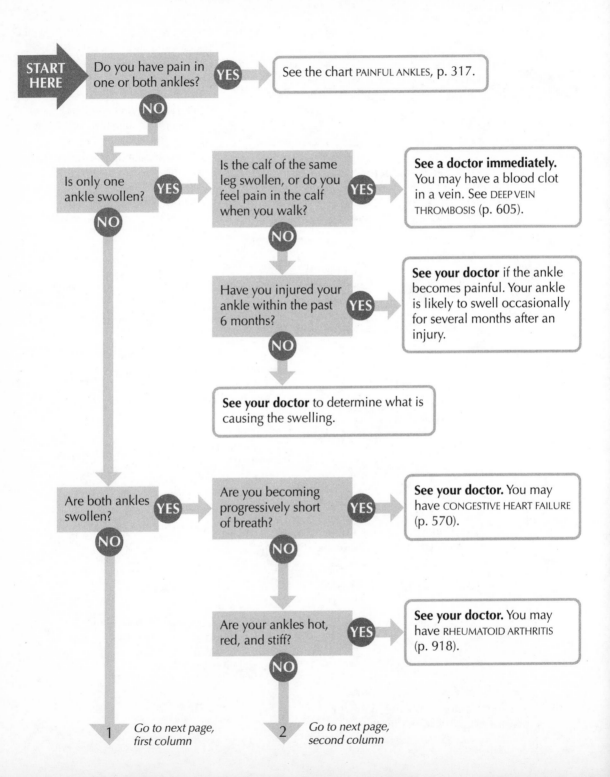

START HERE

Do you have pain in one or both ankles?

YES → See the chart PAINFUL ANKLES, p. 317.

NO

Is only one ankle swollen?

YES → **Is the calf of the same leg swollen, or do you feel pain in the calf when you walk?**

YES → **See a doctor immediately.** You may have a blood clot in a vein. See DEEP VEIN THROMBOSIS (p. 605).

NO

Have you injured your ankle within the past 6 months?

YES → **See your doctor** if the ankle becomes painful. Your ankle is likely to swell occasionally for several months after an injury.

NO

See your doctor to determine what is causing the swelling.

NO

Are both ankles swollen?

YES → **Are you becoming progressively short of breath?**

YES → **See your doctor.** You may have CONGESTIVE HEART FAILURE (p. 570).

NO

Are your ankles hot, red, and stiff?

YES → **See your doctor.** You may have RHEUMATOID ARTHRITIS (p. 918).

NO

1 *Go to next page, first column*

2 *Go to next page, second column*

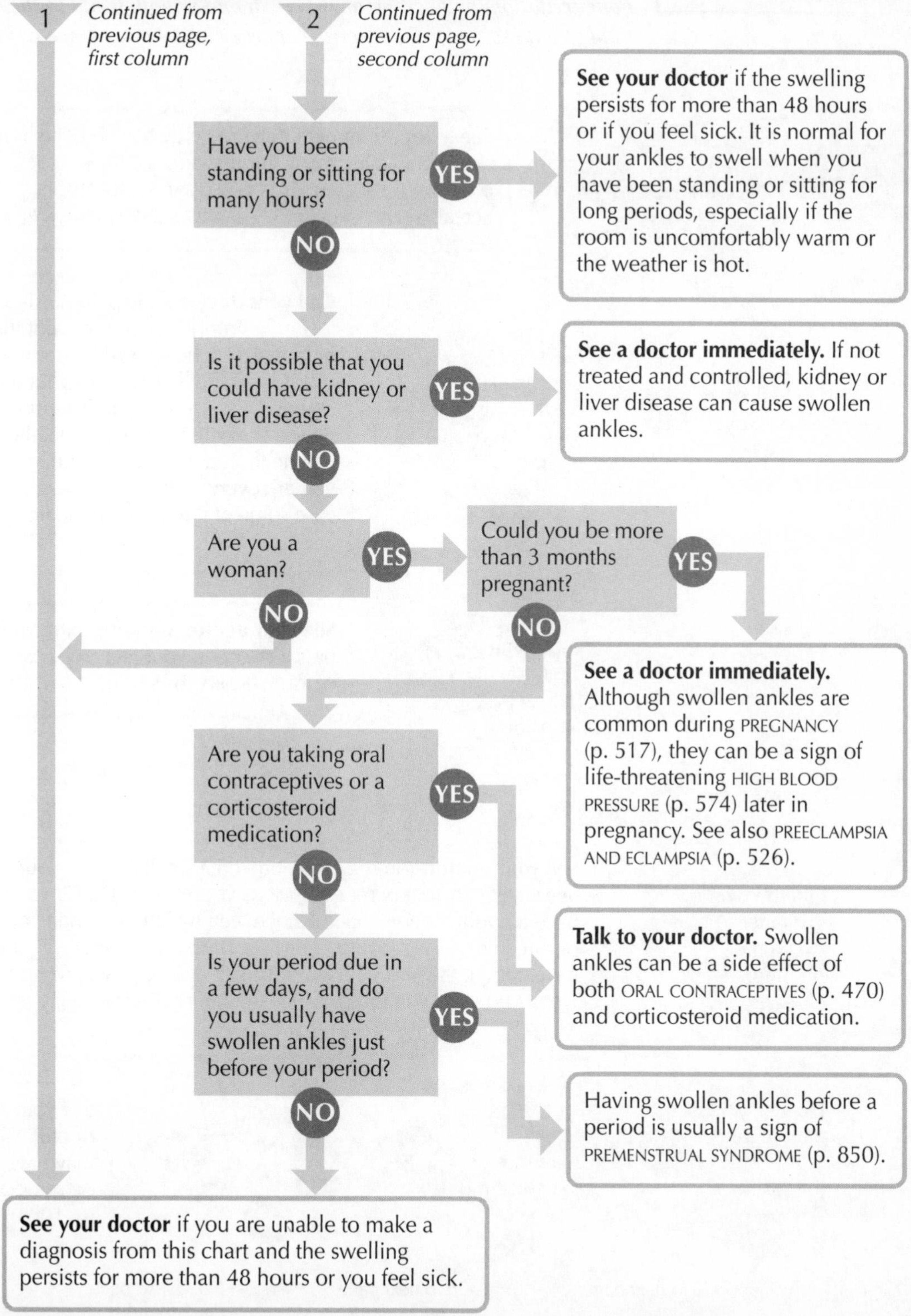

1 *Continued from previous page, first column*

2 *Continued from previous page, second column*

Have you been standing or sitting for many hours?

YES → **See your doctor** if the swelling persists for more than 48 hours or if you feel sick. It is normal for your ankles to swell when you have been standing or sitting for long periods, especially if the room is uncomfortably warm or the weather is hot.

NO ↓

Is it possible that you could have kidney or liver disease?

YES → **See a doctor immediately.** If not treated and controlled, kidney or liver disease can cause swollen ankles.

NO ↓

Are you a woman? **YES** → Could you be more than 3 months pregnant? **YES** →

NO ↓ ← **NO** ↓

See a doctor immediately. Although swollen ankles are common during PREGNANCY (p. 517), they can be a sign of life-threatening HIGH BLOOD PRESSURE (p. 574) later in pregnancy. See also PREECLAMPSIA AND ECLAMPSIA (p. 526).

Are you taking oral contraceptives or a corticosteroid medication?

YES →

NO ↓

Is your period due in a few days, and do you usually have swollen ankles just before your period?

YES → **Talk to your doctor.** Swollen ankles can be a side effect of both ORAL CONTRACEPTIVES (p. 470) and corticosteroid medication.

NO ↓

→ Having swollen ankles before a period is usually a sign of PREMENSTRUAL SYNDROME (p. 850).

See your doctor if you are unable to make a diagnosis from this chart and the swelling persists for more than 48 hours or you feel sick.

Foot problems

Pain, irritation, or swelling anywhere in one or both feet. For the chart
PAINFUL ANKLES, see p. 317. For the chart SWOLLEN ANKLES, see p. 318.

START HERE → Have you injured your foot within the past 24 hours? → **YES** →

See a doctor immediately. You may have broken a bone or strained a ligament. For first aid, see BROKEN OR DISLOCATED BONES (p. 167) and SPRAINS AND STRAINS (p. 176). See also FRACTURES (p. 987) and SPRAINED LIGAMENT (p. 983).

NO ↓

Do both feet ache all over? → **YES** → Have you been walking or standing for long periods of time? → **YES** →

Call your doctor if the pain persists. Your feet may simply be overtired, but the pain may also be caused by stretching or straining of the ligaments of your feet. You may have to wear arch supports and perform exercises to help strengthen the ligaments and muscles of your feet. If you are overweight, losing weight can ease some of the strain on the ligaments. See LOSING WEIGHT SENSIBLY (p. 53).

NO ↓

Are you overweight according to the body mass index chart on p. 11? → **YES** →

See your doctor. Carrying extra weight puts a strain on your feet. See LOSING WEIGHT SENSIBLY (p. 53).

NO ↓

Did the pain start after walking or running? → **YES** →

See your doctor. You may have broken a small bone in your foot. See STRESS FRACTURE IN THE FOOT OR LOWER LEG (p. 982). Or you may have a swollen nerve that rubs between two bones when you walk or run. See PAIN IN THE FRONT OF THE FOOT (p. 981). However, if you have pain in the foot when you walk that disappears promptly when you stop, you may have a circulatory disorder such as ATHEROSCLEROSIS (p. 557).

NO ↓

Do you have pain in one or more toe joints? → **YES** → Is the pain accompanied by redness and swelling? → **YES** → Is only one toe joint affected? → **YES** →

See your doctor. You may have GOUT OR PSEUDOGOUT (p. 1004).

NO ↓ | **NO** ↓ | **NO** ↓

1 *Go to next page, first column*

2 *Go to next page, second column*

3 *Go to next page, third column*

1 *Continued from previous page, first column*

2 *Continued from previous page, second column*

3 *Continued from previous page, third column*

Are you over age 50 and do you also have pain in your ankle, knee, or hip? **YES**

 NO

See your doctor. You may have OSTEOARTHRITIS (p. 996).

Did the pain begin suddenly? **YES**

 NO

Do you also have similar symptoms in your finger joints and other joints? **YES**

 NO

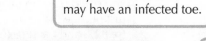
See your doctor. You may have an infected toe.

See your doctor. You may have RHEUMATOID ARTHRITIS (p. 918).

Do you have pain in the sole of your foot, heel pain, thick areas of skin on your toes or on the bottoms of your feet, or a swollen area at the base of your big toe? **YES**

 NO

Do you have a patch of skin on the sole of your foot that is painful when you walk, or thick areas of skin on the bottoms of your feet or on your toes? **YES**

NO

A small spot of thick skin on the sole may be a plantar wart. See WARTS (p. 1060). See also VISUAL AIDS TO DIAGNOSIS (p. 121). Thick skin on the soles of the feet may be calluses, and thick skin on the toes may be corns. See CORNS AND CALLUSES (p. 1061).

Is there an area of redness or swelling on the sole of your foot, heel pain, or a swollen area at the base of your big toe? **YES**

NO

See your doctor. If you have pain in the sole, you may have an infection resulting from a minor cut, or you may have torn the fibrous tissue at the bottom of your foot, which is a common cause of HEEL PAIN (p. 981). A swollen area at the base of the big toe probably is a BUNION (p. 989).

Do you have itching in one or both feet? **YES**

NO

Is the skin between your toes red, soft, and peeling? **YES**

 NO

See your doctor if you are unable to make a diagnosis from this chart.

See your doctor. You may have a fungal infection such as ATHLETE'S FOOT (p. 1073). See also VISUAL AIDS TO DIAGNOSIS (p. 123).

Painful or enlarged testicles

Pain or swelling that may affect one or both testicles or the scrotum (the pouch that contains the testicles).

START HERE

Have you suddenly developed a painful swelling in one or both testicles? **YES** → Have you had an injury to the genital area within the past 48 hours? **YES** →

See a doctor immediately. Painful or swollen testicles after an injury may be a sign of tissue damage. See INJURY TO THE TESTICLES (p. 827).

NO ↓ (from first question)

NO ↓ (from injury question)

See a doctor immediately. Painful, enlarged testicles without an injury may be caused by a twisted spermatic cord. See TORSION OF THE TESTICLE (p. 826). Or you could have an infection inside or just outside the testicle. See EPIDIDYMITIS (p. 827) and ORCHITIS (p. 828).

Do you have a painless swelling in your scrotum? **YES** →

See your doctor. The swelling may result from an INGUINAL HERNIA (p. 762) or from an accumulation of fluid such as from varicose veins around a testicle. See FLUID ACCUMULATION IN THE SCROTUM (p. 829).

NO ↓

Is only one of your testicles enlarged? **YES** →

See a doctor immediately. You may have a harmless cyst. See FLUID ACCUMULATION IN THE SCROTUM (p. 829). However, you could have CANCER OF THE TESTICLE (p. 824).

NO ↓

See your doctor if you are unable to make a diagnosis from this chart.

If you have swelling of a testicle

See a doctor immediately if you notice any swelling of a testicle. A painless swelling of one testicle may be a sign of cancer. See TESTICLE SELF-EXAMINATION (p. 139).

Painful intercourse in men

Pain or discomfort during or just after intercourse.

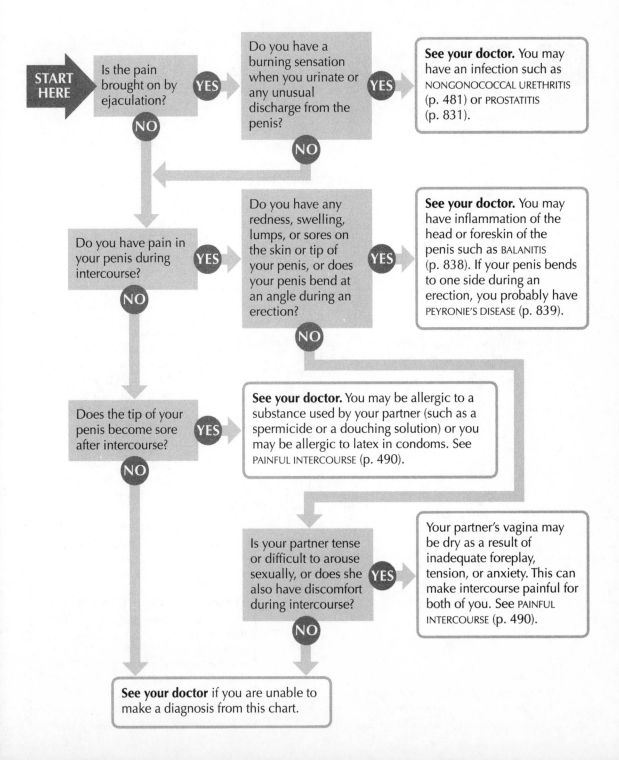

START HERE

Is the pain brought on by ejaculation?

YES → Do you have a burning sensation when you urinate or any unusual discharge from the penis?

YES → **See your doctor.** You may have an infection such as NONGONOCOCCAL URETHRITIS (p. 481) or PROSTATITIS (p. 831).

NO

NO

Do you have pain in your penis during intercourse?

YES → Do you have any redness, swelling, lumps, or sores on the skin or tip of your penis, or does your penis bend at an angle during an erection?

YES → **See your doctor.** You may have inflammation of the head or foreskin of the penis such as BALANITIS (p. 838). If your penis bends to one side during an erection, you probably have PEYRONIE'S DISEASE (p. 839).

NO

NO

Does the tip of your penis become sore after intercourse?

YES → **See your doctor.** You may be allergic to a substance used by your partner (such as a spermicide or a douching solution) or you may be allergic to latex in condoms. See PAINFUL INTERCOURSE (p. 490).

NO

Is your partner tense or difficult to arouse sexually, or does she also have discomfort during intercourse?

YES → Your partner's vagina may be dry as a result of inadequate foreplay, tension, or anxiety. This can make intercourse painful for both of you. See PAINFUL INTERCOURSE (p. 490).

NO

See your doctor if you are unable to make a diagnosis from this chart.

Pain or lumps in the breast

Aches, pain, tenderness, or lumps in one or both breasts. See HOW TO PERFORM A BREAST SELF-EXAMINATION (p. 137).

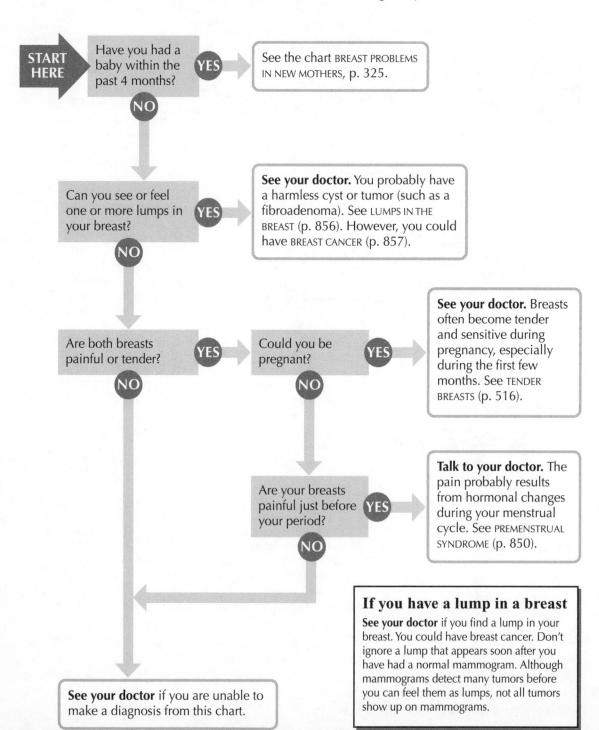

START HERE

Have you had a baby within the past 4 months?

YES → See the chart BREAST PROBLEMS IN NEW MOTHERS, p. 325.

NO ↓

Can you see or feel one or more lumps in your breast?

YES → **See your doctor.** You probably have a harmless cyst or tumor (such as a fibroadenoma). See LUMPS IN THE BREAST (p. 856). However, you could have BREAST CANCER (p. 857).

NO ↓

Are both breasts painful or tender?

YES → Could you be pregnant?

YES → **See your doctor.** Breasts often become tender and sensitive during pregnancy, especially during the first few months. See TENDER BREASTS (p. 516).

NO ↓

Are your breasts painful just before your period?

YES → **Talk to your doctor.** The pain probably results from hormonal changes during your menstrual cycle. See PREMENSTRUAL SYNDROME (p. 850).

NO ↓

See your doctor if you are unable to make a diagnosis from this chart.

If you have a lump in a breast

See your doctor if you find a lump in your breast. You could have breast cancer. Don't ignore a lump that appears soon after you have had a normal mammogram. Although mammograms detect many tumors before you can feel them as lumps, not all tumors show up on mammograms.

Breast problems in new mothers

Pain, tenderness, or lumps in the breasts within 4 months of having a baby.

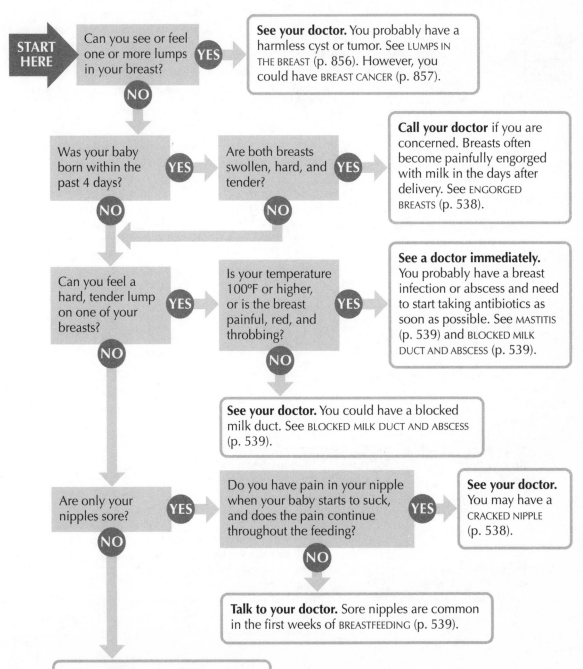

START HERE

Can you see or feel one or more lumps in your breast?

YES → **See your doctor.** You probably have a harmless cyst or tumor. See LUMPS IN THE BREAST (p. 856). However, you could have BREAST CANCER (p. 857).

NO ↓

Was your baby born within the past 4 days?

YES → **Are both breasts swollen, hard, and tender?**

YES → **Call your doctor** if you are concerned. Breasts often become painfully engorged with milk in the days after delivery. See ENGORGED BREASTS (p. 538).

NO ↓   **NO** ↓

Can you feel a hard, tender lump on one of your breasts?

YES → **Is your temperature 100°F or higher, or is the breast painful, red, and throbbing?**

YES → **See a doctor immediately.** You probably have a breast infection or abscess and need to start taking antibiotics as soon as possible. See MASTITIS (p. 539) and BLOCKED MILK DUCT AND ABSCESS (p. 539).

NO ↓   **NO** ↓

See your doctor. You could have a blocked milk duct. See BLOCKED MILK DUCT AND ABSCESS (p. 539).

Are only your nipples sore?

YES → **Do you have pain in your nipple when your baby starts to suck, and does the pain continue throughout the feeding?**

YES → **See your doctor.** You may have a CRACKED NIPPLE (p. 538).

NO ↓   **NO** ↓

Talk to your doctor. Sore nipples are common in the first weeks of BREASTFEEDING (p. 539).

See your doctor if you are unable to make a diagnosis from this chart.

Absent periods

Not getting your menstrual period when it's due.

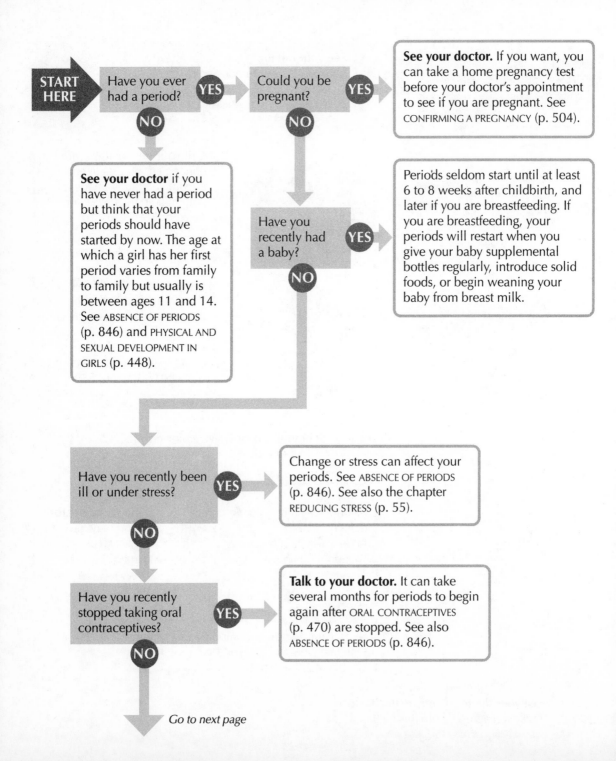

START HERE → Have you ever had a period? — **YES** → Could you be pregnant? — **YES** → **See your doctor.** If you want, you can take a home pregnancy test before your doctor's appointment to see if you are pregnant. See CONFIRMING A PREGNANCY (p. 504).

Have you ever had a period? — **NO** → **See your doctor** if you have never had a period but think that your periods should have started by now. The age at which a girl has her first period varies from family to family but usually is between ages 11 and 14. See ABSENCE OF PERIODS (p. 846) and PHYSICAL AND SEXUAL DEVELOPMENT IN GIRLS (p. 448).

Could you be pregnant? — **NO** → Have you recently had a baby? — **YES** → Periods seldom start until at least 6 to 8 weeks after childbirth, and later if you are breastfeeding. If you are breastfeeding, your periods will restart when you give your baby supplemental bottles regularly, introduce solid foods, or begin weaning your baby from breast milk.

Have you recently had a baby? — **NO** → Have you recently been ill or under stress? — **YES** → Change or stress can affect your periods. See ABSENCE OF PERIODS (p. 846). See also the chapter REDUCING STRESS (p. 55).

Have you recently been ill or under stress? — **NO** → Have you recently stopped taking oral contraceptives? — **YES** → **Talk to your doctor.** It can take several months for periods to begin again after ORAL CONTRACEPTIVES (p. 470) are stopped. See also ABSENCE OF PERIODS (p. 846).

Have you recently stopped taking oral contraceptives? — **NO** →

Go to next page

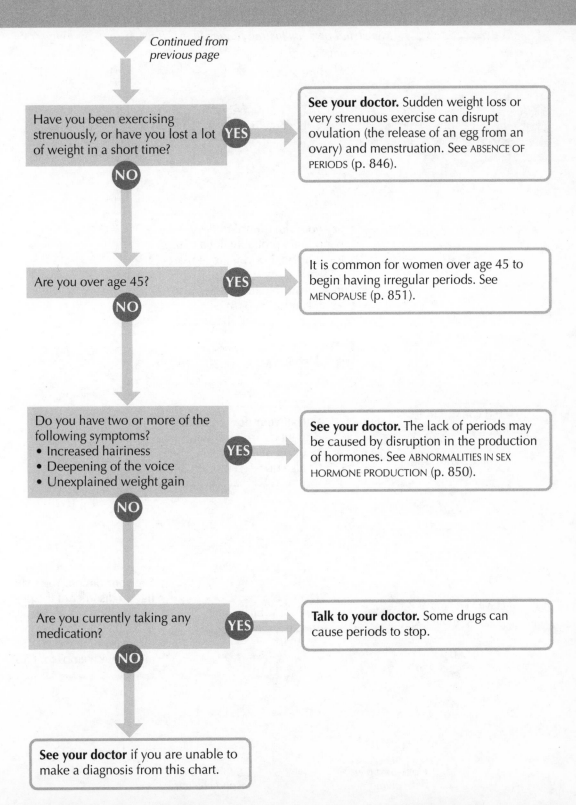

Continued from previous page

Have you been exercising strenuously, or have you lost a lot of weight in a short time?

YES → **See your doctor.** Sudden weight loss or very strenuous exercise can disrupt ovulation (the release of an egg from an ovary) and menstruation. See ABSENCE OF PERIODS (p. 846).

NO ↓

Are you over age 45?

YES → It is common for women over age 45 to begin having irregular periods. See MENOPAUSE (p. 851).

NO ↓

Do you have two or more of the following symptoms?
• Increased hairiness
• Deepening of the voice
• Unexplained weight gain

YES → **See your doctor.** The lack of periods may be caused by disruption in the production of hormones. See ABNORMALITIES IN SEX HORMONE PRODUCTION (p. 850).

NO ↓

Are you currently taking any medication?

YES → **Talk to your doctor.** Some drugs can cause periods to stop.

NO ↓

See your doctor if you are unable to make a diagnosis from this chart.

Heavy periods

Menstrual periods lasting longer than 7 days or that are longer or heavier than usual.

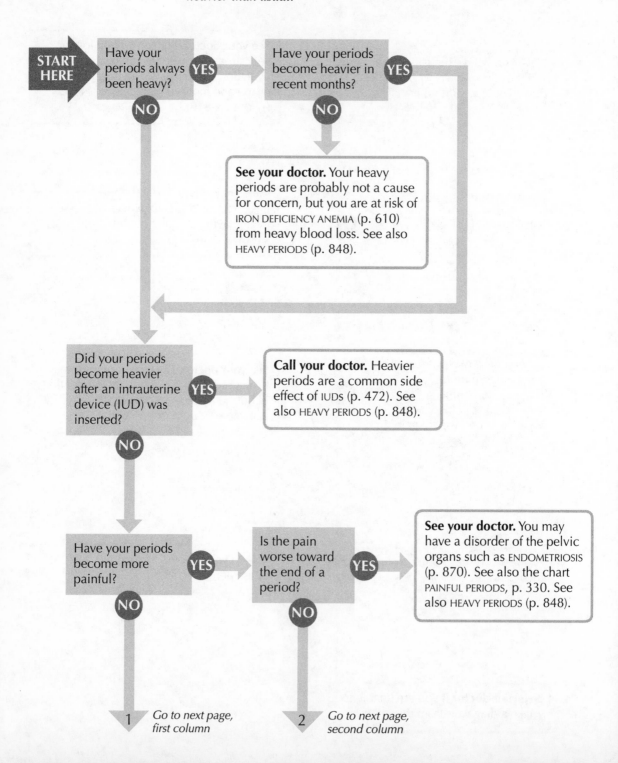

START HERE

Have your periods always been heavy? — **YES** → **Have your periods become heavier in recent months?** — **YES** →

NO ↓

NO ↓

See your doctor. Your heavy periods are probably not a cause for concern, but you are at risk of IRON DEFICIENCY ANEMIA (p. 610) from heavy blood loss. See also HEAVY PERIODS (p. 848).

Did your periods become heavier after an intrauterine device (IUD) was inserted? — **YES** → **Call your doctor.** Heavier periods are a common side effect of IUDs (p. 472). See also HEAVY PERIODS (p. 848).

NO ↓

Have your periods become more painful? — **YES** → **Is the pain worse toward the end of a period?** — **YES** → **See your doctor.** You may have a disorder of the pelvic organs such as ENDOMETRIOSIS (p. 870). See also the chart PAINFUL PERIODS, p. 330. See also HEAVY PERIODS (p. 848).

NO ↓

NO ↓

1 *Go to next page, first column*

2 *Go to next page, second column*

1 *Continued from previous page, first column*

2 *Continued from previous page, second column*

Do you have a vaginal discharge between periods that is unusually heavy or that has an unpleasant odor, or is your temperature 100°F or higher?

 YES → **See your doctor.** You may have an infection of the uterus, fallopian tubes, ovaries, or surrounding tissues. See PELVIC INFLAMMATORY DISEASE (p. 871). See also HEAVY PERIODS (p. 848).

 NO

See your doctor. You may have a benign growth in the uterus. See FIBROIDS (p. 867). See also HEAVY PERIODS (p. 848).

Have you had only one heavy period that was a week or more late? **YES** → **See your doctor.** A delayed period can be heavier than usual and is seldom a cause for concern. However, if there is a possibility that you were pregnant, you could have had an early MISCARRIAGE (p. 522). See also HEAVY PERIODS (p. 848).

 NO

Have you recently started to have a few days of light bleeding at the beginning or end of a period? **YES** → **See your doctor.** These symptoms are common as women approach MENOPAUSE (p. 851). However, they can also be symptoms of FIBROIDS (p. 867) or POLYCYSTIC OVARIAN SYNDROME (p. 865). See also HEAVY PERIODS (p. 848).

 NO

Have you recently had a baby? **YES** → **Talk to your doctor.** The first period after childbirth is often heavier than usual.

 NO

See your doctor if you are unable to make a diagnosis from this chart.

Painful periods

Pain with menstruation.

START HERE

Do you have a vaginal discharge between periods that is unusually heavy or that has an unpleasant odor, or is your temperature 100°F or higher? **YES**

NO

See your doctor. You may have an infection of the uterus, fallopian tubes, ovaries, or surrounding tissues. See PELVIC INFLAMMATORY DISEASE (p. 871). See also PAINFUL PERIODS (p. 848).

Does the pain get worse as your period continues? **YES**

NO

See your doctor. You may have ENDOMETRIOSIS (p. 870). See also PAINFUL PERIODS (p. 848).

Have you started menstruating within the past 3 months? **YES**

NO

Have you had painful periods for most of your adult life, and is the pain the same as usual? **YES**

NO

Talk to your doctor. The pain is unlikely to be caused by an underlying disorder. See PAINFUL PERIODS (p. 848).

Go to next column

Continued from previous column

Have your periods become more painful since you had an intrauterine device (IUD) inserted? **YES**

NO

See your doctor. An increase in menstrual pain is sometimes associated with insertion of an IUD (p. 472). See also PAINFUL PERIODS (p. 848).

Have you recently stopped taking oral contraceptives? **YES**

NO

Talk to your doctor. ORAL CONTRACEPTIVES (p. 470) often reduce menstrual pain, so some women notice an increase in menstrual pain when they stop taking them. See also PAINFUL PERIODS (p. 848).

See your doctor if you are unable to make a diagnosis from this chart.

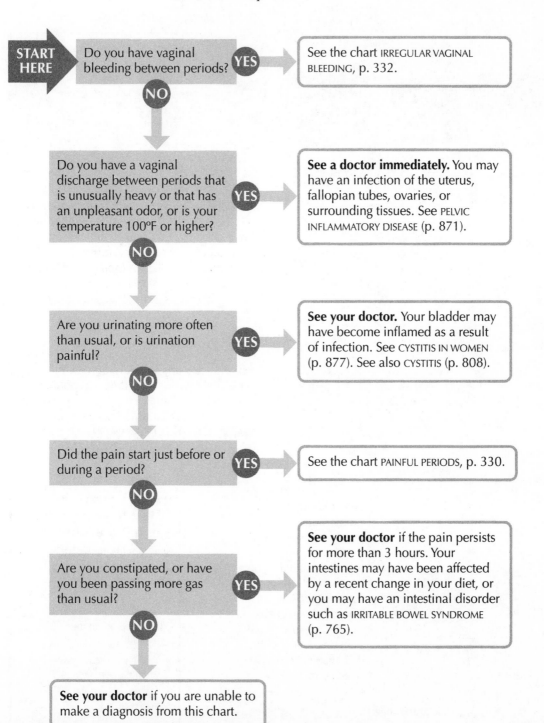

Pelvic pain in women

Pain in the pelvic area. Use this chart only after consulting the chart
ABDOMINAL PAIN, *p. 284.*

START HERE

Do you have vaginal bleeding between periods?

YES → See the chart IRREGULAR VAGINAL BLEEDING, p. 332.

NO ↓

Do you have a vaginal discharge between periods that is unusually heavy or that has an unpleasant odor, or is your temperature 100°F or higher?

YES → **See a doctor immediately.** You may have an infection of the uterus, fallopian tubes, ovaries, or surrounding tissues. See PELVIC INFLAMMATORY DISEASE (p. 871).

NO ↓

Are you urinating more often than usual, or is urination painful?

YES → **See your doctor.** Your bladder may have become inflamed as a result of infection. See CYSTITIS IN WOMEN (p. 877). See also CYSTITIS (p. 808).

NO ↓

Did the pain start just before or during a period?

YES → See the chart PAINFUL PERIODS, p. 330.

NO ↓

Are you constipated, or have you been passing more gas than usual?

YES → **See your doctor** if the pain persists for more than 3 hours. Your intestines may have been affected by a recent change in your diet, or you may have an intestinal disorder such as IRRITABLE BOWEL SYNDROME (p. 765).

NO ↓

See your doctor if you are unable to make a diagnosis from this chart.

Irregular vaginal bleeding

Any bleeding that occurs between menstrual periods, during pregnancy, or after menopause.

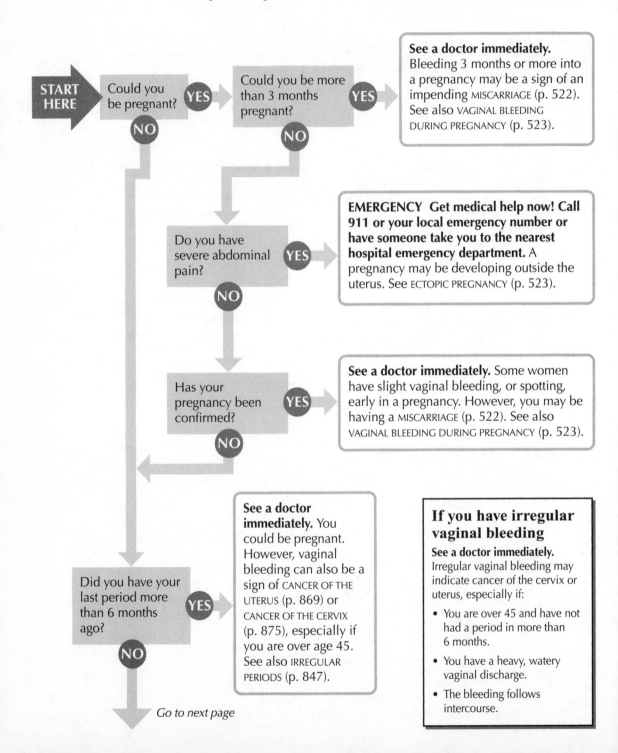

START HERE

Could you be pregnant? — YES →

Could you be more than 3 months pregnant? — YES →

See a doctor immediately. Bleeding 3 months or more into a pregnancy may be a sign of an impending MISCARRIAGE (p. 522). See also VAGINAL BLEEDING DURING PREGNANCY (p. 523).

NO ↓ (from "Could you be more than 3 months pregnant?")

Do you have severe abdominal pain? — YES →

EMERGENCY Get medical help now! Call 911 or your local emergency number or have someone take you to the nearest hospital emergency department. A pregnancy may be developing outside the uterus. See ECTOPIC PREGNANCY (p. 523).

NO ↓

Has your pregnancy been confirmed? — YES →

See a doctor immediately. Some women have slight vaginal bleeding, or spotting, early in a pregnancy. However, you may be having a MISCARRIAGE (p. 522). See also VAGINAL BLEEDING DURING PREGNANCY (p. 523).

NO ↓

Did you have your last period more than 6 months ago? — YES →

See a doctor immediately. You could be pregnant. However, vaginal bleeding can also be a sign of CANCER OF THE UTERUS (p. 869) or CANCER OF THE CERVIX (p. 875), especially if you are over age 45. See also IRREGULAR PERIODS (p. 847).

NO ↓

Go to next page

If you have irregular vaginal bleeding

See a doctor immediately.
Irregular vaginal bleeding may indicate cancer of the cervix or uterus, especially if:

- You are over 45 and have not had a period in more than 6 months.

- You have a heavy, watery vaginal discharge.

- The bleeding follows intercourse.

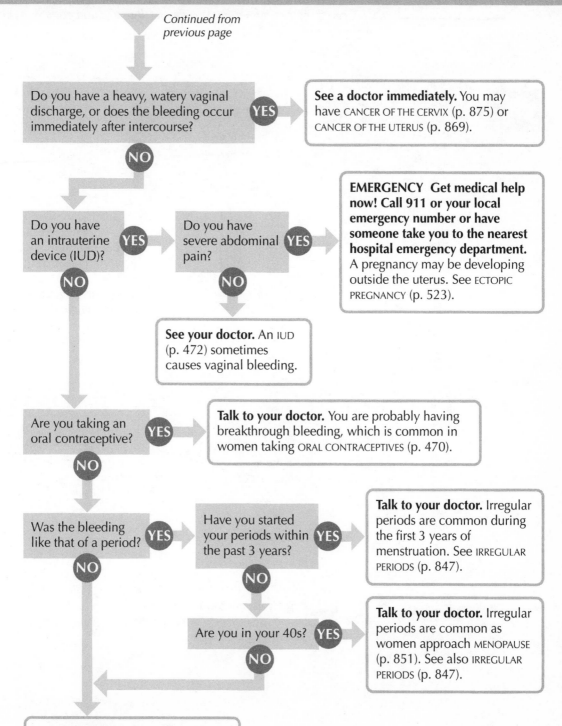

Continued from previous page

Do you have a heavy, watery vaginal discharge, or does the bleeding occur immediately after intercourse? — **YES** → **See a doctor immediately.** You may have CANCER OF THE CERVIX (p. 875) or CANCER OF THE UTERUS (p. 869).

NO ↓

Do you have an intrauterine device (IUD)? — **YES** → **Do you have severe abdominal pain?** — **YES** → **EMERGENCY Get medical help now! Call 911 or your local emergency number or have someone take you to the nearest hospital emergency department.** A pregnancy may be developing outside the uterus. See ECTOPIC PREGNANCY (p. 523).

NO (under IUD) ↓

NO (under severe abdominal pain) ↓ → **See your doctor.** An IUD (p. 472) sometimes causes vaginal bleeding.

Are you taking an oral contraceptive? — **YES** → **Talk to your doctor.** You are probably having breakthrough bleeding, which is common in women taking ORAL CONTRACEPTIVES (p. 470).

NO ↓

Was the bleeding like that of a period? — **YES** → **Have you started your periods within the past 3 years?** — **YES** → **Talk to your doctor.** Irregular periods are common during the first 3 years of menstruation. See IRREGULAR PERIODS (p. 847).

NO (under past 3 years) ↓

Are you in your 40s? — **YES** → **Talk to your doctor.** Irregular periods are common as women approach MENOPAUSE (p. 851). See also IRREGULAR PERIODS (p. 847).

NO ↓

See your doctor if you are unable to make a diagnosis from this chart.

Abnormal vaginal discharge

Discharge from the vagina that is different than usual in color, consistency, or quantity.

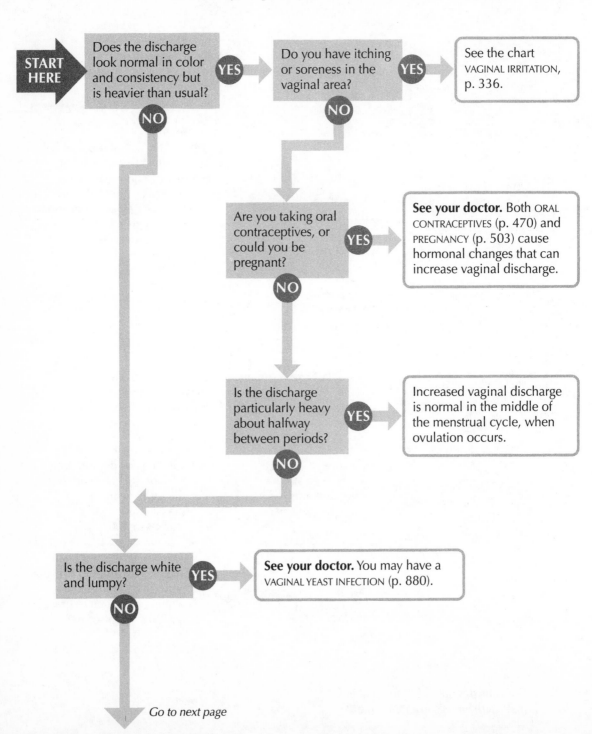

START HERE

Does the discharge look normal in color and consistency but is heavier than usual?

YES → Do you have itching or soreness in the vaginal area?

YES → See the chart VAGINAL IRRITATION, p. 336.

NO ↓

Are you taking oral contraceptives, or could you be pregnant?

YES → **See your doctor.** Both ORAL CONTRACEPTIVES (p. 470) and PREGNANCY (p. 503) cause hormonal changes that can increase vaginal discharge.

NO ↓

Is the discharge particularly heavy about halfway between periods?

YES → Increased vaginal discharge is normal in the middle of the menstrual cycle, when ovulation occurs.

NO ↓

Is the discharge white and lumpy?

YES → **See your doctor.** You may have a VAGINAL YEAST INFECTION (p. 880).

NO ↓

Go to next page

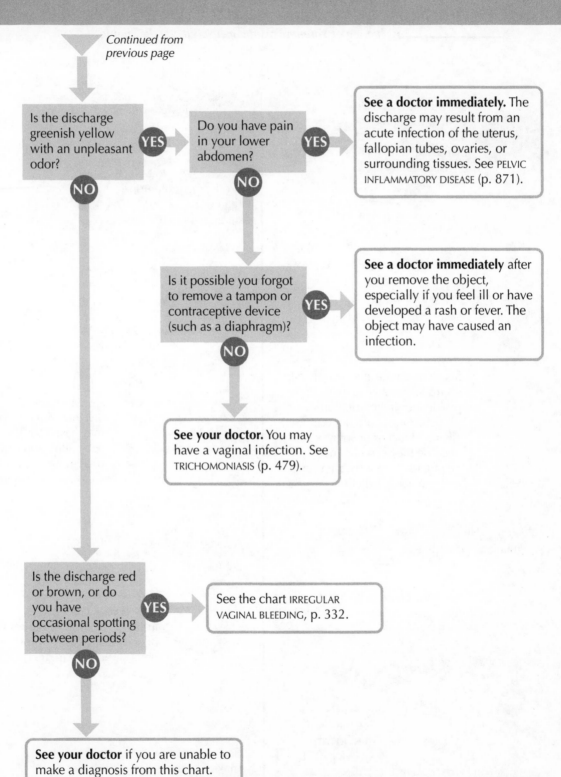

Continued from previous page

Is the discharge greenish yellow with an unpleasant odor?

YES → Do you have pain in your lower abdomen?

YES → **See a doctor immediately.** The discharge may result from an acute infection of the uterus, fallopian tubes, ovaries, or surrounding tissues. See PELVIC INFLAMMATORY DISEASE (p. 871).

NO ↓

Is it possible you forgot to remove a tampon or contraceptive device (such as a diaphragm)?

YES → **See a doctor immediately** after you remove the object, especially if you feel ill or have developed a rash or fever. The object may have caused an infection.

NO ↓

See your doctor. You may have a vaginal infection. See TRICHOMONIASIS (p. 479).

NO ↓

Is the discharge red or brown, or do you have occasional spotting between periods?

YES → See the chart IRREGULAR VAGINAL BLEEDING, p. 332.

NO ↓

See your doctor if you are unable to make a diagnosis from this chart.

WOMEN

Vaginal irritation

Itching or soreness inside or just outside the vagina.

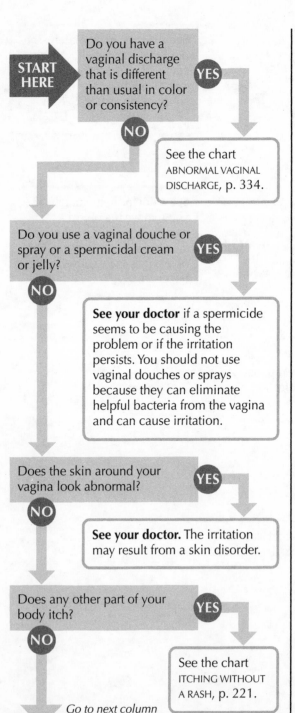

START HERE

Do you have a vaginal discharge that is different than usual in color or consistency?

YES → See the chart ABNORMAL VAGINAL DISCHARGE, p. 334.

NO ↓

Do you use a vaginal douche or spray or a spermicidal cream or jelly?

YES → **See your doctor** if a spermicide seems to be causing the problem or if the irritation persists. You should not use vaginal douches or sprays because they can eliminate helpful bacteria from the vagina and can cause irritation.

NO ↓

Does the skin around your vagina look abnormal?

YES → **See your doctor.** The irritation may result from a skin disorder.

NO ↓

Does any other part of your body itch?

YES → See the chart ITCHING WITHOUT A RASH, p. 221.

NO ↓

Go to next column

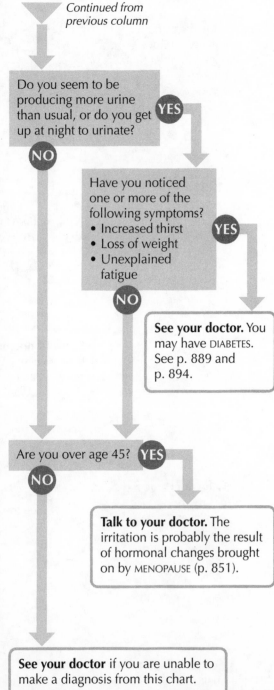

Continued from previous column

↓

Do you seem to be producing more urine than usual, or do you get up at night to urinate?

YES ↓

NO ↓

Have you noticed one or more of the following symptoms?
• Increased thirst
• Loss of weight
• Unexplained fatigue

YES → **See your doctor.** You may have DIABETES. See p. 889 and p. 894.

NO ↓

Are you over age 45?

YES → **Talk to your doctor.** The irritation is probably the result of hormonal changes brought on by MENOPAUSE (p. 851).

NO ↓

See your doctor if you are unable to make a diagnosis from this chart.

Abnormal hair growth in women

Excessive hair anywhere on the body.

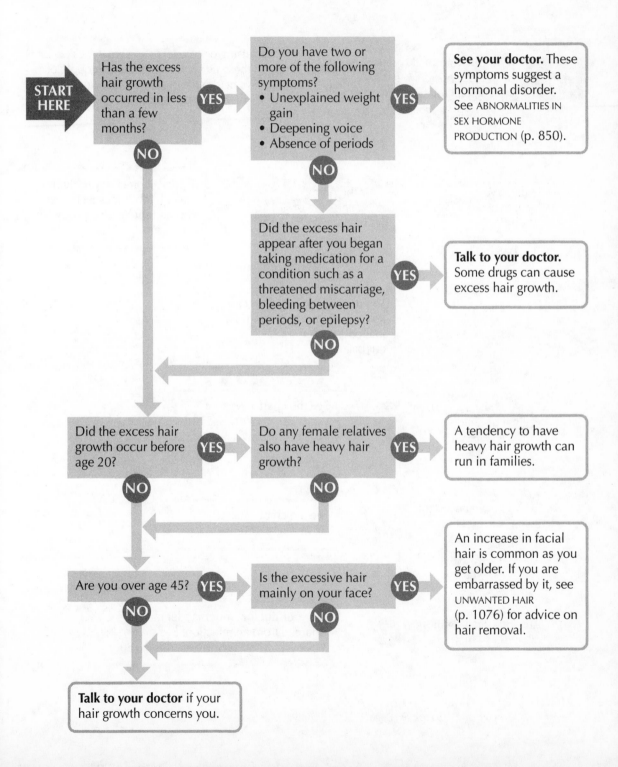

START HERE

Has the excess hair growth occurred in less than a few months?

YES →

Do you have two or more of the following symptoms?
- Unexplained weight gain
- Deepening voice
- Absence of periods

YES →

See your doctor. These symptoms suggest a hormonal disorder. See ABNORMALITIES IN SEX HORMONE PRODUCTION (p. 850).

NO ↓

Did the excess hair appear after you began taking medication for a condition such as a threatened miscarriage, bleeding between periods, or epilepsy?

YES →

Talk to your doctor. Some drugs can cause excess hair growth.

NO

Did the excess hair growth occur before age 20?

YES →

Do any female relatives also have heavy hair growth?

YES →

A tendency to have heavy hair growth can run in families.

NO

NO

Are you over age 45?

YES →

Is the excessive hair mainly on your face?

YES →

An increase in facial hair is common as you get older. If you are embarrassed by it, see UNWANTED HAIR (p. 1076) for advice on hair removal.

NO

NO

Talk to your doctor if your hair growth concerns you.

WOMEN

Painful intercourse in women

Pain or discomfort during or just after sexual intercourse.

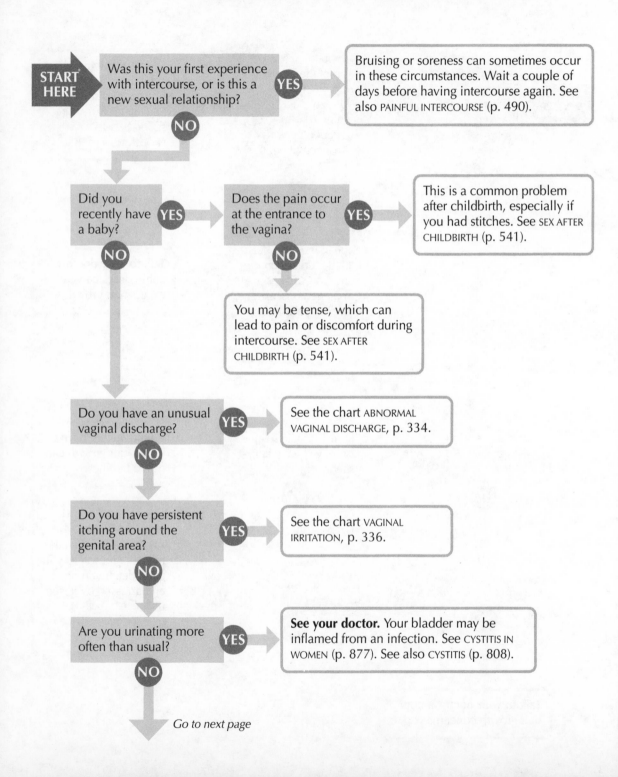

START HERE

Was this your first experience with intercourse, or is this a new sexual relationship?

YES → Bruising or soreness can sometimes occur in these circumstances. Wait a couple of days before having intercourse again. See also PAINFUL INTERCOURSE (p. 490).

NO ↓

Did you recently have a baby?

YES → Does the pain occur at the entrance to the vagina?

YES → This is a common problem after childbirth, especially if you had stitches. See SEX AFTER CHILDBIRTH (p. 541).

NO ↓ (Does the pain occur...) → You may be tense, which can lead to pain or discomfort during intercourse. See SEX AFTER CHILDBIRTH (p. 541).

NO ↓ (Did you recently have a baby?)

Do you have an unusual vaginal discharge?

YES → See the chart ABNORMAL VAGINAL DISCHARGE, p. 334.

NO ↓

Do you have persistent itching around the genital area?

YES → See the chart VAGINAL IRRITATION, p. 336.

NO ↓

Are you urinating more often than usual?

YES → **See your doctor.** Your bladder may be inflamed from an infection. See CYSTITIS IN WOMEN (p. 877). See also CYSTITIS (p. 808).

NO ↓

Go to next page

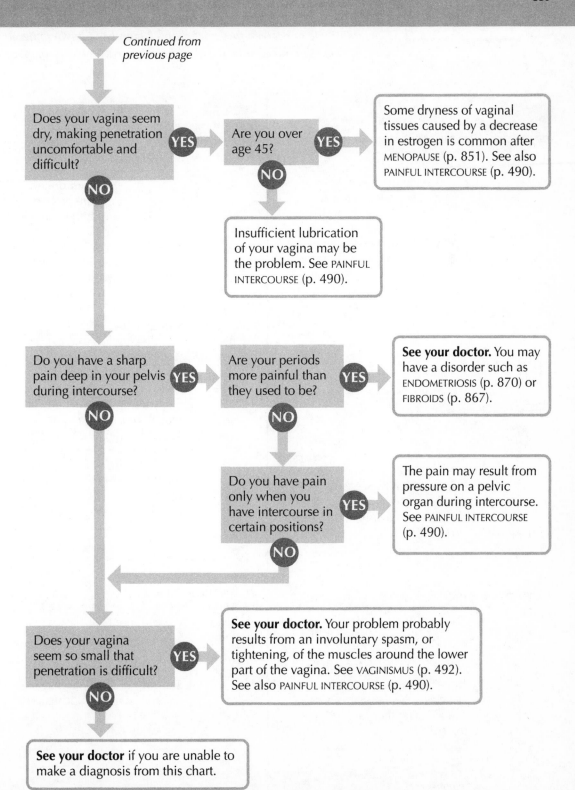

Continued from previous page

Does your vagina seem dry, making penetration uncomfortable and difficult? **YES** → Are you over age 45? **YES** → Some dryness of vaginal tissues caused by a decrease in estrogen is common after MENOPAUSE (p. 851). See also PAINFUL INTERCOURSE (p. 490).

NO (from "Are you over age 45?") → Insufficient lubrication of your vagina may be the problem. See PAINFUL INTERCOURSE (p. 490).

NO (from first question)

Do you have a sharp pain deep in your pelvis during intercourse? **YES** → Are your periods more painful than they used to be? **YES** → **See your doctor.** You may have a disorder such as ENDOMETRIOSIS (p. 870) or FIBROIDS (p. 867).

NO (from "Are your periods more painful") → Do you have pain only when you have intercourse in certain positions? **YES** → The pain may result from pressure on a pelvic organ during intercourse. See PAINFUL INTERCOURSE (p. 490).

NO

NO (from "Do you have a sharp pain deep in your pelvis")

Does your vagina seem so small that penetration is difficult? **YES** → **See your doctor.** Your problem probably results from an involuntary spasm, or tightening, of the muscles around the lower part of the vagina. See VAGINISMUS (p. 492). See also PAINFUL INTERCOURSE (p. 490).

NO → **See your doctor** if you are unable to make a diagnosis from this chart.

Infertility

The inability to conceive after more than 12 months of having intercourse without using contraception. See also the chapter INFERTILITY *(p. 493).*

MEN START HERE

Have you noticed any unusual swelling of your testicles?

YES → **See your doctor.** A disorder of the testicles may be affecting your fertility. See the chart PAINFUL OR ENLARGED TESTICLES, p. 322. See also CAUSES OF INFERTILITY IN MEN (p. 494).

NO ↓

Do you have a discharge from your penis, or have you ever had a sexually transmitted disease (STD)?

YES → **See your doctor.** Some STDs can lead to infertility. See GONORRHEA (p. 480) and CHLAMYDIA (p. 477). See also CAUSES OF INFERTILITY IN MEN (p. 494).

NO ↓

Did you have mumps after age 12?

YES → MUMPS (p. 440) occasionally causes inflammation of the testicles, which, in rare cases, can affect fertility. See ORCHITIS (p. 828).

NO ↓

1 *Go to next page, first column*

WOMEN START HERE

Are your periods infrequent or irregular?

YES → **See your doctor.** You are probably ovulating infrequently. See IRREGULAR PERIODS (p. 847). See also CAUSES OF INFERTILITY IN WOMEN (p. 493).

NO ↓

Have you ever had an infection of the uterus or fallopian tubes or a sexually transmitted disease?

YES → **See your doctor.** The infection may have caused a blockage in your fallopian tubes. See PELVIC INFLAMMATORY DISEASE (p. 871), CHLAMYDIA (p. 477), GONORRHEA (p. 480), and NONGONOCOCCAL URETHRITIS (p. 481). See also CAUSES OF INFERTILITY IN WOMEN (p. 493).

NO ↓

Do you have one or more of the following symptoms?

- Painful periods
- Abnormal vaginal discharge
- Recurring lower abdominal pain

YES → **See your doctor.** You may have a disorder such as ENDOMETRIOSIS (p. 870) or PELVIC INFLAMMATORY DISEASE (p. 871).

NO ↓

2 *Go to next page, second column*

1 *Continued from previous page, first column***

2 *Continued from previous page, second column***

Are you overweight; do you use hot tubs or saunas, wear tight pants, smoke, drink alcohol excessively, use drugs, or eat poorly; are you in poor health; have you had surgery on your reproductive tract; or do you have an abnormality of the reproductive tract? **YES**

NO

See your doctor. Exposing the testicles to consistently high temperatures (as can occur when layers of fat increase the temperature around the testicles or when you use hot tubs or saunas or wear tight pants) reduces sperm count. Smoking, drinking excessively, or using drugs not only lowers sperm count but also reduces sperm motility. Being in generally poor health can also affect your fertility. Having reproductive tract surgery or a structural abnormality of the reproductive tract can obstruct the flow of semen and the passage of sperm.

Are you over age 35? **YES**

NO

See your doctor. Fertility declines as you get older. See CAUSES OF INFERTILITY IN WOMEN (p. 493).

Do you have intercourse less than once a week? **YES**

Your chances of conception will increase if you have intercourse more frequently, especially if you are able to have intercourse around the time of ovulation. To estimate when ovulation occurs, see CONCEPTION (p. 503), the introduction to the section MENSTRUATION (p. 845), and NATURAL METHODS (p. 474).

 NO

Do you or your partner have a sexual problem such as difficulty with erections or pain during intercourse? **YES**

See your doctor. Often, failure to conceive results from sexual difficulties. See the section SEXUAL PROBLEMS (p. 486).

NO

Is either of you ill, or does either of you have a chronic disease? **YES**

See your doctor. Many illnesses (particularly liver and hormone problems) and the medications used to treat them can sometimes cause infertility. See THE CAUSES OF INFERTILITY (p. 493).

 NO

See your doctor if neither of you is able to make a diagnosis from this chart.

Infertility treatment

Infertility in both women and men can often be treated successfully. See TREATING INFERTILITY (p. 498).

CHILDREN
Up to 5 years

Waking at night in children

Difficulty sleeping through the night that causes a child to cry or call out. See also DIFFICULTY FALLING ASLEEP OR SLEEPING THROUGH THE NIGHT (p. 413).

START HERE

Is your child's temperature over 100°F, or does he or she seem ill in any way? **YES**

Call your child's doctor. An illness may be disturbing your child's sleep. See CARING FOR A CHILD WHO IS ILL (p. 435) and the charts FEVER IN YOUNG CHILDREN, p. 354, CRYING IN INFANTS, p. 344, and FEVER IN CHILDREN, p. 356.

NO

Is your child younger than 6 weeks? **YES** → When your baby wakes, do you feed him or her? **YES** → Does your baby go back to sleep after the feeding? **YES**

NO

NO

NO

Your baby is too young to sleep through the night without at least one or two feedings. See also the chart CRYING IN INFANTS, p. 344.

Your baby may have developed an irregular sleep pattern, or the room may be too noisy, bright, warm, or cool. Establish a consistent sleep schedule and BEDTIME ROUTINE (p. 413) and keep the room dark and quiet and the temperature comfortable (68°F to 70°F) to help promote sleep.

Waking at night from hunger is normal at this age. Feed your baby whenever he or she is hungry, at least every few hours.

Is your child younger than 6 months? **YES** → When your baby wakes, do you feed him or her? **YES** → Does your baby go back to sleep after the feeding? **YES**

NO

 NO

 NO

Try feeding your baby when he or she wakes. Your baby may be hungry and may sleep better if fed during the night. See also the chart CRYING IN INFANTS, p. 344.

Babies this age often wake from hunger. Try feeding your baby just before you go to bed.

Go to next page

Continued from previous page

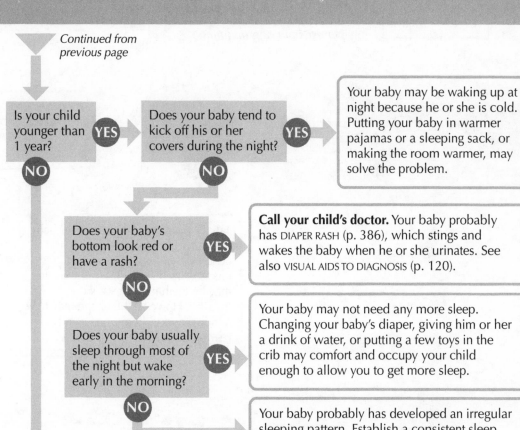

Is your child younger than 1 year? **YES**

Does your baby tend to kick off his or her covers during the night? **YES**

Your baby may be waking up at night because he or she is cold. Putting your baby in warmer pajamas or a sleeping sack, or making the room warmer, may solve the problem.

NO

NO

Does your baby's bottom look red or have a rash? **YES**

Call your child's doctor. Your baby probably has DIAPER RASH (p. 386), which stings and wakes the baby when he or she urinates. See also VISUAL AIDS TO DIAGNOSIS (p. 120).

NO

Does your baby usually sleep through most of the night but wake early in the morning? **YES**

Your baby may not need any more sleep. Changing your baby's diaper, giving him or her a drink of water, or putting a few toys in the crib may comfort and occupy your child enough to allow you to get more sleep.

NO

Your baby probably has developed an irregular sleeping pattern. Establish a consistent sleep schedule and BEDTIME ROUTINE (p. 413).

Does your child seem upset or frightened when he or she wakes up? **YES**

Nightmares may be waking your child. Keep a dim light on in the room if your child seems to be afraid of the dark. See NIGHTMARES, NIGHT TERRORS, and SLEEPWALKING (p. 414).

NO

Does your child have any new experiences that may be a source of stress (such as the arrival of a new baby or starting school), or is there tension in the home? **YES**

Anxiety may be making it difficult for your child to sleep. Extra reassurance and affection during the day and at bedtime may help solve the problem.

NO

Call your child's doctor if you are worried about your child waking at night and you cannot diagnose his or her problem from this chart.

Crying in infants

Any persistent crying in infants.

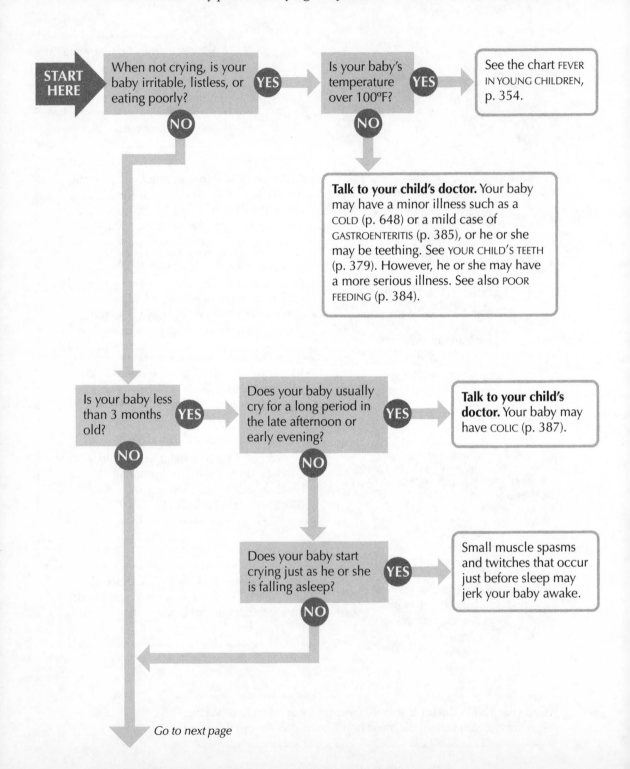

START HERE

When not crying, is your baby irritable, listless, or eating poorly?

YES → Is your baby's temperature over 100°F?

YES → See the chart FEVER IN YOUNG CHILDREN, p. 354.

NO (from temperature) → **Talk to your child's doctor.** Your baby may have a minor illness such as a COLD (p. 648) or a mild case of GASTROENTERITIS (p. 385), or he or she may be teething. See YOUR CHILD'S TEETH (p. 379). However, he or she may have a more serious illness. See also POOR FEEDING (p. 384).

NO (from irritable) → Is your baby less than 3 months old?

YES → Does your baby usually cry for a long period in the late afternoon or early evening?

YES → **Talk to your child's doctor.** Your baby may have COLIC (p. 387).

NO (from cry long period) → Does your baby start crying just as he or she is falling asleep?

YES → Small muscle spasms and twitches that occur just before sleep may jerk your baby awake.

NO (from less than 3 months) and **NO** (from falling asleep) →

Go to next page

345

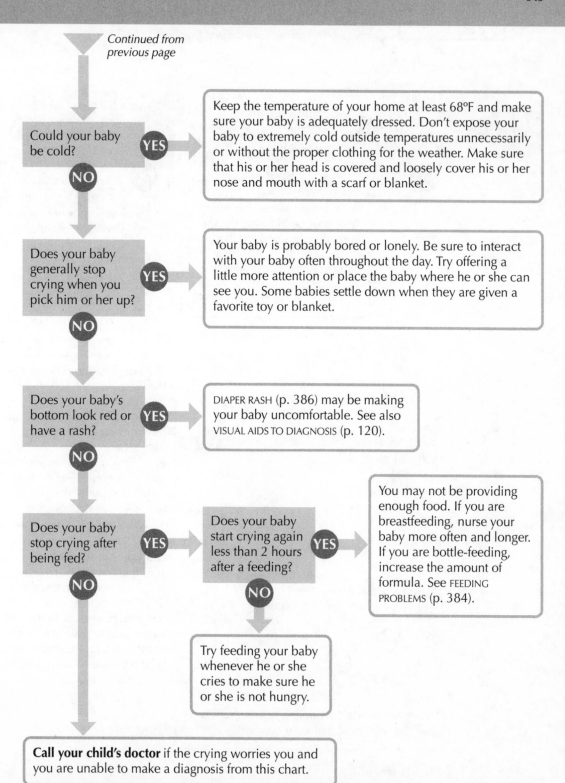

Continued from previous page

Could your baby be cold? YES →
Keep the temperature of your home at least 68°F and make sure your baby is adequately dressed. Don't expose your baby to extremely cold outside temperatures unnecessarily or without the proper clothing for the weather. Make sure that his or her head is covered and loosely cover his or her nose and mouth with a scarf or blanket.

NO

Does your baby generally stop crying when you pick him or her up? YES →
Your baby is probably bored or lonely. Be sure to interact with your baby often throughout the day. Try offering a little more attention or place the baby where he or she can see you. Some babies settle down when they are given a favorite toy or blanket.

NO

Does your baby's bottom look red or have a rash? YES →
DIAPER RASH (p. 386) may be making your baby uncomfortable. See also VISUAL AIDS TO DIAGNOSIS (p. 120).

NO

Does your baby stop crying after being fed? YES → **Does your baby start crying again less than 2 hours after a feeding?** YES →
You may not be providing enough food. If you are breastfeeding, nurse your baby more often and longer. If you are bottle-feeding, increase the amount of formula. See FEEDING PROBLEMS (p. 384).

NO →
Try feeding your baby whenever he or she cries to make sure he or she is not hungry.

NO

Call your child's doctor if the crying worries you and you are unable to make a diagnosis from this chart.

Vomiting in infants

Burping or throwing up after feedings.

START HERE

Does your baby seem healthy except for the vomiting? — **YES** →

Is your baby gaining weight? — **YES** →

Does your baby spit up small amounts of breast milk or formula during or just after feedings? — **YES** →

Spitting up small amounts of breast milk or formula, especially if your baby is very active, is probably not a cause for concern. See SPITTING UP OR VOMITING AFTER FEEDING (p. 385).

NO (Is your baby gaining weight?)

Take your child to the doctor immediately. Vomiting that is severe enough to prevent a baby from gaining weight at the usual rate may indicate an INTESTINAL OBSTRUCTION (p. 405).

NO (Does your baby seem healthy except for the vomiting?)

Are you bottle-feeding your baby? — **YES** →

Have you recently started using a new nipple on the bottle? — **YES** →

The hole in the nipple may be the wrong size. A too-small hole can make your baby swallow air, which can overfill the stomach and cause burping. Or the hole may be too large, causing your baby to gulp the milk or formula. See SPITTING UP OR VOMITING AFTER FEEDING (p. 385).

NO (Are you bottle-feeding your baby?)

NO (Have you recently started using a new nipple on the bottle?)

Is your baby younger than 3 months, and does the vomit shoot forcefully from his or her mouth right after feedings? — **YES** →

Call your child's doctor. Vomiting forcefully (called projectile vomiting) once in a while is usually not a cause for concern. However, if it happens regularly, your baby may have an INTESTINAL OBSTRUCTION (p. 405), which is an emergency.

NO

A single episode of vomiting in an otherwise healthy baby is no cause for concern.

Go to next page

Continued from previous page

Has your baby had three to four watery stools within 24 hours? **YES** → **Call your child's doctor immediately.** Your baby has diarrhea, possibly from an infection of the digestive tract. See the chart DIARRHEA IN INFANTS, p. 348.

NO ↓

Is your baby's temperature over 100°F? **YES** → See the chart FEVER IN YOUNG CHILDREN, p. 354.

NO ↓

Does your baby have a cough or a runny nose? **YES** → **Call your child's doctor** if the vomiting concerns you. However, swallowing mucus from a COLD (p. 648) or other respiratory infection is probably causing the vomiting.

NO ↓

Is your baby crying as if from pain? **YES** → **EMERGENCY Get medical help now! Call 911 or your local emergency number or take your child to the nearest hospital emergency department.** He or she may have an INTESTINAL OBSTRUCTION (p. 405) such as intussusception.

NO ↓

Call your child's doctor if you are unable to make a diagnosis from this chart.

If your child is vomiting repeatedly

Take your child to the doctor immediately. If your baby's vomiting is severe and persistent—for example, if it occurs after all feedings within a 6-hour period—he or she may be losing a dangerous amount of body fluid or may have a serious or life-threatening disorder.

Diarrhea in infants

Having three to four watery bowel movements within 24 hours.

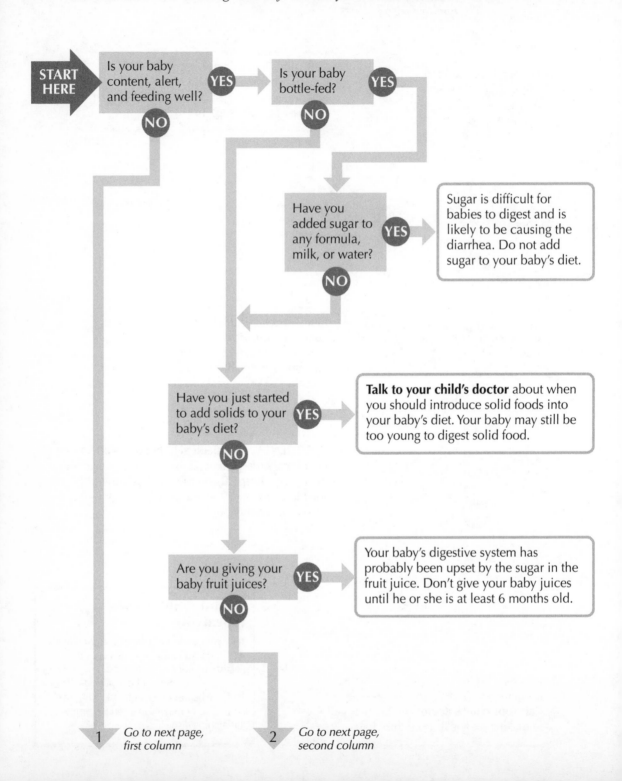

START HERE

Is your baby content, alert, and feeding well? — **YES** → Is your baby bottle-fed? — **YES** →

Have you added sugar to any formula, milk, or water? — **YES** → Sugar is difficult for babies to digest and is likely to be causing the diarrhea. Do not add sugar to your baby's diet.

NO

Have you just started to add solids to your baby's diet? — **YES** → **Talk to your child's doctor** about when you should introduce solid foods into your baby's diet. Your baby may still be too young to digest solid food.

NO

Are you giving your baby fruit juices? — **YES** → Your baby's digestive system has probably been upset by the sugar in the fruit juice. Don't give your baby juices until he or she is at least 6 months old.

NO

1 *Go to next page, first column*

2 *Go to next page, second column*

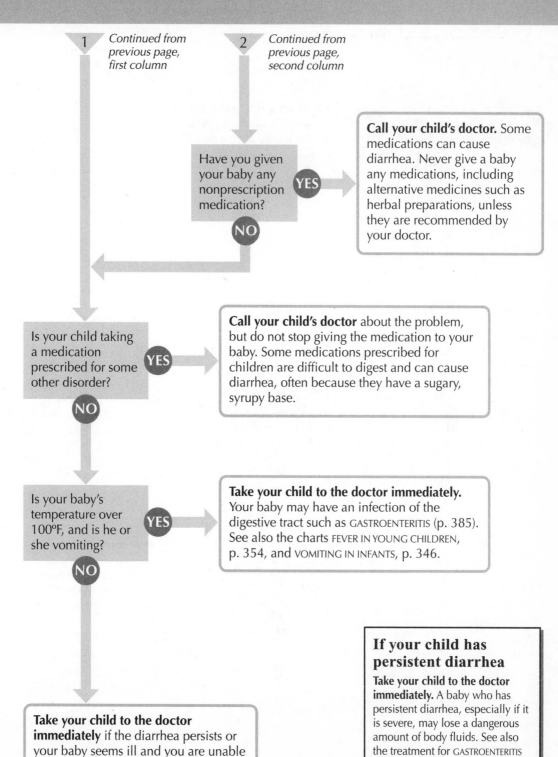

1 *Continued from previous page, first column*

2 *Continued from previous page, second column*

Have you given your baby any nonprescription medication?

YES → **Call your child's doctor.** Some medications can cause diarrhea. Never give a baby any medications, including alternative medicines such as herbal preparations, unless they are recommended by your doctor.

NO

Is your child taking a medication prescribed for some other disorder?

YES → **Call your child's doctor** about the problem, but do not stop giving the medication to your baby. Some medications prescribed for children are difficult to digest and can cause diarrhea, often because they have a sugary, syrupy base.

NO

Is your baby's temperature over 100°F, and is he or she vomiting?

YES → **Take your child to the doctor immediately.** Your baby may have an infection of the digestive tract such as GASTROENTERITIS (p. 385). See also the charts FEVER IN YOUNG CHILDREN, p. 354, and VOMITING IN INFANTS, p. 346.

NO

Take your child to the doctor immediately if the diarrhea persists or your baby seems ill and you are unable to make a diagnosis from this chart.

If your child has persistent diarrhea

Take your child to the doctor immediately. A baby who has persistent diarrhea, especially if it is severe, may lose a dangerous amount of body fluids. See also the treatment for GASTROENTERITIS (p. 385).

Skin problems in young children

Skin discoloration, inflammation, or blemishes.

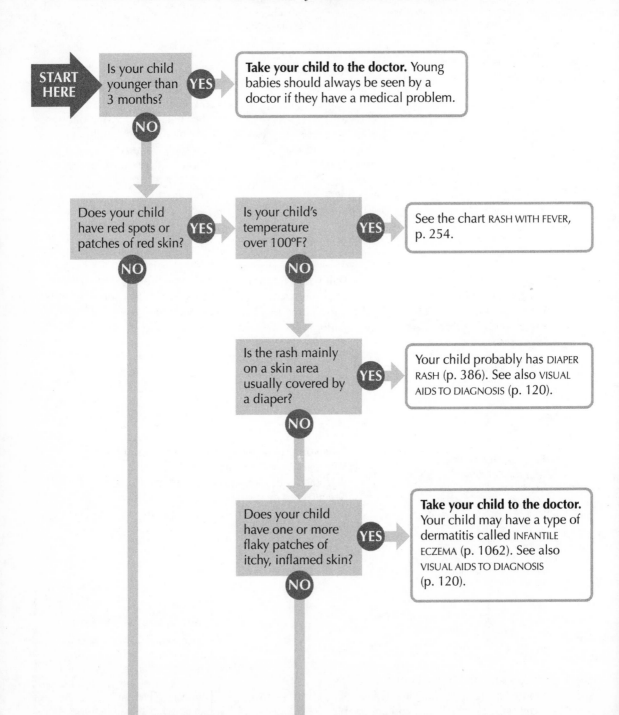

START HERE → Is your child younger than 3 months? — **YES** → **Take your child to the doctor.** Young babies should always be seen by a doctor if they have a medical problem.

NO ↓

Does your child have red spots or patches of red skin? — **YES** → Is your child's temperature over 100°F? — **YES** → See the chart RASH WITH FEVER, p. 254.

NO ↓   **NO** ↓

Is the rash mainly on a skin area usually covered by a diaper? — **YES** → Your child probably has DIAPER RASH (p. 386). See also VISUAL AIDS TO DIAGNOSIS (p. 120).

NO ↓

Does your child have one or more flaky patches of itchy, inflamed skin? — **YES** → **Take your child to the doctor.** Your child may have a type of dermatitis called INFANTILE ECZEMA (p. 1062). See also VISUAL AIDS TO DIAGNOSIS (p. 120).

NO ↓

1 *Go to next page, first column*

2 *Go to next page, second column*

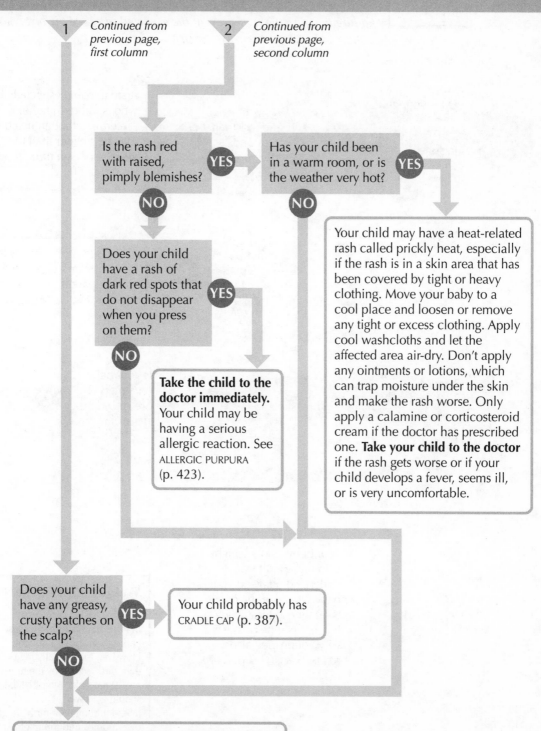

1 *Continued from previous page, first column*

2 *Continued from previous page, second column*

Is the rash red with raised, pimply blemishes?

YES → Has your child been in a warm room, or is the weather very hot?

YES →

NO ↓

Does your child have a rash of dark red spots that do not disappear when you press on them?

YES →

NO ↓

Your child may have a heat-related rash called prickly heat, especially if the rash is in a skin area that has been covered by tight or heavy clothing. Move your baby to a cool place and loosen or remove any tight or excess clothing. Apply cool washcloths and let the affected area air-dry. Don't apply any ointments or lotions, which can trap moisture under the skin and make the rash worse. Only apply a calamine or corticosteroid cream if the doctor has prescribed one. **Take your child to the doctor** if the rash gets worse or if your child develops a fever, seems ill, or is very uncomfortable.

Take the child to the doctor immediately. Your child may be having a serious allergic reaction. See ALLERGIC PURPURA (p. 423).

Does your child have any greasy, crusty patches on the scalp?

YES → Your child probably has CRADLE CAP (p. 387).

NO ↓

Take your child to the doctor if you are unable to make a diagnosis from this chart.

Slow weight gain in young children

Failure to gain weight or grow at the expected rate. See the box below on
WEIGHT GAIN IN THE FIRST YEAR OF LIFE.

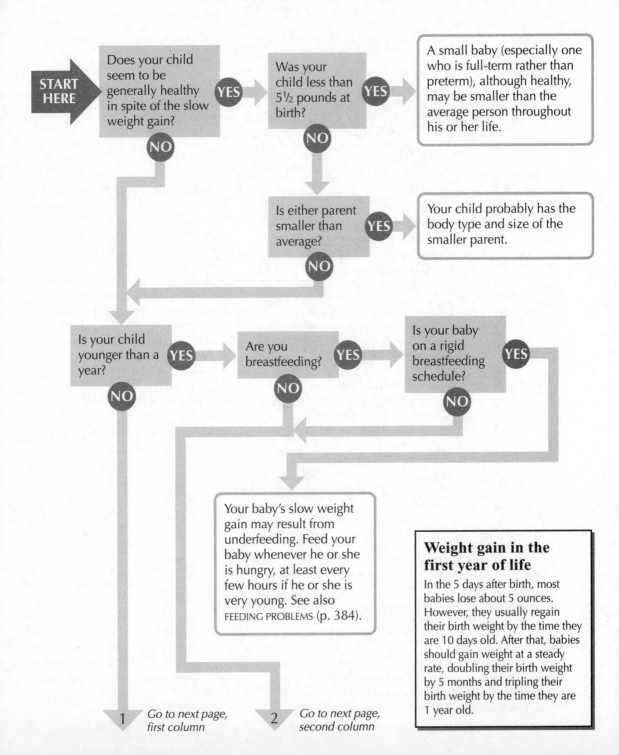

START HERE

Does your child seem to be generally healthy in spite of the slow weight gain?

YES → Was your child less than 5½ pounds at birth?

YES → A small baby (especially one who is full-term rather than preterm), although healthy, may be smaller than the average person throughout his or her life.

NO (from "Was your child less than 5½ pounds at birth?") → Is either parent smaller than average?

YES → Your child probably has the body type and size of the smaller parent.

NO (from "Does your child seem to be generally healthy in spite of the slow weight gain?")

NO (from "Is either parent smaller than average?")

Is your child younger than a year?

YES → Are you breastfeeding?

YES → Is your baby on a rigid breastfeeding schedule?

YES

NO (from "Is your child younger than a year?")

NO (from "Are you breastfeeding?")

NO (from "Is your baby on a rigid breastfeeding schedule?")

Your baby's slow weight gain may result from underfeeding. Feed your baby whenever he or she is hungry, at least every few hours if he or she is very young. See also FEEDING PROBLEMS (p. 384).

1 *Go to next page, first column*

2 *Go to next page, second column*

Weight gain in the first year of life

In the 5 days after birth, most babies lose about 5 ounces. However, they usually regain their birth weight by the time they are 10 days old. After that, babies should gain weight at a steady rate, doubling their birth weight by 5 months and tripling their birth weight by the time they are 1 year old.

1 *Continued from previous page, first column*

2 *Continued from previous page, second column*

Are you bottle-feeding?

YES → **Could you be adding too much water to the formula, or diluting formula that is ready-to-serve?**

YES → Your baby is probably not getting enough nourishment. Read and carefully follow the directions for preparing the formula, and make sure that the formula contains adequate amounts of calories and nutrients.

NO ↓

NO ↓

Does your baby always finish all the formula?

YES → Your baby may still be hungry. As your baby grows, increase the amount of formula you offer.

NO

Does your baby often vomit after feedings?

YES → **Take your child to the doctor.** If your baby is less than 6 months old, see the chart VOMITING IN INFANTS, p. 346. A digestive tract disorder such as an INTESTINAL OBSTRUCTION (p. 405) may be causing the vomiting and preventing your baby from gaining weight. Your baby may also be dehydrated if he or she is not getting sufficient nutrients and fluid (see box below).

NO

Does your child have loose, pale, bulky, and bad-smelling bowel movements?

YES → **Take your child to the doctor.** Your child may have a digestive tract disorder such as CELIAC DISEASE (p. 768) or LACTOSE INTOLERANCE (p. 770).

NO

Is your child taking a corticosteroid medication for a disorder such as asthma?

YES → **Call your child's doctor.** Corticosteroid medications can sometimes affect growth.

NO

Take your child to the doctor if you are unable to make a diagnosis from this chart.

If your baby is dehydrated
Take your child to the doctor immediately. A baby who has dry or wrinkly skin, wets fewer than six diapers a day, or regularly vomits after feedings may be dehydrated.

Fever in young children

An axillary (armpit) temperature over 100°F or a rectal temperature over 102°F.

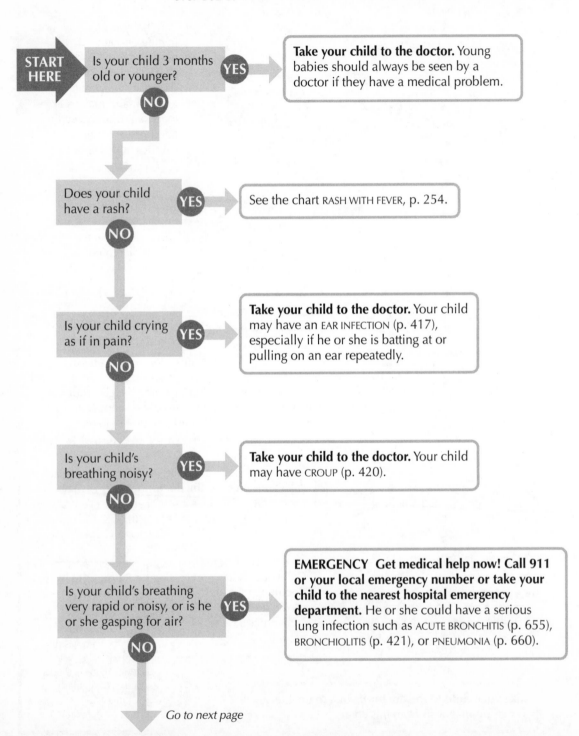

START HERE

Is your child 3 months old or younger?

YES → **Take your child to the doctor.** Young babies should always be seen by a doctor if they have a medical problem.

NO ↓

Does your child have a rash?

YES → See the chart RASH WITH FEVER, p. 254.

NO ↓

Is your child crying as if in pain?

YES → **Take your child to the doctor.** Your child may have an EAR INFECTION (p. 417), especially if he or she is batting at or pulling on an ear repeatedly.

NO ↓

Is your child's breathing noisy?

YES → **Take your child to the doctor.** Your child may have CROUP (p. 420).

NO ↓

Is your child's breathing very rapid or noisy, or is he or she gasping for air?

YES → **EMERGENCY Get medical help now! Call 911 or your local emergency number or take your child to the nearest hospital emergency department.** He or she could have a serious lung infection such as ACUTE BRONCHITIS (p. 655), BRONCHIOLITIS (p. 421), or PNEUMONIA (p. 660).

NO ↓

Go to next page

Continued from previous page

Has your child had three to four watery bowel movements within 24 hours?

YES

Take your child to the doctor. Your child has diarrhea, possibly caused by an infection of the digestive tract such as GASTROENTERITIS (p. 385). See also the chart DIARRHEA IN INFANTS, p. 348.

NO

Does your child have a runny nose?

YES

Call your child's doctor. Your child may have a COLD (p. 648), INFLUENZA (p. 649), or some other infectious disease.

NO

Is the weather hot or the room warm, or is your child dressed in heavy clothing?

YES

Call your child's doctor if the fever doesn't go down after you have moved your child to a cool place, removed some of his or her clothing, and given him or her a drink of water. Your child may be overheated.

NO

Call your child's doctor if you are unable to make a diagnosis from this chart, if your child's temperature remains high for more than 6 hours, or if his or her temperature is higher than 102°F.

Don't give aspirin to children

Do not give aspirin to children who have a fever; use of aspirin by children has been linked with REYE'S SYNDROME (p. 411), a rare but potentially fatal childhood disorder.

If your child has a seizure

EMERGENCY Get medical help now! Call 911 or your local emergency number or take your child to the nearest hospital emergency department. See also FEBRILE SEIZURES (p. 410).

CHILDREN
2 to 12 years

Fever in children

An axillary (armpit) temperature over 100°F, an oral temperature over 101°F, or a rectal temperature over 102°F.

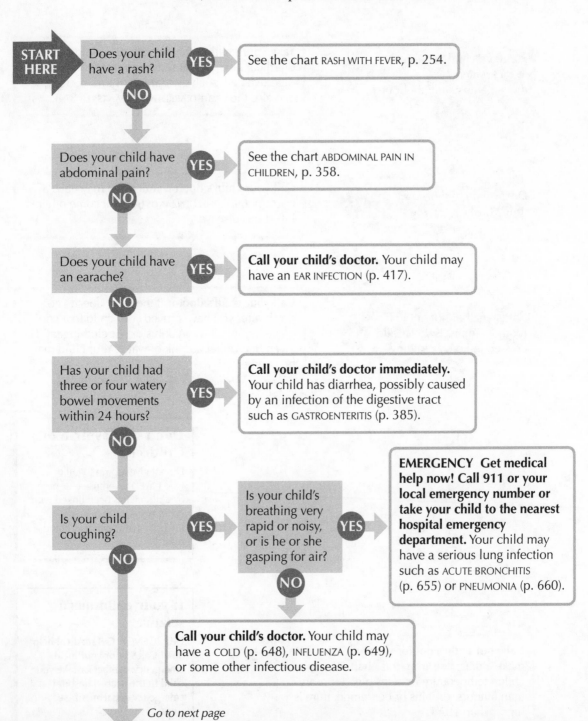

START HERE

Does your child have a rash?
YES → See the chart RASH WITH FEVER, p. 254.

NO ↓

Does your child have abdominal pain?
YES → See the chart ABDOMINAL PAIN IN CHILDREN, p. 358.

NO ↓

Does your child have an earache?
YES → **Call your child's doctor.** Your child may have an EAR INFECTION (p. 417).

NO ↓

Has your child had three or four watery bowel movements within 24 hours?
YES → **Call your child's doctor immediately.** Your child has diarrhea, possibly caused by an infection of the digestive tract such as GASTROENTERITIS (p. 385).

NO ↓

Is your child coughing?
YES → Is your child's breathing very rapid or noisy, or is he or she gasping for air?
YES → **EMERGENCY Get medical help now! Call 911 or your local emergency number or take your child to the nearest hospital emergency department.** Your child may have a serious lung infection such as ACUTE BRONCHITIS (p. 655) or PNEUMONIA (p. 660).

NO ↓

Call your child's doctor. Your child may have a COLD (p. 648), INFLUENZA (p. 649), or some other infectious disease.

NO ↓

Go to next page

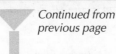
Continued from previous page

Does your child have a sore throat, or is his or her voice faint or hoarse? **YES**

Call your child's doctor. Your child may have an infection of the upper respiratory tract such as TONSILLITIS (p. 653), PHARYNGITIS (p. 653), or LARYNGITIS (p. 654).

 NO

Does your child have a runny nose? **YES**

Call your child's doctor. Your child may have a COLD (p. 648), INFLUENZA (p. 649), or some other infectious disease.

 NO

Is the area between your child's ear and the angle of his or her jaw swollen, painful, or tender? **YES**

Take your child to the doctor. Your child may have MUMPS (p. 440).

 NO

Does your child seem ill, and does he or she have two or more of the following symptoms?
• Vomiting
• Headache
• Sensitivity of the eyes to bright light
• Stiff neck, or pain when trying to bend the head forward

 YES

Take your child to the doctor immediately. Your child may have MENINGITIS (p. 692).

Don't give aspirin to children

Do not give aspirin to children who have a fever; use of aspirin by children has been linked with REYE'S SYNDROME (p. 411), a rare but potentially fatal childhood disorder.

 NO

Call your child's doctor if you are unable to make a diagnosis from this chart, if your child's temperature remains high for more than 6 hours, or if his or her temperature is over 102°F.

If your child has a seizure

EMERGENCY Get medical help now! Call 911 or your local emergency number or take your child to the nearest hospital emergency department. See also FEBRILE SEIZURES (p. 410).

Abdominal pain in children

Pain in the area between the bottom of the rib cage and the groin.

START HERE

Does even the slightest movement seem to hurt so much that your child screams with pain? **YES**

 NO

EMERGENCY Get medical help now! Call 911 or your local emergency number or take your child to the nearest hospital emergency department. He or she could have APPENDICITIS (p. 771).

Has your child overeaten or eaten anything (such as a spicy food) that could have upset his or her stomach? **YES**

 NO

Your child probably has INDIGESTION (p. 749).

Has your child had three to four watery bowel movements within 24 hours or been vomiting? **YES**

 NO

Take your child to the doctor. Your child may have an infection of the digestive tract such as GASTROENTERITIS (p. 385) or he or she could have FOOD POISONING (p. 783).

Has your child not had a bowel movement in 2 or 3 days, or does he or she have difficulty passing stools? **YES**

 NO

Talk to your child's doctor. Your child may be CONSTIPATED (p. 769).

Go to next column

Continued from previous column

Does your child have a runny nose or a sore throat? **YES**

 NO

Children often have abdominal pain when they have a COLD (p. 648) or other respiratory infection because they swallow mucus, which can upset the stomach.

Is your child urinating frequently, or is urination painful? **YES**

 NO

Take your child to the doctor. Your child may have a URINARY TRACT INFECTION (p. 426).

Did your child seem healthy before the abdominal pain started? **YES**

 NO

Does your child often have this type of abdominal pain? **YES**

 NO

Take your child to the doctor. Although many children who are generally healthy get regular attacks of abdominal pain, your child may have an underlying disorder that is causing the pain.

Take your child to the doctor if you are unable to make a diagnosis from this chart.

Itching in children

Skin irritation that makes a child want to scratch.

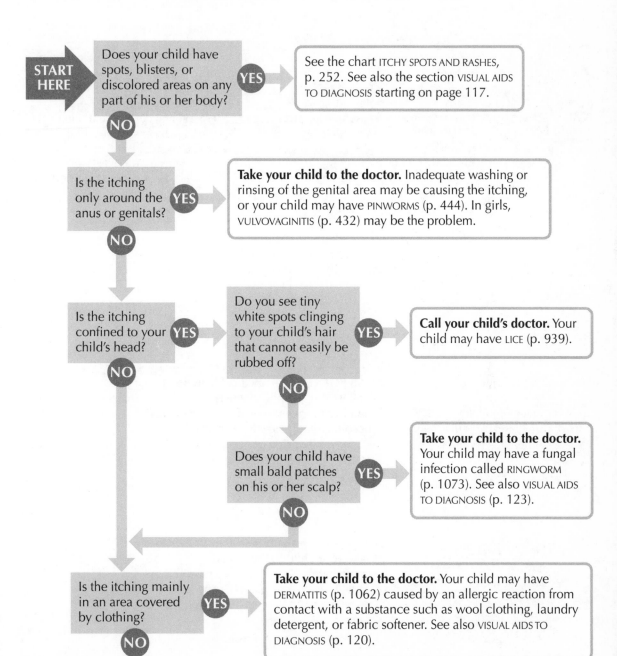

START HERE → Does your child have spots, blisters, or discolored areas on any part of his or her body?

YES → See the chart ITCHY SPOTS AND RASHES, p. 252. See also the section VISUAL AIDS TO DIAGNOSIS starting on page 117.

NO ↓

Is the itching only around the anus or genitals?

YES → **Take your child to the doctor.** Inadequate washing or rinsing of the genital area may be causing the itching, or your child may have PINWORMS (p. 444). In girls, VULVOVAGINITIS (p. 432) may be the problem.

NO ↓

Is the itching confined to your child's head?

YES → Do you see tiny white spots clinging to your child's hair that cannot easily be rubbed off?

YES → **Call your child's doctor.** Your child may have LICE (p. 939).

NO ↓

Does your child have small bald patches on his or her scalp?

YES → **Take your child to the doctor.** Your child may have a fungal infection called RINGWORM (p. 1073). See also VISUAL AIDS TO DIAGNOSIS (p. 123).

NO ↓

NO ↓

Is the itching mainly in an area covered by clothing?

YES → **Take your child to the doctor.** Your child may have DERMATITIS (p. 1062) caused by an allergic reaction from contact with a substance such as wool clothing, laundry detergent, or fabric softener. See also VISUAL AIDS TO DIAGNOSIS (p. 120).

NO ↓

Take your child to the doctor if you are unable to make a diagnosis from this chart.

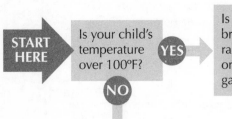

CHILDREN
2 to 12 years

Coughing in children

Coughing in children is usually a symptom of a respiratory infection.

START HERE

Is your child's temperature over 100°F?

YES →

NO ↓

Is your child's breathing very rapid or noisy, or is he or she gasping for air?

YES →

NO ↓

EMERGENCY **Get medical help now! Call 911 or your local emergency number or take your child to the nearest hospital emergency department.** He or she may have a serious lung infection such as ACUTE BRONCHITIS (p. 655), BRONCHIOLITIS (p. 421), or PNEUMONIA (p. 660).

Call your child's doctor. Your child may have a COLD (p. 648), INFLUENZA (p. 649), or some other respiratory infection.

Is your child having difficulty breathing, or is his or her face blue?

YES →

NO ↓

EMERGENCY **Get medical help now! Call 911 or your local emergency number or take your child to the nearest hospital emergency department.** He or she may be having a severe attack of ASTHMA (p. 640) or CROUP (p. 420).

Does your child have episodes of uncontrollable coughing followed by noisy gasping for air?

YES →

NO ↓

Take your child to the doctor immediately. Your child may have WHOOPING COUGH (p. 441), especially if he or she has not been vaccinated against the disease.

Go to next page

Continued from previous page

Is your child's breathing harsh or wheezy? 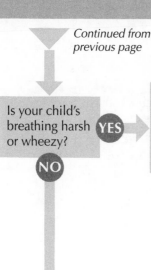 **YES** ➔ Could your child have inhaled a small object or piece of food within the past few days? **YES** ➔ **EMERGENCY Get medical help now! Call 911 or your local emergency number or take your child to the nearest hospital emergency department.** Inhaling an object can partially block the airway, causing wheezing and coughing. For first aid, see CHOKING (p. 155).

NO

NO

Has your child been exposed to any new cleaning products, or do you have a new pet?  **YES** ➔ **Take your child to the doctor immediately.** Your child may be having an allergic reaction. See the section ALLERGIES (p. 912). He or she could also be having an asthma attack. See ASTHMA (p. 640).

 NO

Does your child have a runny or stuffy nose?  **YES** ➔ **Call your child's doctor.** Discharge from the back of the nose may be irritating your child's throat, making him or her cough. Your child may have a COLD (p. 648), INFLUENZA (p. 649), or an ADENOID DISORDER (p. 419).

NO

Has your child had whooping cough within the past 3 months? 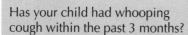 **YES** ➔ Persistent coughing often follows WHOOPING COUGH (p. 441).

NO

Does anyone in the house smoke, or could your child be smoking? **YES** ➔ Smoking or breathing in secondhand smoke can produce a cough. See HOW TO QUIT SMOKING (p. 29).

 NO

Take your child to the doctor if you are unable to make a diagnosis from this chart or if your child's cough persists for more than 2 weeks.

If your child has rapid or noisy breathing
EMERGENCY Get medical help now! Call 911 or your local emergency number or take your child to the nearest hospital emergency department. Rapid or noisy breathing in a child is always a cause for concern, especially if the child is younger than 3 years.

Swellings in children

Any swellings or lumps in the neck or armpits.

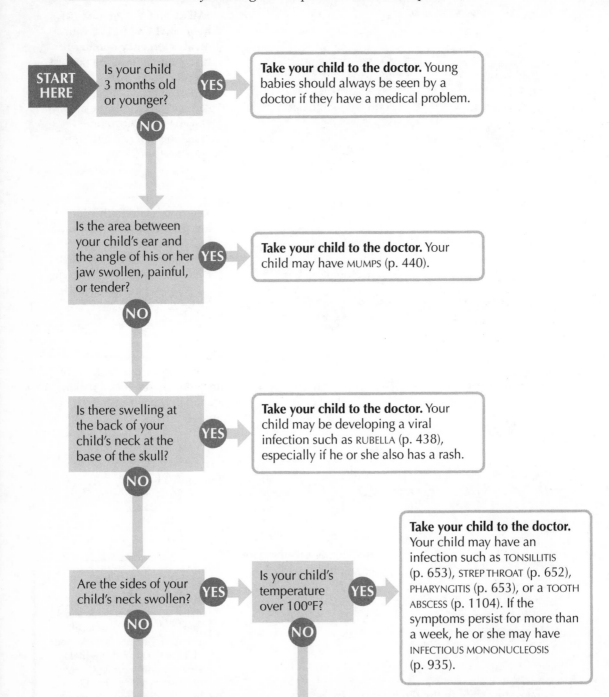

START HERE

Is your child 3 months old or younger?

YES → **Take your child to the doctor.** Young babies should always be seen by a doctor if they have a medical problem.

NO ↓

Is the area between your child's ear and the angle of his or her jaw swollen, painful, or tender?

YES → **Take your child to the doctor.** Your child may have MUMPS (p. 440).

NO ↓

Is there swelling at the back of your child's neck at the base of the skull?

YES → **Take your child to the doctor.** Your child may be developing a viral infection such as RUBELLA (p. 438), especially if he or she also has a rash.

NO ↓

Are the sides of your child's neck swollen?

YES → Is your child's temperature over 100°F?

YES → **Take your child to the doctor.** Your child may have an infection such as TONSILLITIS (p. 653), STREP THROAT (p. 652), PHARYNGITIS (p. 653), or a TOOTH ABSCESS (p. 1104). If the symptoms persist for more than a week, he or she may have INFECTIOUS MONONUCLEOSIS (p. 935).

NO ↓

1 | *Go to next page, first column*

NO ↓

2 | *Go to next page, second column*

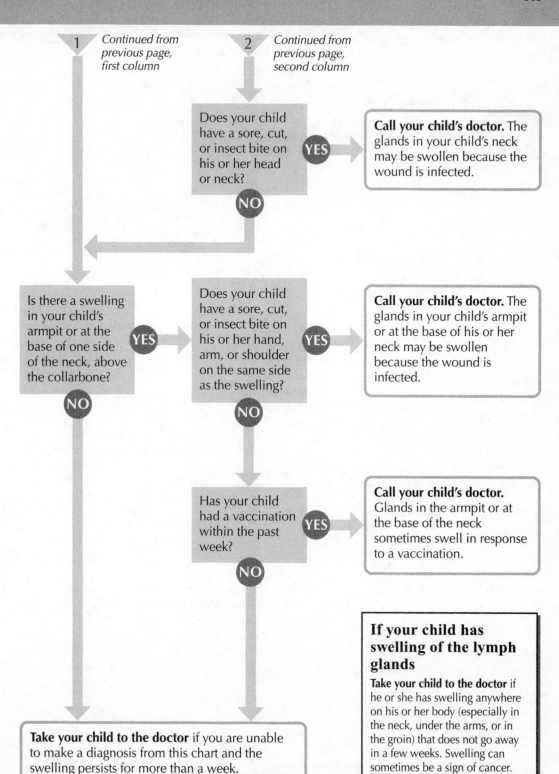

1 *Continued from previous page, first column*

2 *Continued from previous page, second column*

Does your child have a sore, cut, or insect bite on his or her head or neck?

YES → **Call your child's doctor.** The glands in your child's neck may be swollen because the wound is infected.

NO

Is there a swelling in your child's armpit or at the base of one side of the neck, above the collarbone?

YES → Does your child have a sore, cut, or insect bite on his or her hand, arm, or shoulder on the same side as the swelling?

YES → **Call your child's doctor.** The glands in your child's armpit or at the base of his or her neck may be swollen because the wound is infected.

NO

NO

Has your child had a vaccination within the past week?

YES → **Call your child's doctor.** Glands in the armpit or at the base of the neck sometimes swell in response to a vaccination.

NO

Take your child to the doctor if you are unable to make a diagnosis from this chart and the swelling persists for more than a week.

If your child has swelling of the lymph glands

Take your child to the doctor if he or she has swelling anywhere on his or her body (especially in the neck, under the arms, or in the groin) that does not go away in a few weeks. Swelling can sometimes be a sign of cancer.

CHILDREN
Up to 12 years

Limping in children

Difficulty walking (in a young child, a reluctance to walk) that may be accompanied by pain in the affected hip, leg, or foot.

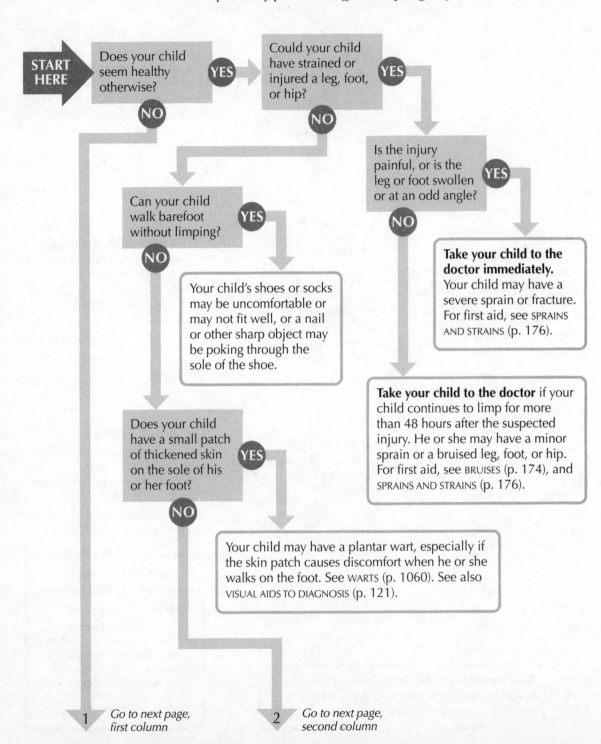

START HERE

Does your child seem healthy otherwise?

YES

Could your child have strained or injured a leg, foot, or hip?

YES

NO

NO

Is the injury painful, or is the leg or foot swollen or at an odd angle?

YES

Can your child walk barefoot without limping?

YES

NO

NO

Take your child to the doctor immediately.
Your child may have a severe sprain or fracture. For first aid, see SPRAINS AND STRAINS (p. 176).

Your child's shoes or socks may be uncomfortable or may not fit well, or a nail or other sharp object may be poking through the sole of the shoe.

Take your child to the doctor if your child continues to limp for more than 48 hours after the suspected injury. He or she may have a minor sprain or a bruised leg, foot, or hip. For first aid, see BRUISES (p. 174), and SPRAINS AND STRAINS (p. 176).

Does your child have a small patch of thickened skin on the sole of his or her foot?

YES

NO

Your child may have a plantar wart, especially if the skin patch causes discomfort when he or she walks on the foot. See WARTS (p. 1060). See also VISUAL AIDS TO DIAGNOSIS (p. 121).

1 *Go to next page, first column*

2 *Go to next page, second column*

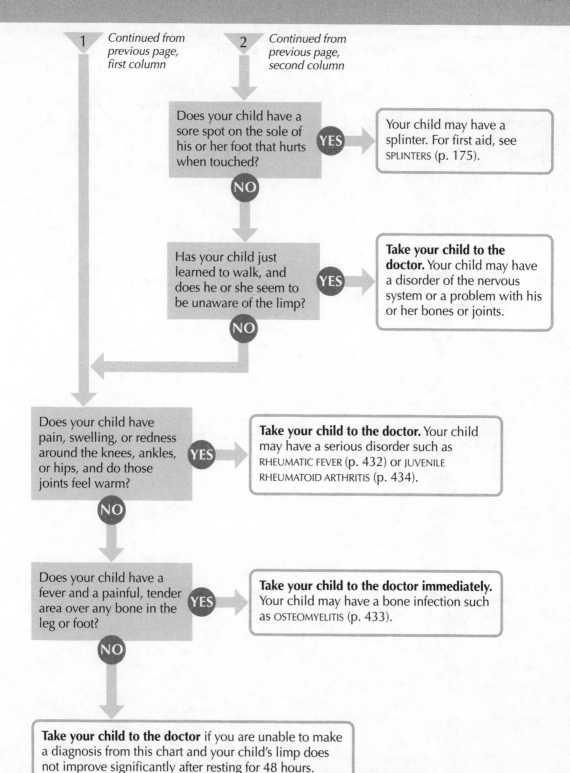

1 *Continued from previous page, first column*

2 *Continued from previous page, second column*

Does your child have a sore spot on the sole of his or her foot that hurts when touched?

YES → Your child may have a splinter. For first aid, see SPLINTERS (p. 175).

NO

Has your child just learned to walk, and does he or she seem to be unaware of the limp?

YES → **Take your child to the doctor.** Your child may have a disorder of the nervous system or a problem with his or her bones or joints.

NO

Does your child have pain, swelling, or redness around the knees, ankles, or hips, and do those joints feel warm?

YES → **Take your child to the doctor.** Your child may have a serious disorder such as RHEUMATIC FEVER (p. 432) or JUVENILE RHEUMATOID ARTHRITIS (p. 434).

NO

Does your child have a fever and a painful, tender area over any bone in the leg or foot?

YES → **Take your child to the doctor immediately.** Your child may have a bone infection such as OSTEOMYELITIS (p. 433).

NO

Take your child to the doctor if you are unable to make a diagnosis from this chart and your child's limp does not improve significantly after resting for 48 hours.

Lack of bladder control in older people

Involuntary urination. Use this chart only after first consulting the chart
LACK OF BLADDER CONTROL, p. 303.

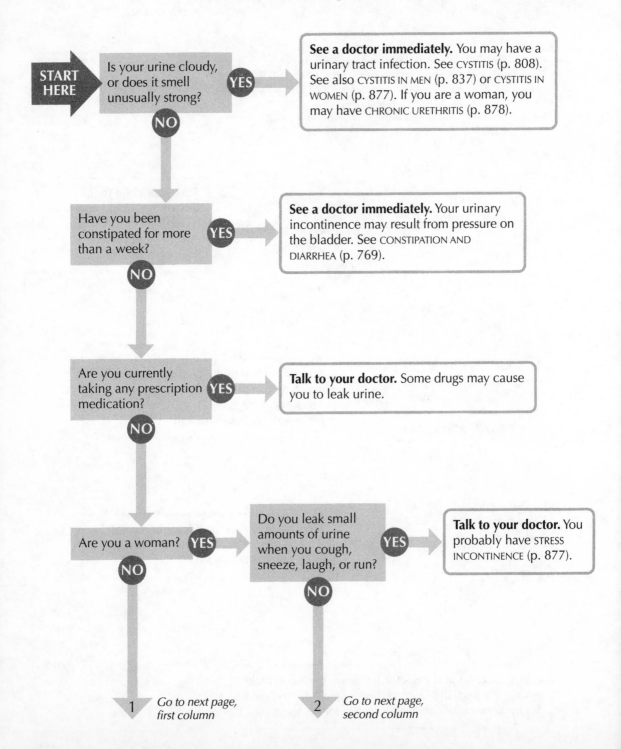

START HERE

Is your urine cloudy, or does it smell unusually strong? **YES** →

See a doctor immediately. You may have a urinary tract infection. See CYSTITIS (p. 808). See also CYSTITIS IN MEN (p. 837) OR CYSTITIS IN WOMEN (p. 877). If you are a woman, you may have CHRONIC URETHRITIS (p. 878).

NO ↓

Have you been constipated for more than a week? **YES** →

See a doctor immediately. Your urinary incontinence may result from pressure on the bladder. See CONSTIPATION AND DIARRHEA (p. 769).

NO ↓

Are you currently taking any prescription medication? **YES** →

Talk to your doctor. Some drugs may cause you to leak urine.

NO ↓

Are you a woman? **YES** →

Do you leak small amounts of urine when you cough, sneeze, laugh, or run? **YES** →

Talk to your doctor. You probably have STRESS INCONTINENCE (p. 877).

NO ↓

NO ↓

1 *Go to next page, first column*

2 *Go to next page, second column*

1 *Continued from previous page, first column*

2 *Continued from previous page, second column*

Do you dribble a little urine after you have finished urinating? **YES**

NO

Does your genital area itch? **YES**

NO

See your doctor. You may have a disorder of the prostate gland. See BENIGN PROSTATIC HYPERPLASIA (p. 832) and PROSTATE CANCER (p. 835).

Talk to your doctor. Genital irritation caused by a VAGINAL YEAST INFECTION (p. 880), as a result of lack of estrogen during MENOPAUSE (p. 851), or from DERMATITIS (p. 1062), can make it difficult to control your bladder.

Do you get to the bathroom in time once you feel the urge to urinate?

NO

See your doctor. If you are a woman, you may have an irritable bladder. See URGE INCONTINENCE (p. 878).

Have you noticed two or more of the following symptoms?
• Change in personality
• Decline in personal appearance or cleanliness
• Impaired ability to remember recent events

YES

See your doctor. These symptoms may indicate the onset of ALZHEIMER'S DISEASE (p. 688). See also OTHER CAUSES OF DEMENTIA (p. 689).

NO

See your doctor if you are unable to make a diagnosis from this chart.

If you lack bowel control

See a doctor immediately.
Occasionally, lack of bowel control accompanies lack of bladder control. If lack of bowel control comes on suddenly, it may result from a spinal cord injury. However, it may also indicate a disorder of the brain and nervous system such as Alzheimer's disease.

OLDER PEOPLE
Over 65 years

Confusion in older people

A loss of clarity about times, places, and events, or a loss of contact with reality. Use this chart only after first consulting the chart CONFUSION, *p. 234.*

START HERE

Have you been feeling confused only recently?

 YES

Have you recently started taking a new medication or changed the dose of one you have been taking?

 YES

Talk to your doctor. He or she may change the dosage or prescribe a different medication or tell you to stop taking the medication.

NO

NO

Did the confusion begin in the days or weeks after a fall or head injury?

 YES

See a doctor immediately. These symptoms suggest the possibility of bleeding inside the skull. See SUBDURAL HEMORRHAGE AND HEMATOMA (p. 678). See also BRAIN INJURY (p. 680).

NO

Have you noticed two or more of the following symptoms?
- Change in personality
- Decline in personal appearance or cleanliness
- Impaired ability to remember recent events

 YES

See a doctor immediately. These symptoms may indicate the onset of ALZHEIMER'S DISEASE (p. 688). You may have had several minor strokes. See TRANSIENT ISCHEMIC ATTACKS (p. 675). Or you may have a BRAIN TUMOR (p. 682). See also OTHER CAUSES OF DEMENTIA (p. 689).

NO

Is the confusion accompanied by signs of illness such as a fever, coughing, or lack of bladder control?

 YES

See a doctor immediately. Many physical illnesses can cause these symptoms along with confusion in older people.

NO

Do you feel very cold or chilled, or does your abdomen feel unusually cold?

 YES

EMERGENCY Get medical help now! Call 911 or your local emergency number or have someone take you to the nearest hospital emergency department. Feeling cold along with being confused can indicate a dangerous drop in body temperature. For first aid, see HYPOTHERMIA (p. 165).

 NO

Go to next page

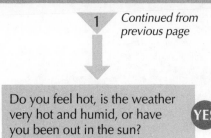

1   *Continued from previous page*

Do you feel hot, is the weather very hot and humid, or have you been out in the sun?

 YES

EMERGENCY Get medical help now! Call 911 or your local emergency number or have someone take you to the nearest hospital emergency department. Your confusion may be the result of exposure to very hot conditions. For first aid, see HEATSTROKE (p. 166).

NO

Have you gone without eating for some time?

 YES

Have something to eat or drink, especially if you have a condition such as diabetes. **See your doctor** if the confusion persists.

NO

See your doctor if you are unable to make a diagnosis from this chart.

Health Issues Throughout Life

1

Children's Health

One of the most important things you can do to make sure that your child is healthy and is developing normally is to take him or her to the doctor for routine examinations, called well-child visits, and all the recommended vaccinations. This chapter describes the developmental steps your child will take during the first few years of life and many of the common problems, such as cradle cap, that occur in young children. The disorder sections are grouped according to the part of the body they affect. Some of the disorders discussed in this chapter occur only in infants and children; others can affect people of all ages but require special diagnostic tests or treatment in infants and children. In addition, the outlook for some disorders is very different for infants and children than for adults.

Routine Health Care

Your child's doctor may be a pediatrician (a doctor who is trained to care for infants, children, and adolescents, usually up to age 18) or a family physician (a doctor who is trained to care for both adults and children). During these visits, the doctor will examine your child, make sure that he or she has all the required vaccinations, and treat any disorders. Take advantage of these visits to talk with the doctor about any concerns or questions you have about your child's health or development.

Examining a Newborn

Immediately after delivery, the doctor and nurses in the delivery room examine a newborn to make sure that he or she is healthy. They use a suction device to remove any mucus from inside the baby's nose and mouth, put antibiotic drops in his or her eyes to prevent infection, and give him or her an injection of vitamin K to help the blood clot normally. The doctor evaluates the infant's heart rate and breathing; measures his or her length, weight, and head circumference; and performs a thorough physical examination to look for any physical abnormalities. All babies are given screening tests for some disorders and an evaluation, called the Apgar score, of their general health status.

The Apgar Score
The Apgar score assesses heart rate, breathing and crying, muscle tone, reflex responses, and skin color (examining the inside of the mouth and lips, palms of the hands, and soles of the feet). Each of these five components is given a number from 0 to 2, and then all five are added up. A score between

7 and 10 is a general indication that the infant is healthy. The score does not, however, predict a baby's development or long-term health.

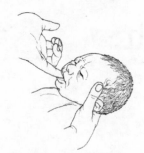

Examining the mouth and face

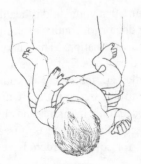

Examining the genitals, navel, feet, and hips

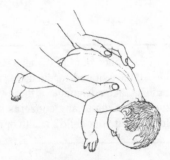

Examining the spine

Physical examination of newborns

A physical examination is performed on newborns immediately after birth to check for birth defects or other abnormalities. In most cases, early detection helps ensure successful treatment. For example, the child's mouth is examined for cleft lip and cleft palate, and his or her face is examined for features of Down syndrome (top). The infant's anus is checked to make sure it is open, the genitals are checked to verify the baby's sex, the navel is examined for swelling (a sign of an umbilical hernia), the feet are examined for clubfoot, and the hips are checked for dislocation (center). The spine is examined for any swelling or opening that could indicate spina bifida (bottom).

Newborn Screening Tests

Every state requires testing of newborns for a variety of disorders 24 hours after birth, before the child is released from the hospital. Some of these disorders cause no symptoms initially but can lead to serious health problems or can be fatal. Testing is done immediately after birth because the risk of complications is reduced significantly when these disorders are diagnosed and treated early. Abnormal results are followed up with more thorough, precise testing.

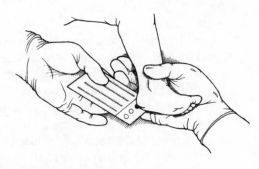

Newborn testing

From a small sample of blood taken from a newborn's heel, doctors can diagnose a number of serious but treatable disorders, including sickle cell disease and phenylketonuria (PKU). The sample is examined in a laboratory and the results are sent to the child's pediatrician.

Vaccinations

Vaccinations, or immunizations, protect against contagious infections, many of which are life-threatening. All children in the United States are required to have vaccinations against a number of infectious diseases, including hepatitis B, measles, mumps, and rubella. Your doctor will tell you when your child needs each vaccination. Keep a record of all your child's vaccinations and bring the record to each visit to make sure your child's immunizations are up-to-date.

All vaccinations are given in shots, usually into the outer, upper part of the thigh or arm. Some vaccinations—such as for measles, mumps, and rubella—are combined and given in a single injection. Some vaccinations cause reactions, but they are usually mild and require no treatment other than applying cold compresses to the injection site

Should I Have My Son Circumcised?

Circumcision is a surgical procedure to remove the foreskin, the loose fold of skin that covers the head of the penis. The procedure is frequently performed for social or religious reasons on newborn boys in the United States, usually by an obstetrician or a pediatrician a day or two after birth. Circumcision is a generally safe procedure when performed by an experienced person under sterile conditions. Possible complications, such as bleeding and infection, are rare. However, only healthy infants should be circumcised shortly after birth, to avoid possible problems with blood clotting.

Circumcision is painful. For this reason, if you decide to have your infant son circumcised, ask the doctor to use a local anesthetic to help prevent pain. Circumcision performed on older boys or men requires general anesthesia. Healing can take up to 10 days.

One advantage of circumcision is a decrease in the number of urinary tract infections during childhood. A circumcised male also may have a decreased risk of cancer of the penis later in life. However, the American Academy of Pediatrics does not recommend routine newborn circumcision. Before making a decision to have your son circumcised, discuss the benefits and risks of circumcision with your pediatrician.

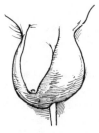
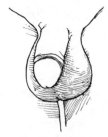

Uncircumcised penis   **Circumcised penis**

Uncircumcised and circumcised penis
A loose fold of skin called the foreskin covers the head of an uncircumcised penis (left). During the first months or years of a boy's life, the foreskin gradually separates from the head of the penis. In a circumcised penis (right), the foreskin has been removed and the head of the penis has been permanently exposed. Healing after a circumcision can take up to 10 days.

Vaccinations

Q. *My friend said she read that there is a link between the mumps-measles-rubella (MMR) vaccination and autism. Is this true?*

A. No. There is no evidence that the MMR vaccination causes autism. Because the incidence of autism is increasing and because autism is often diagnosed at the age at which children receive the MMR vaccination, some parents have suspected that the vaccine caused the disorder. In fact, the health risks of not having the MMR vaccination outweigh any risks associated with the vaccination. For example, mumps can cause permanent hearing loss and can lead to life-threatening complications such as encephalitis and meningitis. Measles can lead to encephalitis and meningitis and can cause pneumonia. A rubella infection in a pregnant woman can cause severe birth defects.

Q. *My doctor recently recommended that I have my 1-year-old son vaccinated against influenza. I thought flu vaccinations were only for children with chronic conditions, such as asthma or diabetes, and older people. Is it a good idea for my son to have a flu shot?*

A. Yes. Influenza is a highly contagious, potentially life-threatening infectious disease, especially for children your son's age. Infants and toddlers with influenza are as likely to be hospitalized for treatment of influenza-related complications (such as pneumonia) as are older people. For these reasons, the CDC recommends that all healthy children between ages 6 months and 23 months (and their family members and caregivers) be vaccinated against influenza. The initial vaccination for children is given in two separate injections about a month apart, because a single dose does not provide enough protection for young children. In addition, all children between 6 months and 18 years who have risk factors such as asthma, heart disease, sickle cell disease, HIV or AIDS, or diabetes should receive a yearly flu shot.

Recommended Schedule of Childhood Vaccinations

The following schedule is a general recommendation for the timing of vaccinations during childhood. Children usually receive the vaccinations during their regular well-child visits to the doctor.

Recommended Schedule of Childhood Vaccinations

Age	Vaccination
Birth–2 months	Hepatitis B (1st dose)
1–4 months	Hepatitis B (2nd dose)
2 months	DTaP, Hib, IPV, PCV
4 months	DTaP, Hib, IPV, PCV
6 months	DTaP, Hib, PCV
6–18 months	Hepatitis B (3rd dose), IPV
6 months–18 years*	Influenza (yearly)
6 months–23 months†	Influenza (yearly)
12–15 months	Hib, MMR (1st dose), PCV
12–23 months	Chickenpox (varicella)
15–18 months	DTaP
2 years–18 years*	PPV, hepatitis A series
4–6 years	DTaP, IPV, MMR (2nd dose)
11–16 years	Td
2–18 years	Hepatitis B series, chickenpox (if not given previously)
11–18 years	MMR (2nd dose, if not given previously)

*Recommended for children who have risk factors such as asthma, heart disease, sickle cell disease, HIV or AIDS, or diabetes.
†Recommended for all healthy children.

Key

DTaP	Diphtheria and tetanus toxoids and acellular pertussis vaccine
Hib	Haemophilus influenzae type b conjugate vaccine
IPV	Inactivated poliovirus vaccine
PCV	Pneumococcal vaccine
PPV	Pneumococcal polysaccharide vaccine
MMR	Measles, mumps, and rubella vaccine
Td	Tetanus and diphtheria toxoids

to relieve swelling or irritation. However, if you notice any unusual symptoms in your child after a vaccination, call your doctor immediately.

Common Childhood Screenings and Tests

At routine visits to the doctor throughout childhood, screening tests are given to children for a number of disorders, including high blood pressure (see page 574) and lead poisoning (see page 425). Early detection of these disorders enables the child to be treated before symptoms develop.

Blood Pressure

The doctor will check your child's blood pressure at each annual checkup starting at age 3. The measurement is compared against the average healthy range for children of the same age and sex. If your child has high blood pressure, the doctor will want to find the cause and will recommend treatment if necessary. High blood pressure can be a sign of a serious disorder such as kidney disease, heart disease, or thyroid disorders. It can also result from being overweight. If your child is overweight, the doctor will recommend a weight-loss program that will include a healthy diet and an increase in exercise; weight loss can significantly lower blood pressure.

Blood Tests

All children are given a blood test at one time or another, either to diagnose a disorder such as an infection or to screen for disorders such as anemia.

Complete blood cell count

A complete blood cell (CBC) count measures the major components of blood, including red cells (which deliver oxygen to cells), white cells (which fight infection), and platelets (which help blood to clot). A CBC count can detect disorders such as anemia (see page 610), which results from a low level of red blood cells, leukemia (see page 621), which affects white blood cells, or the presence of an infection.

Hemoglobin test or hematocrit test

A hemoglobin test measures the level in the blood of the oxygen-carrying protein hemoglobin. A hemocrit test measures the percentage in the blood of red blood cells, which contain hemoglobin. Both tests can be used to screen for anemia. Children usually are given a test at some time in their first year of life and then periodically throughout childhood and adolescence.

Cholesterol

A cholesterol test, which measures the levels of various types of fats in the blood, can help evaluate a child's risk of developing heart disease. Some doctors recommend that all children have a cholesterol screening test at age 6 and a follow-up test at age 8. All doctors recommend a cholesterol test for children who are overweight, who have a parent with a total cholesterol level above 240 milligrams per deciliter (mg/dL), or who have a close relative (parent, grandparent, aunt, or uncle) who developed heart disease or had a heart attack or stroke before age 55. If your child's total cholesterol level is in the healthy range (less than 170 mg/dL) and the level of low-density lipoprotein (LDL; the bad cholesterol) is less than 110 mg/dL, the test should be repeated within 5 years. If the cholesterol levels exceed these numbers, the doctor will recommend steps to bring them down to the healthy range, such as losing weight, exercising more, and eating less saturated fat and cholesterol.

Lead

An elevated level of lead in the blood can stunt a child's physical and mental development; the higher the level, the greater the damage. Doctors recommend that all children have a screening test for lead poisoning (see page 425) between 6 months and 6 years of age, depending on the child's risk factors, such as exposure to lead-based paint in older homes. Many school systems require screening before a child enters school.

Urinalysis

Urine tests can detect potentially serious conditions such as urinary tract infections, kidney disorders, or diabetes, and can evaluate kidney function. A urine test is performed at each checkup, beginning with the child's first checkup after toilet training (at about 3 to 4 years of age). If the child's urine screening test result is abnormal, a sample of urine will be sent to a laboratory for examination under a microscope. Depending on the results of the test, the doctor will recommend appropriate treatment.

Tuberculin Skin Test

Most children in the United States are at low risk of developing tuberculosis (TB; see page 663), a highly contagious bacterial infection of the respiratory system, but many states or schools require regular testing for TB. To administer the tuberculin skin test, a doctor or nurse injects a tiny amount of the TB bacterium protein under the skin of the inner part of the arm. If the skin at the site swells, turns red, or hardens, it indicates that the child has been exposed to or infected with TB. In this case, the child will have a physical examination and a chest X-ray to evaluate his or her condition and determine appropriate treatment.

Developmental Milestones

Generally, all children acquire physical and intellectual skills in the same order. For example, children learn to sit before they learn to stand, and they learn words before they form sentences. However, the rate for acquiring these skills varies from one child to another. For this reason, the ages listed in the following pages for reaching each milestone on childhood development are an average within a wider range and should be used only as a rough guide. Your child may acquire these skills at a faster or slower rate than the average. If you have any concerns about your child's development, talk to your doctor.

At 6 months a child usually:

- Babbles
- Forms simple words such as "dada" or "mama"
- Laughs
- Responds to own name
- Turns in the direction of sounds
- Sits supported
- Rolls over
- Reaches
- Grasps objects
- Transfers objects from hand to hand
- Pushes up on arms

At 12 months a child usually:

- Says first words
- Associates words and meanings
- Recognizes familiar people
- Follows simple commands
- Points to objects
- Uses thumb and fingers to pick up objects
- Plays alone with toys
- Uses both hands well
- Drinks from a cup without assistance
- Feeds self with fingers
- Crawls quickly
- Takes first steps alone

At 18 months a child usually:

- Uses some action words (such as "go" or "come")
- Knows 10 or more words
- Knows some body parts
- Turns pages in a book
- Walks without help
- Runs stiffly
- Feeds self with a spoon
- Scribbles with crayons
- Climbs stairs
- Climbs on furniture
- Looks for hidden objects
- Competes with other children for toys
- Acts anxious when separated from parents

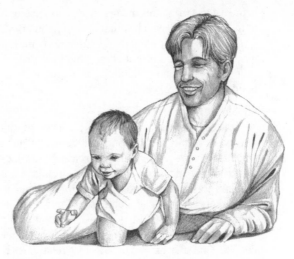

Crawling
Most children begin crawling by about 9 months if they have been given enough "tummy time" on the floor. In addition to exercising a number of muscle groups, crawling gives a child the opportunity to explore. Always supervise your child when he or she is crawling.

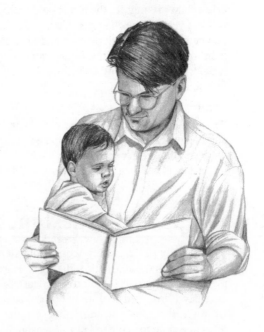

Reading to your child
Reading aloud to your child is a simple and effective way to stimulate the development of his or her brain for learning language and other mental skills. In addition, reading to infants and very young children helps calm, comfort, and entertain them. It also helps them develop their eye muscles. Take time to read to your child every day, and make the experience special and fun.

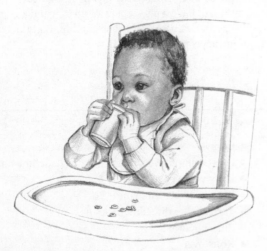

Drinking from a cup
Learning to drink from a cup takes practice. Most children can drink from a cup on their own by about 12 months of age. Start your child out with a cup with a lid to avoid spills.

At 24 months a child usually:

- Knows several hundred words
- Speaks in two- to three-word phrases
- Points to body parts when asked
- Runs and jumps
- Walks backward
- Goes down stairs
- Throws and kicks a ball
- Feeds self with a fork and a spoon
- Drinks from a straw
- Undresses self
- Opens doors, drawers, and boxes

Measuring Your Child's Growth

A child's growth rate is a good indicator of his or her general health. To monitor a child's growth at each visit, a doctor measures and records his or her height and weight and head circumference (if the child is under 2) and compares these measurements with those taken during previous visits. This helps the doctor determine if the child is growing at a healthy rate.

The doctor also compares your child's measurements against the average length and weight ranges for children the same age. Growth rates vary considerably among children and, as long as your child is growing at a steady rate, there usually is no cause for concern.

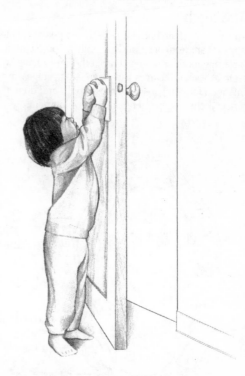

Opening doors
Two-year-olds like to explore and are eager to learn new skills, such as opening doors. To help keep your child safe, install childproof locks on any doors that you don't want him or her to open.

Your Child's Teeth

At about 6 months of age, a child's primary (baby) teeth begin to come in. In most cases, a child has a full set of primary teeth by the time he or she is 2 years old. A baby's first teeth, the incisors, usually appear during the first year and seldom cause problems. The baby may be irritable, cry more than usual, and have difficulty sleeping. Gums may be red and swollen, and the baby may drool more than usual and gnaw on his or her fingers. You may be able to see the teeth coming through the gums. Your baby's feeding, sleeping, and bowel habits may change, but he or she usually has very little pain.

The first and second molars, which usually appear between ages 1 and 3, are much more likely to cause discomfort. Gums may be tender, making eating painful, and the cheek on the affected side of the mouth may feel hot and look flushed. To help relieve your child's discomfort, rub his or her gums gently, give the child a cool drink from a cup, or give him or her a teething ring, teething biscuit, or bagel to chew. To relieve pain, give the child acetaminophen or ibuprofen (not aspirin), or rub his or her gums with an over-the-counter, pain-relieving dental cream or gel for children.

In some cases, a disease or disorder in a child may be overlooked because parents attribute the symptoms to teething. For example, clutching one side of the face may be a sign of an ear infection (see page 417) rather than teething-related discomfort. Therefore, you should talk to your doctor if your child of teething age shows any signs of distress.

The Teeth

The ages at which both baby teeth and permanent teeth appear vary from one child to another. Some children have one tooth or more at birth; others may have no teeth at 1 year. The ages listed here are averages, are intended for comparison purposes only, and do not reflect a child's general health or development.

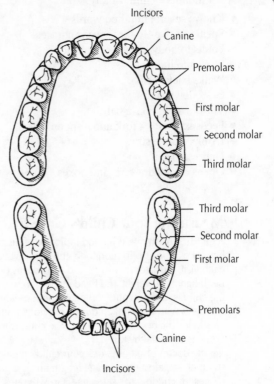

Incisors
Canine
Premolars
First molar
Second molar
Third molar

Third molar
Second molar
First molar

Premolars
Canine
Incisors

Full set of permanent teeth: 32

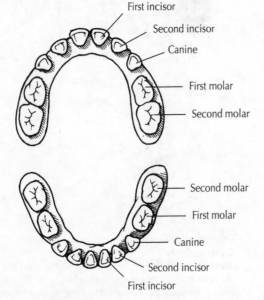

First incisor
Second incisor
Canine
First molar
Second molar

Second molar
First molar
Canine
Second incisor
First incisor

Full set of baby teeth: 20

Ages When Baby Teeth Come In

Age	Baby Teeth
6 months	First incisors
7 months	Second incisors
12 months	First molars
18 months	Canines
2–3 years	Second molars

Ages When Permanent Teeth Come In

Age	Permanent Teeth
6–8 years	First incisors
6–7 years	First molars
7–9 years	Second incisors
9–12 years	Canines
10–12 years	First and second premolars
11–13 years	Second molars
17–20 years (or never)	Third molars (wisdom teeth)

Health Concerns of Newborns and Infants

Most health problems in infants are not life-threatening. Many conditions in infants, such as cradle cap, diaper rash, and colic, are common and are easy to treat at home. As you get to know your child and are familiar with his or her habits and moods, you will quickly recognize any signs or symptoms of possible problems. Serious health problems, such as asphyxia and respiratory distress syndrome, are more likely to occur in babies who are born preterm than in full-term babies.

Asphyxia in the Newborn

Asphyxia is a life-threatening lack of oxygen and carbon dioxide exchange in the lungs that results from poor or absent breathing. The brain controls breathing, and if a baby's brain does not function normally at birth, his or her breathing may be impaired, which can lead to asphyxia. In some cases, a newborn's brain does not function normally because the supply of oxygen from the placenta to the baby during labor was inadequate. This problem may develop when a baby is small for the length of the pregnancy, if delivery is significantly early or overdue, or if the umbilical cord becomes flattened or twisted during labor. In asphyxia, brain damage may occur either before or after the baby is delivered. Infants born to women who smoked during pregnancy are more likely to be small and prone to asphyxia and other respiratory problems.

In hospital deliveries, doctors are prepared to treat babies with asphyxia immediately after birth. For this reason, the risk of brain damage (which can occur after about 4 to 5 minutes without oxygen) or death (which can occur after about 7 to 10 minutes without oxygen) is minimal. In a home birth, the risks of serious complications from asphyxia are significantly greater, even when a doctor is present, because of the lack of special equipment and trained personnel to deal with this medical emergency.

Symptoms

A baby with asphyxia does not breathe or cry at birth. In mild cases, the baby's skin looks blue and his or her arms and legs may feel stiff when you move them. In severe cases, the baby's skin looks gray and he or she is limp and immobile.

Diagnosis

A diagnosis of asphyxia in a newborn is based on the baby's symptoms. In some cases, an obstetrician can identify a baby who is at risk for asphyxia during pregnancy, before labor begins, and can arrange in advance to deliver the baby in a hospital neonatal intensive care unit. However, in most cases, an inadequate supply of oxygen from the placenta is detected during labor, and asphyxia is handled by emergency delivery, sometimes by forceps or cesarean section (see page 534).

Treatment

To treat asphyxia in a newborn, the doctor uses a special tube to quickly suck secretions and other substances that may be blocking the airways—such as amniotic fluid (the fluid that surrounds a fetus during pregnancy) or meconium (the first bowel movement of a newborn)—from the baby's nose, mouth, and throat. In mild cases of asphyxia, as the airways are cleared, the baby will gasp and inhale oxygen, which stimulates the brain to initiate breathing. If the baby does not begin breathing, the doctor maintains an open airway and uses a special bag and mask to breathe for the child. The mask fits over the baby's nose and mouth, and the doctor squeezes the bag to force oxygen into the child's lungs. If the baby does not respond, the doctor threads a tube into his or her airway, and the child is placed on a ventilator (an artificial breathing machine) until he or she can breathe alone and the underlying cause of asphyxia has been treated. The possibility of resulting brain damage depends on the underlying cause of the asphyxia and the length of time the baby's brain has been deprived of oxygen. If the brain has not been deprived of oxygen for more than about 4 or 5 minutes, no permanent damage is likely.

Respiratory Distress Syndrome

Respiratory distress syndrome is a lung disorder in preterm infants (and, occasionally, in full-term infants) that causes increasing difficulty breathing, which can lead to a life-threatening deficiency of oxygen in the blood. A prolonged lack of oxygen in the blood may permanently damage the baby's brain or lungs. The more premature a baby is, the greater the risk of respiratory distress syndrome. The disorder occurs frequently in babies who weigh less than 3 pounds at birth and also is common in infants whose mothers have diabetes (see page 889).

After a baby's first breath has caused his or her lungs to expand, the alveoli (tiny air sacs in the lungs) are kept open by a natural chemical in the lungs called surfactant. Keeping the alveoli open is essential for breathing, because oxygen passes into the bloodstream and carbon dioxide enters the lungs to be exhaled through the capillaries (small blood vessels) that surround the alveoli.

In babies with respiratory distress syndrome, however, the lungs do not contain enough surfactant, and the alveoli start to close again within minutes or hours after birth, leading to increasing difficulty breathing and inadequate exchange of oxygen and carbon dioxide.

Symptoms

In respiratory distress syndrome, a baby's breathing gradually becomes more and more labored and rapid in the first few hours after birth. As the baby breathes in, his or her chest sinks (rather than expands, as it normally would). When breathing out, the baby grunts.

Diagnosis

A diagnosis of respiratory distress syndrome is based on the baby's symptoms and the amount of surfactant in the baby's lungs. In some cases, a doctor may be able to determine the amount of surfactant in a fetus's lungs before delivery by performing amniocentesis (see page 510). If the amount of surfactant appears to be inadequate, it may be increased by giving the pregnant woman an injection of a corticosteroid medication, which stimulates the production of surfactant in the fetus's lungs.

Treatment

A baby who has respiratory distress syndrome or who is at risk of developing it is treated in a hospital neonatal intensive care unit (ICU). Treatment

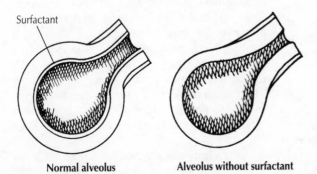

Surfactant

Normal alveolus   **Alveolus without surfactant**

Respiratory distress syndrome
The alveoli produce a substance called surfactant, which normally coats and protects the alveoli and enables them to stay open (left) so they can absorb oxygen from inhaled air. Without surfactant, an alveolus collapses (right), causing the labored breathing that is characteristic of respiratory distress syndrome.

includes placing an inhaler over the baby's face to administer artificial surfactant to open the alveoli and help restore normal breathing. The infant also may be given artificial respiration, in which a tube is threaded into his or her trachea (windpipe) to deliver oxygen to the lungs. The baby's blood will be continuously monitored to determine the levels of oxygen, carbon dioxide, and other body chemicals, including bicarbonate, sodium, potassium, and chloride. After treatment with artificial surfactant, infants who are very premature (born before the 28th week of pregnancy) or who are very small (about 3 pounds or less) remain at risk for respiratory distress syndrome and must be closely monitored in a neonatal ICU for signs of breathing problems.

Neonatal Jaundice

Neonatal jaundice is yellowing of an infant's skin and the whites of the eyes that occurs soon after birth. The condition is caused by an excess of bilirubin (a waste product of the normal breakdown of red blood cells) in the blood. Normally, bilirubin is removed from the blood by the liver. In a newborn, jaundice usually occurs because the liver is not yet fully developed and cannot process the bilirubin fast enough. This type of neonatal jaundice is called physiological jaundice and occurs in more than half of all newborns.

An uncommon form of neonatal jaundice, called hemolytic jaundice, can result from a condition called Rhesus (Rh) incompatibility (see page 508), in which antibodies (infection-fighting proteins) from the mother's blood enter the fetus's blood and combine with the fetus's red blood cells, causing the cells to break down much more quickly than normal. This early breakdown of red blood cells results in excess release of bilirubin into the bloodstream, causing the baby to have severe jaundice at birth or soon after. In some cases, blood type (ABO) incompatibility, in which the blood types (A, B, AB, or O) differ between the baby and the mother, causes a milder form of hemolytic jaundice.

An extremely rare but more serious form of neonatal jaundice, called obstructive jaundice, is caused by malformed or absent bile ducts in an infant's liver. In this disorder, bile (a digestive fluid produced by the liver) and bilirubin cannot pass out

Neonatal Intensive Care Unit

If your baby is born before the 37th week of pregnancy (preterm), weighs less than 5 pounds, or has a serious infection, respiratory problem, or birth defect, he or she may be taken immediately to the neonatal intensive care unit (ICU) of the hospital, or transferred to another hospital that has a neonatal ICU. Immediate care improves the baby's chances for survival and long-term health. Babies born after the 26th week generally do well. Although their development may be delayed, most preterm babies catch up to full-term babies by 2 years of age.

In the neonatal ICU, babies are kept warm in incubators and attached to electronic monitors that check their vital signs. Oxygen may be supplied if a baby's lungs are underdeveloped. Blood samples are taken regularly from a catheter (a thin, flexible tube) placed in the infant's umbilical cord, arm, or leg to make sure the kidneys and liver are functioning properly and the infant is not receiving too much oxygen.

At first, babies are fed breast milk or formula through a tube inserted into their stomach through their nose, or they are fed nutrients intravenously (through a vein). Later, they are fed with a bottle. Your baby will be able to breastfeed as soon as he or she gains strength and his or her sucking reflex improves. In the meantime, express milk from your breasts regularly to provide breast milk for your baby while in the neonatal ICU and to keep your breasts producing milk for when you can breastfeed. Freeze any extra milk for later. A lactation nurse will give you instructions on how to freeze breast milk. Breast milk is especially

beneficial for preterm infants because it provides essential nutrients that promote development and antibodies that help fight infection. If breastfeeding is not possible, formulas are available that provide the nutrients and extra calories that preterm babies need for growth.

Babies usually stay in the neonatal ICU until their weight reaches 4 to 5 pounds and any life-threatening conditions have been treated successfully.

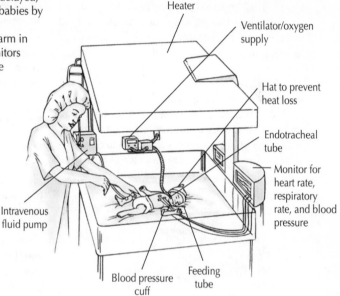

Neonatal intensive care
Inside the incubator, tubes provide essential life support, and sensors help to monitor your baby's condition. Although you cannot hold, cuddle, or breastfeed your baby, spend as much time as you are allowed touching, stroking, and talking to him or her. This stimulation can dramatically improve your baby's breathing and physical development and helps you bond with your baby.

---

of the liver, and bilirubin builds up in the blood, causing jaundice. Other rare causes of neonatal jaundice include neonatal hepatitis (see page 786), hypothyroidism (see page 404), and some rare blood disorders.

All types of jaundice carry a slight risk that the increased level of bilirubin in the blood will cause brain damage. However, brain damage almost never occurs when a baby is treated and the level of bilirubin in the blood is closely monitored.

Symptoms

In all types of neonatal jaundice, a baby's skin and whites of the eyes turn yellow. The yellowing usually occurs within the first day after birth in hemolytic jaundice, after about 3 to 5 days in physiologic jaundice, and after 1 to 2 weeks in obstructive jaundice. In physiologic jaundice and mild hemolytic jaundice, the yellowing is slight and usually disappears after a few days. In severe cases of hemolytic jaundice and in obstructive jaundice, the yellowing gradually becomes more pronounced as bilirubin builds up in the blood.

Diagnosis

To diagnose jaundice, a doctor checks a child's skin and the whites of the eyes for yellowing. If either looks yellow, the doctor will order blood tests to measure the levels of bilirubin, red blood cells, and liver enzymes in the child's blood. In some cases, a doctor will recommend an ultrasound scan (see page 111) or X-rays to examine the child's liver and bile ducts. In addition, a doctor may order blood tests to check for possible underlying causes of jaundice, such as Rh incompatibility.

Treatment

Most cases of physiologic jaundice clear up on their own without treatment. Mild cases of hemolytic jaundice also usually disappear without treatment. Feeding the infant stimulates the passage of meconium (the first bowel movement of a newborn) and

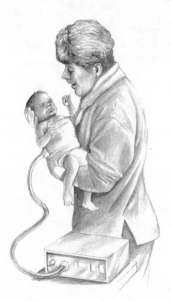

Treating neonatal jaundice
If your baby needs phototherapy for jaundice, you may be able to give the treatment at home. A visiting nurse can teach you how to use the phototherapy equipment and will monitor your baby during daily visits to your home. For the treatment, ultraviolet light is delivered through a fiberoptic panel fitted into a cotton flannel sleeve that wraps around the baby like a wide belt. You can hold, feed, and change your baby while the belt is on. The longer the belt is worn each day, the faster the child's bilirubin reaches a safe level. The process usually takes 3 to 4 days.

the transition to normal stool. Bilirubin is excreted in the stool, which helps lower the levels of bilirubin in the blood.

For obstructive jaundice, surgery to correct the blockage in the outflow of bile and bilirubin from the liver must be performed to prevent fatal liver damage, which can occur within a few months without treatment. In some cases, when the blood level of bilirubin is high, a doctor may perform phototherapy (light therapy), in which the baby is exposed to ultraviolet light to help convert the bilirubin into a form that will pass easily out of the liver, into the urine, and out of the body. Severe cases of jaundice, especially hemolytic jaundice, are treated by an exchange blood transfusion, in which all the baby's blood is replaced with donated blood.

Feeding Problems

Many babies cry for a few minutes after breastfeeding or bottle feeding. If your baby cries after feeding, cuddle and comfort him or her; if your baby has had enough to eat, he or she will soon stop crying and fall asleep. If your baby continues to cry, or cries a lot between feedings, he or she may not be getting enough breast milk or formula. Try giving your baby more but do not force him or her. Babies stop eating when they have had enough. Some babies cry because they are thirsty, especially in hot weather. Try giving your baby some water. If your baby begins to fuss soon after starting a bottle, he or she may be frustrated because the nipple hole is too small or clogged. If this occurs, substitute another nipple.

Poor Feeding

In the first few weeks of life, some babies fall asleep while feeding. Babies this age generally eat small amounts but need to eat frequently throughout the day and night (sometimes as often as every 2 or 3 hours). This is normal. In a healthy baby, this phase usually passes after about a month. Offer the baby the breast or bottle when he or she wakes up or when he or she cries, but don't force the baby to feed if he or she turns away. If this pattern of feeding continues or if the baby seems lethargic or seems to be losing weight, see your pediatrician. Your child's doctor will determine if your baby is getting enough milk or formula by checking his or her weight and growth pattern.

You also should contact your doctor if your baby feeds slowly or does not seem to be eating as much as usual.

Spitting Up or Vomiting After Feeding

Most babies spit up a little milk or formula after feeding, particularly when they burp. Bottle-fed babies are more likely to spit up because they are more likely to swallow air when feeding, which can overfill the stomach. Some very active babies spit up a lot; this is usually not a cause for concern. Most babies gradually stop spitting up when they are about 4 to 6 months old, after they start eating solid food. Spitting up usually stops completely by 9 months. Changing the baby's feeding position and keeping the baby upright after feeding may help.

If your baby is vomiting large amounts, if the vomit contains blood or a greenish brown material, or if the vomit is expelled to some distance (called projectile vomiting) more than two or three times a day, contact your pediatrician right away. An occasional bout of projectile vomiting is usually a symptom of a mild disorder such as a cold, motion sickness, or gastroenteritis (see below). In rare cases, projectile vomiting can be a symptom of a serious problem such as an intestinal obstruction (see page 405).

Beginning Solid Foods

Infants are usually ready to begin gradually eating solid foods when they are between 4 and 6 months old. Your doctor will recommend starting your baby on solid foods by spoon-feeding him or her cereal twice a day. You will then introduce your baby to a variety of puréed vegetables and fruits, one at a time, to detect any allergies or other problems. When your baby is older, you can add finely chopped meat and eggs. Try to start your baby off with good eating habits—only give food at mealtimes, and do not give foods that are high in sugar, fat, or salt, or that are heavily processed or refined. Also, avoid using food to pacify your baby when he or she is fussing or crying.

Gastroenteritis

Gastroenteritis is inflammation of the stomach and intestines, usually as a result of a viral or bacterial infection or from infestation by an intestinal parasite. The infection usually is acquired by eating contaminated food or by sharing food with an infected person, but it also can be spread by coughing, sneezing, or poor hand washing. In most cases, gastroenteritis is mild, easy to treat, and lasts for just a few days. In some cases, however, the disorder may be persistent or severe. If not treated promptly, persistent or severe gastroenteritis can cause dehydration, which can lead to kidney damage or brain damage, or can be fatal.

Symptoms

The main symptoms of gastroenteritis in an infant are mild to severe vomiting and diarrhea. Other possible symptoms include irritability, weakness, slight fever, abdominal cramps or pain, and loss of appetite. The symptoms of dehydration include a dry mouth, sunken eyes, sunken soft spot, lethargy, irritability, decreased tear production, and decreased urination. If the dehydration becomes severe, the baby's skin loses elasticity—if you pinch the child's skin between your thumb and finger, it does not immediately return to its original position. If your baby has symptoms of gastroenteritis, call your doctor. If your baby has symptoms of dehydration and has three large or loose bowel movements and vomits all feedings within a 6-hour period, see your doctor immediately or take your baby immediately to the nearest hospital emergency department.

WARNING!

A Depressed Soft Spot on the Head

If the soft spot on top of your baby's head seems to be sunken, he or she may be dehydrated, possibly because of a digestive problem. Call your doctor immediately or take your baby to the nearest hospital emergency department.

Diagnosis

To diagnose gastroenteritis, the doctor will ask you about your baby's symptoms and perform a physical examination. He or she may order blood tests or may take a small sample of the baby's stool for laboratory analysis to try to identify the organism causing the problem.

Treatment

To treat mild gastroenteritis, continue breastfeeding your baby, and supplement breastfeeding with an over-the-counter rehydration solution. For a baby older than 6 months, you can supplement breastfeeding with a rehydration solution and clear fluids such as broth. Make sure that your baby gets plenty of rest, and give him or her acetaminophen or ibuprofen (not aspirin) to relieve pain.

GERD in Infants

GERD (gastroesophageal reflux disease) occurs when the contents of the stomach (including stomach acid) back up into the esophagus, causing the lining of the esophagus to become inflamed and irritated. In infants, the condition is usually the result of an immature digestive system. Most children outgrow GERD by the time they are 1 year old.

Some common symptoms of GERD include frequent fussiness, irritability, or crying after eating; frequent spitting up or vomiting after eating; frequent spitting up in a child older than 1 year; "wet" burping; sleeping problems; and poor weight gain or weight loss. Some babies with GERD have frequent choking episodes or develop chronic wheezing or aspiration pneumonia when regurgitated stomach contents enter the lungs. Some babies also may experience periods of apnea (cessation of breathing), which can be life-threatening. A child with GERD may refuse to eat, or may gag or choke when trying to swallow.

If the problem occurs regularly, talk to your child's doctor. GERD is usually diagnosed with special X-rays that can show abnormalities in the digestive tract. Sometimes doctors use a test called a 24-hour pH-probed study to measure and monitor the acid levels in the esophagus. Doctors also may perform endoscopy (an examination of the inside of the body using a viewing instrument) to examine the upper part of the digestive tract (the esophagus, stomach, and upper intestine).

To help prevent reflux, feed your baby in an upright position, burp him or her several times during feedings, keep him or her in an upright position for at least 30 minutes after feeding, and avoid feeding him or her within 2 to 3 hours before bedtime. The doctor may recommend that you raise one end of the crib mattress slightly so the baby can sleep with his or her head raised. If you are feeding your baby formula, your doctor may recommend trying a different type of formula. If these changes do not help, the doctor may prescribe medication to reduce the incidence of reflux or help reduce the amount of acid in the child's stomach. In rare cases, doctors recommend surgery to create a valve at the top of the stomach to eliminate reflux.

Your doctor may recommend that you stop the baby's usual feeding for 24 hours and substitute an over-the-counter rehydration solution or sports drink to help restore lost fluids and electrolytes (essential minerals that help regulate various body processes). On the second day, replace the solution or sports drink with breast milk, a soy formula, or a lactose-free formula. Give bland, solid foods if the baby has not vomited for 24 hours and can hold down liquids. Gradually return to the child's usual diet after the diarrhea has stopped.

If a baby has severe gastroenteritis, he or she will be hospitalized and given fluids intravenously (through a vein). In most cases of gastroenteritis, the baby recovers completely, with no lasting effects.

Diaper Rash

Diaper rash (see page 120) is inflammation of the skin on a baby's abdomen, buttocks, thighs, or genital area that usually results from prolonged contact with urine or feces. Diaper rash can also result from chafing or from a bacterial or yeast infection (thrush; see page 539). Sometimes the condition is an allergic reaction to chemical irritants such as soap, detergent, or fabric softener, or to synthetic materials in disposable diapers.

Symptoms

The main symptom of diaper rash is red, spotty, sore, moist skin in the area that is usually covered by a diaper. The rash is painful and can range from mild to severe.

Diagnosis and Treatment

Diaper rash is easily diagnosed by its appearance and is easy to treat at home. Expose the rash area to warm, dry air for as long as possible throughout the day—take the baby's diaper off and lay him or her face down on soft towels placed over a waterproof sheet. Clean up any stool or urine immediately, and bathe the rash with warm water and a mild soap. Change the towels as often as necessary. Afterward, pat the affected area dry with a soft, clean towel. Diaper the baby at bedtime.

Your doctor may recommend gently cleansing the affected area with a cotton ball soaked in mineral oil and applying a nonprescription zinc oxide cream or ointment to the rash. If the affected area becomes soiled again, cleanse it again with mineral oil and reapply the cream.

If the rash is persistent or severe, or if it worsens, talk to your doctor. He or she may recommend other ways to treat the rash at home or may prescribe a cream or ointment to help speed healing. Sometimes diaper rash becomes infected with a fungus called candida. If this occurs, doctors usually recommend a nonprescription antifungal cream or ointment to clear it up.

Cradle Cap

Cradle cap is a common, harmless skin condition that affects an infant's scalp, usually during the first 3 to 6 months of life. Cradle cap, which results from a buildup of oil and dead skin cells, is the most common form of seborrheic dermatitis (see page 1063). The thin, dry scales of cradle cap cause no discomfort for the child.

Symptoms
The initial symptom of cradle cap is the appearance of thin, dry, red, scaly patches on the scalp. The scales eventually become yellow, greasy, crusty patches that can cover the entire scalp and sometimes extend over the eyebrows and behind the ears. Some babies may temporarily lose some hair in the affected area.

Diagnosis and Treatment
To diagnose cradle cap, a doctor will examine the baby's scalp. If your baby has cradle cap, keep the affected area clean and dry by washing it with mild soap and water and drying it gently but thoroughly with a soft, clean towel. If cradle cap is unsightly, your doctor will recommend rubbing the affected areas gently with unscented baby oil or mineral oil and leaving the oil on for a few hours or overnight to loosen the scales. Later, comb the hair gently with a fine-tooth comb to loosen the scales; wash the scales away with a mild shampoo. If the condition recurs, repeat the treatment.

If cradle cap worsens or becomes itchy, or if the scaly patches become soft and begin to ooze yellowish pus, talk to your doctor. These may be symptoms of an infection that requires immediate treatment. Your doctor will prescribe a topical antibiotic ointment to apply to the skin to help relieve the baby's symptoms and clear up the infection.

Colic

Colic is a common condition in which a baby has episodes of loud, continuous, inconsolable crying with no apparent cause. The condition usually begins when a baby is 2 to 4 weeks old and continues for 2 to 3 months. Episodes of colic usually begin suddenly in the late afternoon or early evening, and last for 3 hours or more. The cause of colic is not known.

Symptoms
The main symptoms of colic are daily episodes of loud, inconsolable crying that last for several hours. The baby may also have a swollen, tight abdomen, and he or she may clench his or her hands and bring the knees up to the chest. The baby's face may be flushed, but the area around his or her mouth may be pale. Episodes usually end after the baby falls asleep from exhaustion, or when he or she has a bowel movement or passes gas.

Diagnosis and Treatment
A diagnosis of colic is based on the baby's symptoms. There is no specific treatment for colic, and the condition usually clears up on its own by the time a baby is about 3 months old. Until then, the best way to deal with the problem is to try to

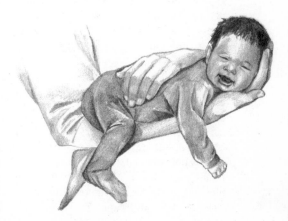

If your baby has colic
Many parents whose baby has colic find that holding their baby in the football position, which puts pressure on the baby's abdomen, often provides some relief. Place your baby facedown on your arm, supporting his or her body with your other hand.

comfort or distract the baby without overstimulating him or her. Some babies with colic seem to feel better if they sleep in a quiet room, are handled very gently, and get a lot of attention from their parents. Your doctor may recommend giving the baby a warm bath and providing a quiet, calm environment. Some babies with colic respond well to soft music or white noise, such as the sound of a washer or dishwasher or radio static. Try singing or humming to the baby. Babies often respond to touch or to gentle rhythmic movement, such as softly massaging their back; rocking, slow dancing, or walking while you are holding him or her; or riding in a car or a stroller.

Changing the baby's diet may help ease the colic or discomfort. If you are nursing, breastfeed your baby smaller amounts more often. Avoid consuming chocolate; caffeine; dairy products; vegetables that cause gas such as broccoli, cabbage, and beans; spicy foods; citrus fruit; and alcohol. These foods may affect your breast milk and cause discomfort in the baby. If you are bottle-feeding, your baby may feel better if you change to a soy or lactose-free formula. Burp your baby frequently, and give him or her a pacifier between feedings.

Trying to cope with the baby's crying can be disturbing and exhausting for parents. Try to avoid becoming frustrated by the baby's crying. Take breaks from caring for the baby whenever you can. Put the baby in his or her crib, close the bedroom door, and let him or her cry for a while. If you feel stressed, talk to your doctor, and don't hesitate to ask friends and relatives for help.

Sudden Infant Death Syndrome

Sudden infant death syndrome (SIDS) is the unexpected, unexplained death of an apparently healthy infant under 1 year old (usually between 1 and 4 months). In the United States, SIDS is the leading cause of death in infants from 1 month to 1 year old, accounting for about 2,500 deaths each year. SIDS occurs somewhat more frequently in boys than in girls, and usually occurs during the fall, winter, or early spring.

Although the exact cause of SIDS is not known, doctors think it may be related to problems in the development and functioning of the child's nervous system or heart, or in breathing patterns. SIDS is not contagious or inherited, is not caused by childhood immunizations, and does not result from child abuse or neglect.

Some factors that increase an infant's risk of SIDS include lack of prenatal care, premature birth, low birth weight, alcohol or drug abuse by the mother during pregnancy, placing a baby on his or her stomach to sleep, and exposure to secondhand smoke. To reduce your baby's risk of SIDS, take the following steps:

- Get early and regular health care throughout your pregnancy.
- Do not smoke cigarettes or drink alcohol during pregnancy.
- Do not use drugs during pregnancy unless your doctor has prescribed them.

WARNING!

Sleep Position

To reduce the risk of SIDS, all babies should sleep on their back unless they have a medical condition that increases the risk of airway obstruction (such as an upper respiratory condition or gastroesophageal reflux). If the baby has an obstructed airway, the side position will help to keep the baby's airways open and make breathing easier. If you put a baby on his or her side, always move the baby's lower arm forward to keep him or her from rolling over onto his or her stomach. If you are not sure what sleep position to use, ask your doctor which is best for your baby.

When your baby is not sleeping, give him or her plenty of supervised time on his or her stomach to build up his or her neck muscles and to prevent flat spots on the head.

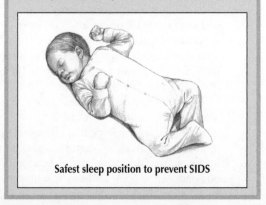

Safest sleep position to prevent SIDS

- Breastfeed your baby.
- Place your baby on his or her back or side to sleep.
- Have your baby sleep on a firm mattress or other firm surface.
- Do not place pillows, fluffy blankets or comforters, or stuffed toys in the crib with your baby.

- Do not allow your baby to become overheated while sleeping.
- Do not allow anyone to smoke around your baby.
- Call your doctor right away if your baby seems ill.
- Make sure your baby receives all of his or her immunizations on schedule.

Congenital Heart Defects

About eight of every 1,000 American children are born with a heart abnormality, making heart abnormalities the most common type of birth defect. A heart defect that is present from birth (congenital) may be so minor that it requires no treatment, and has no effect on a child's health. Other congenital heart defects may be so severe that immediate treatment is necessary to save the child's life.

How Heart Defects Develop

The heart of a fetus starts to develop early in pregnancy and is fully developed by the third month of pregnancy. Any disturbance in development during this critical period (such as a rubella infection; see page 508) can cause a heart defect. The cause of the vast majority of congenital heart abnormalities is unknown. In most cases, both genes and environmental factors are thought to interact to produce the defect, but specific environmental factors usually cannot be identified.

Although most congenital heart defects occur in otherwise healthy infants, they also can be present in children with broader genetic disorders such as Down syndrome (see page 955), Marfan syndrome (see page 967), or Turner syndrome (see page 957). An ultrasound (see page 510) of the fetus is often part of a prenatal examination during the first few months of pregnancy and provides a picture of the internal organs, including the heart. The doctor studies the fetus's heart on the ultrasound and, if he or she suspects an abnormality, will recommend a more specialized test called a fetal cardiac ultrasound to get a more detailed image of the anatomy of the fetus's heart.

Symptoms of Congenital Heart Defects

Many cases of congenital heart defects produce no symptoms, and the defect is detected during a routine examination of the heart. In some cases, symptoms are obvious. Sometimes symptoms are present at birth, and sometimes they don't develop until childhood or much later. Some congenital heart defects that don't produce symptoms early in life require surgery to prevent problems from developing later.

Lack of oxygen in the blood can cause blueness of the skin (cyanosis). Cyanosis is a common sign of congenital heart problems that allow blood lacking oxygen (deoxygenated blood) to circulate through the body. A baby with mild heart failure may have difficulty feeding (because he or she does not have enough energy to suck) and he or she may lose weight and cry less than usual. In severe heart failure, symptoms are more obvious—the child's breathing is rapid and difficult even while resting, and his or her skin may be blue because of the lack of oxygen.

Birth Defects

Abnormalities that are present in a child at birth are called birth defects or congenital abnormalities. Although they are present at birth, their effects may not become apparent until later in life. Birth defects can result from genetic or environmental factors or both. For many, the cause is unknown.

For most birth defects, the earlier a child is treated, the better the outcome for his or her development and physical and emotional health. In addition to medical treatment, a child who has a birth defect can often benefit from counseling by a mental health professional who can help him or her deal with the challenges presented by his or her abnormality. If your child has a birth defect, you might also benefit from counseling; ask your doctor to recommend a counselor or support group that can put you in touch with other parents who have a child with a similar birth defect.

Diagnosing Congenital Heart Defects

A doctor can usually diagnose a congenital heart defect by examining the heart with a stethoscope, which enables him or her to hear the sounds made by the heart when the pumping chambers of the heart (ventricles) contract and the valves open and close. Sounds of blood flow that occur between the sounds of the valves are called murmurs, which can be normal or the sign of a heart abnormality. A harmless murmur is a common, normal sound of blood flow that can be heard in children after 2 to 3 years of age. These normal murmurs (also called innocent murmurs or functional murmurs) do not require any treatment.

If the child's doctor has detected a murmur that suggests an abnormality, he or she will refer the child to a pediatric cardiologist (a doctor who specializes in treating heart disorders in children) to diagnose the specific defect and evaluate its severity. Each type of heart defect usually produces a characteristic murmur, or sound. For this reason, a pediatric cardiologist can usually diagnose a specific heart abnormality with a stethoscope. However, more tests, including one or more of the following, are usually performed to confirm the diagnosis:

- **Chest X-ray**   An X-ray of the chest can show abnormalities in the shape and size of the heart and its chambers and in blood flow to the lungs.
- **Electrocardiogram**   An electrocardiogram (ECG) records the electrical impulses associated with the heartbeat and can detect enlargement of the chambers of the heart or abnormalities of rhythm.
- **Echocardiogram**   An echocardiogram is an ultrasound examination of the heart that can produce images of all four valves, the walls between the chambers, and the function of the pumping chambers. An echocardiogram can often provide enough information to enable a doctor to make an accurate diagnosis of all aspects of a congenital heart defect.
- **Cardiac catheterization**   In rare cases, cardiac catheterization is required to help make a diagnosis. For this procedure, the child is given anesthesia or sedated, and a thin, flexible tube called a catheter is passed into a blood vessel in a leg and threaded up to the heart. The pediatric cardiologist observes the catheter on an X-ray image as it moves through the child's heart, and he or she can see if it passes through any abnormal openings. The catheter also enables the doctor to measure the blood pressure and the amount of oxygen in the blood in each chamber of the heart. An X-ray moving picture is taken while a liquid dye that shows up on X-rays is passed through the catheter into the heart. This film shows the anatomy of the chambers and valves of the heart. With this information, the pediatric cardiologist can diagnose the precise heart defect and recommend appropriate treatment.

Treating Congenital Heart Defects

Many kinds of congenital heart defects do not require treatment. Small holes in the walls between the chambers do not affect the functioning of the heart and do not need to be closed; many eventually close on their own. Minor valve abnormalities also do not require treatment. However, these minor defects can be areas where bacteria that have entered the bloodstream can settle and cause infection. For this reason, a child with one of these minor heart defects will need to take an antibiotic before having any type of dental work (including cleanings or surgery) to prevent bacteria from infecting the heart.

More serious problems can produce symptoms at birth or in early infancy. If the symptoms are severe, immediate treatment will be necessary with a catheterization procedure or surgery to open narrow valves or close abnormal holes. A baby or child with a serious heart defect will be referred to a pediatric cardiologist in a hospital that has the appropriate medical equipment and trained specialists who can perform these procedures. Hospitals that care for a large number of babies and children with congenital heart defects have high success rates for cardiac catheterization and heart surgery, even if the problem is very complex.

Heart transplants (see page 573) are being performed on infants who have major heart defects that cannot be corrected with other forms of treatment. However, there are not enough compatible donor organs available to meet the demand.

Aortic and Pulmonary Stenosis

Aortic stenosis is narrowing of the heart valve that normally allows blood to flow from the heart into the aorta (the main artery in the body) and out to the rest of the body. Pulmonary stenosis is narrowing of the heart valve (or the area around it) that normally allows blood to flow from the heart to the lungs. Both types of stenosis require the heart to work harder to provide normal blood flow to the body or lungs. A child can be born with either type of stenosis.

Symptoms

Mild cases of stenosis do not produce symptoms. Most children with mild or moderate pulmonary stenosis have no symptoms. In severe aortic stenosis, symptoms can include fatigue on exertion, chest pain, and fainting. The severity of the symptoms usually matches the degree of stenosis.

A baby born with severe pulmonary stenosis can have blue skin color (cyanosis) shortly after birth from lack of oxygen in the blood. A baby with severe aortic stenosis can develop heart failure with symptoms such as rapid breathing, difficulty feed-ing, and poor skin color. These symptoms require emergency treatment in a medical center that is equipped for treating children with heart problems.

Diagnosis

If a child has stenosis, with or without symptoms, the doctor can detect it during a physical examina-tion by listening for a heart murmur through a stethoscope. To confirm the diagnosis, the doctor will refer the child to a pediatric cardiologist (a doc-tor who specializes in treating heart disorders in children), who will probably recommend a chest X-ray, an ultrasound examination of the heart (echocardiogram; see previous page), or a record-ing of the electrical activity of the heart (electro-cardiogram; see previous page).

Treatment

If a child has mild stenosis, no treatment is neces-sary, but the doctor will want to monitor the child's condition with regular examinations because steno-sis can worsen over time. If the child develops symptoms or if the stenosis is progressing, the doc-tor will refer him or her to a center that is experi-enced in caring for children with heart problems. A child with either aortic or pulmonary stenosis

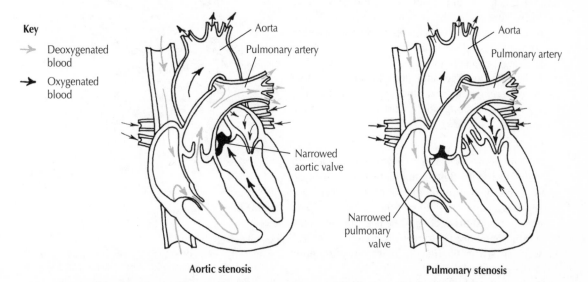

Key

→ Deoxygenated blood

→ Oxygenated blood

Aorta
Pulmonary artery
Narrowed aortic valve

Aortic stenosis

Aorta
Pulmonary artery
Narrowed pulmonary valve

Pulmonary stenosis

Aortic and pulmonary stenosis
A heart with aortic stenosis (left) has a narrowed valve in the aorta. The narrowing obstructs the flow of blood to the child's body, causes the heart to work harder, and thickens the wall of the lower chamber of the heart. A heart with pulmonary stenosis (right) has a narrowed valve in the pul-monary artery (the large blood vessel that transports blood from the heart to the lungs). The narrowing obstructs the flow of blood into the lungs and makes the heart work harder.

needs to take antibiotics before any dental work or surgery to avoid possible bacterial infection of the heart.

To treat severe aortic stenosis, a doctor may recommend heart-valve surgery or balloon valvuloplasty to open the valve and improve blood flow out of the heart to the rest of the body. In balloon valvuloplasty, the doctor threads a small plastic tube with a balloon attached through a blood vessel into the child's narrowed heart valve. He or she then inflates the balloon to open up the abnormal valve. In rare cases, this procedure is unsuccessful and surgery is necessary. Because narrowing at the aortic valve tends to be progressive, more than one balloon valvuloplasty or surgical procedure may be necessary to treat severe aortic stenosis. Balloon valvuloplasty is also recommended for treating severe cases of pulmonary stenosis.

Septal Defects

A septal defect is a hole in the wall, or septum, that separates the left and right sides of the heart. There are two types of septal defects: ventricular septal defects and atrial septal defects. A ventricular septal defect, the most common congenital heart defect, is a hole in the wall between the ventricles (the two lower chambers of the heart). An atrial septal defect is a hole in the wall between the atria (the two upper chambers of the heart).

Septal defects allow blood from the left side of the heart to flow back into the right side. If the hole is large enough, it forces the heart to work harder and can cause congestive heart failure (see page 570).

Symptoms

The symptoms of a ventricular septal defect depend on the size of the hole. Small defects do not cause any symptoms and often close on their own. If a baby has a large ventricular septal defect, he or she may develop signs of congestive heart failure, such as rapid breathing, shortness of breath, excessive sweating while feeding, a heart murmur, poor weight gain, and delayed growth.

Children with atrial septal defects usually have no symptoms, but these defects rarely close on their own. If left untreated, atrial septal defects can progress and cause problems in middle age, including congestive heart failure, arrhythmias (see page 580), and pulmonary hypertension (see page 594).

Key

➡ Oxygenated blood
➡ Deoxygenated blood
➡ Mixed

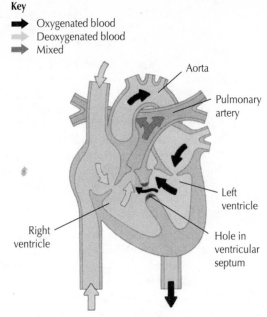

Ventricular septal defect

Aorta
Pulmonary artery
Left ventricle
Hole in ventricular septum
Right ventricle

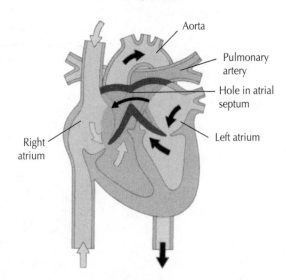

Atrial septal defect

Aorta
Pulmonary artery
Hole in atrial septum
Left atrium
Right atrium

Septal defects
A ventricular septal defect (top) is a hole in the wall (septum) that separates the right and left ventricles. Blood flows abnormally through the hole from the left ventricle into the right ventricle, potentially allowing excess blood to flow to the lungs. An atrial septal defect (bottom) is a hole in the septum that separates the right atrium from the left atrium. This defect also causes the blood to flow abnormally from left to right; if the defect is large enough, too much blood can enter the lungs.

Diagnosis

If a child has a septal defect, the doctor may detect a heart murmur during a physical examination while listening to the child's heart through a stethoscope. To confirm the diagnosis, the doctor will order additional tests, such as a chest X-ray, an ultrasound of the heart (echocardiogram; see page 561), or a recording of the electrical activity of the heart (electrocardiogram; see page 559). Doctors usually refer children with septal defects to pediatric cardiologists (doctors who specialize in treating heart disorders in children).

Treatment

Because children with any kind of heart defect have a slight risk of developing infections at the site of the defect if bacteria enter the bloodstream, the child's doctor will recommend that the child take antibiotics before having any kind of dental work (including cleanings) or surgery.

If a baby has a small ventricular septal defect, no treatment is necessary. More than 80 percent of ventricular septal defects close on their own. If a child has a large ventricular septal defect and signs of congestive heart failure, the doctor will prescribe heart medication and a high-calorie diet (because heart failure uses up calories that are necessary for the child's growth and development). If the baby's condition does not improve or if he or she has pulmonary hypertension (high blood pressure in the lungs) or is not growing at the normal rate, the doctor will recommend open heart surgery to repair the defect in the child's first year of life. Surgery is very effective in correcting these defects, enabling a child to grow and develop normally and lead a full, healthy life.

If an atrial septal defect persists beyond 2 years of age, closure is recommended to avoid future problems. Most defects can be closed using a procedure called catheter device closure. In this procedure a thin flexible tube (catheter) is used to place a metal device in the defect; the device is then locked onto the atrial walls surrounding the defect, closing the hole. Very large defects require open heart surgery. Children who have surgery to close an atrial septal defect can live a full, healthy life and have a normal life span.

Coarctation of the Aorta

Coarctation of the aorta is an abnormal narrowing of the aorta, the major artery leading out of the heart. The narrowing usually occurs just beyond the point where the aorta turns down to supply blood to the lower part of the body, causing blood pressure in the aorta to increase above the narrowing and decrease below the narrowing. As a result, the child develops high blood pressure in the upper portion of the body and low blood pressure in the lower part of the body, and his or her heart has to work harder to pump blood past the narrowing to the rest of the body.

Key

→ Deoxygenated blood

→ Oxygenated blood

Coarctation of the aorta

In a healthy heart (left), the aorta is wide enough to allow normal blood flow. Coarctation of the aorta (right) is a narrowing in the aorta, usually just past the point where the blood vessels that supply blood to the head, neck, and arms branch from the aorta. When the aorta is constricted, the heart must work harder to pump blood to the areas of the body that lie below the narrowed area.

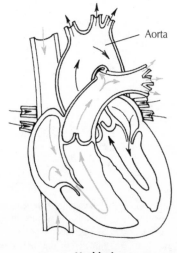

Healthy heart

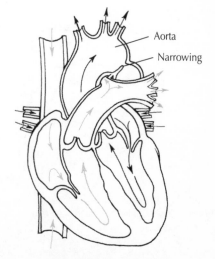

Coarctation of the aorta

Symptoms

If the narrowing of the aorta is severe, symptoms can develop shortly after birth. An infant may feed poorly, become inactive, and have poor skin color. The pulse in the groin area is weak or absent, and the child may have a heart murmur.

Most older children with coarctation of the aorta do not have any symptoms, but some may have throbbing headaches, cold feet or legs, or leg cramps after exercise. They also have high blood pressure in their upper body, low blood pressure in their lower body, and a weak or absent pulse in the groin area. They may also have a heart murmur.

Diagnosis and Treatment

A doctor often detects coarctation of the aorta during a baby's first examination by noticing a weak or absent pulse in the groin. Older children with coarctation have high blood pressure in their arms and often a heart murmur. The diagnosis can be confirmed with an ultrasound evaluation of the aorta and heart (echocardiogram; see page 561).

Surgery to correct the narrowing usually is performed shortly after a diagnosis of coarctation of the aorta is made, even in infants. Surgery relieves the symptoms quickly and prevents high blood pressure and heart damage.

Tetralogy of Fallot

Tetralogy of Fallot is a group of several abnormalities that occur together in the heart. These defects include a large hole in the wall (septum) that separates the ventricles (ventricular septal defect; see page 392), a narrowing at or below the pulmonary valve that opens to send blood from the heart to the lungs, a larger-than-normal right ventricle, and an enlarged aorta (the main blood vessel carrying blood from the heart to the rest of the body), which sits abnormally above both the right and left ventricles. These defects can prevent some of the oxygen-depleted blood from reaching the baby's lungs for a fresh supply of oxygen, causing some oxygen-deficient blood to be pumped out to tissues and preventing the tissues from getting sufficient oxygen.

Symptoms

From birth, or shortly after, the deoxygenated blood gradually turns the baby's skin blue (cyanosis), especially when he or she is crying or feeding.

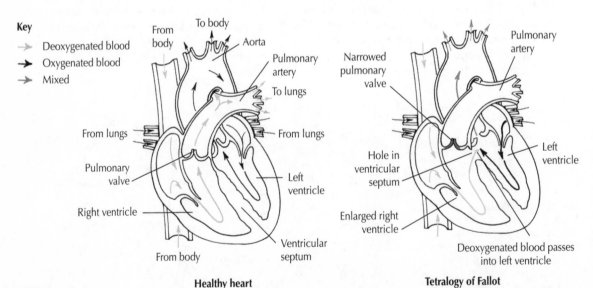

Healthy heart

Tetralogy of Fallot

Key
→ Deoxygenated blood
→ Oxygenated blood
→ Mixed

Tetralogy of Fallot
In tetralogy of Fallot, four heart abnormalities occur together. One of the defects is a large hole in the wall (septum) separating the right and left ventricles, which allows deoxygenated blood to pass from the right ventricle to the left ventricle and be pumped through the aorta to body tissues without receiving a fresh supply of oxygen from the lungs. Another defect is a narrowing at, or just beneath, the pulmonary valve, which partly blocks the flow of deoxygenated blood into the lungs. In addition, the wall of the right ventricle is more muscular and larger than normal, and the aorta lies directly over the hole in the ventricular septum.

Other symptoms include shortness of breath, rapid breathing, a heart murmur, difficulty feeding, failure to gain weight, and slow growth. Without treatment during infancy, a child may develop thickened, clubbed fingers and toes. After exercise, the child is short of breath and squats in a characteristic position to catch his or her breath.

Diagnosis

Tetralogy of Fallot can often be diagnosed shortly after birth when the doctor notices that the baby has bluish skin and detects a heart murmur during a physical examination. A chest X-ray will show an abnormally shaped heart. The doctor will also order an echocardiogram (see page 561) and an electrocardiogram (see page 559) to identify the abnormalities of tetralogy of Fallot and to rule out other heart defects. The doctor will refer the child to a pediatric cardiologist (a doctor who specializes in treating heart disorders in children) for further evaluation and treatment.

Treatment

A child with tetralogy of Fallot will need to have surgery to correct the defects, usually in the first year of life. Before corrective surgery, the doctor may recommend a temporary solution with a surgical procedure using a special shunt that diverts blood flow to the lungs and relieves the child's immediate symptoms. But, as heart surgery for infants evolves, more and more children with tetralogy of Fallot are having the defects repaired early in infancy, eliminating the need for this initial, temporary surgery.

After the defects are repaired, the doctor will prescribe antibiotics for the child to take before having any dental work or surgery to prevent a bacterial infection of the heart. After surgery, the child will grow and develop normally, but he or she will need to be examined regularly throughout life by a cardiologist to detect any problems (such as irregular heart rhythms) that could develop.

Patent Ductus Arteriosus

Patent ductus arteriosus is a heart defect in which a blood vessel called the ductus arteriosus fails to close after birth. This blood vessel connects the pulmonary artery (which transports blood from the heart to the lungs) and the aorta (the main artery that transports blood from the heart to the body) in the fetus. Because this blood vessel stays open (patent) after birth, some of the blood pumped from the left side of the baby's heart flows back to the lungs instead of to the rest of the body. Through a stethoscope, a doctor will be able to hear a murmur of blood flow through the ductus. Patent ductus arteriosus occurs most often in premature infants but also can occur in full-term babies.

Key

→ Oxygenated blood

→ Deoxygenated blood

→ Mixed

Patent ductus arteriosus

A fetus's heart has a channel called the ductus arteriosus, which connects the pulmonary artery and the aorta. Because the fetus receives oxygen from the mother's placenta and umbilical cord, the channel allows blood to bypass the lungs. Normally, the channel closes shortly after birth to allow blood to flow to the lungs to receive oxygen. In patent ductus arteriosus, the channel stays open (patent), allowing oxygenated blood to flow back from the aorta through the pulmonary artery to the baby's lungs, making the heart work extra hard.

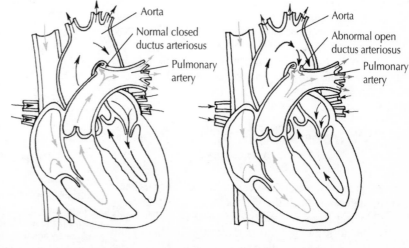

Aorta

Normal closed ductus arteriosus

Pulmonary artery

Aorta

Abnormal open ductus arteriosus

Pulmonary artery

Healthy heart

Patent ductus arteriosus

Symptoms

A small opening in the ductus arteriosus often causes no symptoms or only mild symptoms. A large opening can cause an infant to breathe rapidly and have shortness of breath, a very strong pulse, difficulty feeding, poor weight gain, and frequent chest infections. He or she may also be irritable.

Diagnosis

Doctors can diagnose patent ductus arteriosus by listening for a heart murmur through a stethoscope. To confirm the diagnosis, a doctor will recommend additional tests, such as a chest X-ray, an echocardiogram (see page 561), or an electrocardiogram (see page 559).

Treatment

The doctor will first administer a medication called indomethacin intravenously (through a vein) to close the ductus in a premature infant. He or she will also give the baby diuretics to reduce the fluid levels in his or her body by increasing urination. The baby's intake of fluids will be limited to prevent fluid buildup.

If this treatment is not successful, if the baby is full term, or if patent ductus arteriosus is diagnosed in an older infant or child, the doctor will recommend a cardiac catheterization procedure (see page 592) to close the ductus. In this procedure, the ductus is closed off with coils inserted through a thin, flexible tube (catheter) that is threaded into the heart through an artery or vein. In rare cases, surgery (performed through an incision under the left arm) is necessary to close off the ductus. Both procedures have excellent success rates; the child will have no remaining problems from the defect, and he or she will grow and develop normally.

Transposition of the Great Arteries

Transposition of the great arteries is a serious heart defect in which the two major arteries that carry blood from the heart—the aorta (which carries blood from the heart to the rest of the body) and the pulmonary artery (which carries blood from the heart to the lungs)—are reversed. As a result,

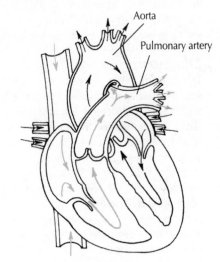

Key

→ Oxygenated blood
→ Deoxygenated blood
→ Mixed

Healthy heart

Deoxygenated blood pumped back to body

Aorta

Pulmonary artery

Transposition of the great arteries

Transposition of the great arteries
Transposition of the great arteries is a heart defect in which the major arteries that carry blood away from the heart—the pulmonary artery and the aorta—are reversed. As a result, deoxygenated blood returning from the body is pumped back to the body without reaching the lungs to receive oxygen.

deoxygenated blood returning from the body to the heart is pumped back to the body without flowing to the lungs to receive a fresh supply of oxygen. Without treatment, a baby with this heart defect is likely to die within the first few weeks of life.

Symptoms
The lack of oxygen in the blood caused by transposition of the great arteries makes the baby's skin turn blue (cyanosis) within the first few hours of life. He or she may breathe rapidly and have difficulty feeding. A doctor can sometimes hear a heart murmur through a stethoscope.

Diagnosis
If a baby's skin turns blue after birth, the doctor will immediately order tests to look for heart defects and determine the cause. Diagnostic tests will include a chest X-ray, a recording of the electrical activity of the heart (electrocardiogram; see page 559), and an ultrasound examination of the heart (echocardiogram; see page 561. The baby will probably be transferred to a neonatal intensive care unit for evaluation by a pediatric cardiologist (a doctor who specializes in treating heart disorders in children).

Treatment
If a baby has been diagnosed with transposition of the great arteries, the doctor probably will recommend cardiac catheterization (see page 592). In this procedure, a thin, flexible tube (catheter) is threaded through an artery to the heart to enlarge the normal opening between the two upper heart chambers (atria). The opening will allow blood that has traveled to the lungs (and received oxygen) to pass to the right side of the baby's heart and out to the body. Within the first 2 weeks of life, the baby also will need to have surgery to switch the positions of the aorta and pulmonary artery. After successful surgery, the child's chances for a full, healthy life are excellent.

Hypoplastic Left Heart Syndrome

Hypoplastic left heart syndrome is a very severe congenital heart defect in which the left side of the heart is underdeveloped. The left ventricle (the pumping chamber), left atrium (the chamber that receives blood from the lungs), aorta (the major blood vessel to the body from the heart), and the valves in the left side of the heart are all absent or are extremely small. As a result, the right side of the heart must do the job of both sides to circulate blood through the body. Within days after birth, the baby's heart begins to fail. Without immediate treatment, a child usually dies within a week.

Symptoms
A newborn with hypoplastic left heart syndrome may look healthy at first, but soon becomes weak and short of breath, has difficulty feeding, and may turn very pale or blue. His or her pulse is weak and the skin is cold, and he or she may have difficulty breathing. Within hours or days, a newborn will become critically ill and die unless he or she is given immediate care.

Diagnosis
If a newborn develops symptoms in the hospital nursery, a doctor usually will diagnose the problem with a chest X-ray, an ultrasound examination of the heart (echocardiogram; see page 561), or a recording of the electrical activity of the heart (electrocardiogram; see page 559). If your baby shows any symptoms of hypoplastic left heart syndrome after leaving the hospital, take him or her to the nearest hospital emergency department immediately. He or she will need to be cared for at a medical center that has extensive experience treating babies with this type of heart defect.

At the hospital, the doctor will stabilize the baby with intravenous heart and blood pressure medications. The baby will need to have surgery within days to enable the right side of his or her heart to pump blood to the rest of the body and to insert a shunt to allow blood to flow to his or her lungs from the pulmonary artery. A second operation is done at about 6 to 12 months of age and a third one between ages 2 and 4. Even after these operations, a child's heart will not be normal; he or she always will need medication to keep the heart functioning well and will need to see a pediatric cardiologist (a doctor who specializes in treating heart disorders in children) regularly. If the three-stage surgery is not recommended in your child's case, a heart transplant to save your child's life is an option, provided a compatible donor heart is available.

Neural Tube Defects

The central nervous system (see page 666), which includes the brain and spinal cord, develops in the fetus within the first 2 months of pregnancy from a strip of cells that runs along the back of the embryo. The edges of the strip gradually curl inward to form a tube of cells. The front part of this tube expands to form the brain; the back part of the tube forms the spinal cord. A liquid (called cerebrospinal fluid) produced by the brain forms inside and around the brain and spinal cord to cushion them. Bone cells develop into the skull and spinal column, which provide more protection for the brain and spinal cord.

Neural tube defects—in which the brain, spinal column, or spinal cord is malformed—are disorders of the central nervous system that are present at birth (congenital). Neural tube defects are linked to a deficiency of the B vitamin folic acid in a pregnant woman. During the first few weeks of pregnancy, which are crucial to the development of the fetus's central nervous system, many women do not know they are pregnant. Most cases of neural tube defects could be prevented if women of child-bearing age who might become pregnant would take 400 micrograms of folic acid (in a supplement or in a multivitamin) every day before they become pregnant and throughout their pregnancy (especially during the early weeks).

Neural tube defects can run in families. If a couple has one affected child, or relatives who have a child with a neural tube defect, they should talk to a genetic counselor (see page 952) about their risks of having another child with the abnormality and to learn how they can prevent it.

Spina Bifida

In a neural tube defect called spina bifida, part of the spinal column does not develop fully, leaving the nerves of the spinal cord in that area exposed and unprotected. The disorder usually affects the bones (vertebrae) in the lower spine and the meninges (the membranes covering the spinal cord). The spinal nerves in that area control the leg muscles, bladder, and intestines. The extent of physical disability depends on the severity of the spinal defect.

Symptoms

The defect in the lower spine and the resulting damage to the spinal cord and symptoms can vary widely. The mildest form of spina bifida, called spina bifida occulta, is not technically a neural tube defect because only the vertebrae are malformed—the spinal cord and meninges remain inside the spinal column. The only visible sign of spina bifida occulta may be a small dimple in the skin, a birthmark, or a wisp of hair over the lower spine. In some children, the spine has an abnormal curve. In rare cases, a child with spina bifida occulta has a physical impairment.

In the most severe and most common form of spina bifida (meningomyelocele), the meninges and spinal cord are exposed on the child's back. In another form, known as a meningocele, a bulging sac containing the meninges appears on the child's back. This sac may or may not be covered by skin but it is fragile and can easily be damaged. An infectious organism can enter the cerebrospinal fluid through a damaged area, causing meningitis (see page 692). When the spinal cord is involved, the cord often is damaged before birth, causing weakness, paralysis, or loss of sensation in the legs and lack of normal bowel and bladder control. Bladder infections are common in a person with spina bifida; they sometimes can lead to kidney damage.

Diagnosis

Spina bifida can be detected before birth by measuring the level of a protein called alpha-fetoprotein (AFP) in a pregnant woman's blood early in pregnancy. If the woman's AFP level is elevated, the doctor will recommend an ultrasound (see page 509) of the fetus and, possibly, amniocentesis (see page 510) to confirm and evaluate the abnormality in the fetus. After birth, doctors can recognize more severe forms of spina bifida during a physical examination. Spina bifida occulta usually is detected by chance on an X-ray of the spine done for another reason.

Treatment

Defects in the formation of the spinal cord cannot be corrected, and any resulting paralysis is permanent. If your child has spina bifida, the doctor will recommend surgery shortly after birth to cover the spinal cord and close the opening on the child's back. A CT scan (see page 112) or an MRI (see page 113) of the brain may be necessary to detect any related brain malformation or excessive accumulation of fluid in the brain (hydrocephalus). If your child has hydrocephalus, he or she may need surgery to place a shunt (a small plastic tube) in the brain to drain excess fluid.

Although it usually is not possible to repair the defective spinal nerves, physical therapy can help develop muscles, enabling a child with spina bifida to learn to move around and become mobile with the help of wheelchairs, braces, or walkers. For your child to develop to his or her full potential,

seek treatment at a children's hospital that has doctors who specialize in neurosurgery and neural tube defects. Many children with spina bifida can attend school in regular classrooms.

In some cases, surgery is recommended to correct deformities of the legs. Some children with spina bifida are able to achieve bladder control with toilet training. If not, the doctor will show you how to place a catheter through your child's urethra into his or her bladder to drain urine. You will need to do this four or five times a day. Treatment with antibiotics may be recommended to reduce the risk of urinary tract infections. If your child has bowel problems, the doctor will recommend a high-fiber diet and may prescribe enemas or laxatives to help your child have regular bowel movements. A neurosurgeon and a urologist should see your child regularly to monitor the effectiveness of the treatment.

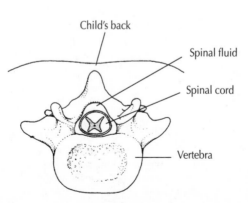

Normal spine

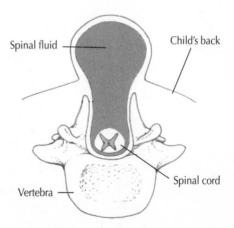

Spine with spina bifida

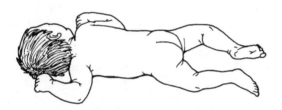

Child's back
Spinal fluid
Spinal cord
Vertebra

Normal spine

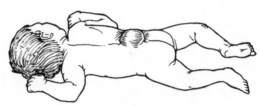

Spinal fluid
Child's back
Spinal cord
Vertebra

Spine with spina bifida

Spina bifida

In a normal spine (left), the spinal cord is protected by the spinal column. In spina bifida, the spine fails to develop completely, leaving part of the spinal cord exposed. In a form of spina bifida called meningocele (right), a bulging sac containing the meninges (the membranes covering the spinal cord) is visible on an infant's back. The sac may be covered by skin.

Hydrocephalus

Cerebrospinal fluid is a fluid inside the brain and around the brain and spinal cord. This fluid is produced by the brain and passes into the space around the brain, where it is absorbed into a membrane surrounding the space. If too much fluid is produced, if the membrane is abnormal in a developing fetus, or if the flow of cerebrospinal fluid is blocked, the fluid builds up in the cavities of the brain. This fluid buildup can put pressure on the brain, which can cause the brain to swell, spreading apart the loosely connected bones of the skull and causing the child's head to become larger than normal.

Hydrocephalus sometimes occurs with spina bifida (see page 398). In premature infants, hydrocephalus can occur from bleeding in the brain. If hydrocephalus is well advanced at birth, the brain can be damaged severely, limiting a child's physical and mental development and, in some cases, resulting in death. Hydrocephalus can occur later in infancy as a result of damage to the brain from an infection or a tumor.

Symptoms

A doctor may suspect that a newborn has hydrocephalus if the circumference of his or her head is significantly larger than average for his or her overall size or if the head is growing too rapidly. If the doctor suspects hydrocephalus, he or she will measure the baby's head periodically. If the rate of growth of the head is greater than normal for the baby's age and size, the doctor probably will order an ultrasound scan (see page 111), an MRI (see page 113), or a CT scan (see page 112) to help make a diagnosis.

Treatment

Hydrocephalus is treated surgically. The infant is given general anesthesia, and the surgeon drills a small hole in the infant's skull. The doctor inserts a tube with a one-way valve into the hole, extending it into the ventricle (a natural space in the brain). He or she then inserts the other end into the child's abdomen or into a major blood vessel leading into the heart. Fluid then drains from the brain through

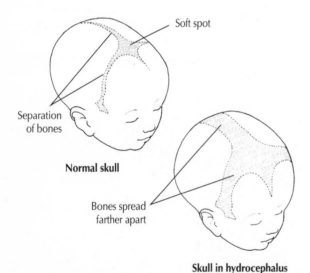

Soft spot

Separation of bones

Normal skull

Bones spread farther apart

Skull in hydrocephalus

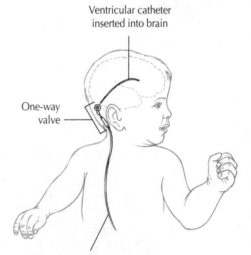

Ventricular catheter inserted into brain

One-way valve

Peritoneal catheter draining fluid from the brain into the abdomen

Hydrocephalus
At birth, the bones of the skull are slightly separated (top left), and you can feel a soft spot called the fontanelle on the top of the child's head. The bones grow together by age 2. In a child with hydrocephalus, the buildup of cerebrospinal fluid in the cavities of the brain causes the brain to swell and spread the skull bones farther apart (bottom right), enlarging the child's head.

Treating hydrocephalus
To relieve pressure on the brain from the accumulation of fluid in hydrocephalus, a surgeon may insert a permanent tube (called a shunt) into the child's head to drain the fluid from the brain into the child's abdomen or into a vein in the neck. The tube usually remains in place for life.

the tube into the abdomen or bloodstream. Placement of the tube is permanent.

After the surgery, the baby's head will gradually return to a normal size. During the first year, he or she will need to have frequent checkups. When children with hydrocephalus have this surgery early in life, their chances of normal mental and physical development are good.

In some cases, as the child grows, the tube becomes blocked, causing pressure to build up in the brain. If this occurs, the child will be irritable, vomit frequently, or develop a headache and fever. If you notice these symptoms in your child, take him or her to the doctor or to a hospital emergency department immediately. If the tube in your child's brain is blocked, he or she will be hospitalized and the blockage will be removed or the tube replaced.

Other Congenital Disorders

S ome birth defects are inherited. Others can result from an abnormality that occurs during fetal development. In most cases, the earlier a child is treated, the more successful the outcome, especially for disorders that can affect a child's development.

For example, congenital dislocation of the hip can interfere with a child's learning to walk, and cleft lip and cleft palate can affect a child's ability to speak and can make eating difficult. Once these disorders are treated, a child can lead a full, healthy life.

Congenital Dislocation of the Hip

Some children are born with a dislocated hip or a hip that becomes dislocated shortly after birth. In a dislocated hip, the head of a thighbone (femur) lies outside of its socket in the pelvis. The socket is shallow and poorly formed. One or both hips may be affected. The cause of congenital hip dislocation (also called developmental dysplasia of the hip) is not known, but about 1 in 60 children is born with a possible hip dislocation. The disorder tends to run in families, and it occurs more frequently in girls than in boys. Babies who were in the breech position (with buttocks or feet down rather than head down) inside the uterus are at increased risk of having a dislocated hip.

Symptoms and Diagnosis

The symptoms of a congenital dislocation of the hip are not obvious. As part of the routine examination of a newborn or infant, the doctor manipulates the child's hip joints and, if one is dislocated, he or she will hear a click. If only one hip is dislocated, the skin folds in the buttocks and legs may be asymmetrical, and the leg on the dislocated side may appear shorter. A more reliable test uses ultrasound imaging (see page 111) to view the hip joints, enabling the doctor to see any underlying defect in the hip socket. Doctors recommend ultrasound at 4 to 6 weeks of age for infants who have risk factors for dislocation of the hip, such as family history, breech birth position, or other abnormalities of the muscles, bones, or joints.

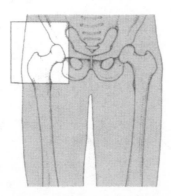

| Normal hip | Dislocated hip |

Hip dislocation
In a normal hip joint (left), the ball at the top of the thighbone fits neatly into the socket in the pelvis. In a dislocated hip joint (right), the ball at the top of the thighbone lies outside the socket.

Treatment

If a hip disorder is detected early in life, an orthopedist (a doctor who specializes in disorders of the bones and joints) will manipulate the baby's thighbone into the correct position and use a special harness or a splint to hold the child's hips in place. Your doctor will give you instructions about any special care your child might need during treatment. This treatment takes about 6 to 8 weeks and is usually successful, enabling the child to walk normally.

If a hip dislocation is not detected until later in childhood, a child will need to have one or more operations to correct the dislocation. The child is hospitalized and given general anesthesia for this surgery. After the surgery, plaster casts are put on the child's legs to stabilize them for several months. This can be an extremely difficult time for a child because the casts restrict movement. Try to engage your child in activities that don't require much movement, such as reading or drawing. If your child doesn't yet know how to read, read to him or her as much as possible to keep his or her mind occupied and to help stimulate brain development. Some children whose hip dislocation is not corrected until later in childhood continue to have problems walking, the length of their legs may differ, and they are at risk of developing arthritis later in life.

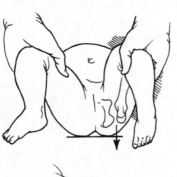
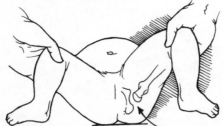

Treating congenital dislocation of the hip
To treat congenital dislocation of the hip, the doctor manually maneuvers the infant's thighbone back into its correct position in the hip.

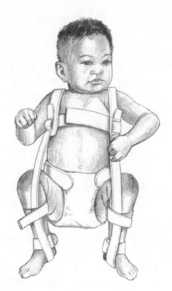

Pavlik harness
After the doctor manipulates the child's thighbone back into its correct position, he or she may place the child in a Pavlik harness to hold the thighbone in place until the hip joint forms properly. The child usually wears the harness continuously for 6 to 8 weeks.

Clubfoot

A baby with clubfoot is born with one or both feet bent either down and in, or up and out. Many babies with normally formed feet persistently turn them inward, but their feet can be manipulated back into the proper position. A clubfoot cannot be placed in the proper position. Clubfoot may run in families and is more common in boys than in girls. In rare cases, clubfoot is linked to other birth defects. Nearly all cases of clubfoot are detected at birth and treated, enabling the child to learn to walk normally.

Symptoms

A clubfoot usually turns down and in. It is seldom painful, but it affects a child's ability to stand and walk. If not treated, the child cannot move the foot normally and walks on the side or top of the foot.

Diagnosis and Treatment

A doctor usually can diagnose clubfoot from a physical examination and X-rays. If a clubfoot is minor, the doctor will show the parents how to manipulate the child's foot regularly each day until,

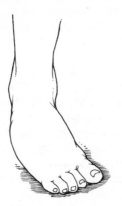

Clubfoot
Clubfoot is a birth defect in which a child's foot is twisted or turned out of its normal position, usually down and in. One or both feet may be affected.

as the bones and ligaments develop, the foot settles into a normal position. In more severe cases, the doctor will refer the child to an orthopedic specialist. The orthopedist will manipulate the foot into as close to normal a position as possible and put a splint or plaster cast on it to hold it in place. Every 2 days, and then at 2-week intervals, the orthopedist will remove the splints or cast, manipulate the child's foot closer to its normal position, and put new splints or a new cast on the foot to hold it in the new position. This treatment takes about 3 to 6 months, after which the child wears corrective shoes. If these measures do not correct the problem, surgery may be necessary.

Cleft Lip and Cleft Palate

A cleft lip is a vertical split in the upper lip that may be partial or extend up to the base of the nose. In some children who have a cleft lip, the nose appears to be flattened. Some children have two splits that can affect both sides of their upper lip, or a gap that continues along the roof of their mouth (the palate). This gap, called a cleft palate, runs along the middle of the palate and extends from behind the teeth to the cavity of the nose. A child with a cleft palate has difficulty eating and swallowing. A newborn may regurgitate milk through the nose. If not treated, the appearance of the cleft lip can cause emotional distress for the child, and an untreated cleft palate can cause serious speech difficulties.

In most cases, the cause of cleft lip and cleft palate is unknown, but both genetic and nongenetic factors appear to play a role. The abnormalities sometimes can run in families and may affect more than one child in a family. For this reason, if you have a child with a cleft lip or palate, or if you have a repaired cleft, it's a good idea to see a genetic counselor (see page 952) to determine your risk of having a child with the same birth defect in the future.

Diagnosis and Treatment

All newborns are checked for cleft lip and cleft palate, which are obvious at birth. If a baby has a cleft, the doctor will examine him or her immediately to determine the extent of the defect.

A baby with a cleft lip or cleft palate will need to have corrective surgery. He or she is likely to receive care from a team of specialists, including a pediatrician, speech therapist, orthodontist (a

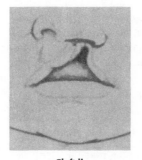 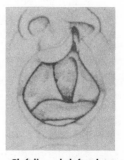

Cleft lip   Cleft lip and cleft palate

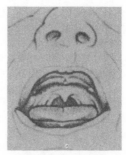

Normal lip and palate

Cleft lip and cleft palate
A cleft lip (above left) can vary in severity from a notch in the upper lip to a split extending to the base of the nose. It can occur on one or both sides of the nose. In some cases, a cleft lip extends into the roof of the mouth (palate), forming a cleft palate (above right). A cleft palate also may occur alone.

dentist who specializes in correcting irregularities of the teeth), pediatric dentist, plastic surgeon, and otolaryngologist (a doctor who specializes in disorders of the ear, nose, and throat).

Surgery to correct a cleft lip is recommended when a child is about 10 weeks old. Treatment from birth until the surgery varies according to the severity of the abnormality. Infants who do not have problems eating do not need any special care during this time. However, some bottle-fed babies may need a special nipple or a nipple with a larger than normal hole. Babies usually stop regurgitating milk through their nose on their own after a few weeks.

Surgery for a cleft palate is more extensive than that for a cleft lip. It is usually done when the child is a little older (usually between 9 and 18 months of age), preferably before he or she learns to talk. Before the surgery, if the baby is having trouble feeding, a dentist will make a device that fits into the roof of the baby's mouth to cover the cleft while he or she is eating. A brace may be placed on the upper gum in the area around the cleft if the gum is out of alignment. Occasionally, a baby may need to be fed through a tube placed in the nose or mouth that extends into the stomach. For long-term tube feeding, the tube may be inserted into the stomach through a small surgical incision in the abdomen.

In some cases, to help prevent ear infections, an otolaryngologist may place a small plastic tube inside each of the child's eardrums at the time of cleft palate surgery. The tubes help air circulate across the eardrum and allow fluid to drain normally. Some children require additional surgery when they get older to improve their appearance. Your child also will need to see an orthodontist to make sure his or her teeth are growing in properly. Depending on your child's situation, your doctor may recommend speech therapy and regular hearing checkups. (Most children have normal speech development after this type of surgery.)

Hypothyroidism

The thyroid gland is a butterfly-shaped gland at the front of the base of the neck that produces the hormones thyroxine and triiodothyronine, which are important for growth and metabolism (the chemical processes that take place in the body). The thyroid also produces calcitonin, which helps regulate the calcium level in the blood and enhances bone formation. Hypothyroidism is a hormonal disorder in which the thyroid gland is underactive and does not produce enough thyroid hormone. As a result, all of the chemical processes in the body slow down.

Hypothyroidism can be congenital, resulting when a child is born without a thyroid gland. Some cases are caused by a genetic defect in the thyroid gland. The disorder often develops later in childhood, usually as a result of damage to the thyroid gland from an abnormal immune response. Without treatment, hypothyroidism can result in serious mental and physical problems, such as mental retardation or short stature.

Symptoms

The symptoms of hypothyroidism in an infant can include poor appetite, constipation, fatigue, slow heart rate, poor circulation, slow growth, and delayed physical and mental development. An infant with hypothyroidism also may have characteristic facial features, including wide-set eyes, a flat nose, and a large tongue. When hypothyroidism develops later in childhood, the symptoms can include muscle weakness and cramps, fatigue, difficulty concentrating, very dry skin, hoarseness, hair loss, and weight gain.

Diagnosis and Treatment

All newborns in the United States are screened soon after birth for thyroid abnormalities. If the test results indicate inadequate blood levels of thyroid hormones, a doctor performs additional tests to determine the cause. In some cases, a doctor may order an MRI (see page 113) to check for a pituitary tumor.

Hypothyroidism is treated with replacement thyroid hormone (in the form of thyroxine) taken orally every day for life. Blood tests are performed regularly to measure the level of thyroid hormone in the blood. The doctor will adjust the dose of thyroid hormone as needed.

When hypothyroidism is detected in the first few days of life, the outlook is excellent. Children treated with replacement thyroid hormone from birth develop normally, both physically and mentally.

Disorders of the Digestive System

While in the uterus, the fetus receives all of its nutrients from the mother through the placenta and umbilical vein. Because a baby does not use its digestive system until after he or she is born, malformations of the digestive system that occur during fetal development do not affect the baby until after delivery.

The two main types of malformations that can affect an infant's digestive system are stenosis (narrowing of a tube or duct, sometimes almost to the point of closing) and atresia (blockage in a tube or duct that separates it into two distinct, sealed-off sections). The causes of these defects are not known.

Although any abnormality in the digestive system can affect an infant's ability to digest food and absorb nutrients, these abnormalities also can pose some other risks. For example, in digestive system disorders that cause vomiting, a baby may inhale the vomit, which can lead to choking or pneumonia. Disorders that cause vomiting and diarrhea can lead to life-threatening dehydration.

Meckel's Diverticulum

Meckel's diverticulum is a congenital (present at birth) disorder in which an abnormal sac, usually lined with gastric (stomach) tissue, forms near the final part of the small intestine (ileum). Meckel's diverticulum occurs in about 1 in 50 children and affects more males than females. The disorder usually does not cause symptoms unless the diverticulum is obstructed, infected, or bleeds from sores in the diverticulum. Stomach acid from the stomach tissue causes the sores, which can bleed severely. If inflammation is severe, the sac can rupture and cause an abscess (a pus-filled cavity) or inflammation of the lining of the abdominal cavity (peritonitis; see page 759). Sometimes Meckel's diverticulum causes a condition called intussusception (see next page), in which the intestine folds back on itself like a telescope. Intussusception occurs more often in infants and young children than in adults.

Symptoms and Diagnosis

The symptoms of Meckel's diverticulum include bleeding from the rectum (the blood is dark reddish brown) and sometimes abdominal pain or vomiting, or, rarely, fever. The condition can be difficult to diagnose because the symptoms are similar to those of other disorders such as an intestinal obstruction (see right), appendicitis (see page 771), or a perforated duodenal ulcer (see page 755).

If a person has symptoms of Meckel's diverticulum, the doctor will order a radionuclide scan (see page 114) to see if stomach tissue is in the diverticulum, and a blood test to check for anemia (see page 610). If the radionuclide scan does not show Meckel's diverticulum, more imaging tests will be done to determine the cause of the symptoms.

Treatment

To treat Meckel's diverticulum, doctors first stop any intestinal bleeding and treat the anemia. Once the bleeding has stopped and the anemia is reduced, the person undergoes surgery to remove the diverticulum and correct any problems such as intussusception. A doctor may prescribe antibiotics to prevent or treat complications such as peritonitis.

Intestinal Obstruction

Intestinal obstruction occurs when the small or large intestine is partially or completely blocked, preventing food and waste from passing through the intestines. The problem can result from a number of disorders of the digestive system.

Pyloric stenosis

Pyloric stenosis is a congenital disorder in which the muscular walls of the pylorus—the outlet from the stomach to the duodenum (the first section of the small intestine)—thicken, which narrows the passageway inside and prevents food from moving from the stomach into the intestines. Pyloric stenosis usually occurs between 2 and 8 weeks after birth and is more common in boys than in girls. The disorder often runs in families. The most common symptoms are choking and vomiting after feeding.

The baby may be irritable and restless and may begin to lose weight. If not treated, pyloric stenosis can lead to dehydration, pneumonia caused by inhaled vomit, or malnutrition, or can be fatal. To treat the disorder, surgery is performed to widen the pylorus to allow food to pass through.

Intestinal atresia

In intestinal atresia, an infant is born with one or more parts of the small intestine missing or shriveled into a useless cord. The main symptom of intestinal atresia is intermittent vomiting of bile (a digestive fluid produced by the liver) beginning within a few hours of birth. The baby has no bowel movements, and his or her abdomen swells as gas builds up in the intestines. To treat intestinal atresia, surgery is performed to join the healthy sections of intestine.

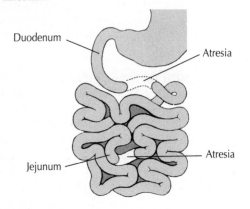

Intestinal atresia
In intestinal atresia, one or more parts of the small intestine are malformed or absent. In some cases, the upper part of the small intestine (duodenum) and the middle or lower part of the small intestine (jejunum or ileum) may be affected.

Volvulus

In volvulus, a loop of intestine becomes twisted, blocking the movement of food and waste. Volvulus may be congenital (present from birth), or it may result from adhesions (scar tissue) that form from chronic inflammation inside the abdomen or as a result of previous surgery. The symptoms of volvulus include severe, intermittent abdominal pain, usually followed by vomiting. Surgery is performed to untwist the affected loop of intestine and prevent strangulation.

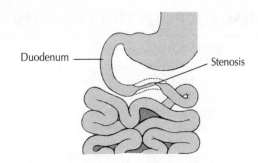

Intestinal stenosis
In intestinal stenosis, the upper intestine, such as the duodenum, is significantly narrowed. To treat this condition, surgery to widen or remove the affected part of the intestine is performed immediately.

Intestinal stenosis

In intestinal stenosis, part of the upper intestine is narrowed almost to the point of closing. The main symptom of intestinal stenosis is intermittent vomiting of bile (a digestive fluid produced by the liver), beginning within a few hours of birth. The baby has no bowel movements, and his or her abdomen swells as gas builds up in the intestines. To treat intestinal stenosis, surgery is performed to widen the narrowed segment of intestine or to remove it and connect the healthy segments.

Intussusception

In intussusception, a segment of the intestine telescopes in on itself, partially or completely blocking the passage of food and waste. Initially, the child may be irritable and lethargic. He or she will experience sudden abdominal pain and vomiting and may have diarrhea, a fever, and blood or mucus in the stool. A doctor may treat this condition with a barium enema, which may push the intestine back into its normal position. If the enema is not effective, surgery is performed to reposition the intestine and remove any damaged tissue.

Hirschsprung's disease

Hirschsprung's disease (sometimes called congenital megacolon) is a rare birth defect in which segments of the lower parts of the large intestine, including the rectum, have no nerve cells to transmit the impulses that stimulate the contractions necessary to move food and waste through the intestines. The defect is more common in boys than in girls and tends to run in families. The main symptom of the disorder is severe constipation.

Other symptoms include a swollen abdomen, gas, abdominal pain, vomiting, poor appetite, and anemia (see page 610). To treat Hirschsprung's disease, surgery is performed to remove the affected part of the intestine and join the healthy sections.

Imperforate anus

Imperforate anus is a birth defect in which the anal canal (the final section of the digestive tract) is closed, either by a membrane stretching across the canal or, in rare cases, because the digestive tract ends at the rectum, with no connection between the rectum and the anus. Imperforate anus is suspected if the baby has not passed meconium (the first bowel movement of a newborn) within 24 hours of birth. The diagnosis is confirmed if a finger or catheter inserted into the anus meets a blockage (the end of the rectum) or if the anal opening is absent. To treat imperforate anus, surgery is performed to remove the membrane or to open the end of the rectum and connect it to the anus.

Diaphragmatic hernia

In diaphragmatic hernia, an infant is born with an opening in the diaphragm (the large sheet of muscle that separates the chest from the abdomen and plays a major role in breathing). Part of the liver, spleen, or stomach or part of the large and small intestines may protrude through the opening into the chest and press on one of the lungs (usually the left lung), causing breathing difficulties. In severe cases, the baby's skin may turn blue (cyanosis) from lack of oxygen and the baby may be placed on a ventilator to assist with breathing until surgery is performed.

Surgery (which is done as soon as possible) involves opening the chest and pushing the protruding organs back into the abdominal cavity and stitching up the diaphragm. Many infants with a diaphragmatic hernia die before or after surgery because their lungs are significantly underdeveloped and they cannot breathe, even with assistance from a ventilator. After surgery, the infant may be placed on a heart-lung machine, which removes carbon dioxide from the blood and supplies adequate oxygen. This procedure enables the diaphragm to rest and heal and improves the infant's chances of survival.

Surgical adhesions

After abdominal surgery, scar tissue called adhesions may form in the abdomen and bind segments of the intestines together, causing an obstruction. The symptoms of surgical adhesions include abdominal swelling, cramping, and pain. The usual treatment for adhesions is surgery to cut the scar tissue to release the segments of intestine that are bound together.

Paralytic ileus

After an infection or surgery, the intestine can become paralyzed, losing its ability to move waste to the rectum. The intestine becomes stretched as it fills with fluid, waste, and air, causing inflammation and pain in the abdomen. Paralytic ileus can lead to fecal impaction, in which hardened stool becomes lodged in the intestine. To treat paralytic ileus, the doctor inserts a flexible tube through the child's nose and down into his or her intestine to remove fluid, waste, and air. The child is given nothing by mouth and is fed intravenously (through a vein) until gas or stool is passed and intestinal function returns to normal.

Esophageal Atresia

Esophageal atresia is a rare birth defect that interferes with an infant's ability to eat and breathe. In esophageal atresia, the part of the esophagus that leads from the mouth is not fully developed and does not reach the stomach. As a result, the infant cannot swallow food or secretions (saliva and mucus), and they can enter the windpipe, partially blocking it.

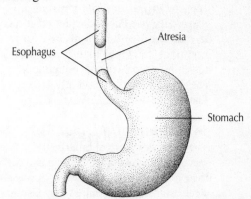

Esophagus — Atresia

— Stomach

Esophageal atresia
In esophageal atresia, the esophagus (which moves food from the mouth to the stomach) is not fully developed, and there is no passageway into the stomach. Surgery is performed as soon as possible to join the separated sections of the esophagus.

Symptoms

The main symptom of esophageal atresia is continuous bubbling noises from the infant's throat. Sometimes, if the airways are obstructed, the baby's skin turns blue from lack of oxygen. When a doctor removes the secretions with a suction tube, the symptoms disappear temporarily, but return as soon as the secretions build up again. When the baby eats, he or she may cough, gag, choke, or vomit. If your child has any of these symptoms, talk to your doctor.

Diagnosis and Treatment

A diagnosis of esophageal atresia is based on the baby's symptoms and a physical examination. The doctor may look for esophageal atresia by trying to pass a soft tube down the baby's esophagus. The diagnosis is confirmed with X-rays. An infant with this disorder cannot be given food or liquids by mouth and is fed intravenously (through a vein) until the condition is corrected. Surgery is performed in one or more stages to open and join the two separate sections of the esophagus, which usually eliminates the problem. After surgery, a tube may be inserted temporarily into the repaired portion of the esophagus to dilate (widen) the esophagus and hold it open.

Biliary Atresia

Biliary atresia (also called bile duct atresia) is a rare congenital (present from birth) disorder in which parts of the bile ducts (the tubes that carry a digestive fluid called bile from the liver to the small intestine) are either malformed or absent. As a result, bile becomes trapped in the liver and damages it. If not treated promptly, the disorder can be fatal before a child is 2 years old.

Symptoms and Diagnosis

The main symptom of biliary atresia is prolonged jaundice (yellowing of the skin and the whites of the eyes), which usually starts during the second week after birth. The infant may also have pale or white stool and dark-colored urine.

A diagnosis of biliary atresia is based on the child's symptoms, a physical examination, and the results of blood tests. The doctor may order an ultrasound scan (see page 111) or a radionuclide scan (see page 114) of the liver to confirm the diagnosis.

Treatment

To treat biliary atresia, doctors usually recommend surgery to bypass the defective or absent bile ducts by connecting the liver to the small intestine. The procedure, which is usually performed when a child is about 2 to 3 months old, enables bile to flow directly from the liver into the small intestine. In other cases, doctors may recommend a liver transplant (see page 790).

Encopresis

Encopresis is a condition in which a child who is toilet trained and has no underlying disease involuntarily passes stool into his or her underpants. In encopresis, large amounts of stool accumulate and harden in the rectum and the lower part of the large intestine, and the child passes liquid stool past the blockage. Possible causes of encopresis include chronic constipation, painful bowel movements, resistance to using the toilet, impaired ability to sense the presence of stool in the rectum, or not taking enough time to use the toilet.

A child may also have involuntary bowel movements because of stress. Parents may (mistakenly) believe that the child is soiling his or her clothing purposely, and react with anger, possibly making the problem worse.

Symptoms

The symptoms of encopresis are usually similar to those of constipation. Bowel movements may be painful, and the child may have only a few bowel movements per week. He or she may strain to move his or her bowels, and some stool may remain in the rectum after a bowel movement. The child may have abdominal pain and bloating and may resist using the toilet. He or she may have no appetite and may be tired and irritable. In some cases, the condition can lead to bed-wetting (see page 427).

Diagnosis and Treatment

A diagnosis of encopresis is based on the child's symptoms and a physical examination. The doctor will feel the child's abdomen to check for the presence of hardened stools in the intestines. He or she may also examine the child's rectum for hardened stools. The doctor may order laboratory tests to rule out an underlying disorder that may be causing the problem.

To treat encopresis, the doctor may prescribe enemas or suppositories to clear the rectum and the lower part of the large intestine and eliminate the blockage. He or she will ask you to encourage your child to sit on the toilet at least once a day, at a specific time. In some cases, a doctor may prescribe enemas, glycerin suppositories, stool softeners, or laxatives for a few days or longer. He or she will recommend dietary changes to prevent constipation, such as drinking eight glasses of water every day and eating a high-fiber diet. If the problem persists, the doctor may recommend that your child see a psychiatrist or other specialist for further evaluation and treatment.

Neurological Disorders

The nervous system consists of the brain, the spine, and nerves throughout the body. Neurological disorders may be congenital (present from birth) or can result from damage to or dysfunction of part of the nervous system caused by injury or disease.

Fetal Alcohol Syndrome

Fetal alcohol syndrome is a group of preventable physical and mental birth defects, which can range from mild to severe, that occur in the children of women who drink alcohol during pregnancy. The syndrome is the leading cause of preventable mental retardation in the United States. When a woman drinks during pregnancy, the alcohol crosses the placenta and enters the fetus's bloodstream. The more alcohol a woman drinks, the greater the potential damage to the fetus. There is no safe amount of alcohol a pregnant woman can drink; any time a woman drinks alcohol during pregnancy, she puts her developing fetus at risk. In some cases, prenatal exposure to alcohol may result in death of the fetus.

Symptoms
Symptoms of fetal alcohol syndrome in a newborn include feeding and sleep difficulties, irritability, and unusual sensitivity to sound. Physical symptoms include facial abnormalities such as narrow, wide-set eyes; protruding, low-set ears; a wider than normal space between the nose and mouth; a thin upper lip; and small teeth. Toddlers with fetal alcohol syndrome may be smaller than other children their age, may have poor coordination, and may be hyperactive. Most children with fetal alcohol syndrome have some degree of mental retardation, delayed development, and learning disabilities. They may also have a small brain, heart defects (see page 389), a cleft palate (see page 403), or dislocation of the hip (see page 401). Adolescents with fetal alcohol syndrome often exhibit inappropriate behavior and emotional responses.

Diagnosis and Treatment
A diagnosis of fetal alcohol syndrome is based on the child's symptoms, a physical examination, and information about the mother's use of alcohol during pregnancy. The effects of fetal alcohol syndrome are not reversible. Treatment focuses on correcting specific physical defects such as a cleft palate, a dislocated hip, or a heart defect. Some children may also need physical therapy, speech therapy, occupational therapy, and special education to help them reach their full potential.

Cerebral Palsy

Cerebral palsy is a disorder of the nerves and muscles caused by faulty development of or damage to the areas of the brain that control muscle movement, resulting in weakness of the arms and legs accompanied by stiffness (called spasticity) or floppiness and, sometimes, unusual body postures. Cerebral palsy may be congenital (present from birth), or it may develop after birth. The disorder cannot be cured, but it does not worsen as the child gets older.

For most children who have cerebral palsy, the exact cause is unknown. The majority of cases result from brain injury during fetal development. Brain injury during delivery, an infection of the brain, or a head injury can also cause cerebral palsy.

Symptoms

The symptoms of cerebral palsy can range from mild to severe, can differ from child to child, and can change over time. In most cases, lack of normal muscle tone and muscle control makes it difficult for an affected child to maintain balance and to coordinate and control his or her movements. A baby with cerebral palsy may have difficulty sucking and swallowing. Normal developmental milestones (see page 377), such as rolling over, sitting, crawling, smiling, speaking, and walking, usually are delayed. Muscle stiffness, spasms, or poor muscle tone in the arms and legs cause many children with cerebral palsy to adopt unusual body postures or to perform involuntary limb, body, mouth, tongue, or facial movements. Because the brain damage that causes cerebral palsy can disrupt the electrical activity of the brain, some children have seizures (see page 686).

Some children with cerebral palsy have vision, hearing, or speech problems. Many affected children have normal intelligence but may have a learning disability. About half of all children with cerebral palsy have some degree of mental retardation.

Diagnosis

To diagnose cerebral palsy, a doctor takes a complete medical history and performs a physical examination that includes testing a child's motor skills and reflexes. The doctor will ask you to describe how well your child can move about and will ask you questions to determine if your child has reached specific developmental milestones, such as sitting, crawling, standing, or walking. The doctor may recommend blood tests, genetic tests, a CT scan (see page 112), or an MRI (see page 113) to help make a diagnosis.

Treatment

Treatment for cerebral palsy focuses on helping the child overcome the disabilities caused by the disorder (or minimizing their effects) so the child can reach his or her full potential. After evaluating the type and extent of a child's disabilities, the doctor will recommend appropriate measures, such as special education, physical therapy, occupational therapy, speech therapy, or counseling.

Speech therapy can improve the child's ability to speak and swallow. In some cases, a feeding tube may be needed to help ensure proper nutrition and to help prevent food from entering and blocking the airway. Surgery is sometimes performed to correct bone and joint deformities, enabling some children to walk with braces, crutches, or a walker. Some doctors prescribe muscle-relaxing medication to control involuntary movements and to make movement easier. These medications can be given by mouth, injected directly into the muscles, or delivered directly into the cerebrospinal fluid (the fluid that surrounds the brain and spinal cord). Doctors also may prescribe anticonvulsants to help prevent seizures. Surgery performed on certain spinal nerves may help decrease stiffness. Hearing problems can be improved with hearing aids (see page 1018). The doctor may recommend prescription eyeglasses or surgery to correct misaligned eyes (see page 1055).

A child who has cerebral palsy should be examined regularly by a doctor to monitor his or her general physical and mental progress. Your doctor can recommend steps you can take to help your child reach his or her full potential and to enhance the quality of his or her life. Caring for a child with cerebral palsy can be demanding and stressful. Ask your doctor or a hospital social worker about support groups and other organizations that can help you and your child.

Febrile Seizures

A febrile seizure is a disturbance in the electrical activity of the brain caused by the rapid onset of a high fever in infants and children. Febrile seizures are very common, affecting 4 to 10 percent of all children between ages 6 months and 5 years. Febrile seizures can be simple or complex. A simple febrile seizure, the most common type, lasts 1 to 5 minutes and affects the entire body. Complex febrile seizures last longer than 15 minutes, affect only one side of the body, and can occur more than once in 24 hours.

Children who have had a febrile seizure have a 30 percent chance of having another one within the next 6 months. Although alarming for parents to watch, febrile seizures usually have no serious, long-term effects on the brain. Children who have had a simple seizure have a 2 to 4 percent chance of developing epilepsy later in life (compared with a 1 percent risk for the general population). If the seizure was complex, if the child has other brain abnormalities, or if epilepsy runs in the family, the child's risk of developing epilepsy rises to 10 percent.

Symptoms

A child with a simple febrile seizure has convulsions that produce a rhythmic jerking of the arms and legs, rolling of the eyes, unresponsiveness, and, sometimes, bluish skin around the mouth and at the tips of the fingers and toes. For the next half hour, the child looks drowsy and confused. As his or her temperature returns to normal, the child may become his or her usual self again. Occasionally, simple febrile seizures produce no convulsions, only a temporary loss of consciousness and stiffening of the body.

Diagnosis and Treatment

If you think your child is having a febrile seizure, take him or her to the doctor or to a hospital emergency department for an evaluation. If your child is older than 18 months, the doctor will probably examine him or her for signs of meningitis (inflammation of the membranes covering the brain and spine; see page 692). If no signs of meningitis are present, your child will not need any treatment, although the doctor may recommend acetaminophen or ibuprofen to reduce the fever.

Children younger than 18 months often fail to show signs of meningitis, so doctors routinely order a lumbar puncture (see page 693) to detect any of the microorganisms that cause meningitis. To perform a lumbar puncture, the doctor inserts a hollow needle into the lower part of the spine and takes a sample of the cerebrospinal fluid for examination under a microscope. There is no specific treatment for viral meningitis, which is usually mild and clears up on its own in about 1 week. Bacterial meningitis requires large doses of antibiotics delivered intravenously (through a vein).

Doctors sometimes prescribe the short-term use of an anticonvulsant medication or the tranquilizer diazepam, given when the child has a fever, to prevent febrile seizures in the future.

Reye's Syndrome

Reye's syndrome is a rare, life-threatening disorder that causes swelling of the brain and liver, most frequently in children between ages 4 and 16 who are recovering from a viral infection such as a cold (see page 648), chickenpox (see page 439), or influenza (see page 649). The swelling damages the brain, liver, and kidneys. Research has shown that Reye's syndrome is often (but not always) linked to taking aspirin or other medications that contain salicylates (such as over-the-counter cold medications) to relieve the symptoms of a viral infection. For this reason, doctors recommend that children younger than 18 years take acetaminophen or ibuprofen instead of aspirin.

Symptoms

The initial symptom of Reye's syndrome is uncontrollable, forceful vomiting that occurs over a period of about 3 hours to 3 days. As the brain swells, it begins to malfunction and the child becomes drowsy, lethargic, confused, and disoriented. Other symptoms that may develop include slurred speech, memory loss, hallucinations (abnormal perceptions not based on reality), and sudden episodes of aggressive behavior. Severe swelling of the brain can lead to seizures, coma, an abnormal heartbeat, and cessation of breathing. Severe swelling of the liver causes jaundice (yellowing of the skin and the whites of the eyes), and damage to the kidneys can lead to kidney failure (see page 817). Reye's syndrome is a medical emergency. If your child has symptoms of Reye's syndrome, take him or her to the nearest hospital emergency department immediately. Early detection and treatment of Reye's syndrome is essential to prevent permanent brain damage or death.

Diagnosis

To diagnose Reye's syndrome, a doctor will order blood tests to measure the child's blood sugar levels and the blood levels of ammonia and liver enzymes to evaluate liver function. A child with Reye's syndrome will have low sugar levels and elevated levels of ammonia and liver enzymes in the blood. The clotting time of the blood also is tested; the blood may take longer than normal to clot. The doctor will feel your child's abdomen to check for swelling of the liver. He or she may order a liver biopsy (in which samples of cells are taken from the liver and examined under a microscope) to see if the liver is damaged, and an electroencephalogram (EEG; see page 687), an examination of the electrical activity of the brain, to evaluate brain function. The doctor also may order CT scans (see page 112) or MRIs (see page 113) to assess swelling of the brain and liver, and a lumbar puncture (see page 693) to examine the spinal fluid to rule out disorders such as meningitis (see page 692).

Treatment

A child with Reye's syndrome is hospitalized and given fluids intravenously (through a vein) to replace those lost from vomiting, to restore the balance of electrolytes (essential minerals that help regulate various body processes) in the blood, and to reduce swelling. Brain swelling is also controlled with medication. Pressure monitors may be implanted in the brain to evaluate brain swelling. The child's electrolyte levels, blood glucose (sugar) levels, and blood clotting also are monitored. If necessary, the child may be given medication to maintain adequate blood pressure. If the child has difficulty breathing, he or she may be placed on a ventilator (an artificial breathing machine).

Recovery depends on the severity of the condition. Children who have a mild episode of Reye's syndrome may recover fully in about a week, with no lasting effects. Children who survive a severe episode of Reye's syndrome may have permanent brain damage.

Tourette Syndrome

Tourette syndrome is a nervous system disorder characterized by sudden, repeated, involuntary movements and vocal sounds called tics. Unlike other tic disorders, the tics of Tourette syndrome often occur along with certain behavior disorders including attention deficit hyperactivity disorder (ADHD; see page 730) and obsessive-compulsive disorder (see page 720). Children with Tourette syndrome often have anxiety (see page 718) or depression (see page 709) and may have a tendency to physically injure themselves. Other behavior disorders that commonly accompany Tourette syndrome are poor impulse control, poor anger control, and antisocial behavior. Such behavior problems can interfere with school performance and social interactions even more than the tics.

Tourette syndrome usually begins between 2 and 15 years of age, and the tics become the most extreme at about age 10. The tics usually lessen as the child gets older; by age 18, half of all affected people no longer have tics. In some people, the disorder is lifelong, and 10 percent of affected people have more severe symptoms in adulthood than in childhood. Estimates of the prevalence of Tourette syndrome range from less than 1 percent to 4 percent of the population, affecting three times as many boys as girls. The disorder tends to run in families.

Symptoms

The tics of Tourette syndrome that involve body movement (motor tics) often include blinking, nose twitching, muscle tensing, mouth opening, shoulder rotation, head shaking, or bending of the trunk. Examples of more extreme motor tics are hitting, jumping, kicking, making obscene gestures, or imitating the gestures of others. Typical vocal tics include sniffing, throat clearing, grunting, or blowing. Some affected children repeat their own words or the words of others or shout profanities or other inappropriate words or phrases. Many children with Tourette syndrome say that these body movements or utterances are preceded by feelings of anxiety or uncomfortable sensations so severe that they can be relieved only by the expression of the tic.

Most children with Tourette syndrome also display the hallmark symptoms of ADHD (inattention, hyperactivity, and impulsiveness) and obsessive-compulsive disorder (intrusive thoughts that trigger compulsive and repetitive actions). Their poor impulse control and inability to control anger can lead to outbursts of temper and aggressive behavior. Some children with the disorder injure themselves by biting, scratching, hitting, or banging their head.

Diagnosis and Treatment

Doctors diagnose Tourette syndrome from a thorough medical history, a physical examination, and the observation of tics. The presence of ADHD and obsessive-compulsive disorder and a family history of related symptoms confirm the diagnosis.

The treatment of Tourette syndrome depends on the child's particular symptoms. Behavior modification techniques may be used to try to reverse the habit of expressing a tic, to correct behavior problems, or to prevent the compulsive behavior triggered by an obsessive thought.

Doctors usually prescribe medications when the child's symptoms are so severe that they interfere with relationships with friends, school performance, or daily activities. In general, doctors target the most bothersome symptoms first. The tics themselves may be treated with medications called neuroleptics (such as haloperidol or pimozide), which block dopamine receptors in the brain. ADHD is treated with central nervous system stimulants such as methylphenidate. Obsessive-compulsive disorder is treated with serotonin reuptake inhibitors (SSRIs) such as fluoxetine, fluvoxamine, or sertraline.

Try to minimize your child's exposure to stress, because stress can make the condition worse. Be careful not to scold your child for his or her uncontrollable behavior, because scolding can increase your child's distress. Talk to your child's teachers to make sure they understand the condition, and ask if they can make any changes in the school environment that would make it easier for your child. For example, educating your child's peers about Tourette syndrome through a video presentation might make your child more accepted in school.

Sleep Problems

In the early weeks of life, many babies wake every 2 or 3 hours to feed, even during the night. But by the time they are 9 months old, most babies sleep through the night without waking. At 1 year of age, babies sleep an average of about 16 out of every 24 hours; about 3 of these 16 hours are used for two daily naps. By the time they are about 15 to 18 months old, many babies go from two naps a day to one.

By toddler stage (about 18 months old), children begin to vary in the amount of sleep they need. Some toddlers wake up very early each morning, are very active during the day, may not take an afternoon nap, and do not become tired until bedtime. Other toddlers may need an afternoon nap to get through the rest of the day. By age 3, many children no longer take an afternoon nap, and by age 5, nearly all children stay awake throughout the day.

Difficulty falling asleep or sleeping through the night

Some children may have difficulty falling asleep or sleeping through the night. If this occurs, try not to make yourself too easily available, because your child could come to expect the attention and have more difficulty falling asleep and staying asleep. For example, if your baby cries after being fed at

night, do not immediately go and pick him or her up. Instead, listen for a few minutes outside the door of his or her room. He or she will probably stop crying after a few minutes and go back to sleep. If the crying continues, go in to check on the baby, but don't play with him or her. Meet the baby's needs (for example, by feeding him or her or changing a diaper) and then leave the room.

Make sure your child isn't sleeping too much during the day. Establish a bedtime routine. Read a bedtime story. Eliminate unnecessary noise such as an older sibling repeatedly entering the bedroom. Sometimes leaving a radio playing music softly or tuned to static (white noise) will help mask disturbing noises. Also avoid sending your child to bed as punishment. If, over a period of time, the child associates going to bed with punishment, he or she may resist going to bed, and, once in bed, sleep poorly.

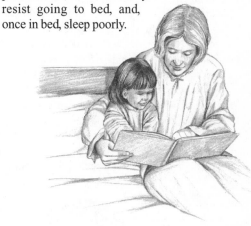

Bedtime routine
To help your child get a good night's sleep, establish a regular bedtime and bedtime routine that includes calming activities such as reading a story. Try to read to your child every night. Not only does it give you a chance to relax and share an experience with your child, it also stimulates the development of your child's brain.

Despite these measures, your child still may find it difficult to fall asleep or may wake often during the night. Ask your child's doctor to recommend ways to help your baby fall asleep and stay asleep. If your child is older and is snoring as well as having difficulty sleeping, he or she may have a disorder such as enlarged adenoids (see page 419). If sleeplessness becomes a persistent, difficult problem for you and your child, the doctor may refer you to a specialist such as a neurologist or a psychiatrist for further evaluation and possible treatment.

Nightmares

Nightmares are frightening dreams that usually occur late at night when a child is in deep sleep. When a child has a nightmare, he or she wakes up frightened and may scream or cry. Although children of all ages have occasional nightmares, children between ages 3 and 6 experience them the most. Nightmares usually occur after a child has witnessed a disturbing incident, heard a scary story, or watched a frightening movie or television program. Occasionally, nightmares signal that a child is experiencing unresolved stress caused by problems at home or at school.

The best way to deal with nightmares is to comfort your child. Turn the lights on to reassure your child that it was only a dream. Hug your child, and

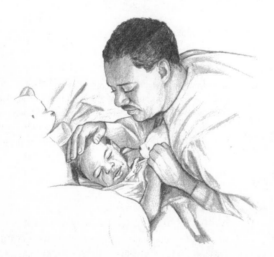

Comfort for nightmares
If your child wakes up frightened and crying from a nightmare, comfort and reassure him or her. Stay with your child until he or she is calm and ready to go back to sleep.

take his or her mind off the disturbance by speaking soothingly about something pleasant. Reassure your child that nothing will harm him or her. If your child has frequent, recurring nightmares, try leaving a night-light on in his or her room. To try to find out what the underlying problem is, ask him or her to talk about it.

Night terrors

A night terror is another type of frightening dream that occurs most often in children between ages 2 and 5. When a child has a night terror, he or she screams or cries out suddenly during sleep and jumps out of bed. The child looks terrified and may be sweating and breathing rapidly. He or she may talk or babble and have wide-open eyes but is still asleep. The child may not recognize familiar people, such as his or her parents, and may be difficult to wake. Doctors do not know what causes night terrors.

If your child has a night terror, check to make sure that he or she is not ill or injured. Because the child is still asleep, he or she may not calm down even when you hold or talk to him or her. The child will usually stop crying or screaming after a few minutes.

Sleepwalking

Sleepwalking is a disorder in which changes in the electrical activity of the brain during sleep cause a child to awaken partially during the night. The child may sit up in bed and perform repetitive movements or may get out of bed and walk around. He or she will not respond to others.

If your child is sleepwalking, do not wake him or her. Instead, silently guide your child back to bed. The child will usually fall back into a deep sleep and will not remember the incident. To protect your child, put a gate in his or her bedroom doorway and across the top of any stairs, and close any accessible windows.

If Your Child Has Sleep Problems

Most children outgrow nightmares, night terrors, and sleepwalking before they reach adolescence. Making sure that your child does not get overtired during the day and that he or she gets enough sleep at night may help eliminate these problems. If your child has persistent sleep problems, see your doctor.

Learning Disabilities

Not all children develop skills at the same rate. Although some children may be slower than others of the same age to develop certain skills, they usually catch up eventually. A learning disability is a significant gap between a person's intelligence and the skills he or she has achieved at each age. Learning disabilities are neurological disorders in which the brain is unable to correctly process, use, or retrieve information that a person reads or hears.

Although the exact cause of learning disabilities is not known, doctors think that they may be caused by disturbances in brain development before birth. Factors that may affect brain development include genes, fetal exposure to drugs (such as alcohol and tobacco) used by a woman during pregnancy, or complications during pregnancy (including preterm delivery; see page 529) that can affect the fetus's developing brain. Exposure to environmental toxins such as lead (see page 425) after birth also can contribute to the development of learning disabilities.

Learning disabilities can affect people of all ages and backgrounds. Many people with learning disabilities are of average or above-average intelligence. The symptoms of learning disabilities can vary greatly from one person to another, and some people have more than one learning disability. Some children with a learning disability also may have an attention deficit disorder (see page 730).

If you are concerned about your child's development or suspect that he or she may have a learning disability, talk to your pediatrician and to teachers (if your child is school age or about to enter school). Federal law guarantees to children who have a learning disability a public education specifically designed to their needs. The earlier a learning disability is diagnosed, the more likely a child is to reach his or her intellectual and academic potential. If your child's school doesn't notice a delay in your child's development, but you do, request an outside evaluation. It is essential to get an accurate diagnosis. If your child is not in school yet, call administrators at the school he or she will attend or the district office to find out what early intervention programs are available for your child.

Developmental Speech and Language Disorders

Developmental speech and language disorders can affect the way a person speaks or understands what is being said. Some children outgrow developmental speech and language disorders. However, in some cases such a disorder may be a sign of a future learning disability. Some subcategories of speech and language disorders include:

Developmental articulation disorders

Developmental articulation disorders are common. A child with a developmental articulation disorder may have difficulty controlling his or her rate of speech or pronouncing certain letters or letter combinations. If diagnosed and treated early, developmental articulation disorders can often be corrected, although children usually outgrow them.

Developmental expressive language disorders

Children who have a developmental expressive language disorder may have difficulty expressing themselves in speech. The child often knows what he or she wants to say but is not able to convert the thoughts into words. Children who have a developmental expressive language disorder may have difficulty answering simple questions or may not be able to combine words to form sentences.

Developmental receptive language disorders

A child who has a developmental receptive language disorder may have difficulty understanding certain aspects of speech because the brain does not recognize certain sounds or words. Children who have a developmental receptive language disorder may seem inattentive, may not follow directions, or may not respond to their name when called.

Diagnosing and treating speech and language disorders

To diagnose a developmental speech or language disorder, a child may be given one or more tests that compare his or her development with what is considered normal development for children of the same age. He or she may also have tests to rule out other problems, such as hearing loss or other ear disorders, or problems with the vocal cords.

Treatment of developmental speech and language disorders depends on the type of disorder, its severity, and the child's individual needs. He or she can be helped by working with trained school professionals, such as speech pathologists.

Academic Skills Disorders

Academic skills disorders may affect a child's ability to read, write, or solve math problems. Academic skills disorders are neurological disorders caused by the brain's inability to process sounds, letters, words, or abstract concepts.

Dyslexia

Dyslexia is a neurological disorder that results from a problem in the way the brain processes written information. A child who has dyslexia may have difficulty distinguishing certain letters, pronouncing words, or spelling. These difficulties can affect the child's ability to read or to understand what he or she is reading.

Dyscalculia

Dyscalculia is a neurological disorder caused by a defect in the way the brain processes information that relates to numbers. Children with dyscalculia may have difficulty recognizing numbers or symbols, remembering information such as multiplication tables, or understanding concepts such as fractions. They also may have trouble telling time, keeping track of time, or reading maps.

Dysgraphia

Dysgraphia is a neurological disorder characterized by the inability to write words on a page. A person with dysgraphia may have difficulty spelling, holding a writing instrument, or forming letters or words on a page. Such difficulties can cause the person's handwriting to be distorted or illegible. A child with dysgraphia also may be unable to organize thoughts on paper even though he or she can convey them verbally.

Dyspraxia

Dyspraxia is a neurological disorder that results from the inability of the brain to properly relay messages to parts of the body. A child who has dyspraxia may seem clumsy or uncoordinated and may have difficulty performing tasks such as dressing or combing his or her hair. He or she may have difficulty reading, writing, or speaking; or may be extremely sensitive to touch. Children with dyspraxia may not be able to understand logic or reason and often behave immaturely.

Diagnosing and treating academic skills disorders

To diagnose an academic skills disorder, a child will take tests to evaluate his or her reading, writing, and math abilities. The child may also have vision and hearing tests to rule out vision and hearing problems.

The treatment of academic skills disorders depends on the disorder. For example, a person who has dyslexia can benefit from a language program that teaches him or her to identify sounds. A person who has dyscalculia may benefit from doing real-life math problems such as counting money. He or she can use a calculator to check his or her work. A person with dysgraphia can benefit from using a computer, using a tape recorder, drawing a picture, or using checklists to organize and express thoughts. A person who has dyspraxia can benefit from physical or occupational therapy to improve his or her coordination and ability to perform daily tasks.

If your child has a learning disability, work closely with his or her teachers and your doctor and other health care professionals to make sure your child gets the needed help. With appropriate intervention and educational programs, most people find ways to compensate for their learning disability and can lead successful, productive lives. Support groups and other organizations are available for people with learning disabilities and their friends and family members.

Common Ear Problems in Children

Ear infections are a common problem in young children, especially between ages 6 months and 1 year. Middle ear infections occur when an upper respiratory infection, such as a cold, spreads to the middle ear cavity by way of the eustachian tube.

Some children have repeated ear infections, which, if left untreated, can lead to serious complications, such as hearing loss. Hearing loss that occurs early in childhood can have a significant impact on a child's speech and language development.

Ear Infections

Infection or inflammation of the middle ear (a condition that doctors call otitis media) can occur in people of all ages but is most common in infants and young children. Otitis media can be either acute (short and severe) or chronic (long-lasting). If a child has three or more acute ear infections within 6 months, or four or more infections within 12 months, the condition is called recurrent acute otitis media.

Otitis media can result when fluid or mucus from a bacterial or viral infection of the nose and throat (such as a cold or flu) or an allergy causes the eustachian tube (the tube that connects the middle ear to the back of the nose and throat) to swell and to drain improperly. Exposure to second-hand smoke can increase the risk of inflammation and infection of the respiratory tract and problems with the eustachian tube in young children. In some children, the adenoids (lymph tissue that lies on each side of the back wall of the nose and the upper part of the throat) can become enlarged and can block drainage from the eustachian tube. If the eustachian tube is blocked, pus can build up in the middle ear, putting pressure on the eardrum and causing severe pain, hearing loss, and, possibly, a ruptured eardrum (see page 1022).

Ear infections and accumulation of middle ear fluid are more frequent in children than in adults because a child's eustachian tubes are smaller and more horizontal than those of an adult, making it more difficult for infected fluid to drain. Children who have a family history of ear infections (who have a parent or siblings with ear infections), a weakened immune system, or some birth defects (such as Down syndrome; see page 955) that change the shape of the eustachian tubes are at increased risk of developing ear infections. For unknown reasons, otitis media is more common in boys than in girls.

Symptoms and Diagnosis

Symptoms of acute otitis media include fever and pressure, pain, or pus in the ear. Other symptoms may include drainage from the ear and hearing loss. A young child may be irritable and pull on the ear that hurts.

To diagnose acute otitis media, a doctor will take a detailed health history and examine the ear with a lighted viewing instrument called an otoscope. The doctor also may take a sample of fluid from the affected ear to check for bacteria.

Treatment

In many cases, an ear infection will go away on its own. However, a doctor may prescribe antibiotics (taken by mouth) to treat acute otitis media caused by bacteria. He or she may also recommend a pain reliever to treat the pain and fever. (Never give aspirin to a child under age 18 because of the risk of a life-threatening condition called Reye's syndrome; see page 411.) The doctor may ask you to return to the office after about 2 weeks to make sure that the infection has cleared up.

In severe cases, the doctor may recommend a procedure called myringotomy, in which a surgeon makes a small incision in the eardrum, suctions out the fluid, and sometimes inserts tiny drainage tubes. Myringotomy usually is done as an outpatient procedure (with general anesthesia) but also can be done in the doctor's office using laser surgery (without general anesthesia). Alternatively, a doctor can treat a persistent case of acute otitis media by suctioning fluid from the middle ear in an office procedure.

Prevention

The following steps can help reduce your child's risk of developing ear infections:

- **Breastfeed your child.** Breastfeeding provides some immunity against ear infections because

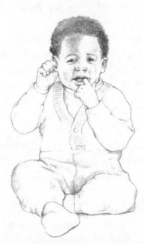

Earache
If your young child has an earache, he or she may not be able to tell you it hurts. You should suspect an earache if you notice your child frequently pulling on his or her ear or being more fussy and irritable than usual.

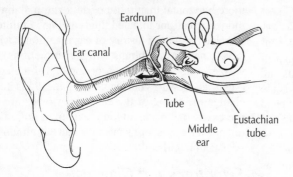

Myringotomy
For children who have frequent ear infections or who have persistent fluid in their ears, doctors sometimes recommend a surgical procedure called myringotomy to drain the fluid. In this procedure, tiny tubes may be placed in the eardrum to ventilate the middle ear. The procedure restores hearing, relieves pain, and helps prevent fluid from reaccumulating and causing more ear infections.

breast milk contains infection-fighting antibodies from the mother.

- **Keep your child upright when bottle-feeding.** If a child drinks from a bottle while lying down, the liquid can pool in the back of his or her throat, blocking the eustachian tubes.
- **Do not smoke around your child.** Secondhand smoke can increase the risk of inflammation and infections in the respiratory tract in young children.
- **Choose a small day care center.** If possible, find a day care setting with no more than six children. Larger numbers of children increase the risk of spreading germs that cause upper respiratory infections, which can lead to ear infections.

Chronic Otitis Media With Effusion

When fluid from an acute middle ear infection remains in the middle ear longer than 6 weeks, doctors call the condition chronic otitis media with effusion (also called chronic middle ear fluid). Chronic otitis media with effusion can also develop without infection—from an anatomical cause such as a cleft palate (see page 403), Down syndrome (see page 955), or a too-narrow eustachian tube. In some cases, the fluid becomes very sticky (which doctors call glue ear). The buildup of fluid can cause mild hearing loss and may delay a child's language development.

Symptoms

Chronic middle ear fluid often does not cause any symptoms. However, sounds may seem muffled or faint, as if heard under water. Some children may have difficulty distinguishing certain sounds in noisy situations.

If untreated, chronic middle ear fluid can result in poor development of language skills in very young children. Less often, the disorder can cause an abnormal growth of the skin of the eardrum (cholesteatoma; see page 1024). Chronic middle ear fluid can also cause the tiny bones of the middle ear (ossicles) to become scarred and bond to the middle ear. If your child is developing language skills slowly or does not respond when you speak to him or her, or if he or she is having trouble paying attention at school, it could be due to partial hearing loss from chronic middle ear fluid.

Diagnosis

Because chronic middle ear fluid usually has no obvious symptoms, doctors often diagnose the disorder while examining a child for another reason or during a well-child visit. However, if you suspect that your child has hearing loss after he or she has had an ear infection, see your doctor. The doctor will take a detailed health history and examine the affected ear with a lighted viewing instrument called an otoscope. He or she may also use a device called a pneumatic otoscope, which blows a puff of air into the ear to check for stiffness of the eardrum.

The doctor may refer you to an otolaryngologist (a doctor who specializes in disorders of the ear, nose, and throat), who may perform special tests such as an impedance test (see page 1016), which can help determine whether your child has fluid in his or her ear. The doctor may refer you to an audiologist (a health care professional who specializes in hearing evaluation and treatment), who will perform hearing tests (see page 1016) to determine if your child has any hearing loss.

Treatment

To treat chronic middle ear fluid that has resulted from a bacterial infection, a doctor may prescribe antibiotics, especially if he or she suspects an underlying sinus infection. Most doctors prefer to wait to see if the fluid clears up on its own, which can take up to 3 months when it affects both ears, and up to

6 months when it affects only one ear. In some cases, a doctor may recommend a procedure called myringotomy (see previous page), to drain the fluid. However, myringotomy is usually done only if the child has significant hearing loss that could interfere with his or her language development.

Disorders of the Respiratory System

The respiratory system delivers oxygen to the body's cells and removes carbon dioxide from the body. The respiratory system consists of the nose, throat, larynx (voice box), trachea (windpipe), and lungs, and a system of blood vessels that carry blood to and from the lungs. In children, infections are the most common cause of respiratory system disorders.

Adenoid Disorders

The adenoids are small masses of lymph (infection-fighting) tissue that lie on either side of the back of the nasal cavity, above the tonsils, and are part of the body's immune system. In most children, the adenoids begin to grow at about age 3, when children are especially vulnerable to infection. At about age 5, the adenoids begin to shrink, and usually disappear by the time a child reaches puberty. In some children, however, the adenoids continue to grow, eventually blocking the airway that leads from the nose to the throat. When this occurs, the flow of secretions at the back of the nose is blocked, and the adenoids become infected. If the infection is not treated promptly, it can spread from the nasal cavity through the eustachian tube to the middle ear, causing a middle ear infection (see page 417).

Symptoms

When the airway that leads from the nose to the throat is blocked, the child usually has a stuffy nose, breathes through the mouth, and snores. In some cases, the child's voice may sound nasal. Infected secretions drip from the child's nose during the day. When the child lies down, these secretions drip down into the throat, causing an irritating cough. The child may have difficulty breathing while asleep, which can lead to restlessness or more serious sleep disturbances such as obstructive sleep apnea (see page 636). If the eustachian tube becomes blocked, the main symptom is a persistent earache. If a chronic middle ear infection develops, hearing loss may result.

Diagnosis

To diagnose an adenoid disorder, the doctor will ask you about your child's symptoms and perform a physical examination. He or she probably will examine your child's adenoids using a tiny mirror with a light attached or a viewing instrument that shines a light on the back of the throat. The doctor may order a side-view X-ray of the child's head to see if the adenoids are enlarged.

The adenoids
The adenoids—small masses of lymphoid tissue (left) that lie on either side of the back of the nasal cavity, above the tonsils—are part of the immune system. The adenoids tend to enlarge (right) when a child has an upper respiratory tract infection.

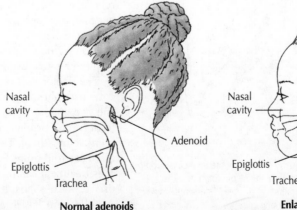

Normal adenoids

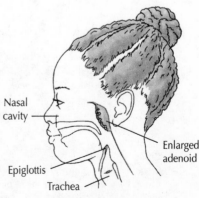

Enlarged adenoids

Treatment

In many cases, an adenoid infection goes away on its own without treatment and the swelling disappears. In other cases, doctors prescribe antibiotics to clear up the infection and relieve the swelling. If the swelling persists after the infection is gone, doctors may prescribe corticosteroid nasal sprays and oral decongestants or antihistamines to help open the airways. When recurring earaches affect a child's hearing, interfere with school attendance, or persist after treatment with antibiotics, a doctor may recommend surgery to remove the adenoids (called adenoidectomy). A doctor also may recommend surgery if the enlarged adenoids cause snoring or obstructive sleep apnea.

Croup

Croup is inflammation and narrowing of the trachea (windpipe) from a respiratory infection caused by a virus called parainfluenza virus, which is prevalent in early fall and in spring. The condition affects children up to about age 5.

Symptoms

The hallmark symptom of croup is a loud, barking cough. Hoarseness also occurs. Older children may experience discomfort at the front of the throat around the larynx (voice box) or at the front of the chest. A child with croup often awakens at night

with an attack of stridor (a shrill wheezing or grunting sound), which usually subsides in a few hours. If stridor develops suddenly and is accompanied by coughing, and the child does not have a respiratory infection, he or she may have inhaled a foreign object. In all cases, rapid, noisy breathing (see next page) is a medical emergency that requires immediate treatment.

Diagnosis and Treatment

A diagnosis of croup is based on a child's symptoms and a physical examination. The doctor may order X-rays to determine if the symptoms are caused by croup or by epiglottitis (see illustration).

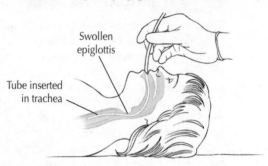
Swollen epiglottis
Tube inserted in trachea

Epiglottitis
Epiglottitis is a life-threatening condition in which the epiglottis (a flap of cartilage at the top of the trachea) becomes infected, swells, and blocks the airway. To treat epiglottitis, a doctor guides a tube through the child's mouth and down the throat to open the airway. The child is admitted to an intensive care unit and given antibiotics intravenously (through a vein).

If your child has an episode of croup, stay calm and reassure him or her. Give your child plenty of fluids and, if he or she has a fever, give acetaminophen or ibuprofen (not aspirin). You may be able to relieve your child's symptoms by exposing him or her to cooler air by using a cool-mist vaporizer in his or her bedroom. Sitting with your child in a bathroom filled with steam from a hot shower can help relieve congestion and make breathing easier.

The doctor will probably prescribe an aerosol corticosteroid medication to relieve inflammation and swelling in the trachea, or aerosol epinephrine (a hormone produced by the adrenal glands) to improve breathing. The doctor may also prescribe corticosteroid drugs to be taken orally or injected. This treatment can be administered in the doctor's office or in a hospital emergency department. A child who has severe difficulty breathing or

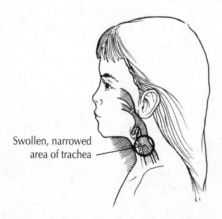
Swollen, narrowed area of trachea

Croup
Croup is inflammation and swelling of the trachea (windpipe) caused by a viral infection of the respiratory tract. The swelling narrows the trachea and causes hoarseness, noisy breathing, and a loud, barking cough.

cyanosis (blueness of the skin caused by lack of oxygen in the blood) will be hospitalized for treatment with supplemental oxygen and medication. If the doctor suspects epiglottitis, the child will be admitted to the hospital intensive care unit immediately for emergency medical treatment.

If a child's airways are severely obstructed by severe croup or epiglottitis, the doctor will pass a tube through the child's mouth down into the throat to open the airway or, in severe cases, make a small incision in the throat and insert a breathing tube. The tube is usually removed within 24 to 72 hours. In rare cases, a child's breathing must be maintained with a ventilator (an artificial breathing machine). Children are admitted to a hospital for this treatment, and recover completely within a few days.

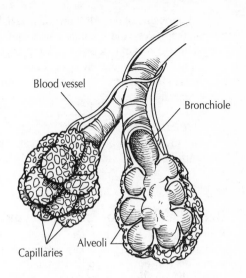

Bronchiolitis
Bronchiolitis is a potentially life-threatening viral infection of the lungs that causes the bronchioles to swell, blocking the exchange of oxygen and carbon dioxide in the alveoli (the tiny sacs in which gas exchange between the lungs and the blood occurs).

WARNING!

Difficult or Noisy Breathing

If a child inhales a foreign object, it can partially or completely block the airway (trachea) and interfere with breathing. If the child's airway is partially blocked, he or she will wheeze or grunt and may cough. In this case, a doctor will perform a procedure called bronchoscopy (an examination of the inside of the lungs with a viewing tube called a bronchoscope) to look for the inhaled object and, if possible, remove it.

If an inhaled object passes farther down into the lungs, it can cause inflammation and infection. In this case, the doctor will use a bronchoscope to locate and remove the object and may prescribe antibiotics to treat or prevent an infection.

If your child has sudden difficulty breathing, if his or her lips look blue, or if he or she is breathing noisily, call 911 or your local emergency number, or take him or her to the nearest hospital emergency department immediately.

Bronchiolitis

Bronchiolitis is a potentially life-threatening viral infection of the lungs in which the lining of the bronchioles (the smallest airways in the lungs) swells and produces secretions that block the passage of air into and out of the alveoli (the tiny sacs through which oxygen and carbon dioxide are exchanged between the lungs and the blood). The infection usually occurs in children under 2 and usually develops during the fall, winter, or early spring. Premature infants have an increased risk of severe bronchiolitis. If your baby has an increased risk of bronchiolitis, the doctor may recommend preventive treatment with monoclonal antibodies (infection-fighting proteins produced in a laboratory to target specific infectious agents) to protect against infection with RSV. Like the common cold, bronchiolitis easily spreads among young children through contact with saliva, mucus, or airborne droplets. The most common cause of bronchiolitis is RSV (respiratory syncytial virus; see page 654).

Symptoms
The symptoms of bronchiolitis include a runny nose, a slight fever, a cough, and shortness of breath. In severe cases, a child may experience rapid (more than 40 breaths per minute), labored breathing, and his or her skin may look blue, especially around the lips and at the fingertips. The child may need to sit up to breathe and may also wheeze. He or she may vomit and be unable to keep liquids down. If your child's skin ever looks bluish, take him or her to the nearest hospital emergency department immediately.

Diagnosis
To diagnose bronchiolitis, the doctor will ask you about your child's symptoms and examine him or

her for signs of dehydration, such as a dry mouth, sunken eyes, and a sunken soft spot. He or she will use a stethoscope to listen to the child's lungs for characteristic wheezing or bubbling noises that indicate the presence of mucus in the bronchioles.

Treatment

In mild cases of bronchiolitis, treatment may not be necessary. Your doctor probably will recom-

mend giving your child plenty of liquids and using a cool-mist vaporizer in the child's bedroom while he or she is sleeping to help relieve congestion. Give your child acetaminophen or ibuprofen (not aspirin) if he or she has a fever. In some cases, a doctor may prescribe liquid medication or nebulizer treatments with a bronchodilator drug to control the coughing and wheezing. A nebulizer is a device that mixes medication with water vapor to produce a mist that the person inhales. To help

---

Recurring Colds or Coldlike Symptoms

It is normal for a child to have a number of coughs and colds, especially during the winter, and usually it is not a cause for concern. Children who are in day care with several children frequently get colds, as do children in their first few years of school, because they are exposed to many new viruses. Gradually, however, they acquire immunity to increasing numbers of cold viruses.

A child's cold is often accompanied by a cough because, instead of blowing his or her nose, a child usually sniffs mucus down into the throat. The mucus irritates the throat, and the child coughs in an attempt to eliminate the mucus. Abdominal pain resulting from swallowing mucus is another common symptom in a child with a cold. In some cases, a child with a cold may complain of abdominal pain, which is actually muscle strain caused by coughing.

When to See a Doctor

Your child may not have a cold, even if he or she has cold symptoms. In some children, coldlike symptoms result from an allergic reaction (see page 912). If your child sneezes and has a runny nose and watery eyes during the warm months, he or she probably has an allergy to pollen. However, if the symptoms occur throughout the year, your child may be allergic to some other allergen, such as mold or dust mites. In some children, recurring coughs result from a serious underlying disorder. For example, a recurring cough that is accompanied by wheezing may be a symptom of asthma (see page 640), sinusitis (see page 651), or enlarged adenoids (see page 419). In rare cases, a recurring cough may be caused by the genetic disorder cystic fibrosis (see page 958). If your child has a persistent cough or frequently has coldlike symptoms, see your doctor.

In some babies, the symptoms of a more serious infection, such as an ear infection (see page 417), bronchiolitis (see previous page), or pneumonia (see page 660), mimic the symptoms of a cold. The baby

may be restless, cry persistently, and refuse to eat. He or she may have a high fever (about 102°F), and his or her skin may feel hot to the touch. The baby may be persistently hoarse and have a dry cough. If your baby has these symptoms, see your doctor.

The doctor will ask about your child's symptoms and examine his or her throat to see if the tonsils are inflamed. Tonsillitis or enlarged adenoids can lead to breathing difficulties. If your child has been wheezing or grunting, the doctor may suspect asthma or a lung infection. The doctor will examine your child's chest to see if the cold is developing into a more serious disorder such as pneumonia or bronchiolitis.

Because a respiratory infection can travel through the eustachian tube to the middle ear cavity and cause a middle ear infection (see page 417), the doctor will examine your child's ears with a lighted viewing instrument called an otoscope. If an ear infection is not treated promptly, it can lead to a ruptured eardrum (see page 1022); chronic ear infections may result in hearing loss.

If Your Child Has a Cold

In some cases, a child with a cold will cough a lot during the night, often because the bedroom is too hot or too cold and the air is irritating his or her throat. Adjusting the room's temperature or humidity may solve the problem.

Infants with colds may have trouble eating, which is not a cause for concern if the problem lasts no more than a few days. You can help restore your baby's appetite by clearing the mucus from his or her nose with a small bulb syringe (available at most drugstores) and using nonprescription saline nose drops.

Try giving an older child liquids before bed to help clear the back of the nasal passage. Wash your face and hands and your child's face and hands frequently to avoid spreading the infection.

prevent the infection from spreading, wash your hands frequently, especially after caring for your child.

In severe cases of bronchiolitis, a child may need to be hospitalized for a few days to receive supplemental oxygen, intravenous fluids to relieve dehydration, and bronchodilator drugs to open the airways. The doctor may prescribe antibiotics to treat any secondary bacterial infection that has developed, such as pneumonia. If a child has severe difficulty breathing, he or she may be put on a ventilator (an artificial breathing machine) until his or her breathing returns to normal. With prompt treatment, the infection usually clears up within a few days and leaves no lasting effects. However, some affected children continue to develop wheezing whenever they have respiratory infections up to about age 5 or 6.

Blood Disorders

B lood disorders can vary greatly in their effects. Because the symptoms are so varied and are often mild at first, these disorders can sometimes go undetected. For a child with iron deficiency anemia or allergic purpura, a delayed diagnosis is not likely to cause any permanent effects.

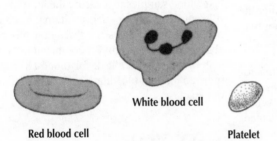

White blood cell

Red blood cell

Platelet

Types of blood cells
Red blood cells are doughnut-shaped cells that carry oxygen from the lungs to tissues throughout the body, where the oxygen is exchanged for carbon dioxide. White blood cells protect the body against infection and fight infection. White blood cells are bigger than red blood cells but not as numerous. Platelets are fragments of blood cells that play an important part in blood clotting.

Allergic Purpura

Allergic purpura (also called anaphylactoid purpura or Henoch-Schoenlein purpura) is an allergic reaction of unknown cause that produces a rash just beneath the surface of the skin. The rash is thought to result from an abnormal reaction between antibodies (infection-fighting proteins) and blood vessels, causing the blood vessels to become inflamed or to burst. In some cases, the antibodies may have been produced to fight a bacterial or viral infection several weeks earlier, or in a reaction to a food or medication.

The condition occurs most often in late fall and winter, affecting mostly children between ages 2 and 7, boys more frequently than girls. Severe cases can lead to kidney failure (see page 817), bleeding into the intestinal tract and other organs, and, rarely, intestinal obstruction (intussusception; see page 406). In some children, allergic purpura can recur for up to 2 years before it finally disappears for good.

Symptoms
Allergic purpura usually starts as an itchy skin rash that is purplish red, irregularly shaped, flat or raised, and can vary in size, resembling bruises. The spots usually appear on the ankles, shins, buttocks, and elbows. The spots tend to come and go and fade after several weeks. In some people, the rash is preceded by a sore throat, headache, fever, and loss of appetite.

Some children also may have swollen joints (usually the ankles or the knees), abdominal pain that is often severe and persistent, and blood in the stool. About half have blood in their urine and a low volume of urine, which, in severe cases, can indicate widespread obstruction of the tiny blood vessels (capillaries) in the filtering structures (glomeruli) of the kidneys (glomerulonephritis; see page 807). Some children may develop high blood pressure.

Diagnosis and Treatment

Allergic purpura is diagnosed by the symptoms, a physical examination, a thorough health history, and blood and urine tests. X-rays or CT scans may be performed to evaluate any complications that develop in the intestines or other organs. In most cases, treatment is not necessary because the condition tends to clear up on its own within a month, but a child may be hospitalized to watch for serious complications. For severe cases, a doctor may prescribe corticosteroids to reduce inflammation, or intravenous gamma globulin (which contains antibodies to fight infection) to alleviate symptoms.

If the kidneys are affected, the doctor will want to see the child for regular checkups to monitor the health of the kidneys. In some cases, a doctor may do a kidney biopsy (microscopic examination of a sample of tissue from the kidney). Elevated levels of blood or protein in the urine may persist for months in some children; these symptoms also require follow-up checkups. If the child develops high blood pressure, the doctor will prescribe medication to control it.

Iron Deficiency Anemia in Children

Iron deficiency anemia, the most common form of anemia in children, results from an insufficient supply of hemoglobin (the oxygen-carrying protein) in the blood. The disorder usually results from an insufficient intake of iron in the diet or from poor absorption of iron by the body. Most full-term babies are born with an adequate supply of iron from their mother during pregnancy and receive iron from breast milk or formula. However, as the child grows and has an increased need for iron, a diet deficient in iron can lead to anemia. Preterm infants, who often are born with an inadequate supply of iron, and children who have a disorder that inhibits iron absorption, such as celiac disease (see page 768), have an increased risk of developing anemia. Infants should not drink cow's milk because it interferes with the absorption of iron and irritates the intestinal lining, causing intestinal bleeding and further contributing to anemia.

Symptoms

Mild anemia usually causes no obvious symptoms. In more severe cases, symptoms can include pale skin (especially on the hands and inside the lower eyelids), fatigue, weakness, or behavioral changes such as irritability or anger. Less often, fainting, breathlessness, and heart palpitations may occur. All of these symptoms are more obvious after physical activity. If your child is less active than usual or if he or she is breathless after even moderate activity, see your doctor. If you suspect that your child may have anemia, do not try to treat it yourself with iron supplements, because too much iron can be dangerous.

Diagnosis

To diagnose iron deficiency anemia, a doctor will take blood samples to measure the level of iron. To rule out other causes, such as internal bleeding or a problem in the digestive tract that blocks iron absorption, a doctor may recommend tests such as a stool analysis to check for blood (which could indicate internal bleeding), or X-rays of the digestive tract.

> **WARNING!**
>
> ### Iron Supplements
>
> Accidental overdose of iron through supplements is the leading cause of poisoning death in children under age 6. If your doctor has prescribed iron supplements for your child, administer them exactly as directed. To prevent an overdose or poisoning, always keep all supplements out of the reach of children.

Treatment

To treat mild iron deficiency anemia, the doctor will make dietary recommendations to help the child get sufficient iron from his or her diet, such as ensuring that the child has an adequate intake of vitamin C, which facilitates iron absorption. To treat severe iron deficiency anemia caused by lack of iron in the diet, the doctor may prescribe iron supplements (usually in liquid form) for your child to take for 2 months or longer. If the anemia results from an underlying disorder, the doctor will recommend appropriate treatment.

Lead Poisoning

Lead is an extremely toxic metal that is easily absorbed by the body. If swallowed or inhaled, lead is absorbed in the intestines or the lungs, enters the bloodstream, and travels to soft tissues such as the liver, kidneys, or brain, where it is stored. Lead also can be stored in the bones and teeth.

Lead poisoning is the No. 1 environmental disease among children in the United States, affecting about one of every five children. Children under age 6 have an increased risk of lead poisoning because their body is able to absorb very high amounts of lead. Lead usually enters a child's body when he or she eats paint chips (from lead-based paints that were available before 1978) or contaminated soil. A child can also be exposed to lead when he or she inhales polluted air outdoors or paint dust in the air at home, or from sucking or chewing on surfaces coated with lead-based paint such as furniture, windowsills, railings, or the slats of window blinds.

Common environmental sources of lead include lead-based paint, soil, tap water, and lead dust brought home from the workplace on clothing. Other, less common sources of lead include lead crystal containers, lead-soldered cans, and lead-glazed pottery.

Symptoms

Although mild lead poisoning often does not cause symptoms, some children may experience irritability, headache, muscle aches, drowsiness, fatigue, poor appetite, constipation, abdominal pain, vomiting, or weight loss. Poor nutrition may lead to anemia (see previous page). Severe lead poisoning may lead to hyperactivity, behavior problems, hearing problems, delayed growth, learning disabilities (see page 415), mental retardation, seizures, or brain damage. The effects of long-term exposure to lead can be severe and usually are irreversible.

Diagnosis

A diagnosis of lead poisoning is based on a child's symptoms and the results of a physical examination. The doctor will order a blood test to measure the amount of lead in the child's blood. A blood level of 10 micrograms or more of lead per 1 deciliter of blood (mcg/dL) indicates lead poisoning. In severe cases, a doctor may order X-rays of the abdomen and the bones in the arms and legs to look for deposits of lead.

Treatment

The main treatment for lead poisoning is to eliminate lead from the child's environment or to remove the child from the contaminated environment. For mild lead poisoning, a doctor may prescribe a drug called a chelating agent, which will bind with the lead and help the body eliminate it in urine. The drug may be taken orally or may be injected into a muscle. To help prevent or reduce absorption of lead, the doctor may recommend a diet that is high in iron and calcium and low in fat. Children with severe lead poisoning (a blood level higher than 20 mcg/dL) may be hospitalized for treatment with intravenous chelating agents and nutritional supplements.

Prevention

Doctors recommend that all children have a screening test for lead poisoning between 6 months and 6 years of age, depending on the child's risk factors, such as exposure to lead-based paint in older homes. You can take a number of steps to limit your family's exposure to lead and help prevent lead poisoning:

- Keep your child away from chipping or peeling paint, and make sure that he or she does not chew or suck on surfaces that could be coated with lead-based paint, such as furniture, railings, windowsills, or the slats of window blinds.
- Have your home tested for lead, and have any lead-based paint removed professionally.
- Keep your home clean and dust-free, especially in areas where your children play.
- Have your local health department or water department test your tap water for lead.
- Run cold water from the tap for at least 1 minute before using it (because water standing in lead pipes can accumulate dissolved lead), and do not drink or cook with hot tap water (because hot tap water dissolves lead in pipes faster than cold water does).
- Do not store beverages in lead crystal containers, and don't cook or store food in lead-glazed pottery.
- Do not let your children play in dirt or mud. Encourage frequent, careful handwashing at

home, especially after playing outdoors, before meals and naps, and at bedtime.

- Check for chipped or peeling paint on playground equipment, and have your local health department test the paint for lead. If the paint is lead-based, it should be removed professionally, or the equipment should be replaced.

- Provide your children a diet that is high in iron and calcium and low in fat to reduce the body's absorption of lead. Good sources of iron include lean red meats, legumes, fortified cereals, and eggs. Good sources of calcium include low-fat or fat-free dairy products such as milk, yogurt, and cheese.

Disorders of the Urinary Tract and Reproductive Organs

The urinary tract consists of two fist-sized organs called the kidneys (which filter the blood and excrete waste products and excess water from the body as urine), two narrow tubes called ureters (which carry urine from the kidneys to the bladder), a hollow, muscular organ called the bladder (which serves as a reservoir for urine), and a narrow tube called the urethra (which carries urine from the bladder out of the body). The reproductive organs are closely linked to the urinary tract.

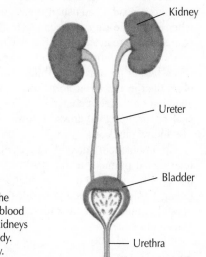

Kidney

Ureter

Bladder

Urethra

The urinary tract
The urinary tract consists of the kidneys, the ureters, the bladder, and the urethra. The kidneys remove waste products and excess fluid from the blood to make urine. The ureters are two tubes that transport urine from the kidneys to the bladder, where the urine is stored until it is expelled from the body. The urethra is a tube that carries urine from the bladder out of the body.

Urinary Tract Infections

In a urinary tract infection, microorganisms (usually bacteria) invade the urinary tract and multiply. Urinary tract infections are common among children. Girls are especially susceptible because the female urethra (the tube that carries urine from the bladder) is fairly short, making it relatively easy for bacteria to move up the urethra and into the bladder.

Few risks are associated with one or two urinary tract infections. However, if the child is a boy or is younger than 2, or if the infection recurs, the child may have an underlying abnormality of the urinary tract that requires treatment to help prevent more serious urinary problems, such as chronic pyelonephritis (see page 806), chronic kidney failure (see page 817), or vesicoureteral reflux (see next page).

Symptoms

Sometimes a urinary tract infection does not cause symptoms. When symptoms occur, they can include a persistent urge to urinate, difficulty urinating, or a burning sensation while urinating. The child may experience pain in the lower back, in the abdomen, or in the groin area. He or she may also have a fever, and his or her urine may be discolored and have a strong, unpleasant odor. If your child has symptoms of a urinary tract infection, talk to your doctor.

Diagnosis

A diagnosis of a urinary tract infection is based on a child's symptoms, a physical examination, and the results of urine tests. If your child is a boy or is younger than 2, has recurring urinary tract infections, or appears to be very ill, the doctor will recommend additional tests, such as an ultrasound (see page 111) or a CT scan (see page 112) of the kidneys, ureters, and bladder; a radionuclide scan (see page 114) of the kidneys; and a voiding cystogram (see page 805). The ultrasound or CT scan shows the shape of the kidneys, ureters, and bladder. The radionuclide scan shows how the kidneys function and detects any infection in the kidneys. The voiding cystogram enables the doctor to examine the bladder during urination to determine the size of the bladder and to check for vesicoureteral reflux.

Treatment

To treat a urinary tract infection, a doctor will prescribe antibiotics in tablets or in liquid form. If the kidneys are affected, the doctor may prescribe antibiotics given intravenously (through a vein).

Any underlying abnormality of the urinary tract can be corrected with surgery. The doctor will recommend giving your child plenty of clear fluids, preferably water, and encouraging your child to empty his or her bladder completely and frequently (at least every 4 to 6 hours). The symptoms usually subside a few days after the child begins taking the antibiotics, but your child still needs to finish all of the prescribed medication or the infection will recur.

Vesicoureteral Reflux

Vesicoureteral reflux is a urinary tract disorder in which the mechanism that prevents the backflow of urine malfunctions, causing urine to flow backward

Bed-Wetting

By age 4 or 5, most children stay dry through the night. Other children may continue to wet the bed at night, and, in rare cases, may also wet themselves during the day. The medical term for this condition is enuresis. If a child begins wetting the bed again after a long period of staying dry through the night, the condition is called secondary enuresis. Enuresis, which can last for several years, occurs slightly more often in boys than in girls and tends to run in families.

In most cases, the cause of bed-wetting is not known. However, in some cases, the cause of enuresis (especially of secondary enuresis) may be psychological, such as stress associated with the arrival of a new baby. In a few cases, an underlying illness—such as a urinary tract infection or undiagnosed diabetes (see page 889)—may be causing the condition. Treating the underlying illness that is causing the bed-wetting usually eliminates the problem.

Dealing With Bed-Wetting

If your child has been wetting the bed, have him or her urinate right before going to bed at night. Then, just before you go to bed, wake your child and have him or her get up and urinate again. If your child is of school age, try setting an alarm clock to go off during the night so he or she can get up and urinate. For an older child, put out dry pajamas and sheets so he or she can change them without waking you for help. If, after a few weeks, this approach has not been effective, have the doctor examine your child to rule out an underlying disorder. The doctor may take a sample of your child's urine for laboratory analysis and, although rare, he or she may order tests to evaluate your child's bladder and kidneys.

Your child must want to deal with his or her bed-wetting problem for treatment to be effective. Use the same principles that apply to toilet training: provide support and encouragement, praise your child for dry nights, and never scold or punish your child for wet nights. A negative, punishing approach to the problem can make it worse. Most children simply outgrow bed-wetting.

If your child is 7 or older and still wets the bed, your doctor may recommend using a special liquid-sensitive pad that sounds a loud alarm as soon as the first drop of urine touches the pad. Most children learn to wake up before the alarm sounds and get up to urinate. A few weeks of this treatment is usually effective; if your child begins wetting the bed again, use the pad again.

The doctor will recommend limiting your child's intake of carbonated and citrus beverages, eliminating caffeine, and not having any dairy products at dinner or after. The doctor will assess the size of the child's bladder by measuring urine output. If the child's bladder is smaller than normal, the doctor may prescribe medication to stretch the bladder and thereby decrease the frequency of urination. Because constipation can contribute to bed-wetting, the doctor will probably recommend measures such as increasing the fiber in your child's diet.

In persistent cases, a doctor may prescribe hormonal treatment to temporarily help control bed-wetting for special occasions such as sleepovers. For some children, treatment with a hormone called desmopressin (a synthetic form of the human hormone that naturally reduces the output of urine) controls bed-wetting.

from the bladder through the ureters and up into the kidneys. This backflow of urine can cause increased pressure on the kidneys or recurring kidney infections, both of which can lead to permanent damage and scarring of the kidneys.

Vesicoureteral reflux often occurs in children who were born with a neural tube defect such as spina bifida (see page 398), and also can occur in children who have a urinary tract abnormality such as a cyst, a stone, or an obstruction. In infancy the disorder is more common among boys; in early childhood it is more common among girls. Vesicoureteral reflux tends to run in families and occurs more often in whites than in blacks.

Symptoms

In many cases, a first-time urinary tract infection (see page 426) is the initial symptom of vesicoureteral reflux. Other possible signs and symptoms of vesicoureteral reflux include recurring urinary tract infections; problems with urination such as urgency, dribbling, and wetting; poor weight gain; and high blood pressure. In some children, swelling of the kidneys can produce a detectable lump in the abdomen.

Diagnosis

A diagnosis of vesicoureteral reflux is based on a child's symptoms and the results of a physical examination. A doctor will order blood tests to evaluate kidney function and may order an X-ray of the urinary tract called a voiding cystourethrogram (see page 805) to check for vesicoureteral reflux and, if the condition is present, determine its severity. The doctor may also recommend an ultrasound (see page 111) of the kidneys to check their size and shape and to look for a cyst, a stone, an obstruction, or another abnormality.

Treatment

The treatment for vesicoureteral reflux depends on the severity of the disorder. Mild cases usually clear up on their own within about 5 years. Doctors often prescribe preventive treatment with antibiotics for children who develop frequent urinary tract infections. In some cases, medication is prescribed to control high blood pressure. In other cases, surgery is performed on the ureters to create a flap of tissue that works like a valve and prevents the backflow of urine. In severe cases the damaged kidney may be removed surgically. The remaining kidney will do the work of both kidneys.

Poststreptococcal Glomerulonephritis

Poststreptococcal glomerulonephritis (also called nephritis) is a rare condition that develops in a child after an infection with streptococcal bacteria. In response to the infection, the body's immune system produces antibodies (infection-fighting proteins) to fight the bacteria, but because of a malfunction in the immune system, the antibodies continue to be active even after the bacteria have been destroyed, and attack the kidneys. The kidneys become inflamed and produce less urine than normal. Blood leaks from the glomeruli (the filtering units of the kidney) into the urine. With prompt treatment, most children recover completely from poststreptococcal glomerulonephritis. However, a few children experience persistent kidney problems and, after many years, may develop chronic kidney failure (see page 817).

Symptoms and Diagnosis

The main symptom of poststreptococcal glomerulonephritis is reduced output of urine. The urine looks smoky or reddish brown because it contains blood. The reduced output of urine leads to edema, an abnormal accumulation of fluid in the body that causes swelling around the eyes and face and sometimes over the entire body. In addition to edema, some children with poststreptococcal glomerulonephritis may gain weight, lose their appetite, have abdominal pain or diarrhea, or develop high blood pressure (see page 574).

A diagnosis of poststreptococcal glomerulonephritis is based on a child's symptoms and the results of a physical examination. If the doctor suspects poststreptococcal glomerulonephritis, he or she will order blood and urine tests to confirm the diagnosis.

Treatment

If your child is very ill, the doctor may recommend bed rest. The doctor will put your child on a special diet that restricts his or her intake of sodium, potassium, liquids, and, possibly, foods that are high in protein (such as meat, fish, and eggs). The diet is designed to reduce strain on the kidneys and prevent the accumulation of fluid.

The doctor may prescribe antibiotics to treat any remaining strep infection and a diuretic to increase the child's output of urine, eliminate excess fluid from the body, and control blood pressure.

If the child's condition worsens, he or she will be hospitalized to treat any complications that could develop, such as kidney failure, heart failure (see page 570), or severe high blood pressure. The doctor will monitor your child's blood pressure and will prescribe antihypertensive medications if the child develops high blood pressure.

Hemolytic Uremic Syndrome

Hemolytic uremic syndrome is a rare complication of a severe gastrointestinal infection, usually with a specific type of E. coli bacteria (E. coli O157:H7). The bacteria can be acquired by eating contaminated food such as meat, poultry, or potatoes; drinking contaminated juice, water, or dairy products; or touching infected people or contaminated surfaces. Hemolytic uremic syndrome occurs when toxins from the bacteria get into the bloodstream and damage red blood cells (which carry oxygen to tissues) and platelets (which help blood to clot). The damaged red blood cells and platelets can then clog the tiny blood vessels in the kidneys, blocking the ability of the kidneys to filter and remove waste products.

Hemolytic uremic syndrome is one of the leading causes of acute kidney failure in children under 10. Although most children have no long-term complications from hemolytic uremic syndrome, some may have permanent kidney damage and may need dialysis (see page 818) or a kidney transplant (see page 820). In severe cases, hemolytic uremic syndrome can be fatal.

Proper food handling and preparation (see page 784) and frequent, thorough washing of hands and utensils can significantly reduce the risk of hemolytic uremic syndrome and other forms of food poisoning.

Symptoms

Symptoms of an E. coli infection, which can last about a week, include vomiting, abdominal pain, and diarrhea that may contain blood. Most children recover fully from an E. coli infection. However, some children go on to develop hemolytic uremic syndrome. The symptoms of hemolytic uremic syndrome include pale skin or jaundice (yellowing of the skin and whites of the eyes), bruising, weakness, lethargy, irritability, and low output of urine. The inability of the kidneys to remove waste can lead to fluid buildup, which can cause swelling of the hands and feet.

Diagnosis and Treatment

A doctor will recommend blood and urine tests and will test stool samples to determine if a child is infected with E. coli and has developed hemolytic uremic syndrome.

To treat an E. coli infection, a child is given fluids to replace lost fluids and help prevent dehydration. Severe cases of hemolytic uremic syndrome may require hospitalization. Treatment for children who develop hemolytic uremic syndrome depends on the severity of the illness and whether it has damaged their kidneys or other organs. Their blood pressure is monitored, and they may need to be given fluids intravenously (through a vein), blood transfusions, or dialysis.

Nephrotic Syndrome

Nephrotic syndrome is an uncommon disorder in which the glomeruli (the filtering units of the kidneys) are damaged, causing protein to leak out of the blood and into the urine. In nephrotic syndrome, the output of urine is significantly reduced, resulting in edema (abnormal accumulation of fluid in the body). About 80 percent of cases of nephrotic syndrome occur in children between ages 1 and 6, mostly ages 2 and 3. Boys are affected more often than girls.

A child with nephrotic syndrome is vulnerable to various infections, including peritonitis (see page 759), urinary tract infections (see page 426), and pneumonia (see page 660). In rare cases, nephrotic syndrome persists after treatment and develops into chronic glomerulonephritis (see page 807), which can lead to kidney failure (see page 817).

Symptoms

Edema is a major symptom of nephrotic syndrome. Over several weeks, the edema causes the child's body to swell; the swelling is usually most noticeable in the face, abdomen, legs, ankles, and feet. The child also has a significant decrease in urine output. If your child has symptoms of nephrotic syndrome, see your doctor right away.

Diagnosis

A diagnosis of nephrotic syndrome is based on a child's symptoms and the results of a physical examination. The doctor takes samples of your child's urine and blood for laboratory analysis. If the test results suggest that your child may have nephrotic syndrome, the doctor will order additional urine and blood tests and, in some cases, a kidney biopsy (in which a small amount of kidney tissue is removed and examined under a microscope) to confirm the diagnosis.

Treatment

A child with nephrotic syndrome is usually hospitalized so treatment can be carefully monitored. He or she is placed on a low-sodium, high-protein diet and given medications such as diuretics (to decrease fluid) and corticosteroids (to reduce inflammation). In some cases, stronger medications such as chemotherapy drugs may be administered. The symptoms usually clear up after 2 weeks of treatment in the hospital, and the child can continue recovering at home.

At home, the child will need to take his or her medication exactly as prescribed and continue eating the special diet. Food should be cooked and served without salt, and the diet should contain plenty of protein—from foods such as fish, meat, eggs, and low-salt cheese—to help restore the body's supply of protein. The doctor also may restrict the child's intake of fluids to reduce edema.

In most cases, children recover completely with no lasting effects. In some cases, the disorder recurs after the child has been free of symptoms for several weeks or months, and treatment must be repeated. Occasionally the disorder continues to come and go, and the child needs prolonged treatment with corticosteroid medications to eliminate the condition. In rare cases, a child develops kidney failure and will need to have a kidney transplant (see page 820).

Renal Dysplasia

Renal dysplasia—also called dysplastic kidneys, multicystic kidneys, or cystic dysplastic renal disease—is a condition in which the cells and structures of the kidneys develop abnormally before birth. Usually only one kidney is affected, although both can be affected. The abnormal kidney may be either small or enlarged, with a number of irregular cysts. Renal dysplasia is one of the most common prenatal developmental abnormalities and is often detected before birth during a routine ultrasound scan. The disorder is not inherited.

Symptoms

The most common sign of renal dysplasia in a newborn is a noticeable mass in the baby's abdomen. The infant may also develop a urinary tract infection, blood in the urine, and high blood pressure. If both kidneys are affected, infants sometimes die if they do not receive a kidney transplant (see page 820). Other developmental abnormalities of the urinary tract—such as an obstructed bladder, ureter, or urethra—are also sometimes present.

Diagnosis

Doctors often identify renal dysplasia during an ultrasound scan before birth. In older children, doctors sometimes detect the possibility of renal dysplasia during a physical examination while taking the child's blood pressure. The diagnosis can be confirmed by an ultrasound scan or a radionuclide scan (see page 114).

Treatment

A child with renal dysplasia may not require treatment because a person can live with only one working kidney. However, if the disorder causes health problems, the doctor may recommend surgical removal of the affected kidney. If both kidneys are affected, the doctor will probably recommend a kidney transplant.

Wilms' Tumor

Wilms' tumor is a rare, life-threatening cancer in which a malignant growth forms in one of the kidneys. The disorder usually affects children under age 5, boys twice as often as girls. The disorder tends to run in families. Prompt treatment is needed to prevent the cancerous cells from spreading to other parts of the body, such as the lungs, liver, brain, or the other kidney.

Symptoms

The main symptom of Wilms' tumor is a hard lump that can be felt in the child's abdomen. Other symptoms may include a slight fever, loss of appetite, constipation, nausea, vomiting, and weight loss. A child with Wilms' tumor may also have the blood disorder anemia (see page 610), which can cause weakness and fatigue, and he or she may develop high blood pressure (see page 574). If your child has any of these symptoms, see your doctor right away.

Diagnosis and Treatment

To diagnose Wilms' tumor, the doctor will ask about your child's symptoms and perform a physical examination. The doctor will order a CT scan (see page 112) or MRI (see page 113) to locate and evaluate the tumor and to determine if the cancer has spread. He or she may order a biopsy (a microscopic examination of tissue from the tumor) to confirm the diagnosis.

If Wilms' tumor is diagnosed, surgery will be performed to remove the affected kidney and prevent the cancer from spreading. The remaining kidney is able to take over the work of the one that is removed. The doctor will prescribe anticancer medication and, in some cases, radiation therapy to destroy any remaining cancer cells.

Undescended Testicles

In boys, the testicles develop inside the abdomen from the same embryonic tissue that becomes the ovaries in girls. In most boys, both testicles descend through the abdominal wall and into the scrotum (the pouch of skin that surrounds the testicles) about a month before birth. In a small number of boys, for reasons that are not known, one testicle or, less frequently, both testicles do not descend into the scrotum by birth. In these cases, the testicle or testicles usually descend by 1 year of age. If the testicles do not descend by age 1, surgery is necessary to bring them down into the scrotum. If the condition is not corrected, the child has an increased risk of being infertile and of developing testicular cancer (see page 824) in either testicle after puberty. For these reasons, early treatment is essential.

Symptoms

Undescended testicles do not cause pain or interfere with urination. Some boys who have an undescended testicle may also have an inguinal hernia (see page 763). If either or both of your son's testicles have not descended by age 1, see the child's doctor.

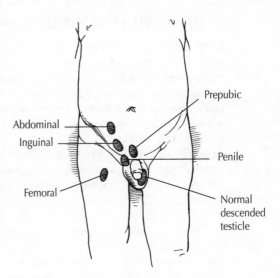

Undescended testicles
In some boys, a testicle may fail to descend from the abdomen into the scrotum before birth. An undescended testicle can be in the abdomen (abdominal), the groin area (inguinal), the upper thigh (femoral), or just above the pubic bone (prepubic) or penis (penile). Although an undescended testicle usually descends on its own by the time a boy is 1 year old, surgery may be performed to move the testicle into the scrotum if it does not descend on its own.

Diagnosis and Treatment

A diagnosis of undescended testicles is based on the results of a physical examination. If both testicles are undescended, the doctor may order a kidney ultrasound (see page 111) to determine the size of the kidneys and to check for possible defects.

Treatment of an undescended testicle should be performed when the child is between ages 1 and 2 and depends on where the testicle is. For example, if the testicle is very near the scrotum, injections of male hormones may cause it to descend into the scrotum. If the testicle is in the groin area, a surgical procedure called orchiopexy can be performed in which the surgeon makes a small cut in the groin area and then lowers the testicle into the scrotum. This procedure takes about an hour and the child usually goes home the same day. If the child also has an inguinal hernia, the surgeon will repair it at the same time. Once the testicles are in place inside the scrotum, children seldom have any more problems. However, some boys may have decreased fertility.

Vulvovaginitis

Vulvovaginitis is inflammation of the vulva (the outer, visible genital area around the vagina). The condition affects only a small number of girls, usually those whose vulva is especially sensitive to irritation. In many cases, the cause of the condition is unknown. In other cases, vulvovaginitis is caused by microorganisms in stool or is an allergic reaction caused by contact with wool, nylon, soap, bubble bath, baby wipes, fabric softener, or detergent. Bedwetting (see page 427) or pinworms (see page 444) also are possible causes of vulvovaginitis. In rare cases, the condition occurs after a child has inserted a foreign object into her vagina. In some cases, vulvovaginitis is a sign of child sexual abuse resulting from someone inserting a finger, penis, or other object into the child's vagina. Vulvovaginitis can occur at any age.

Symptoms

The symptoms of vulvovaginitis include redness, itching, and soreness in the genital area; a foul-smelling discharge from the vagina; painful urination; and a frequent urge to urinate. Because of symptoms such as the frequent urge to urinate and painful urination, vulvovaginitis may be mistaken for a bladder infection. If your daughter has symptoms of vulvovaginitis, see the doctor right away.

Diagnosis and Treatment

A diagnosis of vulvovaginitis is based on the child's symptoms and the results of a physical examination. The doctor will examine your daughter's vagina. If the doctor finds a foreign object, he or she will remove it. If the doctor suspects sexual abuse, he or she is required by law to contact the local department of public health, the department of social services, or the police department.

In most cases, careful hygiene eliminates the problem. Girls should be taught to wipe themselves from front to back after a bowel movement to help prevent bacteria from the anal area from reaching the vaginal area. Bathe the child every day with mild soap, but do not allow her to sit in soapy water, and do not use bubble bath or other potentially irritating bath additives. After bathing, dry the affected area thoroughly but gently and apply a zinc oxide paste or other protective medication the doctor has recommended. Wash the child's genital area carefully after each bowel movement. Make sure your child wears clean underpants each day. Underpants should be loose-fitting and made of cotton or have a cotton insert or panel in the crotch.

Disorders of the Muscles, Bones, or Joints

Injuries are the most common cause of muscle, bone, or joint problems in children, and in most cases, these injuries heal quickly and completely. However, some disorders that affect the muscles, bones, or joints in children—such as rheumatic fever, osteomyelitis, and juvenile rheumatoid arthritis—can be life-threatening and often result in permanent impairment.

Rheumatic Fever

Rheumatic fever is an inflammatory disease that can develop after an infection with streptococcal bacteria, such as strep throat (see page 652). Rheumatic fever can affect the heart, brain, joints, and skin. The disease can occur at any age but usually affects children between ages 5 and 15.

If untreated, rheumatic fever can damage the heart, in a condition called rheumatic heart disease. The inflammation that characterizes rheumatic heart disease can cause heart muscle damage (myocarditis), an irregular heart rate (arrhythmia), or heart valve injury. Damage to the heart valves can prevent the valves from completely opening or closing, which forces the heart to work harder to pump blood. If the heart valves are damaged permanently, health problems such as congestive heart failure (see page 570) can develop.

Symptoms

The symptoms of rheumatic fever can resemble those of other illnesses and usually develop 1 to 6 weeks after a strep throat infection. (In some people, a strep infection can be so mild that it is not noticed.) Symptoms of rheumatic fever include fever; joint pain and swelling that moves from joint to joint (called migratory arthritis); a ring-shaped rash on the chest, back, or abdomen; or abnormal writhing movements of the body and limbs. The child may develop chest pain, changes in heart rate, and symptoms of congestive heart failure (such as fatigue, shortness of breath, and swelling of the legs, ankles, and feet). To prevent rheumatic fever and rheumatic heart disease, see the doctor if you or your child has symptoms of strep throat, such as swollen tonsils, swollen lymph nodes in the neck, and fever. Strep spreads easily among family members.

Diagnosis

To diagnose rheumatic fever, a doctor will take a detailed health history, listen to the child's heart and lungs with a stethoscope, and examine the skin for a rash and the joints for pain and swelling. The doctor may take a sample from the child's throat to check for strep throat and order blood tests to look for evidence of a streptococcal infection. He or she may order an electrocardiogram (see page 559), which records the electrical activity of the heart, and an ultrasound examination of the heart (echocardiogram; see page 561) to check for heart damage.

Treatment

In most cases, treating a strep throat promptly with antibiotics will prevent rheumatic fever. To treat rheumatic fever, a doctor may recommend drugs such as corticosteroids to reduce the inflammation, and he or she will prescribe antibiotics if streptococcal bacteria are present. He or she may also prescribe long-term treatment with antibiotics to prevent recurring strep infections, which can reactivate rheumatic fever.

Scoliosis

Scoliosis is an abnormal curvature of the spine that develops or becomes apparent during the growth spurt of puberty, between ages 10 and 12. The condition affects girls more often than boys. In most cases, the cause is unknown, but some forms can be present at birth, inherited, or related to muscle and neurologic disorders.

Symptoms and Diagnosis

In many children, the curvature of the spine is so slight that it is not noticeable. In some cases, the curvature causes the shoulders, hips, or waist to be uneven. The legs may appear unequal in length and the shoulder blades may be more prominent than usual. In severe cases, the curvature can affect the heart and lungs.

Doctors screen for scoliosis as part of a routine physical examination. If your child has scoliosis, the doctor will refer you to a bone specialist (orthopedist), who will examine your child and order X-rays to confirm the diagnosis.

Treatment

Treatment of scoliosis depends on the degree of the curvature. For a curvature of less than 20 degrees, no treatment is necessary, but a child's spine should be examined at regular intervals. A curvature between 20 and 40 degrees is usually treated with a lightweight brace (worn under clothing) to prevent the curvature from worsening. The child may also need physical therapy to help strengthen his or her back muscles. If the brace is not effective or the curvature is more than 40 degrees, the doctor may recommend surgery to correct it.

Osteomyelitis

Osteomyelitis is a rare bacterial infection of the bone that can develop when bacteria from a contaminated wound or an infection in another part of the body enter the bloodstream and travel to the bone, usually near a joint in one of the long bones of the arms or legs. In rare cases, the infection develops in more than one bone. In children, osteomyelitis usually develops between ages 5 and 14 and affects boys more often than girls.

If osteomyelitis is left untreated or if treatment with medication does not clear up the infection, the bacteria can spread and multiply in the bloodstream and cause blood poisoning (see page 937).

Symptoms and diagnosis

The symptoms of osteomyelitis, which develop gradually over 2 or 3 days, usually include redness, swelling, and pain in the affected bone. Other symptoms include fever, chills, fatigue, and nausea. A diagnosis of osteomyelitis is based on the symptoms and the results of a physical examination. To confirm the diagnosis, the doctor may order X-rays or a bone scan and blood tests to check for infection. In some cases, the doctor may recommend a bone biopsy.

Treatment

To treat acute osteomyelitis, the doctor may admit your child to the hospital for bed rest and to immobilize the affected arm or leg with splints or a cast. He or she will also prescribe a 6-week course of oral antibiotics (which may be given intravenously at first). In some cases, a doctor may recommend minor surgery to drain and clean out the infection in the bone. Rarely, surgery may be necessary to remove infected or damaged bone or surrounding tissue.

Juvenile Rheumatoid Arthritis

Juvenile rheumatoid arthritis is an autoimmune disorder in which the immune system mistakenly produces antibodies (infection-fighting proteins) that attack and damage joints and other tissues throughout the body. The disorder may be mild or severe and occurs more often in girls than in boys. The cause is not known.

Juvenile rheumatoid arthritis can develop at any time between ages 6 months and 16 years, but it often begins between ages 2 and 5. Episodes of juvenile rheumatoid arthritis can come and go for years and they frequently disappear by the time a child reaches puberty. Each episode lasts a few weeks and tends to be less severe than the previous one. In some cases, juvenile rheumatoid arthritis leads to partial or disabling deformities. If the irises (the colored part of the eyes) become inflamed, partial or complete blindness can result.

With treatment, most children and young adults with juvenile rheumatoid arthritis are able to lead full, active lives.

Symptoms

The symptoms of juvenile rheumatoid arthritis include redness, swelling, warmth, stiffness, and pain in the affected joints. The child's temperature usually fluctuates, often from normal (98.6°F) in the morning to about 103°F in the evening. The child may have a poor appetite and may lose weight. A blotchy, red rash may break out over the trunk, arms, and legs. Mild anemia (see page 610)

often develops because the disorder blocks production of blood cells by the bone marrow. The child may have redness and pain around one or both eyes and may be sensitive to bright light.

The areas of inflammation in rheumatoid arthritis can vary widely from child to child. In addition to the area around the eyes, the lymph glands in the neck and armpits may swell, or the outer membrane of the heart may become inflamed (called pericarditis; see page 596), causing chest pain. The joints—usually the knees, ankles, elbows, and neck—can become swollen, stiff, and painful. In some cases, the joints become deformed over time. If your child has symptoms of juvenile rheumatoid arthritis, see the doctor right away.

Diagnosis

To diagnose juvenile rheumatoid arthritis, the doctor will ask about your child's symptoms, take a detailed health history, and perform a physical examination. He or she also may order blood tests, X-rays of the affected areas, and a biopsy of the membrane that encloses one of the affected joints. In a biopsy, a small amount of tissue is removed from the membrane for examination under a microscope. The doctor also may recommend laboratory analysis of the fluid inside the joints (synovial fluid).

The doctor may refer your child to a rheumatologist (a doctor who specializes in treating joint disorders) for further evaluation and treatment. He or she will recommend that your child see an ophthalmologist (a doctor who specializes in treating eye disorders), who can evaluate your child's eyes for signs of inflammation.

Treatment

Treatment for juvenile rheumatoid arthritis focuses on reducing the inflammation. The doctor may recommend giving your child acetaminophen or ibuprofen to reduce the fever and relieve pain, or he or she may prescribe a stronger anti-inflammatory medication to reduce pain and inflammation. The doctor will recommend a combination of physical therapy and regular exercise to slow progression of the disease, help restore and maintain mobility and flexibility in the joints, and build strength and endurance. Because fatigue can trigger a flare-up, help your child learn to balance exercise and other activities with periods of rest. Regular eye examinations are needed to check for signs of vision loss.

Childhood Infections

Infectious diseases occur when infectious microorganisms enter the body through the thin membranes that line the respiratory system or digestive tract. After the microbes enter the body, they start multiplying and can spread through the bloodstream and lymphatic system, causing symptoms.

The immune system attempts to fight the infection by producing proteins called antibodies to neutralize or destroy the microbes. Each microbe triggers production of a specific antibody that recognizes it. Once you have had a particular childhood infection, your immune system is able to recognize the infection-causing germ the next time and destroy it before symptoms develop.

Infectious diseases are contagious, which means that they can be spread from one person to another. Childhood infectious diseases can be contracted by inhaling airborne droplets that have been sneezed or coughed into the air by an infected person, or by direct contact with infected secretions. After recovering from some childhood infections—such as measles, rubella, chickenpox, or mumps—a child becomes immune to them, which means that he or she cannot be reinfected. This process is called natural immunity. Today, these infectious diseases are prevented with immunization, injections of harmless forms of the infectious agents to produce immunity.

Caring for a Child Who Is Ill

When a child is ill, he or she may be fussy and irritable or seem withdrawn and mopey. A sick child needs to be comforted. If your child is sick, pay special attention to his or her needs. Keep a record of his or her symptoms and, if you are unsure about anything, call your child's doctor.

Giving Medications to Children

If your child has difficulty taking medication, ask the doctor for tips. A child 3 years old or older may be able to swallow a tablet or capsule whole with the help of a drink. If the child can't swallow a tablet, ask your doctor if you should crush it and mix it with a food the child likes, such as applesauce or pudding. Don't open a capsule and mix its contents with food, because you could alter the timed-release properties of the medication. Remember that some medications should only be taken on an empty stomach. If you have any questions, ask the doctor.

Because small children often cannot swallow pills easily, doctors usually prescribe medication for them in liquid form. Give the medication exactly as prescribed, shaking the bottle if it is required. Special medication spoons are available that measure doses accurately. Measuring spoons for cooking, dosing cups, and oral syringes are also accurate, but make sure the unit of measurement is the same as the unit of the dose you want to give. Never use silverware spoons to give medicine to a child because the sizes of spoons can vary.

It is important for a child who is ill to take all the medication exactly as prescribed. If you are giving medicine to a sick child, keep the following in mind:

- **Immediately remove and dispose of the cap on a medicine syringe.** Children can choke on these caps.
- **Never share prescription medications.** Although two children may have the same illness, they may have different medication needs.
- **Never give a child leftover medication.** If a child who is sick has finished his or her medication as prescribed and there is medication left over, dispose of the leftover medication properly.
- **Dispose of old prescriptions safely.** Keep the medication in its original container with a child-resistant cap, put it in a sealable plastic bag, and throw it in the trash.
- **Store all medications as directed.** Some medicines can lose their effectiveness if not stored properly.

If Your Child Has a Fever

If your child is sick or you think he or she has a fever, use a thermometer to take his or her temperature. A variety of thermometers is available; however, not all of them are accurate. Types of available thermometers include glass mercury, digital, and

Acetaminophen Poisoning

Children can be unintentionally harmed by overly high doses of common, over-the-counter medications containing acetaminophen. Acetaminophen usually is prescribed for children as an alternative to aspirin (which can cause Reye's syndrome in children; see page 411). When taken as prescribed, acetaminophen is a safe medication. However, in even slightly higher doses than recommended, acetaminophen can damage the liver and cause it to shut down, leading to permanent disability and death.

Acetaminophen overdoses can occur for the following reasons:

- Acetaminophen is sold in a concentrated liquid form for infants (because infants cannot swallow as much liquid as older children). This concentrated form for infants can easily be confused with the standard liquid form for children because the bottles are almost indistinguishable. However, the infant formula is three times stronger than the children's formula.
- The medication is not given exactly as instructed.
- More than one person administers the medication to a child.
- Children are more vulnerable than adults to having serious side effects from medications.
- Some children drink the sweet, fruit-flavored liquid thinking it is fruit juice or a fruit drink.

To prevent an accidental overdose of acetaminophen:

- Make sure you are using the correct strength prescribed.
- Don't substitute one type of acetaminophen for another.
- Follow directions carefully, giving the exact dose at the correct time.
- Never double a dose, even if you miss one.
- Verify that no one else has given the medication to the child.
- Always keep all medicines out of the reach of children.

---

temperature strips. Glass thermometers use mercury that rises when heated to measure temperature. Although glass thermometers are the most traditional method, concerns about possible exposure to mercury have led doctors to recommend using digital thermometers. Though slightly more expensive than glass thermometers, digital thermometers are safe and accurate. Ear thermometers (which measure temperature through the ear) and strip thermometers (which can be placed on the forehead) can measure a child's temperature quickly but are not as accurate as glass or digital thermometers.

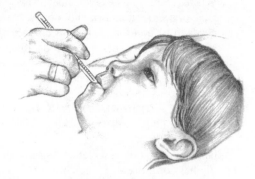

Taking a temperature by mouth

Taking a child's temperature

You can use a digital or glass thermometer to take a child's temperature by mouth, rectally (in the rectum), or in the armpit.

Taking a temperature by mouth

If you are taking your child's temperature by mouth, wait 20 to 30 minutes after he or she has finished eating or drinking anything. Make sure the child doesn't have anything in his or her mouth. Tell him or her not to bite down as you place the thermometer under his or her tongue. Ask the child to close his or her mouth. A glass thermometer usually registers temperature in 3 to 5 minutes. A digital thermometer will beep when the temperature is registered. If the child's oral temperature is above 99.5°F, he or she has a fever.

Taking a temperature rectally

A temperature taken rectally is always 1°F or 2°F higher than a temperature taken orally. To take a rectal temperature, lubricate the bulb end of the thermometer and your child's anus with a water-soluble lubricating jelly. Place the child, stomach down, across your lap or on a sturdy surface (such as a changing table or bed). Press the palm of one hand against the child's lower back, just above the buttocks. Use your other hand to gently insert the

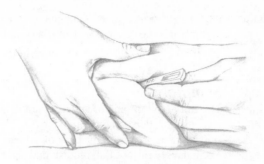

Taking a temperature rectally

thermometer ½ inch to 1 inch into the anus. Stop if you feel resistance. A glass thermometer usually registers a temperature in 2 to 3 minutes. A digital thermometer will beep when the temperature is registered. If the child's rectal temperature is above 100.5°F, he or she has a fever.

Taking a temperature in the armpit

To take an armpit temperature, remove the child's clothing above the waist and make sure his or her armpit is cool and dry. Place the thermometer under the armpit and fold the child's arm across his or her chest, or hold the arm securely to his or her side to keep the thermometer in place. A glass thermometer should remain in the armpit for at least 4 minutes for children under age 2 and for 5 or 6 minutes for children over 2. A digital thermometer will beep when the temperature is registered.

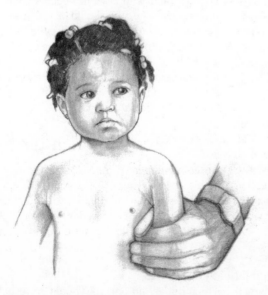

Taking a temperature in the armpit

A fever is seldom dangerous and rarely has any harmful effects. In some children, however, a fever may cause febrile seizures (see page 410). If your child's fever is lower than 102°F (a low-grade fever) and he or she has no other symptoms, the only treatment necessary may be giving plenty of fluids and rest.

If a child has a fever above 102°F (a high-grade fever), ask your doctor to recommend a fever reducer (such as acetaminophen or ibuprofen). Do not give aspirin to children or adolescents because they can develop Reye's syndrome (see page 411), a potentially fatal condition. Give your child the medication at regular intervals as recommended by your doctor, but take the child's temperature before doing so. When the child's temperature starts to fall, discontinue the fever reducer. If your child is asleep, do not wake him or her; sleep is helpful when you have a fever.

If, after your child has been given a fever reducer, his or her temperature continues to rise and reaches 104°F or higher, call your doctor immediately. If your child has had a previous febrile seizure, make sure your doctor knows.

To relieve discomfort caused by a fever, take the following steps:

- Sponge the child's face, neck, arms, and legs with lukewarm water, and let them air-dry. Evaporation cools the skin. Do not use a fan, ice, cold water, or rubbing alcohol on the skin to reduce a fever; they can cause shivering, which can raise the temperature even more.
- Keep the child's room at a comfortable temperature. Do not turn up the heat.
- Dress the child in light, comfortable clothing.
- Do not cover the child with heavy blankets. Using heavy blankets to try to get a child to sweat out a fever can cause his or her temperature to rise even higher.
- Do not let the child get overexerted.

Measles

Measles (also called rubeola) is a highly contagious viral infection that affects primarily the respiratory system. The disease is contracted by inhaling airborne droplets that have been coughed or sneezed into the air by an infected person. Possible complications of measles include croup (see page 420), bronchiolitis (see page 421), bronchitis (see page

655), pneumonia (see page 660), and encephalitis (see page 694).

Symptoms

The initial symptoms of measles include irritability; fever; a runny nose; red, watery eyes; a dry, hacking cough; swollen glands; and, sometimes, diarrhea. In some cases, tiny white spots (called Koplik's spots) that resemble grains of salt appear inside the mouth. Within about 4 to 5 days, a rash of flat, pink spots (each about $\frac{1}{10}$ inch in diameter) begins to develop, first on the forehead and behind the ears, and then on the face, neck, trunk, arms, legs, and feet. A few days after it appears, the rash begins to fade and the fever breaks.

Some children with measles may be sensitive to bright light. Although this symptom is usually no cause for concern, tell your doctor because, in rare cases, it can be a sign of meningitis (see page 692), which can be life-threatening.

Diagnosis and Treatment

A diagnosis of measles is based on the child's symptoms and the results of a physical examination. The doctor will recommend having your child rest and giving him or her plenty of fluids, such as water, lemonade, fruit juice, or clear broth. He or she will recommend acetaminophen or ibuprofen (not aspirin) to help relieve the pain or reduce the fever. If your child is sensitive to bright light, dim the light in his or her room, or have him or her wear sunglasses. If your child develops a secondary bacterial infection such as a sore throat, an ear infection, or pneumonia, the doctor will prescribe antibiotics. Most children recover from measles within 10 to 14 days.

Prevention

To prevent measles, have your child vaccinated (see page 376) when he or she is 12 to 15 months old, and again between ages 4 and 6. A doctor may give an unvaccinated child who has been exposed to measles an injection of antibodies called immunoglobulin to fight the infection, or a measles vaccination within 72 hours of exposure to the virus.

Rubella

Rubella (also called German measles) is a mild viral infection that affects the skin and the lymph glands. The disease is usually contracted by inhaling airborne droplets coughed or sneezed into the air by an infected person. Rubella is slightly less common than measles (see previous page) and is not as contagious.

Symptoms

The initial symptoms of rubella include a slight fever and swollen glands behind the ears, down the side of the neck, and on the back of the neck. After 1 or 2 days, a rash of flat, reddish pink spots (each about $\frac{1}{10}$ inch in diameter) appears on the head or elsewhere on the body. Gradually, the spots may merge to form patches. The rash does not itch, and it lasts for about 3 days. Other possible symptoms include a runny or stuffy nose, red eyes, pain and swelling in the joints, and, in boys, pain and swelling in the testicles.

Diagnosis and Treatment

A diagnosis of rubella is based on the symptoms and the results of a physical examination. The doctor may recommend rest, plenty of fluids, and acetaminophen or ibuprofen (not aspirin) to reduce fever and relieve pain. Most children recover completely from rubella in about 1 week.

Prevention

A combined vaccine for measles, mumps, and rubella is available, and all children should be vaccinated (see page 376). Women who could become pregnant and who have not been vaccinated for rubella (see page 508) should be vaccinated to prevent a group of birth defects called congenital rubella syndrome, which includes cataracts, congenital heart disease, and low birth weight. Because the vaccination can cause birth defects, a woman should not get pregnant for at least 3 months after having the vaccination.

Roseola Infantum

Roseola infantum is a mild viral infection caused by one of two types of herpesvirus (type 6 or type 7). The infection is spread through contact with infected respiratory secretions or saliva. Roseola usually affects children between ages 6 months and 3 years.

Symptoms

The initial symptoms of roseola are usually irritability and a sudden high fever (between 101°F and 105°F). In some children, the fever may cause seizures (see page 410). After about 2 to 5 days, the child's temperature suddenly returns to normal (98.6°F). As the fever subsides, a raised rash of pink or red spots appears on the child's trunk and may quickly spread to his or her neck, face, arms, and legs. The rash usually lasts for no more than 3 to 5 days. Once the rash appears, the infection is no longer contagious. Along with the rash, the child may have flulike symptoms, including a sore throat, cough, swollen lymph glands in the neck, and diarrhea. He or she may refuse to drink when offered fluids. Except for the sudden high fever, the symptoms of roseola are usually mild.

Diagnosis and Treatment

A diagnosis of roseola infantum is based on the child's symptoms and a physical examination. In some cases, a doctor may order tests to rule out other possible causes of the symptoms.

Treatment for roseola focuses on reducing the fever. Give your child a sponge bath with lukewarm water and dress him or her in lightweight clothing. Do not use ice, cold water, rubbing alcohol, or a fan to lower your child's temperature; they can cause shivering, which can raise the temperature even more. The doctor will recommend that your child rest and drink plenty of fluids, including water, over-the-counter electrolyte solutions, sports drinks, or clear broth. The doctor also will recommend giving your child a nonprescription fever-reducing medication such as acetaminophen or ibuprofen. (Do not give aspirin to a child or adolescent who has a fever because aspirin has been linked to a potentially fatal disorder called Reye's syndrome; see page 411.)

Most children recover from roseola infantum in about a week. There is no vaccine available to prevent roseola, but having the disease usually provides lifelong immunity.

Fifth Disease

Fifth disease (also called erythema infectiosum or "slapped cheek" disease) is a highly contagious infection caused by a type of virus called a parvovirus. The infection spreads easily among children through direct contact. Outbreaks of fifth disease occur most often in the spring and early summer, affecting mostly children between ages 5 and 15. A possible complication of fifth disease is acute bone marrow failure, a life-threatening condition in which the bone marrow stops producing red blood cells (which deliver oxygen to tissues), white blood cells (which fight infection), and platelets (which enable blood to clot).

Symptoms

The main symptom of fifth disease is a rash of flat red spots, rings, or patches that make the face look like it's been slapped (because the sides of the face are bright red). However, the rash also may appear on the trunk, arms, legs, and buttocks and sometimes is accompanied by joint pain. Exercise or bathing can make the rash worse. Once the rash appears, the infection is no longer contagious. Other symptoms include a slight fever, a sore throat, swollen lymph glands in the neck, a headache, red eyes, a stuffy or runny nose, and diarrhea.

Diagnosis and Treatment

A diagnosis of fifth disease is based on a child's symptoms and a physical examination. In some cases, the doctor may order a blood test to detect the parvovirus. To treat fifth disease, doctors recommend rest, plenty of fluids, and acetaminophen or ibuprofen to reduce fever and relieve pain. (Do not give aspirin to a child or adolescent who has a fever because aspirin has been linked to a potentially fatal disorder called Reye's syndrome; see page 411.) Apply a soothing cream or lotion to the rash if it itches. Recovery usually takes about 10 days, although the rash can last for up to 3 weeks. If joint swelling occurs, it can last for months or even years.

Prevention

There is no vaccine available to prevent fifth disease, but having the disease usually provides lifelong immunity. Good hygiene, especially frequent handwashing, can help prevent the infection. Pregnant women who have been exposed to fifth disease should contact their doctor right away; an infection in the fetus can block fetal red blood cell production, which can lead to anemia or heart failure in the fetus, or can be fatal to the fetus.

Chickenpox

Chickenpox (also called varicella) is a very contagious viral infection caused by a type of herpesvirus called the varicella zoster virus, the same virus that, after years of dormancy, can cause shingles (see page 936) in adults. The infection usually occurs in late winter or early spring and primarily affects the skin and the membrane lining of the mouth and throat. A chickenpox vaccination is required for all children between 12 months and 23 months of age.

Symptoms

The main symptom of chickenpox is a rash of small, red, fluid-filled blisters that appears initially on the trunk and then spread to the face, arms, and legs. The rash may also appear on the scalp and genitals and inside the nose, ears, and mouth. After a few days, the blisters break open, dry out, crust over, and form scabs. Once the scabs have formed, the infection is no longer contagious. The rash is very itchy. Scratching is difficult to resist, but scratching the rash can produce scars. A child with chickenpox may also have a slight fever and abdominal pain, and may feel generally ill. Possible complications include pneumonia (see page 660), encephalitis (see page 694), and severe infections of the blisters.

Diagnosis and Treatment

A diagnosis of chickenpox is based on a child's symptoms and the results of a physical examination. Applying calamine lotion to the rash will help relieve itching. Oatmeal soaps or bath preparations and warm compresses can be helpful. Bathwater should be cool or lukewarm. If the rash occurs in the genital area, an anesthetic cream can be applied to relieve pain; ask the doctor to recommend one. If the rash becomes infected from excessive scratching, your doctor may prescribe a topical antibiotic ointment or an oral antibiotic. In some cases, doctors prescribe an antihistamine such as diphenhydramine to relieve itching. Trimming your child's nails if necessary can help prevent scratches.

Doctors sometimes recommend an injection of chickenpox antibodies called zoster immunoglobulin to prevent or reduce the severity of the disease in children who have an increased risk of complications, such as those with immune system disorders or who are undergoing chemotherapy for cancer. An antiviral drug called acyclovir, taken by mouth, is sometimes prescribed to reduce the severity of the infection or shorten it.

Give your child cold fluids and soft, bland foods.

Avoid salty or acidic foods and drinks. The doctor may recommend giving your child acetaminophen or ibuprofen to reduce fever and relieve pain. (Do not give aspirin to a child or adolescent who has a fever because aspirin has been linked to a potentially fatal disorder called Reye's syndrome; see page 411.) Most children with chickenpox recover within about 7 to 10 days.

Mumps

Mumps is a viral infection that causes inflammation and swelling of the saliva-producing (salivary) glands between the ear and the jaw. In some cases a child's joints, pancreas, testicles, or ovaries also may be affected. Mumps occurs most often in the spring and usually is spread through contact with infected saliva. The disease usually occurs in children ages 10 or older; having the infection provides lifelong immunity. Possible complications of mumps include encephalitis (see page 694), meningitis (see page 692), acute pancreatitis (see page 798), and orchitis (swelling of the testicle) in older boys. Doctors recommend that all children be vaccinated (see page 376) against mumps between 12 months and 15 months of age, and again between ages 4 and 6.

Symptoms

The main symptoms of mumps are swelling and tenderness on the sides of the face under the ears, which may be accompanied by an earache. In most cases, both sides of the face become swollen, one side of the face a few days before the other. A child can have difficulty talking, chewing, and swallowing. In most cases, he or she also has a headache, a fever (up to 103°F), loss of appetite, and diarrhea. If a child's testicle becomes swollen, symptoms include pain in the affected testicle, chills, a high fever (up to 106°F), nausea, and vomiting. Swelling of the ovaries or pancreas can cause discomfort or pain in the lower abdomen.

Diagnosis and Treatment

A diagnosis of mumps is based on a child's symptoms and the results of a physical examination. Have your child rest, and give him or her plenty of fluids, including water, fruit juice, sports drinks, tea, or decaffeinated soft drinks. Your doctor will recommend giving your child acetaminophen or ibuprofen (not aspirin) to relieve the pain and fever. You can also help relieve pain in the affected area by applying an ice pack wrapped in a towel. If the testicles are swollen, the doctor will prescribe medication to relieve the pain and swelling. Applying warm or cool packs to the testicles can often be helpful. A child with mumps usually recovers completely within about 10 to 12 days.

Whooping Cough

Whooping cough (also called pertussis) is a serious bacterial infection of the respiratory system caused by the bacterium Bordetella pertussis, which makes the air passages become inflamed, narrowed, and clogged with thick mucus. The infection is spread by inhaling droplets that have been sneezed or coughed into the air by an infected person. The severe coughing bouts that are characteristic of the infection, which can cause permanent damage to an infant's lungs or brain, are the body's attempts to clear the lungs of mucus. Young infants (6 months old or younger) can contract the disease from adolescents or adults who have not been vaccinated or whose vaccine protection has weakened over time.

All children are required to be vaccinated against whooping cough (in a combined vaccine with diphtheria and tetanus) starting at 2 months of age, and four more times up to age 6. A child who has been immunized against whooping cough may still develop a mild case of the infection. Having had whooping cough once does not provide lifelong immunity.

Symptoms

The early symptoms of whooping cough are coldlike symptoms, including a runny nose, dry cough, and slight fever. Unlike a cold, however,

---

WARNING!

Don't Give Cough Medicine for Whooping Cough

Do not give over-the-counter cough medications to a child with whooping cough. Your child needs to cough to prevent mucus from clogging his or her airways. Some over-the-counter cough medications contain ingredients that can suppress the cough and cause the airways to become blocked with mucus. If your child has a severe cough, talk to your doctor before giving him or her any medication.

---

the symptoms worsen after a few days. The nasal discharge thickens, and the coughing becomes more severe, occurring in episodes lasting up to 1 minute. During a bout of coughing, a child's face turns deep red, or even blue, from lack of oxygen. At the end of each coughing episode, as the child gasps for air, he or she makes the whooping sound that gives the disease its name. Infants with whooping cough tend to whoop more quietly than older children, or may not whoop at all.

After a bout of coughing, the child often vomits. The severe coughing phase of the disease can last from 2 to 10 weeks. Gradually the coughing and vomiting become less severe and less frequent, although a mild cough can persist for several months.

If your child has symptoms of whooping cough or has a cough that does not clear up within a few days and seems to be getting worse, talk to your doctor. If your child has symptoms of whooping cough, turns blue around the mouth or at the fingertips during a bout of coughing, or has difficulty breathing, call 911 or your local emergency number, or take him or her to the nearest hospital emergency department immediately.

Diagnosis

A diagnosis of whooping cough is based on a child's symptoms and the results of a physical examination. The doctor may order a blood test or a microscopic examination of secretions from the child's nose and throat to check for the infection-causing bacteria. He or she may recommend X-rays of the lungs to confirm the diagnosis. An infant with whooping cough may need to be hospitalized so the doctor can evaluate the severity of the disease and monitor it.

Treatment

To treat whooping cough, a child may need to be hospitalized and isolated from other children for a few days to help prevent the infection from spreading. Doctors monitor the child's breathing, suction out any secretions that are blocking the airways, and prescribe antibiotics to kill the bacteria. In some cases, doctors recommend supplemental oxygen to assist breathing and intravenous fluids to prevent dehydration.

When caring for your child at home, have him or her rest in bed. The doctor probably will recommend using a cool-mist vaporizer in the child's room at night to ease breathing during sleep. Keep your home free of environmental irritants, such as tobacco smoke, cooking smoke, aerosol sprays, and fireplace fumes. To help prevent vomiting, serve smaller, more frequent meals. To prevent dehydration, give your child plenty of fluids, such as water, fruit juice, or clear broth. Full recovery can take 5 to 10 weeks or longer.

Hand-Foot-and-Mouth Disease

Hand-foot-and-mouth disease is a mild viral infection caused by a type of virus called the coxsackievirus. The infection tends to occur during the summer and early fall, and usually affects children under age 10, especially those in preschool or day care.

The infection can be spread when a child inhales infected droplets coughed or sneezed into the air. The virus also can spread when an infected child touches the infected secretions in his or her nose or mouth or does not wash his or her hands properly after using the bathroom and then touches other children or shares toys, cups or glasses, eating utensils, or food.

Hand-foot-and-mouth disease is not related in any way to foot-and-mouth disease, which is caused by a different virus and occurs only in livestock such as cattle and sheep.

Symptoms

The initial symptoms of hand-foot-and-mouth disease include a sudden fever (a temperature between 101°F and 103°F), sore throat, and runny nose. A day or two after the fever begins, small red blisters appear inside the mouth—usually on the tongue and gums, inside the cheeks, and down the throat. The blisters break open and form open sores. Chewing and swallowing may become painful, and the child may lose his or her appetite. He or she may also avoid drinking, which can cause dehydration. A painful, red, blistery rash that is not itchy appears on the palms of the hands and the soles of the feet. The rash also may occur between the fingers and toes and on the thighs or buttocks or in the groin area.

Diagnosis and Treatment

To diagnose hand-foot-and-mouth disease, the doctor will ask about your child's symptoms and perform a physical examination. In some cases, a doctor may take a throat swab or a stool sample for laboratory analysis to detect the virus and confirm the diagnosis.

To treat hand-foot-and-mouth disease, give your child acetaminophen or ibuprofen (not aspirin) to relieve the pain and reduce the fever, and plenty of fluids to prevent dehydration. If he or she has trouble swallowing, try giving him or her ice chips to suck. Cold foods such as frozen yogurt or ice cream can help numb the inside of the mouth and relieve pain. Most children recover from the infection within about 10 days.

Prevention

To prevent hand-foot-and-mouth disease, wash your hands frequently and thoroughly, especially after using the bathroom or changing diapers. Teach your child to wash his or her hands carefully after using the bathroom. If your child has hand-foot-and-mouth disease, do not let him or her share cups, glasses, or eating utensils. Disinfect potentially contaminated surfaces in your home with a household cleaner. Wash your child's soiled clothing in detergent and hot water. Keep your child home from school or day care and away from other people until the fever is gone and the sores have healed.

Polio

Polio (poliomyelitis) is a viral infection that affects the brain and spinal cord. The infection can be spread through contact with an infected person or by ingesting food or water that is contaminated with the virus. Thanks to routine vaccination (see page 374), polio is now rare in the United States. Children are vaccinated against polio when they are 2 months, 4 months, 6 to 18 months, and 4 to 6 years of age.

Symptoms

In most cases, a polio infection is mild, does not affect the nervous system, and does not produce symptoms. In some cases, symptoms—such as a slight fever, sore throat, upset stomach, and headache—develop suddenly and disappear after a few days.

In rare cases, the virus causes a severe infection that produces muscle aches and twitching, and pain and stiffness in the neck, legs, and back. About a week after these initial symptoms, a person can develop paralysis, especially in the lower part of the trunk and in the legs. In severe cases, a person may have difficulty swallowing and breathing as a result of paralysis of the muscles in the throat and chest. The paralysis may be temporary or permanent. Some children have long-term muscle weakness that continues into adulthood, while others have no lasting effects. In some cases, the infection may be fatal.

Post-Polio Syndrome

Post-polio syndrome is a condition that affects about 25 percent of people who have recovered from polio. The syndrome, which occurs from 10 to 40 years after having polio, results from the death of motor neurons (nerve cells in the brain and spinal cord that control muscle activity) that did not die in the initial infection.

The symptoms of post-polio syndrome can include fatigue, slowly progressing muscle weakness, muscle and joint pain, difficulty swallowing, difficulty breathing, and, sometimes, muscle atrophy (shrinking or wasting of the muscles). The severity of the symptoms depends on the severity of the initial polio infection. Post-polio syndrome usually is not life-threatening unless a person's breathing becomes severely impaired.

To diagnose post-polio syndrome, a doctor usually orders tests such as an MRI (see page 113) to look for changes in the brain or spine or to rule out other possible neurological disorders, an examination of the electrical activity of the brain (electroencephalogram; see page 687), and a muscle biopsy (microscopic examination of small samples of muscle tissue). He or she may order a lumbar puncture, in which a hollow needle is inserted into the lower back to remove a small sample of cerebrospinal fluid (the fluid that surrounds the brain and spinal cord) for examination under a microscope.

There is no treatment for post-polio syndrome, and the condition cannot be prevented. For some people, a healthy diet and regular moderate exercise may help reduce the severity of the symptoms. People with impaired breathing may need a ventilator (an artificial breathing machine) to assist with breathing. Research to develop medications to relieve symptoms or to slow or reverse progression of the disease is ongoing.

Diagnosis and Treatment

A diagnosis of polio is based on the symptoms and the results of a physical examination. The doctor may take a small sample of stool for microscopic examination to check for the virus. He or she may recommend a lumbar puncture (see page 693) to detect the virus in cerebrospinal fluid (the liquid that surrounds the brain and spinal cord).

There is no effective treatment for polio. If a child has paralysis, he or she may be hospitalized and undergo physical therapy. If a child has difficulty breathing, he or she may be placed on a ventilator (an artificial breathing machine) to assist with breathing.

Scarlet Fever

Scarlet fever is a contagious bacterial infection of the throat that is caused by group A streptococci. Without prompt treatment with antibiotics, the bacteria multiply and produce a toxin that circulates in the blood. The two main complications of scarlet fever are rheumatic fever (see page 432), an inflammatory disease that affects tissues and organs throughout the body, and poststreptococcal glomerulonephritis (see page 428), inflammation of the filtering units of the kidneys (glomeruli).

Symptoms

The symptoms of scarlet fever can vary from child to child. However, in most cases, on the first day of the infection, a child develops a high fever (a temperature up to 104°F) and a red, sore throat and tonsils. Other possible symptoms include chills, body aches, loss of appetite, nausea, and vomiting. A whitish or yellowish coating may cover the tongue and tonsils.

On the second day, a bright red (scarlet), sometimes itchy rash that looks and feels like sandpaper appears on the child's face, except for the area just around the mouth. By the third day, the rash spreads to the child's neck, chest, back, arms, and legs. At the same time, the child's temperature begins to return to normal (98.6°F), and his or her tongue turns bright red. By the sixth day, the rash fades, and the skin and the tongue may begin to peel, exposing a red, raw surface underneath. The peeling process can last another 10 to 14 days.

Diagnosis and Treatment

A diagnosis of scarlet fever is based on a child's symptoms and the results of a physical examination. The doctor may also order a laboratory analysis of samples of secretions from the child's throat to check for group A streptococcal bacteria.

To treat scarlet fever, doctors prescribe either oral or intravenous antibiotics. It is very important for your child to take the entire prescription as instructed. The child may need to be isolated from other family members for the first 48 hours, when the infection is contagious. The doctor will recommend giving your child plenty of fluids, such as water, fruit juice, and clear broth. He or she also may recommend providing soft, bland foods or a liquid diet. Try using a cool-mist humidifier at night in the child's bedroom to help make breathing easier. A warm, moist towel applied to the child's neck can help soothe swollen glands.

There is no vaccine to prevent scarlet fever, and having the disease does not provide immunity. Most children with scarlet fever recover completely with no lasting effects.

Diphtheria

Diphtheria is a highly contagious, life-threatening bacterial infection that affects the nose and throat and usually occurs in children younger than 5. The bacteria that cause diphtheria can be spread by sneezing, coughing, or laughing. If not treated promptly, the infection can damage the heart, kidneys, and nervous system and can cause permanent disability or death. Diphtheria rarely occurs in the United States because of widespread childhood immunization against the disease. The vaccination is given in a combined vaccine with tetanus and whooping cough (DTaP; see page 376), beginning at 2 months of age and four more times up to age 6 years. Having diphtheria does not provide immunity.

Symptoms

The symptoms of diphtheria include sore throat, a slight fever, rapid heartbeat, swollen lymph glands in the neck, difficulty swallowing, difficulty breathing, and, occasionally, a thick, yellow discharge from the nose. In the advanced stages, symptoms can include double vision, slurred speech, paralysis, or shock (see page 579). The most dangerous symptom of diphtheria is a grayish membrane that forms on the throat and tonsils. The membrane may become large enough to cause croup (see page 420) or obstruct breathing. Contact your doctor immediately if your child has symptoms of diphtheria.

Diagnosis and Treatment

A diagnosis of diphtheria is based on a child's symptoms and the results of a physical examination. The doctor may order a blood test or a microscopic examination of secretions from the nose and throat to detect the diphtheria bacteria.

To treat diphtheria, a child is hospitalized and isolated from other patients to prevent the infection from spreading. He or she is given injections of antibiotics to kill the bacteria, and antitoxins to neutralize the toxins the bacteria produce. In some cases, these medications may be given intravenously (through a vein). If a child's breathing is blocked, a temporary tracheotomy (an airway opening cut into the windpipe) may be necessary to restore breathing, or a child may be put on a ventilator to assist breathing. Supplemental oxygen may also be necessary. If the bacterial toxin spreads to the kidneys, heart, or nervous system, the doctor may prescribe intravenous fluids or nonsteroidal anti-inflammatory drugs to reduce inflammation and assist breathing. The child will need to rest in bed for about 4 to 6 weeks or until he or she has recovered fully.

Pinworms

Pinworms are tiny white worms that frequently infest the intestines of young children. The eggs of pinworms can easily enter a child's body when he or she touches contaminated food or contaminated clothing, toys, or a sandbox. The eggs hatch in the intestines, and young worms quickly begin to grow into adults. About 2 weeks later, a mature female worm lays eggs around the child's anus during the night. This may cause irritation. If the child scratches the area, he or she can pick up some of the eggs on his or her fingers. If the child sucks his or her fingers or eats without washing them thoroughly, he or she can become reinfested. The pinworms can spread to other family members if the child touches food, drinking glasses, sheets, towels, or other shared household items.

Symptoms

Some children who have pinworms do not have any symptoms. Others experience itching between the buttocks and around the anus, usually at night. Some girls with pinworms may have vaginal itching and may experience pain when urinating. In many children, pinworms interfere with normal sleep.

Diagnosis

A diagnosis of pinworms is based on a child's symptoms and the results of a physical examination. Pinworms are sometimes visible in stool or may be visible around the child's anus, especially at night. You can confirm the presence of pinworms by briefly placing a strip of transparent tape across your child's anus in the early morning (before he or she has a bowel movement). Any eggs in the area will stick to the tape. Put the egg-infested tape in a plastic bag and take it to the doctor's office. The doctor can examine it under a microscope to confirm the diagnosis.

Treatment

Because pinworms spread easily, the doctor may recommend treating the entire family with prescription medications (antihelmintics) that kill worms. To relieve anal inflammation, the doctor may recommend applying a nonprescription ointment that contains a substance that kills pinworm eggs.

Because it is relatively easy to become reinfested with pinworms, the doctor will recommend that everyone in the household wash their hands thoroughly and frequently, especially after going to the toilet or handling a pet, and before touching food. All family members should cut their fingernails short and keep them short to reduce the risk of spreading the eggs. To kill the pinworm eggs, change all bed linens and underwear daily, wash them in very hot water, and dry them on high heat. Because pets can also be infested with pinworms, your doctor will recommend taking your pets to a veterinarian for evaluation and treatment.

2

Adolescent Health

Adolescence is the transition period from childhood to adulthood. Changes associated with adolescence normally begin soon after age 10 in girls and after 12 in boys. Adolescence is generally considered to last to age 18 or 20, although there are individual variations. Growth toward physical maturity tends to level off soon after age 17 in both sexes. During these developmental years, a person undergoes physical, mental, and emotional changes that can make adolescence an especially difficult time.

Physical and Sexual Development at Puberty

A person experiences physical changes during puberty that transform him or her from a child into an adult who is capable of reproducing. Puberty is relatively short, usually lasting about 5 to 7 years.

Although the hormonal changes that signal the beginning of puberty usually start at about age 10 in girls and 12 in boys, there are wide variations in adolescent growth patterns. While both boys and girls grow taller and gain weight during puberty, girls generally start their growth spurt much earlier than boys. Body weight can double during this period, usually because of a hormone-influenced increase in muscle mass in boys and fat in girls. Heredity is an important factor in sexual development—a girl usually starts menstruating at about the same age as her mother or a grandmother. A boy's physical and sexual development is likely to follow the pattern of his father or grandfathers.

Whether an adolescent develops earlier or later than his or her peers can also depend on factors such as general health. For example, poor nutrition or illness during childhood may delay the onset of puberty. In addition, a child who is smaller or thinner than average is likely to develop relatively late. Girls who are overweight tend to start puberty earlier than girls of normal weight, probably because fat cells produce the female hormone estrogen.

Most adolescents are preoccupied with their changing body and concerned about being and appearing normal. Boys may worry about their height and the size of their penis, and girls about their breasts and weight. The age at which body hair begins to grow and menstruation begins varies. Many boys and girls begin to develop earlier or later than the average ages. But if your child's development is unusually early or late, see your pediatrician.

Physical and Sexual Development in Girls

Puberty can begin as early as age 8 or 9 in girls, with breast development as the first sign. It is not uncommon for one breast to begin to grow before the other. Breasts usually do not grow much beyond the age of 16. A girl should see her pediatrician if breast development has not begun by age 13.

Development of body hair varies greatly and depends largely on heredity. Pubic hair usually is noticeable at the start of puberty, while underarm hair begins to grow a year or two later (around age 12 or 13) and darkens and thickens as puberty progresses. An increase in perspiration under the arms and in the groin contributes to a body odor that does not occur in younger children.

Menstruation (see page 845) begins 2 to 3 years after the onset of puberty in girls at an average age of about 12 years. Menstruation often begins with extremely irregular menstrual periods (that are sometimes months apart) but periods usually become regular (about 3 to 7 days of menstrual flow every 28 days) about 2 to 3 years after a girl's first period. Girls who have painful periods (see page 848) or who are extremely uncomfortable before their periods (premenstrual syndrome; see page 850) should see their doctor, who can recommend medication to prevent or lessen the discomfort associated with menstruation. Delayed periods (called primary amenorrhea) are usually the result of a naturally late onset of puberty, but it may be caused by a hormonal disorder or by an abnormality of the reproductive system.

A girl who is 14 years old and has not yet had a period, has not begun to develop breasts or pubic hair, and has not had a growth spurt should see her doctor. He or she will do a thorough evaluation that includes a health history, physical examination, and laboratory tests. If a girl has not started to

Precocious Puberty

Normal sexual development in children varies widely, mostly depending on heredity. Most girls start to go through puberty at about age 11 and boys at age 12 or 13. Precocious puberty is defined as the onset of sexual development before age 8 in girls and 9½ in boys. It occurs in about one out of every 5,000 children and is much more common in girls than in boys.

In most cases of precocious puberty (especially in girls), sexual development simply occurs earlier than expected, with no known cause. Some boys inherit a gene that brings on early puberty. About 15 percent of cases of precocious puberty result from underlying medical conditions such as central nervous system tumors (see page 682), Albright's syndrome (a disorder characterized by a group of abnormalities including irregular skin-color patches, bone deformities, and early puberty), an underactive thyroid gland (hypothyroidism; see page 903), or adrenal gland disorders.

Some children who start puberty prematurely rapidly grow taller than their peers at first but end up being shorter because the hormonal changes stop their growth before they have reached a normal adult height. Children who develop early often feel different from their peers, which can sometimes cause emotional distress. A child who develops prematurely should be evaluated by his or her doctor.

To diagnose precocious puberty, doctors use blood tests to measure hormone levels, along with observation of a child's physical changes and a complete physical examination. They may also order X-rays of the hand and wrist, taken in succession over time, to calculate bone growth. An ultrasound examination of the ovaries may be used to help compare the size of a girl's ovaries with the standard size for girls her age. A CT scan or MRI of the brain and abdomen may be done to rule out a brain or abdominal tumor as the cause of precocious puberty.

The goal of treatment for precocious puberty is to stop and possibly reverse the premature sexual development; the treatment varies depending on the cause. For example, if precocious puberty has resulted from an adrenal gland tumor, removal of the tumor will correct the condition. In most cases, a doctor prescribes a hormone (given by injection or nasal spray) that suppresses the body's production of sex hormones (estrogen in girls; testosterone in boys). Once the hormone treatment is stopped, the body's own hormone function gradually returns and the process of puberty continues normally.

menstruate by age 16 but is fully developed physically, she should see her doctor.

Female hormones stimulate an increase in fat all over the body, but mostly on the hips, thighs, and buttocks. Girls have a normally higher proportion of fat to muscle and bone than boys do. Also, a girl's pelvis widens during puberty.

Physical and Sexual Development in Boys

In boys, puberty begins at about age 12 or 13 (and continues until 17 or 18). Puberty can begin as early as $9\frac{1}{2}$ years of age, and continue until 21 years of age in boys who start puberty late. A boy's testicles and scrotum (the pouch of skin and tissue that holds the testicles) usually start to enlarge by age 11 or 12 and stop by age 16 or 17. One testicle may appear to be larger or hang lower than the other; this is normal. As the testicles grow, the skin of the scrotum darkens.

The penis lengthens before it grows broader at about age 12 or 13; growth stops at about 15 or 16. The ability to ejaculate semen (a fluid produced by the male reproductive organs that contains sperm) begins about a year after the penis starts to grow. At about the time that a boy's penis starts to lengthen and widen, he usually starts having more frequent erections. It is normal to have erections for no apparent reason, although erections usually occur with sexual excitement or physical stimulation. Spontaneous erections generally go away after a few minutes and are not noticeable to anyone else. Some boys (but not all) have erections and ejaculate during their sleep when they are dreaming (nocturnal emissions, or wet dreams), which is a normal part of sexual development. Many boys worry about the size (or shape) of their penis. If changes in the testicles or penis are not noticeable in a boy by age 15, he should see his pediatrician.

Pubic hair is visible by age 11 or 12, but underarm hair may not appear until 13 or even 15. As in girls, the development of hair on the body varies from person to person and depends on heredity. Although pubic and underarm hair usually stop growing noticeably by about age 16 (depending on when growth started), hair on the chest and abdomen usually continues growing into adulthood. Sweating and underarm odor, along with the development of sweat glands in the groin, usually are first noticeable between ages 13 and 15.

In boys and young men, the larynx enlarges, making the Adam's apple more prominent, and the vocal cords become longer and thicker, causing the voice to deepen at about age 14. During this time a boy's voice may fluctuate between high and low, cracking or breaking (changing pitch) unexpectedly. The deepening may occur gradually or rapidly. If a boy still has a childlike voice at age 16, he should see a doctor. A boy usually starts growing a beard at about the time his voice changes. Beards grow slowly at first and get heavier with age.

The male hormone testosterone makes muscles grow larger in most boys, especially the muscles in the shoulders and upper chest. Testosterone also causes the bones to lengthen, giving most boys a heavier bone structure and longer arms and legs than girls.

Health Concerns During Adolescence

Adolescence is a good time for teens to begin taking responsibility for their health by adopting a healthy lifestyle. Along with disorders that can occur at any age, some health problems are common in adolescents. For example, acne (see page 1065) is a chronic skin disorder affecting the face and back that almost always begins at puberty. Sports injuries (see page 978) are common among teenagers. Headaches, particularly migraines (see page 684), may appear for the first time during adolescence. Infectious mononucleosis (see page 935) is a viral infection that often develops during the teen years. Some forms of cancer—such as Hodgkin's disease (see page 626) or leukemia (see page 621)—often first appear in adolescents and young adults.

Stages of Puberty in Girls and Boys

Stages of Puberty in Girls

Puberty starts in the brain when the hypothalamus stimulates the pituitary gland to signal the ovaries to produce hormones. These hormones stimulate the ovaries to produce estrogen. Girls have a significant growth spurt starting at about age 10, brought on by sex hormones such as estrogen. Because of estrogen, girls have a higher ratio of fat to muscle and bone than boys do. Girls grow and develop earlier than boys and are usually taller and bigger than boys of the same age. By age 18, girls have usually reached their full adult height and often weigh nearly double what they weighed when puberty began.

Prepuberty

In the period immediately preceding puberty, there are no visible signs of sexual development, but the ovaries are getting ready to produce female sex hormones.

Early puberty

The first outward signs of puberty appear. Girls have a slight increase in the size of their breasts and, sometimes, more prominent nipples caused by the growth of breast tissue beneath. Girls start to grow quickly at this stage, not only getting taller but also rapidly putting on weight. Pubic hair grows in sparsely.

Middle puberty

Breasts become slightly larger, and pubic hair starts to fill in. Underarm hair and an increase in perspiration under the arms occur about a year or two after the appearance of pubic hair. Skin, particularly on the face, becomes more oily, possibly causing acne.

Late puberty

Girls grow taller and their weight increases. The breasts become fuller and nipples more prominent. Pubic hair is almost completely grown in. A white discharge from the vagina will appear from 6 to 12 months before a girl's first menstrual period. Ovulation (the development and release of an egg from an ovary) may begin at about this time but usually does not become regular for a few years. Even with irregular periods and infrequent ovulation, it is possible to become pregnant at this time.

Maturity

Girls reach their full physical and sexual maturity at an average age of about 18. They reach their full adult height, and their breasts reach their adult size. Ovulation and menstrual periods usually become regular.

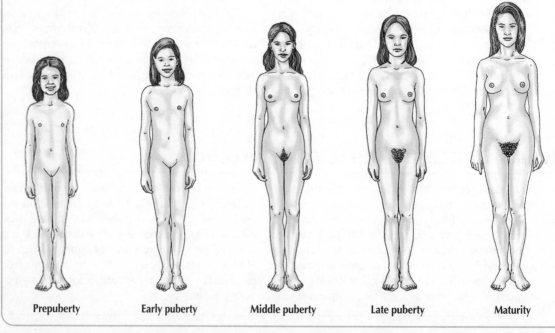

| Prepuberty | Early puberty | Middle puberty | Late puberty | Maturity |

Stages of Puberty in Boys

In boys, puberty starts when the hypothalamus produces sex hormones that are then excreted by the pituitary gland in the brain. These hormones act on the testicles to increase the secretion of the male sex hormone testosterone and other sex hormones. Testosterone increases muscle and bone mass. Boys may be temporarily shorter and smaller than girls of the same age but usually will be taller and heavier than most girls their age by the time they are 21.

Prepuberty

No signs of sexual development are visible before puberty, but the testicles are preparing to release sex hormones.

Early puberty

During this stage, the first signs of puberty appear. Boys will notice an enlargement of their testicles and scrotum.

Middle puberty

Pubic hair begins to grow during this stage. The penis grows longer, and boys may be able to ejaculate. Perspiration increases, and underarm hair may start to grow. The testicles continue to grow. Skin is oily, possibly causing acne. Because the vocal cords are starting to grow, the voice may crack or change pitch.

Late puberty

Pubic hair fills in during late puberty. The penis grows longer and thicker, and the skin of the scrotum and penis darkens. Facial hair starts to grow, mostly on the upper lip and chin. At this stage, a growth spurt takes place, and boys get noticeably taller.

Maturity

At this stage, boys reach physical and sexual maturity (usually between ages 18 and 21). The dramatic growth in height slows considerably. Pubic hair may have spread to cover the inner thighs. Hair may start to grow on the chest.

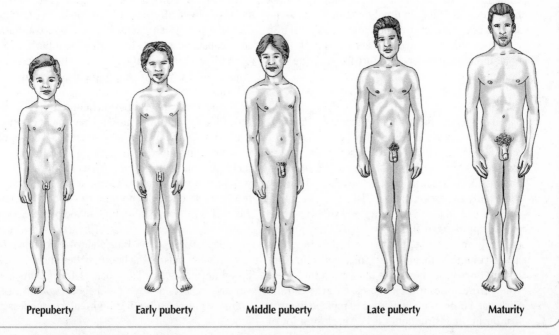

| Prepuberty | Early puberty | Middle puberty | Late puberty | Maturity |

Nutrition

Not eating the right foods, eating too much, or not eating enough during adolescence can lead to life-long health problems or life-threatening diseases such as obesity, cancer, diabetes, heart disease, and osteoporosis. The tremendous physical growth that occurs during puberty requires good nutrition. To meet their energy needs throughout the day, teens should eat at least three healthy meals, including a good breakfast. Teens often eat on the run. A wide variety of healthful foods available at home—such as fresh fruits, low-fat cheeses and yogurt, and cut-up raw vegetables with a low-fat bean dip or salsa—may help keep teens from eating the high-fat, high-sugar, high-calorie foods they normally reach for first. Sodas and diet sodas have little or no nutritional value.

Calcium

Teens, especially girls, need to eat foods that are high in calcium, such as low-fat dairy products, fish with edible bones (such as salmon and sardines), and dark green vegetables (such as collard greens, broccoli, and kale). They should have three or more servings a day of calcium-rich foods. Nearly all of a person's total bone mass is formed by the end of the teen years. Children who don't take in enough calcium may not develop their maximum potential bone mass. Building optimal bone mass by doing weight-bearing exercise and eating foods high in calcium can help prevent or delay the onset of the bone-thinning disorder osteoporosis (see page 989) later in life.

Iron

The daily requirement for iron increases dramatically starting at age 10, especially between ages 11 and 18, because of increased muscle mass and an expanded volume of blood. Iron can be found in animal foods such as beef, chicken and turkey (especially the dark meat), or fish. Strict vegetarians (see page 43) can get their daily supply of iron from plant foods such as dried beans, leafy greens, nuts, and dried fruits, but they will have to eat a larger volume of them to get sufficient iron. Adolescent boys need more iron than when they were younger because of their increased growth rate. Girls need even more than boys to replace the iron lost during menstruation. Girls who lose a lot of blood during heavy menstrual periods are at risk of developing iron deficiency anemia (see page 610). Symptoms of iron deficiency anemia include fatigue, irritability, headaches, and tingling in the hands and feet.

Folic Acid

Folic acid, a B vitamin, is an essential nutrient, especially for girls and women of childbearing age. A deficiency of folic acid during pregnancy can cause neural tube defects such as spina bifida (see page 398) in a fetus. All adolescent girls should get at least 400 micrograms of folic acid every day, either in a supplement (all multivitamin supplements include folic acid) or in food. Good sources of folic acid include green, leafy vegetables; fruit; cheese; legumes; liver; and fortified breakfast cereals and other grain products.

Calorie Intake

Calorie needs depend on a teen's individual growth rate and physical activity level. During the rapid growth spurt between ages 15 and 19, some boys are able to eat up to 4,000 calories a day without gaining weight. However, once this growth spurt ends, they can quickly gain unwanted pounds that will be difficult to lose as they get older. Girls usually stop growing by age 15 and tend to be less physically active than boys. Girls (and inactive boys) can easily become overweight if they consume more calories than they burn. Most of the beverages (including soda, fruit juices, and whole milk) that teens drink are also very high in calories.

Many teens have busy schedules that allow little time for nutritious meals. They find it easier to eat fast-food meals and processed snacks, which tend to be high in calories and fat. As a result, an increasing number of American teenagers are overweight and beginning to have many of the health problems associated with obesity—including type 2 diabetes (see page 894), high blood pressure (see page 574), and early signs of heart disease (see page 559). Parents have little control over their adolescent's diet outside the home so they should stock up on nutritious snacks—such as fresh fruits and vegetables, low-fat yogurt and cheeses, and whole grains—and resist buying high-calorie processed foods.

Body Image

Being obsessed with their weight or appearance leads some girls, and an increasing number of boys, to develop eating disorders (see page 724) such as anorexia or bulimia. Some teens think they need to be thinner than they should be based on their body build and height. During adolescence, girls often start dieting to lose the additional fat that comes with puberty. Boys usually develop eating disorders as a result of a desire to succeed in sports or to meet a sport's weight requirements. Most eating disorders start during adolescence. Having an eating disorder can lead to changes in the body's metabolism, damage to internal organs, and skin and dental problems. Symptoms include fainting, anxiety, dry skin, and fine hair all over the body. In girls who have bulimia, scars may form on the hands or knuckles. Girls who become too thin can stop having menstrual periods.

Some teens (usually boys) will grow into their body and lose weight as they get taller. If a child is concerned about his or her weight or unsure what it should be, a doctor can evaluate it and determine whether the teen needs to lose weight. The doctor can work with him or her to develop a weight-loss plan (see page 53) and help the teen learn the basics of a healthy diet (see page 36).

Exercise

Along with overeating, lack of exercise is a major factor in the epidemic of obesity among young people in the United States. Only about one out of three American adolescents gets enough exercise. Many children spend more time sitting in front of a TV or computer than engaging in physical activities. Teens who play sports and are physically active are less likely than their less active peers to have medical problems such as diabetes and obesity. They are also less likely to smoke, drink, have an unplanned pregnancy, or commit suicide, possibly because exercise improves mood and lowers stress and anxiety. Organized sports have the added benefit of instilling discipline and teamwork and developing skills.

Weight-bearing exercise (such as walking, running, aerobics, and lifting light weights) makes bones strong and helps them take in the bone-building mineral calcium, which is especially important for adolescent girls. However, young people should not aggressively train with weights until their bodies are fully physically mature, usually between ages 15 and 18. Lifting weights that are too heavy and lifting incorrectly (for example, lifting the weights with a jerk, as professional power lifters do) can cause injuries. In addition, lifting weights that are too heavy can inhibit (rather than strengthen) bone growth in adolescents by putting pressure on still-growing bones.

A teen should pick a sport or physical activity that he or she enjoys. Interacting with people who have the same interests can help teens stick with an exercise program. The most successful activities are those that help them develop skills while having fun. Ideally, teens should try to exercise 6 days a week for at least 60 minutes, but any amount of

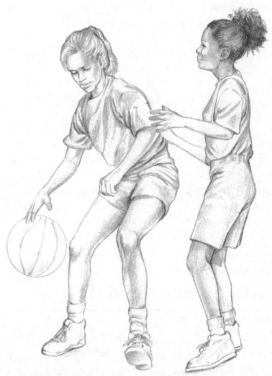

Participating in a sport
Belonging to a team or playing a sport not only contributes to overall physical health but also can build self-confidence and make teens less likely to be bored and have the spare time that can lead to risky behavior.

exercise is better than none. Exercising longer and harder has additional health benefits. However, adolescent girls who exercise too much and eat too little can develop a disorder called female athlete triad (see page 847).

Getting Enough Sleep

Sleep problems (see page 703), such as not getting enough sleep and falling asleep and waking at unusual hours, are common among teenagers. Teenagers require more sleep—9 to 10 hours a day—than children who are even slightly younger, and more than most adults. It is normal for teenagers to have difficulty falling asleep in the evening and difficulty waking in the morning because their biological clock is "off" in the daytime when they should be awake, and "on" in the evening when they should be sleeping. Adolescents who get 6 to 7 hours of sleep a night fall asleep more often during the day, especially during sedentary activities (such as sitting in a classroom or driving). Cutting back on sleep, even by 1 or 2 hours, has been linked to poor school performance, irritability, and vehicle collisions. Over time, increased levels of the stress hormone cortisol (brought on by lack of sleep) can damage brain cells directly and cause memory and learning problems.

Exposure to bright light (about 30 to 40 minutes first thing in the morning) as well as going to bed and waking up at the same time every day can help reset an adolescent's biological clock. It also helps if teens leave a little time at the end of the day to unwind. They should also limit their intake of caffeine during the day and avoid exercising right before going to bed.

Staying Healthy: What Can Parents Do?

● Provide nutritious, well-balanced meals (see page 36). Girls especially need to get enough calcium (1,200 to 1,500 milligrams a day) during adolescence to build strong bones.

● Encourage your child to be physically active with activities such as walking, dancing, or sports.

● Try to see that your child goes to bed and wakes up at about the same time on weekdays and weekends, and that he or she gets 9 to 10 hours of sleep every day.

● Make sure that your teen does not take on too many activities. Think of ways to make his or her schedule more manageable, such as working fewer hours or dropping an activity. School, homework, sports, after-school activities, and a job may not provide time for an adequate amount of sleep, time with family, or nutritious meals.

● Make appointments for your teenager for regular medical checkups. Girls need to start having regular pelvic examinations (see page 140) and Pap smears at age 18—younger if they are or are about to become sexually active, or if they have menstrual problems.

● Make sure your child is aware of health self-examinations he or she should be performing regularly. Girls should begin doing monthly breast self-examinations (see page 138) by age 18. Boys should begin doing testicle self-examinations (see page 139) at puberty.

Adolescent Sexuality

Parents often have unrealistic views of their children's sexuality and are unaware that their children are sexually active. However, most adolescents experiment with relationships and sex and, by the time they graduate from high school, many have had sexual experiences. It is important for parents to talk with their children about relationships, including the roles of sex, self-respect, and love. The more knowledge adolescents have about sex (including about contraception and safer sex), the less likely they are to engage in irresponsible or early sexual activity. Parents who find it difficult to talk about sex (or are not sure what to say) should ask their doctor to talk to their teen for them or ask the doctor to recommend a book to give to the teenager on the subject. However, parents should be available and willing to discuss any questions their children (of any age) have.

Pregnancy: A Responsibility of Both Partners

Adolescents who are having sex should actively prevent an unwanted pregnancy. Each year in the United States, nearly 800,000 unintended pregnancies occur in girls 15 to 19 years old. A boy and a girl should both use contraception (see page 470)—including for their first experience with sexual intercourse. It is possible for a girl to become pregnant even if she has not begun menstruating because the first egg could be released from an ovary (and fertilized by the boy's sperm) in the days before she has her first period.

Most teenagers are not adequately educated about their reproductive potential and the risk of unintended pregnancy. Timing sex based on a girl's menstrual period, either by having intercourse only during a girl's period or by using the rhythm method (see page 474), is not reliable; sperm can live for up to 7 days after intercourse and the release of an egg may not occur at the same time every month (or may occur more than once in a cycle).

Some teens think that a girl will not get pregnant if she does not have an orgasm during sex or if they have sex in particular positions (such as while standing up or with the girl on top). These misconceptions frequently lead to unexpected pregnancies. If a teen is ready to have sex, he or she should seek information in advance about sex, reproduction, and contraception. Teens can get information about contraception from their doctor or a family planning clinic such as Planned Parenthood; all inquiries are confidential and will not be shared with parents or anyone else without the teen's permission.

If a pregnancy occurs, both partners should talk to their parents as soon as possible. The earlier they talk to someone and get help, the more options they will have. The girl should see her doctor right away—girls younger than 16 who are pregnant are at high risk for disorders such as anemia (see page 610), high blood pressure (see page 574), sexually transmitted diseases (STDs; see page 477), and difficult labor.

The girl will have to decide whether to continue with the pregnancy (and raise the child or arrange for an adoption) or have an abortion (see page 506). If she decides to have an abortion, it is safer and easier to do so as early in the pregnancy as possible. Because there are legal restrictions on the availability of abortion to minor children in some states, talk to your doctor or call your local chapter of Planned Parenthood for information.

Boys and girls are equally responsible for supporting a child. Either can be held legally responsible for child support until the child is 18 years old. When a pregnancy occurs in very young teenagers, legal issues may need to be explored, such as the possibility of incest or sexual assault.

Practicing Safer Sex

Each year, more than 3 million new cases of sexually transmitted diseases (STDs; see page 477) occur in children between ages 10 and 19. Chlamydia and gonorrhea, two of the most common STDs, occur more often in teenagers than in any other age group. One in five people over age 12 has genital herpes, which is incurable. Most people who develop AIDS in their 20s were infected with HIV (the virus that causes AIDS) in their teens. The more people a teen has sex with, the greater the risk of acquiring an STD. Many teens are infected with STDs and don't know it. The most reliable way to protect against STDs if you are having sex is to use a latex condom correctly every time you have sex—although condoms are not 100 percent reliable in preventing STDs. If you are diagnosed with an STD, your partner should also be treated.

Abstinence

The only sure way to avoid STDs is not to have sex. Teenagers benefit from putting off sex and learning other ways to be involved in a close relationship. Having sex does not solve relationship problems, and is often the cause of new problems. Teens who abstain from sex—that is, who avoid oral, anal, or vaginal contact—eliminate the risk of an unwanted pregnancy or an STD. Without the maturity that a healthy sexual relationship requires, teenagers can more safely and easily develop a trusting relationship based on friendship and mutual understanding and respect.

Each person in a relationship should expect his or her feelings to be respected. If they are not, the teen should get out of the relationship. Teens who don't want to have sex should not allow themselves to be pressured into having sex with coercive statements such as "Everyone is doing it," "If you loved me, you would," or "If you don't have sex with me, someone else will." Even if teens have already had sexual experiences, it isn't too late to abstain from sexual activity until they feel they are ready to accept the emotional commitment and responsibility that a sexual relationship involves.

Sexual Activities Other Than Intercourse

While the percentage of teenagers having intercourse is falling, the percentage of teens who engage in other sexual activities seems to be on the rise. Many adolescents think that having oral sex or "outercourse" (mutual masturbation) rather than vaginal or anal intercourse is not actually having sex and will prevent them from being infected with STDs. Oral sex is not necessarily safer than sexual intercourse—any STD can be transmitted through oral sex. Using a condom or a dental dam for oral sex may help prevent some STDs, but few teenagers use these methods of protection. Sexual activities that involve mutual masturbation or mechanical sex enhancers (such as vibrators) pose a risk for some STDs such as herpes (see page 482), genital warts (HPV; see page 480), or scabies (see page 938).

Homosexuality

Most homosexual people realize that they are attracted sexually to people of the same sex during adolescence. A person's sexual orientation is established in childhood through a combination of genetic, biological, psychological, and environmental influences. Although biology plays a major role, no specific hormonal or psychological influences have been identified. Parents have little influence on their children's sexual orientation—and children raised by homosexual parents are no more likely to be homosexual than children raised by heterosexual parents. Kissing or holding hands or having sexual experiences with a person of the same sex during adolescence may simply be sexual experimentation and does not necessarily indicate that a person is homosexual.

Homosexual teenagers have an especially difficult time during adolescence because they fear the rejection of their family and friends. The biggest problems with their homosexuality are often social and emotional issues. A network of friends, especially from within the homosexual community, can give a gay teen the support he or she needs. If a teen is having a difficult time accepting his or her sexuality, he or she can benefit from talking to a counselor who specializes in helping people accept their sexual orientation and learn positive, healthy ways to deal with it.

Sexuality: What Can Parents Do?

The single most important thing you can do as a parent to help your child develop a healthy understanding of sex and sexual relationships is to be available and open in discussing the topic and answering questions. Having this knowledge can give your teen self-confidence and enable him or her to make responsible decisions about sex. Here are some tips:

- Make sure your children are well informed about sex.

- Encourage your children to ask questions about sex, and give them honest answers.

- Stress that there are other ways than sex to have a close relationship with someone. Suggest going dancing or to movies, plays, or sporting events; participating in sports; or going out with a group of friends.

- Explain the risks of oral sex. Many teenagers think they are "abstaining" from sex by engaging in nonintercourse sexual activities. They don't realize that they can contract many sexually transmitted diseases (STDs)—including chlamydia, gonorrhea, herpes, genital warts, and HIV—through oral sex.

- Explain the risks of sexual intercourse, including pregnancy and STDs. Teenagers also need to know where they can be treated for STDs, and that not all STDs can be cured. Emphasize the importance of reporting an STD to a doctor so that all of their sexual contacts can be located and treated. Stress that they themselves would want to know if they had been exposed to an STD, and that all such reports are kept confidential.

- Inform your teen about all available contraceptive techniques (see page 470). Condoms help prevent pregnancy and provide some protection against STDs. If you are not sure about the facts, refer your child to a family planning clinic such as Planned Parenthood. Reassure your child that all health visits and records are confidential.

- Accept your child's sexuality; if your child tells you that he or she is homosexual (or if you think he or she may be), accept the possibility and get information and support from a support organization such as Parents, Families and Friends of Lesbians and Gays (PFLAG).

Psychological, Emotional, and Behavioral Development

The physical, mental, and emotional changes that take place during adolescence can make it an especially difficult time for both the adolescent and his or her parents. At the same time that relationships are getting more complicated, classes are getting harder and peer pressure is at its peak.

Independence is necessary for healthy growth, and it helps teens learn to make good choices. Most teens get through these years safely by learning through experience, sometimes making some bad choices that have no long-term, harmful consequences. Adolescents learn to become independent by expressing their individuality in a number of ways, such as through music, clothes, or hairstyles. These forms of rebellion are often part of a teenager's growth toward independence and maturity. In some cases, however, teens make poor choices, or their life experiences become too difficult for them to handle. Other teens may develop psychological or emotional problems that require treatment by mental health professionals.

The severity of a teen's behavior or emotions is usually what distinguishes the average teen from one who has psychological or emotional problems. Here are some ways to tell if your teen's behavior is normal or if he or she is having problems coping. Most teens:

- Are sad sometimes or cry easily—but their mood eventually improves.
- Worry about their appearance and experiment with diets or exercise programs—but don't jeopardize their health.
- Skip a class or two—but not enough to fail a class or get poor grades.
- Worry about their popularity—but not to the point where they are unable to deal with everyday life.

Mental and Emotional Health in Teens: What Can Parents Do?

Although their friends and peers are of increasing importance, for most teenagers, parents and family are the most important influences. Use your influence to help your children face the many choices and decisions they have to make at this time in their lives.

- Be available, both physically and emotionally. Spend as much time as you can with your children.
- Show affection. Hug or kiss your children or use words to show that you care about them.
- Compliment teenagers often and tell them you are proud of them.
- Set clear, reasonable expectations for your children.
- Be a good role model. Behave in the way you want your children to behave.
- Spend more time listening than talking. Showing an interest in what your children have to say makes them feel important and boosts their self-esteem.
- Don't be judgmental. Accepting your children's ideas and feelings will make them more likely to confide in you.
- Do not compare your child to other children.
- Never ridicule your child.

- Give advice, not orders. Avoid nagging. Teens need reliable information from someone they trust, but they have to learn many things for themselves.
- Take an interest in your children's activities.
- Get to know your children's friends. Are they people you want your child to be around? Your teen is likely to drink alcohol or smoke cigarettes if his or her friends do. Having a friend who has attempted suicide is strongly associated with a teen's own risk of suicide.
- Stay in contact with your children's teachers. Keep an eye on school performance. Poor performance in school is linked to smoking, alcohol and drug use, violent behavior, and suicide.
- Keep track of how your children spend their free time, and know where they are. Children with too much free time away from adults can get into trouble and are at increased risk of smoking, drinking alcohol, and using drugs. Encourage bored teens to join an activity, sport, or club (or start one of their own). You can also suggest activities such as household chores, reading, tutoring, or doing volunteer work in the community.

- Spend a lot of time by themselves in their room—but not for days at a time.
- Are often frustrated with home life or their parents—but not enough to run away from home.
- May be distracted—but not to the extent that they do poorly in school or get fired from a job.
- Get moody or irritable—but are pleasant most of the time.
- Argue or lose their temper—but will not become physically violent.

Tattoos and Body Piercings

During adolescence, every generation finds ways to make itself different from the previous generation. Creating a separate identity through body modification is often part of the process. If a teen changes his or her appearance as a form of self-expression, it usually is not harmful. Some teens get tattoos or piercings to make a social statement, fit in with their friends, emulate a favorite celebrity, or rebel against the standard forms of beauty. However, it is illegal in most states for anyone under 18 to get piercings or tattoos without a parent's consent.

Some parents find it hard to accept tattoos and piercings because they worry about what other people might think and because tattoos are permanent. If your child wants to get a tattoo or piercing, discuss the short- and long-term consequences. Tattoos and piercings pose the risk of a bacterial or viral infection such as hepatitis B or C (see page 786) from unsterile conditions or contaminated needles. A person can't give blood for a year after getting a tattoo or piercing because of the risk of transmitting hepatitis.

A piercing can take up to 2 years to heal. Piercings around the mouth or in the tongue can cause cracked teeth, nerve damage or paralysis, or difficulty speaking—and can be swallowed accidentally. Piercings also can get caught on clothes and other objects and rip the skin.

Tattoos are expensive and difficult to remove. If your teen decides to get a tattoo or piercing, make sure it is done by a highly skilled, licensed professional.

If a teen gets more and more tattoos or piercings and never seems satisfied, or if tattoos are large or in highly visible places (such as the forehead) or are obscene or violent, the teen may have a psychological or emotional problem. Some teens like to provoke a reaction in other people. If you think your teen's behavior is harming him or her, or is disturbing to others, discuss the situation with your doctor or a mental health professional. Your teen could probably benefit from counseling.

Smoking and Using Tobacco

Almost all adults who smoke cigarettes (see page 27) became addicted by the time they were 17. The

What Teens Should Know About Smoking and Tobacco

Teens who smoke rarely respond to warnings about the health effects of smoking because most problems develop only after many years of smoking. Try to get your teen to stop smoking or using other tobacco products (or not to start) by stressing the negative effects that are most important to him or her now:

- **Attractiveness**   Few teens want to date someone who smokes. They say that seeing someone smoke turns them off and that they don't like being around smokers.

- **Image**   Smoking causes bad breath; stained teeth; smelly hair and clothes; wrinkled, dry skin; and red, itchy, watery eyes. Smokeless tobacco can cause cracked lips and sores around the mouth. Teens who smoke produce more than twice as much phlegm as nonsmokers.

- **Enjoyment**   Smoking ruins the smell and taste of food, for the smoker and for others.

- **Endurance**   All forms of tobacco, including smokeless tobacco and cigars, can affect endurance and overall athletic performance by narrowing blood vessels, straining the heart, and reducing oxygen to the muscles and lungs.

- **Poison factor**   Cigarettes contain poisons such as nicotine (which is also used in insecticides to kill insects), formaldehyde (the chemical used in biology classes to preserve dead animals), and cyanide (the same chemical found in rat poison).

- **Cost**   It's expensive to smoke.

average smoker starts by age 12 and smokes daily by age 14. Teens usually start smoking because their friends do, they think it's cool, and it makes them seem older. Boys often think it makes them look manly, and many girls do it to look glamorous and to control their weight.

For some teens, using tobacco can be an early warning sign of other problems. Smoking is associated with high-risk behaviors such as fighting and having unprotected sex. Teens who smoke are more likely than nonsmokers to drink alcohol, smoke marijuana, or use cocaine.

Alcohol and Other Drugs

Alcohol is the drug most commonly abused by teens. Many teens drink alcohol regularly and, of those who do, many drink heavily. Binge drinking (having more than five drinks in a session for males or four drinks in a session for females) is a serious problem on most college campuses. Almost half of teens have tried marijuana. Other drugs less frequently abused by teens include amphetamines, heroin, and cocaine (see page 737).

Problems with alcohol and other drugs are occurring at increasingly younger ages. Teens whose parents use alcohol or other drugs are more likely to use them too. Teens use alcohol and other drugs for some of the same reasons adults do—they think it will relax them, give them self-confidence, or help them feel better temporarily. Some teens try alcohol and drugs out of curiosity, or because their friends do and they want to fit in. Many teens who abuse alcohol or drugs have behavioral problems or learning disabilities (see page 415).

The average teen may experiment with alcohol or marijuana but will not use it regularly. If drug use progresses beyond the stage of experimentation, the teen's behavior will be affected as getting high becomes more and more important. Young people are especially vulnerable to the effects of drug use because their body and brain are still developing. As teens become psychologically or physically dependent on drugs, they tend to spend a lot of time alone or disappear for long periods, and their friends and interests change. They often become depressed and unmotivated and their grades fall. Drug use can also lead to hostility, violence, and delinquency.

It's hard for teens to deal with drug or alcohol abuse problems by themselves. They might think that they don't drink much or that addictions happen only to other people. Here are some steps you can take to help a teen realize that he or she may have a substance abuse problem:

- Find out before you talk to the teen where he or she could go for help. Be prepared to offer the information.
- Tell the teen at an appropriate time (preferably when he or she is not under the influence) that you think alcohol or other drugs are causing problems for him or her and you are worried and want to help.
- Don't accuse the teen of being an alcoholic or drug addict, and don't blame him or her for the problem.
- Don't show pity or be condescending.
- Give examples of what you've seen him or her do when he or she is high.
- Be prepared for the teen's anger and denials.
- Encourage the teen to talk to other people who have recovered from substance abuse problems.
- Try to get the teen to see a counselor who specializes in substance abuse problems. The child's safety, health, and life may depend on it.

Inhalants

An increasing number of teens inhale substances such as common household products because they are inexpensive, easy to obtain, and have a legal intended use. Using inhalants is extremely dangerous because these chemicals can make the heart beat rapidly and irregularly and cause cardiac arrest (make the heart stop) even in a young person. Inhalants can also cause sudden death by suffocation or by choking (on vomit). If your teen is using inhalants, he or she needs immediate help; call your doctor right away.

Anabolic Steroids

Some teenagers—both boys and girls—use anabolic steroids to improve their athletic performance. Make sure your teen is aware of the harmful (and sometimes irreversible) side effects of steroids, such as (in boys) shrunken testicles, breast development, impotence, and baldness, and (in girls) facial hair, reduced breast size, irregular menstrual periods, and a deep voice. Steroid use also can cause acne, jaundice (yellowing of the skin and whites of the eyes), infertility, depression, and aggression.

Ecstasy and Other Club Drugs

Ecstasy (also called XTC, MDMA, Adam, or the hug drug or love drug) and other club drugs are popular with teens at bars, dance clubs, and raves (all-night dance parties). Ten percent of American teens say they have tried ecstasy. Club drugs are popular with teens because they are relatively inexpensive, increase stamina, create a high, and heighten sensitivity to touch.

Most teens think that these drugs are harmless, low-risk ways to get high. But deaths from club drugs are on the rise. People 25 years or younger make up 80 percent of ecstasy-related hospital emergency department visits. Ecstasy can cause brain damage that can persist for years or be permanent. When taken together, alcohol and ecstasy can dangerously boost each other's effects.

Temporary side effects include hallucinations (abnormal perceptions not based on reality), paranoia (excessive or irrational suspiciousness), and amnesia (loss of memory). Users may act impulsively and aggressively. Chronic users sometimes wear retainers or use pacifiers or lollipops to try to prevent the cracked or worn teeth or jaw problems caused by jaw clenching or teeth grinding, which are common side effects of ecstasy.

People 25 years or younger also make up the majority of emergency department visits involving the date rape drug GHB (gamma-hydroxybutyrate). Because GHB is colorless, somewhat tasteless (it can be slightly bitter), and odorless (like other club drugs), it can be added to drinks without being detected. GHB puts a person into a stupor and sometimes into a coma, which can be fatal.

Prescription Drugs

Increasing numbers of young people are abusing prescription drugs that have been prescribed for another person for a legitimate purpose. One of the prescription drugs most frequently abused by young people is methylphenidate (known primarily by the brand name Ritalin and popularly as Vitamin R and R-Ball), a mild stimulant prescribed for treating attention deficit disorders (see page 730). Some young people take methylphenidate without a prescription to try to improve their concentration, enable them to study all night, or boost their

alertness during a test. The drugs are often made available by people who get them or steal them from someone who has a legitimate prescription, and then sell them or give them to friends, which is illegal.

> **WARNING!**
>
> ### Monitor Your Child's Medicine
>
> As a parent, consider yourself responsible for all medications your child takes. Hold them and administer them to your child inside the home, and do not allow your child to take medicine to school unless your doctor has told you it is necessary. If your child must take his or her medicine at school, make sure the medicine is held by the school nurse and administered in his or her presence or in the presence of a school official. If your child is attending day care, camp, or a sleepover, give his or her medicine to a responsible adult to give to your child when needed.

Methylphenidate can be dangerous if snorted, injected, or taken in large doses. The drug can increase heart rate and blood pressure and, in severe cases, cause an irregular heartbeat (arrhythmia; see page 580) that can result in sudden death. Complications from injecting the drug include overdose, blood clots, infections, lung problems, and skin and circulatory problems. Injecting crushed tablets of the drug can cause permanent lung damage.

Irresponsible Driving

Motor vehicle crashes are the leading cause of death of teenagers in the United States. Most teens believe they are good drivers. The main reasons for irresponsible driving are immaturity and lack of driving experience—the crash risk for a 16-year-old is more than twice that of an 18- or 19-year-old. Two out of three teens killed in motor vehicle crashes are boys. However, the crash rate for teenage girls is approaching that of boys.

The majority of motor vehicle deaths are caused by driving while under the influence of alcohol. One out of five teenage drivers has driven while drunk, and one out of five teens involved in fatal crashes had been drinking. Other factors in addition to drinking that contribute to motor vehicle injuries

Safe Driving: Tips for Parents of Teens Who Drive

To reduce collisions and injuries, many states are establishing graduated licensing systems in which full driving privileges are phased in for 16-year-olds. In the initial phase, the teen may be allowed to drive only with adult supervision, and parents must certify that their child has driven a specified number of hours (usually 25 to 50 hours) under supervision. In the next phase, the teen is able to drive without adult supervision but may be restricted from driving at night or from driving with nonadult passengers. These phases usually last about 6 months, but may last longer depending on the state. Many states require driver education as part of their graduated licensing system.

- Have your teen drive under supervision (with an adult in the car as a passenger) for at least 50 hours before letting him or her get a driver's license. Observe his or her driving in all kinds of weather conditions and traffic situations.
- Establish rules early for safe driving. Take away your child's driving privileges if he or she breaks a rule, especially if he or she gets a speeding ticket or causes a collision.
- Set a good example by following all traffic rules and by controlling your anger on the road.

- Have your teen drive a nonflashy, nonsporty car. He or she will be less likely to show off or speed.
- Tell your teen to call for a ride any time he or she (or another driver) is not capable of driving, no matter the circumstances, including drinking. Assure him or her that there will be no consequences or punishment.
- Remind your teen to follow all traffic rules—such as wearing a seat belt at all times, not speeding, not weaving in and out of traffic, and especially not drinking any alcohol before getting behind the wheel. He or she also should insist that all passengers wear seat belts.
- Remind your teen of the importance of focusing on driving and of avoiding unnecessary distractions such as talking on the phone, adjusting the radio or CD player, putting on makeup, eating, or looking at a map. He or she should pull over to use the phone or study maps or notes for directions.
- Discourage your child from driving or riding on a motorcycle. If he or she does, insist that he or she wear a helmet and other proper equipment or clothing.

or deaths are speeding, not wearing a seat belt, and being distracted while driving. Three out of four teens admit to speeding while driving, and many teens say they rarely or never wear a seat belt. Being distracted can contribute to or cause a collision; cars carrying two or more teens are four times more likely to be involved in a collision than cars carrying only the teen driver.

Depression

Feeling sad or down every once in a while is normal, but being depressed is not a normal part of adolescence. Depression (see page 709) results from an imbalance of chemicals in the brain. Some people are genetically susceptible to developing depression, while others may become temporarily depressed in response to a stressful situation. For example, depression sometimes develops during the teen years when a teen feels ostracized as peer pressure escalates and social cliques form. A teen may have serious depression if any of the following symptoms lasts longer than a few weeks or is

severe, or if the teen has more than one symptom. Your child may have depression if he or she:

- Is sad or cries, is irritable or restless, or is tired or forgetful most or all of the time.
- Has lost confidence in himself or herself, has a negative attitude, or feels worthless.
- Feels as if nothing good will ever happen again or feels numb, showing little interest in anything.
- Wants to be left alone.
- Thinks or talks about dying or suicide (see next page).
- Has trouble falling asleep, wakes up earlier than usual in the mornings, or sleeps more than 10 hours a day.
- Eats a lot more than usual or has no appetite.
- Feels sick or has aches and pains that don't respond to treatment.
- Has started to drink alcohol or abuse drugs.

Depression will not go away on its own. If your teen has more than one of the above symptoms, or if any symptom lasts longer than a few weeks or is especially severe, get help immediately. Start by

Suicide

Suicide is the third-leading cause of death among people under age 24 in the United States. Untreated depression is the major cause of suicide.

Risk factors for suicide (and depression) include:

- Losing a friend or family member
- Going away to school or to a new school, or moving to a new city or neighborhood
- Having problems in school such as truancy, failing to pass an important test, failing a class, or being teased or bullied
- Committing crimes or being a member of a gang
- Breaking up with a boyfriend or girlfriend
- Having family problems such as an unexpected or unwanted pregnancy, parents who are getting a divorce, or family members who are depressed or who abuse drugs or alcohol
- Being involved in a life-changing tragedy such as a vehicle collision, a house fire, or a serious injury or illness

Teens who talk about suicide or who have suicidal thoughts need to get help right away.

Warning signs of suicide include:

- Talking or joking about committing suicide
- Having a drastic personality change such as suddenly seeming at peace or happy after weeks of being depressed
- Giving away possessions
- Being preoccupied with death and dying
- Visiting good friends or relatives after not showing an interest in them for a long time
- Seeming to be getting things in order, such as by making lists

calling your child's doctor. Most teens with depression can be helped with counseling by a trained psychologist or therapist, and often with medication prescribed by a psychiatrist. Counseling may be helpful for family members also. If teens take medication for depression, they need to take it consistently and exactly as prescribed, even if they are feeling better.

Self-Mutilation

Self-mutilation is the act of injuring yourself seriously enough to cause harm in an attempt to relieve stress, anxiety, or depression. Forms of self-mutilation include cutting, burning, scratching, bruising, or biting. A large number of teen girls and an increasing number of boys practice self-mutilation in some form. Teens who do it say that it gives them a sense of control over their life or body. Self-mutilation is not the same as tattooing or piercing (see page 458) because it is not performed for body decoration or to fit in with peers. The injuries are done in private and usually are kept secret.

Some signs that a teen is engaged in self-mutilation include new injuries, scars or wounds from old injuries, or blood or burn stains on clothing. He or she may insist on doing his or her own laundry and not want to take gym class or change clothes in front of others. He or she has knives, razor blades, matches, or lighters for no apparent purpose.

Self-mutilation is not a sign of a failed suicide attempt, but it can be a symptom of depression that needs to be treated. Some teens who self-injure eventually attempt or commit suicide if their depression is not treated. Self-mutilation usually is treated with psychotherapy and antianxiety and antidepressant medication. Psychotherapy helps the teen learn new, positive ways to cope with stress.

Violence and Teens

Children are harmed emotionally and developmentally, as well as physically, when they are exposed to or experience violence. Exposure to violence (either actual or through media such as movies) can rewire a child's brain in ways that can make him or her more prone to aggressive behavior later in life. There is no precise profile of someone who will commit acts of violence but, in addition to exposure to violence, risk factors include alcohol or drug abuse, being a victim of child abuse or neglect, being a gang member, and having access to a gun. In the United States, guns are responsible for most of the deaths of people between ages 15 and 24. Violent behavior usually peaks by age 16 or 17, but the vast majority of teens who have been violent stop committing violent acts by the time they are 21.

It is usually the interaction of a number of influences over time that can make a teen violent. Good parenting and the love and acceptance of even just one caring adult can often help teens gain confidence and social skills, set positive goals to

WARNING!

Could Your Child Become Violent?

Violent teens may show signs of having emotional or behavioral problems long before they behave violently. Consult a doctor or mental health professional if a child or teen:

- Damages property
- Hurts animals
- Frequently loses his or her temper or gets into fights
- Carries a weapon or is a member of a gang
- Bullies another child (or is being bullied)
- Abuses alcohol or other drugs
- Is easily frustrated and feels that he or she is being treated unfairly
- Has low self-esteem and seems depressed
- Seems to have no friends and is often alone
- Is verbally abusive or threatens others
- Is truant or has a history of discipline problems in school
- Has extreme mood swings or has talked about committing suicide

strive for, and serve as buffers against potentially harmful biological or environmental influences.

Bullying

Nearly half of all schoolchildren are bullied by another student at some time during their education. Bullying is defined as a pattern of repeated aggression against or negative behavior toward a person. Boys are more likely to be bullies than girls, and boys usually bully other boys; girls tend to bully other girls. Bullying can take the form of physical attacks (such as hitting, kicking, or pushing), verbal attacks (such as name-calling, insults, or teasing), or psychological attacks (such as intimidation, spreading rumors, or persuading other children to reject or exclude the child). Boys who are bullies usually use physical force or threats, while girls are more likely to use verbal or psychological attacks.

Bullies are usually children who have themselves been victims of physical abuse or bullying, usually at home. They tend to be aggressive, controlling, and dominating, and often have an inflated self-image and difficulty empathizing with other people. By contrast, the victims of bullying tend to be introverted, passive, and easily intimidated, and frequently are seen by classmates as being different in some way (such as by race, ethnicity, sexual orientation, academic ability, or unusual haircut or clothing).

If you think that your child is a victim of bullying, or if you are concerned that your child may be a bully, quickly take steps to stop it. Bullying can have long-term consequences for both victims and bullies. Victims of bullying often try to avoid going to school, and their academic performance may suffer. Many victims have difficulty socializing, have low self-esteem, and frequently become isolated and depressed. In extreme cases, victims may consider or attempt suicide (see previous page). Children who are bullies are more likely than other children to be truant from school, drop out of school, or get into fights. They also are more likely than other children to commit a crime (such as vandalism, shoplifting, or drug-related offenses) by the time they are 24.

If your child is being bullied:

- **Believe your child.** Reassure your child and make sure he or she knows that you care. Listen to what he or she has to say, and ask questions so you can get a clear understanding of the situation.
- **Get help.** Talk to your child's teacher and the school principal, and ask them to investigate the situation. They may be able to reduce the incidence of bullying by increasing supervision in areas where it is most likely to occur, including hallways, bathrooms, locker rooms, playgrounds, and school buses.
- **Encourage your child to be assertive.** Tell your child to get immediate help from an adult when he or she is confronted by a bully. Help your child gain self-confidence by getting him or her involved in an activity he or she enjoys and is good at, such as sports or playing a musical instrument. Children who appear self-confident are less likely to become victims of bullies.
- **Make sure your child has a friend.** Children who are isolated are more likely to be victims of bullying. Encourage your child to invite a classmate home to play or study, and talk to your child's teacher about intervening to find a classmate to be your child's buddy.

If your child is a bully:

- **Get help at school.** Talk to your child's teacher, the school principal, or a school counselor; ask them to monitor your child's behavior at school and let you know right away about any problems.

- **Seek professional help for your child.** If your child's aggressive behavior does not stop, talk to your child's doctor, who can recommend a mental health professional to help your child learn positive ways of dealing with his or her negative feelings and behavior. Ask your child's teacher if the school has a social worker available who can work with your child.

- **Consider your own attitude toward bullying.** Do you think it is an inevitable part of growing up? If so, you could be unknowingly sending the message to your child that bullying is acceptable. Make sure your child knows you disapprove of bullying and will not tolerate it.

Dating Violence

One in five high school girls has been physically abused or forced to have sex on a date. The abuse can also take the form of emotional mistreatment, which is less likely to be detected by parents or friends. Girls may not report the abuse because, like many women who are victims of domestic violence (see page 79), they may feel they deserve it, they don't want to give up the relationship, they are ashamed, or they are afraid of making their boyfriend angry. Some girls may feel that abuse is part of a normal relationship (especially if they see it at home), or that jealous outbursts or attempts to control their behavior or appearance prove that their boyfriend cares about them.

Girls who are in abusive relationships are at risk of having eating disorders (see page 724), abusing alcohol or other drugs, or engaging in risky sexual activities such as early intercourse or having sex with multiple partners. In addition, their risk of suicide is high.

Boys who abuse their dates may have been physically or verbally abused at home or have parents who are involved in an abusive relationship. These boys believe they have to use violence to control their girlfriend. Boys frequently are not held accountable for the violence because young women seldom report the abuse.

Helping teens (both boys and girls) understand the difference between healthy and unhealthy relationships can help prevent dating violence. If a girl is in an abusive relationship, she should confide in someone she trusts. With the help of parents and friends, she should be encouraged to end the relationship, report the assault, and receive counseling by a mental health professional who can help her learn to avoid abusive relationships in the future.

Acquaintance Rape

Acquaintance rape, or date rape, accounts for 60 percent of all rapes. These sexual assaults occur not only on dates but also at parties and in college dormitories and are usually committed by a friend, classmate, or coworker. There seems to be a strong association between alcohol and acquaintance rape: more than half of women and two out of three men involved in sexual assault had been drinking when the assault occurred. Sexual assault by an acquaintance shatters trust, and the victim (usually a female) does not always get the support she needs from friends, coworkers, classmates, or school officials, who may side with the attacker. Victims may become depressed or anxious, may abuse alcohol or other drugs, and may attempt suicide. As with dating violence, victims of any kind of sexual assault should report it as soon as possible to authorities and get counseling from a trained mental health professional.

3

Sexuality

Sexuality is the way in which we experience and express affectionate or erotic feelings, which are influenced by biological, psychological, social, and cultural factors. A satisfying sexual relationship is one of the most important aspects of life. The shared intimacy of sex can be a physically and emotionally rewarding experience. Sexual arousal is influenced by our feelings of attraction to another person and involves physical responses such as an erection or vaginal lubrication.

Sexual arousal affects the whole body. The skin is highly sensitive to arousal, especially the skin over the upper and inner thighs, the lower back, and the buttocks. During arousal, the genitals, earlobes, and nipples in both men and women become erect, and the lining of the nose becomes swollen and engorged with blood. The contractions of orgasm affect many muscles in the body, including those in the legs, back, neck, face, and toes.

Because the female sex organs are more interior than the male sex organs, some women may be unfamiliar with their own genitals. If you are a woman who has never seen her external genitals, you can look at them with a small mirror held between your legs. Your pubic hair covers the protective tissue known as the mons pubis, which lies over the external genitals. Underneath are two folds of skin called the outer lips or labia. Inside the outer labia are two inner lips, which cover the openings to the urinary tract and the vagina. The clitoris, the principal site of female sexual stimulation, is at the top, where the inner lips meet; the clitoris, like a man's penis, becomes erect and swollen during sexual arousal. The vagina is a long, muscular canal that extends (at an angle) from the outside of the body up to the uterus. At the upper end of the vagina is the cervix, which is the opening of the uterus. During arousal, the vagina produces

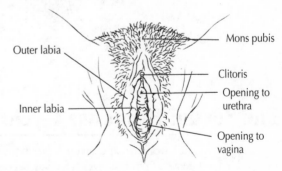

The female sex organs
Most of the female reproductive system is internal—and only the genitals are visible. The outer, visible area is called the vulva, which includes the mons pubis (the hair-covered mound over the pubic bone); the outer, hair-covered lips (labia majora); and the smaller, inner lips (labia minora), which protect the opening to the vagina. The clitoris is a tiny, sexually sensitive mound of tissue. During sexual arousal, the clitoris, the labia minora, the vagina, and the network of connecting blood vessels and muscles swell with blood.

a fluid that lubricates it and makes penetration by the penis easier.

For the most part, the male sex organs are external. The penis passes urine out of the body and expels semen (a mixture of sperm and secretions from the seminal vesicles and prostate gland) at orgasm. When a male is unaroused sexually, the penis is soft, but during arousal, blood rushes into the penis, making it swollen and erect. Sperm are produced in the testicles, two round, firm spheres enclosed in a pouch of skin called the scrotum. The testicles are outside the body because they must be cooler than body temperature to produce sperm. The left testicle usually hangs slightly lower than the right testicle.

On top of each testicle is a coiled tube called the epididymis, in which sperm develop.

From the back of each testicle, a long, thin tube called the vas deferens extends up into an organ called the ampulla of the vas deferens, which is behind the bladder. The ampulla of the vas deferens stores sperm for up to several months. Right before ejaculation, sperm exit the ampulla and mix with secretions from the seminal vesicles. As the mixture enters the urethra (the tube inside the penis through which urine passes out of the body), it combines with secretions from the prostate gland. This final mixture is called semen. The penis ejects semen as orgasm begins.

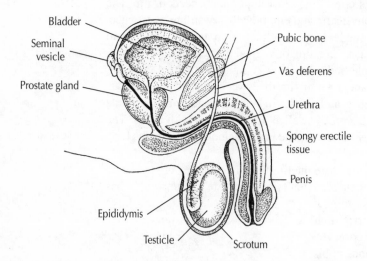

Bladder
Seminal vesicle
Prostate gland
Epididymis
Testicle
Scrotum
Pubic bone
Vas deferens
Urethra
Spongy erectile tissue
Penis

The male sex organs
The penis and the testicles are the most visible parts of the male reproductive system. The testicles are suspended in a pouch of skin called the scrotum. The testicles produce sperm and the male sex hormone testosterone. During sexual arousal, spongy tissue inside the penis becomes engorged with blood. Sperm travel from the testicles through a duct called the vas deferens into a pair of sacs called the seminal vesicles. The prostate gland and seminal vesicles produce a fluid that combines with the sperm to create semen—the fluid that is ejaculated at orgasm.

The Sexual Response Cycle

Men and women experience a predictable sequence of physical events as they become sexually aroused and begin to engage in sexual intercourse or masturbation. This sequence of events is called the sexual response cycle. The human sexual response cycle occurs in four stages—excitement, plateau, orgasm, and resolution. Men and women go through the same four stages, but the timing of the stages differs. For example, women usually take longer to become aroused during the excitement stage, although this is not always true. From beginning to end, a woman's arousal and response cycle lasts almost four times longer than that of a man. This difference in timing is completely normal, but it can lead to sexual problems and misunderstanding if the partners are unaware of it. At the end of the sexual response cycle, men go through an additional phase, called the refractory period, during which they can no longer respond to sexual stimuli.

Excitement

Becoming sexually aroused depends on our ability to allow ourselves to focus on and experience effective sexual stimulation, which can be in the form of sexually stimulating touch, thoughts, or imagination. During the excitement, or arousal, stage, a woman's vaginal lining secretes a lubricating fluid after erotic stimulation begins, making insertion of the penis easier and penetration more pleasurable. Her breasts, nipples, and labia swell, and her clitoris becomes engorged with blood. The man's penis becomes erect, and his nipples also swell. Both men and women experience an accelerated heart rate and breathing as well as increased blood pressure. As arousal increases, blood flow to the sex organs increases. Late in this stage, many women and some men experience flushing on their chest. The excitement stage can last from a few minutes to several hours.

Plateau

The plateau stage is an advanced state of arousal preceding orgasm. This stage involves an acceleration of breathing, heart rate, and blood pressure experienced during the excitement stage. The outer third of the woman's vagina swells and becomes longer, and the clitoris retracts to avoid direct stimulation by the penis. The man's testicles enlarge and are drawn up into the scrotum, which tightens. A few drops of fluid that can contain sperm may appear at the tip of the penis. In both sexes, muscle spasms may occur in the face, hands, and feet. Muscle tension increases throughout the body. Men and women can move from the plateau phase to the resolution phase without having an orgasm.

Orgasm

Orgasm is the climax stage of the sexual response cycle and usually lasts only a few seconds. During

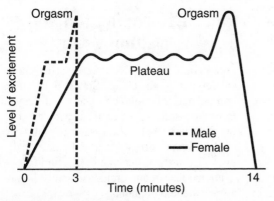

Male and female sexual responses
Male and female sexual responses proceed through four stages—excitement, plateau, orgasm, and resolution. Women usually take longer to become aroused during the excitement phase and, generally, a woman's sexual response cycle lasts about four times longer than that of a man. During the resolution stage, men go through a refractory period during which they do not respond to sexual stimuli and cannot have another orgasm for a certain length of time. Unlike men, women can have multiple orgasms or go directly from the plateau to the resolution stage.

What Happens During Orgasm?

Orgasm can be defined as a peak of pressure in the blood vessels and tissues of the genitals that is characterized by pleasurable muscle contractions in the genitals and over the entire body.

When a woman reaches orgasm, the muscles in the lower third of the vagina contract repeatedly, while those in the upper third expand. The uterus also contracts during orgasm. To achieve orgasm, a woman must get sufficient stimulation at the base of her clitoris, but only 20 to 30 percent of all women are able to reach orgasm during intercourse with penetration of the penis alone. For a woman, having an orgasm during intercourse depends on the anatomy of both partners and the activity they engage in. Some couples fit together and move in a way that stimulates the clitoris; others do not. If you are a woman who has difficulty having an orgasm during intercourse, ask your partner to stimulate your clitoris with a finger, the mouth, or a vibrator beforehand so you can be sufficiently aroused. You can also try different positions to see if they are more stimulating, or masturbate during penetration. Many women can achieve orgasm more easily when they are on top.

When a man becomes sexually aroused, his brain sends signals to relax the muscles in his penis so blood can rush in and fill the penis sufficiently to produce an erection. Just before orgasm, the muscles around the base of the penis contract to help eject semen from the penis. After these pleasurable muscle contractions, he enters a period of relaxation in which he cannot respond to sexual stimulation.

orgasm, heart rate, breathing, and blood pressure reach their highest levels. The skin may become flushed or appear to have a rash. In women, the muscles in the vagina contract rhythmically, producing pleasurable sensations. The uterus also contracts during orgasm. Women are capable of having multiple orgasms.

The male orgasm occurs in two parts. First, semen collects in the urethra and the man feels that orgasm is inevitable. Then the penis contracts and expels the semen. Each ejaculation contains from 300 million to 500 million sperm, but only a few hundred will reach the woman's fallopian tubes.

Resolution

During the resolution stage, the heightened state of arousal reverts to normal. The sex organs return to their normal size. Breathing, heart rate, and blood pressure decrease to their normal levels. This process usually takes longer for women, and women can be stimulated to reach another orgasm during this stage. Men go through a refractory period during which they cannot have another orgasm until a certain amount of time has passed. This refractory period can last from minutes to hours depending on the man's age and physical condition.

Sexual Orientation

Sexual orientation is a term that refers to a person's emotional, romantic, and sexual attraction to a person of a particular gender. People who are attracted to members of the opposite sex are called heterosexual, while those who are attracted to people of the same sex are called homosexual, gay (men and women), or lesbian (women). Some people are attracted to both men and women; they are called bisexual. It is difficult to determine the exact number of people in the United States who identify themselves as homosexual or bisexual.

Bisexuality and Homosexuality

The factors that influence a person's sexual orientation are not completely understood, but they appear to encompass a complex combination of biological, psychological, and social influences. What is clear is that sexual orientation is not a lifestyle choice that can easily be changed. Most people discover at a very early age—in childhood or adolescence—before they have had any sexual experiences, that they are attracted to people of a certain gender.

To avoid the social stigma sometimes attached to being homosexual, some gay people try hard to change their sexual orientation, usually without success. No scientific evidence shows that trying to alter one's sexual orientation is an appropriate goal of psychological or psychiatric treatment. Homosexuality and bisexuality are not mental disorders or emotional problems. Doctors view homosexuality and bisexuality as normal variations of human sexual expression. Most emotional problems that occur in homosexuals are caused by a sense of alienation from living in an unaccepting environment.

Discrimination and Coming Out

Gay people frequently face discrimination and stereotyping in the United States. Hate crimes and similar acts of violence pose a genuine threat. Between 5 and 10 percent of gay people report having experienced physical assault or abuse because of their sexual orientation, and almost half have been victims of some type of discrimination. This irrational fear of and prejudice against homosexuals is called homophobia.

Still, many gay people feel uncomfortable keeping their sexual orientation hidden. The process of recognizing and accepting being gay or lesbian and then telling other people about it is called coming out. This process can be difficult emotionally, not only for the gay person but also for his or her family and friends. The person's parents may be alternately shocked, angry, and concerned for their child's welfare as the child faces the difficulties of being part of a group that may be stigmatized. The gay person may fear rejection by his or her parents and other family members, friends, or coworkers. But for most gay people, coming out is a positive and healthy emotional experience because they no longer have to keep an important part of their life a secret.

If you have recently learned that a relative or friend is homosexual or bisexual, get information and emotional support from a group such as Parents, Families and Friends of Lesbians and Gays (PFLAG).

Health Issues

Some medical conditions are more prevalent among gay men than among the general population. For example, the incidence of some sexually transmitted diseases (STDs) such as gonorrhea (see page 480) and genital warts (see page 480) is higher in homosexual men who engage in unprotected anal intercourse. Infection with gonorrhea can increase the risk of infection with HIV (the virus that causes AIDS; see page 909) because infected tissue is more easily injured, allowing the virus to enter through tiny breaks in the tissue. Although most HIV-infected people worldwide are heterosexual, the majority of new cases in the United States are among gay men, especially young black men between ages 15 and 29. Many of these men do not know they are at risk for HIV infection and engage in unsafe sex—that is, they do not use condoms consistently or correctly (see page 478). Many young men who become infected do not know it—and they continue to practice unsafe sex, putting their sex partners at risk of infection.

Gay men are also at increased risk of infection with the hepatitis A and B viruses (see page 786). Hepatitis A can be transmitted in infected fecal matter during oral-anal intercourse (which also can transmit some bacterial infections and intestinal parasites). Hepatitis B can be transmitted in infected blood during unprotected anal or oral intercourse. Hepatitis B can become chronic (long-term), causing damage to the liver, including scarring (cirrhosis; see page 790) and liver cancer (see page 792). Effective vaccines are available against hepatitis A and B, but many gay men are unaware of their risks of contracting the viruses and also are unaware of the availability of the vaccines.

Some types of cancer—such as Kaposi's sarcoma and some kinds of lymphoma (see page 625)—disproportionately affect people who are HIV-positive or who have AIDS because the virus attacks and weakens the body's immune defense system. For this reason, the risk of anal cancer is also increased in men who are HIV-positive. The human papillomavirus (HPV), which causes genital warts (and cervical cancer in women), can cause anal cancer in men who engage in anal intercourse.

Lesbians also are at risk of acquiring STDs during sexual activity. Herpes (see page 482), HPV, and bacterial vaginosis (see page 879) are especially easy to transmit, while HIV, gonorrhea, and chlamydia are more difficult to transmit. Additionally, some lesbians have sex with men, from whom they can contract an STD and then transmit it to a female partner. An HPV infection can lead to cancer of the cervix (see page 875), although women can also develop another type of cervical cancer that is unrelated to sexual intercourse or HPV exposure. For this reason, lesbians need to have regular Pap smears (see page 140) to detect precancerous changes in the cells of the cervix at an early stage, when they are easiest to treat.

Staying Healthy

If you are gay, you can take positive steps to protect yourself from sexually transmitted diseases and more serious medical conditions such as HIV infection and cancer by following these guidelines:

- **Practice safer sex.** Use a latex condom every time you have any type of sex, and make sure you know how to use it correctly (see page 478).
- **Get vaccinated.** Ask your doctor about getting vaccinated against hepatitis A and B.
- **Drink alcohol only in moderation, and don't use other drugs.** Unprotected or irresponsible sexual activity is more likely to occur when you are under the influence of alcohol or other drugs.
- **Get tested.** Ask your doctor to test you for STDs if you have had unprotected intercourse so you can be treated right away.

Contraception

A wide range of reliable contraceptives is available, and each contraceptive has advantages and disadvantages. Some contraceptives require a prescription, while others are available over the counter. Be sure to talk with your doctor about the risks and benefits of each method of birth control before choosing one. Consider reliability, side effects, and protection against sexually transmitted diseases (STDs; see page 477) when making your decision. Remember that hormonal and barrier methods of birth control do not protect against STDs. Doctors strongly recommend that women who use these birth-control methods and are not in a mutually monogamous relationship also use condoms during sexual intercourse to protect themselves from STDs.

Oral Contraceptives

The contraceptive pill (birth-control pill) is currently the most effective method of reversible birth control. The most frequently prescribed birth-control pills are called combined pills because they blend synthetic versions of estrogen and progesterone (progestin). Estrogen and progesterone are the major hormones that control the female reproductive cycle.

Birth-control pills work primarily by preventing ovulation, the monthly release of an egg by the ovaries. The pills also make it difficult for sperm to enter the uterus by making the mucus produced by the cervix thicker and harder to penetrate. Birth-control pills regulate a woman's menstrual cycle by providing a controlled dose of hormones daily. Most women notice changes in their menstrual cycle when they take birth-control pills—their periods occur precisely every 28 days and usually are shorter and lighter. Many women take birth-control pills specifically to regulate their cycle and reduce menstrual flow, not just for contraception.

In addition to preventing pregnancy, birth-control pills have other beneficial effects. A woman who takes birth-control pills is much less likely to have ovarian cysts (see page 864), breast lumps (see page 856), iron deficiency anemia (see page 610), rheumatoid arthritis (see page 918), or pelvic inflammatory disease (PID; see page 871) than a woman who does not take birth-control pills. Birth-control pills also protect against cancer of the ovary, uterus, and colon. The combined pill, because it contains estrogen, helps maintain bone density in women who are at risk for osteoporosis (see page 989) and can prevent ectopic pregnancies (see page 523).

Birth-control pills are packaged in 21-day or 28-day packs. The pills you take for the first 3 weeks contain the hormones that prevent pregnancy and regulate your menstrual cycle. The pills you take during the fourth week are inactive (placebo) pills. You take one pill every day at the same time. After you take the last of the hormone-containing pills, the hormone levels in your blood fall quickly, and menstrual bleeding occurs. If you miss a pill, you should take it as soon as you remember. If you miss two or more pills from one package, take two pills a day until you catch up, but use an additional method of birth control until you begin a new package of pills. When you miss a pill, the sudden withdrawal of the hormones can cause menstrual bleeding. Birth-control pills do not have any effect on your ability to become pregnant after you stop taking them.

If your doctor has recommended against taking the combined pill, you may be able to take the minipill. The minipill contains only the hormone progesterone (progestin) and may be safer if you smoke and are over age 35. (Women over 35 who smoke cigarettes should not take estrogen because it can increase their risk of blood clots and stroke.) Because the minipill does not contain estrogen, it can cause breakthrough bleeding (bleeding between periods), especially if you miss a pill or take one late. Some women who take the minipill do not have regular menstrual periods for a long time. Minipills are slightly less effective than combined birth-control pills; on average, about 2 of every 100 women who use the minipill for a year become pregnant.

Your doctor probably will tell you to begin taking the minipill on the first day of your period, and to take one each day for as long as you want contraception to continue. It is especially important that you take the minipill at the same time each day and use a backup method of birth control, such as a condom, if you take a pill more than 4 hours late.

Some women experience bleeding between periods when starting birth-control pills. Breakthrough bleeding is common during the first few months of using the pill and requires no treatment. Breakthrough bleeding is less likely to occur if you take the pill at the same time every day and don't skip any. If the bleeding continues, your doctor may prescribe a different dosage of the pills to try for several months. Mild breast tenderness also may occur temporarily. One rare but serious potential side effect of taking birth-control pills is the formation of blood clots in the veins, which can travel to the lungs and cause sudden death.

Emergency Contraceptives

Emergency contraceptive pills (sometimes called morning-after pills) are available in two-pill packets to prevent pregnancy after unprotected intercourse. The pills, like birth-control pills, are either a combination of estrogen and progestin, or progestin alone. The first pill must be taken as soon as possible within 72 hours of unprotected intercourse (it is most effective when taken within 24 hours); the second pill must be taken 12 hours after the first pill. The pills work in the same way as regular birth-control pills and have similar side effects. You should not consider emergency contraceptives a regular form of birth control.

Male and Female Condoms

A condom is a thin rubber sheath (usually made of latex and closed at one end) that is rolled onto the erect penis before intercourse. When a man ejaculates, his sperm are trapped in the closed end of the condom. For maximum reliability, you should use condoms along with a spermicide. Some available condoms are already lubricated with spermicide.

Condoms are up to 98 percent effective in preventing pregnancy when used correctly. Not only do condoms prevent pregnancy, they also prevent the transmission of most sexually transmitted diseases (STDs), reducing the risk by 99.9 percent. But condoms reach these levels of effectiveness only when they are used consistently and correctly (see page 478)—every time you have sex, including oral and anal intercourse.

A variation of the condom is the female condom.

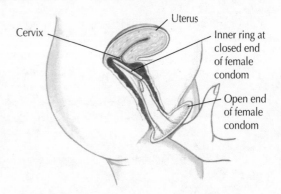

Female condom
The female condom is a thin rubber sheath that fits inside the vagina. The condom has soft, flexible rings at both ends. A small ring at the closed end of the condom holds the condom in place against the cervix. A larger ring at the other, open end of the condom remains outside the vagina. To insert the condom, you squeeze the smaller inner ring on the closed end and insert it into your vagina. Using your index finger, push the condom up as far as you can until it reaches the cervix. About 1 inch of the open end stays outside the vagina and rests against the external genitals.

This thin rubber sheath fits inside the vagina and has an outer rim that remains outside to protect the labia and the clitoris. Like the male condom, the female condom provides both contraception and protection against many STDs.

Spermicides

Spermicides are chemicals that kill sperm. They are available over the counter as cream, jelly, or foam and are inserted into the vagina shortly before intercourse. Follow the package directions and reinsert more spermicide before each time you have intercourse. Always use a spermicide with a condom, a diaphragm, or a cervical cap. Very rarely, spermicides can cause mild allergic reactions, producing itching and redness in either partner's genital area.

Diaphragm

The diaphragm is a rubber cup fitted over a flexible wire frame that blocks sperm from entering the uterus. A trained health care professional fits a diaphragm to a woman's vagina to cover the cervix (the opening to the uterus) and shows her how to use it. A diaphragm must be inserted correctly and

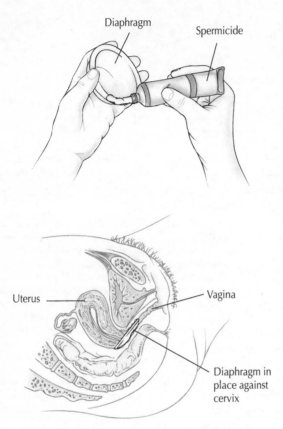

Using a diaphragm
Before using your diaphragm, place some spermicide around the rim and in the center of the cup (top). When inserted properly, the diaphragm completely covers the cervix, and the rim of the diaphragm lies behind your pubic bone (bottom).

no more than 6 hours before intercourse. You must put a ring of spermicidal cream or jelly around the edge of the diaphragm and about half a teaspoon in its center before you insert it. To insert it, you squeeze it together into a half circle. Check immediately after insertion to make sure that the rubber of the diaphragm covers your cervix and that the edge of the diaphragm is behind your pubic bone. If the diaphragm does not cover your cervix, it will not block sperm from the uterus and you can become pregnant.

After intercourse, you must leave the diaphragm in place for at least 6 hours to allow the spermicide to kill any sperm. If you have intercourse again within 6 hours, put more spermicidal cream or jelly in your vagina, using the plastic applicator that comes with the spermicide. For intercourse after 6

hours, remove the diaphragm, wash it, put spermicidal cream or jelly on it again, and reposition it in your vagina. The diaphragm can be a highly effective method of birth control if you use it carefully and consistently.

Cervical Cap

The cervical cap, like the diaphragm, blocks sperm from the uterus. The cap is much smaller than the diaphragm and fits tightly over the cervix (the opening to the uterus) rather than extending to the walls of the vagina. A trained health care professional fits the cervical cap to each woman and instructs her in how to insert it. The cervical cap should be used in the same way as a diaphragm, with spermicidal cream or jelly, following the same precautions. Used in this way, a cervical cap is about as effective as a diaphragm in preventing pregnancy. However, the smaller size of the cap can make it trickier to place correctly, especially for women who have short fingers.

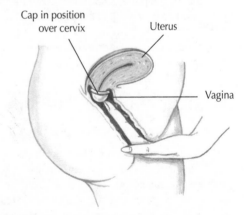

Cervical cap
The cervical cap is a barrier method of birth control. Like a diaphragm but smaller, the cap completely covers the cervix, blocking sperm from entering the uterus.

IUD

The intrauterine device (IUD) is a tiny contraceptive device made of copper or a hormone-containing plastic that your doctor inserts into your uterus. An IUD prevents pregnancy by blocking sperm from the fallopian tubes, where fertilization normally takes place. An IUD is usually inserted during a woman's menstrual period, when the cervix (the opening to the uterus) is more open, but it can be inserted at any time of the menstrual cycle once the doctor determines that the woman is not pregnant.

The insertion takes only a few minutes, but it sometimes causes brief cramping pain. Once inserted, the IUD protects against pregnancy. An IUD can be accidentally expelled at any time, so you should check frequently to make sure it is still in place. A good time to check is toward the end of your period (because both menstrual cramps and tampon insertion and removal can increase the risk of expulsion). You can check for the IUD by inserting your finger inside your vagina; if you can feel the string, the IUD is in place. If you feel the hard plastic of the IUD, it is being expelled. See your doctor so he or she can remove the IUD and replace it with a new one.

The most common problem with copper IUDs is the slight risk of increased menstrual bleeding and intensified menstrual pain, although most users do not experience these problems. The copper IUD prevents pregnancy for 10 to 12 years. But the copper IUD may not be the best contraceptive method for you if you already have long and painful periods. An IUD that releases timed doses of progestin (a form of the female hormone progesterone) causes less menstrual bleeding—but it prevents pregnancy for only 5 years.

If you are not in a mutually monogamous sexual relationship and you have an IUD, you are at an increased risk of developing pelvic inflammatory disease (PID; see page 871) from a sexually transmitted disease (STD; see page 477). Untreated, PID can lead to ectopic pregnancy (see page 523) and infertility. To protect against pelvic infection, use a latex condom each time you have intercourse.

Hormone Injections

Injection of progestin (a form of the female hormone progesterone) every 3 months provides highly effective birth control. The hormone blocks ovulation and increases the thickness of the mucus secreted by the cervix, making penetration of sperm more difficult. An alternative injectable contraceptive—which is 99 percent effective—combines progesterone and estrogen to prevent ovulation but lasts only 28 days. Both injections are given in a woman's arm or buttocks during the first 5 days of her period.

Hormone injections lessen menstrual cramping and protect against cancers of the ovary and uterus. Common side effects include irregular bleeding, lighter periods (which may eventually stop altogether), longer and heavier periods, bleeding between periods (breakthrough bleeding or spotting), sore breasts, or weight gain. Women with unexplained vaginal bleeding, a history of blood clots, liver disease, or breast cancer should not use hormone injections for birth control. Regular ovulation and fertility usually resume about 6 to 9 months after the last injection of progesterone, somewhat sooner if the combined hormone injection is used.

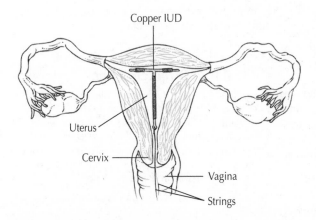

How an IUD prevents pregnancy
When correctly positioned in the uterus, an IUD prevents an egg from being fertilized by preventing sperm from reaching the fallopian tubes. Hormone-releasing IUDs thicken the mucus produced by the cervix, blocking sperm from the uterus, and also may make the uterine lining thinner and less favorable for implantation of a fertilized egg. Both types of IUD have plastic strings attached to the lower end to make removal easier.

Contraceptive Patch

The contraceptive patch prevents pregnancy by releasing the hormones estrogen and progestin (a form of the female hormone progesterone) directly into the skin. The hormones prevent ovulation and cause the mucus released by the cervix to thicken, inhibiting penetration by sperm. A patch is applied to the skin (on the upper, outer arm; the back; the lower abdomen; or the buttocks) every week for 3 weeks in a row. No patch is worn the fourth week, triggering menstruation. The cycle is repeated as long as birth control is desired. The patch stays adhered to the skin even during showering, bathing, and swimming.

The side effects of the contraceptive patch are similar to those of the birth-control pill (see page 470), including breast tenderness. A rare but serious risk is the development of blood clots that can travel to the lungs and cause sudden death. Women who cannot take the pill (such as smokers over age 35) should not use the patch.

Vaginal Ring

The vaginal ring, which is available only by prescription, is a pliable, transparent ring that is inserted into the vagina to prevent pregnancy. The ring continuously releases estrogen and a form of progesterone (progestin) to inhibit ovulation and block implantation of a fertilized egg. The ring stays in place for 3 weeks, and you remove it for the week that you have your period. You insert a new ring at the end of the fourth week. The ring is easier to insert and remove than a diaphragm (see page 471) because it does not require special positioning over the cervix. It is 99 percent effective in preventing pregnancy (but check regularly to make sure it has not been accidentally expelled).

Side effects of the vaginal ring include vaginal discharge or discomfort, or the sensation of a foreign body inside the vagina. Like the birth-control pill, the vaginal ring can increase the risk of blood clots, heart attack, and stroke, especially in women over age 35 who smoke cigarettes.

Natural Methods

The natural method of contraception, sometimes called the rhythm method, attempts to prevent pregnancy by predicting the day in the menstrual cycle when a woman will ovulate and abstaining from intercourse on the potentially unsafe days before and after. Intercourse on the day of ovulation and 3 to 4 days before and after carries a high risk of conception because sperm can live in a woman's body for as long as 6 days after intercourse (an average of 4 days). A sperm can fertilize an egg during the first 24 hours after ovulation.

Natural birth-control methods are the least reliable form of contraception because they depend on an estimate of the time of ovulation; each woman's menstrual cycle can vary from month to month, and some women may ovulate more than once during a cycle. You will need to keep records over several months to be able to accurately estimate the pattern of your cycle. There are several ways to calculate the time of ovulation, which occurs in most women about 14 days before the first day of their period.

Temperature Method

In most women, morning temperature (called basal body temperature) rises slightly just after ovulation and does not fall again until shortly before their period begins. Take your temperature each day as soon as you wake up—before you get out of bed or eat or drink anything—using a special thermometer designed to record small changes in temperature. Keep a chart of each temperature recording to determine your pattern of ovulation. Avoid intercourse from the first day of a period until 3 full days after the temperature rise. The disadvantages to this method are that you have no warning when ovulation will occur, and temperature readings can be inaccurate.

Ovulation-Predictor Kits

Ovulation-predictor kits are available over the counter to help you determine when you are ovulating. To use, hold a test strip under your stream of urine and check the strip's change of color according to the package directions. To prevent pregnancy, avoid having intercourse for 3 to 4 days before and after ovulation.

Mucus-Inspection Method

About 4 days before ovulation, the mucus from the cervix becomes thin, clear, sticky, and plentiful, similar to the consistency of egg whites. To prevent pregnancy, avoid intercourse from the time the wet mucus appears until 4 days after the mucus becomes noticeably reduced and drier after ovulation.

Mucothermal Method

The mucothermal method combines the temperature method and the mucus-inspection method (see previous page). It is the most reliable natural method, especially when performed with the guidance of a trained health care professional. But you must avoid intercourse for at least 3 days after your temperature rises and for 4 days after your mucus thins.

Calendar Method

The calendar method is the least reliable natural method. To detect ovulation, you keep an accurate record of the lengths of your cycles for at least 12 months. Count the first day of your period as day 1. Subtract 20 days from your shortest menstrual cycle to determine the first day of your fertile time and then subtract 10 days from your longest cycle to find the last day of your fertile time each month. The calendar method is impractical if you have an irregular menstrual cycle; you would need to abstain from intercourse most days of the month.

Sterilization

If you are certain that you do not want children in the future, sterilization is an almost completely safe and reliable form of birth control. Most doctors recommend male rather than female sterilization because it carries less risk and is simpler to perform. Because both sterilization procedures seal off only the tubes that carry sperm or eggs, they have no effect on the production of sex hormones. If you are a man, you will produce a sperm-free seminal fluid. If you are a woman, you will produce eggs, but they will not be able to reach the uterus. Menstrual periods are not affected in most cases.

Male Sterilization

A vasectomy is a simple procedure that usually involves no hospitalization. It is performed in a doctor's office or in an outpatient surgical center. A vasectomy requires only a local anesthetic and takes about 20 minutes to complete. During a conventional vasectomy, the doctor makes an incision over each side of the scrotum. He or she then cuts the two vas deferens (the tubes that carry sperm from the testicles) and blocks the tubes by tying them,

burning (cauterizing) them, or clipping them. He or she then stitches the incision in the scrotum. In a nonsurgical technique called the no-scalpel or no-suture vasectomy, the doctor makes only a tiny puncture in the skin to reach each vas deferens. As

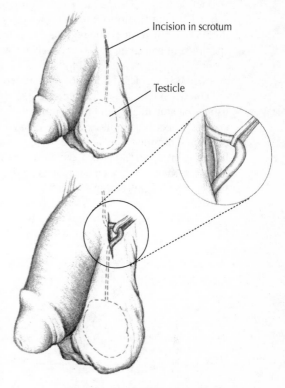

Vas deferens pulled through incision

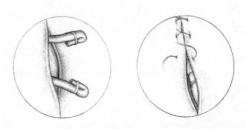

Cut ends of vas deferens sealed   Incision closed

Vasectomy
During a conventional vasectomy, the doctor makes a small ($^1/_4$" to $^1/_2$") incision in the scrotum (top) and pulls the vas deferens through the incision (center). He or she then cuts the vas deferens and ties, burns, or clips the ends to seal them off (bottom left). The incision is then closed with three or four stitches (bottom right).

in a conventional vasectomy, he or she then cuts and clips the tubes to seal them. You will still be able to ejaculate after the surgery, but your semen will not contain sperm.

Some sperm may have been stored in the seminal vesicles before the procedure, so your doctor will tell you to use some other method of contraception for the first 6 to 8 weeks after the procedure. During that time, you will have to bring in a specimen of semen at least twice. When two consecutive specimens are found to be free of sperm, you will be considered infertile. Your surgeon will tell you when it is safe to have intercourse without using a backup method of birth control. Vasectomy does not affect your ability to have an erection or an orgasm. Complications are rare but can include bleeding, bruising, and infection at the surgical site. Vasectomy is considered a permanent sterilization procedure, although surgical reversal is sometimes possible.

Female Sterilization

Female sterilization, or tubal ligation, is usually done in outpatient surgery while the woman is under general or spinal anesthesia. The operation takes less than half an hour to complete and can usually be performed through small incisions using a laparoscope (a viewing tube equipped with blades for cutting).

In the most commonly performed tubal ligation procedure, two tiny cuts that leave virtually no scars are made just below the navel. Through these cuts, the surgeon inserts the laparoscope and surgical instruments. An attachment to the laparoscope seals off the fallopian tubes, using electrocautery (application of heat using electric currents), tiny metal or plastic clips, rubber rings, or surgical cuts. Tubal ligation is often performed immediately after a vaginal delivery or as part of a cesarean section (see page 534), through the cesarean incision in the abdomen. The procedure is considered irreversible.

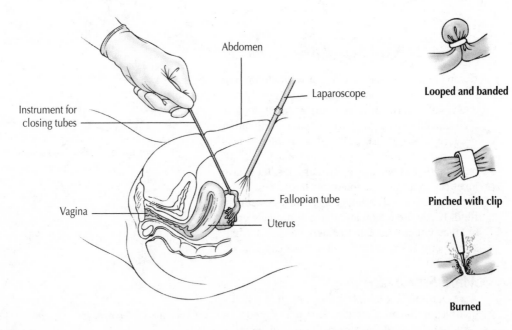

Looped and banded

Pinched with clip

Burned

Cut and tied

Tubal ligation
To perform a laparoscopic tubal ligation, the doctor makes two tiny incisions in the lower abdomen and inserts a lighted viewing instrument called a laparoscope into one of the incisions. He or she inserts another instrument into the other incision to permanently close off the fallopian tubes. The tubes are closed off by either looping and banding them with rubber rings, pinching them closed with metal or plastic clips, burning them with an electric current, or cutting and tying them off with stitches.

Sexually Transmitted Diseases

Sexually transmitted diseases (STDs) are infections that usually spread from one person to another through sexual contact. Although most STDs are transmitted through vaginal or anal intercourse, other forms of sexual contact, such as oral sex, can also transmit some STDs. Although anyone who is sexually active can contract an STD, about two thirds of people who have STDs are age 25 or younger. About 15 million new STD cases occur each year in the United States.

Factors that increase your risk of contracting an STD include having more than one sex partner, having a sex partner who has more than one sex partner, not using condoms (see next page), and having a history of other STDs. To reduce your risk of contracting an STD, abstain from sex or limit the number of sex partners you have and use a latex condom every time you have vaginal, oral, or anal sex.

All STDs can be treated, and most can be cured. If you have symptoms or think that you may have been exposed to an STD, contact your doctor, your local health department, or an STD or family planning clinic (such as Planned Parenthood) for confidential testing and treatment. If you are sexually active and are not in a monogamous relationship with an uninfected partner, you should be tested for STDs regularly. Because STDs often occur together, people who have one STD should be tested for others.

While you are being treated for an STD, you still can pass the infection to a sex partner. And even after successful treatment, you can easily become reinfected through sexual contact with an infected partner. For these reasons, your doctor will recommend that you and your partner be treated at the same time and that you both avoid all sexual contact until your treatment has been completed and you have no symptoms. Your doctor will tell you when it is safe to resume sexual activity.

Safer Sex

Abstinence (not having sex) is the only sure way to protect yourself from STDs. However, if you are sexually active, taking the following precautions will significantly reduce your risk of contracting an STD:

- Have sex with only one partner who has sex only with you. Ask all potential sex partners about their sexual history and intravenous (IV) drug use before becoming physically intimate.

- Use a latex condom every time you have vaginal, oral, or anal sex. Use only water-based lubricants. Do not use a condom after its expiration date or if it has been damaged in any way. Never reuse a condom.

- Keep in mind that STDs can be transmitted during sex using sexual aids or body parts other than the penis, such as fingers.

- Note that although spermicides kill some infectious microorganisms, they are formulated to kill sperm and are meant to be used along with condoms, not as a substitute. In addition, spermicides (including those containing nonoxynol-9) are not effective in preventing STDs, including HIV infection.

Although condoms provide effective protection against most STDs, they cannot always completely block contact with the bacteria or viruses that cause STDs. For this reason, always look for any signs of STDs, such as sores on the penis or around the vagina, in your sex partner. Because STDs do not always produce obvious signs, ask your partner directly. If you still have any doubts, don't have sex.

Chlamydia

Chlamydia is the most common sexually transmitted disease in the United States. It is caused by infection with the bacterium Chlamydia trachomatis, which is usually transmitted during vaginal or anal sex and, less frequently, during oral sex. In women, the bacteria can infect the urethra, the uterus and cervix, the fallopian tubes, the anus, and the conjunctiva (the mucous membrane that covers the white of the eye and lines the inside of the eyelids). In men, the bacteria can infect the urethra, the epididymis, the prostate gland, the anus, and the conjunctiva.

In women, untreated chlamydia can lead to pelvic inflammatory disease (see page 871), which can cause infertility. The infection can also cause inflammation of the urethra (nongonococcal urethritis; see page 481) in women. In men, chlamydia is one of the leading causes of urethritis. If not treated, the infection can lead to inflammation of the prostate gland (prostatitis; see page 831), narrowing of the urethra (urethral stricture; see page 837), inflammation of the epididymis (epididymitis; see page 827), an autoimmune disorder called Reiter's syndrome, or infertility (see page 494). In

How to Use a Condom Correctly

A condom is a sheath of latex that fits over an erect penis and protects against sexually transmitted diseases (STDs) by blocking the exchange of body fluids. However, condoms cannot protect against STDs unless they are used consistently and correctly. The following guidelines will help you to use condoms correctly:

- Use only latex condoms, and store them in a cool, dry place, out of direct sunlight.
- Never use a condom after its expiration date.
- Use a new condom each time you have vaginal, anal, or oral sex. Never reuse a condom.
- To avoid tearing a condom, do not use your fingernails, teeth, or any other sharp object to open a condom wrapper. If you tear a condom, throw it away and use a new one.

Opening a condom wrapper
Always open a condom wrapper carefully to avoid damaging the condom. Never open a condom wrapper with your teeth, fingernails, or other sharp object. If you damage a condom, throw it away.

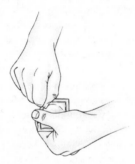

- Do not unroll the condom before placing it on the penis.
- Put the condom on after the penis is erect and before any contact is made between the penis and any part of your partner's body.
- If the condom does not have a reservoir tip, pinch the tip enough to leave $1/2$ inch of space for semen to collect. Always squeeze the tip of the condom to get the air out, which will help prevent the condom from breaking.
- If you are uncircumcised, pull back the foreskin before putting on the condom.
- If the condom is not prelubricated, place a couple of drops of water-based lubricant inside the condom.

WARNING!

Use Only Water-Based Lubricants With Latex Condoms

Never use creams, lotions, oils, or petroleum jelly to lubricate a condom; these products can weaken the latex and cause the condom to break.

- Holding the condom rim, place the condom over the tip of the penis. Then, continuing to hold it by the rim, unroll the condom to the base of the penis. If the condom is not prelubricated, lubricate the outside of the condom with a couple of drops of a water-based lubricant. (Lubricating the condom will increase sensitivity and help avoid tearing the condom.)

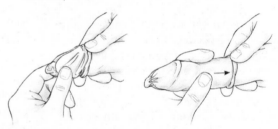

Putting on a condom
Hold the rim of the condom and place the condom over the tip of the erect penis (left). Continue to hold the rim of the condom and unroll the condom all the way down to the base of the penis (right). Pinch the tip of the condom to get the air out and to leave $1/2$ inch of space for semen to collect.

- If you feel the condom break during intercourse, stop immediately, withdraw carefully, and put on a new condom.
- After ejaculation and before the penis gets soft, grip the rim of the condom and carefully withdraw to make sure the condom doesn't slip off.
- To remove the condom, gently pull it off the penis, being careful that semen does not spill out.
- Wrap the condom in a tissue and throw it away. Wash your hands thoroughly with plenty of soap and hot water.

both men and women, the infection can be transmitted to the eye during sex or by hand-to-eye contact, where it can cause inflammation of the conjunctiva (conjunctivitis; see page 1038).

People who have chlamydia have an increased risk of becoming infected with HIV, the virus that causes AIDS (see page 909). Chlamydia can cause CD4 cells (the infection-fighting white blood cells that are targeted by HIV) to go to the infected area to fight the infection. If HIV is present in the infected area, it will target and infect the CD4 cells, which can then spread HIV throughout the body.

Symptoms

Because most people who have chlamydia have no symptoms, they do not seek treatment, which puts their sex partners at risk. If symptoms develop, it is usually within 1 to 3 weeks after exposure to the bacteria. In men, possible symptoms can include pain during urination, burning or itching around the urethra, a discharge from the penis, or swelling of the testicles. In women, possible symptoms can include pain in the lower abdomen, pain during sexual intercourse, vaginal discharge, and bleeding between menstrual periods. Women are less likely to have symptoms than men, but are more likely to experience long-term complications—such as infertility—as a result of the infection. Also, a pregnant woman who has chlamydia can pass the infection to her baby during delivery, which can cause pneumonia or conjunctivitis in the newborn.

Diagnosis

To diagnose chlamydia, a doctor uses a swab to obtain a sample of discharge from a man's urethra or a woman's cervix, for examination under a microscope. The doctor probably will order laboratory tests of a sample of urine and samples of cells taken from the penis, cervix, urethra, or anus.

Treatment

To treat chlamydia, a doctor may prescribe an antibiotic such as azithromycin or doxycycline. Because people with chlamydia may also have an STD called gonorrhea (see next page), doctors frequently prescribe a combination of antibiotics to treat both infections at the same time. In some cases, the antibiotics may be administered intravenously (through a vein) in the hospital. Both you and your partner should be treated to help ensure that the infection is eliminated. Your doctor

will ask you to avoid all sexual contact until treatment is completed and you have no symptoms. Ask your doctor when you can safely resume sexual activity.

Trichomoniasis

Trichomoniasis is a common sexually transmitted disease (STD) caused by Trichomonas vaginalis, a tiny, one-cell parasite. In women, the microorganism infects the vagina. In men, it can infect the urethra, the epididymis, the prostate gland, or the bladder. Five million new cases of trichomoniasis occur each year in women and men in the United States. Because the infection is usually transmitted through intercourse, it is likely that your sex partner also has the infection if you have it.

Symptoms

In women, trichomoniasis produces a frothy, yellow-green vaginal discharge, often with a strong odor. Itching and irritation may develop in the vaginal area. The infection can also cause discomfort during intercourse or urination. In a pregnant woman, trichomoniasis can cause preterm delivery (see page 529). Although most men with trichomoniasis do not have symptoms, some men may experience irritation inside the urethra, a mild discharge from the penis, or a mild burning sensation after ejaculation or urination. If the infection spreads to the epididymis, it can cause pain in the testicles. Even without symptoms, men with trichomoniasis can infect their sex partner.

Diagnosis

To diagnose trichomoniasis in a woman, a doctor will perform a pelvic examination and take a sample of vaginal secretions for laboratory analysis. To diagnose trichomoniasis in a man, a doctor will take a sample of secretions from the urethra for laboratory analysis. The doctor may also order urine tests.

Treatment

The usual treatment for trichomoniasis is the antibiotic metronidazole, given by mouth in a single dose. Both partners should be treated at the same time to help ensure that the parasite is eliminated. Your doctor will ask you to avoid sexual contact until both you and your partner complete treatment and have no symptoms. Ask your doctor when you can safely resume sexual activity.

> **WARNING!**
>
> ## Do Not Drink Alcohol When Taking Metronidazole
>
> When taking metronidazole, do not drink alcohol or take nonprescription medications that contain alcohol (for example, some over-the-counter cold medications). The combination of metronidazole and alcohol can cause serious side effects such as abdominal cramping, flushing, headache, nausea, or vomiting.

Genital Warts

Genital warts are a common and highly contagious sexually transmitted disease (STD) caused by infection with the human papillomavirus (HPV). More than 5 million people are infected with HPV each year in the United States. There are more than 100 types of HPV, 30 of which can infect the genital area. Some strains of HPV can produce genital warts and cause precancerous changes in cells. Some strains of HPV have been linked to cervical cancer in women and other genital cancers in both men and women.

Genital warts are spread during vaginal, anal, or oral sex and usually develop in warm, moist areas of the body, including the vagina, vulva, cervix, penis, scrotum, urethra, anus, or rectum. The warts usually develop within 6 weeks to 6 months after exposure to HPV. In rare cases, genital warts may develop on the lips, the tongue, the roof of the mouth, or in the throat.

There is no cure for genital warts, but most outbreaks clear up on their own after a few months. The warts frequently recur, even after they have been removed, requiring repeat treatment.

Symptoms
Genital warts usually begin as tiny, soft, flesh-colored swellings that eventually become hard and rough-surfaced and often develop stalks. Multiple warts often grow in a cluster that resembles a small cauliflower. Genital warts are usually painless, but they can cause itching. The warts tend to grow more rapidly during pregnancy or when the immune system has been weakened by diseases such as diabetes

(see page 889), HIV infection or AIDS (see page 909), or Hodgkin's disease (see page 626), or by having chemotherapy (see page 23) or taking anti-rejection drugs after transplant surgery.

Because many people who are infected with HPV never develop genital warts, they do not know they are infected. However, even without warts, they can transmit the virus to others. If left untreated, genital warts can cause sores and bleeding, which can increase the risk of becoming infected with HIV by providing a site for the virus to enter the bloodstream.

Diagnosis
A diagnosis of genital warts is based on the symptoms and a physical examination. In women, genital warts are often detected during a pelvic examination (see page 140). A doctor will remove and examine any wart that looks unusual or that persists for an unusually long time, to make sure it is not cancerous.

Treatment
An outbreak of genital warts can be treated by applying a prescription cream or gel, such as imiquimod or podofilox, directly to the affected area. Other topical treatments, such as podophyllum, trichloroacetic acid, or biochloroacetic acid, are applied to the affected area by a doctor or nurse. Because these treatments can harm a developing fetus, they are not prescribed for pregnant women. Genital warts can also be removed by cryosurgery (freezing), electrocauterization (burning), or laser surgery using a highly concentrated beam of light. Warts inside the urethra can be treated with medication or removed surgically. In some uncircumcised men, circumcision may be recommended to help prevent repeated outbreaks of genital warts.

Gonorrhea

Gonorrhea is a common sexually transmitted disease (STD) caused by the gonococcal bacteria Neisseria gonorrhoeae. In men, the bacteria usually infect the urethra (the tube that carries urine from the bladder out of the body); in women, the bacteria usually infect the cervix (the opening to the uterus). Gonorrhea can also infect the rectum or the throat through anal or oral sexual contact.

In men, untreated gonorrhea can spread up the urethra and cause painful inflammation of the prostate gland and the epididymis, which, if not treated promptly, can lead to infertility. In some men, gonorrhea can lead to a painful condition called urethral stricture (see page 837), in which scar tissue forms in the urethra, making urination difficult.

In women, untreated gonorrhea can cause pelvic inflammatory disease (see page 871), a condition that can damage the lining of the fallopian tubes or the uterus, causing infertility. The bacteria can also spread to the uterus and the abdominal cavity, causing abscesses (collections of pus) to form around the fallopian tubes and the ovaries. If the abscesses are not treated, they can rupture and spill into the abdomen, causing inflammation of the lining of the abdominal cavity (peritonitis; see page 759). If not treated, gonorrhea can increase the risk of ectopic pregnancy (see page 523) or miscarriage (see page 522). A pregnant woman with gonorrhea can pass the infection to her baby during delivery, causing the eye infection conjunctivitis (see page 1038).

In rare cases, untreated gonorrhea can spread through the bloodstream and cause inflammation in other parts of the body, such as the joints, heart valves, or brain. In some people, the condition causes skin lesions.

People who have gonorrhea have an increased risk of becoming infected with HIV, the virus that causes AIDS (see page 909). Gonorrhea can cause CD4 cells (the infection-fighting white blood cells that are targeted by HIV) to go to the infected area to fight the infection. If HIV is present in the infected area, it will target and infect the CD4 cells, which can then spread HIV throughout the body.

Symptoms

The symptoms of gonorrhea usually develop about 2 to 5 days after sexual contact with an infected person, but can take as long as 30 days. In the early stages of the infection, the symptoms are often mild and may go unnoticed. Frequently, women with gonorrhea have no symptoms, but some women develop symptoms about 2 to 8 days after sexual contact with an infected person or at the beginning of their next period. Possible symptoms include a mild fever, burning or pain during urination, cloudy discharge from the vagina, discomfort or pain in the lower abdomen, or abnormal bleeding from the vagina. In some cases, a woman with gonorrhea experiences painful urination, inflammation of the bladder (cystitis; see page 877), or vaginal bleeding with sexual intercourse. If gonorrhea has led to pelvic inflammatory disease, symptoms can include abdominal cramps and pain, bleeding between periods, vomiting, or fever.

Men who have gonorrhea often have no symptoms, or they may urinate more often than usual or have severe pain and burning during urination or a cloudy, pus-filled discharge from the penis.

When gonorrhea infects the rectum, a person may experience anal itching, a cloudy discharge from the anus, and painful, bloody bowel movements. When gonorrhea infects the throat, most people have no symptoms, but some can have a sore throat.

Diagnosis

A diagnosis of gonorrhea is based on the symptoms, a physical examination, the results of blood and urine tests, and laboratory analysis of the discharge. The doctor uses a swab to obtain a sample of discharge from the man's urethra or the woman's cervix for examination under a microscope.

Treatment

Gonorrhea can be treated with antibiotics such as cefixime (taken orally) or ceftriaxone (injected directly into a muscle). Because people who have gonorrhea often also have an STD called chlamydia (see page 477), doctors usually prescribe a combination of antibiotics to treat both infections at the same time. If gonorrhea has spread through the bloodstream, a doctor will admit the person to a hospital and prescribe intravenous antibiotics.

To prevent conjunctivitis in a newborn whose mother has gonorrhea, a doctor will apply medication such as silver nitrate to the infant's eyes immediately after delivery. If untreated, gonorrhea in an infant can lead to arthritis (see page 996) or a life-threatening condition called sepsis (bacteria in the blood).

Nongonococcal Urethritis

Nongonococcal urethritis (NGU) is a sexually transmitted disease (STD) that causes inflammation of the urethra (the tube that carries urine from the bladder out of the body). Nongonococcal means that the infection is not caused by the type of bacteria that causes gonorrhea (see page 480). Most cases are caused by the bacterium Chlamydia trachomatis.

NGU is usually transmitted through contact with the mucous membranes in the penis, vagina, mouth, or anus of an infected person during sexual activity. Other possible causes of NGU include urinary tract infections (see page 803), inflammation of the prostate gland (bacterial prostatitis; see page 831), narrowing of the urethra (urethral stricture; see page 837), tightening of the foreskin (phimosis; see page 839), and having a urinary catheter (a thin, flexible tube used to drain urine from the bladder).

In men, untreated NGU can lead to inflammation of the epididymis (epididymitis; see page 827), which can result in infertility (see page 494), arthritis (see page 996), conjunctivitis (see page 1038), and skin lesions. In women, untreated NGU can cause pelvic inflammatory disease (see page 871), which, in turn, can lead to ectopic pregnancy (see page 523), infertility, chronic pelvic pain, chronic inflammation of the urethra (urethritis; see page 878), inflammation of the vagina (vaginitis; see page 879), or, in a pregnant woman, miscarriage (see page 522). In both men and women, untreated NGU resulting from anal sex can cause severe inflammation of the rectum.

Symptoms

Often, NGU does not produce symptoms, but an infected person can still pass the infection to his or her sex partner. In men, possible symptoms can include a discharge from the penis, pain or burning when urinating, and itching, irritation, and tenderness. In women, possible symptoms include a painful, burning sensation during urination, and a frequent need to urinate that produces only a small amount of urine. Other symptoms in women include abdominal pain, a heavy vaginal discharge, bleeding between periods, or heavy menstrual bleeding. In both men and women, an anal infection can cause rectal itching and a discharge or pain during bowel movements. An oral infection usually does not produce symptoms, but some people can have a sore throat.

Diagnosis

A diagnosis of NGU is based on the symptoms, a physical examination, the results of urine tests, and laboratory analysis of any discharge. A doctor uses a swab to obtain a sample of discharge from a man's urethra or a woman's cervix for examination under a microscope. He or she usually orders a blood test to rule out gonorrhea.

Treatment

NGU is usually treated with an antibiotic such as azithromycin or doxycycline. You and your sex partner should be treated at the same time to help ensure that the infection is eliminated. Your doctor will ask you to avoid sexual contact until you have completed treatment and have no symptoms. Ask your doctor when you can safely resume sexual activity. Note that even after successful treatment, NGU may recur. If symptoms return, see your doctor immediately.

Genital Herpes

Genital herpes is a common, incurable sexually transmitted disease (STD) caused by the herpes simplex virus. One out of five Americans over age 12 has genital herpes. A similar virus that causes cold sores (see page 744) in the mouth also causes about 15 percent of cases of genital herpes, usually as a result of oral-genital contact. Genital herpes can be transmitted from one person to another through touching, kissing, and vaginal, oral, or anal sex.

In a person whose immune system has been weakened, such as from undergoing chemotherapy (see page 23), the herpes virus can spread throughout the body via the bloodstream and infect other organs and tissues. If a pregnant woman has an outbreak of genital herpes near the time of delivery, an obstetrician will recommend cesarean section (see page 534) to avoid infecting the baby.

People who have genital herpes have an increased risk of becoming infected with HIV, the virus that causes AIDS (see page 909), because genital herpes can cause sores and bleeding, which can increase the risk of HIV infection by providing a site for the virus to enter the bloodstream.

Symptoms

Because genital herpes often produces no symptoms, most people who have the disease do not know they are infected. In other cases, pain, tenderness, and itching may develop near the penis or vulva about 2 to 6 days after exposure to the virus. The person may also have a fever, a headache, or feel generally ill. The first episode of genital herpes symptoms, called primary herpes, usually occurs within 2 to 3 weeks of exposure to the virus.

In primary herpes, groups of blisters begin to appear in the area that was exposed to the virus on an infected person. In women, blisters may form inside the vagina or on the cervix, where they are not visible. In both men and women, blisters can also develop on the thighs or buttocks. Eventually the blisters break open to form extremely painful, shallow, open sores, which last about 2 weeks. Some people experience severe symptoms in primary herpes, including sore, swollen lymph glands in the throat, armpits, and groin, and flulike symptoms including fever, chills, headache, and fatigue.

Because the virus remains in the body after the blisters subside, about half of people who develop genital herpes have recurring outbreaks over the following months or years. Stress, sexual intercourse, surgery, menstruation, other infections, and skin irritations such as sunburn or a rash may trigger outbreaks. The subsequent outbreaks are usually mild, last about a week, and often can be suppressed by taking daily doses of an antiviral medication. Some people have frequent outbreaks, while others have none. Outbreaks usually last longer and are more painful in women than in men and in people who have a weakened immune system, such as those who are infected with HIV.

The major risk for people who have genital herpes is transmitting the virus to another person. Although genital herpes is most contagious when blisters or open sores are present, a person can still spread the virus between outbreaks. The virus can infect the skin if the skin is cut, chafed, or burned, or if a rash or other sores are already present.

Diagnosis

A diagnosis of genital herpes is based on the symptoms, a physical examination, and the results of laboratory tests performed on samples of fluid taken from the open sores. Because people who are infected with the herpes simplex virus have an increased risk of contracting other STDs, doctors may also order tests for other STDs. To confirm the diagnosis, a doctor may order blood tests to check for antibodies (infection-fighting proteins) produced by the immune system to fight the herpes virus.

Treatment

There is no cure for genital herpes, but your doctor may prescribe an antiviral drug such as acyclovir, famciclovir, or valacyclovir, which may speed healing and reduce the period of time during which the disease is most contagious. Your doctor will recommend that you keep the affected area clean and dry during outbreaks, avoid touching the sores, wash your hands thoroughly if you touch the sores, and avoid sexual contact from the moment symptoms begin until the last sore has fully healed. If you have another STD, the doctor will recommend treatment for that infection as well. Ask your doctor when you can safely resume sexual activity.

Syphilis

Syphilis is a sexually transmitted disease (STD) caused by the bacterium Treponema pallidum. The bacteria are transmitted by direct contact with a syphilis sore during vaginal, oral, or anal sex, and the infection spreads throughout the body in the blood and lymphatic vessels. A pregnant woman can transmit the infection to her fetus, potentially causing serious birth defects or stillbirth.

People who have syphilis have an increased risk of becoming infected with HIV, the virus that causes AIDS (see page 909). Syphilis can cause CD4 cells (the infection-fighting white blood cells that are targeted by HIV) to go to the infected area to fight the infection. If HIV is present in the infected area, it will target and infect the CD4 cells, which can then spread HIV throughout the body.

Symptoms

Syphilis progresses through three distinct stages, each with its own symptoms. If not treated promptly, the infection can persist for years.

● **First stage**   In the first stage, called primary syphilis, the disease is confined to one area of the body. From 10 days to 3 months after exposure to the bacteria (but usually within 2 to 6 weeks), a small, painless sore called a chancre develops. A chancre is usually red and solid and protrudes above the skin. The initial chancre usually appears in the genital area, such as on the penis or vulva or inside the vagina, but can also develop on the lips, tongue, cervix, rectum, or other parts of the body. Chancres on the penis are usually visible, but when they develop in a woman's vagina or cervix they are not easily detected. A chancre heals in 1 to 5 weeks, leaving a thin scar. During this stage, the bacteria circulate in the bloodstream.

- **Second stage**   During the second stage, called secondary syphilis, the bacteria spread and cause symptoms throughout the body. About 6 weeks after the chancre has healed, you may feel generally ill and have a sore throat, fever, and headache. You may have swollen glands in your neck, armpits, and groin, and a skin rash of small, red, scaly bumps that do not itch. You may experience patchy hair loss. Spots may appear on the palms of your hands and on the soles of your feet. Gray patches of skin, which are different from chancres, can develop in the mucous membranes of the mouth, vulva, and penis. A rash may also develop around the rectum. These skin conditions, which are highly infectious, usually heal within 2 to 6 weeks.

- **Third stage**   For several years during the third stage, called tertiary syphilis, a person has no symptoms. Then, without warning, the disease flares up, producing a variety of symptoms depending on the part of the body that has been infected. For example, if the infection has spread to the brain and nervous system, it can cause paralysis, dementia, loss of equilibrium, loss of sensation in the legs, and, rarely, blindness. If the aorta (the main artery in the body) is infected, its walls may weaken and balloon out, forming an aneurysm (see page 599). The infection can interfere with the functioning of the aortic valve, causing inflammation of the aorta or aortic insufficiency (see page 593). During this stage, syphilis can also affect the liver, the stomach, the eyes, and other organs and tissues throughout the body.

Diagnosis and Treatment

A diagnosis of syphilis is based on the symptoms, a physical examination, and the results of blood tests. A doctor may remove a sample of tissue from a sore for examination under a microscope, to look for the syphilis bacteria. If the doctor suspects damage to the brain and nervous system, he or she may test a sample of cerebrospinal fluid.

Syphilis is easy to treat in the first stage (and sometimes in the second stage) with injections of antibiotics (usually penicillin). If you are allergic to penicillin, the doctor will either prescribe another antibiotic or have you undergo a desensitization procedure in the hospital so you will be able to take penicillin. Desensitization involves giving the drug in a series of small doses, which helps prevent an allergic reaction. Treatment in the third stage of syphilis can prevent the disease from progressing but cannot reverse existing damage to tissues and organs.

If you are diagnosed with syphilis, you and your sex partner will be treated at the same time. Your doctor will ask you to avoid all sexual contact until treatment is complete and you have no symptoms. Ask your doctor when you can safely resume sexual activity. Remember to practice safer sex (see page 477 can be reinfected with syphilis after the disease has been cured.

Chancroid

Chancroid, also called soft chancre and soft sore, is a highly contagious sexually transmitted disease that is caused by the bacterium Haemophilus ducreyi. The infection causes painful, persistent ulcers (open sores), usually in the genital area. Chancroid is transmitted by skin-to-skin contact with an ulcer or by contact with the discharge from an ulcer. The infection is contagious only when ulcers are present.

People who have chancroid have an increased risk of becoming infected with HIV, the virus that causes AIDS (see page 909), because chancroid can cause sores and bleeding, which can provide a site for the virus to easily enter the bloodstream.

Symptoms

The symptoms of chancroid usually develop about 3 to 10 days after contact with an infected person. Initially, small, tender, pus-filled blisters form in the genital area and around the anus. The blisters quickly rupture to form soft, shallow ulcers, which may expand and join together to form larger ulcers. Although ulcers in the genital area can be very painful in men, women often are not aware that they have them. In some cases, the lymph glands in the groin become tender and swollen and a shiny, red-surfaced abscess forms. The abscess may rupture and release pus.

Diagnosis

A diagnosis of chancroid is based on the symptoms and an examination of the ulcers. Because a chancroid ulcer may initially be mistaken for a skin lesion caused by syphilis (see page 483) or genital herpes (see page 482), a doctor usually examines a sample of discharge from the ulcer under a microscope to confirm the diagnosis.

Treatment

To treat chancroid, doctors prescribe antibiotics such as azithromycin or ceftriaxone. In some cases, a doctor uses a hollow needle and a syringe to remove pus from an abscess. The doctor will monitor the infection for at least 3 months after treatment is completed to make sure it has been eliminated. Healing time is directly related to the size of the ulcer; larger ulcers can take several weeks or longer to heal completely. In severe cases, deep scarring can result.

Pubic Lice

Pubic lice (also called crab lice or crabs) are tiny, wingless, parasitic insects the size of fleas. An adult pubic louse has a small, flat body and is either gray, white, or brown, so it blends into its surroundings and is difficult to see. The lice lay shiny white eggs, called nits, at the bottom of hair shafts, where they hatch 7 to 10 days later.

Pubic lice need blood to survive, but can live for up to 48 hours without a human host. The lice usually infest pubic hair, but they occasionally attach themselves to armpit hair, beards, mustaches, eyebrows, eyelashes, or the hair on a person's head. In some cases, pubic lice infest the area around the anus and the hair on the hands, arms, legs, or trunk. An infestation usually involves fewer than a dozen lice.

Pubic lice can be transmitted by skin-to-skin contact with an infested person, sleeping in an infested bed, using an infested towel, wearing infested clothing, or, in some cases, by sitting on an infested toilet seat.

Symptoms

The symptoms of pubic lice usually develop about 5 days after infestation and include itching and skin irritation in the affected area (usually the pubic area) that worsens at night. The itching and skin irritation are an allergic reaction to the bites. (Resist the urge to scratch; scratching can spread the lice to other parts of the body.) If lice infest the eyebrows or eyelashes, the eyes may become itchy, watery, and reddened. If the infested area becomes infected, it can cause redness, swelling, tenderness, or drainage.

Diagnosis and Treatment

A diagnosis of pubic lice is based on the symptoms and an examination of the affected area. The lice and their nits may be visible to the naked eye or with a magnifying glass. A doctor may look at the lice under a microscope to confirm the diagnosis.

You can treat pubic lice at home by washing the affected area with a nonprescription medicated shampoo or lotion that contains a pesticide such as permethrin, lindane, or pyrethrins with piperonyl butoxide. Ask your doctor to recommend one. Follow the package directions carefully, because the chemicals in these products can be toxic if not used correctly. A single application is usually effective. Because itching and skin irritation can persist for a few days after treatment, your doctor may recommend applying a nonprescription hydrocortisone cream to the area. If you develop any symptoms of an infection, see your doctor, who will probably prescribe antibiotics.

Because pubic lice can survive without a human host for up to 2 days, you must also wash your clothes and bedding in very hot water and dry them on a high-heat setting to kill both the lice and their nits. Because pubic lice are spread by sexual contact, the affected person's sex partner or partners also must be treated, to avoid reinfestation. The affected person should avoid intimate contact with others until he or she is sure that the lice have been eliminated. The nits can survive for up to 6 days without a human host, so it is important to complete the entire course of treatment, according to package instructions, to kill all of them.

Not having sex and limiting the number of sex partners you have can help keep you from becoming infested (or reinfested) with pubic lice. Latex condoms are not an effective barrier against lice.

Sexual Problems

Sexual problems can prevent you from having a satisfying and fulfilling sexual relationship. These problems can be caused by or made worse by such factors as a lack of sexual knowledge and experience, inhibition, fatigue, interpersonal conflict, boredom, dissatisfaction with the appearance of your body, performance anxiety, guilt, or previous sexual abuse or assault. Sexual problems also can signal the presence of an underlying medical condition, such as diabetes. Sometimes physical problems such as an infection or inflammation can produce symptoms that prevent you from enjoying sex. Once diagnosed and treated by a doctor, these problems often disappear.

The symptoms of most sexual problems can be reversed with increased knowledge about sex and your own sexuality or simple techniques you can learn in sex therapy. The most common sexual problems in men include erection problems and premature ejaculation. In women, the most common sexual problems are the inability to achieve orgasm, lack of arousal or desire (which can also affect men), painful sex (medically known as dyspareunia), and vaginismus (involuntary spasms of the vagina). Differences in the level of sexual desire is a problem that can affect both men and women in a relationship when one partner wants to have sex more often than the other.

Erection Problems

An erection problem (which doctors call erectile dysfunction) refers to the inability to achieve and maintain an erection adequate for sexual intercourse. Erection problems are the most common sexual problem seen by doctors. Most men experience erection problems at some time in their life, but for 30 million American men (about 10 percent of the entire male population and 35 percent of men over age 60), erection problems are a chronic, recurring condition. Most erection problems are treatable and, with increased awareness of the problem, more men are seeking and responding to treatment.

Most erection problems are caused by physical factors. The ability to achieve and maintain an adequate erection depends on a combination of healthy nerves, blood vessels, muscles, and fibrous tissues, as well as on adequate levels of hormones such as testosterone. Damage, injury, or malfunction in any of these areas can interfere with the ability to achieve or maintain an erection.

Inflammation or infection of the prostate gland or bladder can make urination, erection, or ejaculation painful and difficult. In uncircumcised men, neglecting to clean under the foreskin increases the risk of an infection. The foreskin can become so tight over the swollen tip of the inflamed penis that it cannot be drawn back (phimosis; see page 839). Sexually transmitted diseases (STDs; see page 477) such as gonorrhea, chlamydia, or herpes also can affect a man's ability to have an erection.

Medical conditions that damage nerves and blood vessels—such as diabetes (see page 889), heart disease (see page 558), brain or spinal cord injuries, multiple sclerosis (see page 696), or Parkinson's disease (see page 691)—can cause erection problems. In some cases, prescription medications—such as drugs used to treat high blood pressure and heart disease, and drugs that affect the nervous system such as antidepressants, tranquilizers, and sedatives—contribute to erection problems. Cigarette smoking, over-the-counter medications, alcohol, or illicit drugs such as marijuana, heroin, and cocaine also can play a role. Peyronie's disease (see page 839), a condition in which scarring of the penile tissues produces a curvature of the penis and pain during an erection, is another possible cause. Smoking adversely affects blood flow and can affect a man's ability to have an erection.

In some men, psychological factors such as anger, stress, anxiety, or depression can contribute to erection problems. Being unable to maintain an erection can make a man feel inadequate, embarrassed, or guilty, and consider himself unattractive to his partner. These feelings may cause him to avoid intimate situations or withdraw from his partner, which can increase tension in the relationship. The psychological effects of erection problems can also affect other areas of his life, such as social interactions and job performance.

Symptoms

Men who have erection problems may be unable to achieve an erection, may be able to achieve an erection only occasionally, or may be unable to maintain an erection. If you have symptoms of erection problems, your doctor may refer you to a urologist (a doctor who specializes in treating disorders of the urinary tract).

Diagnosis

To help diagnose erection problems, a doctor will take a detailed health history and a sexual history. He or she will ask about your ability to achieve and maintain erections and ask you when and how often they occur. The doctor also will want to know about other diseases or conditions you have that could be contributing to the problem. He or she will ask questions about your use of prescription medications and other drugs (including alcohol), which can affect sexual performance. The doctor will perform a physical examination and may recommend blood and urine tests to measure levels of hormones, cholesterol, and glucose, and to evaluate pituitary, liver, kidney, testicle, and thyroid function.

In some cases, the doctor orders specialized tests to evaluate erectile function by examining the blood vessels, nerves, muscles, and other tissues of the penis and surrounding areas. The doctor also may evaluate blood flow in the penis using ultrasound (see page 111) images, which are pictures of blood flow in the penis during an erection induced by injecting a drug that dilates the blood vessels in the penis. The blood pressure in the penis is evaluated with a special cuff. A series of X-rays using a contrast medium (dye) may be performed to evaluate blood flow in the penis.

The doctor will probably evaluate your secondary sexual characteristics, such as breast development, to determine if you have a testosterone deficiency or an excess of the female hormone estrogen, either of which can interfere with the ability to have an erection. Penile nerve function tests can determine if there is sufficient sensation in the penis and surrounding area. Some doctors perform biothesiometry, a diagnostic technique that uses vibration to measure the perception of sensation. A decreased perception of vibration can indicate nerve damage in the pelvic area, which can result in erection problems. Erections during sleep can be measured at home by using either a snap gauge or a strain gauge, devices that are wrapped around the penis to monitor and measure nocturnal erections.

Treatment

If you have erection problems, your doctor will describe the available treatments. For any method to be effective, you must be committed to the option you select and have realistic expectations about the outcome. Because treatment will affect both you and your partner, your partner's involvement, commitment, and support are essential for success.

Medication

Sildenafil (also known by the brand name Viagra) is oral prescription medication used for treating erection problems. The drug does not produce erections, but improves erections already induced by sexual stimulation. For this reason, foreplay is essential for this drug to be effective. Sildenafil works by inhibiting the enzyme responsible for diminishing an erection by breaking down a chemical called cyclic guanosine monophosphate (cGMP). The action of sildenafil in the body increases the levels of cGMP, relaxing the smooth muscles in the penis and increasing blood flow into the penis.

Sildenafil is absorbed and processed rapidly by the body. It must be taken at least 30 minutes to 1 hour before sexual intercourse and should not be used more than once a day. Effectiveness depends on the cause of the erection problem, but the drug is effective in 50 to 75 percent of men who use it. Possible side effects include headaches, flushing, indigestion, and seeing some colors differently.

Vardenafil (brand name Levitra) and tadalafil (brand name Cialis) are other oral medications used to treat erection problems. Both drugs work in the same way as sildenafil to help men with erection problems achieve and maintain an erection in response to sexual stimulation.

Self-injection drug therapy

In self-injection drug therapy for erection problems, a man or his partner uses a tiny needle to inject a small amount of medication directly into the side of the penis. The drug relaxes the smooth muscle and widens the main artery that supplies blood to the penis, increasing blood flow to the penis. The injections are relatively painless and produce an erection that begins about 5 to 15 minutes after the injection and lasts from 30 minutes to 2 hours. No foreplay is needed to produce an erection.

Medications for Erection Problems

Q. *Can sildenafil or another medication improve my sex life?*

A. Yes and no. These drugs are prescription medications used for treating the inability to achieve and maintain an erection adequate for sexual intercourse. If you can achieve an erection through sexual stimulation but cannot maintain it, these drugs can help you. Keep in mind, however, that they are not aphrodisiacs, do not arouse or increase sexual desire, and are not substitutes for working on a relationship. Nor do they improve or prolong erections in men who have normal erections.

Q. *How do I obtain one of these drugs?*

A. These medications are available only by prescription. See your doctor if you have an erection problem. The doctor will give you a thorough examination to diagnose your sexual problem to determine if medication would be helpful. Some Web sites offer prescriptions for these drugs without obtaining sufficient medical information from the person.

Q. *I have heart disease and, several months ago, my doctor prescribed nitroglycerin for my chest pain. I use it every day to prevent chest pain. Lately I've been having some problems getting erections. I've heard that medication could help with this problem. Should I ask my doctor for a prescription?*

A. No. You cannot safely use sildenafil, vardenafil, or tadalafil for your erection problem if you are taking heart medications such as nitroglycerin or alpha blockers. The combination can cause dangerously low blood pressure. Make sure your doctor knows about all medications you are taking.

Urethral suppositories

Urethral suppositories are sometimes recommended for treating erection problems. A urethral suppository is a single-use applicator filled with the drug alprostadil, a vasodilator that causes an erection by relaxing the smooth muscle of the penis and widening the main artery that supplies blood to the penis. To use a urethral suppository, insert the applicator about an inch into the urethral opening of the penis. The drug is released, absorbed by the urethra, and transported to the surrounding tissues. An erection begins within 8 to 10 minutes and may last as long as 30 to 60 minutes.

Vacuum devices

Vacuum devices produce erections by pulling blood into the penis and trapping it. You insert your penis into a hollow plastic tube that is closed at one end and press the tube against your body to form a seal. A vacuum is created in the tube with a small hand- or battery-driven pump, drawing blood into the penis and causing the penis to engorge, enlarge, and become rigid. After 1 to 3 minutes in the vacuum, an adequate erection develops and you place a soft rubber O-ring around the base of

the penis to trap blood and maintain the erection until you remove the O-ring after sex. The O-ring should be left in place for no more than 30 minutes, or the blood supply to the penis could be blocked.

Penile implants

An implantable penile prosthesis (artificial device) is another treatment option for erection problems. All penile implants place prosthetic tubes inside the penis to produce engorgement similar to that of a natural erection. Most implants are inflatable and

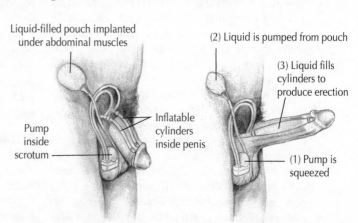

Penile implant
The inflatable penile implant is a device that is surgically implanted in the penis, scrotum, and lower abdomen. The implant contains cylinders that fill with fluid in the penis to mimic the natural engorgement process that occurs during an erection. The cylinders are attached to a pump that is activated by squeezing the scrotum.

are flaccid when not in use. These devices are very effective for treating all types of erection problems but, because they are mechanical, they can occasionally malfunction.

Vascular reconstructive surgery

Vascular reconstructive surgery is used only to treat erection problems caused by specific blood vessel abnormalities that block the flow of blood to the penis. Only a very small percentage of men are candidates for this surgery. Experimental techniques include revascularization (rerouting blood vessels to renew and increase blood flow to the penis) and venous ligation (sealing off the veins in the penis that leak blood and prevent erections).

Premature Ejaculation

Premature ejaculation is ejaculation with minimal sexual stimulation or too rapidly to allow full enjoyment of sexual relations. Most men have premature ejaculation from time to time, but it becomes a problem when it persists or recurs. The problem occurs most often in young, inexperienced men during their first sexual experiences, but it can affect men of any age. Many men with the condition are able to postpone orgasm and ejaculation while masturbating but cannot do so during intercourse.

Some affected men can delay ejaculation in a long-term relationship but find that it recurs when they are with a new partner. In these cases, the problem is likely to be caused by the lack of intercourse for a long period or by performance anxiety. Other men may have had early sexual experiences, such as masturbating hastily to avoid being caught by their parents, that programmed them to ejaculate quickly. But for most men with persistent premature ejaculation, the problem occurs because they have not learned how to regulate the amount of sexual stimulation and control the increase in sexual arousal before it reaches the point at which ejaculation is inevitable. Premature ejaculation can also be caused by withdrawal from alcohol or some illicit drugs such as heroin.

Diagnosis and Treatment

Premature ejaculation is often a temporary problem affecting sexually inexperienced men that resolves on its own over time, especially with an understanding partner. Your doctor will be able to diagnose premature ejaculation after listening to a description of your problem. He or she may prescribe a selective serotonin reuptake inhibitor, a medication usually used to treat depression, which is often effective for the treatment of premature ejaculation.

The doctor also may refer you to a sex therapist or suggest techniques that can help you delay ejaculation. Most of these techniques teach you how to identify and control the sensations that precede orgasm. For example, the start-stop technique is a series of progressive exercises beginning with masturbation and ending with intercourse that provide greater and greater control over ejaculation. In the squeeze technique, your partner squeezes just below the head of your penis or at the base of your penis to delay orgasm. Having intercourse with your partner on top can make you more relaxed and better able to guide your partner's actions.

Desensitizing creams and condoms can diminish the amount of sensation you experience during intercourse, but they do not provide a long-term solution to the problem and can cause irritation in your partner. Trying to concentrate on something else during intercourse generally does not help.

Inability to Achieve Orgasm

Many women have never experienced an orgasm, but lack of orgasm is rare among men. Only about 20 to 30 percent of all women regularly reach orgasm through vaginal penetration alone, without additional stimulation of the clitoris. Up to 10 percent of women cannot reach orgasm even with stimulation of the clitoris by themselves or their partner.

The inability to reach orgasm may be lifelong or can begin at any time. A common factor contributing to the inability to achieve orgasm (medically known as anorgasmia) is lack of adequate sexual information. Reaching orgasm requires sufficient stimulation of the clitoris, and many women may never have learned how to get enough stimulation to reach orgasm. Some women have never allowed themselves to be fully sexual, possibly because of a strict or religious upbringing. They may consider their sexuality embarrassing, making sex difficult because of their beliefs and feelings. A lack of sexual awareness, self-exploration, and self-stimulation is a common characteristic of women who are seeking treatment for anorgasmia.

The inability to achieve orgasm also can result from a lack of sexual interest that began with a physical problem such as damage to the vagina after childbirth, thyroid disease, or a side effect of drugs such as antidepressants.

Diagnosis and Treatment

If you are unable to achieve orgasm during sexual activity, talk about the problem with your doctor. He or she will perform a physical examination and will probably order a variety of tests to rule out a physical cause of your problem.

Treatment of an inability to achieve orgasm depends on the underlying cause. If your doctor cannot identify an underlying physical condition, he or she may be able to suggest ways to help you achieve orgasm or may refer you to a sex therapist for treatment. Sex therapy usually requires both partners to participate in therapy sessions and perform recommended exercises at home.

The most successful treatment prescribed by sex therapists for anorgasmia is sexual self-exploration through masturbation, combined with sexual fantasy. Masturbation is a normal, healthy activity that can help a woman learn how to become aroused and find the kind of sexual stimulation she needs to reach orgasm. Then she can use self-stimulation to reach orgasm when she is with her partner, showing her partner the techniques that work best.

Sometimes trying a new position during intercourse can help. If your partner is willing, experiment with some new positions. Many women find it easier to attain orgasm when they are on top, astride their partner. In this position, a woman can control the intensity and exact location of her clitoral and vaginal stimulation.

Painful Intercourse

Pain during sexual intercourse, also called dyspareunia, can affect both men and women and is usually caused by a physical condition. In women, causes of frictional pain at the vaginal opening include inadequate vaginal lubrication, a vaginal or bladder infection, a sexually transmitted disease (STD) such as genital herpes (see page 482), or

soreness after childbirth. Deep pelvic pain can result from conditions such as endometriosis (see page 870), a disorder of the ovaries, or allergic reactions. Chronic pain in the lower back also can cause deep pelvic pain during intercourse.

Common causes of painful intercourse in men include a tight foreskin, an STD, infection of the prostate gland or bladder, an anatomical abnormality of the penis, or inflammation. Cancer of the penis or testicles and musculoskeletal conditions such as arthritis in the lower back also make thrusting uncomfortable. Some spermicides (see page 471) can cause a burning sensation in both men and women.

Symptoms, Diagnosis, and Treatment

In women, symptoms of dyspareunia include pain or discomfort in the external part of the genitals or deep inside the pelvic area. Men usually experience pain in the penis.

Your doctor will be able to find the cause of your discomfort by performing a physical examination of your reproductive organs and ordering tests to detect an infection or an underlying medical condition. Treatment of dyspareunia depends on the underlying cause.

Lack of Interest in Sex

A lack of interest in sex is the second most common sexual problem (after erection problems) and affects both men and women. The problem can involve both a lack of desire for one's partner and the inability to become sexually aroused during sexual activity. Fatigue and stress are common causes of lack of interest in sex. Physical causes include a hormonal imbalance, infection, anemia, genital pain, or a long-term illness such as cancer or heart disease. Disinterest in sex sometimes masks another sexual problem, such as premature ejaculation (see previous page) or a woman's inability to have an orgasm (see previous page). After the birth of a baby, some women feel a lack of desire for sex. Pain and bleeding from a recent delivery, sleep deprivation, postpartum depression (see page 540), and fear of another pregnancy can contribute to a decreased desire for sexual activity at this time. Other causes of decreased desire in both men and women include:

- Anxiety after a traumatic life event, such as death of a family member, financial problems, or losing a job
- Anger
- Depression
- A traumatic sexual experience in childhood
- Use of alcohol or other drugs such as narcotics or tranquilizers

The male sex hormone testosterone stimulates the male sex drive. If your testosterone levels are low, your sexual interest and capacity for arousal are also likely to be low. The condition underlying a drop in testosterone level may be physical, such as liver, kidney, or pituitary disease, or it may be a side effect of a drug you are taking. Other sexual disorders, such as erection problems (see page 486), can interfere with the enjoyment of intercourse and cause a man to lose interest in sex or avoid sex.

In some cases, poor communication causes a woman to receive less than adequate sexual stimulation from her partner. In other cases, a partner may forget or ignore a woman's request for a certain type of foreplay. All of these factors can contribute to a loss of sexual desire in women.

Diagnosis and Treatment

Your doctor will examine you to rule out any physical cause for your lack of interest in sex. If no obvious physical cause is found, your doctor probably will recommend sex therapy for you and your partner. Sex therapists usually prescribe psychological therapy sessions and progressive exercises to do at home, to teach both partners how to get more in touch with their body. The goal of the process is to resolve old conflicts and rekindle a desire for sexual activity.

| MY STORY | **Lack of Interest in Sex** |

I'm 36 years old and haven't been interested in having sex with my husband since our second baby was born 1 year ago. At first I thought I was just recovering from the delivery and pain from my episiotomy. Also, my husband, Pete, and I felt like zombies because we were getting along on very little sleep. He was traveling a lot on business, so sometimes I felt like a single parent when I was here alone with the kids. I told myself that when things settled down, my sex drive would return to normal. But after 6 months or so I still felt no desire for sex.

Having an infant and a toddler raises the stress level incredibly. The same thing happened with our first child, but my sex drive didn't disappear after I had my first baby the way it did after the second one. It's funny, but before we had this baby I couldn't wait to go to bed with Pete. After the baby, I would wait until Pete was asleep before going upstairs to bed, even though I was exhausted. I began to feel guilty about turning him away, and I knew that we couldn't go on this way forever. Finally we had a big argument about it that seemed to clear the air. We decided to seek help.

I told my gynecologist about the problem and she surprised me by saying that a lack of desire for

Little by little, I began to feel desire for my husband again.

sex happens to a lot of women after childbirth. She suggested that Pete and I see a sex therapist.

During sex therapy, we did a lot of soul-searching as we completed each stage of the therapy. I found the guided imagery—using my imagination to go through each part of my body—especially helpful because it helped me realize that part of my problem was that I had a lot of anxiety about getting pregnant again. We want only two children, and the more anxious I became about a possible third pregnancy, the less I wanted to have sex with Pete.

Pete felt terrible when I told him my fears. Being so emotional made me realize how much I love him and how badly I had been treating him. Little by little, I began to feel desire for my husband again. We're having sex two or three times a month now. That may not seem like much, but with all of our pressing responsibilities, it feels like a honeymoon. My gynecologist recommended a very effective method of birth control, so my pregnancy worries have diminished. It's wonderful to have resolved our problem so we can have a healthy relationship again—both physically and emotionally.

Differences in Sex Drive

People have different levels of sexual desire. Many—if not most—couples experience a difference in their sex drives. When misunderstood, these differences can cause friction and resentment in a relationship. Often, couples do not need counseling or treatment to find a solution to their problem—they simply negotiate their differences. For example, if your partner wants to have sex more often than you do, you can suggest having intercourse the same number of times each week and adding oral stimulation once or twice a week. If this type of negotiation is not possible, you may benefit from seeing a qualified therapist or counselor.

If you think that a physical problem—such as genital pain, extreme fatigue, or a hormonal imbalance—may be lowering your or your partner's desire for sex, see your doctor for a physical examination. Other medical conditions that can affect sexual desire include depression (see page 709) and anxiety (see page 718). Drinking too much alcohol, taking sleeping pills or tranquilizers, or using illegal drugs can lower sexual desire. Some prescription drugs, such as those used for treating seizures and high blood pressure, also can have a dampening effect on sex drive. Talk to your doctor if your interest in sex has declined so much that it is causing problems in your relationship.

Vaginismus

Vaginismus is the involuntary spasm of the muscles in the lower third of a woman's vagina. This condition prevents intercourse because the muscles around the opening of the vagina tighten so much that the penis cannot penetrate. Women who have vaginismus may not even be able to insert a tampon into their vagina. The inability to reach orgasm (see page 489) often accompanies this disorder.

Vaginismus is an exaggeration of a natural protective vaginal reflex, similar to the action of closing your eyes in a dust storm. The most common causes of vaginismus are emotional factors such as shame, guilt, or anxiety over a possible pregnancy, or the anticipation of painful intercourse. Inadequate education or misinformation about sexuality can produce fear that results in the disorder.

Temporary vaginismus sometimes occurs when a woman has a physical problem that affects the genitals, such as an abscess or severe inflammation of the vagina. Any traumatic sexual experience, such as rape or sexual abuse, can cause temporary or permanent vaginismus.

Diagnosis and Treatment

Your doctor can diagnose vaginismus from your description of the symptoms and an examination of your genital area. If the doctor suspects a physical cause, he or she will order any tests necessary to diagnose it. If no physical cause is detected, the doctor probably will refer you to a sex therapist for treatment. The therapist will work with you to find the underlying cause of the problem and help you overcome it.

4

Infertility

Infertility is a medical condition that impairs a person's ability to have children. Doctors diagnose infertility when a couple has failed to achieve a pregnancy after having unprotected intercourse for several months. Doctors also consider women infertile who have become pregnant but have not been able to have a live birth because of repeated miscarriages or stillbirths. Infertility affects more than 6 million people nationwide, occurring in both men and women.

Coping with infertility can be a difficult, life-changing process that produces strong feelings of loss and disappointment. Both women and men may feel helpless, angry, or guilty; men may feel that it diminishes their masculinity and women their femininity. Couples who undergo treatment for infertility often experience hope followed by disappointment.

Diagnostic techniques, innovative drugs, and surgical procedures are available to help many infertile couples. Most cases of infertility are treated with medication or surgery. However, about 5 percent of cases require more sophisticated assisted reproductive techniques, such as in vitro fertilization.

The Causes of Infertility

Infertility is a problem usually experienced as a couple. There are many causes of infertility, and a couple can have more than one medical condition that affects their fertility. About 40 to 50 percent of cases of infertility result from a difficulty with the woman's reproductive system and about 30 to 40 percent from a difficulty with the man's. In approximately 10 to 30 percent of couples, infertility results from either factors related to both the man and the woman or is considered unexplained. Many causes of infertility are reversible with treatment, but some are not. If the cause of infertility cannot be corrected, techniques exist that can bypass it and result in a pregnancy. However, there are no guarantees of success from infertility treatment and, in spite of repeated attempts, some couples never conceive.

Causes of Infertility in Women

The causes of infertility in women are numerous and range from a deficiency of eggs, to infection that causes obstructive scarring in the reproductive system, to medical conditions such as diabetes or thyroid disorders that alter metabolism. The most common causes of infertility in women are:

- **Lack of ovulation** Failure to ovulate (release an egg from the ovary during the menstrual cycle) is usually caused by a hormonal imbalance.
- **Polycystic ovarian syndrome** Polycystic ovarian syndrome (see page 865), a metabolic

disorder characterized by abnormal hormone levels, affects up to 10 percent of all women. An imbalance of the ovulation-stimulating hormones, follicle-stimulating hormone (FSH), and luteinizing hormone (LH) blocks ovulation.

● **Infection** Sexually transmitted diseases (STDs; see page 477) or peritonitis (inflammation of the membrane lining the wall of the abdominal cavity) can cause scarring and blockage of the fallopian tubes.

● **Endometriosis** The growth of uterine tissue in the pelvis can either block an egg's passage from the ovary through a fallopian tube or form ovarian cysts.

● **Pelvic surgery** Surgery in the pelvic area can result in adhesions (bands of fibrous scar tissue) that obstruct or misshape a woman's reproductive organs, preventing an egg from reaching a fallopian tube or the uterus.

● **Abnormal growths in the uterus** Fibroids (see page 867) or polyps inside the uterus can prevent a fertilized egg from implanting in the uterine wall.

● **Medical conditions** Some disorders, such as diabetes (see page 889) or hypothyroidism (see page 903), can inhibit ovulation and the production of the hormones needed to sustain a pregnancy.

● **Scant or thick cervical mucus** Mucus secreted by the cervix normally eases the passage of sperm, but in rare cases in which the amount of mucus is either insufficient or the mucus is too thick, sperm cannot enter the uterus.

Causes of Infertility in Men

Most causes of infertility in men result from the inability of sperm to fertilize an egg. A man may not produce enough sperm, the sperm may not be mobile enough to reach an egg and fertilize it, or the sperm may be abnormal in shape or size. Blockage of the vas deferens (one of the tubes that carry sperm from the testicles to the urethra) also can prevent sperm from leaving the body during ejaculation. Erection problems (see page 486) have a similar effect. The most common causes of male infertility include:

● **Chronic infection** Some STDs, such as chlamydia (see page 477) and gonorrhea (see page 480), and other infections (such as an infection in the prostate gland) can produce a blockage in the vas deferens or lower the number of sperm produced (sperm count).

● **Exposing the testicles to high temperatures** The testicles are outside of the body, in the scrotum, because they need to be in a temperature lower than body temperature to work properly. Soaking for a long time in a tub of very hot water, wearing tight clothing, or sitting for long periods can raise the temperature of the testicles, reducing sperm count.

● **Cigarettes, alcohol, and drugs** Smoking more than a pack of cigarettes a day, drinking excessively, or using marijuana or cocaine can lower sperm count and reduce sperm motility (movement).

● **Varicose veins in the testicles** Called varicoceles (see page 829), varicose veins in the testicles decrease sperm production and affect about 40 percent of infertile men.

● **Reproductive tract surgery** Hernia repair, prostate surgery, or a vasectomy can produce scar tissue or damage nerves, affecting the functioning of the vas deferens and obstructing the flow of semen.

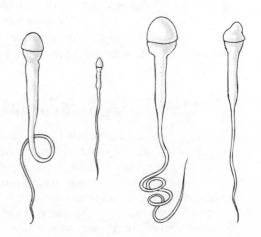

| Healthy sperm | Abnormally small sperm | Abnormally large sperm | Abnormally shaped sperm |

Abnormal sperm
All men have some abnormal sperm that cannot fertilize an egg. Abnormal sperm can be too small, too large, or misshapen. A man is considered fertile if at least half of his sperm are healthy. (All illustrations are magnified.)

- **Prescription drugs**   Medications used to treat depression or high blood pressure can make it difficult to achieve an erection.
- **Medical conditions**   Some disorders—such as diabetes (see page 889), heart disease (see page 558), multiple sclerosis (see page 696), and Parkinson's disease (see page 691)—can affect blood vessels and nerves and cause erection problems.
- **Structural abnormalities in the reproductive tract**   Structural abnormalities, which may be congenital (present at birth) or develop from infection or surgery, can obstruct the passage of sperm or semen.

- **Injury to the groin**   An injury to the testicles can produce scar tissue that obstructs the passage of sperm.
- **Disorders of the immune system**   Conditions that affect the immune system, which may be hormonal or may occur when a man's immune system mistakenly produces infection-fighting antibodies that attack his own sperm, can prevent sperm from reaching and penetrating an egg.
- **Ejaculation problems**   If a man has erection problems or a condition in which semen is ejaculated backward into the bladder (called retrograde ejaculation), sperm cannot fertilize an egg.

Lifestyle Factors That Affect Fertility

The causes of infertility are numerous, and many can be traced to a treatable medical condition, but some lifestyle factors also can affect your chances of conceiving a child. If you are trying to conceive, keep the following in mind:

- **Delayed childbearing**   A woman's fertility starts to decline after about age 30. Advancing maternal age coupled with a medical cause of infertility significantly increases a woman's risk of infertility.

- **Smoking**   Cigarette smoking decreases the amount of estrogen a woman's ovaries produce for ovulation and increases the risk of genetic abnormalities in her eggs. Smoking also increases the risk of miscarriage and can bring on early menopause. In men, smoking seems to increase the production of abnormally shaped or genetically altered sperm.

- **Weight problems**   Overweight women produce excessive amounts of estrogen and underweight women produce too little estrogen, both of which can disrupt ovulation. Obese women have an increased risk of miscarriage, which can result from a hormonal imbalance. Obese men can become infertile when layers of fat increase the temperature around the testicles, producing a low sperm count.

- **Alcohol consumption**   Having even one alcoholic drink per week can lower a woman's chances of conceiving by about 7 percent. Excessive drinking (consuming more than two drinks a day) lowers a man's sperm count. The more you drink, the lower your chances of conceiving.

- **Sexually transmitted diseases**   STDs such as chlamydia can cause scarring of the fallopian tubes, blocking them and preventing eggs from traveling to the uterus.

- **Caffeine**   Consuming more than two caffeine-containing beverages per day may decrease fertility.

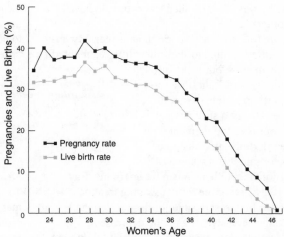

Age and success rates for assisted reproductive technologies
A woman's age has the biggest influence on the success of an assisted reproductive technology using the woman's own eggs. The success rates are defined by pregnancies and live births. The success rates are highest for women in their 20s and start to decline after about age 30, reflecting the normal gradual decline in a woman's fertility with age. The chart above is based on 1999 figures from the US Centers for Disease Control and Prevention (CDC).

Diagnosing Infertility

During the time you are trying to conceive, keep track of the length of your menstrual cycles for a few months and use a home ovulation-predictor kit to predict when you ovulate. Recording this information in a log will help you determine the best time to have intercourse, and the information can help your doctor later if you seek help trying to conceive. In the past, many doctors told their patients to try to conceive for 12 months before seeking medical help, but because many women are waiting until they are older to have a baby, this may be too long.

If you have not conceived after 6 months of trying, you and your partner should see your doctor, especially if you are over age 30, have a history of pelvic inflammatory disease (PID; see page 871), or have irregular periods. Your doctor will take a complete medical history from both you and your partner, including asking questions about the frequency and timing of your sexual intercourse. He or she may order some initial infertility tests. Depending on the findings of these tests, your doctor may then refer you to a reproductive endocrinologist (a doctor who specializes in diagnosing and treating fertility problems).

Infertility Testing in Women

Infertility testing is usually much more extensive for women than for men. The initial tests will determine if you are ovulating and can evaluate the quality of your eggs. At your first appointment with the infertility specialist, he or she can test your baseline levels of follicle-stimulating hormone (FSH) and estrogen. FSH stimulates the growth of follicles

---

MY STORY   **Secondary Infertility**

My husband and I had our first child, Shelby, when I was 34. I had no trouble getting pregnant, and the pregnancy went very smoothly. When Shelby was 3, we decided it was time to have another child.

We tried to conceive for about a year. My husband, Ray, wanted to start infertility treatment after a few months, but I was sure I would get pregnant if we just kept trying. After 18 months, I agreed to see a specialist. During our first appointment with the infertility specialist, the doctor said that my age was part of the problem. When we got home, Ray started blaming me for not seeking treatment sooner. I felt responsible for the problem and became defensive, angry, and depressed.

Our marriage began to suffer, and I didn't get much support from my family or friends—especially those who were having problems conceiving their first child. They thought I should stop complaining and be thankful for the child I have. They didn't seem to understand that you can be extremely grateful for a child and still yearn for another. Special occasions that used to be happy now triggered sadness. I declined invitations to friends' baby showers and stopped going to my

They didn't seem to understand that you can be extremely grateful for a child and still yearn for another.

sister-in-law's house because I couldn't bear to see her children playing together.

Shelby could feel the tension between Ray and me even though we never talked about it in front of her. She became anxious and clingy and didn't want to be away from us. She seemed to think we were upset with her. I felt guilty about not giving her a sibling.

The doctors eventually discovered a blockage in one of my fallopian tubes that must have been caused by an infection that occurred during my first pregnancy. By then, I was 38 and my biological clock was sounding an alarm. To save our relationship, Ray and I started seeing a marriage counselor and began attending a support group of infertile couples sponsored by a national infertility association. Through these resources, we learned to cope with the fact that the large family we had hoped for might never become a reality. People in the group who had gone through a similar situation helped us mourn our loss and move on, a process that took several months.

Now I'm 41 and Shelby is a happy, healthy 7-year-old. I went back to work when she entered first grade, and I love my job. Ray and I are content with our family and cherish Shelby.

(fluid-filled sacs that contain the developing eggs) in the ovaries. If you have an ovulation problem, measuring the level of luteinizing hormone (LH) also can be helpful. LH stimulates the follicles to release an egg and causes the lining of the uterus to thicken in preparation for a pregnancy. The doctor can compare these initial hormone levels with levels found at other times in your cycle.

The doctor will ask you about your medical history and current health status to determine if any medical problems could be affecting your ability to conceive. He or she will ask about your menstrual history; any past pregnancies, miscarriages, or abortions; any medications you are taking; and the type of birth control you use. Tell the doctor if you have ever had any STDs or abdominal surgery; surgery or pelvic infections from some STDs can scar and block the fallopian tubes, preventing pregnancy.

The doctor will perform a complete physical examination, including checking your thyroid gland for any abnormalities and looking for unusual hair growth on your face and body that could indicate high levels of male hormones. During the breast examination, the doctor may gently squeeze your nipples to see if any liquid comes out, a sign of increased levels of prolactin, a hormone that prevents ovulation. The doctor will then perform a pelvic examination to look for any growths, sores, or signs of infection.

Your second appointment will take place just before you ovulate so the doctor can perform an ultrasound examination to detect any abnormalities of your uterus and ovaries and to monitor the development of the egg-releasing follicle. More hormone tests will be done to screen for abnormal hormone levels.

Depending on the results of these tests, your doctor may also order some of the following tests:

● **Hysterosalpingogram**   A hysterosalpingogram is an X-ray procedure that uses a dye that is injected into the cervix and travels up the uterus and into the fallopian tubes. The dye looks black on the X-ray, allowing the doctor to see any abnormalities in your reproductive organs, such as a fibroid (see page 867) in the uterus or scar tissue blocking the fallopian tubes.

● **Hysteroscopy**   Doctors perform a hysteroscopy (see page 849) using a lighted viewing tube (hysteroscope) inserted into the cervix to see any

abnormality or growth in the uterus more clearly.

● **Laparoscopy**   In laparoscopy, a doctor inserts a viewing instrument (laparoscope) into your abdomen to evaluate the condition of the ovaries, fallopian tubes, and uterus. With laparoscopy, a doctor can detect conditions such as endometriosis (see page 870), adhesions (scar tissue), and abnormalities of the ovaries.

● **Endometrial biopsy**   Doctors do an endometrial biopsy (see page 849) to determine if the lining of the uterus is thickening enough in preparation for pregnancy. If the lining is too thin, you may not be producing enough of the hormone progesterone, which is needed to maintain a pregnancy. The doctor will take a small sample of tissue from the lining of your uterus shortly before your next period and send it to a laboratory for analysis.

Infertility Testing in Men

At your first appointment, the infertility specialist will ask you about your health history to find out if any past medical problems—hernia repair, groin injuries, STDs, or inflammation of the prostate—could be affecting your fertility. He or she will ask about your current health and lifestyle to determine if excessive smoking, drinking, or other drug use could be affecting your sperm. The doctor will then perform a thorough physical examination, including an examination of the hair growth in your genital area to determine if you are producing a sufficient amount of testosterone, and an examination of your penis, scrotum, and prostate (to look for abnormalities).

The semen analysis is the most important test for male fertility. The doctor will ask for at least one semen sample, obtained by masturbation. Before producing a sample, you will have to wait at least 48 hours (but not more than 5 days) after your last ejaculation. Among the factors the doctor will consider when evaluating your semen sample are the appearance and consistency of the semen, the total sperm count, the shape and structure of the sperm, and the motility (movement) and speed of the sperm. If any of these factors fall outside the normal range, the doctor will probably order a second sperm analysis for confirmation and a hormone evaluation to screen for more specific abnormalities.

In a small number of couples with otherwise unexplained infertility, doctors sometimes order specialized tests, such as a sperm penetration assay, which measures the sperm's ability to penetrate an egg by pairing the sperm with the egg from a hamster using in vitro fertilization (see page 500). Infertile men who have very low or absent sperm counts may undergo genetic testing to determine if they have a chromosome abnormality (see page 955). The results of the initial tests determine what other tests you will need.

If the results of your semen analysis are abnormal, the infertility specialist will probably refer you to a urologist (a doctor who specializes in treating disorders of the male urinary and reproductive system) who is trained in male infertility for a more extensive evaluation.

Unexplained Infertility

About 10 to 30 percent of all infertile couples are told that their infertility cannot be explained. Doctors reach a diagnosis of unexplained infertility after ruling out other possible causes through a standard battery of tests. The diagnosis does not mean that no cause for the infertility exists, but rather that the cause cannot be identified using the initial screening tests.

After 1 to 3 years of unexplained infertility, many couples conceive on their own. The age of the woman is usually the key in this process. Spontaneous conception is much more likely in a woman under age 35 than in a woman who is over 40. But treatment for unexplained infertility has been shown to improve pregnancy success rates over unprotected intercourse alone.

Many infertility centers recommend the following course of treatment: three to six cycles of ovulation-inducing drugs combined with intrauterine insemination (see page 500), followed by in vitro fertilization. Using this treatment regimen, pregnancy rates for couples with unexplained infertility are equal to or higher than those of couples with a diagnosed cause of infertility.

How to Choose an Infertility Treatment Center

Selecting an infertility treatment center can be confusing because different centers provide different services and produce varying success rates. When you are searching for infertility treatment, ask whether the centers you have selected offer the following basic services:

- **Seven-day availability** The center's staff and services should be available every day of the week, on weekends, and on holidays so you can call with information about your menstrual cycle and find out your test results quickly.
- **Psychological support** The center should have mental health professionals available to provide support during this difficult time.
- **On-site laboratory** The clinic should be able to perform semen analysis, postcoital tests, and blood and hormone tests on site to save critical time. The laboratory should be fully certified.
- **Ultrasound equipment** Transvaginal ultrasound monitoring, in which an ultrasound scan of your ovaries is performed through the vagina, helps to determine if the prescribed medication is stimulating ovulation and if your ovaries are releasing eggs.

Ask whether the doctors who will be caring for you are board-certified in reproductive endocrinology, how many live births have occurred in their program, and what the costs will be. Insurance coverage for infertility treatment varies by state and type of health insurance. Check with your employer to find out exactly what kind of coverage you have.

The US Centers for Disease Control and Prevention (CDC) collects and reports the success rates of all assisted reproductive technology programs in the country that belong to the Society for Assisted Reproductive Technologies. You can access this information on the Internet at http://www.cdc.gov/nccdphp/drh/art.htm. To obtain a printed copy, call the CDC's division of reproductive health at 770-488-5372.

Treating Infertility

Once the doctor has determined the cause of your infertility, he or she will recommend the most effective treatment. Many doctors try one therapy, such as ovulation-inducing drugs, for several months before changing to another. Infertility treatment can be stressful, so be sure to ask your doctor how realistic your chances are of conceiving using a given method before trying it. Remember that you have control over whether to continue treatment, stop treatment temporarily or permanently, or explore other options, such as adoption.

Treating Infertility in Women

Infertility treatment for women depends on the cause. Doctors usually try to treat infertility using conventional methods, such as drugs and surgery, before trying more advanced assisted reproductive techniques, such as in vitro fertilization (see page

500). However, some infertility problems, such as blockage of the fallopian tubes, have a better outcome using treatments such as in vitro fertilization, and doctors often recommend using them right away.

Drugs that induce ovulation

If failure to ovulate is the reason for your infertility, the first step is to look for easily treatable causes such as thyroid disease, which can often alter a woman's hormonal balance enough to affect ovulation. Otherwise, your doctor may recommend starting you on an ovulation-inducing drug such as clomiphene citrate (in pill form), which can stimulate the ovaries to release mature eggs. Women usually take one to four pills a day from the third to the seventh day of their menstrual cycle. Your doctor may take several blood samples to measure estrogen levels while you are taking the drug, and ultrasound scans to monitor your eggs. If this drug regimen is not effective in stimulating ovulation, the doctor may start you on a series of human menopausal gonadotropin hormones, taken by injection. This treatment may continue for several months and may be repeated.

While taking drugs to induce ovulation, you will be examined with vaginal ultrasound scans to check the growth of the developing ovarian follicles. This monitoring also helps reduce the risk of the drug overstimulating the ovaries, which could result in a multiple pregnancy (see page 525) or side effects such as hot flashes, headache, nausea, and fatigue.

Surgery

Doctors perform surgery to remove fibroids (see page 867) and to remove tissue deposits caused by endometriosis (see page 870). They can sometimes surgically repair blocked fallopian tubes using one of three procedures—tubal cannulation, adhesiolysis, or tubal reanastomosis. In tubal cannulation, the surgeon inserts a thin tube (called a cannula) into the obstructed fallopian tube to open it. In adhesiolysis, the doctor removes scar tissue near the obstructed fallopian tube and ovary. Tubal reanastomosis joins the two severed ends of a fallopian tube after a blockage has been surgically removed; this procedure is also used to try to reverse a tubal ligation (see page 476). In women who have a structural defect such as a wall in the center of their uterus, surgeons can correct the defect, improving the chances of pregnancy. Some

of these surgical procedures can be performed with laparoscopy, using a lighted viewing instrument (laparoscope) and other instruments inserted through small incisions in the abdomen, which minimizes recovery time and scarring.

If a health condition such as diabetes (see page 889) or obesity is affecting your ability to become pregnant, your doctor will recommend treating the condition before trying infertility treatments.

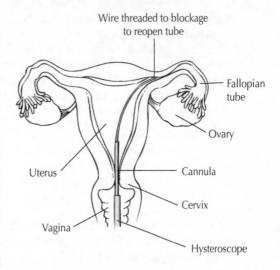

Tubal cannulation

Tubal cannulation is a procedure to open a blocked fallopian tube. In this procedure, a wire is threaded through a thin tube (cannula) that is moved through a hysteroscope inserted through the vagina and uterus into the blockage in the fallopian tube.

Treating Infertility in Men

As with women, the infertility treatment a man receives depends on the cause of the infertility. For example, if your sperm count has been lowered by an infection or a medical condition, your doctor will provide appropriate treatment. The doctor also will strongly recommend that you discontinue any activities—including excessive smoking, drinking, or other drug use—that might be contributing to your infertility. In general, a healthy lifestyle promotes good sperm production.

Surgery

If infertility is the result of a blockage in the vas deferens (one of the tubes that carry sperm from the testicles to the urethra), surgeons can sometimes open the blockage. Doctors can correct a varicose vein in a testicle (varicocele; see page 829), which can lower sperm production, by performing surgery to tie off the affected vein.

An outpatient procedure called percutaneous embolization is as effective as traditional surgery in correcting a varicocele without the need for general anesthesia and has fewer complications. During percutaneous embolization, the surgeon inserts a small tube into a vein in the groin area through a tiny incision. He or she then injects a dye into the vein and, guided by X-ray imaging, inserts tiny metal coils or a balloon into the vein to block the flow of blood, which shrinks the varicose vein. Recovery takes less than 24 hours. Treating a varicocele improves sperm production and increases the chances of conception.

Medications

A low sperm count or poor sperm motility (movement) can sometimes result if a man's testicles are not being stimulated enough naturally by the hormones FSH (follicle-stimulating hormone) and LH (luteinizing hormone). In this case, a doctor may recommend taking the hormone human chorionic gonadotropin (HCG) for several months to improve sperm production and motility.

Assisted Reproductive Technologies

If treatment with medication or surgery has not helped you and your partner conceive, you may want to consider additional infertility techniques known collectively as assisted reproductive technologies. These techniques use high-tech methods to fertilize an egg and transfer it to a woman's uterus. This technology, which has helped many couples achieve a pregnancy, has improved steadily over the past several years, and the success rate may soon be approaching 50 percent for each attempt.

Assisted reproductive techniques such as in vitro fertilization (see right) are the most stressful of all infertility treatments. The woman must give herself frequent injections of drugs and have blood tests and ultrasound scans regularly. Both partners usually approach each attempt with hope and can be disappointed if the procedure fails. Feelings of depression, frustration, and hopelessness are common after a failed in vitro fertilization. Then the process starts over again the next month, and may be repeated several times. Before undergoing assisted reproductive techniques, educate yourself about

them thoroughly, ask for support from your family and friends, and take good care of yourself by getting enough rest and exercise and by eating well. It can be helpful to talk to a mental health professional who has been recommended by your infertility clinic.

Intrauterine insemination

In intrauterine insemination, often called artificial insemination, a doctor uses a thin tube (catheter) and syringe to introduce sperm from the woman's partner (or from a donor) directly into the uterus, close to the time of ovulation. Intrauterine insemination is designed to make it easier for sperm to reach the fallopian tubes to fertilize an egg. It is used when the man's sperm count is only marginally low or when the woman's cervical mucus prevents sperm from entering the uterus.

Donor Sperm

Couples sometimes choose to use donated sperm if the man cannot produce enough normal sperm to fertilize his partner's egg. Single women who want to conceive also may choose to use sperm from a donor. Sperm donation is extremely safe when it is done at a reliable infertility center by an experienced and board-certified reproductive endocrinologist and following the established national guidelines. Sperm donors are carefully screened for medical problems and STDs before they can donate. Anonymous donors are registered by age, race, hair and eye color, and build so that women or couples can choose a preferred genetic background. If the donor is known, a couple should consult an attorney before undergoing insemination with donated sperm to resolve any potential paternity issues.

In vitro fertilization

In vitro fertilization (IVF) is the most widely used assisted reproductive technology. It is the standard treatment for women with obstructed fallopian tubes. During IVF, the ovaries are stimulated to produce multiple eggs, which are removed from the ovaries through the vagina, with ultrasound guidance. The eggs are then fertilized in a laboratory by sperm from the male partner or from a donor. The fertilized eggs are allowed to undergo cell division until they are viable enough to be introduced into the woman's uterus and possibly to produce a pregnancy.

The IVF process consists of four stages: ovulation induction, egg retrieval, fertilization in a laboratory, and embryo transfer (into the uterus). At the beginning of an IVF cycle, you will be asked to give yourself injections of a drug that stops your body's production of estrogen, allowing the doctors to create a new monthly cycle in which they can control exactly when ovulation will occur. Then you will take other drugs to stimulate multiple ovulation. During this time you will need to undergo regular vaginal ultrasound scans to monitor the progress of your ripening ovarian follicles.

When it is time to retrieve your eggs, you will go to a hospital or outpatient facility for the procedure. You will be given a light sedative and pain medication. Guided by vaginal ultrasound, the doctor harvests your eggs using a long, thin needle inserted through the vagina and into each of your ovaries. After your partner provides a fresh semen sample, his sperm (or sperm from a donor) is mixed with your eggs in a plastic dish and allowed to incubate for 14 hours or more. Then the fertilized eggs are examined, and the most viable ones are implanted in your uterus within a few days. Some couples who produce a large number of embryos can choose to have some of them frozen for implantation later.

During embryo transfer, the doctor uses a soft rubber tube to transfer the embryos into your uterus. You will have to stay in bed for 1 to 4 hours after the procedure, possibly in a position in which your lower body is elevated above your head. You will need to take the hormone progesterone to help stabilize the lining of your uterus for implantation of the embryo. You will have a pregnancy test 10 to 14 days after the transfer. If you are pregnant, you will continue to take progesterone for up to 12 weeks. The average success rate for IVF is about 38 percent per attempt, but the rate is much lower for women over age 40.

Because up to four or more embryos are transferred during each attempt, IVF carries the risk of a multiple pregnancy. Most multiple pregnancies result in twins, but triplets, quadruplets, and even higher numbers of fetuses can occur. The decision about how many embryos to transfer is made by you and your doctor. The more embryos that are transferred, the greater the chances of having a multiple pregnancy with three or more fetuses. For this reason, many countries limit the number of embryos that can be transferred. In the general population,

the risk of multiple pregnancy is only 1 to 2 percent.

Multiple pregnancies carry risks to both the woman and the fetuses. Fetuses are at risk of miscarriage, premature birth, birth defects, and mental or physical problems such as cerebral palsy (see

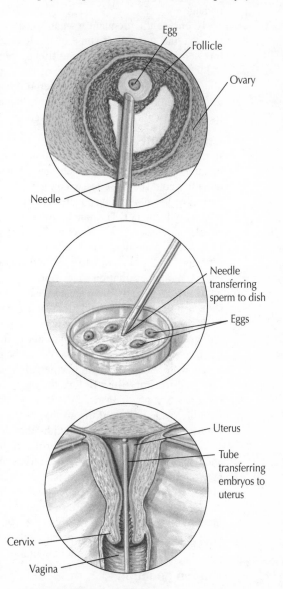

In vitro fertilization

In vitro fertilization is a process in which a needle is inserted through the wall of the vagina along the outside of the uterus to retrieve eggs from the woman's ovaries (top). Fluid from the follicles is removed along with the eggs. The eggs are fertilized in a plastic dish in the laboratory with sperm from the male partner (center). After a few days, the embryos are transferred to the woman's uterus with a soft rubber tube (bottom).

page 409) that can occur from a preterm delivery (see page 529). Risks to the woman include pregnancy-induced high blood pressure (preeclampsia; page 526), gestational diabetes (see page 521), anemia (see page 610), and vaginal or uterine hemorrhage.

To ensure the pregnant woman's health and to improve the survival of some of the fetuses, doctors sometimes recommend multifetal pregnancy reduction, in which one or more of the fetuses is aborted. Deciding whether to undergo this procedure is an emotionally difficult process that may be made easier with professional counseling.

Egg donation

If a woman's ovaries have stopped functioning prematurely, she is over age 40, or she has a genetic disorder that could be passed on to children, she and her partner may explore using donated eggs to achieve a pregnancy using IVF. The donor may be a person the couple knows, such as a sister, or may be anonymous. Either way, each donor is carefully screened for infectious and genetic diseases and must undergo a psychological evaluation. The donor should be between ages 21 and 35 and must have blood tests to show that her ovaries are still producing eggs.

If you are considering using egg donation, you will need to have a thorough physical examination to make sure that your health would not be endangered by pregnancy. Your partner also will be screened for infertility. Before the egg donation takes place, you will receive IVF drugs so that your monthly cycle will conform to that of the donor, whose cycle will be controlled with other drugs.

After the eggs are retrieved, fertilized in vitro, and one or more embryos have been transferred to your uterus, you will need to take estrogen and progesterone until your pregnancy test on the 28th day of your cycle. If you are pregnant, the hormones will be continued until about the 10th week of pregnancy. Egg donation increases the success rate of IVF to about 40 percent per attempt.

Embryo donation

Couples who have a successful in vitro fertilization usually have some unused embryos left over, which are frozen. An increasing number of couples are choosing to donate their embryos to another infertile couple. Embryo donation is an option for the same reasons as egg donation. In addition, it may be used by single women whose own eggs would not otherwise be used or by couples in which both the male and female are infertile and who choose not to (or cannot afford to) undergo a complete cycle of IVF.

The process is similar to the final step of IVF, in which embryos are introduced into the woman's uterus to produce a pregnancy. Before undergoing the procedure, the woman who is receiving the donated embryos will have a thorough physical examination and tests to make sure that a pregnancy would not compromise her health. She will be given hormones, including estrogen and progesterone, to prepare the lining of her uterus to accept an embryo. In some cases, the timing of implantation is based on the woman's own menstrual cycle. When the uterus is ready, the frozen embryos are thawed and transferred to the uterus. If pregnancy results, the woman continues to take the estrogen and progesterone for 8 weeks.

If you are considering embryo donation (either as a donor or as a recipient), talk to a mental health professional and a lawyer about the ethical and legal issues concerning the procedure. For example, you will need to consider issues such as disclosure—whether the donor wants to be named, whether you want the donor to know you, and what you will tell your prospective child. Each state has different laws that apply to embryo donation.

Gestational carrier

Some women cannot carry a pregnancy because they have had a hysterectomy (see page 870), were born without a uterus, or have had multiple miscarriages. In these cases, some infertile couples ask another woman to serve as a gestational carrier—also known as a surrogate mother. This agreement is a legal contract in which the woman consents to have a fertilized egg from the couple implanted into her uterus and to carry the pregnancy to term. The woman further agrees to turn the baby over to the couple upon delivery.

Having a baby with a gestational carrier has a number of medical and legal consequences, so be sure to discuss the topic thoroughly with both your doctor and an attorney before going ahead with it.

5

Pregnancy and Childbirth

A healthy pregnancy starts before a woman gets pregnant. If you are planning to get pregnant, make an appointment with your doctor. He or she will perform a thorough examination to evaluate your health and determine if you have any medical conditions or inherited disorders that could complicate a pregnancy or make it inadvisable for you to get pregnant. In addition, if you have a chronic disorder—such as a heart disorder (see page 520), epilepsy (see page 686), diabetes (see page 889), kidney disease, or an autoimmune disease such as lupus (see page 920) or rheumatoid arthritis (see page 918)—your condition must be carefully monitored throughout your pregnancy.

Pregnancy

The healthier you are during your pregnancy, the more likely your child will be born healthy. If you are trying to become pregnant, take steps now to help ensure a healthy pregnancy. Stop smoking cigarettes and drinking alcohol, avoid potentially harmful drugs or chemicals, eat healthfully (lots of vegetables, fruits, whole grains, and legumes), and exercise regularly. Taking 400 micrograms (0.4 milligram) of folic acid every day in a supplement will reduce your risk of having a child with abnormal development of the spine or brain (neural tube defect; see page 398). Depending on your health history, higher doses of folic acid may be recommended.

Conception

Conception begins with the fertilization of one of a woman's eggs. Fertilization can occur shortly after a mature egg is released from an ovary, which usually occurs about halfway through the menstrual cycle. If a woman has sexual intercourse during this time, she can get pregnant as sperm ejaculated from her male partner travel through her vagina and uterus up to the fallopian tubes. Fertilization occurs if a sperm penetrates the cell wall of an egg inside one of the fallopian tubes. The fertilized egg reaches the uterus 2 to 7 days later and embeds itself in the lining of the uterus, at about the time a woman's period is due. By the time most women suspect they may be pregnant, the egg has become an embryo that is developing inside the uterus.

A full-term pregnancy lasts about 40 weeks from the time of conception to delivery. Although conception usually occurs halfway through a woman's menstrual cycle, the delivery date is calculated from the first day of her last period because the exact day the egg is fertilized is difficult to know.

Confirming a Pregnancy

If you have missed a menstrual period and want to know if you are pregnant, you can use a home pregnancy test. Home pregnancy tests work by detecting the hormone human chorionic gonadotropin (HCG), which is present in the urine of a pregnant woman about 2 weeks after her first missed period. The results are most accurate when you follow the manufacturer's instructions exactly and test your urine first thing in the morning before you drink anything. The results of a home pregnancy test may not be reliable if you are taking antidepressants (see page 712), are approaching

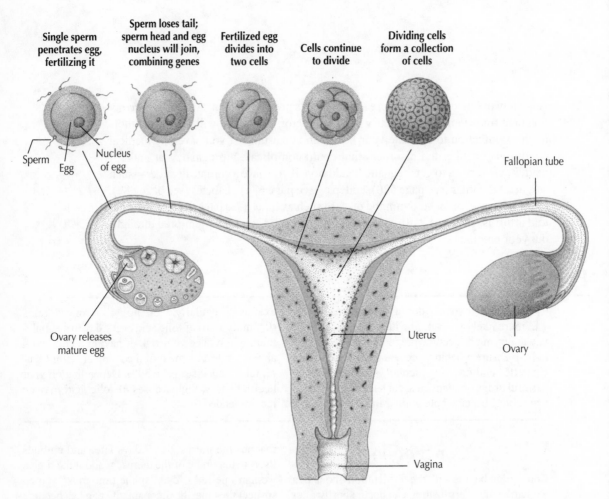

Single sperm penetrates egg, fertilizing it

Sperm loses tail; sperm head and egg nucleus will join, combining genes

Fertilized egg divides into two cells

Cells continue to divide

Dividing cells form a collection of cells

Sperm

Egg

Nucleus of egg

Fallopian tube

Ovary releases mature egg

Uterus

Ovary

Vagina

Eggs, sperm, and fertilization

A woman's ovaries, one on each side of her uterus, contain thousands of immature eggs, with which she was born. After puberty, one of the eggs matures each month in one of the ovaries and, about halfway through the menstrual cycle, it is released into the adjacent fallopian tube. In males, sperm are produced continuously inside the testicles and are stored in the seminal vesicles until ejaculation.

Fertilization of an egg by a sperm takes place in one of the fallopian tubes shortly after the egg is released into the fallopian tube. The sperm's nucleus joins with the egg's nucleus, combining their genes, and the cell divides into two cells. Each of these cells then divides into two, which divide again, and so on. The group of dividing cells travels along the fallopian tube toward the uterus and, about 2 to 7 days after fertilization, is implanted in the lining of the uterus. In a few weeks, the fertilized egg develops into an embryo and placenta.

Stages of embryo development

The fertilized egg is called an embryo until about the 12th week of pregnancy, when it is called a fetus. At 6 weeks, the embryo is about the size of a grain of rice and the most developed organ is the heart. At 7 weeks, the arms and legs can be seen as limb buds. The eyes and ears are more obvious by 9 weeks. At 10 weeks, the embryo is about 1$\frac{1}{4}$ inches long and growing rapidly. The detailed features of an embryo and its actual size are shown here at different stages of development.

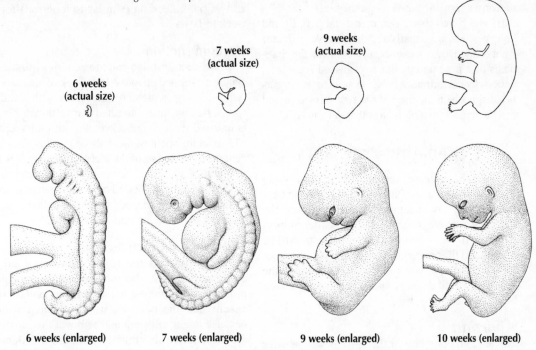

10 weeks (actual size)

9 weeks (actual size)

7 weeks (actual size)

6 weeks (actual size)

6 weeks (enlarged) **7 weeks (enlarged)** **9 weeks (enlarged)** **10 weeks (enlarged)**

Placenta: The fetal lifeline

Inside the uterus, the fetus is attached to the placenta by the umbilical cord. Fetal blood flows to and from the placenta, absorbing nutrients from and expelling waste into the pregnant woman's blood. Tiny fingerlike projections called villi provide a large surface area in the placenta to help maximize the exchange of these substances.

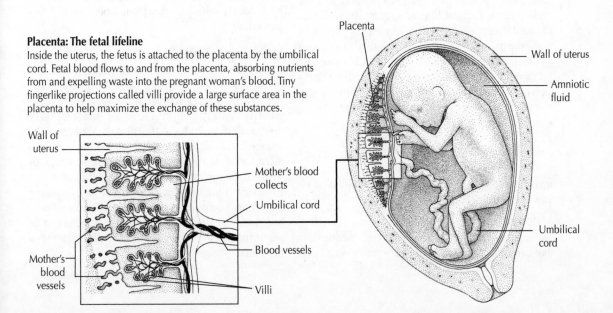

Placenta

Wall of uterus

Amniotic fluid

Umbilical cord

Wall of uterus

Mother's blood collects

Umbilical cord

Blood vessels

Mother's blood vessels

Villi

menopause, or have irregular or infrequent periods. Also, a negative result (indicating you are not pregnant) is less reliable than a positive result (indicating you are pregnant). You should see your doctor if you have a negative result on a home test but still suspect that you are pregnant. Your doctor, a family planning clinic, or your local health department can perform a more accurate pregnancy test.

If you have missed two menstrual periods and your periods are usually regular, see your doctor right away. Doctors can usually confirm the diagnosis of a pregnancy after two missed menstrual periods by performing a pelvic examination. An earlier diagnosis at the time of the first missed period can be made with a blood test that detects HCG.

Terminating Pregnancy

Learning that you are pregnant may require you to make some serious decisions. You may want to consider having a medical or surgical abortion if the fetus has a severe or fatal genetic disorder or birth defect or if your life or the life of the fetus will be in danger if the pregnancy progresses. If you cannot raise a child now, you can choose to continue the pregnancy until delivery and arrange to have your baby adopted.

Abortion

Talking to a counselor or therapist as well as your doctor may be helpful during this time. If you are under age 18, find out from an organization such as Planned Parenthood if the law in your state requires that your parents be notified before you have an abortion. After age 18 and until the 12th week of pregnancy, an abortion is a private medical decision made by a woman and her doctor. Some states have enacted laws to govern termination of a pregnancy after the 12th week.

Although the risks from an early abortion are fewer than the risks involved in carrying a pregnancy to term, complications of abortion can include infection, bleeding, and continuation of an unwanted pregnancy.

Mifepristone

Mifepristone is a synthetic hormone medication that can induce an abortion in a woman who is up to 9 weeks pregnant when it is taken with medications called prostaglandins, which cause the uterus to contract. The success rate is higher if it is taken earlier than 6 weeks. Mifepristone induces abortion by making the lining of the uterus shed. It can take several days to terminate a pregnancy using mifepristone. You will have cramps for a few days and vaginal bleeding (similar to a period) for 1 week to 10 days.

Vacuum suction

Vacuum suction (also called vacuum aspiration) can be performed up to the 16th week of pregnancy. After dilating (widening) the cervix with slender rods, a flexible tube connected to a suction machine is inserted through the cervix and into the uterus. The machine suctions the embryo or fetus, the placenta, and the lining of the uterus out of the uterus. Sometimes a D and C (see page 869) is performed at the same time or instead of vacuum suction. In a D and C, a spoon-shaped instrument called a curet is used to remove any remaining tissue.

Dilation and evacuation

Between weeks 13 and 16 of pregnancy, dilation and evacuation is the most common abortion procedure. It is similar to vacuum suction (above) except that the cervix must be opened wider because larger grasping and removal instruments are used after the initial suctioning. Dilation and evacuation is a safe method when performed by a doctor who has experience performing this procedure.

Late-stage abortion

From the 16th to the 24th week, termination of a pregnancy is possible using surgical methods similar to dilation and evacuation or by using nonsurgical methods such as the use of a saline solution or medication to induce abortion. Labor may be induced with vaginal suppositories or medications introduced intravenously (through a vein) or injected through the uterine wall into the amniotic fluid (the fluid that surrounds the fetus). Inducing labor may be preferable to surgically terminating a pregnancy at this stage if an autopsy needs to be performed to look for structural malformations in the fetus.

Prenatal Care

It is important to start prenatal care early, even before you get pregnant, to make sure that both you and your baby are healthy by the time of delivery. Besides regular checkups with your doctor to monitor the progress of your pregnancy and to receive information about how to have a healthy pregnancy, prenatal care may involve tests to detect genetic diseases or birth defects in the fetus such as congenital heart disease (see page 389), neural tube defects (see page 398), or chromosome abnormalities such as Down syndrome (see page 955). A woman and her partner may also want to sign up for childbirth preparation classes to prepare themselves for labor and delivery.

Regular Prenatal Checkups

Once your pregnancy has been confirmed, your doctor may refer you to an obstetrician (a doctor who specializes in the care of a woman during pregnancy, labor, delivery, and the period immediately after delivery), or schedule you for subsequent checkups and tests. Prenatal checkups are usually scheduled monthly until the third trimester, when they are scheduled more frequently.

Prenatal care helps prevent complications of pregnancy and childbirth and provides both the pregnant woman and the fetus with any necessary medical care before birth. Because fetal development is affected by environmental factors inside the uterus and by the woman's state of health (especially during the crucial first 3 months), a woman's doctor may make some lifestyle recommendations. For example, doctors usually recommend that pregnant women not smoke cigarettes (smoking increases the risk of having a baby with a low birth weight or of having a preterm delivery) and avoid alcohol because it can cause a number of serious problems in the fetus, including mental retardation (fetal alcohol syndrome; see page 409). Also avoid taking any unnecessary drugs or exposing yourself to radiation or environmental substances such as lead, mercury, pesticides, or solvents, which can cause complications during pregnancy and delivery. Stay away from saunas, steam baths, hot tubs, and extremely hot baths, which can raise your body temperature to a level that could be harmful to the fetus.

At your first visit, your doctor will perform a physical examination (including measuring your blood pressure and weight) and establish your due date (which usually is set 40 weeks from the first day of your last menstrual period, but may be adjusted based on the size of the fetus shown on an ultrasound or the size of your uterus felt on a pelvic examination). The doctor will examine your cervix to make sure it can support a pregnancy. He or she will take your medical history and ask if there is a possibility that you could have a sexually transmitted disease (all pregnant women are tested for gonorrhea and syphilis).

At your initial visit or during subsequent visits, you will have blood tests for blood type (see page 145), Rh factor (see next page), and anemia (see page 610); for infections (see next page) such as rubella, hepatitis B (see page 786), and toxoplasmosis; and for excess levels of protein (which can indicate preeclampsia; see page 526) and glucose (a sign of gestational diabetes; see page 521).

Smoking and Pregnancy

Smoking is especially harmful during pregnancy. Seriously consider quitting if you are pregnant because:

- Smoking increases your risk of having an ectopic pregnancy or miscarriage.
- Smoking doubles your risk of having serious pregnancy complications involving the placenta.
- Smoking makes you twice as likely as a nonsmoking woman to have a baby with a low birth weight, and more likely to have a preterm delivery.
- Smoking may increase your baby's risk of having birth defects such as clubfoot, cleft lip, or cleft palate.
- Smoking triples your baby's risk of dying of sudden infant death syndrome (SIDS) compared with children of mothers who did not smoke during pregnancy.
- Smoking increases your child's risk of having an attention deficit disorder or learning disability.

Ask your doctor about a quit-smoking strategy (see page 29) that would be safe and effective for you.

Infectious Diseases and Pregnancy

Some infections that a woman develops during pregnancy can cause birth defects or can be fatal to the fetus. It is best to talk to your doctor about infections before you get pregnant, but if you are already pregnant, ask your doctor about any precautions you should take during your pregnancy to avoid infections.

Childhood infections

If you are pregnant and have not had common childhood diseases such as chickenpox (see page 439) or fifth disease (see page 439) or have not had or been vaccinated against measles (see page 437) or German measles (rubella; see page 438), talk to your doctor. Having these infections during pregnancy can harm the fetus. Most adults have been vaccinated against measles (or had it during childhood) or have had chickenpox (and are therefore immune), and about half are immune to fifth disease. In the United States, all children are required to have vaccinations against rubella and chickenpox. Because there is no vaccination against fifth disease, avoid contact with anyone who has it. You are at increased risk of exposure to the virus that causes fifth disease if you have children at home or if you work around children.

Vaccinations Before Pregnancy

If you are not sure if you have been vaccinated against rubella or measles or had chickenpox during childhood, ask your doctor about having a blood test before you become pregnant to determine if you are immune to these diseases. If the test shows that you have not had these infections (and you definitely are not pregnant), you still can be immunized. You should then wait at least 3 months before getting pregnant because the risk of heart defects in the fetus caused by these viruses is greatest in the first 3 months of pregnancy.

Cytomegalovirus

Cytomegalovirus is an infection that usually causes no symptoms; most people have had the infection and have not known it. However, if a pregnant woman is infected during pregnancy, especially during the first trimester, the virus can be transmitted to the fetus and can cause birth defects such as blindness or mental retardation, or can be fatal. Still, only a small percentage of babies who are born with the infection have any problems. If you think you may have been exposed to an infected person during your pregnancy, or if you have a flu-like illness during pregnancy, see your doctor.

Toxoplasmosis

Toxoplasmosis (see page 940) is an infection caused by a parasite that lives in raw meat and in some animals, including cats. Although the infection causes only flulike symptoms in adults, it can infect a fetus and cause severe birth defects or can be fatal. If you have a cat, your doctor will recommend having a test to see if you are immune to toxoplasmosis. If you are immune, your fetus cannot become infected. If you are not immune, your doctor will tell you what precautions to take to avoid infection, such as not changing the cat's litter box, wearing gloves when gardening, and washing fruits and vegetables before eating them.

Rh Incompatibility

Rh (Rhesus) incompatibility is a mismatch between the blood of the pregnant woman and the blood of the fetus. Rh incompatibility occurs only when the mother's blood is Rh negative and the fetus's blood is Rh positive. Complications from Rh incompatibility are rare because it is usually diagnosed and treated immediately with a blood product called Rh immunoglobulin, which is given to the pregnant woman to prevent her immune system from attacking the fetus's blood.

The blood of an Rh-positive fetus may enter the bloodstream of an Rh-negative woman anytime during the pregnancy but usually occurs at birth. Recognizing the Rh-positive blood as a foreign substance, the mother's immune system produces antibodies to attack the Rh-positive red blood cells. This is usually not a problem for a first Rh-positive fetus because the number of antibodies produced initially is not great enough to harm the fetus. However, if the woman does not receive the Rh immunoglobulin, her body will continue to produce antibodies against Rh-positive blood. If she has a fetus with Rh-positive blood in a subsequent pregnancy, the antibodies will attack the fetus's red blood cells, possibly causing a potentially fatal (to the fetus) form of Rh incompatibility called hydrops fetalis. If the fetus does not die before birth, after birth a child can develop symptoms of hydrops fetalis such as anemia, heart failure, severe swelling, and respiratory distress.

The Rh immunoglobulin is usually given at about the 28th week of pregnancy and again within 72 hours of delivery. In addition to preventing the mother's immune system from producing antibodies to Rh-positive blood, the immunoglobulin destroys any red blood cells from the fetus that may have entered her circulation before her body started developing antibodies. If the mother's antibodies have begun to destroy the fetus's red blood cells, a doctor may induce labor if the pregnancy is close to term. If the fetus is not mature enough to be delivered, a fetal blood transfusion may be given inside the uterus, which will allow time for the fetus to mature sufficiently for delivery. In general, the health outlook for infants with Rh incompatibility is good.

Prenatal Testing

A number of pregnancy tests and procedures are available to help doctors evaluate the health of the pregnancy and the fetus. Some of the tests, such as amniocentesis, can determine if a fetus has a genetic abnormality or a malformation. Other tests, such as ultrasound, can evaluate the development of the fetus, detect any structural abnormalities, and date the pregnancy. For various reasons, pregnant women may choose not to have the tests. For example, some women would never consider terminating a pregnancy even if a severe or lethal defect were found in the fetus. During your pregnancy, discuss your feelings with your doctor, who can help you evaluate the benefits and risks of having the tests.

Ultrasound

Ultrasound (see page 111) is an imaging procedure that uses sound waves to produce pictures of the developing fetus on a monitor. Ultrasound does not involve radiation or X-rays and is harmless, painless, and noninvasive. Ultrasound is offered to most women at least once during their pregnancy and more frequently to women who may be at risk of

Rh Disease in Pregnancy

When a woman with Rh-negative blood has a fetus with Rh-positive blood, some of the fetus's blood may enter the woman's bloodstream at birth, or during pregnancy. If the woman is not given Rh immunoglobulin within 72 hours of delivery, her immune system will develop antibodies to fight the Rh-positive blood, which it recognizes as foreign. These antibodies don't cause problems in a first Rh-incompatible pregnancy, but if the woman does not receive the Rh immunoglobulin and has a subsequent Rh-positive fetus, her antibodies could cross the placenta and destroy the fetus's red blood cells, possibly causing anemia or even death. After a miscarriage or the termination of a pregnancy, Rh immunoglobulin should always be administered to an Rh-negative woman.

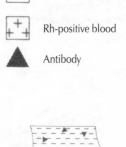

Key

$\boxed{-}$ Rh-negative blood

$\boxed{+}$ Rh-positive blood

▲ Antibody

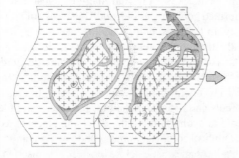

Rh-negative woman with Rh-positive fetus

Rh-positive blood from fetus moves into woman's bloodstream

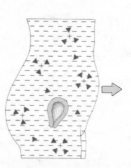

Woman develops antibodies to fight the Rh-positive blood

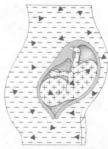

Woman's antibodies cross placenta and destroy fetus's red blood cells

having problems. During the first trimester, ultrasound is often used to confirm and date a pregnancy by determining the size and shape of the fetus. Many doctors recommend an ultrasound between the 17th and 19th weeks of pregnancy to evaluate fetal growth and development and to rule out some structural abnormalities such as neural tube defects (see page 398) or cleft lip or cleft palate (see page 403). Ultrasound can also detect twins and, after the

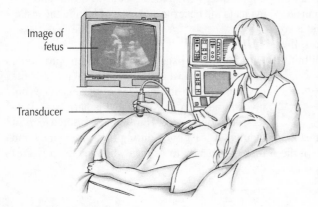

Abdominal ultrasound
In an abdominal ultrasound, a device called a transducer is moved along the surface of the pregnant woman's abdomen, emitting sound waves that reflect off the fetus and the woman's internal organs. The sound waves are electronically translated into an image on a computer screen.

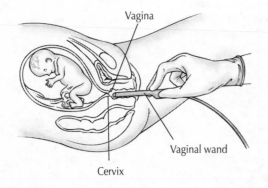

Vaginal ultrasound
In a vaginal ultrasound, a narrow transducer (called a vaginal wand) is inserted into the vagina to produce images on a monitor. Vaginal ultrasounds may be used in the first trimester of pregnancy for a number of reasons, such as to see a fetus more clearly or to confirm (or rule out) a pregnancy or an abnormality such as an elongated cervix (which can indicate an impending miscarriage) or an ectopic pregnancy.

16th week, can sometimes determine a fetus's gender. During late pregnancy, ultrasound may be used to evaluate the health, size, and position of the fetus and the placenta in preparation for delivery.

AFP and Triple Screen Blood Tests

All women are offered one of two blood tests between the 15th and 20th weeks of pregnancy to measure the level of alpha-fetoprotein (more familiarly known simply as AFP), a protein produced by the developing fetus. AFP is present in amniotic fluid and, in smaller amounts, in a pregnant woman's blood. One test measures just AFP. The triple screen blood test measures AFP and two hormones, human chorionic gonadotropin (HCG) and estriol (a form of estrogen), which are produced by the placenta during pregnancy. The interpretation of these measurements is based on factors such as a woman's age, race, and weight.

These blood tests help evaluate the risk that the fetus has a chromosome abnormality such as Down syndrome (see page 955) or a spinal cord or brain abnormality (neural tube defect; see page 398). These tests are not conclusive, however—3 to 5 percent of women have an abnormal result that is later proven false 90 percent of the time in more precise testing. If the AFP or triple screen test results are abnormal, a doctor usually recommends more accurate testing such as amniocentesis (below) to determine if the fetus has a genetic abnormality.

Amniocentesis

Amniocentesis is a prenatal diagnostic test that is performed between the 14th and 18th weeks of pregnancy. In the procedure, a doctor inserts a hollow needle through the pregnant woman's abdomen into the uterus to withdraw a sample of amniotic fluid, which surrounds the fetus and contains some fetal cells. The doctor uses ultrasound imaging to locate the fetus and determine the best place to insert the needle to avoid harming the fetus, the placenta, or the umbilical cord. The woman's abdomen is numbed with a local anesthetic before the needle is inserted.

The fetal cells are grown in the laboratory for up to 2 weeks and then examined for chromosome abnormalities such as Down syndrome, some genetic disorders such as cystic fibrosis and sickle cell disease, and neural tube defects.

Amniocentesis is offered to all pregnant women age 35 or older, whose age puts them at increased risk of having a baby with a chromosome abnormality. Women are also offered amniocentesis if they have a child with a severe birth defect, if someone in their family has a genetic disorder, or if the results of an ultrasound (see page 509) or AFP test (see previous page) show an increased risk of a chromosome abnormality. If you are having amniocentesis and you do not want to know the sex of your fetus, let your doctor know before the procedure because the test can determine sex. Amniocentesis carries a small (1 in 200 to 1 in 400) risk of miscarriage.

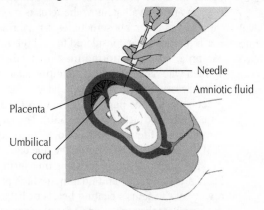

Amniocentesis

In amniocentesis, a sample of amniotic fluid is withdrawn from the amniotic sac surrounding the fetus. Doctors use ultrasound imaging to position the needle to avoid the fetus, placenta, and umbilical cord. Amniotic fluid contains cells from the fetus, which are examined to diagnose many disorders, including chromosome abnormalities and open neural tube defects.

Chorionic Villus Sampling

Chorionic villus sampling (CVS) is a procedure performed during pregnancy to diagnose chromosome abnormalities such as Down syndrome and some genetic disorders in the fetus. The test is offered to women who are at increased risk of having a child with a genetic abnormality, such as women 35 or older, women who have a child with a genetic disorder, and women who have a family history of genetic abnormalities. CVS can be performed earlier in pregnancy than amniocentesis (see previous page)—between the 10th and 12th weeks.

Chorionic villi are threadlike projections that form part of the developing placenta and contain the same genetic material as cells of the fetus. In CVS, a small sample of tissue is removed from the placenta through a thin tube (catheter). The sample is removed under ultrasound guidance, either through the vagina and cervix using a minor suction procedure or through the abdomen. CVS poses a small (1 in 100) risk of miscarriage.

First Trimester Screening Test

A newer prenatal screening test is available that can detect Down syndrome (see page 955) and another chromosome abnormality called trisomy 18 syndrome during the first trimester by analyzing a blood sample from a pregnant woman and measuring the thickening of the back of the fetus's neck with ultrasound imaging. A fetus with abnormal thickening of the back of the neck is at increased risk of having a chromosome abnormality. This test is performed between the 10th and 14th weeks of pregnancy. Because the results of the test are not conclusive, however, more accurate testing, such as amniocentesis (see previous page), is recommended for women whose test results indicate an abnormality.

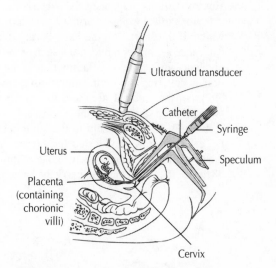

CVS

In CVS, a thin tube called a catheter is inserted through the vagina into the uterus. (An alternative method is to insert a hollow needle through the abdomen into the uterus.) A syringe attached to the catheter is used to withdraw a small sample of tissue containing chorionic villi (small, fingerlike projections) from the placenta. The path of the catheter or needle is guided by ultrasound. The vagina is held open with a vaginal speculum.

Glucose Screening Test

Glucose screening is offered to all pregnant women during pregnancy, usually between the 24th and 28th weeks, to screen for gestational diabetes (see page 521), a form of diabetes that develops during pregnancy and goes away after delivery. With early diagnosis and careful control of blood glucose during pregnancy, gestational diabetes seldom causes problems for either the pregnant woman or the fetus. Untreated, however, the condition can cause the fetus to be larger than normal (resulting in a more complicated delivery) or to have a low glucose level and chemical imbalances after delivery.

During glucose screening, you are given a glucose solution to drink, and a blood sample is taken 1 hour later. If the test shows that your glucose level is elevated, you will have another, more accurate test called the glucose tolerance test (see page 895) to make a diagnosis.

Group B Strep Test

Most pregnant women are screened for group B streptococcal bacteria that live in the reproductive and urinary systems and seldom cause symptoms. However, during pregnancy, the bacteria can cause infections in the woman's urinary tract and uterus, which, if transmitted to the baby during delivery, can cause serious complications such as pneumonia, blood infection, or inflammation of the membranes covering the brain (meningitis; see page 692). For the group B strep test, the doctor uses a swab to take a sample from the woman's vagina and rectum. The sample is sent to the laboratory, and the cells are grown and tested for the presence of the bacteria. Test results are available within 24 to 48 hours. If you are found to carry the bacteria, you will be given antibiotics intravenously (through a vein) during labor and delivery to prevent your baby from being infected. Although one out of three pregnant women carries the bacteria, only 1 out of 200 babies actually develops an infection. The infection can usually be treated effectively by giving the baby intravenous antibiotics for about 10 days after delivery.

Fetal Monitoring

Throughout pregnancy and labor, doctors can evaluate the health of the fetus by measuring the fetal heart rate. Fetal monitoring is most frequently used during labor to make sure the fetus is getting enough oxygen and to evaluate how the fetus is reacting to the stress of labor, but sometimes is performed earlier in pregnancies considered to be high risk. For example, fetal monitoring may be performed in women who have a medical condition such as high blood pressure or diabetes, who have symptoms of preeclampsia (see page 526), or who have had a fetus die before birth (see page 530). The fetus also is monitored if fetal growth is slower than expected or if the pregnancy has passed the due date.

The simplest techniques for measuring fetal heart rate are ultrasound imaging (which provides a view of the fetus's beating heart) or listening to the heartbeat through a type of stethoscope (called a fetoscope) placed on the women's abdomen.

Nonstress test

A nonstress test is a noninvasive test done to evaluate the health of the fetus, usually during the last 3 to 4 months of pregnancy. Doctors measure the fetus's heart rate as the fetus moves inside the uterus, making sure that the fetal heart rate increases in response to environmental factors,

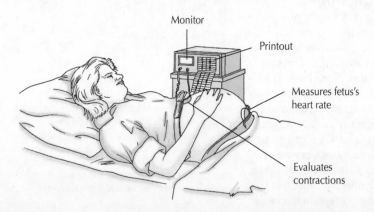

Monitor

Printout

Measures fetus's heart rate

Evaluates contractions

Nonstress test
In a nonstress test, one or two instruments attached to belts are placed on the pregnant woman's abdomen. One of the instruments records the fetus's heart rate; the other instrument measures the length, frequency, and relative intensity of contractions.

indicating that the fetus is healthy. If the fetus's heart rate stays the same or decreases, the doctor may recommend further testing, such as a biophysical profile (see below). A nonstress test can also be used to measure the frequency of contractions later in a pregnancy.

Biophysical profile

A biophysical profile is an evaluation of the fetus's health using the results of a nonstress test (which assesses the fetus's heart rate) and an ultrasound (which assesses the fetus's breathing, movements, and muscle tone, and the amount of amniotic fluid). This information helps the doctor determine if an early delivery is necessary, if more testing is needed, or if the pregnancy can continue naturally with frequent monitoring.

Contraction stress test

A contraction stress test may be performed in high-risk pregnancies or when a nonstress test or biophysical profile has produced abnormal results. The contraction stress test measures the fetus's heart rate during uterine contractions to determine if the fetus will be able to handle the stress of labor. In a stress test, ultrasound is used to evaluate the fetus's heart rate during uterine contractions, which briefly decrease the flow of blood to the placenta. To stimulate contractions, the pregnant woman is given a carefully controlled dose of a drug called oxytocin. If the fetus responds normally, the pregnancy is allowed to continue naturally. If the doctor sees signs of stress in the fetus, such as a decreased heart rate, he or she may recommend early delivery by inducing labor (see page 533) or by cesarean delivery (see page 534).

Prenatal Classes

If you are pregnant, it is important to learn not only about pregnancy but also about labor and delivery. Many organizations (such as hospitals, doctors' offices, and community organizations) sponsor childbirth education classes such as Lamaze. Ask your doctor to recommend one. Have your partner (or a family member or close friend you have chosen to be your labor coach) attend classes with you. He or she can provide encouragement, support, and comfort during your labor and possibly during the delivery.

Natural childbirth and psychoprophylaxis are terms used for childbirth in which the pregnant woman and her labor coach learn relaxation techniques and breathing exercises to lessen the pain of uterine contractions during labor. For many women, these techniques can reduce or eliminate the need for anesthesia and pain medications. The classes usually begin during the seventh month of pregnancy. Women who attend these classes tend to have a more positive childbirth experience because they know what to expect and are more relaxed during delivery.

Planning Ahead for Labor and Delivery

Before making a decision about where and how you want to deliver your baby, discuss all the possibilities with your doctor. Most women deliver in a hospital, and some hospitals offer alternatives to traditional labor and delivery rooms. One of these hospital-based alternatives is a birthing room or center (a private room with a more homelike atmosphere than a standard hospital room) where you, with the help of your labor coach, go through both labor and delivery. If problems arise, you can easily be moved into a labor and delivery suite, which has the staff and equipment to manage complications. However, to qualify for an alternative birthing experience such as a birthing room, you must have no medical problems that could complicate your pregnancy. Some centers also require that the pregnant woman have regular prenatal care and that she and her coach attend prenatal classes.

Some women prefer home childbirth. Nurse-midwives provide a valuable service to any woman who chooses to deliver at home. However, if any complications arise that require emergency treatment, home childbirth can be risky for both the mother and baby. To minimize the potential risks involved with home births, the pregnant woman should be healthy, the pregnancy uncomplicated, and a medical doctor on call to handle any complications that could arise during labor and delivery.

Discuss with your doctor his or her recommendations or thoughts about nurse-midwives, nurse practitioners, pain management during delivery (see page 532), episiotomy (see page 533), cesarean delivery (see page 534), and other methods of assisting during labor.

Health Concerns During Pregnancy

Some women can tell right away that they are pregnant; others can tell only if they experience some of the early symptoms of pregnancy. The early signs of pregnancy can include missing a period (when you previously have had regular periods); having an unusually light period; having tender, swollen breasts with darkened nipples; feeling nauseated or vomiting (especially in the morning); urinating frequently; having a heavier than usual vaginal discharge; or feeling unusually tired. Some women have cravings or lose their taste for particular foods or have increased sensitivity to odors. The topics discussed in this section can occur at any time during a pregnancy.

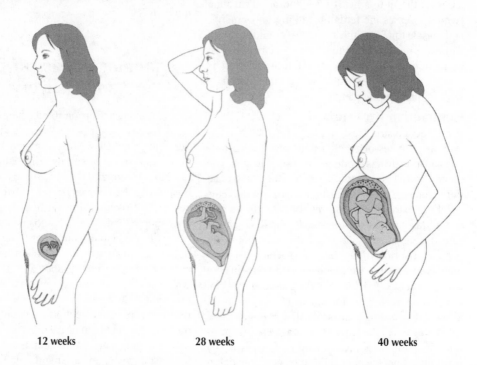

12 weeks   28 weeks   40 weeks

How a woman's body changes during pregnancy
During the first weeks of pregnancy, a woman's body changes very little, although her breasts may look somewhat larger. By the 12th week, her enlarging uterus may make her abdomen protrude slightly. By the time she is 28 weeks pregnant, her abdomen may be very prominent and her navel may bulge out. Toward the end of the pregnancy, the head of the fetus may move down into the woman's pelvic cavity, making her abdomen appear somewhat less prominent.

Diet

What you eat when you're pregnant provides nutrition for your fetus. Eat regular, well-balanced meals that are rich in vegetables, fruits, whole grains, and legumes. To nourish your developing fetus, eat foods that contain essential nutrients such as protein (for cell growth and blood production), calcium (for building strong bones and teeth and developing muscle, heart, and nerve tissue), iron (for producing red blood cells), folic acid (for developing the brain and spinal cord and preventing neural tube defects; see page 398), and zinc (for normal growth and development of the reproductive organs).

Meat, fish, cheese, dried peas and beans, and eggs are excellent sources of protein. Low-fat dairy products are rich in calcium. Good sources of iron include eggs, liver, kidneys, whole-grain or enriched breads and cereals, dried fruit, and green, leafy vegetables. Folic acid is added to breakfast cereals and other grain products and can be obtained from liver, raw green vegetables, and foods that contain yeast. Lean red meat, whole-grain cereals, nuts, peas, and beans are good sources of zinc. Your doctor will probably prescribe vitamins specially formulated for pregnant women. If you are a vegetarian, talk to your doctor and possibly a dietitian to make sure you are getting enough protein and vitamins (particularly vitamins B12 and D) in your diet.

Many women have cravings for particular foods during pregnancy. It's OK to indulge a craving if it's for a nutritious food. High-fat or high-calorie foods can make you gain too much weight, and salty foods can make you retain water. Aversion to certain foods usually is accompanied by nausea or indigestion (see next page). Doctors usually recommend that pregnant women gain about 20 to 30 pounds; gaining too much or too little weight can harm a fetus.

Stay well hydrated by drinking plenty of water. Eating fiber-containing foods (such as fresh fruits and vegetables and legumes) can help prevent constipation that can develop from the extra iron you are consuming.

Cut back on your caffeine consumption during pregnancy because it can affect sleep and cause cardiac palpitations. Some foods to avoid during pregnancy (because they could harm the fetus) include raw meat, raw eggs, raw fish, and shellfish; unwashed or unpeeled fruits and vegetables (because of pesticide residue); and unpasteurized cheeses and apple juice. No safe level of alcohol consumption during pregnancy has been established, so you should avoid alcohol entirely throughout your pregnancy.

Exercise

Exercising regularly will keep you in good physical condition and improve your mental state during your pregnancy. It can help control your blood pressure, reduce stress, prevent constipation, tone your muscles, and help you fall asleep. In general, you can continue any exercise you did before you were pregnant as long as it doesn't overtire you or cause excessive straining. Maintain a heart rate of less than 140 beats per minute during exercise. Walking and swimming are good exercises for pregnant women. Avoid strenuous sports and sports in which you or the fetus might be injured. If you are an athlete, your doctor will closely monitor the growth of the fetus and your weight.

Work

Many pregnant women continue to work up until labor and delivery. If your doctor thinks that your job is too strenuous, he or she may recommend that you take a medical leave of absence if it is contributing to complications in your pregnancy. However, you probably can continue to work if you are healthy and have not been diagnosed with a condition that could cause complications during the pregnancy. Take a break a few times a day to stretch and walk, and don't strain or lift heavy objects.

Travel

If you are traveling, bring your medical records with you, along with any special instructions your doctor has given you. Don't take medications for motion sickness because they can trigger uterine contractions. Ask your doctor what you can do for motion sickness.

Discuss with your doctor the safety of any vaccinations you may need to have for foreign travel. Avoid traveling far from home or a hospital if you have had any problems with your pregnancy such as bleeding or if you are within 4 to 6 weeks of your due date. Traveling can tire you more than usual. If you are sitting for long periods, such as when flying, get up and walk around the cabin whenever you can, at least every 2 hours. Check with your doctor and the airline before making reservations for a trip. Most airlines will not allow women to fly during their last few weeks of pregnancy because of the risk of delivery.

Sex

You can safely have sexual intercourse while you are pregnant—it does not harm the fetus. Some women feel increased desire for sex during pregnancy, while others lose interest. As your uterus enlarges, you may want to experiment with more comfortable positions for intercourse, such as with you on top. If you or your partner finds that intercourse is less enjoyable or more difficult during pregnancy, find other ways of giving each other pleasure. Keep in mind that toward the end of pregnancy, nipple stimulation can trigger labor contractions.

Your doctor will advise you not to have intercourse if you are at risk of miscarriage (see page 522), premature rupture of the membranes (see page 528), preterm labor (see page 529), placenta previa (see page 527), or vaginal bleeding, or if you have been diagnosed with an incompetent cervix (see page 524).

Tender Breasts

Breast tenderness (caused by increased production of the hormone progesterone) is often one of the earliest signs of pregnancy. Your breasts become swollen and tender, and your nipples may be sore. Your nipples may also become more prominent. Breast tenderness usually subsides as pregnancy progresses. If you plan to breastfeed, buy several nursing bras, and wear them in your last trimester to provide extra support and minimize soreness.

Nausea

Nausea (sometimes accompanied by vomiting) occurs in about half of all pregnant women in the first 3 months of pregnancy. Some women are nauseated throughout their pregnancy. The feeling of nausea often comes on in the morning right after waking (called morning sickness), but can occur at any time of the day or night. Nausea usually begins during the first month of pregnancy and continues until about the 14th to 16th week.

The exact cause of nausea during pregnancy is unknown, but some doctors think that it may result from the rapid rise in the level of the hormone estrogen during pregnancy. Nausea and a mild amount of vomiting usually are harmless. However, in a small percentage of pregnant women, vomiting is so severe that it drains their body of fluids and minerals, harming their health and possibly the health of the fetus.

Prevention and Treatment

To avoid or treat nausea, nibble on crackers, dry toast, or an apple as soon as you wake up (or whenever you feel nauseous). Get out of bed slowly and sit on the edge of the bed for a minute or two. Try to keep something in your stomach throughout the day. Tell your doctor about the extent of your nausea, especially if it continues or if vomiting is severe. He or she will want to examine you to rule out an underlying condition.

Drinking lots of fluids, especially water, can prevent dehydration. Don't take an antinausea medication unless your doctor has prescribed it. If your vomiting is severe, you may have to be hospitalized and be given fluids and minerals intravenously (through a vein) to replace those you have lost.

Indigestion

Indigestion, often called heartburn, is a burning pain in the center of the upper chest. It is common during pregnancy and affects almost half of all pregnant women. Indigestion occurs during pregnancy because a woman's enlarged abdomen presses on her stomach and esophagus and because the increased level of the female hormone progesterone during pregnancy relaxes the muscles in the esophagus that usually prevent the backup of stomach acid. In rare cases, indigestion may be a symptom of polyhydramnios (excess amniotic fluid; see page 526), which puts even more pressure on the abdomen and esophagus. The symptoms of indigestion usually disappear after childbirth unless the indigestion is not related to the pregnancy.

Prevention and Treatment

To prevent indigestion, don't eat too much at one time, and avoid highly spiced, greasy, or acidic foods. Eat small, frequent meals. Avoid bending over or lying flat. Try some of the suggestions on page 750 for relieving and preventing indigestion. If these steps don't help, see your doctor. He or she may prescribe an antacid or recommend changes in your diet. If the indigestion persists or is severe, the doctor may order tests to rule out the possibility of a more serious condition.

Abdominal Pain

See your doctor immediately about any abdominal pain during pregnancy. Many women have pain in their abdomen during pregnancy (called round ligament pain) that results from stretching of the ligaments that attach the uterus to the abdominal wall. The pain usually is most severe from the fourth through the sixth month of pregnancy (when the uterus expands most rapidly), but the pain can occur at any time. You can relieve round ligament pain by lying on the aching side. This type of pain usually disappears after childbirth.

Urinary Problems

Problems with urination are common in pregnant women. You may urinate more often than usual during pregnancy or feel a strong urge to urinate, which could be caused by hormonal changes and the pressure of your enlarging uterus on the bladder. You may also be thirsty and drink more liquids and therefore excrete more urine than you did before pregnancy. Some pregnant women leak urine (urinary incontinence; see page 877) when they cough or sneeze. Urinary incontinence during pregnancy can result from pressure of the uterus on the bladder and the relaxation of the muscles in the pelvis in preparation for birth.

Relaxation of the pelvic muscles during pregnancy can also lead to urinary tract infections (see page 877), possibly because bacteria can more easily travel up the ureters to the bladder. But urinary tract infections during pregnancy are more likely to be caused by the uterus pressing on the bladder, which makes it more difficult for the bladder to empty completely. If you have symptoms of a urinary tract infection such as painful urination, cloudy urine, or a sore abdomen or back, see your doctor.

Fatigue

Sometimes the first sign of pregnancy is extreme fatigue, which can result from hormonal changes, but may also be caused by anemia (see next page). In addition, as the pregnancy progresses, you are carrying more weight than usual, which can make you more tired. Fatigue is most common during the first and third trimesters. Being pregnant can also cause sleep problems, especially in the last few months, because of discomfort from an enlarging abdomen. Try to rest whenever you can, and get at least 8 hours of sleep every night.

Leg Cramps

Some women get sharp pains or cramps in their legs during pregnancy (especially during the last 3 months), possibly from increased pressure of the uterus on the blood vessels that carry blood to the legs, or from a calcium deficiency. These cramps may be followed by dull aching that can last several hours.

To prevent muscle cramps, take in 1,500 milligrams of calcium every day (either in your diet or in supplements), and stretch your calf muscles before going to bed and first thing in the morning. To treat muscle cramps, massage the sore area, straighten and flex your ankle and toes upward, and try to get up and walk around slowly.

Swollen Ankles and Hands

During pregnancy, your shoes may feel tight and your rings may no longer fit your fingers because of swelling (edema) caused by the increased fluid that is retained during pregnancy. To relieve some of the swelling, avoid salty foods (and don't add salt to food), elevate your legs while resting, and try not to stand for long periods. Because swelling can also be caused by a serious condition called preeclampsia (see page 526), see your doctor if the swelling is severe or if you have other symptoms of preeclampsia, such as headaches or blurred vision.

Dental Problems

The increased level of the hormone progesterone during pregnancy makes your gums swollen and spongy, which allows bacteria to grow more easily between your teeth and gums. Some women have noticeable swelling of the gums that disappears without treatment after delivery. Your teeth and gums may also be more susceptible to infection during pregnancy because your dentist may postpone some treatments and procedures (if they involve general anesthesia, for example) until after childbirth. Although dental X-rays are usually considered safe (a lead apron draped over the woman's abdomen protects the fetus from radiation), routine X-rays are usually postponed until after pregnancy.

Brush and floss your teeth at least twice a day. And be sure to have regular dental cleanings and checkups during pregnancy to try to prevent tooth and gum problems.

Skin Changes

Your skin may change in a number of ways during pregnancy. Changes in hormone levels result in increased production of pigment-producing cells. Pigmentation may darken in already pigmented skin areas such as freckles, moles, and birthmarks. Your nipples and the areolas (the pigmented areas surrounding the nipples) may become darker. In some women, a line of darker skin may extend down the middle of the abdomen. Patches of dark skin (medically called chloasma or melasma) may appear on your face. These darkened skin patches usually fade over time after delivery. Because sunlight can intensify the pigment changes, stay out of the sun or use a sunscreen with a sun protection factor (SPF) of at least 15.

The skin of your abdomen may itch because the skin is stretched tight as the uterus enlarges. Apply a moisturizer to relieve dry, itchy skin. Red lines called stretch marks may appear on your breasts, abdomen, and thighs, especially if you gain weight rapidly or put on too much weight during your pregnancy. Because stretch marks can be permanent, try not to gain too much weight.

Hormone changes may cause excessive perspiration by widening blood vessels, which increases blood flow to the skin. Sweating may be more apparent at night because it can wake you up. To relieve heavy perspiration, wear loose-fitting clothes; drink plenty of liquids, especially water; and keep your bedroom cool at night.

Anemia

One of the most important components of blood is a protein called hemoglobin, which carries oxygen to tissues. If hemoglobin in your blood falls below an adequate level, you can develop a condition called iron deficiency anemia (see page 610). Another possible cause of anemia during pregnancy is inadequate intake of the B vitamin folic acid (see page 514), which the fetus needs for development. Women are most likely to develop anemia in about the fifth month of pregnancy, when the fetus uses more iron and folic acid. If you have a family history of the inherited blood disorder sickle cell disease (see page 613), see your doctor before you become pregnant to determine if you have the sickle cell gene, which can be transmitted to a child.

The symptoms of anemia may not be obvious, but you might look pale; feel faint, tired, and weak; be breathless; or have heart palpitations. Because anemia can make you more vulnerable to infection and more likely to have a preterm delivery or a baby with a low birth weight, your doctor will perform a blood test early in your pregnancy to find out if you have anemia.

Prevention and Treatment

To prevent anemia, eat foods that are rich in iron such as liver, beef, whole-grain bread, eggs, and dried fruits. Eat citrus fruits and fresh vegetables that contain vitamin C, which helps the body absorb iron more efficiently. Take your prenatal vitamins every day to help ensure that you are getting sufficient amounts of folic acid. Your doctor may prescribe an iron supplement if you are diagnosed with anemia.

Constipation and Hemorrhoids

Constipation (see page 769) is common during pregnancy because the increase in hormones can slow the movement of food through the digestive tract. In about the fourth month, constipation sometimes results from pressure on the intestines by the enlarging uterus. Constipation can cause hemorrhoids (see page 777). If you already have hemorrhoids, constipation can worsen them by making you strain harder during bowel movements.

Prevention and Treatment

To prevent constipation, eat plenty of fresh fruits and vegetables, legumes, whole grains, and other foods that are high in fiber (see page 37). Drink at least eight glasses of water a day. Some people find prune juice helpful. Don't wait to move your bowels; go whenever you have the urge, but don't strain. Regular exercise can also help keep you regular.

Before taking any medications for constipation, talk to your doctor. You probably can safely use milk of magnesia or glycerin suppositories while you are pregnant, but don't use other over-the-counter laxatives.

If none of these measures work, your doctor may prescribe medication to soften your stools. If you have hemorrhoids, take warm baths. Check with your doctor before using any hemorrhoid creams or suppositories.

Varicose Veins

Many women develop swollen veins in their legs (varicose veins; see page 602) during pregnancy, especially during the last 3 months. During pregnancy, the veins are carrying an increased volume of blood to supply to the developing fetus. In addition, as the uterus enlarges and presses on some major veins, blood flow from the leg veins up to the pelvis can slow down. This combination of factors sometimes produces enough pressure to cause the veins in the calves and thighs to become swollen and painful. The same kinds of pressure can also affect the veins around the entrance to the vagina and rectum.

You are more likely to develop varicose veins during pregnancy if you have a family history of the condition. Varicose veins that develop during pregnancy usually become significantly less swollen or disappear within 12 weeks of delivery.

Prevention and Treatment
To reduce your risk of developing varicose veins, don't wear clothes that fit tightly around your waist or upper legs. Avoid standing for long periods, but take regular walks every day. Rest with your feet up (preferably higher than the level of your heart) as much as possible. Don't gain too much weight during your pregnancy because the excess weight can put more strain on your veins. Your doctor may recommend wearing elastic support stockings to help improve your circulation. Put the stockings on in the morning before you get out of bed.

Sleep Problems

Many women find it difficult to get to sleep or stay asleep while they are pregnant. Sleep problems can result from changes in hormone levels, a need to urinate more often, or emotional stress (for example, worrying about your health or the health of your baby). Toward the end of pregnancy, you may find it difficult to find a comfortable position for sleeping. Sleep is essential for good health—for both you and your fetus. Lack of sleep can make you susceptible to infections and can lead to irritability.

Prevention and Treatment
If you have trouble falling asleep at night, avoid napping during the later part of the day. Take a warm bath and drink a glass of warm milk before going to bed. Because caffeine is a stimulant, cut back on or eliminate coffee, tea, or other caffeine-containing foods or beverages from your diet. Get plenty of exercise during the day, but don't exercise within a few hours of going to bed. Try performing some relaxation exercises (see page 59) at bedtime.

If you are losing a lot of sleep, talk to your doctor. Most doctors prefer not to prescribe sleep medications such as sedatives because of the possibility of affecting the fetus. This is especially true during the critical first 14 weeks, when the fetus's organs are developing, and in the days closer to the due date, when the medication could suppress the baby's nervous system and affect his or her breathing during labor and delivery. Don't take any medications—including over-the-counter or alternative sleep aids such as the hormone melatonin—unless your doctor has prescribed them.

Back Pain

During pregnancy, the ligaments and fibrous tissue that normally support a woman's joints become slightly more elastic. This elasticity allows the pelvis to expand during delivery but also makes the joints more susceptible to strain. In addition, the joints of the spine are under increased strain because of the additional weight of a pregnancy and because the growing uterus shifts the woman's center of balance and can put strain on her lower back.

In the first few months of pregnancy, severe back pain can be a sign of a miscarriage (see page 522) or an ectopic pregnancy (see page 523). Later in pregnancy, back pain can be a symptom of labor (see page 531), especially if it is accompanied by other symptoms, such as bleeding or vaginal discharge.

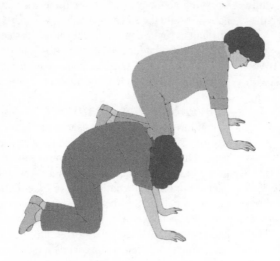

Relieving backache
A gentle exercise for relieving backache is to get on your hands and knees, keeping your head straight and in line with your spine (don't let your spine sag). Curve your back up, tightening the muscles in your abdomen and buttocks and lowering your head. Gradually raise your head and return your back to its original position. Repeat several times.

Prevention and Treatment
To reduce the risk of back pain, try not to gain too much weight during your pregnancy. Wear low-heeled shoes, and don't lift heavy objects. Don't cross your legs or slouch when you sit; sit in a firm, high-backed chair and use a small cushion to support your lower back. Sleep on a firm mattress, and don't use a pillow under your head if you sleep on your back (but putting a pillow under your knees can relieve pressure on your lower back). If you sleep on your side, rest your head on a pillow and support your upper leg with a pillow to keep your spine straight.

Stress can sometimes cause or worsen a backache, so try to relax. Don't use a pain reliever for back pain unless it has been prescribed by your doctor. Before having massage therapy or using hot or cold applications, talk to your doctor. A pelvic support belt, found in most maternity departments, can be helpful. Your doctor or prenatal class teacher can recommend exercises that can help strengthen your back and abdominal muscles, which may relieve your back pain.

High Blood Pressure
Some women are found to have high blood pressure (see page 574) at routine checkups during pregnancy. The high blood pressure may have been present before pregnancy, or it could be related to the pregnancy. It is common for blood pressure to fall slightly during the middle weeks of pregnancy and to rise slightly toward the end.

High blood pressure usually has no symptoms, but a serious form of pregnancy-induced high blood pressure (called preeclampsia; see page 526) can cause swelling of the face and hands, changes in vision (such as seeing spots), and severe and persistent headaches. Most women with high blood pressure have a normal delivery. However, extremely high blood pressure can result in serious complications during pregnancy, such as hemorrhage, and can inhibit the fetus's growth or even cause fetal death.

Treatment
The earlier high blood pressure is diagnosed, the better your chances of having a healthy pregnancy. If you have mildly elevated blood pressure, your doctor will want to monitor it closely to make sure it is under control during your pregnancy. If your blood pressure is high, your doctor will prescribe medication to lower it. He or she may also order regular blood and urine tests to monitor the function of your kidneys, and ultrasound scans (see page 509) to make sure the fetus is developing at the normal rate.

Heart Disorders
Pregnancy puts an extra workload on your heart. If you have an underlying heart defect such as a congenital heart defect (see page 389), or a heart valve disease caused by rheumatic fever, you have a risk of heart failure. Your doctor should know about any heart conditions before you get pregnant—or at least as soon as the pregnancy is confirmed. Your doctor may refer you to a cardiologist (heart specialist) for additional care during your pregnancy. The cardiologist will monitor your health throughout your pregnancy for any possible complications related to the heart disorder.

Sometimes a heart disorder such as a murmur (abnormal heart sounds) shows up for the first time during pregnancy from the extra demands placed on the heart. Most heart murmurs discovered in the first 3 months of pregnancy are insignificant, but the doctor may order tests such as an ultrasound image of the heart (echocardiogram; see page 561) or a recording of the electrical activity of the heart (electrocardiogram; see page 559) to evaluate the condition.

If you have a heart condition, you will have to deliver in a hospital. If you have no complications, your pregnancy should be healthy and you should go into labor normally at full term. When you go into labor, your doctor will help make sure that the delivery is as easy as possible for you—with a minimum of pushing, which puts a strain on the heart and deprives it of oxygen.

Treatment

The main treatment for a heart disorder during pregnancy is rest to reduce strain on the heart, which is already working harder than usual. When you are lying down, keep shifting your position and relaxing and contracting your muscles to keep the blood moving through your legs to prevent blood clots. Restrict your intake of salt and salty foods to prevent fluid retention. Many standard antihypertensive medications have potentially harmful effects on the fetus and usually are not recommended during pregnancy.

Gestational Diabetes

Gestational diabetes is a form of diabetes that can develop during pregnancy. The condition can occur because the placenta produces hormones that can block the effects of the hormone insulin, which moves glucose into cells for energy. This insulin-blocking effect usually develops between the 20th and 24th weeks of pregnancy. The pancreas can usually overcome this effect by producing more insulin, but if it cannot make enough insulin to overcome the effects of the insulin-blocking hormones, glucose builds up in the pregnant woman's blood, causing gestational diabetes. The condition goes away after pregnancy because there is no placenta to produce the insulin-blocking hormones.

You are at increased risk of having gestational diabetes if you are obese, have a family history of diabetes, previously gave birth to a very large infant (weighing more than 9 pounds, 14 ounces), had gestational diabetes in a previous pregnancy, had a

stillbirth (see page 530) or a child with a birth defect, or are older than 25.

When diagnosed and treated, gestational diabetes usually does not cause problems for either the pregnant woman or the fetus. If not treated, however, gestational diabetes can produce an excessive amount of amniotic fluid in the uterus (which can stretch the uterus into the abdomen, making breathing difficult) and life-threatening high blood pressure (preeclampsia; see page 526) in the pregnant woman. The fetus may grow very large from the excess glucose in the woman's blood (which can make delivery difficult); after birth, a baby may have low blood sugar, respiratory problems, or neonatal jaundice (see page 382).

Symptoms

Gestational diabetes seldom causes symptoms in the early stages. For this reason, all women are offered a glucose screening test (see page 512) during pregnancy. If your blood glucose level is found to be elevated on the screening test, you will then have a more accurate diagnostic test called the glucose tolerance test. For this test, you will be asked to eat a high-carbohydrate diet for 3 days and then to fast overnight (for 10 to 14 hours) before the test. You will be given a strong solution of glucose to drink, and blood samples will be taken and evaluated every hour for 3 hours to determine if you have a high glucose level, indicating gestational diabetes.

Treatment

Gestational diabetes is usually treated with a carefully controlled diet. If you are diagnosed with gestational diabetes, your doctor will prescribe a diet to help keep your blood glucose level in the normal range. The doctor will probably refer you to a registered dietitian, who can help you plan meals to meet your needs. Most women with gestational diabetes require three meals a day and a bedtime snack. Meals should be evenly spaced, and calories should be distributed evenly throughout the day. Avoid high-fat foods and cooking methods such as frying, which can make you gain too much weight (excess weight can raise blood glucose levels). Regular exercise can also help keep your glucose level, as well as your weight, down.

Your doctor will want to test your glucose level regularly and will ask you to test it frequently at home to see if your diet is keeping your glucose level in the healthy range. If your blood glucose cannot be controlled with diet, you will need to have insulin injections throughout the rest of your pregnancy and labor. Most women do not need the insulin after delivery because their blood glucose level returns to normal immediately. However, you are at increased risk of developing gestational diabetes in a future pregnancy and of developing type 2 diabetes (see page 894) later in life. For this

reason, your doctor will recommend a glucose screening test 2 months after delivery and early in any subsequent pregnancies as well as routine blood tests at future checkups to monitor your glucose level.

In addition to monitoring your health, the doctor will monitor the fetus's condition throughout your pregnancy and labor to make sure that no complications develop.

Complications During Pregnancy

Some infections that a woman has during pregnancy, and lifestyle factors such as her drinking alcohol or smoking cigarettes, can harm a fetus. A severe genetic abnormality in the embryo or a disorder of a woman's reproductive system that can affect implantation of a fertilized egg can cause serious complications, including miscarriage. During the first 3 months after conception (the first trimester), the fetus is especially vulnerable because it is going through many major developmental changes. In the fourth through the sixth month (the second trimester), most pregnancies continue smoothly, and women usually feel

generally well because the physical changes associated with the development of the fetus proceed more slowly at this time.

Most fetuses have a better chance of survival the closer the pregnancy is to full term when they are born. Some women may receive treatment during the final 3 months of pregnancy (third trimester) to prevent them from going into labor too soon (preterm labor; see page 529). If a doctor thinks that a baby has a better chance of survival outside the uterus before the pregnancy is full term, he or she will induce labor (see page 533) or deliver the baby by cesarean (see page 534).

Miscarriage

Miscarriage (also called spontaneous abortion) occurs when a pregnancy ends naturally before the fetus is developed enough to survive outside the uterus. About 20 percent of all pregnancies end in miscarriage, usually during the first 8 weeks. During a miscarriage, the developing fetus and the placenta separate from the inner wall of the uterus. This separation may occur because of a developmental or genetic defect in the fetus or because the placenta is not attached properly to the uterus. More than half of miscarriages result from a chromosome abnormality (see page 955) in the fetus. Other causes of miscarriage include an abnormally shaped uterus, scar tissue in the uterus, or fibroids (see page 867), all of which can interfere with a fertilized egg's ability to implant in the membrane that lines the inside of the uterus. Often the cause of a miscarriage is unknown. It is rare for miscarriages to result from falls or other injuries because the fetus is well protected inside the uterus.

Symptoms

The first symptom of a threatened, or possible, miscarriage early in a pregnancy is slight bleeding from the vagina. If the miscarriage occurs later in the pregnancy, the bleeding can range from a few drops of blood to a heavy flow. The bleeding may start with no warning or may be preceded by a brownish discharge. A threatened miscarriage is often painless.

If the fetus has died, a miscarriage is usually unavoidable (called an inevitable miscarriage). An inevitable miscarriage is usually accompanied by cramping pain in the lower abdomen or back. The pain can be either dull and constant or sharp and intermittent. If you pass any solid tissue from your vagina, save it in a jar to bring to your doctor for examination. The doctor can tell by looking at the tissue if you have eliminated all of the fetus and placenta. He or she will also send the tissue to a laboratory for microscopic examination to try to determine the cause of the miscarriage.

If any parts of the fetus or placenta remain in the

uterus, it is called an incomplete miscarriage. If a miscarriage is incomplete, you may have constant or intermittent bleeding and pain for several days. If an incomplete miscarriage is not diagnosed, the bleeding can continue and the tissue left in the uterus can become infected.

In rare cases, a fetus dies in the uterus but the woman has no symptoms of miscarriage (called a missed miscarriage). Although you do not have symptoms of a miscarriage in a missed miscarriage, you will no longer experience any of the symptoms of pregnancy. Missed miscarriages are often discovered on a prenatal visit when the doctor notices that the uterus has not increased in size.

Keeping a Kick Chart

An active fetus is usually a healthy fetus. Your doctor may ask you to keep a record of how active your fetus is with a kick chart. He or she may give you a chart (or you can make a chart yourself) to log the movements of your fetus for a day or two. He or she will ask you to record the kicks at the time of day when your fetus is most active. Discuss the results of the kick chart with your doctor. Healthy fetuses may kick only 10 times a day or kick eight or more times in their most active hour. Keep in mind, however, that the number of movements can vary, and some perfectly healthy babies may not kick much. Also, fetuses move less toward the end of pregnancy, when space is more limited inside the uterus.

Diagnosis and Treatment

If the vaginal bleeding stops or is not very heavy, your doctor may recommend that you rest in bed at home. If the pregnancy seems to be continuing despite the bleeding, your doctor may arrange for you to have a series of blood tests to measure the level of human chorionic gonadotropin (HCG) to confirm that the pregnancy is continuing, and an ultrasound to make sure that the developing fetus is still alive. Don't have sexual intercourse for a few weeks after you have vaginal bleeding because sex can stimulate labor contractions. Ask your doctor about other precautions to take.

No known medical treatment can stop a threatened miscarriage. If you are having a miscarriage, the doctor may recommend that you rest in bed, or at least stay close to home, until the fetus is expelled. In the case of an inevitable or missed miscarriage, your doctor may remove the fetus and placenta by suction or by a D and C (see page 869). For an incomplete miscarriage, he or she will remove any tissue that remains in the uterus. These procedures are usually performed in a hospital but may be done in the doctor's office or in a clinic.

Some women benefit from short-term psychological counseling after a miscarriage, especially if they were trying to get pregnant. After a miscarriage, you can safely start trying to conceive again in about 6 to 8 weeks. The doctor will probably recommend waiting before trying to conceive until you have had at least one normal period because it makes it easier to estimate a due date. If you have more than one miscarriage, your doctor may recommend examinations and tests to determine the cause.

Ectopic Pregnancy

In an ectopic pregnancy, an egg is fertilized by a sperm but develops outside the uterus, usually in one of the fallopian tubes (called a tubal pregnancy). In rare cases, an ectopic pregnancy develops in an ovary or in the abdominal cavity or cervix. The fertilized egg continues to divide and grow even though the space is too small to accommodate it. When the space, such as a fallopian tube, can no longer contain the growing embryo, the tube ruptures.

About 1 in 100 pregnancies is an ectopic pregnancy; most are discovered within the first 2 months. It is essential to diagnose an ectopic pregnancy as early as possible because a ruptured fallopian tube can be life-threatening. You are more likely to have an ectopic pregnancy if you were born with an abnormality of one or both of your fallopian tubes; if you have ever had an infection in your fallopian tubes, such as a sexually transmitted disease (see page 477) or pelvic inflammatory disease (see page 871); if you have ever had surgery on a fallopian tube; or if you are using an intrauterine device (IUD; see page 472).

Symptoms

In an ectopic pregnancy, you may have cramping abdominal pain, often on one side, which may be accompanied by vaginal bleeding. You may not have any other symptoms of pregnancy and you may not even know that you are pregnant. If the internal bleeding is severe, it can lead to shock (see page 579), which is life-threatening.

Diagnosis and Treatment

If you experience abdominal pain that lasts for more than a few hours, your doctor will perform a thorough physical examination, including a pelvic examination, to rule out other disorders, such as a miscarriage (see page 522), appendicitis (see page 771), or an infection of the fallopian tubes. To diagnose an ectopic pregnancy, a doctor may use ultrasound, laparoscopy (an examination of the inside of the abdomen using a viewing tube inserted through a small incision in the abdomen), and possibly a series of blood tests to measure the level of the hormone human chorionic gonadotropin (HCG), which is present during pregnancy. In an ectopic pregnancy, the level of HCG does not increase as quickly as it does in a normal pregnancy.

If your doctor confirms that you have an ectopic pregnancy, you will be hospitalized immediately and given fluids intravenously (through a vein), and possibly a blood transfusion if you have lost a lot of blood. If the fallopian tube is ruptured or bleeding, part or all of it may have to be removed. If the remaining fallopian tube is healthy, you still will be able to get pregnant, although the chances of conception are slightly reduced. Sometimes more extensive surgery of the abdominal cavity is necessary to remove the fetus, placenta, surrounding tissue, and any damaged blood vessels.

If an ectopic pregnancy is diagnosed early and has not ruptured, and if the woman is not bleeding

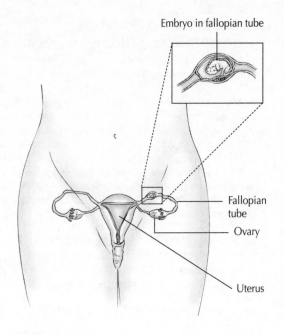

Embryo in fallopian tube

Fallopian tube

Ovary

Uterus

Tubal pregnancy
A tubal pregnancy is a pregnancy that occurs in a fallopian tube when the fertilized egg does not make it all the way into the uterus and instead remains inside the tube. If the fertilized egg continues to grow inside the tube, it eventually can cause the tube to burst, which can be life-threatening.

or having any pain, the doctor may treat the ectopic pregnancy with one or more injections of the powerful anticancer medication methotrexate and perform a series of blood tests to ensure that the drug is working. Methotrexate breaks down the abnormal tissue, allowing the body to absorb it.

If you have had an ectopic pregnancy, your doctor may recommend waiting until you have had one or two periods before trying to get pregnant again to give your body a chance to heal. Because a woman who has had an ectopic pregnancy is at increased risk of having another one, you will need to have the pregnancy confirmed as early as possible to make sure it is progressing normally (inside the uterus).

Incompetent Cervix

If a woman has an incompetent cervix, her cervix is weak and dilates (widens) under the weight of the fetus and placenta during pregnancy. The fetus and placenta can drop down out of the uterus, resulting in miscarriage (see page 522), usually

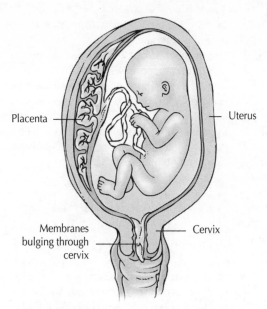

Placenta

Uterus

Membranes bulging through cervix

Cervix

Incompetent cervix
If a woman's cervix is weak, the increasing weight of the developing fetus can cause the cervix to open and widen prematurely. As a result, the membranes that surround the fetus may bulge down through the cervix and rupture, causing a miscarriage.

after the 14th week of pregnancy. The cause of incompetent cervix is usually unknown, but the cervix sometimes can be weakened from past medical procedures such as a biopsy in which a large amount of tissue was taken from the cervix (cone biopsy). Incompetent cervix also can occur in women whose mothers took the drug diethylstilbestrol (DES) when they were pregnant to prevent miscarriage. (DES was prescribed from the 1940s to the 1970s.)

If you are pregnant and have had a miscarriage because of an incompetent cervix, or if your doctor thinks that you may have an incompetent cervix, he or she may perform surgery early in your pregnancy to correct the weakness. For this procedure, you will be given spinal or general anesthesia, and the doctor will tighten your cervix using a piece of strong thread. Your doctor may prescribe medication to reduce the risk that the surgery will stimulate preterm labor (see page 529). He or she may recommend that you rest as much as possible and abstain from sexual intercourse until the delivery. At about the 37th week of pregnancy or when you go into labor, the thread is cut to allow the fetus and placenta to pass through the cervix.

Multiple Fetuses

Twins occur as a result of either the splitting of a single fertilized egg or the parallel development of two fertilized eggs. Twins account for 1 in 90 births in the United States (triplets, by contrast, are uncommon and occur in only 1 in 8,000 births). Two out of three sets of twins are fraternal (nonidentical), which means that two different eggs from the woman were fertilized by two different

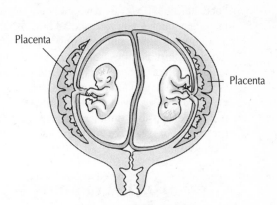

Placenta

Placenta

Fraternal (nonidentical) twins

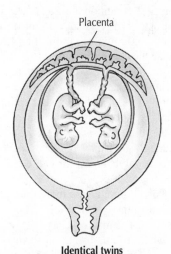

Placenta

Identical twins

Fraternal and identical twins
Fraternal twins result when two separate eggs are fertilized by two different sperm. Each twin gets nourishment from his or her own placenta. Identical twins result when a single egg that has been fertilized by one sperm divides into two identical embryos. Identical twins share a placenta.

sperm from the man. Identical twins develop from one egg, fertilized by one sperm, that splits shortly after fertilization. Fraternal twins each have a placenta; identical twins share a placenta. Identical twins have identical genetic makeup, while fraternal twins are no more alike genetically than other siblings.

A multiple pregnancy is usually discovered by a doctor during a routine prenatal examination and confirmed by ultrasound. The outlook is usually good for both the pregnant woman and the fetuses if the woman has adequate prenatal care, rest, and good nutrition. If you are having twins, your doctor may recommend that you take additional vitamin and mineral supplements throughout your pregnancy. Complications from multiple births can include anemia (see page 518), high blood pressure (see page 520), gestational diabetes (see page 521), preeclampsia (see below right), placenta previa (see next page), postpartum bleeding (see page 537), preterm labor (see page 529), and babies with low birth weight.

Polyhydramnios

Polyhydramnios (sometimes called simply hydramnios) is excess amniotic fluid in the uterus, a usually harmless condition that can occur in the middle to late stages of pregnancy. In most cases, the uterus swells only slightly more than normal and may cause no symptoms or only slight abdominal discomfort. The woman may feel slightly more breathless than usual or may have indigestion. In some cases, the abdominal swelling may be pronounced, stretching the skin over the abdomen. If polyhydramnios is severe, symptoms may begin suddenly and may be accompanied by nausea. Severe polyhydramnios can cause preterm labor (see page 529).

Polyhydramnios is more common in pregnancies that involve multiple fetuses (see previous page), in a woman who has diabetes (see page 889), or when a fetus has a malformation of the gastrointestinal system (such as a diaphragmatic hernia; see page 407) or of the spine or brain (such as a neural tube defect; see page 398).

Diagnosis and Treatment
If you have symptoms of polyhydramnios, your doctor may order a detailed ultrasound (see page 509) to rule out a fetal malformation or to detect a multiple pregnancy.

For a mild case of polyhydramnios, a doctor may recommend rest and may prescribe medication to relax the uterus and reduce the risk of preterm labor. In rare, severe cases, amniocentesis (see page 510) is performed to withdraw some of the excess fluid through a needle to reduce the pregnant woman's discomfort; however, amniocentesis can bring on preterm labor.

Oligohydramnios

Oligohydramnios is a rare condition in which an abnormally small amount of amniotic fluid surrounds and cushions the fetus. The condition can result from severe preeclampsia (see below) in the woman, urinary abnormalities in the fetus, or a postterm pregnancy (see page 530). Early in pregnancy, oligohydramnios can cause a miscarriage. Late in pregnancy, it can cause deformities in the fetus or can be fatal to the fetus. If the amniotic fluid is not sufficient to cushion the fetus from pressure from the woman's abdominal organs, the fetus can squeeze the umbilical cord against the wall of the uterus, cutting off its supply of oxygen and nutrients. In rare cases, the pressure of the uterus on the fetus can cause structural birth defects such as clubfoot (see page 402).

Treatment
If your doctor thinks you may have oligohydramnios, he or she will first try to treat the underlying disorder that has caused it, which is easier if it has resulted from preeclampsia rather than from an abnormality in the fetus. If your pregnancy is past the 37th week, your doctor may induce labor or perform a cesarean delivery (see page 534).

Preeclampsia and Eclampsia

Preeclampsia (also called toxemia of pregnancy or pregnancy-induced high blood pressure or hypertension) is a disorder that usually occurs late in pregnancy. In preeclampsia, a woman's blood pressure rises, she retains excess fluid, and she has protein in her urine. The cause of preeclampsia is unknown. It is common in pregnancies that involve multiple fetuses (see previous page). Preeclampsia seems to occur more often in the first pregnancies of women between ages 18 and 30 and in women who have (or have a family history of) high blood pressure or diabetes.

Because high blood pressure reduces the efficiency of the placenta (which provides the fetus with oxygen and nutrients), some doctors think that high blood pressure may retard the growth of the fetus and may lead to preterm delivery. High blood pressure during pregnancy can also damage the woman's kidneys, brain, eyes, and liver.

In some cases, preeclampsia leads to an even more serious condition called eclampsia. In eclampsia, blood pressure gets so high that it decreases oxygen to the pregnant woman's brain and causes seizures, which can be life-threatening to her and to the fetus. Seizures have been linked to stroke, the most common cause of maternal death from eclampsia.

Symptoms

Because the symptoms of preeclampsia are not noticeable at first, make sure you go to all of your prenatal checkups so that preeclampsia can be diagnosed early and treated. The symptoms of severe preeclampsia include headaches, blurred vision, intolerance to bright light, upper abdominal pain, nausea and vomiting, and bloating.

Treatment

If you have preeclampsia, your doctor will recommend that you get lots of rest and reduce your salt intake to help lower your blood pressure. He or she may prescribe a medication to control your blood pressure. The doctor will order ultrasound scans regularly to monitor the fetus's growth and to watch for a buildup of amniotic fluid. If you have symptoms of severe preeclampsia or of eclampsia, you will be admitted to a hospital immediately and will be given medication to lower your blood pressure and remove excess fluid from your body. Your doctor may recommend immediate delivery by inducing labor (see page 533) or performing a cesarean delivery (see page 534).

Placenta Previa and Placental Abruption

Normally, the placenta is attached to the top portion of the uterus. Any part of the placenta that is near the cervix (the opening into the uterus) is poorly supported and vulnerable to damage. In placenta previa, the placenta develops low in the uterus, either partially or completely covering the cervix and blocking the entrance to the vagina. The weight of the fetus puts pressure on the part of the placenta that covers the cervix, sometimes causing bleeding if part of the placenta detaches from the wall of the uterus. Placenta previa occurs in about 1 in 200 pregnancies after the 28th week.

The cause of placenta previa is unknown. It occurs more frequently in women who have given birth to several children and in pregnancies with multiple fetuses (see page 525). In some cases, the placenta is low in the uterus early in pregnancy but then moves up the wall of the uterus to a more normal position as the pregnancy progresses, where it usually does not interfere with delivery.

If the placenta ruptures or tears, causing heavy bleeding, it can cut off the blood supply to the fetus. In placental abruption, a placenta that is positioned normally in the uterus separates prematurely from the uterine wall. Placental abruption is more common in women who have high blood pressure (see page 520). Placental abruption may be linked to a deficiency of the B vitamin folic acid.

Symptoms

Placenta previa may cause no symptoms. If the placenta becomes partly detached from the uterus, the woman will have sporadic bleeding but usually no pain. Placental abruption may cause some pain along with the bleeding. However, in some cases, placental abruption causes no bleeding because the blood is trapped between the wall of the uterus and the placenta. This collection of blood can trigger preterm labor (see page 529).

Diagnosis and Treatment

If the placenta is only partially blocking your cervix, your doctor may recommend resting in bed, avoiding sexual intercourse, and limiting other physical activity. He or she will use ultrasound (see page 509) to monitor the health of the fetus and the position of the placenta.

If you have vaginal bleeding, call your doctor immediately. (Don't try to stop the bleeding by putting in a tampon.) If the bleeding is light or stops on its own and the fetus is not in any danger, your doctor will probably monitor your condition with ultrasound. If the bleeding is severe, you may need to have a blood transfusion, and the baby will be delivered as

Placenta previa

The normal placement of the placenta is near the top of the uterus. In placenta previa, the placenta is attached at the bottom of the uterus, where it can partially or completely cover the cervix. If the placenta reaches to the edge of the cervix but does not cover it, the condition is called marginal placenta previa (left). In partial placenta previa (center), the placenta blocks part of the cervix. In complete placenta previa (right), the placenta covers the entire cervix.

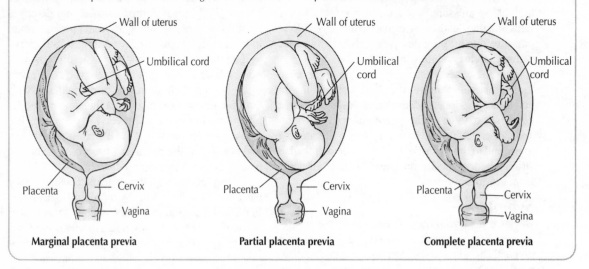

Marginal placenta previa   Partial placenta previa   Complete placenta previa

soon as possible by cesarean (see page 534). Severe bleeding is dangerous but rarely fatal to the pregnant woman, but it can be fatal to the fetus.

Premature Rupture of the Membranes

When labor begins, the membranes surrounding the fetus rupture, releasing amniotic fluid (often referred to as the water breaking). The amniotic fluid may leak out slowly through the vagina or in a sudden rush. Occasionally, the membranes rupture before labor has begun. The main risks of premature rupture of the membranes containing the amniotic fluid are infection and preterm labor (see next page).

Diagnosis and Treatment

If your membranes have ruptured prematurely, you probably will be admitted to the hospital. Your doctor will collect any remaining fluid and perform amniocentesis (see page 510) to determine if the fetus's lungs are developed enough for delivery. Sometimes a small tear in the membranes surrounding the fetus heals and the pregnancy can continue. Because there is a risk of infection, you may have to stay in the hospital so your condition and the health of the fetus can be monitored carefully. If the fetus is mature enough (usually after the 36th week) or if there is sign of an infection, labor will be induced (see page 533).

Chorioamnionitis

Chorioamnionitis is infection of the chorion and amnion membranes of the placenta and the amniotic fluid that surrounds the fetus. The infection, caused by bacteria that enter the uterus from the vagina, usually occurs at the end of pregnancy when more than 24 hours elapse between the time the membranes rupture and delivery. In rare cases, the infection develops earlier, before the 37th week of pregnancy, and causes preterm labor (see next page). The symptoms of chorioamnionitis include tenderness in the uterus and a fever. The fetus may have signs of infection such as an unusually high heart rate.

Treatment

Chorioamnionitis is treated with antibiotics given intravenously (through a vein) to the mother and immediate delivery (because the antibiotics given to the mother don't reach the fetus). If the baby is born with a severe infection, he or she is given antibiotics intravenously to prevent or treat other, more serious infections, such as pneumonia or meningitis.

Preterm Labor

Labor is considered to be preterm (or premature) if it occurs between about the 24th and 36th weeks of pregnancy. About 5 percent of pregnancies result in preterm labor. Severe preeclampsia or eclampsia (see page 526) account for about a third of all cases of preterm delivery. High blood pressure (see page 520), placenta previa and placental abruption (see page 527), vaginal bleeding (see page 523), and other factors, such as cigarette smoking and drug abuse, account for some cases of preterm labor.

The earlier in a pregnancy a baby is born, the lower his or her chances of survival. Preterm infants who survive run the risk of having respiratory distress syndrome (see page 381), neonatal jaundice (see page 382), and other medical and developmental problems. The risk of having these disorders increases the earlier in pregnancy the baby is born.

Diagnosis and Treatment

If you think you are starting labor prematurely, contact your doctor immediately. If your doctor is not available, call the hospital where you plan to deliver your baby, tell the staff what the problem is, and ask for their advice. They will probably tell you to come to the hospital right away. Arrange to have someone drive you if possible. If you don't think you will be able to make it to your hospital in time, call 911 or your local emergency number and arrange to be taken to the nearest hospital emergency department.

When you arrive at the hospital, you will be examined to see if you have started labor. A doctor may perform amniocentesis (see page 510) to evaluate the fetus's lung development. If you are having contractions, you may be given medication to control them to allow the pregnancy to continue until the fetus is more mature. If the doctor decides to let the labor proceed, you may have an episiotomy (see page 533) to allow easier passage of the baby's head, which is more fragile than that of a full-term baby.

Depending on your infant's health status, he or she will be sent to either the nursery or the neonatal intensive care unit (see page 383), where his or her heartbeat, breathing, and temperature will be monitored and any problems treated promptly.

Retarded Growth of the Fetus

In some pregnancies, the placenta does not supply enough nourishment to the fetus, resulting in stunted development (called intrauterine growth retardation or retarded fetal growth). A fetus's growth is determined to be retarded if the fetus's weight falls below the fifth percentile. The inability of the placenta to supply nourishment can result from scarring in areas of the placenta where tissue has died from lack of blood. The obstruction of blood flow can result from preeclampsia (see page 526), high blood pressure (see page 520), vaginal bleeding (see page 523), or placenta previa or placental abruption (see page 527). Retarded fetal growth can also occur when the pregnant woman has a heart disorder (see page 520) or diabetes (see page 521), or when she smokes cigarettes, drinks alcohol or uses other drugs, or is malnourished during pregnancy.

A newborn whose growth is stunted has less body fat (and therefore is less able to resist cold) and is more susceptible to having low blood sugar (hypoglycemia; see page 897) than an infant who is at a normal weight. Low-birth-weight babies have more medical and developmental problems, some of which can be life-threatening. If the infant is preterm (see left), he or she may have complications such as respiratory distress syndrome (see page 381).

To help ensure that your baby is born healthy, go to all of your scheduled prenatal appointments. If you are beyond the 30th week of your pregnancy and think that your fetus is not moving as much as before, your doctor may recommend that you keep a kick chart (see page 523) to record fetal movements. To monitor the fetus's condition, your doctor may recommend that you have an ultrasound and tests that measure the fetus's heartbeat.

If your doctor thinks that your fetus's growth may be stunted, he or she will discuss moving up the delivery date by inducing labor (see page 533) or by performing a cesarean (see page 534). A fetus that is not growing normally inside the uterus may do better in a neonatal intensive care unit. Your doctor will recommend that you deliver in a hospital that has a neonatal intensive care unit so that any problems your baby has can be treated promptly by trained neonatal specialists.

Postterm Pregnancy

Ideally, labor starts when the fetus is fully mature and able to survive outside the uterus. Most women give birth between the 37th and 42nd weeks of pregnancy. A pregnancy that goes beyond the 42nd week is called a postterm pregnancy, or postmaturity. Postterm pregnancies occur most frequently in women who have gestational diabetes (see page 521) or a family history of diabetes (see page 894).

A placenta that has been providing nourishment to a fetus for longer than 42 weeks may not be able to provide a large fetus with a sufficient amount of oxygenated blood, which can cause an abnormal heart rate or brain damage. The placenta can also stop functioning normally, reducing the amount of oxygen and nutrients to the fetus or causing the fetus to secrete less urine, thereby reducing the volume of amniotic fluid. Because amniotic fluid provides cushioning between the fetus and the uterine wall, a deficiency of fluid (oligohydramnios; see page 526) can cause the umbilical cord to be squeezed, cutting off the fetus's supply of oxygen and nutrients. Postterm fetuses may be too large to deliver vaginally. In addition, they may be so mature that they excrete their first bowel movement (called meconium) into the amniotic fluid, which

can be life-threatening if they inhale the meconium and it blocks their air passages. The death rate of infants who are delivered long after the due date is almost double that of infants who are delivered closer to term.

If your doctor thinks that your pregnancy is postterm, he or she will use ultrasound and fetal monitoring (see page 533) to ensure that the fetus is healthy. Your doctor will induce labor (see page 533) only if there are medical reasons to do so or if your cervix has started to dilate (widen). He or she will monitor your labor and delivery carefully and, if your baby seems to be in distress, may use forceps or other techniques to assist the delivery or may perform a cesarean delivery (see page 534).

Stillbirth

Death of the fetus, or stillbirth, is the death of a fetus after the 18th week of pregnancy. In many cases, stillbirth results from a severe abnormality in the fetus, severe preeclampsia or eclampsia (see page 526), vaginal bleeding (see page 523), or postterm pregnancy (see left). It is also linked to gestational diabetes (see page 521), high blood pressure (see page 520), Rh incompatibility (see page 508), and infections in the pregnant woman. In many cases, the cause of death is unknown.

In most cases, the only indication that a fetus has died inside the uterus is lack of fetal movement. A doctor will listen for a heartbeat and will use ultrasound (see page 509) and an electrocardiogram (see page 559) to determine if the fetus is alive. If labor has not begun, the doctor will induce labor (see page 533).

Childbirth

As you near your delivery date, you may experience some signs of approaching labor. The first signs of normal labor are contractions of the uterus. Initially, these contractions may seem like irregular bursts of pain resembling indigestion or twinges of pain in the lower back. The closer you get to delivery, the contractions occur at more regular intervals and are closer together and more intense.

However, contractions are not always a reliable sign that labor has started. Throughout pregnancy,

the uterus contracts in preparation for labor. These contractions, called Braxton Hicks contractions or false labor, are usually not noticeable until the last weeks of pregnancy. If you have contractions that do not increase in frequency or intensity and you have no other signs of labor, you probably are not in labor.

As labor starts, the mucus plug that has formed a protective barrier between the uterus and vagina during pregnancy may be expelled as a mucus discharge tinged pink or brown with blood (called bloody show). This discharge is a normal part of childbirth.

Another sign of labor is the rupture of the membranes that surround the amniotic fluid. This rupture may occur as a small trickle or a sudden gush of fluid from your vagina (usually referred to as the water breaking).

Call your doctor if you have any of these signs.

He or she will probably tell you to go directly to the hospital where you are planning to give birth. Or he or she may tell you to wait before going to the hospital until your contractions are more regular and frequent. After you arrive at the hospital, the doctor will perform a vaginal examination to see if (and how much) your cervix has dilated (widened), check the fetus's position and heart rate, and evaluate your contractions.

Stages of Labor

Labor can be divided into three general stages. In the first stage, contractions of the muscles of the uterus open the cervix to allow the baby to pass into the vagina. In the second stage, the baby moves through and then out of the vagina (delivery), aided by contractions and some pushing by the mother. In the third stage, the placenta is expelled from the uterus.

First Stage: Dilation and Effacement

The first stage of labor begins with the first contractions, which help widen (dilate) the cervix. With each contraction, the cervix dilates and becomes thinner, or effaced. Effacement is given in percentages, with 100 percent effacement indicating that the cervix is ready for delivery. Dilation is measured in centimeters, with a diameter of 10 centimeters (about 4 inches) indicating full dilation. At full dilation, contractions are intense and occur 2 to 3 minutes apart. This is called the transition phase, and it is the most difficult, painful stage. By the end of this stage, the baby has begun to enter the vagina, and the mother may feel a strong urge to push.

The average duration of the first stage of labor is 12 hours for a first baby and 4 to 8 hours for a subsequent delivery. For some women who are having their first baby, the first stage can last longer than 24 hours. For women who have had several babies, this stage may last only a few minutes.

Second Stage: Delivery

During the second stage, contractions move the baby down the birth canal with the help of the mother's pushing, or bearing down. You will be told to push only when you are having a contraction, because the contractions double the effect of your pushing,

allowing you to rest between contractions, which helps you conserve energy. An episiotomy (see page 533) may be performed toward the end of the second stage of labor, before the baby's head emerges.

The second stage of labor ends when the baby is completely out of the vagina. Immediately after birth, the umbilical cord (which has connected the

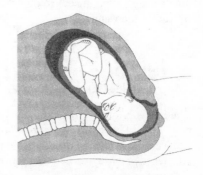

Contractions move the baby's head through the pelvis

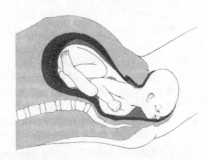

Baby's head emerges through the vaginal opening

Labor and delivery
During the first stage of labor, uterine contractions increase in strength and frequency and move the baby down into the birth canal (top). When the cervix is fully dilated, the contractions become stronger, pushing the baby farther down the birth canal and out of the vagina (bottom).

baby to the placenta) is tied and cut. The second stage can last up to 3 hours for a first baby and 2 hours for a subsequent delivery.

Third Stage: Expelling the Placenta

In the third stage of labor, after delivery of the baby, the placenta detaches from the uterine wall and is expelled from the uterus (afterbirth). Contractions (usually less painful than those of labor) help the uterus expel the placenta. Doctors often assist the delivery of the placenta by massaging the woman's abdomen and pulling gently on the umbilical cord during contractions.

The third stage can last from a few minutes to half an hour. After the placenta has been expelled, the mother may be given medication to prevent excessive bleeding. The doctor cleans and stitches any incisions from the episiotomy (see next page) or tears in the vagina.

Pain Relief During Labor and Delivery

The intensity of pain during labor varies significantly from woman to woman and is partly influenced by a woman's expectations. If you are frightened or tense, you may feel pain more acutely. If you attended childbirth classes with your labor coach, you will know what to expect and probably will be better prepared to deal with the pain. You can help ease contractions by staying upright and active as long as possible (without tiring yourself out); in addition, gravity helps the baby descend and speeds up dilation of the cervix. Breathe slowly and deeply during and after each contraction. Try a variety of positions to find the ones that are most comfortable.

You may not need pain relief during labor but, if you do, several options are available. Because some pain relievers can affect the baby's breathing if given late in labor, your doctor may give you pain medication only if the first stage of labor is very painful and if he or she is sure that delivery is not imminent. Medications for pain relief are carefully chosen so that if a baby is delivered soon after the medication is administered, the baby can be given another medication to reverse the effect of the pain medication.

Pudendal Block

Vaginal pain can be relieved by an anesthetic called a pudendal block, which is injected into the tissue of the vagina. A pudendal block is often used just before a forceps delivery (see page 534), or before an episiotomy (see next page), in which an incision is made in the perineum (the skin between the opening of the vagina and the anus) to allow the baby to pass through the vagina more easily.

Epidural and Spinal Anesthesia

If your pain is severe, the doctor may recommend epidural (see below) or spinal anesthesia for pain relief. For an epidural, the doctor or an anesthesiologist injects an anesthetic into the space surrounding the spinal cord at the base of the spine (epidural space). The anesthetic is infused through a thin, flexible tube (catheter) to provide small doses of the anesthetic as needed during labor and delivery. An epidural numbs the body from the waist down.

Spinal anesthesia is similar to an epidural except that it is given in one injection, and it paralyzes, not just numbs, the body from the waist down. Spinals are used mostly for cesarean deliveries (see page 534) because vaginal deliveries require the mother to be able to help push the baby through the birth canal.

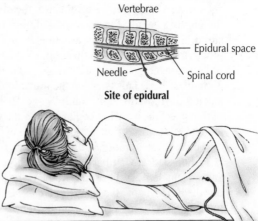

Site of epidural

Epidural anesthesia
Epidural anesthesia during pregnancy is given between contractions, with the pregnant woman lying on her side. The needle (which is attached to a catheter) is inserted between the vertebrae of the spine into the epidural space surrounding the spinal cord. An epidural causes numbness from the waist down, but the woman is fully conscious.

Complications from epidurals are rare. An epidural may prevent a woman from feeling when to push with contractions, possibly making labor longer. Sometimes an epidural relaxes the pregnant woman's blood vessels, causing her blood pressure to drop, which may slow the baby's heart rate. To prevent this potential problem, women are given intravenous fluids before and during administration of the epidural.

Techniques Used to Aid Delivery

Doctors can use a number of techniques and procedures to assist women during labor and delivery. These techniques can help ensure that childbirth is as comfortable as possible for the woman and safe for the baby. Doctors are able to continuously monitor the fetus's health throughout labor, if necessary, and ease delivery using instruments such as forceps.

Fetal Monitoring During Labor

Fetal monitoring is performed routinely during labor when there is some reason to evaluate the fetus's health more closely than usual. In external fetal monitoring, two belts are placed on the woman's abdomen, one to measure the fetus's heartbeat and the other to measure the length, frequency, and relative intensity of uterine contractions during labor. If complications such as bleeding occur

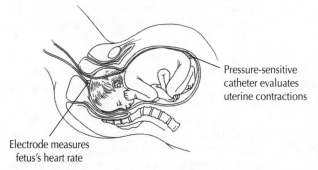

Pressure-sensitive catheter evaluates uterine contractions

Electrode measures fetus's heart rate

Internal monitoring of uterine contractions
If complications develop, internal monitoring is sometimes performed during labor to evaluate uterine contractions and the health of the fetus. In internal monitoring, an electrode is inserted through the vagina and attached to the fetus's scalp to measure the fetus's heart rate. Usually, a long thin tube (a pressure-sensitive catheter) is also inserted through the vagina into the uterus to measure the actual intensity, length, and frequency of the contractions.

during labor, a doctor may recommend internal fetal monitoring, which can be done only after the membranes of the amniotic sac have been broken.

To perform internal fetal monitoring, the doctor inserts an electrode through the woman's vagina into her uterus and attaches it to the fetus's scalp to measure fetal heart rate. A long, thin tube called a pressure catheter also may be inserted through the vagina into the uterus to measure the actual intensity, length, and frequency of the contractions. Internal monitoring usually continues until delivery to ensure that the fetus is not under stress. If the fetus is having difficulty, the doctor may recommend a cesarean (see next page).

Inducing Labor

Inducing labor is the act of starting labor mechanically or medically. Labor is usually induced when the risks of allowing the pregnancy to continue—such as retarded growth of the fetus (see page 529), extremely high blood pressure in the pregnant woman (see page 520), or a postterm pregnancy (see page 530)—are greater than the risks of inducing labor. Labor is seldom induced before the baby's lungs are sufficiently developed to survive outside the uterus. Before inducing labor, your doctor will evaluate the health of the baby and examine you internally to see if your cervix has begun to dilate.

One way to induce labor is to drain the amniotic fluid (the liquid that surrounds the fetus). To "break the bag of water," the doctor will make a small, painless incision in the membranes of the amniotic sac.

If draining the fluid does not trigger labor, you may receive an injection of the hormone oxytocin, which stimulates uterine contractions. However, 1 in 50 injections of oxytocin fails to stimulate labor.

If your due date has passed, your doctor may try to induce labor by separating the amniotic membranes from their attachments in the cervix and lower wall of the uterus (called stripping the membranes). There is no risk involved, but you may feel mild cramps or contractions after the procedure.

Episiotomy

An episiotomy is a surgical incision that is sometimes used during labor to enlarge the opening of the vagina, usually to avoid putting unnecessary pressure on the baby's head during delivery, especially during a forceps delivery. An episiotomy is also sometimes performed to avoid irregular tearing of the vagina, which can be more difficult to stitch up than a straight cut. Episiotomies are usually performed toward the end of the second stage of labor, before the baby's head emerges.

After injecting a local anesthetic, the doctor usually makes a small, straight cut in the perineum (the area of skin between the opening of the vagina and the anus) from the vagina to the anus; this is called a midline episiotomy. For a mediolateral episiotomy, the cut is made at an angle from the vagina to the left or right of the anus. After delivery, the incision is closed with stitches that gradually dissolve. The incision usually heals rapidly, although the scar may cause discomfort for up to 3 months.

To relieve discomfort in the area around the incision, your doctor will recommend periodically using an ice pack for a few minutes, sitting in a shallow tub of warm water, or sitting on a doughnut-shaped pillow. To help prevent infection, rinse the area with warm water and pat it dry each time you use the toilet.

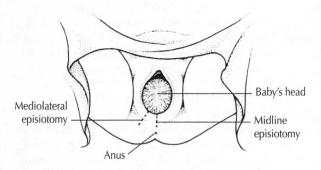

Episiotomy
In a midline episiotomy, the incision is made straight from the vagina toward the anus. In a mediolateral episiotomy, the incision is made to the side and at an angle to the anus. A midline incision is the most common type of episiotomy because it cuts through less tissue and usually causes less discomfort than a mediolateral episiotomy. A mediolateral episiotomy may be necessary if a baby is very large or if forceps are used for delivery.

Forceps

Obstetrical forceps are two wide, blunt, curved blades designed to fit around a baby's head to assist delivery. There are several different types of forceps used for different circumstances. For example, they may be used to protect the baby's head in a breech (buttocks first) presentation (see next page) or in a preterm delivery (see page 529). When epidural anesthesia (see page 532) has been used toward the end of labor, forceps are often used to assist delivery because a woman may not feel the urge to push. Forceps also are frequently used if the woman is unable to push or if the baby is showing signs of distress.

An episiotomy (see previous page) is usually performed before forceps are used, and the woman is usually given a local anesthetic or epidural anesthesia. The doctor inserts the forceps into the vagina along both sides of the baby's head and gently pulls the baby out as the woman pushes with her contractions. The risks of using forceps range from temporary marks on the baby's cheeks or ears to nerve damage or injury to the woman's vagina. Most nerve damage is temporary. A forceps delivery is usually less risky than a cesarean (see below) for both the woman and the baby.

Vacuum Extraction

Vacuum extraction is sometimes performed as an alternative to forceps delivery. The doctor places a suction cup (which is attached to a vacuum pump) on the baby's head in the birth canal. The pump is turned on to secure the baby's head to the cup, and the doctor gently pulls the baby out of the vagina with each contraction.

Vacuum extraction poses less risk of vaginal injury than a forceps delivery, although you may still have an episiotomy before delivery. The baby may have slight swelling of his or her scalp from the vacuum cup, but this will disappear in a few days.

Cesarean Delivery

Cesarean delivery (also called cesarean section or, for short, C-section) is a surgical procedure in which the baby is delivered through incisions in the wall of the uterus and in the lower abdomen. A cesarean delivery is usually done when it would be safer or easier than a vaginal delivery. Reasons for having a cesarean delivery include having a large baby or multiple babies, prolonged labor or failure of labor to progress, fetal distress, a breech presentation (see next page), or a medical condition the woman has.

If you have previously delivered a baby by cesarean, you and your doctor will weigh the benefits and risks of having another cesarean delivery. Many women who have delivered a baby by cesarean can later have a successful vaginal delivery. However, there is a risk of uterine rupture at the site of the cesarean incision.

The preparation for a cesarean delivery is similar to that for other surgical procedures. The incision area is washed and may be shaved, a catheter is inserted into the woman's bladder, and an intravenous line is inserted to allow her to receive medication and fluids if necessary. Most cesareans are performed using epidural or spinal anesthesia (see page 532). General anesthesia is usually used for cesarean deliveries only in emergency situations.

Your doctor will make either a low horizontal incision (called the bikini incision) that may be hidden by your pubic hair, or a vertical incision from below the navel to the top of the pubic hairline. The incision into the uterus itself may be either horizontal or vertical and is not always in the same direction as the skin incision. The doctor will remove the baby from the uterus and cut the umbilical cord before removing the placenta. Both incisions will be closed with dissolvable stitches; in some cases, the skin incision is closed with staples that will be removed later.

Most cesarean deliveries pose no problems, but possible complications include infection, excessive bleeding, blood clots, and injury to the woman's bladder. As with a vaginal delivery, a woman will probably be able to hold her baby very soon after delivery.

Possible Problems With Delivery

Labor and delivery usually progress with very little difficulty. However, sometimes unexpected problems develop. Hospitals are well equipped to handle these problems as they arise. Make sure your doctor and other health care professionals who are assisting you are aware of any unusual signs or symptoms you have.

Abnormal Presentation

A fetus usually rotates naturally into the normal, head-down position for birth. The part of the fetus that is positioned at the opening of the cervix immediately before birth is called the presenting

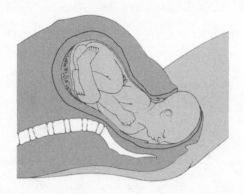

Normal presentation
In a normal presentation, the baby's head is down and facing the mother's back. This position allows for the easiest passage through the birth canal.

part. In most cases, the part that presents is the top of the baby's head, with the baby facing toward the mother's back. This position allows for the easiest passage through the birth canal. However, a fetus can be in another position (called abnormal presentation, or malpresentation), which may make delivery more difficult.

Breech presentation
In a breech presentation, the baby is positioned with the buttocks down, usually with the buttocks against the cervix. Breech presentation is common in cases of preterm labor (see page 529) because the fetus hasn't had time to assume the normal position for delivery, which usually occurs later in pregnancy. Babies in a breech presentation can often be delivered vaginally (usually with the aid of forceps), but a cesarean (see previous page) is frequently performed to avoid complications.

During the last few weeks of pregnancy, a doctor may be able to manipulate the fetus into the normal presentation using his or her hands on the woman's abdomen, usually guided by ultrasound. This manual manipulation, called external version, is done only when the baby is mature enough for delivery. If the baby is still in the breech position when labor begins and you have no other problems, your doctor may recommend allowing labor to continue while preparing for a cesarean delivery if labor becomes difficult.

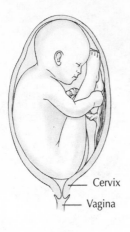

Cervix

Vagina

Frank breech

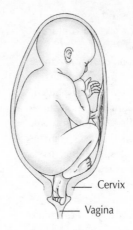

Cervix

Vagina

Footling breech

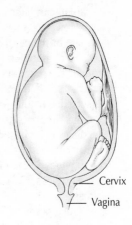

Cervix

Vagina

Complete breech

Breech presentation
In a breech presentation, the fetus passes through the birth canal with the head up and either the buttocks or feet against the cervix. A vaginal delivery is possible with a baby in the breech position, but a doctor may use forceps to aid the delivery or perform a cesarean delivery. In a frank breech (left), the baby's hips are bent and the legs extend upward, toward the head. In a footling breech (center), one or both of the baby's feet are over (or protrude into) the cervix. In a complete breech (right), both the baby's hips and knees are bent.

Prolonged Labor

Prolonged labor is defined as labor that lasts longer than 20 hours for a woman's first delivery and longer than 14 hours for a subsequent delivery. Labor can be prolonged if the muscles of the uterus do not produce sufficiently strong or regular contractions to dilate the cervix. Having epidural or spinal anesthesia (see page 532) can interfere with muscle contraction. In some cases, the fetus's head is too large to pass through the woman's pelvis, or the fetus is in an abnormal position that makes delivery difficult.

Your doctor may induce labor (see page 533) by giving you the hormone oxytocin intravenously (through a vein) to stimulate uterine contractions. Depending on the stage of labor and the position of the fetus, your doctor may perform a cesarean delivery (see page 534) or use forceps (see page 534) to assist delivery.

Disproportion

The term disproportion means that the woman's pelvis is too narrow for the passage of the baby's head. Disproportion can occur in women of any size or height but is more common in small-boned women and in women who are shorter than 5 feet. In some cases, a woman's pelvis is disproportionately small because of a previous injury. Disproportion can also occur if the baby's head is abnormally large, as with babies who have hydrocephalus (see page 400).

If your doctor suspects that your pelvis may be too small for the baby's head to pass through, he or she will perform an ultrasound of your pelvis. If the disproportion seems severe, the doctor will probably recommend a cesarean delivery (see page 534). If the disproportion is not too severe, he or she may decide to proceed with a vaginal delivery but closely monitor the baby's condition throughout labor.

Prolapse of the Umbilical Cord

A prolapsed umbilical cord occurs during (and in rare cases before) delivery when the umbilical cord drops down into the cervix or vagina. A compressed cord can cut off the fetus's blood and oxygen supplies, causing severe damage to or death of the fetus within minutes. A prolapsed cord can occur with conditions such as polyhydramnios (see page 526),

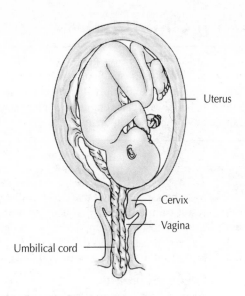

Prolapsed umbilical cord
A prolapsed umbilical cord is an umbilical cord that has moved into the vagina before the baby's head. A prolapsed cord can become compressed or squeezed and cut off the baby's supply of blood and oxygen. An emergency cesarean delivery is usually necessary.

breech presentation (see page 535), or premature rupture of the membranes (see page 528). Pressure on the umbilical cord must be relieved immediately, usually by cesarean delivery (see page 534).

Excessive Bleeding After Delivery

Postpartum hemorrhage is excessive loss of blood from the uterus or vagina after delivery. Bleeding often occurs when the uterine contractions are not strong enough to enable the uterus to shrink back to its original shape and compress the blood vessels in the uterus. (The contractions limit bleeding caused by the separation of the placenta from the uterus.) The muscles of the uterus may be weakened by an unusually long labor or stretched excessively by multiple fetuses or by multiple previous deliveries. Bleeding also can result when fragments of the placenta remain inside the uterus and prevent it from contracting sufficiently after childbirth. Excessive bleeding can also occur if the vagina was torn during delivery.

Bleeding from the uterus can be controlled with medications that stimulate the uterus to contract. If fragments of placenta remain inside the uterus, they will be removed. If the bleeding has resulted from torn vaginal tissues, the tear will be closed with stitches after the area has been numbed with a local anesthetic. Bleeding that is life-threatening may require surgical removal of the uterus (hysterectomy; see page 870).

Retained Placenta

The placenta usually separates easily from the wall of the uterus after delivery. The doctor may assist the separation of the placenta by pressing on the woman's abdomen (which helps the uterus contract) while at the same time pulling gently on the umbilical cord. Massaging the abdomen not only helps the uterus contract but also helps stop bleeding. Occasionally the placenta becomes trapped inside the uterus if it doesn't separate completely from the uterine wall. A retained placenta is a placenta that hasn't been expelled within 30 minutes of delivery.

A retained placenta is removed by the doctor. After giving you an anesthetic, the doctor will reach inside your uterus with his or her hand and remove the placenta. You will then be given medication to help your uterus contract and prevent excessive bleeding.

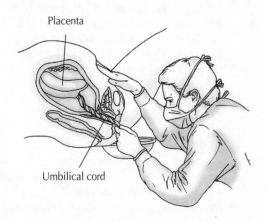

Delivering the placenta
The uterus continues to contract after delivery until the placenta (afterbirth) is delivered, completing the third and final stage of labor. To help expel the placenta, the doctor massages the woman's abdomen and, while the uterine contractions push the placenta out, the doctor gently pulls on the umbilical cord (which is attached to the placenta).

Adjusting After Pregnancy and Childbirth

Although the dramatic physical changes you experienced over the 9 months of your pregnancy occurred gradually and slowly, they reverse themselves relatively quickly after delivery. Your body will undergo other changes during this transition time as you get to know your newborn and take on the challenges and joys of parenting. Be flexible and enjoy this special time with your baby. Always call your doctor or pediatrician about any problems that arise.

Common Problems

After delivery, your body will be readjusting from the demands placed on it during pregnancy and childbirth. You will probably experience one or more of the following common problems or discomforts in the weeks after delivery.

Uterine Contractions

After the delivery and over a period of about 6 weeks, you will have mild contractions of your uterus that will help it return to its normal size. Breastfeeding helps to stimulate these contractions. If the contractions are painful, your doctor can prescribe a pain reliever.

Vaginal Discharge

For the first few days after delivery, most women have a vaginal discharge that consists of blood and some remaining tissue of the placenta. The discharge is heavy at first, but after 2 to 6 weeks it gradually tapers off and stops. You should not use tampons during this time because of the risk of infection. Avoid sexual intercourse for as long as your doctor recommends, usually for about 4 to 6 weeks after delivery.

Vaginal Soreness

If you had a vaginal delivery, your vaginal area will be sore and swollen because the skin around the vaginal opening (perineum) was stretched and may have torn or been surgically cut (episiotomy; see page 533) during delivery. Urination can be painful for a couple of days after delivery. Your doctor may recommend applying cold packs periodically for the first few hours after delivery to help relieve the pain. Many women find that using a doughnut-shaped pillow can make sitting more comfortable. You will be given instructions for cleaning your vaginal area to reduce the risk of infection.

Breast Conditions

Most breast conditions that develop after pregnancy result from breastfeeding, usually during the first weeks. Most of these problems are temporary, can be treated easily, and do not require you to stop breastfeeding, so don't be discouraged.

Engorged breasts

As your body begins to produce breast milk (about 2 to 4 days after delivery), your breasts will become engorged with milk and may be swollen and painful. If you are breastfeeding, the best solution for engorgement from the buildup of milk is to feed your baby frequently. However, if your nipples are swollen and difficult for the baby to latch on to, you may need to express some milk with a breast pump before putting the baby to your breast. Hot showers can also help soften the breasts. A good support bra can help relieve some of the discomfort, which usually subsides within a few days.

If you are not breastfeeding, try applying ice packs to your breasts to relieve the pain. Don't pump your breasts to relieve the engorgement—doing so will produce more milk and cause more engorgement. After about 3 days without stimulation from a nursing infant, your breasts will stop producing milk. If the pain is severe, ask your doctor about taking a pain reliever.

Cracked nipples

When you are breastfeeding, your nipples can become dry and cracked, which you can feel as a sharp pain in a nipple while your baby is nursing. Prevent dry, cracked nipples by using only warm water (no soap) to wash your nipples and by drying your nipples thoroughly after each feeding. Also, make sure the baby has the whole nipple and areola (the surrounding pigmented area) in his or her mouth, not just the nipple (because it puts too much pressure on the nipple). Your doctor may recommend a soothing cream to apply to a sore nipple between feedings. The crack should heal in a few days; feed your baby from the other breast more frequently until the sore nipple heals.

Mastitis

Mastitis is infection of the milk ducts, which is a common problem in women who breastfeed. The infection usually occurs when bacteria from the nursing child's mouth enter the milk duct. Symptoms include soreness, hardness, redness, and swelling of the breast, and sometimes chills and a fever. See your doctor if you have any of these symptoms; he or she will prescribe an antibiotic if you have an infection. Continue to breastfeed during treatment, because this can help relieve the pain and clear up the infection. Have the baby start feeding on the unaffected breast first because he or she sucks hardest at the beginning, when hungriest. If the baby doesn't empty the breast completely, pump it after each feeding until it is empty.

Blocked milk duct and abscess

If you feel a small, hard lump in your breast, you may have a blocked milk duct. Try massaging your breast and taking hot showers. If the lump does not disappear in a day or two, see your doctor right away; you could have a breast abscess (see page 855). The doctor will examine your breast and may give you antibiotics to treat the infection. If the abscess is not treated quickly enough, you may need to have it drained with a needle or small incision, which is done in the doctor's office using a local anesthetic. You can continue to breastfeed from the affected breast during treatment.

Thrush

Some women who are breastfeeding develop a yeast infection called thrush, which the nursing baby also has (it appears on the baby's tongue as white patches). The infection can make the nipples sore and cracked. Your doctor will prescribe an antifungal cream to apply to your nipples several times a day and oral drops for the baby. If the infection spreads through the baby's digestive tract, it can cause a form of diaper rash, which can be treated with an antifungal cream. Treatment can take several weeks, but you can continue to breastfeed during treatment.

Feeding Your Baby

During your pregnancy, you probably decided whether you wanted to breastfeed or bottle-feed your baby. Both methods have advantages and disadvantages. Your choice will be based mostly on your personal preferences and your lifestyle. Feeding your baby, whether by breast or bottle, is an important time for you to form a strong emotional attachment to your baby, which is just as essential to your baby's growth and development as nutrition.

Breastfeeding

For various reasons, not all women want to (or can) breastfeed. However, breastfeeding has many benefits for both mother and child. Doctors recommend breastfeeding as the most beneficial nutrition for babies in their first year of life. Breast milk provides the perfect mix of nutrients that

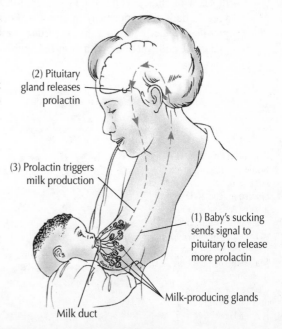

Breastfeeding
The hormone prolactin, which stimulates milk production, is produced by the pituitary gland in the brain. After childbirth, the pituitary gland releases prolactin into the mother's bloodstream, where it stimulates milk production. When a baby sucks on the breast, the stimulation from the sucking sends a signal to the pituitary gland to release more prolactin to trigger milk production. Milk flows from the milk-producing glands at the back of the breast into tiny sacs called milk ducts under the woman's areola (the darker area surrounding the nipple). The pressure of the baby's mouth on the areola squeezes milk from the milk ducts out through the nipple. Feeding a baby alternately from both breasts helps ensure that both breasts receive equal stimulation to produce an equal amount of milk.

(2) Pituitary gland releases prolactin

(3) Prolactin triggers milk production

(1) Baby's sucking sends signal to pituitary to release more prolactin

Milk-producing glands

Milk duct

infants need to develop properly, and it causes fewer food allergies and fewer digestive problems (such as constipation) than formula. Breast milk also provides a newborn with infection-fighting antibodies from the mother's body and reduces the incidence of ear, respiratory, and digestive tract infections during the first few years of life. Breast-feeding is convenient because breast milk is always available and requires no preparation, and you can feed your baby whenever he or she is hungry. Breastfed babies do not gain weight as quickly as bottle-fed babies, and breastfed babies seldom become overweight.

For the mother, breastfeeding helps the uterus get back to its normal size more quickly. Also, because you are burning calories when you breast-feed, you will lose weight faster. Breastfeeding longer than 3 months confers some protection to women against developing breast cancer later in life.

If you have any problems in the first few days of breastfeeding, don't be discouraged. Talk to your doctor and to friends who have breastfed and ask for tips. Call or attend group meetings of the local La Leche League, a volunteer group that offers practical advice and encouragement to women who are breastfeeding.

Bottle-Feeding

Many women choose to bottle-feed their babies. If this is your choice, you should not feel guilty that you are depriving your baby in any way. Formula provides the nutrients your infant needs to develop and grow, and you bond with your baby when you

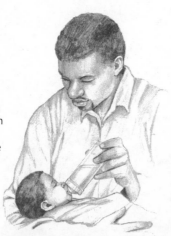

Bottle-feeding
Bottle-feeding can give other people, particularly fathers, a chance to feed and bond with a baby. A baby who fusses soon after sucking on a bottle may be having trouble with the nipple or formula. Make sure that the hole in the nipple is not clogged or too small and that the formula is not too hot.

hold him or her for feedings. Make sure that you prepare the formula according to the package instructions. Some people prefer the convenience of bottle-feeding because other people can help out with feedings. It also gives the father and older siblings an opportunity to participate in feedings and form their own attachment to the baby.

Postpartum Depression

Many women feel blue during the first few days after childbirth. This is normal. New mothers usually are very tired. First-time mothers may be afraid, anxious, or overwhelmed by their new responsibilities and challenges. Some women may have a sense of letdown after anticipating the birth for so many months. These blues usually go away in a few days or weeks.

However, some women continue to feel depressed to such an extent that they cannot function. This condition, called postpartum depression, is serious. Postpartum depression may result from a combination of factors such as a genetic susceptibility, the sudden change in hormone levels, and chronic lack of sleep.

Tips for Preventing New-Mother Blues

One of the most important (and difficult) things you can do after your baby is born is to avoid becoming overtired. You need all the sleep you can get because lack of sleep can influence your hormone levels, which can interfere with your ability to function. Keeping your baby in the same bedroom with you at night is usually not a good idea because you can be awakened not only when the baby is hungry but also when the baby moves even slightly in his or her sleep or makes noises.

Make a shift schedule with your partner, so that you are not the only one taking care of the baby every time he or she needs attention. Even if you are breastfeeding, your partner can get up at night and change a diaper or attend to the baby in other ways when necessary. In addition, don't hesitate to accept offers from family or friends to help out by shopping for you or taking care of the baby while you get some rest during the day.

You may have postpartum depression if you have any of the following symptoms:

- Feelings of anxiety or hopelessness that last longer than 2 weeks
- Panic attacks
- Inability to sleep even when you're tired
- Sleeping too much, even when the baby is awake
- Having little interest in your baby or other family members
- Thoughts of harming yourself or the baby

If you have any of these symptoms, talk to your doctor right away. He or she may prescribe an antidepressant medication or refer you to a mental health professional who has experience treating women with postpartum depression. He or she may also recommend a support group of women and families who have experienced what you are going through. In rare, severe cases, a woman may need to be admitted to a hospital for treatment.

Sex After Childbirth

Your doctor will tell you when you can safely resume having sexual intercourse after delivery. Most doctors recommend waiting about 4 to 6 weeks, until after the postnatal checkup. Because you can become pregnant again after childbirth, talk to your doctor about birth control. Your periods will resume about 6 to 8 weeks after delivery; if you are breastfeeding, they will resume when you start giving your baby solid foods or supplemental bottles or when you start weaning your baby from breast milk.

You should not consider breastfeeding a reliable form of contraception. Your doctor will probably recommend using a barrier method of birth control (such as a diaphragm) instead of birth-control pills during the first 6 weeks after delivery because the hormones can interfere with your milk production. If you want to become pregnant again soon, talk to your doctor about any potential risks.

Your vagina may be extremely tender for the first 10 days or so after childbirth, or for a couple of weeks if you had an episiotomy (see page 533) or if the skin around your vagina was torn during labor. If intercourse is painful, see your doctor.

Your vagina may have lost some elasticity. To strengthen the muscles around the vagina, perform pelvic-floor strengthening exercises (see page 874)—squeezing the muscles periodically to a count of 10, as though you are interrupting and resuming the flow of urine in midstream.

Taking care of a new baby can be exhausting both physically and emotionally and can leave you no energy for sex. Try the tips on the previous page for avoiding new-mother blues. Especially with a first baby, your partner may feel left out and may seek reassurances of your affection. Your partner may also feel anxious about the new responsibilities and challenges of being a parent. Talk to your partner openly and honestly about your feelings, and encourage your partner to bond with your baby and participate in all parenting tasks.

6

Dying and Death

Most people hope for a long, healthy life, and increasing numbers of Americans are living longer and healthier. At the turn of the 20th century, life expectancy in the United States was only 46. Today, life expectancy is approaching 80, an astounding 75 percent increase in one century, greater than at any other time in history.

Still, death is inevitable, and for many of us, it is a process that occurs slowly over a period of weeks or months. Unlike a sudden, unexpected death, a slow death can give a dying person and his or her family and friends the opportunity to come to terms with death (and to prepare for it).

The 10 Leading Causes of Death in the United States

Following are the 10 leading causes of death in the United States in 2000. The information comes from the Centers for Disease Control and Prevention (CDC).

1. Heart disease
2. Cancer
3. Stroke
4. Chronic lower respiratory disease
5. Accidents
6. Diabetes
7. Pneumonia and influenza
8. Alzheimer's disease
9. Kidney disease
10. Blood poisoning

Terminal Illness

A terminally ill person should decide the timing and extent of any discussion about death, including organ donation or funeral arrangements. If a terminally ill person asks questions about dying, he or she may have, to some extent, already come to terms with it. Once the person has brought up the subject of death, it can be easier to talk about specific aspects of his or her death. Some terminally ill people want to know the facts about their condition, while others prefer to know as little as possible. Try to gauge how much the dying person wants to know.

The person's doctor, family, and friends need to be compassionate when talking about death because it is essential to maintain a degree of hope. This does not mean, however, that you should encourage false hopes of recovery, which could cause the person to lose confidence in his or her doctors or miss the opportunity to say good-bye to loved ones or put his or her affairs in order.

Sometimes a person who is terminally ill or his or her family members or friends may find it easier to talk about death with someone who is not emotionally involved in the situation. In such cases, it can be helpful to seek counseling from a mental health professional such as a psychiatrist or from a member of the clergy.

Organ Donation

The need for donated organs far surpasses the supply, and the waiting lists are long. But only a fraction of people who could donate organs actually do. The decision to donate vital organs after death for transplantation is a difficult one. Organ donation, however, ensures that the donor will make a lasting and meaningful gift that can help a critically ill person live a longer, healthier life.

Agreeing to the surgical removal of one or more organs or parts of organs after death can be done by the dying person or his or her family members. Most organs are removed immediately after death. The heart, lungs, liver, pancreas, kidneys, eyes, and skin are some of the organs that can be successfully transplanted after death. A person may also want to donate his or her whole body for medical education or research.

If you decide to donate your organs or body after death, you must sign a donor card, which you can obtain from a local hospital, health department, library, driver's license facility, or an organization such as the Red Cross. Ask a family member to also sign the donor card. You should make your intentions about organ donation clear to your relatives and doctor because a signed donor card alone is not enough to guarantee that your wishes will be carried out. All states require the permission of a close family member after death (even if the deceased person has a signed donor card).

The acceptability of a body or organ can be determined only at the time of death. Older people may be able to donate only parts of their body (such as their eyes), but medical schools accept bodies of any age for research. To be a donor, the person has to be of sound mind and 18 years old or older, although, with parental consent, a person under 18 can be a donor. Donations are considered gifts; it is illegal to pay for a donated body or body part. However, transporting the body after death is the financial responsibility of the family or estate, whether the body is transported to a hospital or medical school for donation or to a funeral parlor.

Organ donation is performed with respect for the donor's body, using standard surgical practices. It does not violate the beliefs of most religions, or affect funeral practices, including the option of an open casket. And in the case of whole-body donation, not having the body at a memorial service can change the emphasis of the ceremony to the person's life (rather than his or her death).

Advance Directives

At some point, a person may become unable to make decisions about his or her medical treatment. Advance directives, legal documents that provide guidance and instructions to the person's family, friends, or doctors or other health care providers, can help ensure that any health care decisions that are made on the person's behalf are consistent with his or her wishes. Advance directives may be general statements about a person's attitudes toward extraordinary lifesaving measures and end-of-life medical treatment. They may also be specific directives such as a do-not-resuscitate order or detailed instructions about specific types of medical treatment a person does or does not want to receive. Living wills and durable powers of attorney for health care are the most common types of advance directives.

Ideally, advance directives should be prepared and signed before the need for them arises. The person seeking an advance directive should talk with his or her doctor, family, friends, and clergy, to help sort out his or her feelings about life-sustaining medical treatments and to make his or her wishes known. The person can continue to make his or her own decisions about medical treatment as long as he or she is competent. Advance directives can be withdrawn by the person at any time.

Legal forms for advance directives are usually available through hospital social services departments or from local or state medical societies or bar associations. A lawyer can create a living will and durable power of attorney for health care that will suit the person's needs. Although not necessary, it is a good idea to consult an attorney when preparing or filling out forms for a living will or durable power of attorney for health care because laws and requirements regarding advance directives vary from state to state.

A person should tell his or her doctor and close

family members or friends about the advance directives. The person's doctor and appointed health care agent (also referred to as proxy, attorney-in-fact, or representative) should receive copies of the directives. If health care institutions are involved, they should also receive copies of the advance directives so they are aware of the person's wishes regarding medical treatment. In addition, the person should keep copies where they can be found easily. The person or his or her health care agent should review these documents regularly and keep them up-to-date.

Living Will

A living will is a legal document that contains written instructions about a person's wishes regarding medical treatment when he or she is terminally ill or unable to make decisions. A living will may be written in general or specific terms. For example, it may state simply that the person does not want any extraordinary measures taken to prolong his or her life when he or she is terminally ill, or it may list the specific types of medical treatments he or she does or does not want to receive. These treatments can include measures such as cardiopulmonary resuscitation (CPR), dialysis, surgery, artificial breathing with the assistance of a ventilator, blood transfusions, artificial feeding through tubes, and chemotherapy for cancer.

A living will is prepared when a person is still able to make decisions about medical care. However, it is activated only when the person can no longer make decisions or communicate his or her preferences about treatment. A living will may be changed or withdrawn (revoked) by the person whenever he or she chooses. The requirements for and legal authority of living wills vary from state to state; a living will that is legally binding in one state may not be binding in another. Therefore it is a good idea to consult a lawyer when preparing a living will.

Do-not-resuscitate order

A do-not-resuscitate (DNR) order is a doctor's order stating that CPR should not be initiated if a person's heart stops beating. A DNR order can be included in a living will. Without a written DNR order signed by a doctor, all medical personnel are required to begin CPR and take other lifesaving measures (such as attaching the person to a ventilator, which takes over breathing) if the person's heart stops beating.

If a person is no longer competent, a family member (or health care agent) can request a DNR order. A DNR order can be prepared and issued by a doctor after discussions with the person who is ill and his or her family members or health care agent. In a hospital setting, only the person's doctor signs the DNR order. A DNR order can be withdrawn at any time by the doctor. Copies of the doctor's written DNR order should be kept in the person's medical record at a hospital, nursing facility, or home health care agency.

Durable Power of Attorney for Health Care

A durable power of attorney for health care is a legal document in which a competent person gives another person (called a health care agent) the authority to make medical decisions on his or her behalf. The agent may be a relative, friend, lawyer, or guardian. A durable power of attorney for health care may also name a second and third alternate agent. The health care agent has the right to make all decisions about the person's health care, to access medical records, to consent to or refuse any treatment, and to withdraw life-sustaining treatment. The health care agent also has the authority to donate the person's organs or tissues (see previous page). A health care agent is required to exercise good judgment in accordance with the person's wishes.

The person can withdraw the durable power of attorney for health care at any time. A durable power of attorney for health care goes into effect only after the person is no longer competent to make his or her own medical decisions.

A durable power of attorney for health care is different from a durable power of attorney. A durable power of attorney is a legal document in which a competent person gives an agent the authority to make legal or financial (rather than medical) decisions on his or her behalf.

Palliative Care

It is rarely true that nothing can be done for a terminally ill person when curative treatment is no longer appropriate. Along with understanding and comfort, a dying person needs relief from symptoms, especially pain. This type of care is called palliative care. Some hospitals have palliative care programs or trained staff members who can help keep a terminally ill person comfortable and try to fulfill the wishes and needs of the person and his or her family. Palliative care can take place in the terminally ill person's own home or in a homelike setting (called hospice) within or affiliated with a hospital.

Hospice Programs

Hospice programs are palliative care programs that relieve the symptoms of a dying person, allowing him or her to die as comfortably as possible, surrounded by family and friends, in a secure, homelike environment. A doctor's authorization is required to place a person in a hospice program. In most cases, a person is eligible for hospice when a doctor has determined that he or she is not expected to live longer than 6 months.

Various types of hospice programs offer different types of care—from basic emotional support to complex medical services. Most hospice programs are Medicare-certified and are licensed and regulated by the state in which they operate. Regardless of the level of care provided, trained professionals work closely with the dying person and his or her loved ones and are available to assist the family 24 hours a day. Some hospice programs may also provide grief counseling for family members after the person has died.

Medicare covers the full cost of Medicare-certified hospice care. Medicaid programs in many states, most private health insurance plans, and some health maintenance organizations and other managed care plans also cover the cost of hospice care. The dying person or his or her family may pay out-of-pocket expenses for hospice care if the person is not eligible for Medicare or Medicaid hospice benefits or if his or her health insurance plan does not cover the cost. Because most hospice programs provide care based on need rather than on a person's ability to pay, cost is determined on a sliding scale. In some cases, hospice care may be available at no cost to people who have limited resources. Find out about a particular hospice program's payment policies in advance.

Caring for a Terminally Ill Person at Home

In many cases, palliative care is best provided at home (rather than in a nursing facility or hospital).

This is especially true if the caregiving is not excessively demanding or complicated. For people who may require complex care, the family may still want to care for the person at home during the last few weeks of his or her life. In general, hospitals are better equipped to treat people who are acutely ill than people who are terminally ill. At home, a terminally ill person can remain more independent, participate in family life, and avoid feelings of loneliness and isolation.

If a family member plans to care for a terminally ill relative at home, regular visits from the doctor, along with support from other family members and friends, are essential. The family should consider using the services of visiting nurses if they are available in their community. Many hospitals offer palliative services that provide support for people who are caring for a terminally ill person at home.

Controlling Pain

Pain is the most feared symptom associated with terminal illness. Continuous pain over a long period can wear a person down emotionally and physically and undermine his or her ability to cope. Pain control, which is the responsibility of a person's doctor and caregivers, enhances the quality of the person's life during the terminal phase of an illness.

Although some families express concern that a terminally ill person will become addicted to pain medication, drug addiction is not a realistic concern in the last few weeks of a person's life. Cutting back on pain medication can result in inadequate pain relief and needless suffering. Keeping a terminally ill person as pain-free as possible should be the major goal.

Doctors often prescribe long-acting morphine to control the pain of a terminal illness such as cancer. If pain recurs between doses, the doctor may also prescribe a shorter-acting form of the drug or another pain reliever to use between doses of the longer-acting medication. If pain medication is prescribed on an as-needed basis, the medication should be given as soon as the person becomes uncomfortable. It is important to give pain medication on a regular basis to ensure continuous pain relief. Once pain begins to worsen, it is more difficult to control. To keep pain under control, medication is usually given around the clock, not just when a person asks for it. If the person is taking pain medication and is still in pain, talk to the doctor or the visiting nurse about adjusting the dosage.

Other pain-relief methods (including relaxation techniques such as deep breathing, meditation, guided imagery, and massage) can be used along with medication to help control pain and improve a dying person's sense of well-being. In general, the earlier a person begins to use relaxation techniques and massage for pain relief, the more effective these methods are likely to be.

The Process of Dying

The term dying refers to the process in which the body's systems shut down and prepare for death. It is difficult to estimate how long the dying process will take. The actual moment of death is often very peaceful.

Nutrition and Elimination

One sign of dying is decreased food consumption and increased weight loss. If the person can (and wants to) eat, give him or her soft foods that won't cause choking. The person may not be hungry or thirsty and may gradually withdraw from food or may refuse to eat or drink. Moisten his or her mouth by giving ice chips to suck on or by wetting his or her mouth with a wet cloth. Don't force the person to eat or drink. Swallowing may be difficult. Urine output will start to decrease because the person is not drinking enough fluid, and he or she will have few bowel movements because of decreased food intake and movement. Keep the dying person clean and dry by using incontinence pads or disposable briefs and changing them when they are soiled.

Circulation

Circulation will slow, and the person's pulse will grow weaker. The underside of the body may become darker in color as blood begins to pool. The person's arms and legs may be cold and look bluish purple. If the dying person feels chilled, keep him or her covered with blankets. (Don't use electric blankets because of the possibility of causing burns.) Keep the room comfortable and not too warm.

Agitation

A person who is dying may become agitated, especially just before death. The agitation may be a sign not of pain but of discomfort. The person may become more and more restless. He or she may pull at the sheets, have trouble sleeping, continuously fidget, and even groan. Although reassuring the person can be helpful, the agitation is often a physical response that cannot be relieved by reassurance alone. In this case, the doctor may prescribe a medication such as alprazolam or lorazepam to help calm the person.

Anxiety and Depression

Depression is a normal emotional response to dying. Depression may be relieved somewhat by antidepressants and counseling. If a dying person is anxious, the anxiety may be the result of unresolved personal or religious issues. If the person cannot be comforted by a friend or relative, ask a member of the clergy or another person to whom the dying person looks for comfort to try to provide guidance and reassurance.

Breathing

A dying person may breathe rapidly (sometimes more than 30 breaths per minute). At times the periods of rapid breathing may be mixed with periods of no breathing that may last up to 15 seconds. Breathing may also become shallower. An increase in the amount and thickness of secretions in the back of the throat (caused by decreased fluid intake and decreased ability to cough up saliva) can produce a rattlelike sound while breathing. If breathing becomes difficult, elevate the person's head by putting pillows under it or by raising the head of the bed. Repositioning the dying person on his or her side may also help relieve a breathing problem.

Responsiveness

The person may begin to spend more and more time sleeping and may become difficult to arouse. He or she may stop communicating with people. If your loved one is no longer able to speak, communicate through the sense of touch. Holding your loved one or stroking his or her head or hand can convey your love and help you reassure him or her. During the time a person is dying, caregivers, family members, and friends should sit close to the person and talk softly. Visitors should be cautioned not to talk about the person because he or she can hear, and probably understand, what they are saying (even if he or she is unresponsive).

At the Time of Death

Hospital or hospice personnel will help you as the death occurs. If the death is taking place at home and you think death is very near, call the doctor for assistance and support. If the person dies before the hospice team arrives, do not call 911 (which sends emergency personnel to save lives). If the person was planning to donate organs for transplantation, or if the family wants to donate any organs, the organs are removed before life-support systems are disconnected, immediately after a doctor certifies that the person is brain-dead.

You will know that death has occurred by the following signs:

- Breathing and heartbeat stop.
- Bowel and bladder control stop (resulting in soiling of the bed linens).
- The person is completely unresponsive.
- Jaw relaxes; mouth may open slightly.
- The eyelids are slightly open and the eyes are fixed on a certain spot.

A hospice team or the person's doctor can instruct you on what to do after the person dies. The doctor may ask you to arrange to have the person brought to the hospital to be pronounced dead; most funeral directors will take the body to a hospital if directed to do so by a doctor. If the body is to be donated for research, contact the appropriate medical school or organization as soon as possible.

Brain Death

Brain death is the irreversible cessation of all functions of the brain. The recognition of brain death has allowed doctors to certify death based on the absence of brain function in situations in which the lungs and heart continue to function with artificial assistance. If a person has severe brain damage, doctors can maintain a person's heartbeat, breathing, blood pressure, and other vital functions in the hope that, with time, the person's brain will recover. In some circumstances, the person may be breathing on his or her own, but the brain is damaged so extensively that it will never recover its function and the person will remain in a permanent state of unconsciousness (coma).

Practicalities of Death

Practical matters to deal with after a person dies include contacting a funeral director to make funeral and burial arrangements and to transport the body. Although a body does not legally have to be embalmed or sealed in a particular type of casket or vault, some cemeteries have specific requirements. The funeral director can provide this information.

You will need to make additional arrangements if the body or parts of the body are to be donated for research or transplantation (see page 658) or if the body is to be cremated. After cremation, the crematorium will offer you the ashes to keep, bury, or scatter; or you can ask the crematorium to scatter the ashes for you.

Legal matters that need to be taken care of after a death has occurred include pronouncing the person dead and certifying the cause of death. In some cases, a doctor may be required to report a death to the police for investigation by the medical examiner or coroner.

Death Certificate

A death certificate is a medical document that states the cause and time of a person's death. Although in some circumstances a justice of the peace, a nurse, or a physician's assistant can pronounce a person dead and record the time of death, only a licensed doctor can certify a death and sign a death certificate.

If the person's doctor is present at the time of death, he or she may examine the body before filling out a death certificate. If the doctor is not present at the time of death but has seen the person within an amount of time specified by state law, he or she does not have to examine the body before signing a death certificate. However, the doctor is required to examine the body if it is to be cremated. After a doctor has completed a death certificate, the certificate is given to the funeral director, who contacts authorities to register the death.

Autopsy

An autopsy (also called a postmortem examination) is a detailed examination of a body after death that may be performed for a variety of reasons. For example, if no doctor cared for the person during his or her final illness, if the cause of death is not known, or if a death may have been caused by violence, an autopsy is usually required. Depending on where you live, either a medical examiner or a coroner is authorized to investigate unexplained or violent deaths.

Autopsies are usually performed before a body is embalmed, and a body cannot be cremated until a cause of death has been determined. A death certificate is issued only after a cause of death has been determined.

If an autopsy does not reveal a cause of death or if the death was violent, unnatural, or resulted from an injury, there may be an inquest (public court hearing). After the inquest, the medical examiner or coroner issues a death certificate and releases the body to the funeral director.

Medical/legal autopsy

A medical/legal autopsy is ordered by legal authorities to establish a cause of death and to determine if a death was the result of a crime. Medical/legal autopsies are also sometimes performed to investigate possible industrial hazards or contagious diseases that may endanger public health or to establish a cause of death for insurance purposes.

A medical/legal autopsy can range from a simple examination of the appearance of a body and the situation in which it was found to a study of the entire body and all its parts (including the structure of individual cells), depending on what is being investigated. A pathologist (a doctor who performs autopsies and studies tissues and organs) makes detailed notes and keeps a record of everything that is done during an autopsy in case the information is needed as evidence.

Medical/educational autopsy

A medical/educational autopsy may be requested by a hospital staff member or by the person's family and is usually performed in the hospital where the person died. The family's permission is required. In most cases, a medical/educational autopsy is performed to determine the exact cause of death or to provide the family with information about any contagious diseases or inherited medical conditions. Sometimes information about genetic diseases (see page 953) can be obtained from an autopsy. Medical/educational autopsies are sometimes performed so doctors can learn more about a particular disease or condition.

In some cases, medical/educational autopsies are performed to check the accuracy of a diagnosis or the appropriateness of medical treatment. If a person died unexpectedly or if his or her symptoms were puzzling, a doctor or the person's family may request an autopsy to look for a possible cause of death.

If you are asked to give permission to perform a medical/educational autopsy, you can agree to a limited autopsy (that is, you can specify that only particular parts of the body can be studied).

The Mourning Process

Immediately after the death of a loved one, many people feel numb. Some may, for a time, go on with their life as if nothing has happened, until they are eventually overcome by intense grief. Grief is an essential process that cannot be rushed.

During the period immediately following a death, delusions of seeing the person are common. There is a tendency to forget that the person is dead and even act as if he or she were still alive. It is also common to idealize the dead person and feel guilty for not doing more for the person when he or she was alive. Guilt and intense grief occur frequently when a person has died unexpectedly. When death occurs after a long illness, the bereaved person has usually been able to anticipate the loss and may have been able to provide care, which can lessen feelings of guilt and grief. Also, it is normal for close friends or family members to feel relief once the death has occurred, especially if the death was a long, difficult, or painful one. This sense of relief is normal, and they should not feel guilty about it.

The intensity of grief lessens over time, although the amount of time varies from person to person and depends on the closeness of the relationship. Usually after about 6 weeks, grief will slowly be replaced by a more general lack of feeling or depression that will become much less intense after a year or so. By then, most bereaved people have recovered from their loss and have returned, more or less, to their previous life. However, feelings of grief may reappear at unpredictable times in the years that follow.

Coping With Grief

Some people think that no one ever really gets over a death but that we just learn to adapt to the loss. If someone close to you has died, try to acknowledge the loss. Don't try to forget about the death or put it out of your mind. Talk about the dead person to relatives and friends. Express your feelings openly; cry if it helps.

To help yourself recover from the loss of someone close to you, try to meet new people and continue to engage in your favorite activities. Stay involved with groups or organizations that have been sources of support. Reading books about the grieving process may help you cope. For many people, sorting out the person's possessions can help them come to terms with the death. For others, the task is very painful and they delay it for as long as possible.

Give yourself time to accept your loss, acknowledge your feelings of grief, and then begin to rebuild your life through positive interests and new relationships. You will begin to think less about your loss and focus more on happy memories of your loved one.

Physical Symptoms of Grief

People tend to forget that there is a physical side to grief as well as an emotional one. Some physical manifestations of grief can include insomnia or sleeping excessively, upset stomach or lost appetite, headache, fatigue, and muscle aches.

Losing sleep and not exercising or eating properly can jeopardize your health. Try to get sufficient sleep and eat regular, nutritious meals. Don't use medication for depression or sleep loss unless it has been prescribed by your doctor, and never use drugs or alcohol to cope with the stress of losing a loved one. Exercise not only benefits your physical health but also helps relieve depression by releasing hormones called endorphins, which have a pain-relieving and soothing effect on the body.

Coping With the Death of a Child

The death of a child can cause more anger and grief than the death of an adult. We experience extreme distress, partly because we may feel that the child has not experienced enough of life. If the child died suddenly, it is often even more difficult to bear than if the death occurred after a long illness. Professional counseling is almost always necessary for parents, siblings, and other close relatives such as grandparents. Support groups or group therapy with other parents and children who have had similar experiences can be a great comfort.

The Dying Child

A child may be able to face the prospect of his or her own death better than his or her parents can. A child may fear pain and, if admission to the hospital is necessary, separation from his or her parents more than he or she fears death. It will usually help a child come to terms with death if he or she is told about the illness. Death should not be treated as a forbidden subject. The most important thing that parents can give their child is security—physical security by their presence, and emotional security by their loving support.

It is important for a terminally ill child to lead as normal a life as possible for as long as possible. Avoid treating the child in a way that will make him or her feel different from his or her siblings or friends. Discipline the child as you normally would. The child should go to school, do homework, see friends, and participate in normal family activities for as long as possible.

Whenever possible, it is comforting for a terminally ill child to be cared for at home rather than in a hospital, although it is necessary for parents who take on home care to be sure they can reach their child's doctor at all times. However, the child should be admitted to a hospital if the parents can no longer cope with the situation at home or if the child needs more complex or specialized medical care.

When a Child Loses a Loved One

Until about age 3, children have no concept of death. By age 9, most children are at least partially able to understand that death is the end of life and is inevitable. Children experience the same feelings about death as adults. However, children should be allowed to grieve in their own way and not be forced to conform to adult ideas about grieving.

Young children often appear to recover from bereavement very quickly, especially if they become attached to a substitute for the person who has died. However, they may be unable to articulate their emotions and may suppress grief because they don't want to cause any more pain for their grieving parents or other relatives. Some children find relief for their emotions through play, as adults might throw themselves into their work.

Do not suppress your own grief in front of a child in a false attempt to shield the child. It is better to give the child a role model for grieving and for how to cope with trauma. Children often sense unexpressed feelings, which can make them feel even more uneasy. Give the child opportunities to ask questions about death and to express his or her grief. Some children may feel that a death is somehow their fault, and need reassurance that this is not the case.

Some mental health specialists think that not allowing children to attend funerals prevents them from actively participating in the grieving process. Funerals provide a place for children to see how people comfort each other, mourn a loved one, honor a life, and show respect for the deceased. They also give the child an opportunity to say good-bye. In addition, children who have not been allowed to see the body or attend a funeral sometimes imagine far worse things than the reality.

Even if a child appears to show few signs of grief after the death of a close relative, it is best to try to avoid any major changes in the child's life for about 6 months, if possible. Too much change may be more than the child can handle. Stability and a feeling of security are important to a child who has lost a loved one.

Helping a Person Who Is Grieving

A person who is grieving will need practical help at first (such as help with children, meal preparation, cleaning, and running errands) to continue with his or her daily life. Apart from helping with practical matters, it may seem that there is little real comfort you can offer a person who has lost a spouse or other close family member, or a friend. However, this is not true. Be a good listener. By allowing the person to talk about his or her loss, you provide an outlet for the person's grief that can be highly beneficial. Let the person cry. When appropriate, share your positive memories of the deceased.

Do not limit your help to only the first few days or weeks after the death. The grieving person will need support throughout the months and years that follow. The first anniversary of a death or the first holiday spent without the person can be an especially difficult time. Try to make sure that the person is not alone at these times. Don't wait for him or her to call you—a visit or a call from you will be welcome.

In some cases, grief is prolonged or intense and cannot be relieved without help from a mental health professional such as a psychiatrist. Support groups are available for people who are grieving to find comfort in sharing their feelings with others who have had similar experiences. Ask the person's doctor to recommend a support group. Those most likely to benefit from counseling are people who may have strong feelings of guilt or anger and those who are socially isolated.

Diseases, Disorders, and Other Problems

Disorders of the Heart and Circulation

1

The circulatory system (also called the cardiovascular system) consists of the heart and blood vessels (arteries and veins). The heart is a muscular pump about the size and shape of a fist. As it beats, the heart moves blood continuously around the body through the blood vessels. About once every minute, the heart pumps at least 9 pints of blood through the entire circulatory system.

The arteries carry oxygen-rich blood away from the heart to the tissues. The main arteries branch into smaller arteries called arterioles, which branch to form tiny capillaries, the smallest blood vessels in the body. Capillary walls are only one cell thick, allowing oxygen and other vital nutrients in the blood to pass through the walls to nourish the tissues and allowing waste to be taken up by the capillaries for removal. The capillaries returning to the heart gradually become larger, forming tiny blood vessels called venules, which gradually become larger and form veins. The veins carry oxygen-depleted blood through organs such as the kidneys and liver, which remove waste, and through the lungs, which provide a fresh supply of oxygen. From the lungs, the veins carry the blood back to the heart, where the cycle of circulation begins again.

Heart Disorders

To function properly, your heart requires a constant supply of blood, which provides oxygen and other nutrients to the heart muscle. Three major coronary arteries and a network of smaller blood vessels on the surface of the heart supply blood to the heart muscle. The walls of healthy arteries are muscular, smooth, and elastic to allow blood to flow through them easily. Heart disease, also called coronary artery disease, develops when the coronary arteries become narrowed, reducing or blocking the flow of blood (and oxygen and other nutrients) to the heart. This narrowing of the arteries is usually caused by atherosclerosis, a gradual thickening and hardening of artery walls caused by buildup of a fatty substance called plaque. Over a lifetime, plaque can grow larger and the artery walls can become thicker, making the channel inside the artery narrower and potentially blocking blood flow.

In atherosclerosis, the heart has to pump harder and faster to push blood through the narrowed arteries, causing high blood pressure (see page 574). The reduced supply of oxygen to the heart muscle can cause pain in the chest called angina. In some people, the heart muscle is damaged and its pumping action weakened, causing heart failure (see page 570).

The Heart and Blood Vessels

The Heart

The heart is a muscular organ made up of two pumps, each divided into two sections that are linked by valves. The larger section is the left ventricle, which pumps oxygen-rich blood through the aorta to all parts of the body. The blood then returns to the heart, entering the right atrium through two large channels (superior vena cava and inferior vena cava). From the right atrium the blood passes through the tricuspid valve into the right ventricle. It is then pumped through the pulmonary artery into the lungs, where it eliminates carbon dioxide and takes up oxygen. The oxygen-rich blood flows back to the left atrium of the heart through the pulmonary veins. From the left atrium it passes through the mitral valve into the left ventricle, where the cycle begins again.

Pulmonary artery (carries oxygen-depleted blood from right ventricle to lungs)

Aorta (sends oxygen-rich blood from heart to rest of body)

Pulmonary valve (controls flow of oxygen-depleted blood from right ventricle into pulmonary artery)

Superior vena cava (returns oxygen-depleted blood from head and upper body to heart)

Pulmonary veins (carry oxygen-rich blood from lungs to left atrium)

Left atrium (receives oxygen-rich blood from lungs through pulmonary veins)

Right atrium (receives oxygen-depleted blood from superior vena cava and inferior vena cava)

Aortic valve (controls flow of oxygen-rich blood from left ventricle into aorta)

Tricuspid valve (allows oxygen-depleted blood to flow from right atrium to right ventricle)

Mitral valve (allows oxygen-rich blood to flow from left atrium to left ventricle)

Left ventricle (pumps oxygen-rich blood from heart into aorta)

Inferior vena cava (brings oxygen-depleted blood from lower body and legs to heart)

Right ventricle (pumps oxygen-depleted blood from heart into pulmonary artery)

Coronary arteries

Oxygen-rich blood is pumped out of the aorta and flows into the coronary arteries, a branching network of blood vessels on the surface of the heart that supply oxygen- and nutrient-rich blood to the heart muscle.

Aorta

Left main coronary artery

Left circumflex coronary artery

Right coronary artery

Left anterior descending coronary artery

The Blood Vessels

Blood vessels transport blood to and from the heart and throughout the body. Arteries carry fresh, oxygen-rich blood away from the heart to the tissues; veins return used, oxygen-depleted blood from the tissues back to the heart and lungs for a new supply of oxygen.

Artery walls are very strong because blood is pumped through them under pressure from the heart. Arteries have three layers: a fibrous outer layer, a middle layer of strong muscle and tough elastic tissue, and a membrane inner lining.

Veins run parallel to arteries. Because the blood that veins carry is under much less pressure than the blood in the arteries, veins have thinner, less elastic, less muscular walls. Squeezing of the walls by routine muscle activity—such as walking—helps to move blood back to the heart. Veins have three layers: a fibrous outer layer, a thin middle layer of muscle, and a membrane inner lining.

Capillaries are tiny, thin-walled blood vessels that form a network (see below) between the smallest arteries (arterioles) and the smallest veins (venules). They carry blood to the cells and remove waste products. Nutrients and oxygen in the blood pass through the tiny spaces in the thin capillary walls into tissues; wastes such as carbon dioxide are taken up in the blood and carried to organs that break them down and eliminate them.

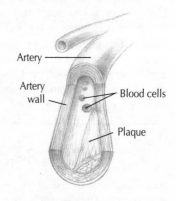

Atherosclerosis

Atherosclerosis is the buildup of hardened fatty deposits called plaque inside arteries. A buildup of plaque can reduce or block the flow of blood to tissues supplied by an artery.

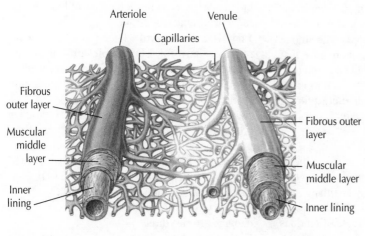

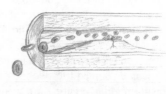

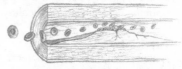

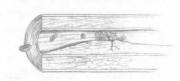

Valves in the veins

The veins contain one-way valves that open to allow used, oxygen-depleted blood to be pumped back to the heart, and close to keep blood from flowing backward. When you are physically active, your muscles contract and squeeze your veins, the valves open, and blood is pumped back toward your heart.

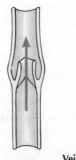
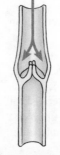

Veins

Open valve   Closed valve

How plaque causes blood clots to form

A buildup of plaque in an artery can cause blood clots to form. Cracks develop in the roughened surface of plaque (top). The body reacts as though the cracks are an injury and forms blood clots to seal them and promote healing (center). If a clot grows large enough (bottom), it can block blood flow in the artery and cause a heart attack or stroke.

A large plaque deposit causes turbulence in the bloodstream, which may cause blood clots to form. Plaque also is prone to cracking. Your body may react as though the cracks are an injury and form blood clots around them. If a clot grows large enough or breaks loose, or if a small bit of plaque breaks loose, it can block blood flow in the artery, causing a heart attack or stroke.

If atherosclerosis reduces or blocks blood flow in arteries elsewhere in the body, tissues receiving blood from these arteries can be damaged or destroyed. For example, if an artery in the brain is blocked, a stroke results. Blocked blood flow in an arm or leg can lead to gangrene (tissue death). Reduced blood flow to the kidneys can result in kidney failure.

Heart Disease

Heart disease is the No. 1 killer of American men and women. The disease kills more women each year than all cancers combined and 10 times more women than breast cancer. A woman's risk increases sharply after menopause. Doctors call heart disease a lifestyle disease because it generally results from things we do to ourselves, such as getting too little exercise, eating too much and too many of the wrong kinds of foods (those high in fat and calories and low in nutrients) and too few of the right kinds of foods (those rich in antioxidants and fiber), and weighing more than we should. People who smoke increase their risk even more. Doctors believe that nearly all cases of heart disease could be eliminated if people adopted lifestyle measures such as exercising regularly, eating a nutritious diet, quitting smoking, and staying at a healthy weight.

Risk Factors

A number of factors can increase your risk of heart disease. Although you cannot control risk factors such as age, gender, race, and family health history, you can control other risk factors by following a healthy lifestyle. Because heart disease often does not cause symptoms, especially in the early stages, many people who died of heart disease were not aware that they had it. The following factors can increase your risk of heart disease:

- **Age** Your chances of developing heart disease increase with age. In men, the risk increases at age 45; in women, the risk increases at age 55.
- **Gender** Men are generally at greater risk of developing heart disease than women up to age 55; a woman's risk increases significantly after menopause.
- **Family history of heart disease** A family history of heart disease increases your risk, especially if your father or brother had heart disease

before age 55, or your mother or sister had heart disease before age 65.
- **High blood pressure** High blood pressure makes the heart pump harder, increasing both the size of the heart muscle and the chances of heart failure.
- **High total cholesterol and LDL cholesterol** An excess of cholesterol in the blood, especially LDL (bad) cholesterol, leads to the formation of fatty deposits called plaque on artery walls (atherosclerosis). Plaque can rupture, producing blood clots that can block the flow of blood, causing a heart attack or stroke.
- **Low HDL cholesterol** HDL (good) cholesterol removes harmful LDL cholesterol from the blood, reducing plaque buildup in artery walls.
- **High C-reactive protein levels** Inflammation (which contributes to atherosclerosis) leaves a chemical by-product in the blood called C-reactive protein (CRP); the higher a person's CRP level, the greater his or her risk of a heart attack or stroke.
- **Smoking** Smoking raises blood pressure. Free radicals from cigarette smoke damage LDL cholesterol, making it more likely to collect as plaque on artery walls. Also, toxic chemicals in smoke damage arteries directly.
- **Diabetes** Most people who have diabetes die of some form of blood vessel disease or heart disease.
- **Race** Blacks have a higher risk of heart disease than people of other races.
- **Being overweight** Being overweight makes the heart work harder, increases the chances of developing high blood pressure and type 2 diabetes, and worsens blood cholesterol levels.
- **Lack of exercise** An inactive lifestyle leads to weight gain, obesity, high cholesterol levels, and type 2 diabetes.
- **Stress** Although the precise mechanism is unclear, in some people unmanaged stress can lead to heart disease.

- **High homocysteine levels** Too much of a body chemical called homocysteine in the blood may damage artery walls and promote formation of blood clots, significantly increasing the risk of heart attack and stroke. Taking 400 micrograms of the B vitamin folic acid every day can help keep homocysteine at a healthy level.

Warning Signs of Heart Disease

The main symptom of heart disease is temporary mild to severe chest pain (angina). See your doctor as soon as possible if you have any of the following symptoms:

- Pain or pressure in the chest while resting
- Pain or pressure in the chest during physical activity (such as climbing stairs or running)
- Shortness of breath during physical activity
- Chest pain that stops after a brief rest
- Dizziness, nausea, sweating, or difficulty breathing

Symptoms

Heart disease often does not produce symptoms, and for some people the first sign of heart disease is a heart attack. Others, however, may experience angina, a type of chest pain that results from an inadequate supply of oxygen to the heart muscle. Healthy coronary arteries can easily supply the heart with as much oxygen as it needs. Arteries that have been narrowed or damaged by atherosclerosis cannot provide sufficient oxygen, especially during times of increased demand, such as when a person exercises or is under emotional stress.

Angina can be temporary moderate to severe pain or pressure in the center of the chest that sometimes radiates to the left shoulder and down the left arm or to the throat, jaw, and lower teeth. Sometimes the pain spreads to the right shoulder and down the right arm. Angina usually occurs when a person is active and subsides when he or she stops and rests. Other symptoms that sometimes occur along with angina include difficulty breathing, sweating, nausea, and dizziness.

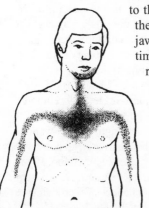

Location of angina pain

Chest Pain

If an episode of chest pain lasts longer than about 15 minutes and does not subside with rest (or with medication if you have been diagnosed with heart disease), you could be having a heart attack (see page 567). Call 911 or your local emergency number, or go to the nearest hospital emergency department immediately.

Although angina is usually a symptom of heart disease, it can also result from other health problems. For example, a defect in the aortic valve may reduce blood flow to the coronary arteries, thereby reducing the supply of oxygen to the heart muscle. Arterial spasm, which causes sudden temporary narrowing of a coronary artery, can also cause angina. Severe anemia (see page 610), which may decrease the supply of oxygen to the heart, is another possible cause of angina.

In some people, symptoms of congestive heart failure (see page 570) such as shortness of breath; persistent coughing up of sputum; or swollen legs, ankles, and feet are the first signs of heart disease. Heart failure occurs when the heart muscle is too weak to pump an adequate supply of blood to body tissues. Occasionally, symptoms of conditions that do not involve the heart and blood vessels, such as indigestion or gastroesophageal reflux disease (GERD; see page 750), can be mistaken for angina. If your doctor determines that you do not have heart disease, he or she will perform additional tests to find the cause of your symptoms and provide appropriate treatment.

Diagnosis

If you have symptoms of heart disease or if you think you may have angina, see your doctor as soon as possible. He or she will examine you and may recommend that you see a cardiologist, a doctor who specializes in treating heart problems. To determine the condition of your heart and blood vessels, the cardiologist will probably perform one or more of the following tests:

Electrocardiogram

An electrocardiogram (ECG) measures the electrical activity of the heart muscle and enables the doctor to detect a number of heart problems, including early signs of heart disease such as arrhythmias (abnormal heartbeats) or episodes of ischemia (inadequate blood flow to the heart). During an ECG, electrodes are placed on specific areas of your chest, arms, and legs, and a machine records the electrical activity of your heart. Continuous ECG monitoring is done using a portable device called a Holter monitor. The monitor, which you wear around your neck, over your shoulder, or at your waist, records an ECG over a period of 24 hours or longer.

Exercise stress testing

Exercise stress testing measures the electrical activity of the heart with an ECG while you walk or run on a treadmill or ride a stationary bicycle. This test helps evaluate the severity of heart disease and the ability of the heart to

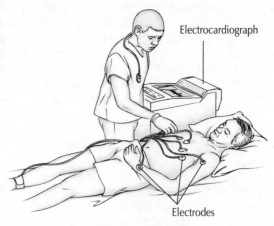

Electrocardiograph

Electrodes

Electrocardiogram

| MY STORY | ## Heart Attack

I had been having chest pains off and on, and was feeling anxious and having trouble sleeping for a couple of months. I thought it was just heartburn. The idea of heart disease didn't occur to me because I assumed it happened mainly to men. I hadn't had a physical exam in a few years. Then one morning, while I was making breakfast at my son's house, the pain started again. This time it got really bad. It hurt in the center of my chest, as it usually did, but then the pain and pressure spread to my left arm and jaw. I broke out in a cold sweat and started feeling light-headed and nauseous. While I was telling my son how I was feeling, I became short of breath.

I learned in the hospital that heart disease is the country's No. 1 killer—not only of men but of women, too.

My son seemed to know what was happening right away. "Mom, you could be having a heart attack!" he said, and ran to the phone and called 911. Then he gave me an aspirin tablet and told me to chew it up and swallow it. The paramedics came about 10 minutes later and attached some wires to my chest. They told me it was a test called an ECG that shows the heart's electrical activity. The ECG showed that I was having abnormal heartbeats and that the blood flow to my heart was partially stopped. They rushed me to the hospital.

In the emergency room, the hospital workers tested my blood, and the test confirmed that I was having a heart attack. So the emergency room doctor gave me a drug that he said would dissolve the blood clot that was blocking one of my arteries. Then they transferred me to a hospital room.

I had to stay in the hospital for 4 days. While I was there, I received a number of different drugs—blood thinners, a blood pressure medication, and something to control the rhythm of my heart. I learned in the hospital that heart disease is the country's No. 1 killer—not only of men but of women, too.

After I came home from the hospital, I started going to a cardiac rehab center near my home. The staff at the center taught me how I could change my lifestyle to prevent another heart attack. I started a regular walking program, which I still enjoy. A dietitian at the center gave me a sensible, low-fat eating plan that is easy to follow. (Now my husband follows it too.) And a very nice counselor at the center met with me several times to help me control the fear and anxiety I was feeling about having another heart attack.

Now I feel better than ever. I have lost 20 pounds and both my cholesterol level and blood pressure have gone down quite a bit. I was so lucky that I got medical help right away. I want every woman to know that heart attacks don't happen just to men; they affect women too. If you think you might be having a heart attack, get help as soon as you can. Your chances of recovering completely will be so much better.

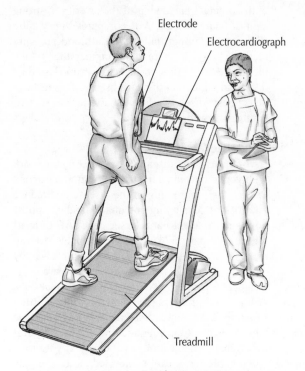

Electrode

Electrocardiograph

Treadmill

Exercise stress test

respond to an inadequate blood supply. If this test reveals arrhythmias or ischemia, the doctor may recommend drug treatment. If the ischemia persists even with drug treatment, the doctor may recommend a coronary angiogram (see right) to determine if angioplasty (see page 565) or bypass surgery (see page 564) is needed to restore blood flow to the heart. The test may also be performed before or shortly after a person leaves the hospital after a heart attack to help determine how well he or she is doing and whether the ischemia is continuing.

Thallium exercise stress testing

Thallium exercise stress testing combines radionuclide scanning (see page 114) with exercise stress testing. While you walk or run on a treadmill or ride a stationary bicycle, the doctor injects a small amount of a radioactive substance called thallium into your bloodstream, which carries it to the coronary arteries and heart muscle. After exercising, you lie on an examining table and the doctor uses a scanner called a gamma camera to produce images of blood flow through the

coronary arteries to the heart. The doctor performs a second scan a few hours later while you are resting. The test shows if blood flow through the coronary arteries is normal during both exercise and rest and if the arteries are narrowed or blocked. Absence of thallium in part of the heart muscle is a sign of damage (dead heart muscle tissue) from a previous heart attack.

Echocardiogram

An echocardiogram is a procedure in which images are obtained by bouncing ultrasound waves off the heart. In this test, the technician places a handheld ultrasound transducer (a device that transmits sound waves that are converted to images on a video monitor) on the left side of your chest, below the rib cage. The image on the monitor shows the size of your heart, movement of the heart muscle, blood flow through the heart valves, and valve function. If you have ischemia, the pumping motion of the wall of the left ventricle appears abnormal on the echocardiogram. An echocardiogram can be performed while you are at rest or while you walk or run on a treadmill or ride a stationary bicycle.

Coronary angiogram

A coronary angiogram (also called an arteriogram or cardiac catheterization) allows doctors to examine the coronary arteries on film. A catheter (a thin, flexible tube) is usually inserted into the femoral artery (a large blood vessel in the groin area) and moved up through the aorta (the main artery in the body) into the coronary arteries. A contrast medium (dye) is injected through the catheter into the artery under examination, and rapid-sequence X-rays (like a

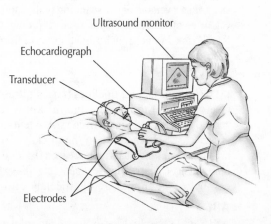

Ultrasound monitor

Echocardiograph

Transducer

Electrodes

Echocardiogram

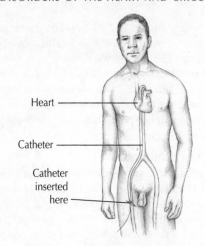

Heart

Catheter

Catheter
inserted
here

Coronary angiogram

movie) are taken of the artery. Narrowing and blood flow inside the arteries are clearly visible, allowing the doctor to determine if the arteries can be treated with bypass surgery or angioplasty. Occasionally, an angiogram is performed to detect spasms in coronary arteries that do not have any plaque (hardened fatty deposits in artery walls). In this case, medication is given to stimulate a spasm during the procedure to help diagnose heart disease.

CT scan

A CT (computed tomography) scan is a diagnostic procedure in which you lie on a table as it slides through a ring-shaped machine. Detectors inside the scanning ring send signals to a computer, which constructs cross-sectional X-ray images of the heart and coronary arteries. This test detects calcium deposits in the arteries resulting from atherosclerosis. A faster version of CT scanning (called ultrafast CT or electron beam CT) is used to predict heart attack risk in people who have no symptoms of heart disease.

IMT

IMT (intimal-medial thickness) uses ultrasound (see page 111) to measure the thickness of the carotid arteries and to determine the extent of atherosclerosis. An increase in the thickness of the carotid arteries indicates an increased risk of developing heart disease. This test can detect heart disease before the arteries are significantly narrowed.

ABI

ABI (ankle-brachial index) uses Doppler ultrasound (see page 111) and standard blood pressure

cuffs to detect narrowing of the arteries, a strong sign of heart disease. ABI compares the systolic (the first, or upper, number in a blood pressure reading) blood pressure in the ankle to the systolic blood pressure in the arm. A low ratio (less than 0.9) is an indication of heart disease. This test can detect heart disease before the arteries are significantly narrowed.

Treatment

If you have heart disease, your doctor will work with you to develop a treatment program designed to slow the progression of the disease and reduce your risk of developing potentially fatal complications such as a heart attack (see page 567) or heart failure (see page 570). You will probably need to make lifestyle changes such as following a healthy diet (see page 35), losing weight if you are overweight (see page 51), exercising regularly (see page 45), managing stress (see page 55), and quitting smoking if you smoke (see page 29). If you have high blood pressure, your doctor will prescribe antihypertensive medication (see below). If your total blood cholesterol level is elevated, he or she may prescribe a cholesterol-lowering medication (see page 564). Your doctor may also recommend surgery (see page 564) to bypass or clear an obstructed or blocked artery.

Medications for heart disease

If you have heart disease, your doctor may prescribe medication to improve blood flow and relieve your symptoms. You may need to take this medication for the rest of your life. If you experience any unpleasant side effects from the medication, talk to your doctor but keep taking the medication until he or she tells you to stop. Your doctor will probably prescribe another medication that does not cause the side effects. Medications used to treat heart disease include the following:

- **Beta blockers**   Beta blockers interfere with the effects of hormones in the body that normally increase heart rate and blood pressure. Beta blockers reduce the resting heart rate and, during exercise, limit the increase in heart rate, decreasing the body's demand for oxygen. Beta blockers lower the risk of heart attack and sudden death in people who have heart disease and can significantly reduce the risk of death from heart disease in people who have had a heart attack. The more severe the heart attack, the more benefit these drugs provide. Possible side effects include slow heartbeat, fatigue, or erectile dysfunction (in men).

- **Diuretics** Diuretic drugs lower blood pressure by causing the kidneys to eliminate more water and sodium from the body, reducing the heart's workload. Possible side effects include a rash, muscle cramps, fatigue, or erectile dysfunction (in men).

- **ACE inhibitors** ACE (angiotensin-converting enzyme) inhibitors block the production of an enzyme (angiotensin II) that causes blood vessels to constrict. These drugs are often prescribed to treat high blood pressure in people who have diabetes or heart failure. The most common side effect is a dry, irritating cough.

- **Angiotensin-receptor blockers** Angiotensin-receptor blockers prevent the arteries from constricting and prevent the kidneys from retaining excess sodium and water. These drugs are usually prescribed for people who cannot use ACE inhibitors. Possible side effects include dizziness, fatigue, or stomach pain.

- **Calcium channel blockers** Calcium channel blockers prevent blood vessels from constricting and interfering with blood flow. Because some of these drugs can slow the heart rate, they are also used to treat some types of arrhythmias. Possible side effects include dizziness, nausea, headache, flushing of the skin, ankle swelling, or fatigue.

- **Nitrate drugs** Nitrate drugs such as nitroglycerin dilate (widen) the blood vessels, improving blood flow. Both short-acting and long-acting nitrates are available. A small tablet of nitroglycerin placed under the tongue usually relieves an episode of angina (chest pain) in 1 to 3 minutes. The effects of this short-acting nitrate drug last about 30 minutes. People who have chronic (long-lasting) stable angina are usually advised to carry nitroglycerin with them at all times. Some people learn to take the nitroglycerin just before they reach the level of exertion they know can induce their angina. Long-acting nitrate drugs are taken one to four times daily. They are available as skin patches and a paste, which allow the medication to be absorbed through the skin over many hours. Over time, long-acting nitrates lose their ability to provide relief. Doctors often recommend that people try to go 8- to 12-hour periods without taking the drug as a way to help maintain its effectiveness. Possible side effects include headache, flushing of the skin, or dizziness.

- **Digitalis drugs** Digitalis drugs strengthen the force of the heart's contractions by increasing the supply of calcium to the heart muscle. These drugs are used to treat heart failure and arrhythmias. Possible side effects include nausea, loss of appetite, fatigue, or disturbed vision.

- **Anticoagulants, antiplatelet agents, and thrombolytics** Anticoagulants, antiplatelet agents, and thrombolytics are anticlotting drugs that help prevent the formation of blood clots. Aspirin and other anticlotting drugs bind to platelets (cell fragments that enable blood to clot) and keep them from clumping on blood vessel walls, significantly reducing the risk that a blocked artery will cause a second heart attack. Thrombolytics such as streptokinase or tPA (tissue plasminogen activator) are often given intravenously (through a vein) during a heart attack to dissolve an existing clot that is blocking a coronary artery. These drugs can cause bleeding in some people.

Additional classes of medications used to also treat high blood pressure include the following:

- **Alpha blockers** Alpha blockers help lower blood pressure by preventing the blood vessels from constricting. These drugs also interfere with the effects of hormones in the body that normally raise blood pressure. Alpha blockers are often prescribed in combination with other types of antihypertensive medications. Possible side effects include dizziness, headache, or mild fluid retention.

- **Vasodilators** Vasodilators widen the arteries by acting directly on the smooth muscle of the artery walls. These medications are usually given only in emergencies, when blood pressure cannot be controlled with other drugs. Possible side effects include headache, increased fluid retention, and an unusually strong, rapid heartbeat (more than 100 beats per minute).

- **Centrally acting drugs** Centrally acting drugs lower blood pressure by acting directly on the brain and nervous system to reduce heart rate and prevent blood vessels from constricting. These drugs may be used in combination with diuretic drugs. Possible side effects include dry mouth, dizziness, drowsiness, or fatigue.

- **Peripheral adrenergic antagonists** Peripheral adrenergic antagonists widen blood vessels and lower blood pressure by blocking the effects of the stress hormone epinephrine. They may be used with diuretics. They can cause drowsiness when taken in high doses.

Cholesterol-lowering medications

If your cholesterol levels are high or if you have heart disease, your doctor may prescribe cholesterol-lowering medication to reduce your risk of developing heart disease or of having a heart attack. You may need to take this medication for the rest of your life. Cholesterol-lowering medications include the following:

- **Statins**   Statin drugs (HMG CoA reductase inhibitors) block the action of an enzyme called HMG CoA reductase in the liver, causing the liver to produce less cholesterol. Possible side effects include occasional muscle aches and nausea. In rare cases, liver damage may result. Currently available statin drugs include lovastatin, simvastatin, provastatin, fluvastatin, and atorvastatin.

- **Bile acid binding resins**   Bile acid binding resins prevent absorption of cholesterol into the blood and stimulate the liver to remove cholesterol from the bloodstream. Possible side effects include bloating, cramping, and diarrhea. Examples of bile acid binding resins include cholestyramine, colestipol, and colesevelam.

- **Fibrates**   Fibrates (also called fibric acid derivatives) decrease blood levels of triglycerides (a type of fat in the blood). These drugs can also decrease LDL (bad) cholesterol and mildly increase HDL (good) cholesterol. People who take fibrates have a slightly increased risk of developing gallstones (see page 793) and gallbladder disease. Examples include clofibrate, fenofibrate, and gemfibrozil.

- **Niacin**   Niacin (nicotinic acid) is a vitamin that decreases production of LDL (bad) cholesterol in the liver. Depending on the dosage, it can also increase HDL (good) cholesterol. Possible side effects include bloating, cramping, or diarrhea. In rare cases, niacin may cause liver damage. A number of nonprescription niacin supplements are available over the counter.

Surgery for heart disease

A number of surgical procedures can be performed to treat heart disease, primarily by rerouting blood vessels around a blockage or reopening a blocked artery. These procedures include coronary artery bypass surgery, balloon angioplasty, and stent placement.

Coronary artery bypass surgery

Coronary artery bypass surgery is very effective for people who have angina and whose heart muscle has not been damaged by a heart attack. Bypass surgery is the procedure most widely used to treat heart disease caused by atherosclerosis (see page 557). The procedure can improve endurance, reduce symptoms, and decrease the amount of medication a person needs to take. Bypass surgery is most likely to benefit people who have severe angina that cannot be controlled with medication, who have a normally functioning heart, and who have not had a heart attack. About 85 percent of people who have bypass surgery experience complete or significant relief from their symptoms.

Bypass surgery involves grafting veins or arteries from another part of the body onto the coronary artery to reroute blood flow around the obstruction. The surgeon usually uses veins from the person's leg. Most surgeons also use at least one artery, usually taken from the person's chest wall. Atherosclerosis seldom develops in the treated arteries, and most treated arteries stay open for at least 10 years after the surgery. However, if the grafted veins become obstructed, the procedure may need to be repeated.

For bypass surgery you are given general anesthesia, your heart is stopped, and you are placed on a heart-lung machine, which takes over your circulation and breathing. The machine oxygenates your blood and pumps it throughout your body. If

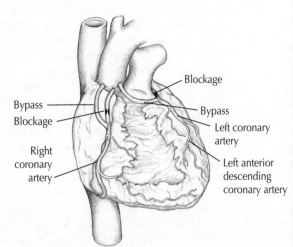

Coronary artery bypass surgery
This illustration shows blood vessels that were taken from other parts of the body and grafted onto the right and left coronary arteries to allow blood flow to bypass two blockages.

necessary, more than one bypass can be performed during the same procedure.

A day or two after surgery, you will probably begin a cardiac rehabilitation program to help you recondition your heart, lungs, and muscles, and control your cholesterol levels. The rehabilitation program usually includes eating a low-fat diet, exercising regularly, and having lifestyle counseling designed to help you keep your heart healthy and prevent future blockages in your arteries.

Coronary angioplasty and other procedures to open arteries

Doctors perform a number of procedures to open narrowed or blocked arteries. These procedures are often used instead of bypass surgery, which is riskier and has a longer recovery time. Your doctor may recommend this type of surgery if you have angina that cannot be controlled with medication or if only one or two of your arteries are significantly blocked. Coronary angioplasty can be used to control heart disease successfully over the long term. Before any of these procedures, you will be given medication to relax you and a local anesthetic to numb the area where the medical instrument will be inserted.

● **Balloon angioplasty**   In balloon angioplasty, the surgeon inserts a hollow needle into the femoral artery in the groin area and threads a long guide wire through the needle, up to the heart, through the aorta, and into the obstructed artery. A catheter (a thin, flexible tube) with a tiny balloon at its tip is then threaded over the guide wire and into the obstructed

artery. When the catheter reaches the obstruction, the balloon is inflated and deflated several times, for several seconds each time. The inflated balloon squeezes the plaque against the artery wall, reopening the artery and restoring blood flow. The catheter and guide wire are then withdrawn.

● **Stent placement**   Stent placement is essentially coronary angioplasty with one additional step. After the surgeon opens the obstructed artery with the balloon, he or she places a tiny metallic or plastic wire mesh (stent) inside the artery to keep it open. This procedure may cut the risk of reblockage (restenosis) in half.

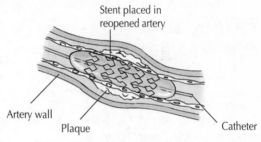

Stent placed in reopened artery

Artery wall

Plaque

Catheter

Stent placement

● **Radiation therapy**   Radiation therapy (also called vascular brachytherapy) may be used in addition to stent placement when an artery becomes blocked again within 6 months of angioplasty. In this case, after the stent is in place, the surgeon inserts a series of tiny radioactive pellets into the artery through the catheter. The pellets emit low-dose radiation, which helps prevent scar tissue from forming and reblocking the artery. After 5 minutes or less, the pellets are withdrawn through the catheter.

● **Atherectomy**   In atherectomy, a catheter with a tiny surgical instrument is inserted into the femoral artery in the groin area and guided to the blocked

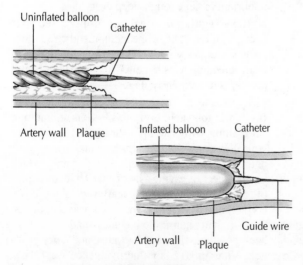

Uninflated balloon

Catheter

Artery wall   Plaque

Inflated balloon

Catheter

Artery wall   Plaque

Guide wire

Balloon angioplasty

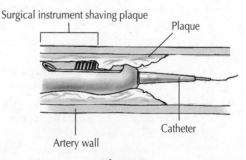

Surgical instrument shaving plaque

Plaque

Catheter

Artery wall

Atherectomy

artery. The surgical instrument shaves the plaque away in very thin layers. The shavings are then removed through the catheter.

- **Laser angioplasty** In laser angioplasty, the doctor uses a highly concentrated beam of light (laser) to vaporize the blockage.

After any of these procedures, you will need to carefully monitor the area where the catheter was inserted into your artery. If you notice any swelling or bleeding, or if you have any numbness, tingling, or a feeling of coolness in your toes, foot, or leg, contact your doctor as soon as possible. You may have a blood clot or a bleeding problem that requires immediate treatment.

> **WARNING!**
>
> ## Bleeding After Angioplasty
>
> If bright, red blood flows from the area where the catheter was inserted, lie down and press down firmly on that area for 20 minutes and then carefully release the pressure. If another person is with you, have him or her apply pressure to the area instead. If the bleeding does not stop, call 911 or your local emergency number.

The success rate for angioplasty procedures is about the same as that for bypass surgery. Like bypass surgery, angioplasty may have to be repeated if the blood vessels become blocked again.

Preventing Heart Disease

Although heart disease can begin to develop early in life, symptoms usually do not appear until the disease has caused irreversible damage to the heart and blood vessels. Because of this, the best treatment for heart disease is prevention. Take the following steps to reduce your risks:

- **Quit smoking now.** Smoking reduces the amount of oxygen in the blood, damages blood vessel walls, and raises the level of LDL (harmful) cholesterol, increasing your risk of heart disease.
- **Exercise regularly.** Regular, moderate exercise—such as brisk walking, jogging, or swimming—helps you control your weight, improves your cholesterol profile, and lowers your blood pressure. To gain the most benefit, you need to exercise for at least 60 minutes most days of the week.
- **Eat a healthy diet.** A diet that is low in fat and cholesterol and includes plenty of fresh fruits and vegetables can help lower your risk of heart disease by improving your cholesterol profile and keeping

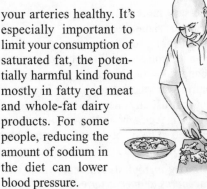

your arteries healthy. It's especially important to limit your consumption of saturated fat, the potentially harmful kind found mostly in fatty red meat and whole-fat dairy products. For some people, reducing the amount of sodium in the diet can lower blood pressure.

- **Know your cholesterol profile.** If your total cholesterol is above 200 or if your LDL (harmful) cholesterol is above 100 or your HDL (beneficial) cholesterol is below 60 (for men) or 50 (for women), you need to take steps—such as eating a healthy diet, exercising more, quitting smoking, and losing weight if you are overweight—to improve these numbers. Depending on your health history and heart disease risk factors, your doctor may prescribe a cholesterol-lowering medication (see page 564).
- **Control your blood pressure.** High blood pressure is the main risk factor for heart disease. Work with your doctor and follow a healthy lifestyle to help keep your blood pressure at a heart-healthy level.
- **Manage your stress.** Find positive ways to cope with or reduce stress in your life. If you are not able to relax, try techniques such as deep breathing, meditation, yoga, or biofeedback. It is also important to get enough sleep every day.
- **Have regular medical checkups.** See your doctor as often as he or she recommends. Your doctor will monitor your blood pressure and may perform screening tests to help detect and treat health problems in their early stages.
- **Consume at least 400 micrograms of the B vitamin folic acid every day.** Consuming folic acid, along with vitamins B6 and B12, either in your diet or in vitamin supplements, lowers your homocysteine level (see page 559) and may reduce your chances of having a heart attack. Good sources of folic acid include green, leafy vegetables; broccoli; orange juice; eggs; and dried peas and beans. Foods rich in vitamin B6 include bananas, chicken, beef, potatoes, fish, whole grains, and dairy products. Vitamin B12 is found in chicken, beef, fish, eggs, and dairy products.

Heart Attack

The heart needs a continuous supply of oxygen-rich blood from the coronary arteries to function properly. A heart attack occurs when a coronary artery is blocked, depriving part of the heart muscle of blood. The resulting damage to the heart muscle is the most common cause of death in people who have heart disease.

A blocked coronary artery usually results from long-term atherosclerosis (see page 557), a condition in which arteries are narrowed by hardened fatty deposits called plaque. Most heart attacks occur when a plaque ruptures and a blood clot forms on the rough surface of the ruptured plaque and blocks blood flow through the artery suddenly and completely. In rare cases, a heart attack can result when a blood clot from another area of the heart breaks loose and blocks a coronary artery. Another rare cause of a heart attack is a spasm in a coronary artery that stops blood flow to the heart muscle. Using a stimulant drug such as cocaine can trigger this type of spasm.

Once a coronary artery has been blocked, damage to the heart muscle occurs quickly and can become permanent within minutes. In general, the longer the blockage lasts, the more extensive the damage to the heart muscle. Immediate medical treatment is essential to limit damage to the heart muscle and increase a person's chances of survival.

In some cases after a heart attack, a blood clot may form inside one of the four chambers of the heart. If the clot breaks loose, it can travel through the bloodstream and cause damage to tissues elsewhere in the body. For example, if the clot blocks an artery that supplies blood to the brain, the result is a stroke (see page 669). Sometimes damage caused by a heart attack weakens and stretches one of the walls of the heart chambers, causing a bulge in the wall called an aneurysm (see page 599). An aneurysm can grow and burst without warning, causing uncontrolled bleeding (hemorrhage). Inactivity during bed rest may cause blood clots to form in the veins of the legs (deep vein thrombosis; see page 605). These clots can break off, travel through the bloodstream, and block an artery that supplies blood to the lungs (pulmonary embolism; see page 606).

Risk Factors

The following risk factors increase your chances of having a heart attack. While some of these can't be changed—such as family health history, race, and gender—others can be modified or eliminated through lifestyle changes.

- **Family health history** If siblings, parents, or grandparents had heart attacks at an early age, you are also at risk.
- **Gender** Men are at greater risk of having a heart attack than women before age 55. After menopause, a woman's risk is the same as a man's.
- **Undesirable cholesterol profile** An unhealthy cholesterol profile (see page 146) promotes atherosclerosis, which increases your risk of having a heart attack.
- **High blood pressure** Uncontrolled high blood pressure promotes atherosclerosis (see page 557).
- **Smoking** Smoking (including exposure to secondhand smoke) raises blood pressure, damages artery walls, and increases the risk of blood clot formation.
- **Diabetes** Uncontrolled diabetes promotes atherosclerosis and increases blood levels of LDL (harmful) cholesterol.
- **Race** Blacks are at greater risk of having a heart attack than people of other races.
- **Lack of exercise** A sedentary lifestyle often results in weight gain and a poor cholesterol profile.
- **Being overweight** Weighing more than your ideal body weight (see page 51) increases your

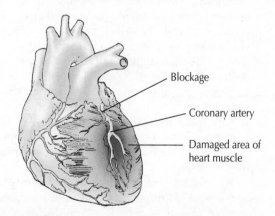

Heart attack
A blood clot is more likely to block an artery if the artery walls have been narrowed by a buildup of plaque. A blood clot in a coronary artery—a condition called coronary thrombosis—can block blood flow to the heart muscle and cause a heart attack. The area of the heart muscle normally supplied by the artery becomes damaged.

Blockage

Coronary artery

Damaged area of heart muscle

risk for high cholesterol, high blood pressure, and diabetes.

- **Alcohol consumption** Drinking excessive amounts of alcohol can lead to high blood pressure and can raise blood levels of triglycerides (a potentially harmful type of fat in the blood).
- **Stress** In some people, long-term stress can contribute to high blood pressure.

Symptoms

Symptoms of a heart attack vary in type and intensity from one person to another and from one heart attack to another in the same person. Some people may have a heart attack and have no symptoms. However, in most cases, the main symptom of a heart attack is sudden pain in the center of the chest. Some people describe the pain as a feeling of tightness, pressure, or fullness, or a squeezing sensation. The pain is usually severe and may spread to the back, left arm, neck, jaw, upper abdomen, and sometimes to the right arm. The pain may be continuous or may last for a few minutes, fade, and then return.

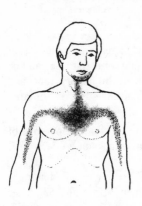

Location of heart attack pain

Most people who have a heart attack have recurring chest pain, shortness of breath, and fatigue for a few days before the attack. In some people, arrhythmia (irregular heartbeat) may also precede a heart attack. Unlike angina, the pain of a heart attack is not relieved with rest or after taking nitroglycerin (a medication prescribed to relieve angina). Also, heart attack pain is usually more severe and longer-lasting than angina.

Other common symptoms of a heart attack include dizziness, shortness of breath, sweating, chills, nausea, restlessness or anxiety, fainting, or weakness. Sometimes the lips, hands, or feet turn slightly blue. Women are more likely than men to have these symptoms in addition to chest pain. In rare cases, a heart attack does not cause symptoms and is detected by chance on an electrocardiogram (ECG; see page 559), a recording of the electrical activity of the heart, performed for another purpose.

Some people may ignore their symptoms or assume they are caused by some other condition, such as indigestion or overexertion. However, because most deaths from a heart attack occur within an hour of the onset of symptoms, it is crucial to be able to recognize the symptoms and act quickly. The sooner treatment begins, the less damage to the heart muscle and the better the long-term prognosis.

Diagnosis

After you arrive at the hospital emergency department, a doctor or nurse will check your temperature, pulse, and blood pressure and ask you to describe your symptoms. Because other conditions—such as indigestion, pneumonia, a blood clot in a lung, or gastroesophageal reflux disease—can imitate the symptoms of a heart attack, the doctor will order an ECG and blood enzyme tests to make a diagnosis. An ECG will often show heart muscle damage caused by a heart attack. However, if several ECGs performed over the course of several hours appear normal, the doctor will probably use the blood enzyme tests to make the diagnosis.

An elevated blood level of heart muscle enzymes called troponins indicates heart muscle damage caused by a heart attack. The level of troponins in the blood increases about 4 to 6 hours after a heart attack, peaks about 10 to 24 hours after the attack, and can be detected in the blood for about a week. Troponin levels are usually measured soon after a person is admitted to the hospital with

CPR Can Save Lives

Cardiopulmonary resuscitation (CPR) is a lifesaving technique that is performed to restart a person's breathing and heartbeat after they have stopped. The procedure involves keeping the person's airway open, performing rescue breathing, and doing chest compressions to pump blood through the heart. Because of the potential for serious injury, only people who have been fully trained in CPR should attempt this procedure. Before starting CPR, call 911 or your local emergency number. Once you have started CPR, do not stop until emergency medical personnel have taken over.

Ask your doctor about the availability of CPR classes in your community. Your local hospital or fire department may offer a class. If not, contact the local chapter of the American Red Cross or the American Heart Association. CPR training can mean the difference between life and death.

WARNING!

Signs of a Heart Attack

A heart attack is a medical emergency. If you have symptoms of a heart attack, call 911 or your local emergency number immediately. The sooner treatment begins, the greater your chances of survival, so act quickly, even if you are not sure you are having a heart attack. The most common symptoms of a heart attack include:

- Sudden squeezing pain or a feeling of tightness, pressure, or fullness in the center of the chest that lasts for more than several minutes
- Chest pain that extends to the shoulders, arms, back, neck, or jaw
- Indigestion or persistent pain in the upper abdomen
- Shortness of breath
- Dizziness or fainting
- Weakness or fatigue
- Heavy sweating
- Chills
- Nausea and vomiting
- Backache
- Arm or jaw numbness
- Restlessness or anxiety; sleeplessness
- Paleness
- Blueness of the lips, hands, or feet

   While waiting for emergency help to arrive, take an aspirin tablet; aspirin reduces blood clotting and helps limit damage to the heart muscle, improving your chances of survival. Keep warm and calm. If you are with a person who is having a heart attack and he or she loses consciousness, use a portable defibrillator (see page 581), if one is available, to restart the heart. Or perform cardiopulmonary resuscitation (CPR; see previous page) if you have been trained in this lifesaving technique.

chest pain and a possible heart attack and at 8-hour intervals over a 24-hour period.

Another heart muscle enzyme, called CK-MB, is also released into the blood after a heart attack. Elevated CK-MB levels appear within 6 hours of a heart attack and last for 36 to 48 hours. CK-MB levels usually are measured soon after a person is admitted to the hospital and at 6- to 8-hour intervals over the next 24 hours.

If you have had or are having a heart attack, treatment will begin immediately. The doctor may

order additional tests, such as a chest X-ray (see page 109), an echocardiogram (see page 561), a radionuclide scan (see page 114), or a coronary angiogram (see page 561). A chest X-ray allows the doctor to evaluate the size and shape of your heart and coronary arteries. An echocardiogram may show damage to the left ventricle (the pumping chamber of the heart). A radionuclide scan may show reduced blood flow to a specific area of the heart that has been damaged by a heart attack. A coronary angiogram can show if the arteries that supply blood to the heart are narrowed or blocked.

Before you leave the hospital, you will probably have tests to evaluate the extent of any underlying heart disease. These tests—an ECG and, perhaps, a coronary angiogram or an echocardiogram—will help the doctor accurately determine the extent of the damage to the heart muscle and whether any narrowed or blocked sections in the coronary arteries might need to be opened with surgery. The severity of the disease will determine if surgery is necessary.

Treatment

The sooner treatment for a heart attack begins, the better your chances of survival. Treatment may include medication, surgery, or both, depending on your overall health and the amount of damage to the heart muscle.

Medication

You may be given nitroglycerin to improve blood flow to and from your heart and to relieve pain. If your pain is severe, you may be given a strong pain reliever such as morphine. You will probably be given antiplatelet drugs (such as aspirin) or anticoagulant drugs (such as heparin) to help prevent blood clots from forming again in the coronary arteries or new clots from forming in the veins, especially in the legs (see page 605). Beta blockers (see page 562) may be given to help reduce the heart's workload by slowing the heartbeat and lowering blood pressure.

You may be given thrombolytic (clot-dissolving) drugs (see page 563) to dissolve the blood clot that is blocking the coronary artery. However, this treatment is effective only if no more than 6 hours have passed since the onset of symptoms. In most cases, thrombolytic drugs are given (usually by injection directly into a vein) as soon as the diagnosis of a heart attack is confirmed.

Surgery

You will have additional tests, such as a coronary angiogram (see page 561), to determine whether the clot has dissolved and blood flow has been restored. If the tests show that the coronary artery is still blocked, a procedure such as angioplasty (see page 565) may be performed to reopen the artery. If the artery becomes blocked again after surgery, the procedure may be repeated a few days later.

As an alternative to treatment with a thrombolytic drug, your doctor may perform immediate angioplasty of the blocked blood vessel using specially designed instruments to remove the blood clot from the artery. Balloons and stents may be used to open the artery. In many cases, immediate angioplasty for a heart attack can be as effective as treatment with thrombolytic drugs in limiting the damage caused by a heart attack and improving a person's chances of survival. In rare cases a doctor may perform emergency coronary artery bypass surgery (see page 564) at the time of a heart attack.

Preventing Another Heart Attack

If you have had a heart attack, you are at risk of having another. Treatment after a heart attack focuses on healing the heart and preventing another heart attack. The following steps can help you reduce your chances of having another heart attack:

- Have regular medical checkups to help ensure early detection and treatment of health problems.
- Keep your blood pressure under control and have your blood pressure checked as often as your doctor recommends.
- Have your blood cholesterol levels checked as often as your doctor recommends.

- Do not smoke or use other tobacco products.
- Maintain a healthy weight.
- Eat a low-fat diet that includes plenty of whole grains and fresh fruits and vegetables.
- Exercise regularly.
- Resume sexual activity when it is safe to do so (ask your doctor for advice).
- Manage your stress.
- Drink alcohol only in moderation.
- Take all medication exactly as prescribed.

Before you leave the hospital, your doctor will refer you to a cardiac rehabilitation program designed to help you recondition your heart, lungs, and muscles, and improve your cholesterol profile. Cardiac rehabilitation begins in the hospital and continues for weeks or months after you return home. The program usually includes diet, exercise, and lifestyle counseling. You also may need to take medication that reduces strain on your heart, improves its efficiency, and prevents irregular heartbeats. Medications may include:

- Antiplatelet agents or anticoagulants (see page 563)
- Beta blockers (see page 562)
- Angiotensin-converting enzyme (ACE) inhibitors (see page 563)
- Cholesterol-lowering medications (see page 564)
- Calcium channel blockers (see page 563)

Congestive Heart Failure

Congestive heart failure develops when the heart is weakened and is no longer able to pump an adequate supply of blood to the lungs and other body

---

After a Heart Attack

After you have had emergency treatment for a heart attack, you may be admitted to the hospital's coronary care unit (CCU) or intensive care unit (ICU), where specially trained nurses will monitor your condition continuously for signs of any complications. If you had a minor heart attack, without complications, you will probably be encouraged to get out of bed after 48 hours. Even if the attack was severe, you will probably be encouraged to get out of bed and use a bedside commode. Doctors think that even a little exercise helps to reduce the risk of blood clots. Before leaving the hospital, you will probably have an exercise stress test (see page 560) to see if your

heart muscle is getting enough oxygen. If not, your doctor will discuss possible treatment options with you.

Many people are anxious or depressed after a heart attack, and some people may hesitate to resume sexual activity. If you are feeling anxious or depressed, or if you are having sexual problems, talk to your doctor. He or she can diagnose and treat any underlying disease or condition or refer you to a support group or mental health professional who can help you deal with your feelings. By making an effort and maintaining a positive outlook, most people are able to lead full, active lives after a heart attack.

tissues. Heart failure does not mean that the heart stops pumping, but that it is not pumping efficiently. A number of disorders can lead to heart failure, including heart disease, heart attack, high blood pressure, heart valve disorders, arrhythmias (irregular heartbeats), anemia (a condition in which the oxygen content in the blood is reduced), or cardiomyopathy (a degenerative disease of the heart muscle). Heart failure can occur when the heart muscle is not able to contract effectively (called systolic, or left-sided heart failure) or when the heart muscle is not able to relax (called diastolic, or right-sided heart failure). Other risk factors include smoking, a poor cholesterol profile, high blood pressure, and being overweight.

Heart failure occurs more frequently in men than in women and is twice as common among blacks as among whites. Up to 3 million Americans have heart failure, and the risk of developing the condition increases with age.

In systolic heart failure, blood backs up in the veins that carry blood from the lungs to the heart, increasing blood pressure in the lungs. The lungs become swollen and congested with fluid. This condition is called pulmonary edema. In diastolic heart failure, blood accumulates in the veins that lead to the heart from other parts of the body. These parts of the body, especially the legs, ankles, and feet, may become swollen. Some people who have diastolic heart failure also have lung congestion.

Despite its name, heart failure is not always life-threatening. The outcome depends on the severity of the underlying disorder that is causing heart failure and on how soon treatment begins. Although there is no cure for heart failure, it can be controlled with medication and a healthy lifestyle.

Symptoms

Heart failure usually develops slowly. The main symptom of heart failure is shortness of breath as a result of lung congestion. You may become short of breath while active or while resting. You may have difficulty breathing when you lie down, and your breathing problems may become severe enough to disturb your sleep. At times you may wake up gasping for air. Although episodes of severe shortness of breath usually last less than an hour, the experience can be frightening.

Your lungs may become so swollen and congested that your breathing may be raspy or you may wheeze. You may also have chest pain and a persistent cough that produces frothy, blood-flecked phlegm. The fluid in your lungs decreases your resistance to infection; pneumonia (see page 660), for example, is a frequent complication of heart failure.

Fatigue is another common symptom of heart failure. Because your body tissues are not receiving enough oxygen and nutrients, you may feel weak or tire easily. Fluid accumulation may cause the lowest part of your body to swell. For example, if you are confined to bed, the lower part of your back may become swollen. If you are standing, your legs, ankles, or feet may become swollen. Your liver may also become swollen, causing abdominal pain.

Other possible symptoms of congestive heart failure include low blood pressure, dizziness, and confusion. You also may lose your appetite but experience rapid weight gain from the accumulation of fluid.

For some people, symptoms may not develop until the condition is at an advanced stage. The heart muscle attempts to compensate for its decreased pumping ability by growing larger and thicker and contracting more often. However, the effects of this adjustment are only temporary, and symptoms develop eventually.

Diagnosis

Diagnosis of heart failure is based on your symptoms and risk factors and a physical examination. The doctor will listen for lung congestion and abnormal heart sounds with a stethoscope. He or she may order a chest X-ray to look for lung congestion and check the size and shape of your heart. The doctor may order an echocardiogram (see page 561) to examine the heart valves and determine how much blood the heart pumps out when it contracts, and an electrocardiogram (ECG; see page 559) to determine how well the heart is functioning. He or she may also recommend a coronary angiogram (see page 561) to evaluate the condition of the coronary arteries. The doctor may order additional tests to rule out possible causes of your symptoms other than heart disease, such as anemia (see page 610) or an overactive thyroid gland (hyperthyroidism; see page 901).

Treatment

Treatment of congestive heart failure focuses on the underlying disease or condition that is causing it. Your doctor will recommend lifestyle changes you will need to make to improve the quality of your life and control your risk factors for heart disease. For example, if you smoke, your doctor will recommend that you quit smoking. He or she also will recommend that you lose weight if necessary and reduce the amount of fat in your diet. Your doctor also may recommend reducing your intake of caffeine and sodium and eating smaller, more frequent meals, which can help keep you from overeating and can improve your body's absorption of nutrients. Caffeine can temporarily raise blood pressure and heart rate. For some people, consuming large amounts of sodium (more than 2,400 milligrams a day) can lead to fluid retention, which can increase blood pressure. If you have severe heart failure, you may need to limit your fluid intake to avoid fluid retention. Your doctor will probably recommend that you begin a program of regular, moderate exercise under his or her supervision.

Your doctor is likely to prescribe medication to help relieve your symptoms. Diuretic drugs will help your body eliminate excess fluid and sodium, thereby decreasing blood volume and lowering your blood pressure. Because diuretic drugs increase the body's output of urine, always take them in the morning to avoid having to get up during the night to urinate.

Other medications frequently prescribed to treat heart failure include digitalis drugs (usually digoxin) and vasodilators such as ACE (angiotensin-converting enzyme) inhibitors. Digitalis drugs slow the heart rate while increasing the strength of the heartbeat and the heart's output of blood. ACE inhibitors widen both small arteries and veins and counteract some of the substances produced by the kidneys that can narrow small arteries and cause the body to retain fluid. ACE inhibitors reduce the heart's workload and significantly prolong life in many people. They are powerful drugs, and you and your doctor may need to work together to find the appropriate dosage for you. If you cannot take ACE inhibitors, your doctor may prescribe a nitrate drug or hydralazine, both of which relax smooth muscle to widen blood vessels and improve blood flow. Doctors often prescribe beta blockers (see page 562) to treat heart failure. Like ACE inhibitors, they can relieve symptoms and prolong life in people who have heart failure.

If your doctor prescribes a long period of bed rest, he or she may also prescribe an anticoagulant medication to help prevent the formation of blood clots. If your doctor prescribes an anticoagulant, he or she will carefully monitor the effect of the drug in your blood to help prevent possible complications such as bleeding in the intestines, skin, brain, or other organs.

Drug treatment should relieve your shortness of breath and swelling. By following a low-sodium diet and taking your medication as prescribed, you can expect to lead an active life. However, if your heart failure does not respond to treatment with rest, lifestyle changes, and medication, you may need to have a heart transplant (see next page). Heart transplantation has a high success rate. However, because of a severe shortage of donor hearts, the availability of this option is limited. Most people who need a heart transplant are placed on a waiting list until a donor heart becomes available.

Some people with severe heart failure who are waiting for a heart transplant are able to use a small mechanical pump called a left ventricular assist device (LVAD). An LVAD is attached to the heart to help the heart pump blood. In many people who have heart failure, an LVAD improves the heart's ability to pump blood, eliminating the need for a heart transplant. Research continues on longer-term use of these devices.

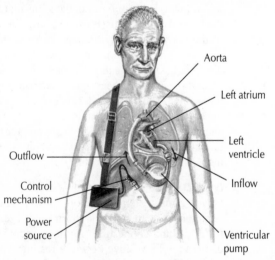

Left ventricular assist device

A left ventricular assist device consists of an air-driven pump, a control mechanism, a power source, and connective tubing. The pump and tubing are surgically implanted in the body and attached to the heart. The control mechanism and power source are worn outside the body and are connected by wires to the pump. A tube inserted into the left ventricle draws blood into the pump (inflow). The blood is then pumped out to the tissues through a tube inserted into the aorta (outflow).

How a Heart Transplant Is Done

In heart transplant operations, surgeons remove the entire damaged heart, except for the back walls of the upper chambers (the atria). Most of the connections to the major blood vessels are left intact, making it easier to connect the donated heart tissue. Before the recipient's heart is removed, surgeons connect him or her to a heart-lung machine, which bypasses the blood flow to the lungs and heart. The machine temporarily takes over for the heart, pumping blood throughout the body, until the donor heart is implanted and attached to the blood vessels. As the donor heart gets warm, it begins to beat. If the heart does not start to beat, the surgeons stimulate it with an electric shock to trigger beating. All of the new connections in the blood vessels and heart chambers are checked for leaking before the heart-lung machine is disconnected.

Heart transplant recipients usually get out of bed a few days after the operation and can go home within 2 weeks if no problems arise. Eventually, about 85 percent of people with heart transplants go back to work or have the ability to do so, and many engage in swimming, running, or other physical activities.

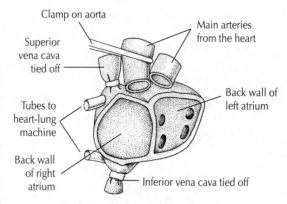

Damaged heart ready for transplant

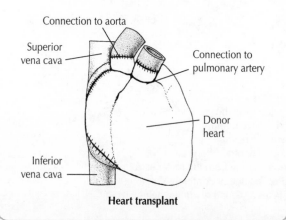

Heart transplant

Heart transplants

The first human heart transplant was performed in 1967. Since that time, the procedure has become an established treatment for advanced heart disease. Surgeons perform nearly 2,300 heart transplants nationwide each year. Doctors usually recommend a heart transplant only when a person has irreversible, long-term heart failure that cannot be controlled with other medical or surgical treatments. (The artificial hearts now available are still experimental and cannot offer a reliable, long-term solution to the problem of a diseased heart.) Heart transplants can be performed at any age, including infancy and childhood, but the procedure is usually not recommended for people over age 65. The most common causes of heart failure are:

- Coronary artery disease (blockage in the arteries leading to the heart)
- Cardiomyopathy (weakness of the heart muscle, affecting its ability to pump blood)
- Heart disease that is present at birth
- Damage to the heart muscle or valves
- Failure of an earlier transplant

After surgery, early symptoms of rejection (see page 821) of the donor heart are not always apparent, so doctors must regularly take tiny samples of the heart muscle and examine them under a microscope (a procedure called a biopsy) to check for signs of rejection. To obtain samples of the tissue, a doctor inserts a small tube into an incision in the neck, down the jugular vein, and into the heart. If the doctor finds signs of rejection, he or she will give the person higher doses of immune-suppressing drugs.

After the person goes home from the hospital for recovery, he or she will have to visit the doctor for regular follow-up visits and more biopsies. Some of the early complications (in addition to rejection) that can arise after heart transplant surgery include kidney failure (which is usually temporary), wound infection, pneumonia, and stroke. Irregular heartbeats called arrhythmias (see page 580) sometimes occur.

Heart transplants now have a high success rate: about 85 percent of those who receive a new heart are alive after 1 year, 79 percent after 3 years, and 74 percent after 5 years. These survival rates continue to improve. Without this lifesaving procedure, the vast majority of heart transplant recipients would have died within 2 years.

High Blood Pressure

Blood pressure is produced by the heart as it pumps blood through the arteries and as the arteries resist blood flow. It is measured in millimeters of mercury (mm Hg) with an instrument called a sphygmomanometer. Blood pressure is highest when the heart contracts (beats) and pumps blood into the arteries. This is the systolic pressure. Between beats, when the heart is resting, the pressure falls. This is the diastolic pressure. A blood pressure reading is given as a combination of these two pressures; the systolic pressure is written above or before the diastolic pressure. For example, if your blood pressure reading is 130 over 80, it is written as 130/80 mm Hg; 130 is the systolic pressure and 80 is the diastolic pressure.

In healthy people, blood pressure varies throughout the day, depending on factors such as physical activity and stress. In people who have high blood pressure, the heart always pumps with greater force than necessary, regardless of other factors, and blood pressure is never within the normal range. The medical term for high blood pressure is hypertension.

High blood pressure is a very common condition, affecting about 50 million adults in the United States. Because it seldom causes symptoms, many people who have high blood pressure do not know that they have it. However, in most cases, high blood pressure is easy for doctors to detect and treat.

The cause of high blood pressure is usually unknown. This is called primary or essential hypertension. Most people who have high blood pressure have essential hypertension. Although essential hypertension can't be cured, it can be controlled. Hypertension that results from an underlying disease or condition—such as long-term kidney disease, thyroid disease, adrenal gland abnormalities, or use of illicit drugs—is called secondary hypertension. Secondary hypertension can be cured by successfully treating the underlying disease or condition.

In most people who have hypertension, blood pressure continues to rise over time unless it is treated. Sometimes, however, significantly high blood pressure develops very quickly. This life-threatening condition, which can result from either essential hypertension or secondary hypertension, is called malignant hypertension. Untreated malignant hypertension can lead rapidly to stroke, kidney failure, or heart failure.

Risk Factors

Although the cause of high blood pressure is usually unknown, a number of factors can increase your chances of developing high blood pressure or worsen existing high blood pressure:

- You have close family members (parents or siblings) who have high blood pressure.
- You are male.

Testing Blood Pressure

The Meter

Blood pressure is measured with an instrument called a sphygmomanometer, which consists of an inflatable rubber cuff and a special type of pressure gauge. Because the earliest devices for measuring blood pressure used a mercury-filled glass column, blood pressure is expressed as millimeters of mercury (mm Hg).

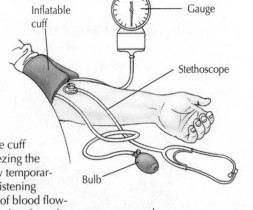

Inflatable cuff

Gauge

Stethoscope

Bulb

Measuring Blood Pressure

To measure your blood pressure, the doctor or nurse wraps the cuff securely around your upper arm and inflates the cuff by squeezing the attached rubber bulb until it is tight enough to stop blood flow temporarily. He or she then begins to gradually deflate the cuff, while listening through a stethoscope placed inside your elbow to the sound of blood flowing through the main artery in your arm. The doctor takes a reading from the meter as soon as he or she hears the first heartbeat. This is the systolic pressure. The doctor continues deflating the cuff until blood flows steadily through the artery. The doctor takes a second reading when he or she hears the last heartbeat. This is the diastolic pressure.

- You are female and past menopause.
- You are black.
- You are overweight.
- You do not exercise regularly.
- You use any tobacco products (including smokeless tobacco).
- You regularly consume more than two alcoholic drinks per day.
- You have diabetes or long-term kidney disease.
- You are not able to cope with stress.

Symptoms

In the early stages, high blood pressure usually does not produce symptoms. By the time symptoms such as severe headaches, palpitations (heartbeats that you're aware of), or shortness of breath occur, the disease has already caused organ damage. Therefore, it is vital to monitor your blood pressure and have it checked every time you visit your doctor, especially if you have any of the risk factors for hypertension described above.

If not treated, high blood pressure can lead to the following health problems, even if you don't have any symptoms:

- **Atherosclerosis**   Uncontrolled high blood pressure causes the artery walls to thicken and lose elasticity, which promotes formation of hardened fatty deposits (plaque) in artery walls. Plaque narrows the channel inside the artery and interferes with blood flow throughout the body. Over time, atherosclerosis can lead to a heart attack or stroke.
- **Enlarged heart**   High blood pressure makes the heart work harder. Over time, this extra effort causes the heart muscle to thicken. The heart becomes less efficient and has to work harder and harder to pump blood through the body, potentially leading to heart failure.
- **Kidney damage**   The kidneys filter waste from the blood. Over time, high blood pressure can cause the blood vessels in the kidneys to narrow and thicken. The kidneys then filter less blood, and waste builds up in the bloodstream, sometimes leading to kidney failure. A person with kidney failure may need dialysis (a technique to remove waste from the blood) or a kidney transplant.
- **Stroke**   High blood pressure can weaken the walls of the arteries or cause them to thicken. A weakened artery wall in the brain may break, causing a hemorrhage. A blood clot may block one of the narrowed arteries in the brain, causing a stroke.

- **Eye damage**   High blood pressure can damage blood vessels in the eyes, causing them to thicken, narrow, or tear. This damage can lead to loss of vision.

Diagnosis

High blood pressure is usually detected during a routine checkup. When you visit your doctor, he or she will take a health history (see page 130), perform a physical examination, and measure your blood pressure. Because factors such as physical activity or stress can cause a temporary increase in blood pressure, your doctor will need to take a number of blood pressure readings over a period of several weeks or months to determine whether you have high blood pressure. If your blood pressure readings are occasionally above normal, your doctor may recommend that you monitor your blood pressure at home. If your blood pressure readings are consistently above normal, you have high blood pressure.

The doctor will probably examine your eyes with a viewing instrument called an ophthalmoscope. The condition of the blood vessels in the retina (the light-sensitive membrane that lines the back of the eyes) can provide valuable information about the extent of damage caused by high blood pressure.

Your doctor may perform additional tests to determine if you have essential hypertension or secondary hypertension. He or she may perform a chest X-ray (see page 109), an echocardiogram (see page 561), and an electrocardiogram (ECG; see page 559) to see if your heart is enlarged. The ECG will also reveal any previous damage to the heart muscle, such as damage caused by a heart attack. You will have blood and urine tests to determine if your kidneys are functioning properly. Some people may also need to have intravenous urography, a test in which the doctor injects a harmless dye into an artery and examines the kidneys on an X-ray image. Other people may have tests to evaluate blood flow, such as a CT scan (see page 562), an MRI (see page 113), a radionuclide scan (see page 114), or a coronary angiogram (see page 561).

A blood pressure reading of less than 120/80 mm Hg is generally considered normal. A category called prehypertension—120-139/80-89—indicates that a person is at risk of eventually developing high blood pressure. Blood pressure is classified according to increasing level of health risk, as reflected in the guidelines on the next page.

Treatment

When the underlying cause of secondary hypertension is treated successfully, blood pressure usually returns to normal levels. However, if the underlying cause cannot be cured, treatment is usually the same as that for essential hypertension.

Lifestyle changes

For many people, lifestyle changes such as giving up tobacco, following a healthy diet, exercising regularly, losing weight, and managing stress not only decrease the risk of developing high blood pressure but also significantly reduce existing high blood pressure. However, if lifestyle changes do not lower blood pressure to within the normal range, the doctor will probably recommend treatment with antihypertensive drugs.

Medication

Doctors usually prescribe antihypertensive medication when high blood pressure cannot be controlled with lifestyle changes. Most people who take antihypertensive medication need to take it for the rest of their life.

The following list provides a brief description of the most frequently prescribed types of antihypertensive medications. (For additional information about these medications, see page 562.)

- **Diuretics** Diuretics increase the kidneys' excretion of water and sodium, reducing the volume of blood the heart has to pump, thereby reducing blood pressure.

Blood Pressure Classifications for People Age 18 or Older		
Category	Systolic	Diastolic
Normal blood pressure	Lower than 120 mm Hg	Lower than 80 mm Hg
Prehypertension	120 to 139 mm Hg	80 to 89 mm Hg
Stage 1 hypertension	140 to 159 mm Hg	90 to 99 mm Hg
Stage 2 hypertension	160 mm Hg or higher	100 mm Hg or higher

A diagnosis of hypertension is based on two or more blood pressure readings taken at separate visits to the doctor's office or clinic. If your systolic pressure falls into one category and your diastolic pressure into another, the higher reading is used to classify your blood pressure.

- **Beta blockers** Beta blockers slow the heart rate and block the output of an enzyme that raises blood pressure.
- **Alpha blockers** Alpha blockers prevent arteries from constricting and block the effects of the stress hormone epinephrine, which raises blood pressure.
- **ACE inhibitors** ACE (angiotensin-converting enzyme) inhibitors block production of an enzyme (ACE) that causes blood vessels to constrict.
- **Angiotensin-receptor blockers** Angiotensin-receptor blockers prevent the arteries from constricting and prevent the kidneys from retaining sodium and water, which can raise blood pressure.
- **Centrally acting drugs** Centrally acting drugs work directly on the brain and nervous system to

---

WARNING!

Sudden, Rapid Drop in Blood Pressure

Hypotension is the medical term for low blood pressure. Postural hypotension is a rapid drop in blood pressure that occurs when you sit up or stand too quickly. When you change position suddenly, your body usually makes a quick adjustment in blood pressure. But in postural hypotension, your blood pressure falls and blood flow to your brain is temporarily reduced, causing dizziness and sometimes fainting.

Postural hypotension may be a side effect of antihypertensive medication. Occasionally, postural hypotension occurs during pregnancy or as a symptom of a disease or condition such as diabetes (see page 889), atherosclerosis (see page 557), Addison's disease (see page 899), or dehydration.

If you often feel dizzy or faint when getting up from a sitting or lying position, try to move more slowly. If this does not help, talk to your doctor. If you are taking antihypertensive medication, he or she will probably adjust the dosage or prescribe a different drug. If this does not relieve your symptoms, you may need to have a physical examination and tests to determine the underlying cause of the problem.

Checking Your Blood Pressure at Home

Your doctor will probably recommend that you check your blood pressure at home with a home blood pressure monitor. Both mechanical and electronic blood pressure monitors are available at drugstores and medical supply companies. Ask your doctor which type of monitor you should buy.

A home blood pressure kit should include an easy-to-read pressure gauge, cuffs in various sizes, a stethoscope (for mechanical monitors), and easy-to-understand instructions. Your doctor or a nurse can teach you how to use the monitor correctly.

The following guidelines will help you take an accurate reading with a mechanical blood pressure monitor:

- Check your blood pressure at the same time every day.
- Avoid caffeine and nicotine for at least 30 minutes before checking your blood pressure.
- Relax in a quiet place for several minutes before beginning.
- Rest your arm on a tabletop at heart level.
- Press gently yet firmly with your fingertips on your inner elbow to find the pulse in the main artery in your arm.
- Wrap the cuff snugly around your upper arm. The cuff should extend from just below the armpit to just above the elbow.
- Place the gauge where you can easily read it.
- Place the bell of the stethoscope directly and firmly over the artery in your inner elbow.
- Place the earpieces of the stethoscope lightly in your ears.
- Look at the gauge and inflate the cuff to at least 30 mm Hg above your most recent systolic pressure

(you should not hear a beating sound through the stethoscope at this time).
- Deflate the cuff slowly (about 2 mm Hg per second) by turning the release valve. Watch the gauge and listen closely.
- As soon as you hear a beating sound, record the number on the gauge. This is the systolic pressure.
- Continue deflating the cuff. As soon as the beating sound stops, record the number on the gauge. This is the diastolic pressure.
- Repeat the procedure to check for accuracy.

Practice taking your blood pressure until you are confident and comfortable performing the procedure. If you have any problems, ask your doctor or a nurse to check to see that you are doing it properly. If you are using an electronic blood pressure monitor, follow the manufacturer's instructions.

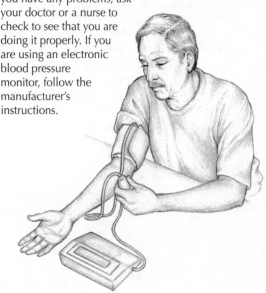

---

prevent arteries from constricting, lowering heart rate and blood pressure.

- **Calcium channel blockers** Calcium channel blockers prevent the smooth muscle of the artery walls from contracting and narrowing the blood vessels; calcium channel blockers may also slow or block the development of plaque, which can build up on artery walls and narrow them.

Take your medication exactly as your doctor prescribes it; follow his or her instructions carefully and completely. If you experience any unpleasant side effects, talk to your doctor right away. He or she will work with you to fine-tune your drug treat-

ment program so that your blood pressure is controlled without unpleasant side effects. Never change the dosage or stop taking any medication until your doctor tells you to do so. If the cost of your medication is a concern, ask your doctor or pharmacist if less expensive alternatives are available.

After your blood pressure is under control, you may be tempted to stop taking your medication. But keep in mind that there is no cure for essential hypertension and that normal blood pressure readings are a sign that the medication is working. If you stop taking it, your blood pressure will rise again.

Preventing High Blood Pressure

You can lower your risk of developing high blood pressure or lower existing high blood pressure by doing the following:

● **Maintain a healthy weight.**   As your body weight increases, your blood pressure rises. Being overweight can make you more likely to develop high blood pressure than a person who is at a healthy weight (see page 11). You can reduce your risk of high blood pressure by losing weight. Even a small weight loss can reduce your risk significantly. And if you are overweight and already have hypertension, losing weight can help you lower your blood pressure.

● **Exercise regularly.**   Regular exercise is an effective way to lose weight and control blood pressure. When combined with a healthy diet, regular exercise can help you lose more weight and keep it off longer than with either diet or exercise alone. Aerobic exercise—such as walking, cycling, swimming, stair-climbing, or jogging—helps improve the fitness of your heart, blood vessels, and lungs, which, in turn, helps lower your blood

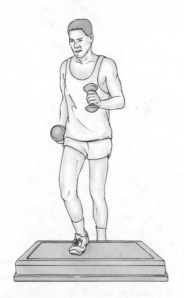

The benefits of exercise
Regular aerobic exercise, such as step aerobics and jogging, and strength training, such as lifting weights, provide many health benefits—including protection against high blood pressure, heart disease, type 2 diabetes, and osteoporosis. Regular exercise helps you condition your heart and lungs, improve your strength and endurance, and maintain a healthy weight.

pressure and protect you against heart disease. (For more information on the health benefits of regular exercise, see page 45.)

● **Cut down on salt.**   Most Americans take in more sodium than they need. Excess salt causes your body to retain water, which raises blood volume and therefore blood pressure. If you are salt-sensitive, which means that your blood pressure rises when you eat salt, eating less salt—no more than 1 teaspoon per day—will benefit your health.

● **Limit alcohol.**   Drinking too much alcohol will raise your blood pressure temporarily and, over time, may also lead to high blood pressure. Limit yourself to one drink a day if you are a woman or two drinks a day if you are a man. A drink is defined as $1\frac{1}{2}$ ounces of 80-proof liquor, 5 ounces of wine, or 12 ounces of beer.

● **Do not use tobacco.**   Smoking puts you at risk of developing high blood pressure or having a heart attack or stroke. Smoking also worsens a person's cholesterol profile, which is a factor in heart disease. Chemicals in smokeless tobacco can also raise blood pressure. (For helpful tips on how to quit smoking, see page 29.)

Other factors that may help prevent high blood pressure in some people include:

● **Potassium**   Having an adequate level of potassium in the body may help prevent high blood pressure by balancing the amount of sodium in the body. Good sources of potassium include fresh fruits and vegetables (especially bananas, oranges, melons, and potatoes), low-fat or fat-free dairy products, and fish. Do not take potassium supplements unless your doctor recommends them. Too much potassium can cause an irregular heartbeat.

● **Calcium**   Too little calcium in the diet may lead to high blood pressure (as well as weak bones). You can get the calcium you need—1,200 to 1,500 milligrams per day for adults—from low-fat and fat-free dairy products such as milk, yogurt, and cheese, and green leafy vegetables. Doctors do not recommend taking calcium supplements to help prevent high blood pressure.

● **Magnesium**   A diet low in magnesium may increase blood pressure. The best sources of magnesium are whole grains, green leafy vegetables, seeds, nuts, and dried peas and beans. Doctors do not recommend taking magnesium supplements to help prevent high blood pressure.

High Blood Pressure

Q. *My friend said that her doctor told her she could stop taking her medication for high blood pressure. She did it by losing only 10 pounds and exercising more. How can that be?*

A. Even a weight loss of as few as 10 pounds can help lower blood pressure. Exercise is also a proven blood-pressure reducer. As long as your friend keeps her weight at a healthy level by eating a nutritious, low-fat diet rich in fruits and vegetables and by exercising regularly, she should be able to continue to control her blood pressure without medication. However, she needs to continue to have her blood pressure measured to make sure it is staying at a healthy level.

Q. *Why is it taking so long to find the right combination of medications to control my high blood pressure?*

A. Blood pressure is a highly complex biochemical process that is influenced by many different factors. Because your body is a unique biological system, it will not respond in exactly the same way to a particular medication as another person's system will. An antihypertensive medication or combination of medications that works for one person may not work for another. Until drugs are developed that can be tailored to our unique genetic makeup, finding the right medication will continue to be a matter of trial and error. I'm sure your doctor will soon find a medication that is effective for you.

- **Fish oils** Omega-3 fatty acids are a type of fat found in fatty fish such as mackerel and salmon. These oils help protect the lining of arteries, prevent irregular heart rhythms, and reduce the formation of blood clots. Eating fish two or more times a week can also help reduce high blood pressure and improve your cholesterol profile.

- **Fat and cholesterol** To help prevent heart disease, limit the amount of fat in your diet, especially the saturated fat found in foods such as fatty meats and full-fat dairy products. Too much saturated fat raises your blood cholesterol level, which increases your risk of developing heart disease. High-fat foods are usually high in calories.

- **Caffeine** Although caffeine in coffee, tea, and soft drinks may raise blood pressure temporarily in some people, it quickly returns to its usual level. Limit your caffeine intake if your doctor recommends it.

- **Stress management** Stress can raise blood pressure temporarily and can aggravate existing high blood pressure, making it more difficult to control. Although stress management techniques—such as biofeedback, meditation, or relaxation training—do not help prevent high blood pressure, they may help you deal positively with the stress in your life. Getting enough sleep can also be helpful.

Shock

Shock is a life-threatening condition in which blood flow throughout the body suddenly becomes inadequate or is blocked, depriving body tissues of oxygen and other vital nutrients. Shock is usually caused by extremely low blood pressure, which prevents the heart muscle from pumping an adequate supply of blood to the tissues. If not treated quickly, shock can be fatal.

Very low blood pressure can result from conditions—such as a heart attack or arrhythmia—that interfere with the ability of the left ventricle of the heart to pump effectively. Another possible cause of extremely low blood pressure is severe blood loss resulting from an injury or from a disorder that causes internal bleeding, such as a perforated peptic ulcer (see page 755) or a ruptured aneurysm (see page 599). Tissue damage from a severe burn or severe dehydration caused by persistent vomiting, diarrhea, or inadequate fluid intake can decrease blood volume, resulting in very low blood pressure. Sometimes toxins from a severe infection get into the bloodstream and cause shock. Shock can also develop when a severe allergic reaction causes blood vessels to dilate (widen) and leak fluid, decreasing blood volume.

WARNING!

Shock

Shock is a medical emergency. Symptoms of shock are very low blood pressure combined with sweating, faintness, nausea, shallow breathing, rapid pulse, or pale, cold, clammy skin. Reduced blood flow to the kidneys causes urine production to stop. Inadequate blood supply to the brain leads to drowsiness, confusion, and loss of consciousness.

If you are with someone who has symptoms of shock, call 911 or your local emergency number, or take the person to the nearest hospital emergency department immediately. (For information on what to do while waiting for emergency help to arrive, see page 162.)

Heart Rate and Rhythm Disorders

The heart has four chambers: the left atrium and right atrium at the top, and the left ventricle and right ventricle at the bottom. Valves between the chambers keep blood moving in the proper direction, and electrical impulses produced by a group of cells in the right atrium help control the frequency and regularity of heart muscle contractions (the heartbeat). These electrical impulses move rapidly along specialized muscles that function like nerve pathways, branching out in all directions in all four chambers of the heart. For the heart to pump efficiently, all areas of the heart muscle must contract (beat) at the same time. If a problem develops anywhere along these pathways, the regular rhythm of the heartbeat is disrupted. A single irregular heartbeat is called an ectopic heartbeat (see page 583). A persistently irregular heartbeat is called an arrhythmia.

Arrhythmias

A normal heart rate for a person who is resting is between 60 and 100 beats per minute, with some minor variations. The two major types of arrhythmias are bradycardias, in which the resting heartbeat is slower than 60 beats per minute, and tachycardias, in which the resting heartbeat is faster than 100 beats per minute. An arrhythmia may be mild to severe and it may be continuous or alternate with periods in which the heart beats normally. A sudden, very rapid or very slow arrhythmia can reduce blood flow to the brain and may cause fainting or dizziness.

Risk Factors
In some cases, an arrhythmia may develop without an obvious underlying cause. Factors that increase the risk of arrhythmia include:

- Heart disease
- Congestive heart failure
- Heart valve disorders
- Overactive or underactive thyroid gland
- Chemical imbalances in the body
- Smoking
- Excessive intake of alcohol
- Excessive intake of caffeine

Symptoms
Arrhythmias, whether mild or severe, do not always cause symptoms. Because of this, even a life-threatening arrhythmia can go undetected. Possible symptoms of an arrhythmia include palpitations (heartbeats that you're aware of), dizziness, fainting, shortness of breath, and angina (chest pain).

An arrhythmia can sometimes be a symptom of a serious underlying disorder. If you have symptoms of an arrhythmia, see your doctor.

Diagnosis
Your doctor will examine you, check your pulse, and listen to your heart through a stethoscope. He or she will probably order an electrocardiogram (ECG; see page 559) to evaluate your heart rate and rhythm. If the arrhythmia seems to come and go, you may need to wear a Holter monitor for 24 hours or longer. A Holter monitor is a portable ECG device that you wear over your shoulder, around your neck, or at your waist, with electrodes attached to specific areas of your chest. While you go about your daily routine, the monitor records your heart's electrical activity on a special cassette tape. After 24 hours, the doctor reviews the recorded information to make a diagnosis.

Sometimes a person may use a smaller device called an event recorder, which is used only at the time the arrhythmia occurs. A person who has a severe arrhythmia may need to be hospitalized for continuous ECG monitoring. In some cases, a person is placed on a table that tilts from horizontal to vertical while an ECG is performed to diagnose some forms of arrhythmia.

The cause of some arrhythmias can be determined by examining the heart in a cardiac catheterization procedure (see page 592), in which a thin, flexible tube is inserted into the heart through an artery or vein in the groin or in the arm. When diagnosing arrhythmias, doctors may also perform blood tests to check for chemical imbalances or thyroid problems.

Treatment

Mild arrhythmias often do not require treatment. More severe arrhythmias and those that produce intolerable symptoms may be treated with beta blockers (see page 562), calcium channel blockers (see page 563), or medications that slow the heart's electrical impulses. You may need to try several drugs before finding the medication that works best for you.

Some severe arrhythmias are treated surgically. Coronary artery bypass surgery (see page 564) and coronary angioplasty (see page 565) are sometimes used to treat arrhythmias that result from heart disease. A procedure called catheter ablation uses radiofrequency energy to destroy or remove a spot on the heart that is causing an arrhythmia. This procedure is similar to cardiac catheterization (see page 592); a catheter is threaded into the heart, and the radiofrequency therapy is delivered through the catheter.

Many severe arrhythmias are treated by temporarily or permanently implanting an electronic pacemaker (see page 584) beneath the skin of the chest. A pacemaker is a battery-powered device that produces electrical impulses that regulate the heartbeat.

Cardiac Arrest

Cardiac arrest means that the heart is beating ineffectively or has stopped beating. Possible causes of cardiac arrest include ventricular tachycardia (a rapid, ineffective heartbeat originating in the ventricles), ventricular fibrillation (a disorganized, ineffective attempt by the ventricles to contract), or cardiac asystole (cessation of heartbeat). When cardiac arrest occurs, the heart cannot beat effectively, the brain does not get enough blood, and loss of consciousness occurs immediately. Cardiac arrest in a person who seems healthy usually results from undetected heart disease (see page 558). Cardiac arrest can begin with ventricular tachycardia and degenerate into ventricular fibrillation.

Treatment

If cardiac arrest is caused by ventricular fibrillation, the person's heartbeat can often be restored with a portable defibrillator (see below).

In people who have recurring episodes of ventricular tachycardia that does not respond to treatment with drugs, a device called an implantable defibrillator (see page 584) may be recommended. The device senses the onset of an arrhythmia and automatically provides a potentially lifesaving electrical shock to the heart muscle. Some implantable defibrillators also function as pacemakers (see page 584).

WARNING!

Cardiac Arrest

Cardiac arrest is a medical emergency. Call 911 or your local emergency number immediately if someone you know goes into cardiac arrest. If you are alone with the person, call for emergency medical assistance first, and then use a portable defibrillator if one is available. Or begin cardiopulmonary resuscitation (CPR) if you are trained to perform CPR. These techniques can stimulate the heart and keep the brain alive until emergency medical help arrives. It is possible to recover from cardiac arrest if the heartbeat and circulation are restored within a few minutes. The chances of recovering from cardiac arrest are good if emergency treatment is prompt and effective. If emergency treatment is delayed, damage to the heart and brain can be permanent.

Portable Defibrillators Can Save Lives

An automatic external defibrillator is a portable electronic device that can be used to restore the heartbeat of a person whose heart is beating irregularly (fibrillating) or has stopped beating. With the push of a button, a person who has been trained to use the device can administer an electric shock to another person's heart through conductive adhesive pads placed directly on his or her chest. The device also analyzes the person's heart rhythm. Increasing numbers of public facilities, such as airports, shopping malls, hotels, and workplaces, have portable defibrillators available for use in an emergency. These devices come with easy-to-understand instructions, so even people who have not been trained can use them effectively.

Atrial Fibrillation and Flutter

In atrial fibrillation and flutter, the atria (the two upper chambers of the heart) contract (beat) irregularly and are not synchronized with the contractions (beating) of the ventricles (the two lower, pumping chambers of the heart). These uncoordinated heartbeats impair the heart's ability to pump blood to the tissues.

Atrial flutter is similar to atrial fibrillation, except that in atrial flutter the muscles contract more regularly and at a somewhat slower rate. Both fibrillation and flutter tend to come and go, alternating with periods of normal heart rhythm.

Atrial fibrillation and flutter are usually the result of heart disease (see page 558). The fibrillation or flutter can also be caused by an overactive thyroid gland, high fever, or excessive consumption of alcohol. Any disease that causes heart failure and enlargement of the right or left atrium can cause atrial fibrillation and flutter. In about 10 percent of cases, especially among older people, the condition has no obvious cause. People who have atrial fibrillation or flutter have an increased risk of embolism (see page 601), seizures (see page 686), heart failure (see page 570), or stroke (see page 669).

Symptoms

Atrial fibrillation and flutter often do not cause symptoms. When symptoms occur, they can include palpitations (heartbeats that you're aware of), weakness, dizziness, angina (chest pain), or fainting. Some people also have symptoms of heart failure such as shortness of breath or fatigue. If you have symptoms of atrial fibrillation or flutter, see your doctor right away.

Diagnosis

To diagnose atrial fibrillation or flutter, your doctor will probably order an electrocardiogram (ECG; see page 559) and an echocardiogram (see page 561) to evaluate the condition of your heart. Because atrial fibrillation or flutter often comes and goes, you may need to wear a portable ECG device called a Holter monitor (see page 580) for 24 hours or longer. The doctor also may order blood tests to rule out thyroid problems.

Treatment

Treatment for atrial fibrillation or flutter usually depends on the underlying cause of the problem. The doctor will probably recommend lifestyle changes such as eating a heart-healthy diet; cutting back on sodium, caffeine, and alcohol; exercising regularly; losing weight if you are overweight; quitting smoking if you smoke; and managing stress.

Doctors frequently prescribe digitalis drugs to help improve the efficiency of the heart by slowing the contractions of the ventricles. The doctor may prescribe beta blockers to improve the efficiency of the ventricles by slowing the electrical impulses from the sinoatrial node (the heart's natural pacemaker). Antiarrhythmic drugs can help return the heart rhythm to normal. The doctor may also prescribe an anticoagulant drug to help prevent blood clots from forming.

If your heart is basically healthy, or if the underlying cause of atrial fibrillation or flutter persists despite treatment, your doctor may recommend a treatment called cardioversion (see below). In this procedure, the doctor administers an electrical shock to your heart while you are under mild anesthesia. Cardioversion is frequently successful in restoring normal heart rhythm.

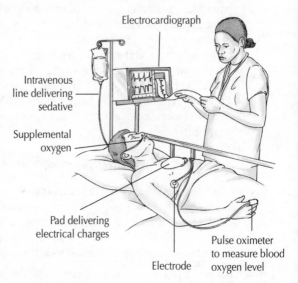

Electrocardiograph

Intravenous line delivering sedative

Supplemental oxygen

Pad delivering electrical charges

Electrode

Pulse oximeter to measure blood oxygen level

Cardioversion

Cardioversion is a procedure that is used to restore normal heart rhythm. During the procedure, you are connected with electrodes to an ECG and are given medication intravenously (through a vein) to help you relax. You are given supplemental oxygen through a nasal catheter. A device called a pulse oximeter is attached to your finger to monitor the oxygen content of your blood. Two large pads are attached to your chest; the pads are connected to a machine called a defibrillator. The defibrillator delivers a series of electrical charges through the pads to your heart in an attempt to correct the arrhythmia. Because you are sedated, you do not feel the electrical charges. The procedure lasts about 30 minutes. After the procedure, you will rest in bed until you are fully awake.

Ectopic Heartbeats

Ectopic heartbeats are irregular beats among otherwise normal heartbeats that feel as though the heart has either missed or gained a beat. This condition is common and usually does not require treatment.

If you are bothered by an occasional irregular heartbeat, your doctor may prescribe medication to treat the condition. Frequent ectopic heartbeats may result from using too much caffeine, alcohol, or nicotine. If you use these substances, quit smoking and cut down on alcohol and coffee, tea, soft drinks, and other beverages that contain caffeine.

Heart Block

The heart rate is controlled by a natural pacemaker called the sinoatrial node, a group of specialized cells in the wall of the right atrium (the upper right chamber of the heart). The sinoatrial node transmits electrical impulses between the atria and ventricles (the lower chambers of the heart), causing rhythmic contractions of the heart muscle, or heartbeats. If the sinoatrial node malfunctions, the beating of the atria is not coordinated with the beating of the ventricles.

In first-degree heart block, the electrical impulses take longer to travel from the atria to the ventricles. In second-degree heart block, some of the electrical impulses fail to reach the ventricles, causing an irregular heartbeat. In third-degree heart block, electrical impulses do not reach the ventricles, which continue beating slowly, independently of the sinoatrial node and the atria.

In healthy people, the heart rate increases during times of increased demand on the circulatory system, such as during exercise or periods of emotional stress. But in people who have heart block, heart rate does not increase despite an increased demand for blood, and the brain and other body tissues do not receive enough blood and oxygen to function properly.

Heart block often occurs as a result of heart disease (see page 558) or a heart attack (see page 567). An overdose of a digitalis drug used to treat an irregular heartbeat can also cause heart block. In some people, heart block occurs for no obvious reason. The risk of heart block increases with age, and the disorder occurs most often in older people.

Symptoms

In most people, first-degree and second-degree heart block usually do not produce symptoms. Third-degree heart block may cause sudden loss of consciousness, seizures, or stroke. In some people, third-degree heart block may produce symptoms of heart failure (see page 570), such as shortness of breath or fatigue. If you are an older person and you have episodes of dizziness, weakness, or confusion, see your doctor as soon as possible. Although these symptoms have many possible causes, early detection and treatment of heart block may save your life.

Diagnosis

To diagnose heart block, your doctor will examine you and will probably order an electrocardiogram (ECG; see page 559), an examination of the electrical activity of the heart. You may need to wear a portable electronic ECG device called a Holter monitor (see page 580) to record the electrical activity of your heart for 24 hours or longer.

Treatment

If the doctor has determined that your heart's natural pacemaker is causing your symptoms, he or she may recommend temporary or permanent insertion of an artificial pacemaker (see next page) to regulate the heartbeat.

Paroxysmal Atrial Tachycardia

In healthy adults, the heart beats from 60 to 100 times per minute, and increases to about 160 beats per minute during physical activity. In an episode (or paroxysm) of atrial tachycardia, the heart rate suddenly jumps to 160 or more beats per minute without physical exertion. An episode of paroxysmal atrial tachycardia can last from about 1 minute to several days.

Symptoms

Palpitations (heartbeats that you're aware of) are the main symptom of paroxysmal atrial tachycardia. If you suddenly become aware of your rapid heartbeat, you may become anxious or frightened. Some people who have paroxysmal atrial tachycardia say they have a feeling of impending death. Other symptoms can include shortness of breath,

Pacemakers and Implantable Defibrillators

An electronic pacemaker is a battery-operated device that is often used to treat severe arrhythmias. A pacemaker may be temporary or permanent. A temporary pacemaker is usually inserted under the skin of the chest after a heart attack has disturbed the heart's normal rhythm. The pacemaker produces electrical impulses that keep the heart beating at a normal rate. In most people, the heart rate returns to normal in a few days and the temporary pacemaker is removed.

A permanent pacemaker is implanted under the skin of the chest to regulate an abnormally slow heart rate. When the heart rate slows, or when the heart misses a beat, the pacemaker produces electrical impulses that restore a normal heart rate. After the heart rate returns to normal, the pacemaker stops producing the impulses until they are needed again. The pacemaker also can produce electrical impulses at a constant rate, depending on a person's needs.

During the Procedure

Implanting a pacemaker is a minor surgical procedure that is performed while the person is awake. To implant a pacemaker, the doctor numbs the chest with a local anesthetic, makes a 2-inch incision just below the collarbone, and inserts a catheter (a thin, flexible tube) through a large vein called the subclavian vein. While watching a video monitor, the doctor then threads one or more electrodes through the catheter into one of the chambers of the heart. The electrodes, which will provide electrical impulses to the heart, are attached by very thin wires to a small, battery-operated power source. The doctor then creates a small pocket just under the skin of the chest below the collarbone, places the pulse generator inside, and stitches the incision closed.

After the Procedure

You will leave the hospital the day of the procedure or the following day. You will be asked to keep the incision dry for about a week. For at least 8 weeks after the procedure, you will need to limit your movement, particularly on the side where the pacemaker is implanted, to prevent the wires from disconnecting. Your doctor will ask you to avoid making sudden, jerking arm movements or raising your arms above your head. You will also need to avoid all strenuous activities that involve the use of your arms, such as tennis, swimming, sweeping, raking, scrubbing, or lifting and carrying heavy or bulky objects. After 8 weeks, when the wires will be set in place, you can resume your usual activities.

The pacemaker's power source operates like a tiny computer. By placing an external control device on your chest over the pacemaker, your doctor can examine the pacemaker and reprogram it if necessary. Some pacemakers provide information about how the heart is functioning. A person can also transmit information from his or her pacemaker over the telephone to the doctor's office. Your doctor will examine your pacemaker about 2 weeks after surgery and

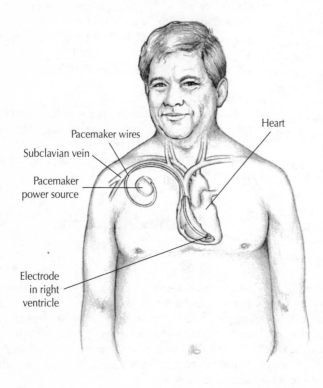

Pacemaker

A pacemaker is an electronic device that is implanted just beneath the skin and attached to the heart with very thin wires. The device delivers an electrical impulse (at a fixed rate or whenever it is needed) to an electrode placed in one of the ventricles of the heart. A pacemaker is powered for 8 to 10 years by a tiny battery that a doctor can easily replace in a minor surgical procedure.

Pacemaker wires
Subclavian vein
Pacemaker power source
Electrode in right ventricle
Heart

again about 3 and 6 months after surgery. After that, he or she will continue to examine your pacemaker at regular intervals, at least once a year, to help ensure that it is functioning properly.

A pacemaker is powered by a tiny battery that is designed to last 8 to 10 years. When the battery begins to run low, it gives off a warning signal that can be detected by an external control device or over the telephone many months before it actually fails. Your doctor can replace the battery quickly and easily in a minor surgical procedure.

Most household appliances do not affect newer pacemakers, but cellular phones, MRI (magnetic resonance imaging) scanners, and diathermy (a form of physical therapy that uses heat) machines can interfere with a pacemaker and may cause it to stop functioning. Ask your doctor what devices and situations you need to avoid to protect your pacemaker.

Implantable Defibrillators

Implantable defibrillators are used to treat ventricular fibrillation (see Cardiac Arrest; page 581). Surgery to implant a defibrillator is similar to the implantation of a permanent pacemaker.

Your doctor will monitor the defibrillator at regular intervals to ensure that it is working properly and to check the battery. When the battery signals that it is running low, the doctor removes the old defibrillator and implants a new one.

The same precautions and restrictions that apply to pacemakers apply to implantable defibrillators. However, if you have an implanted defibrillator, you should not drive a car or operate heavy machinery because of the risk that you could briefly lose consciousness when the defibrillator sends an electrical impulse to your heart.

Living With a Pacemaker or Implantable Defibrillator

Once you have recovered from the implantation surgery, you can return to your usual daily routine. Most people do not have any problems as long as they follow all their doctor's instructions, which usually include eating a prescribed diet, taking medication, and keeping all follow-up appointments.

Your doctor will give you a card that indicates that you have a pacemaker or implantable defibrillator. Always carry this card with you so that emergency medical personnel will know what treatment to provide in case of an emergency. Most people who have a pacemaker or implantable defibrillator become very aware of their heart and how it is supposed to function. If you notice that your heart is suddenly beating more slowly, more rapidly, or irregularly; if you feel dizzy or faint; or if you are short of breath, call 911 or your local emergency number, or go to the nearest hospital emergency department immediately.

Implantable defibrillator
An implantable defibrillator is an electronic device that is implanted just beneath the skin of the abdomen and attached with very thin wires to the heart. Whenever it is needed, the defibrillator delivers an electrical charge to the heart to slow a potentially dangerous rapid heartbeat and return the heartbeat to normal.

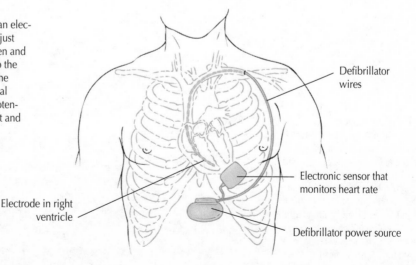

Defibrillator wires

Electronic sensor that monitors heart rate

Electrode in right ventricle

Defibrillator power source

fainting, angina (chest pain), or frequent urination. Despite the anxiety or fear it may cause, paroxysmal atrial tachycardia is not life-threatening, although sometimes it can lead to congestive heart failure (see page 570). If you have recurring symptoms of paroxysmal atrial tachycardia, see your doctor.

Diagnosis

To diagnose paroxysmal atrial tachycardia, your doctor will examine you, and may order an electro-cardiogram (ECG; see page 559) to evaluate the electrical activity of your heart. If your symptoms come and go, you may need to wear a portable elec-tronic ECG device called a Holter monitor (see page 580) to record the electrical activity of your heart over a period of 24 hours or more.

Treatment

If you have palpitations, try to slow your heart rate by holding your breath, taking a slow drink of cold water, or rinsing your face with cold water. If these measures do not help, try bearing down as if having a bowel movement. This is called the Valsalva maneuver and can sometimes correct an arrhythmia.

To help prevent further episodes, your doctor will probably recommend that you cut down on alcohol and caffeine and quit smoking (if you smoke). He or she may massage the carotid artery in your neck to try to slow your heart rate. The doc-tor may prescribe medication that decreases the excitability of the heart muscle and prevents the heart rate from increasing. In some cases, the doc-tor may inject a medication that helps slow a rapid heartbeat. In severe cases of persistent atrial tachy-cardia, the doctor may recommend cardioversion (see page 582), a procedure in which an electrical shock is administered to the heart while the person is under mild anesthesia.

Heart Valve Disorders

The heart has four valves. The mitral valve con-trols the flow of blood from the left atrium (the filling chamber on the upper left side of the heart) into the left ventricle (the pumping chamber on the lower left side of the heart). The tricuspid valve per-forms the same function between the right atrium and right ventricle. The pulmonary valve controls the opening from the right ventricle into the pul-monary artery, which carries blood into the lungs. The aortic valve controls the movement of blood from the left ventricle into the aorta (the main artery in the body).

How heart valves work
With each heartbeat, the left ventricle contracts and pumps fresh, oxygenated blood out of the heart. The aortic and pulmonary valves open to let blood flow out of the heart and into the arter-ies. Between heartbeats, the ventricles relax and the aortic and pulmonary valves close. The mitral and tricuspid valves then open to allow blood to flow into the ventricles from the atria. The constant and regular repetition of this cycle keeps blood circulating throughout the body.

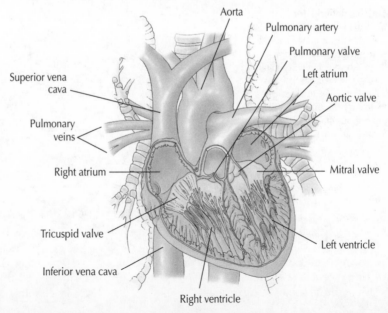

- Aorta
- Pulmonary artery
- Pulmonary valve
- Left atrium
- Aortic valve
- Superior vena cava
- Pulmonary veins
- Mitral valve
- Right atrium
- Tricuspid valve
- Left ventricle
- Inferior vena cava
- Right ventricle

When a valve does not open wide enough, the heart must work harder to pump out an adequate supply of blood to the rest of the body. When a valve does not close completely, some of the blood leaks back into the heart, which must then pump it out again. Both of these conditions increase the heart's workload and can lead to thickening of the heart muscle and eventually to heart failure.

Inflammation of a valve or other changes such as scarring can eventually lead to stenosis or insufficiency. Stenosis is thickening of a valve, which narrows its opening. Insufficiency results when a change in a valve prevents it from closing fully, allowing blood to flow back into the chamber.

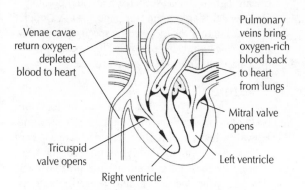

Blood flow to the heart
The veins bring oxygen-depleted blood back to the heart from body tissues for a fresh supply of oxygen. The tricuspid valve opens to allow the oxygen-poor blood into the right ventricle of the heart, which sends it to the lungs for oxygen. When the oxygen-rich blood returns to the heart from the lungs, the mitral valve opens to allow the blood into the left ventricle, the pumping chamber of the heart.

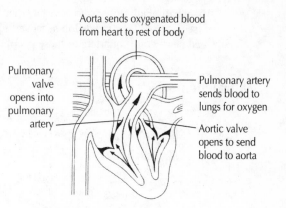

Blood flow from the heart
When the heart receives oxygen-depleted blood from the rest of the body, the pulmonary valve opens to send the blood from the heart into the lungs for a fresh supply of oxygen. The lungs send the oxygen-rich blood back to the heart, and the aortic valve opens to allow the blood into the aorta, which sends it to the rest of the body.

Mitral Stenosis

Mitral stenosis occurs when the mitral valve, which is located between the left atrium (one of the two upper chambers of the heart) and the left ventricle (one of the two lower, pumping chambers of the heart), becomes scarred, the valve flaps (leaflets) stick together, and the channel becomes abnormally narrow. To pump blood through the narrowed opening, the atrium enlarges, and pressure inside the chamber gradually rises. This pressure is passed back through the pulmonary veins and capillaries to the lungs, which, over a period of years, become congested. To keep blood flowing through the lungs at a normal rate, the right ventricle also pumps harder and becomes enlarged.

Symptoms

The main symptom of mitral stenosis is shortness of breath. Shortness of breath occurs most often after exercise, but it also can occur during the night or whenever you lie down. When you are sleeping, you may awaken suddenly, feeling as though you can't breathe. You may cough up small amounts of blood or blood-flecked, frothy phlegm. You may begin to wheeze, and breathing may become more difficult. These symptoms can be mistaken for bronchitis (see page 655).

As pressure builds throughout the circulatory system, you may experience fatigue, swollen ankles, or other symptoms of congestive heart failure (see page 570). Shortness of breath and fatigue can be disabling, especially if you are pregnant or if you have a chest infection, an overactive thyroid gland, or any condition that increases cardiac output. The main complication of mitral stenosis is atrial fibrillation (see page 581), which can cause heart failure and formation of a blood clot in the left atrium. A blood clot may break loose, travel through the bloodstream, and block a distant blood vessel, often in the brain, where it causes a stroke (see page 669).

About half of all people who have had rheumatic fever (see page 432) later develop heart valve damage, and nearly three quarters of these people have mitral stenosis. However, because rheumatic fever is rare today, mitral stenosis occurs much less frequently.

Diagnosis

In some cases, a doctor detects mitral stenosis during a routine physical examination when listening to the heart through a stethoscope. If additional testing is needed, your doctor may order a chest X-ray, an electrocardiogram (ECG; see page 559), and possibly a Doppler echocardiogram (see page 561). A Doppler echocardiogram can measure the speed of blood flow through the mitral valve, allowing the doctor to determine how much the valve has narrowed.

Treatment

Your doctor may prescribe a diuretic to help your body eliminate excess fluid and decrease swelling. However, because diuretics may also cause loss of potassium (a mineral that is essential for the heart muscle to contract and maintain a normal heart rhythm), your doctor also may prescribe a potassium supplement. If you have atrial fibrillation, your doctor will prescribe medication to control it. He or she also may prescribe anticoagulants to prevent the formation of blood clots in the left atrium.

If your mitral stenosis is severe and interferes with your daily activities, your doctor may recommend a surgical procedure called balloon valvuloplasty. In this procedure, the doctor guides a catheter (a thin, flexible tube) through an artery to the damaged valve. He or she then guides a tiny deflated balloon through the catheter to the valve and then inflates the balloon, opening the valve. This procedure is highly effective in relieving symptoms of mitral stenosis.

Doctors may recommend surgery for pregnant women who have severe symptoms of mitral stenosis. In an open-heart procedure called mitral valvotomy, the surgeon widens the valve. In many cases, symptoms do not return, or return years later. If your symptoms return, you may need to have a second mitral valvotomy, or your doctor may recommend heart valve replacement surgery (see page 590). Most people who have a heart valve replacement survive for at least 5 years.

If your symptoms are not severe, you should be able to lead an active life without treatment. However, you will need to take prescription antibiotics as a precaution before having any dental treatment or surgery, to protect you from developing infective

Mitral Stenosis

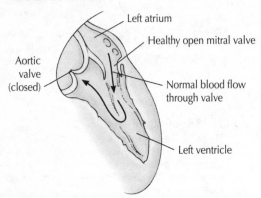

Healthy mitral valve
A healthy mitral valve allows oxygen-rich blood to flow from the left atrium into the left ventricle, the main pumping chamber of the heart.

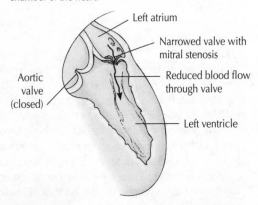

Mitral stenosis
In mitral stenosis, the mitral valve narrows, restricting blood flow from the left atrium into the left ventricle and causing pressure to rise in the atrium. This pressure can lead to increased pressure and congestion in the lungs, eventually resulting in congestive heart failure.

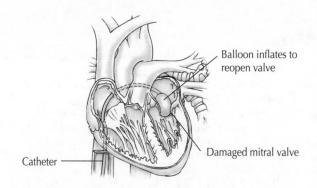

Catheter

Balloon inflates to reopen valve

Damaged mitral valve

Balloon valvuloplasty
In balloon valvuloplasty, the surgeon inserts a catheter (a thin, flexible tube) into an artery in the groin area and threads the catheter to the damaged heart valve. He or she then guides a tiny deflated balloon through the catheter to the valve and inflates the balloon, opening the valve. The balloon is then deflated and withdrawn along with the catheter.

endocarditis (see page 593), a potentially life-threatening infection of the inner lining of the heart muscle.

Mitral Regurgitation

If the mitral valve does not close properly, the blood circulating through the heart may leak back into the left atrium (one of the two upper chambers of the heart) from the left ventricle (one of the two lower, pumping chambers of the heart). This condition, called mitral regurgitation or mitral insufficiency, increases the heart's workload, causing the muscular heart wall to enlarge. The left atrium also becomes enlarged.

Mitral regurgitation often results from an abnormality of the mitral valve called mitral valve prolapse (see page 591), which causes the valve to move abnormally when the ventricles contract. When the valve flaps do not meet to close, blood leaks back through the opening. Mitral regurgitation may be congenital (present at birth), or it may result from infective endocarditis (see page 593), a potentially life-threatening infection of the inner lining of the heart muscle, or from any heart muscle disorder that causes the left ventricle to enlarge and widen.

Symptoms

Many people who have mitral regurgitation have no symptoms. Others may experience shortness of breath, fatigue, or other symptoms of congestive heart failure (see page 570). The increased

workload on the heart can permanently damage the left ventricle, preventing it from contracting properly and interfering with its ability to pump blood. If this occurs, the doctor will probably recommend replacing the valve. As the left atrium becomes enlarged, atrial fibrillation (see page 581) usually occurs.

Treatment

Treatment for mitral regurgitation is not necessary unless a person has symptoms. If you have mitral regurgitation, your doctor will prescribe antibiotics for you to take before having surgery or dental treatment to protect you from infective endocarditis.

Your doctor may prescribe a diuretic to help your body eliminate excess fluid and decrease swelling. However, because diuretics may also cause loss of potassium (a mineral that is essential for the heart muscle to contract and maintain a normal heart rhythm), your doctor also may prescribe a potassium supplement.

If your symptoms are severe, your doctor may recommend surgery to repair or replace the damaged valve (see next page). Although repairing the valve is preferable, it is not always possible. Replacement heart valves are either mechanical valves made of metal and plastic, or tissue valves made of human or animal tissue. The surgeon decides which type of replacement valve is appropriate. Mechanical replacement valves are efficient, but can cause blood clots to form that can break loose, travel through the bloodstream, and block an artery in the brain or elsewhere in the body. If you have a mechanical valve replacement, your doctor will prescribe an anticoagulant to help prevent the formation of blood clots. The opening and closing of a mechanical heart valve can also cause red blood cells to break down (hemolysis). Tissue valves are much less likely to cause clots to form, but they may be less durable than mechanical valves.

> **WARNING!**
>
> ### Heart Valve Replacement
> If you have had heart valve replacement surgery and you suddenly become short of breath, dizzy, or faint; if your urine looks abnormally dark; or if your chest begins to ache, see your doctor right away. These symptoms may indicate that the replacement valve is not working.

Heart Valve Replacement Surgery

Doctors perform heart valve replacement surgery to replace damaged heart valves with either mechanical valves made of metal and plastic, or tissue valves made of human or animal tissue.

During Surgery

During the procedure, you are under general anesthesia, and a heart-lung machine takes over your circulation and breathing. An anesthesiologist monitors your breathing and vital signs. The surgeon makes an incision, either along your breastbone or along a lower rib on your left side. Your ribs are parted, your heart is opened, and the damaged valve is removed. The new valve is then stitched in place. The procedure takes from 2 to 4 hours.

After Surgery

You will spend the first few days after surgery in the hospital's CCU (cardiac care unit) or ICU (intensive care unit). One or two drainage tubes will be placed in your chest and attached to suction bottles. You will breathe oxygen through a tube leading into your nose and you may need to use a ventilator (a device that assists with breathing). Your bladder will be drained with a catheter. You will receive fluid and blood through intravenous tubes, and your heart and vital signs will be monitored constantly.

Choice of Valves

The best type of valve for you depends on factors such as your age and general health. Mechanical valves last a long time, but you will need to take anticoagulant drugs to help prevent blood clot formation. Tissue valves made from animal or human tissue may need to be replaced after a period of years, but people who have tissue valves often do not need to take anticoagulants. The risk of complications is low with both types of valves.

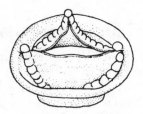

Heart valve made of tissue

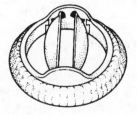

Mechanical heart valve

Replacement heart valves
Replacement heart valves may be mechanical or made of tissue. Mechanical valves are made of metal and plastic; tissue valves are made from animal or human tissue. A mechanical heart valve allows blood to flow in one direction by forcing the metal valve flaps (leaflets) apart. If blood begins to flow in the opposite direction, it forces the leaflets together firmly against the ring, closing the valve. A tissue heart valve functions like a natural heart valve.

Aorta
Pulmonary artery
Left atrium
Mitral valve
Right atrium
Left ventricle
Right ventricle

Replacement valve

Replacement heart valve in position

Mitral Valve Prolapse

Mitral valve prolapse is a deformity of the mitral valve that can sometimes produce mitral regurgitation (see page 589). Mitral valve prolapse produces a sound called a heart murmur that a doctor can hear through a stethoscope. This condition affects about 5 percent of Americans and is much more common in women than in men.

The cause of mitral valve prolapse is usually not known, but it may result from an inherited weakness in the connective tissue of the valve that allows the valve to bulge. Occasionally, mitral valve prolapse results from rheumatic fever (see page 432), heart disease (see page 558), or cardiomyopathy (a degenerative disease of the heart muscle).

Symptoms

Symptoms of mitral valve prolapse may include chest pain, arrhythmias (irregular heartbeats), shortness of breath, or fatigue. However, most people who have mitral valve prolapse have no symptoms.

Treatment

Treatment for mitral valve prolapse is usually not necessary. However, people who have both mitral valve prolapse and mitral regurgitation need to take antibiotic drugs before having any type of dental treatment or surgery to help prevent infective endocarditis (see page 593), a potentially life-threatening infection of the inner lining of the heart muscle. When mitral valve prolapse is severe enough to cause heart failure, a doctor may prescribe heart disease medications such as beta blockers, diuretics, or digitalis drugs, or he or she may recommend heart valve replacement surgery (see previous page).

Aortic Stenosis

Aortic stenosis occurs when the aortic valve (the valve between the aorta and the left ventricle) becomes abnormally thick or the valve flaps (leaflets) become stuck together, narrowing the opening. The aorta is the artery through which the left ventricle of the heart pumps blood to the body tissues. If the opening becomes narrowed, the volume of blood that the heart can pump decreases. In an effort to squeeze more blood through the valve and keep the volume of blood pumped by the heart normal, the muscular wall of the left ventricle thickens. This thicker, harder-working tissue requires more and more blood to keep working. The blood squirting past the obstructed valve produces a sound called a heart murmur that a doctor can hear through a stethoscope.

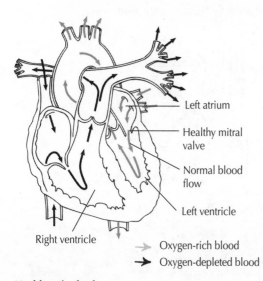

Healthy mitral valve
A healthy mitral valve allows oxygen-rich blood to flow from the left atrium into the left ventricle, the main pumping chamber of the heart.

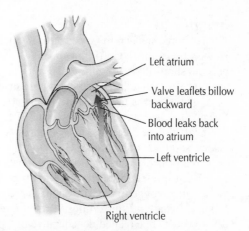

Mitral valve prolapse
In mitral valve prolapse, the valve leaflets can become thickened and elongated and may not close properly, causing blood to leak back into the left atrium from the left ventricle. This condition, called mitral regurgitation or mitral insufficiency, increases the heart's workload, causing the muscular heart wall and the left atrium to enlarge.

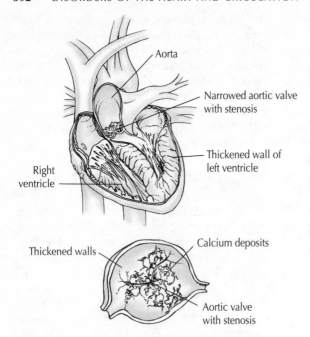

Aorta

Narrowed aortic valve with stenosis

Thickened wall of left ventricle

Right ventricle

Thickened walls

Calcium deposits

Aortic valve with stenosis

Close-up of valve with stenosis

Aortic stenosis
In aortic stenosis, the aortic valve becomes thickened and narrowed, allowing less blood to flow through. Because the left ventricle must then work harder to pump the same volume of blood, the ventricle wall gradually thickens and the ventricle becomes enlarged. Aortic stenosis can lead to irregular heart rhythms, heart failure, or a heart attack.

Symptoms
At first, aortic stenosis may produce no symptoms. However, as the condition worsens, you will become short of breath during and after physical activity. You may experience chest pain or dizziness, or you may faint when you exert yourself. Eventually, you may develop symptoms of congestive heart failure (see page 570) such as swollen ankles, shortness of breath, or fatigue.

Three possible causes of aortic stenosis are a congenital (present at birth) malformation of the valve called congenital aortic stenosis (see page 591), scarring and thickening of the valve that develops with age (called degenerative or calcific aortic stenosis), or narrowing of the valve as a result of rheumatic fever (see page 432). For unknown reasons, men are about three times more likely to develop aortic stenosis than women.

As the workload of the left ventricle increases, the blood supply to the heart muscle is reduced,

which can cause chest pain, a heart attack, ventricular fibrillation (see Cardiac Arrest; page 581), or sudden death. Once symptoms develop, the risk of dying increases significantly. About half of people who develop symptoms of aortic stenosis die within 3 years. If you have symptoms of aortic stenosis, see your doctor as soon as possible.

Diagnosis
A doctor can detect aortic stenosis during a routine physical examination. A chest X-ray may show whether your heart is enlarged. An electrocardiogram (ECG; see page 559) can help the doctor determine the source of the problem. A Doppler ultrasound scan (see page 111) can also help the doctor evaluate the stenosis. The diagnosis can be confirmed with cardiac catheterization (see below).

Treatment
If you have mild aortic stenosis, you will need to avoid strenuous activity. Your doctor will probably recommend regular, moderate exercise such as walking. When you have sexual intercourse, let your partner be the more active participant. You will need to take antibiotics before having any kind of dental treatment or surgery to protect against infective endocarditis (see page 593), a potentially life-threatening infection of the inner lining of the heart muscle. You will also need to see your cardiologist for a yearly heart examination.

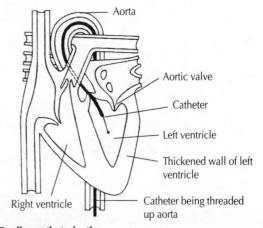

Aorta

Aortic valve

Catheter

Left ventricle

Thickened wall of left ventricle

Right ventricle

Catheter being threaded up aorta

Cardiac catheterization
Aortic stenosis can be confirmed with cardiac catheterization. In this procedure, a catheter (a thin, flexible tube) containing an electronic device that measures pressure is guided through an artery to the heart to measure the pressure in the left ventricle and in the aorta.

Surgery is the usual treatment for aortic stenosis that is causing symptoms. If the doctor thinks that surgery may be necessary to repair the stenosis, you will probably have a coronary angiogram (see page 561) to evaluate the severity of the aortic stenosis and determine if there are any blockages in the coronary arteries.

The type of surgery performed most often is heart valve replacement surgery (see page 590). Balloon valvuloplasty (see page 589), a procedure in which a catheter containing a balloon is passed through a blood vessel to the valve to enlarge the valve opening, may be performed on people who are not good candidates for heart valve replacement surgery.

Aortic Insufficiency

If the aortic valve (the valve between the aorta and the left ventricle) does not close properly, aortic insufficiency (also called aortic incompetence or aortic regurgitation) may develop. The left ventricle of the heart pumps blood through the aorta (the main artery in the body) to body tissues. If the aortic valve does not close properly, blood can leak back into the left ventricle, causing a sound called a heart murmur, which a doctor can hear through a stethoscope. A congenital (present at birth) abnormality of the valve is usually the cause of aortic insufficiency. Other possible causes include infective endocarditis (a potentially life-threatening infection of the inner lining of the heart muscle; see right), syphilis (see page 483), or stretching of the tissues that support the aortic valve.

In severe cases of aortic insufficiency, the left ventricle enlarges and its walls thicken as the heart responds to an increased workload. The large volume of blood pumped into the aorta may cause the arteries to pulsate abnormally, which is a sign of severe aortic insufficiency. In some cases, the aortic valve ruptures as a result of damage caused by infective endocarditis.

Symptoms

In most cases, symptoms do not occur until many years after the problem begins to develop. However, if the valve suddenly ruptures or if the heart muscle loses its effectiveness, a person can have shortness of breath, fatigue, or other symptoms of congestive heart failure (see page 570).

Diagnosis

To diagnose aortic insufficiency, a doctor performs a physical examination and will order diagnostic tests such as an echocardiogram (see page 561), an ultrasound examination of the heart, or an electrocardiogram (ECG; see page 559), a recording of the electrical activity of the heart. The doctor also may order blood tests to rule out rheumatoid arthritis (see page 918), ankylosing spondylitis (see page 1002), or syphilis.

Treatment

The treatment for aortic insufficiency is the same as the treatment for aortic stenosis (see page 591). Heart valve replacement surgery (see page 590) is usually required.

Infective Endocarditis

The endocardium is the inner lining of the heart muscle and covering of the heart valves. If the endocardium is damaged, such as from mitral regurgitation (see page 589), bacteria or other germs can infect the damaged area. As the microorganisms multiply, they cause more damage to the endocardium and may travel through the bloodstream to other parts of the body. The microorganisms can form infected blood clots that can lodge in small arteries and block blood flow. Gradually, the multiplying microorganisms cause severe damage to the heart valves, resulting in heart failure (see page 570).

Most people who develop infective endocarditis have an underlying heart valve disorder, such as mitral valve prolapse (see page 591) or congenital (present at birth) lesions of the heart valves. Heart valve replacement surgery (see page 590) can sometimes lead to infective endocarditis. Bacteria also can enter the bloodstream during minor surgery, tooth extractions, teeth cleaning, endoscopy (an examination of the inside of the body using a viewing instrument), or by injecting illicit drugs with contaminated syringes or needles. To prevent infective endocarditis, people who have heart disease need to take antibiotics immediately before surgery or dental treatment or promptly after any skin infections develop. This precaution helps destroy any bacteria that might otherwise enter the bloodstream and cause infective endocarditis.

Symptoms

A person with infective endocarditis usually has a fever of less than 102°F. Other possible symptoms include sudden chills (especially after the bacteria have spread through the bloodstream), headaches, aching joints, fatigue, and loss of appetite. If the heart valves are affected, symptoms of heart failure (see page 570) may occur eventually.

If blood clots form, symptoms depend on their location. For example, if clots form in the hands or feet, you may have painful lumps in the tips of your fingers or toes, or small bruises behind your nails. A clot that lodges in the brain can cause a stroke (see page 669). Clots from bacterial endocarditis can lodge anywhere in the body, sometimes causing small abscesses (pus-filled cavities surrounded by inflamed tissue) to form. Bacterial endocarditis can also cause anemia or kidney disease, both of which usually clear up after the infection is treated successfully. If you have any of the symptoms described above, see your doctor as soon as possible.

Diagnosis

Because the symptoms of infective endocarditis can be caused by a number of diseases and conditions, tell your doctor if you have had a heart valve disorder or a heart murmur, or any of the symptoms described above.

If your doctor thinks you may have infective endocarditis, he or she will admit you to a hospital and will order blood tests to identify the type of microorganism that is causing the infection. You will also have a Doppler ultrasound scan (see page 111) to help determine the location and severity of damage to the valve.

Treatment

To treat infective endocarditis, a doctor will prescribe an antibiotic to fight the microorganism that is causing the infection. If bacterial endocarditis is diagnosed and treated effectively within 6 weeks of infection, there is a 90 percent chance of eliminating the infection. Long-term effects depend on the valve that is damaged and the severity of the damage.

Pulmonary Hypertension

Pulmonary hypertension is elevated blood pressure in the lungs. The disorder can result from any disease that blocks the flow of blood or oxygen through the lungs, such as congenital (present at birth) heart disease (see page 389), chronic bronchitis (see page 655), and emphysema (see page 656). People who live for many years at high altitudes have an increased risk of pulmonary hypertension. Whatever the cause, the main result is increased pressure inside the pulmonary arteries. Over time, this pressure leads to thickening of the arteries, which obstructs blood flow. In an attempt to compensate for poor circulation, the right side of the heart becomes enlarged. The increased workload can eventually cause heart failure (see page 570). Women are five times more likely than men to develop pulmonary hypertension.

Symptoms

Pulmonary hypertension often causes no symptoms until the condition is advanced, when the main symptom is swollen ankles. Your skin may have a bluish tinge because your blood does not contain enough oxygen. The low oxygen content of the blood stimulates the production of more red blood cells, a condition called polycythemia (see page 627). As the number of red cells increases, the blood becomes thicker and harder to push through the small blood vessels in the lungs, further increasing blood pressure in the pulmonary arteries and decreasing the volume of blood pumped by the heart. If you already have shortness of breath because of underlying lung disease, pulmonary hypertension is likely to make breathing even more difficult. You also may experience other symptoms of heart failure, such as fatigue.

Diagnosis

To diagnose pulmonary hypertension, a doctor will take a medical history and perform a physical examination. He or she will order blood tests to determine blood count (see page 145) and to evaluate kidney and liver function. The doctor also will order a chest X-ray to check for an enlarged pulmonary artery, and an echocardiogram (ECG; see page 561), a recording of the electrical activity of the heart, to determine if the heart is enlarged or if it is not pumping efficiently.

Treatment

Treatment of pulmonary hypertension depends on the underlying disorder that is causing it. Daily home treatment with oxygen (which reduces spasms in the pulmonary arteries) sometimes helps lower pulmonary blood pressure. If pulmonary hypertension is caused by chronic lung disease, the goal of long-term treatment is to stop further deterioration of the lungs. Your doctor may prescribe antibiotics and will make sure you get yearly flu shots (see page 145) and a vaccination against pneumonia (see page 145) every 5 to 7 years to help prevent chest infections.

Heart failure caused by pulmonary hypertension can be relieved with rest and treatment with oxygen and diuretics (which eliminate excess fluid from the body). In some cases, vasodilator drugs are effective in reducing blood pressure in the pulmonary arteries by widening the blood vessels.

People who have pulmonary hypertension and progressive heart and lung disease can be treated successfully with a heart and lung transplant (see page 658) or, if the heart has not been damaged, a lung transplant (see page 658). Major surgery of this kind carries substantial risks and is performed only after all other treatments have been unsuccessful.

Heart Muscle and Pericardium Disorders

The walls of the heart are made of muscle that contracts rhythmically about 100,000 times a day. If heart muscle is diseased or damaged, the force of the heartbeat decreases and reduces blood circulation. The term cardiomyopathy is used to refer to several forms of heart muscle disease. In cardiomyopathy, the tiny muscle fibers of the heart are damaged, often from an unknown cause. Over time, this damage decreases the ability of the heart muscle to contract, leading to widening of the ventricles (the pumping chambers of the heart) and eventually to heart failure (see page 570). In some people, the damage is confined to the heart. In other people, other organs are affected as well. Cardiomyopathies generally occur less often than most other types of heart disorders. Although some types of cardiomyopathy run in families, the cause is usually unknown.

Myocarditis

Myocarditis, or inflammation of the heart muscle, is a type of cardiomyopathy that occurs as a rare complication of an infection, usually caused by a virus. In mild cases, the only symptoms may be slight chest pain, shortness of breath, and a rapid pulse. In more severe cases, such as those caused by diphtheria, myocarditis can lead to heart failure (see page 570), third-degree heart block (see page 583), or death.

Diagnosis
If your doctor thinks you may have myocarditis, he or she may order a chest X-ray; an electrocardiogram (ECG; see page 559), a recording of the electrical activity of the heart; and an echocardiogram (see page 561), an ultrasound examination of the heart. You may also have a heart muscle biopsy, in which a small amount of tissue is removed from the heart muscle in a cardiac catheterization procedure (see page 592) and examined under a microscope.

Treatment
Myocarditis is usually caused by a virus, for which there is no specific treatment. The doctor will recommend complete rest. In some cases, a doctor will prescribe a corticosteroid drug to reduce inflammation.

Nutritional Cardiomyopathy

Heart muscle can be damaged by toxins. In the United States, the most severe form of cardiomyopathy caused by toxins occurs among people who drink alcohol heavily. Excessive intake of alcohol can poison the heart muscle. In rare cases, inadequate intake of vitamin B1 (which is often deficient in heavy drinkers) causes cardiomyopathy.

Symptoms
The symptoms of nutritional cardiomyopathy vary greatly from one person to another. Symptoms may include palpitations (heartbeats that you're aware of) or an irregular or very rapid heartbeat, or

swollen hands and feet. Because damage to the heart muscle can lead to disorders such as atrial fibrillation (see page 581) and heart failure (see page 570), a person also may have symptoms of these disorders.

Treatment

A doctor will recommend that a person with nutritional cardiomyopathy stop drinking alcohol. The doctor may also prescribe dietary changes or vitamin supplements. The condition improves in about one third of the people who give up alcohol. In the remaining two thirds, treatment is the same as that for heart failure.

Hypertrophic Cardiomyopathy

Defective cells in the heart muscle, possibly as a result of a congenital (present at birth) abnormality, may cause the heart muscle to weaken. To compensate for the weakened heart muscle, the walls of the heart may thicken. In severe cases, the thickened walls can interfere with blood flow into and out of the heart.

Symptoms

Symptoms of hypertrophic cardiomyopathy include fatigue, chest pain, shortness of breath, and palpitations (heartbeats that you're aware of).

Diagnosis

To diagnose hypertrophic cardiomyopathy, a doctor will order diagnostic tests such as a chest X-ray; an electrocardiogram (ECG; see page 559), a recording of the electrical activity of the heart; and an echocardiogram (see page 561), an ultrasound examination of the heart.

Treatment

There is no cure for hypertrophic cardiomyopathy, but symptoms can be relieved with heart disease medications such as beta blockers, which help slow the heart rate, and diuretics, which help eliminate excess fluid from the body. Calcium channel blockers help the heart fill with blood more efficiently. If symptoms become severe, especially if blood flow from the heart is obstructed, surgery to remove some of the excess heart muscle can significantly improve symptoms. Some people who have heart failure as a result of hypertrophic cardiomyopathy will need a heart transplant (see page 573).

Acute Pericarditis

Pericarditis is inflammation of the pericardium, the membrane that surrounds the heart. When the pericardium becomes inflamed, fluid can collect in the space between the membrane and the heart (called pericardial effusion). The inflammation in acute pericarditis is usually caused by a viral infection, but it can also result from tuberculosis (see page 663), rheumatic fever (see page 432), a disease of connective tissue such as lupus (see page 920), or chronic kidney failure (see page 817). In rare cases, acute pericarditis follows a heart attack (see page 567) or a chest injury. Pericarditis often occurs along with more serious illness and occasionally can follow open-heart surgery.

Symptoms

The main symptom of acute pericarditis is severe pain, usually in the center of the chest, that may radiate to the left shoulder. The pain of acute pericarditis becomes worse if you breathe deeply, cough, or twist your body. Chest pain, especially if it occurs along with breathing difficulty, can be a symptom of a serious illness such as pneumonia (see page 660), pulmonary embolism (see page 606), and heart attack.

You may also be short of breath and have a slight fever. As fluid collects around the heart, it creates pressure that can interfere with the normal filling of the heart with blood and cause a severe decrease in the volume of blood pumped by the heart, which can lead to death.

WARNING!

Chest Pain

Chest pain can be a symptom of a heart attack. If you have severe chest pain that lasts longer than 10 to 15 minutes, call 911 or your local emergency number immediately.

Diagnosis

After examining you, your doctor will probably order diagnostic tests such as a chest X-ray; an echocardiogram (see page 561), an ultrasound examination of the heart; an electrocardiogram (ECG; see page 559), a recording of the electrical activity of the heart; or blood tests. The doctor may insert a needle into your chest to remove some of the fluid for examination in a laboratory. These tests will help determine if you have acute pericarditis and, if you do, will help determine the cause of the inflammation.

Treatment

Acute pericarditis caused by a viral infection usually clears up without treatment. If the pain is severe, the doctor will probably prescribe a nonsteroidal anti-inflammatory drug such as aspirin, ibuprofen, or indomethacin. The doctor may insert a needle into the chest to remove some of the fluid and relieve pressure on the heart.

The inflammation usually subsides within 10 to 14 days and leaves no aftereffects. In rare cases, such as when acute pericarditis occurs a few weeks after a heart attack, a doctor may prescribe a corticosteroid drug to reduce inflammation. When acute pericarditis results from a connective tissue disorder or a metabolic disorder, the underlying disease must be treated.

Constrictive Pericarditis

Pericarditis is inflammation of the pericardium, the membrane that surrounds the heart. The course of constrictive pericarditis is different from that of acute pericarditis (see previous article). Constrictive pericarditis results from long-term inflammation, frequently of unknown cause, but sometimes from a chronic infection such as tuberculosis (see page 663) or from radiation therapy (see page 565), which can thicken, scar, and shrink the pericardium until the heart cannot fill with blood normally. Because tuberculosis is no longer widespread and radiation techniques have improved, constrictive pericarditis is not common.

Symptoms

The main symptoms of constrictive pericarditis are swollen legs and a swollen abdomen caused by fluid accumulation in those areas. Symptoms of heart failure (see page 570) such as shortness of breath and fatigue may also occur. Without surgical treatment, severe heart failure is likely to develop.

Diagnosis

If you have symptoms of heart failure, your doctor will probably recommend diagnostic tests such as a chest X-ray; an echocardiogram (see page 561), an ultrasound examination of the heart; and an electrocardiogram (ECG; see page 559), a recording of the electrical activity of the heart. Your doctor may also recommend cardiac catheterization (see page 592), a procedure to measure the pressure in the arteries and ventricles and to check for possible underlying diseases. The doctor may also order a CT scan (see page 562) or an MRI (see page 113) to evaluate the thickness of the pericardium. He or she will probably order tests of the skin and of phlegm to rule out tuberculosis.

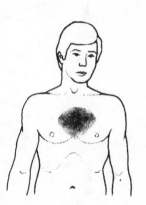

Location of constrictive pericarditis pain

Treatment

Constrictive pericarditis can be treated with a surgical procedure called pericardectomy. In this procedure, the surgeon carefully removes the thickened pericardium from the surface of the heart, which relieves the symptoms significantly.

Disorders of the Circulation

Blood follows two distinct circuits as it flows through the body. In the longer circuit (called the systemic circulation), the heart pumps oxygen-rich blood throughout the body to supply the tissues with oxygen and nutrients and to pick up carbon dioxide and other waste products. In the shorter circuit (called the pulmonary circulation), the heart pumps oxygen-depleted blood through the lungs to receive a fresh supply of oxygen and discard carbon dioxide. The blood then returns to the heart, and the cycle begins again.

The arteries that carry blood away from the heart have thick, muscular walls to absorb the peaks of blood pressure that occur every time the heart beats. The aorta (the main artery in the body) has an internal diameter of about 1¼ inches. It branches into smaller arteries, then into tiny arterioles, and finally into microscopic capillaries with thin, porous walls that allow easy exchange of oxygen and nutrients for carbon dioxide and other waste products. Gradually the capillaries combine to form small veins called venules, and the venules combine to form soft-walled, flexible veins, which return oxygen-depleted blood to the heart.

Blood does not flow at a constant rate to all parts of the body. The rate varies according to the amount of blood the tissues need at a given time.

For example, when you are running, your leg muscles receive more blood than they do when you are resting. When you feel cold, less blood flows in superficial blood vessels near the chilled skin, and more blood flows in deeper vessels, to conserve heat. This pattern reverses when you feel hot, making you perspire to avoid becoming overheated.

The circulatory system is complex, and it can stop working if the heart malfunctions or if problems develop inside the blood vessels. For example, artery walls may weaken or harden, causing circulation problems or high blood pressure. Blood clots can form and block blood vessels, and a number of other disorders, some mild and some severe, can affect circulation.

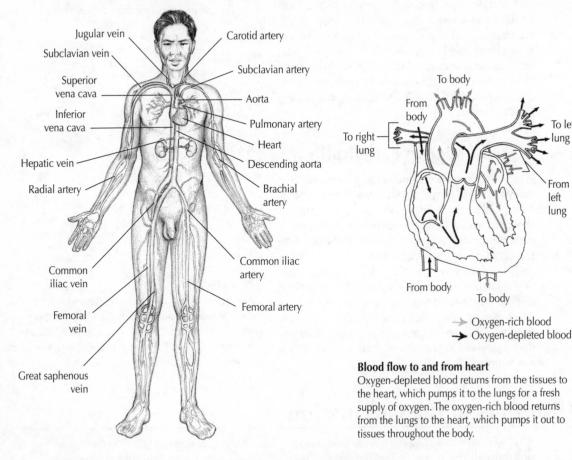

Blood flow to and from heart
Oxygen-depleted blood returns from the tissues to the heart, which pumps it to the lungs for a fresh supply of oxygen. The oxygen-rich blood returns from the lungs to the heart, which pumps it out to tissues throughout the body.

The circulatory system
The circulatory system, which consists of the heart and blood vessels, continuously transports oxygen and other nutrients to all the cells of the body and removes carbon dioxide and other waste products. Arteries carry oxygen-rich blood away from the heart; veins return oxygen-depleted blood to the heart to receive a fresh supply of oxygen.

Aneurysms

An aneurysm is an abnormal ballooning of a damaged or weakened area in an artery wall. If part of an artery wall is damaged or weakened, the force of blood flowing through the artery may cause the affected area to balloon outward. Although aneurysms can form in any artery, they usually form in the aorta (the main artery in the body) or in arteries in the brain. An aneurysm can develop for any of the following reasons:

- **Defective artery wall** An artery wall has an outer, middle, and inner layer of tissue. In some people, the muscular middle layer, which provides support and strength to the artery, has a congenital (present at birth) defect that makes it thin and weak. As blood flows through the defective artery, it may produce a saclike swelling (called a saccular aneurysm) at the weakened area. This type of aneurysm occurs most often in men and in people who have close relatives (especially parents or siblings) who have had an aneurysm, indicating a genetic component. Aneurysms caused by congenital defects usually form in the arteries at the base of the brain.

- **Inflamed artery** Inflammation caused by disorders such as infective endocarditis (see page 593), polyarteritis nodosa (see page 927), or syphilis (see page 483) may weaken part of an artery wall. If the cause of the inflammation is unknown, the condition is called arteritis. Normal blood flow through the inflamed artery can cause the weakened section of the artery wall to bulge.

- **Damaged artery wall** A portion of the muscular middle layer of an artery wall may slowly weaken as a result of a chronic (long-lasting) condition such as atherosclerosis (see page 557). An aneurysm caused by atherosclerosis is usually a ballooning of both artery walls along a short length of the artery (called a fusiform aneurysm). High blood pressure can accelerate damage to artery walls and is often a factor in the formation of aneurysms. Increased blood pressure in an artery can stretch the artery wall in various ways. In some cases, the layers of the artery wall split and blood flows between them, causing a bulge (called a dissecting aneurysm) in the artery wall.

The main risk of an aneurysm is that it might rupture and cause severe internal bleeding, depriving tissues and organs of oxygen and vital nutrients. If the bleeding significantly reduces the volume of blood in the body, the entire circulatory system could stop functioning. Without immediate medical help, a ruptured aneurysm in the aorta is usually fatal.

Three Types of Aneurysms

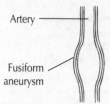

Fusiform aneurysm
A fusiform aneurysm forms when the artery wall is weakened all the way around the artery, like a spindle. This type of aneurysm is more common than saccular or dissecting aneurysms.

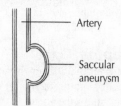

Saccular aneurysm
A saccular aneurysm develops when part of the muscular middle layer of an artery wall is damaged. This type of aneurysm occurs most often in men and in people with close relatives who have had an aneurysm.

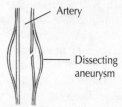

Dissecting aneurysm
High blood pressure may cause the inner and outer layers of an artery wall to split apart. Blood is then forced between the layers, causing the outer wall to stretch. Blood trapped between the layers tends to form clots, which may fill the aneurysm and seal it off. This dissected aneurysm can then become chronic without causing any problems. However, there is a risk that the aneurysm will grow or rupture.

An aneurysm that does not rupture can disturb blood flow, creating turbulence that can lead to the formation of a thrombus (blood clot). Tiny pieces of a thrombus (called emboli) can break away and travel through the bloodstream, blocking smaller arteries and damaging tissues and organs. An aneurysm that forms in the ascending aorta may stretch the aortic valve in the heart, causing aortic insufficiency (see page 593). Aneurysms can also grow and press on and damage nearby organs, nerves, blood vessels, and other tissues.

Risk Factors

Because atherosclerosis (see page 557) and high blood pressure (see page 574) damage artery walls, people who have these conditions have an increased risk of developing aneurysms. Following a healthy lifestyle—including eating a low-fat diet, exercising regularly, not smoking, and managing stress—and taking cholesterol-lowering drugs or antihypertensive medications can help prevent or slow the progression of atherosclerosis and help keep blood pressure under control, thereby decreasing the risk of aneurysms.

Symptoms

Symptoms of aortic aneurysms depend on the type of aneurysm, the section of the aorta affected, and the structures the aneurysm presses on. Saccular or fusiform aneurysms usually do not cause symptoms. However, if a large aneurysm forms in the thoracic aorta (the portion of the aorta that passes through the chest), it may cause chest pain, back pain, hoarseness, shortness of breath, difficulty swallowing, or a persistent cough. A dissecting aneurysm in the thoracic aorta usually causes severe chest pain and shortness of breath, and may be mistaken for a heart attack.

A large saccular or fusiform aneurysm in the abdominal aorta (the portion of the aorta that passes through the abdomen) is often visible as a pulsating lump on the surface of the abdomen. If the aneurysm is toward the back, it may press on the spine and cause severe backache, especially if the aneurysm expands or ruptures. Dissecting aneurysms of the abdominal aorta are rare. When they develop, the main symptom is severe abdominal or intestinal pain.

Although aneurysms in the peripheral arteries of the arms and legs are not common and are not considered dangerous, an aneurysm that forms in the artery behind the knee can suddenly clot, blocking blood flow and causing gangrene (see page 601) of the leg.

If you have symptoms of an aortic aneurysm or if you notice an unexplainable lump anywhere on your body, especially on your abdomen, and particularly if it throbs, see your doctor right away. Most people who have a ruptured aneurysm die before they can get emergency medical treatment.

Diagnosis

Aneurysms are often detected during a routine physical examination or when a person has an ultrasound (see page 111), a CT scan (see page 112), an MRI (see page 113), or conventional X-rays for another purpose. If a person has symptoms of an aneurysm, these imaging procedures are often used to confirm the diagnosis.

Treatment

The usual treatment for an aneurysm is surgery to repair or replace the affected portion of the artery with a tiny plastic tube. In people who do not have other health problems, most elective surgical procedures performed on aneurysms in either the thoracic (chest) or abdominal aortas are successful.

If an aneurysm in the thoracic aorta can be treated with surgery, chances of recovery are very good. If the aneurysm cannot be treated surgically, chances of survival are poor. In general, small aneurysms in the abdominal aorta are not life-threatening and usually do not require immediate treatment. Aneurysms in the abdominal aorta are removed surgically only if they are large or are expanding. Before recommending surgery, a doctor will usually monitor the aneurysm with ultrasound or CT scanning to determine how rapidly it is expanding. If a person is in generally good health, elective surgery on a large or rapidly expanding aneurysm carries far less risk than emergency surgery performed after the aneurysm has ruptured.

In a procedure called stent grafting, the doctor inserts a thin, flexible wire into an artery in the groin area and, observing the aorta on a video monitor, threads the wire to the aortic aneurysm. He or she then guides a tiny tube called a stent along the wire to the aneurysm. Once the stent is inside the aneurysm, the doctor expands it until it bridges the area of the aneurysm. By providing a sturdy new channel for blood flow, the stent relieves pressure on the weakened artery walls.

Arterial Embolism

An embolus is usually a fragment of clotted blood or a piece of a fatty deposit (plaque) that is carried along in the bloodstream. The embolus may be very small, but, because the arteries branch into smaller and smaller blood vessels as they deliver blood to the tissues, the embolus will eventually get stuck and create a blockage (called an embolism) that prevents blood from reaching the tissues beyond the blockage. An embolus may develop in the heart after a heart attack (see page 567) or from another heart disorder. It may be a fragment of bacterial growth resulting from bacterial endocarditis (see page 593). In rare cases, an embolus may be a tiny foreign object that entered an artery through a wound, or a gas bubble that formed in the tissues.

The severity of an arterial embolism depends on its size and location. Some organs, such as the brain, kidneys, and heart, are extremely sensitive to sudden decreases in blood supply. Other organs have multiple sources of blood and may not be affected significantly by an embolism. Although arterial embolisms most often affect the brain and legs, they can occur anywhere in the body.

Symptoms

A small embolism usually goes unnoticed unless it blocks the blood supply to a large area or to a very sensitive organ such as the heart or brain. An embolism in the intestine may cause loss of function in the affected part of the intestine and may produce symptoms of an intestinal obstruction (see page 759). To learn about the symptoms of a cerebral embolism, read the articles on stroke (see page 669) and transient ischemic attacks (see page 675). To learn about the symptoms of an embolism that affects the heart muscle, read the article on heart attack. In other parts of the body, especially the arms and legs, pain may be the earliest symptom, followed by a tingling or prickling sensation. The affected area eventually becomes numb, weak, and cold. If the embolism is in an arm or leg, the skin appears pale at first but later appears blue as sluggish blood flow depletes oxygen and leaves behind bluish, oxygen-poor hemoglobin. Both legs can be affected if a large embolus blocks the aorta (the main artery in the body) where it divides in two. This type of embolism (called a saddle embolism) can cause severe pain in the abdomen, back, and legs.

If a major artery is blocked, the tissues it supplies with oxygen and nutrients will be damaged if the blockage is not treated promptly, and gangrene (tissue death) may develop (see next article). In the brain, an embolism can cause a fatal stroke. If a blockage occurs in the aorta, the chance of survival without surgery is only 50 percent.

Diagnosis

A doctor makes a diagnosis of arterial embolism based on a person's symptoms and a physical examination. He or she will order an arteriogram (see page 561), an MRI (see page 113), or a Doppler ultrasound (see page 111) to determine the location and size of the embolism before recommending surgery or other treatment.

Treatment

A doctor may prescribe anticoagulants (blood thinners) such as heparin and thrombolytic agents (clot busters) such as streptokinase or tPA (tissue plasminogen activator) to reduce clotting and break up any clots that have formed. The combination of these drugs triggers the body's natural processes to dissolve the blood clot and prevent further clots from forming.

If, despite drug treatment, a major artery remains blocked after a few hours, surgery will be necessary to prevent gangrene. The procedure, called an embolectomy, involves inserting a catheter (a thin, flexible tube) into the affected artery and drawing the embolus out through the catheter. With prompt surgery, a person usually recovers completely.

Gangrene

Gangrene is tissue death. Its characteristic black color is a sign that the skin and, often, underlying muscle and bone are dead. The two basic types of gangrene are dry gangrene and infected (wet) gangrene. Dry gangrene does not involve infection; it occurs when blood flow to the tissues is blocked or reduced. This may result from an arterial embolism (see previous article) or from poor circulation caused by conditions that affect the blood vessels, including diabetes (see page 889), atherosclerosis (see page 557), or severe frostbite (see page 165). The oxygen-deprived tissue dies, but the gangrene does not spread.

Infected gangrene may develop when an area of muscle and overlying skin is killed by toxins produced by bacteria called Clostridia, which multiply in dead tissue. This condition is also called gas gangrene, since the bacteria produce gas in the tissues. Infection with these bacteria may occur when a wound is contaminated. Surgeons can usually prevent infected gangrene by following careful wound hygiene precautions such as removing all of the affected tissue and all contaminated materials. Sometimes, to prevent gangrene, part of an arm or leg must be amputated. The term infected gangrene is also used when dry gangrene becomes infected with a microorganism other than Clostridia.

Symptoms

Dry gangrene may develop in the foot or leg of anyone with poor circulation. In the early stages, the limb is cold, with a dull, aching pain that increases with physical activity. If your foot is painful or unusually pale and you have poor circulation, see your doctor immediately. Pain is also the main symptom of infected gangrene. The area around the wound becomes red, swollen, extremely painful, and oozes pus. The wound may develop an unpleasant odor. The person usually experiences extreme pain while the tissue is dying, but once the tissue is dead, the pain disappears. The tissue slowly turns black, and a visible line separates the dead tissue from living tissue.

Treatment

For dry gangrene, a doctor will treat the underlying disorder that is blocking blood flow to the affected area. He or she may prescribe antibiotics to prevent infection. Doctors treat infected gangrene with antibiotics to kill the bacteria and with surgery to remove the dying and dead skin, muscle, and bone. Usually some healthy tissue next to the dead, gangrenous tissue also must be removed. To prevent the infection from spreading to healthy tissue, the doctor may recommend soaking an affected hand or foot in an antiseptic solution, removing any layer of pus that forms, and elevating the affected hand or foot as often as possible.

Preventing Gangrene

Dry gangrene can be prevented by taking steps to help maintain good circulation, such as exercising regularly and not smoking. If you have diabetes, work with your doctor to keep the disease under control. Take special care of your feet (see page 892) and always wear shoes that fit properly. If you

have symptoms of dry gangrene, see your doctor immediately for treatment.

Varicose Veins

Varicose veins are veins directly beneath the skin that have become stretched and twisted over time. This condition usually occurs in the legs when veins lose their elasticity and widen, causing the edges of the valves inside the veins to separate. The veins are then unable to return blood to the heart, causing blood to collect in the veins, widening them further.

Varicose veins are often visible because they lie directly under the skin. Although they are often unsightly, varicose veins seldom cause serious symptoms or health problems. Some people inherit a

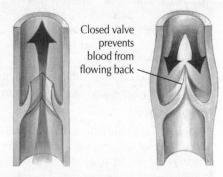

Closed valve
prevents
blood from
flowing back

Normal blood flow in healthy veins

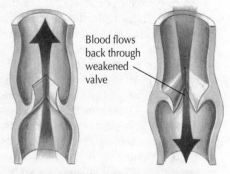

Blood flows
back through
weakened
valve

Abnormal blood flow in varicose veins

Blood flow in normal veins and in varicose veins
Varicose veins occur when the valves in the veins are no longer able to close properly, which interferes with the ability of the veins to return blood to the heart. Blood flows backward through the open valve, increasing pressure inside the vein and causing it to widen and stretch.

tendency to develop severe varicose veins. Varicose veins in the legs often result from excess pressure caused by standing for long periods. In severe cases, blood can clot on the inflamed, roughened walls of varicose veins, which can lead to thrombophlebitis (see next page), a more serious condition.

Symptoms

Varicose veins usually appear bluish and swollen and are more prominent when you are standing. They usually occur at the back of the calf or on the inside of the leg between the ankle and the groin. Varicose veins can also occur in the rectal area (see page 777), in the vagina during pregnancy, or where the esophagus meets the stomach in advanced cases of cirrhosis of the liver (see page 790).

A varicose vein in the leg may gradually enlarge. The vein may become tender to the touch, and the skin above it or at the ankle may begin to itch. The entire leg may ache, especially when you stand for long periods. Your feet may become swollen after standing for a short period and your shoes may seem very tight by the end of the day. During pregnancy, varicose veins may worsen because of increased pressure in the abdomen. Symptoms usually do not worsen if only superficial veins are affected. But when deep veins are also involved, circulation can be impaired, causing persistent leg swelling and a brownish skin discoloration, especially near the ankles. An itchy rash may develop near the affected vein.

In some people, varicose veins can significantly reduce the supply of blood to the tissues, causing the skin to break down and form an ulcer. A varicose ulcer will not heal until the vein has been treated successfully.

Diagnosis

Because varicose veins are frequently visible under the skin, a doctor can usually detect them during a physical examination. To determine the exact location of the veins that have damaged valves, he or she may apply an elastic tourniquet to your leg (see illustration).

Treatment

Your doctor may recommend that you wear elastic support stockings to help improve circulation. You will need to put the stockings on every day, before you get out of bed. Ask your doctor or a nurse to show you the correct way to put them on. Some people find the stockings uncomfortable, especially during hot weather. If your varicose veins are causing discomfort or pain, sit or lie down with your legs elevated above the level of your chest. This will help the blood flow back toward your heart from your ankles and feet.

If you cut the skin over a varicose vein and it begins to bleed, lie down as quickly as possible (no matter where you are), raise the affected leg, and keep it raised. The bleeding should slow immediately. Then, using a clean cloth, place moderate pressure on the wound. After the bleeding has stopped, seek immediate medical attention to have the wound cleaned and bandaged.

Do not attempt to treat a varicose ulcer or a rash on your leg, and never scratch an itching varicose vein. See your doctor for treatment. He or she will probably recommend support stockings or soothing dressings to relieve skin irritation. If you have both deep and superficial varicose veins, your doctor will probably recommend that you wear an elastic stocking on the affected leg and avoid standing for long periods.

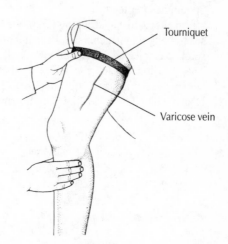

Tourniquet

Varicose vein

Locating varicose veins
To find the damaged valves that are causing your varicose veins, your doctor will apply a tourniquet to your leg to stop the flow of blood through the vein while you are lying down. If a valve is damaged in a section of the vein directly below the tourniquet, blood will leak back through the valve when you stand up, making the vein clearly visible through the skin. To detect other damaged valves in veins, the doctor repeats the procedure by moving the tourniquet to various points down your leg.

Surgery is usually the most effective treatment for varicose veins that are causing symptoms. The most common type of surgery involves removing the affected veins from the leg in a procedure called stripping. After the damaged veins are removed, the remaining small veins quickly enlarge and take over the work of the damaged veins. For surgery to remove varicose veins, a person usually receives epidural anesthesia (see page 532). The procedure may be performed in an outpatient facility, or you may need to stay overnight in the hospital.

For the stripping procedure, the surgeon makes an incision about 2 inches long at the top of the inner thigh and a similar incision at the ankle to expose part of the affected vein. He or she also makes several very tiny incisions down the leg where branches of the main vein go deeper into the leg. The branches are then cut and tied to stop them from bleeding. The surgeon inserts a flexible wire (with a hook at the tip) into the incision at the ankle and passes it through the main vein to the thigh. As the surgeon withdraws the wire, the hook pulls the vein from beneath the skin. At the same time, the doctor or nurse bandages the leg tightly to prevent bleeding. The procedure usually takes about 30 minutes per leg.

An alternative to stripping is a procedure called sclerotherapy, in which a small amount of an irritant solution is injected directly into the damaged veins. The solution causes the walls of the veins to become inflamed and stick together, effectively blocking blood flow. Healthy veins nearby then take over the work of the treated veins. This procedure is usually performed in two or three visits to an outpatient facility or a doctor's office. Sclerotherapy is usually not effective on varicose veins in the thighs. Doctors often recommend stripping the veins first and treating any minor recurrences with sclerotherapy. New varicose veins may develop elsewhere after either treatment.

After undergoing stripping or sclerotherapy, you will need to wear support stockings for about 6 weeks. Your doctor will recommend that you walk as much as possible, avoid standing for long periods, and frequently sit with your legs elevated above the level of your chest.

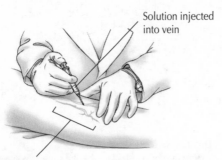

Solution injected into vein

Varicose veins

Sclerotherapy
Sclerotherapy is a nonsurgical treatment for varicose veins in which a doctor injects a small amount of an irritant solution directly into a damaged vein, closing it off to blood flow. The blood then reroutes itself through healthy veins nearby. Treatment is usually completed in two or three visits to an outpatient facility or a doctor's office.

> ### Spider Veins
>
> Spider veins are very tiny veins that are visible under the skin of the thighs and legs. Although they may be unsightly, spider veins do not cause any health problems. Cosmetic laser treatments or chemical injections can make spider veins less visible, but these procedures may not produce permanent results.

Thrombophlebitis

Phlebitis is inflammation of a vein, usually caused by infection or injury. When phlebitis occurs, blood flow through the roughened, swollen vein may become sluggish, encouraging blood clots (thrombi) to develop and adhere to the walls of the vein. This condition, called thrombophlebitis, often occurs in the superficial veins in the legs. In rare cases, thrombophlebitis occurs in the arms.

Women are slightly more likely to develop thrombophlebitis than men. The condition also occurs more frequently in people who have varicose veins (see page 602). In rare cases, people who are undergoing medical treatment that involves piercing the veins with needles (such as inserting an intravenous line) develop thrombophlebitis.

An untreated infection can lead to blood poisoning (see page 937). There is also a very slight chance that blood clots break off, travel through the bloodstream, and block a blood vessel. However, the most serious risk of thrombophlebitis is that the clot may travel to a more vulnerable spot, such as a deeper vein, most likely in the leg or pelvic area (see next article).

Symptoms

The main symptoms of thrombophlebitis are pain, redness, warmth, tenderness, itching, or swelling under the skin along the length of the affected vein. If the area is infected, you may also have a fever.

Diagnosis

A doctor can diagnose thrombophlebitis from a person's symptoms and an examination of the affected area. Tests are usually not needed.

Treatment

If you have thrombophlebitis, your doctor may recommend that you take a nonsteroidal anti-inflammatory drug such as aspirin or ibuprofen to relieve pain and inflammation. If you have an infection, he or she may prescribe an antibiotic. The doctor may also recommend that you rest frequently, elevate the affected leg, and apply warm, moist compresses to the affected area. A nonprescription zinc oxide ointment can help relieve itching; ask your doctor to recommend one. The doctor also may recommend that you wear elastic support stockings. With treatment, thrombophlebitis usually clears up within a few weeks.

Deep Vein Thrombosis

Thrombosis is the formation of a blood clot (thrombus), which can partially or completely block a blood vessel. If a blood clot forms in a deeper vein, the condition is called deep vein thrombosis. Although deep vein thrombosis occurs most frequently in the legs and lower abdomen, it can occur anywhere in the body. The two main causes of deep vein thrombosis are injury to the lining of a vein and sluggish blood flow.

If you are older or are overweight or if you have injured your pelvis or a bone in your leg, you have an increased risk of deep vein thrombosis. The condition often develops during periods of immobility, especially while recovering from surgery or serious illness. Thrombosis also frequently occurs when an arm or leg is immobilized in a cast to stabilize a broken bone, or in the legs after a long trip on a plane or train. In these situations, blood flow tends to become sluggish. The disorder may also affect people whose blood clots more easily than normal, such as those who have a genetic defect in blood-clotting factors or a disease such as systemic lupus

erythematosus (see page 920) or polycythemia (see page 627). Women over age 35 who smoke cigarettes and also take birth-control pills are at increased risk of thrombosis.

Symptoms

In deep vein thrombosis, the area drained by the vein, usually the calf or thigh, becomes swollen and painful as blood flow to it is obstructed. The pressure in the veins and capillaries in the leg increases, causing swelling. If the thrombosis is not in the leg, there may be no symptoms unless pieces of the clot break off, enter the bloodstream, and travel to the lungs, causing a pulmonary embolism (see next article). If the swelling is long-lasting, the skin may develop a brownish discoloration and may injure easily and develop frequent sores. If you have symptoms of deep vein thrombosis, see your doctor.

Diagnosis

Your doctor may order a Doppler ultrasound examination (see page 111) of the affected leg or a venogram, in which a contrast medium (dye) is injected into a vein in the foot and a series of X-rays of the affected leg is taken. The doctor also may recommend a radionuclide scan (see page 114) of the lungs to determine if any blood clots have traveled to the lungs through the bloodstream.

Treatment

If you have deep vein thrombosis, especially if blood clots have traveled to your lungs, your doctor will prescribe an anticoagulant drug to prevent clotting. The drugs are usually injected initially and then taken in pill form. Treatment is usually done on an outpatient basis. Because these drugs can cause bleeding if used incorrectly, you must take them exactly as prescribed, usually for about 6 months. Most clots are gradually reabsorbed into the bloodstream. In rare cases, surgery is necessary to remove blood clots.

If you are scheduled to have surgery, and your doctor thinks you may be at risk of developing deep vein thrombosis, he or she may give you injections of an anticoagulant drug such as heparin, either before or after surgery, to help prevent the formation of blood clots.

If you are confined to bed, your doctor will probably encourage you to flex your leg muscles,

Preventing Blood Clots When You Fly

Deep vein thrombosis can develop during long-distance air travel because you are forced to sit for long periods. You are at increased risk of developing deep vein thrombosis from inactivity if you are over-weight, a smoker, an athlete, or pregnant; have already had blood clots in a leg or have varicose veins; or have recently had pelvic surgery or a leg injury. To prevent yourself from developing deep vein thrombo-sis on a plane, exercise your leg muscles often during the flight.

Here are some other tips to minimize your risk of circulation problems during air travel:

- Wear loose, comfortable clothing. Don't wear any-thing such as knee-length stockings or an elastic knee brace that could hinder the circulation of blood in your legs.

- To get more legroom, ask for a seat in an emergency-exit row, at the bulkhead (the area in front of the first row in a section of a plane), or on the aisle.
- Don't sit with your legs crossed.
- Extend your legs straight out if you can, and flex your ankles up and down. If you can't extend your legs, try curling your toes while you lift your heels off the floor. Slide your feet forward and back a few inches to exercise your thigh muscles.
- Massage your feet and legs to propel blood out of your legs and toward your heart.
- Get up and walk in the aisle as often as you can.

Some doctors recommend taking half an aspirin before a long flight to reduce the risk of clotting and to maxi-mize blood circulation; ask your doctor if taking aspirin before flights would be helpful for you.

wiggle your toes, and bend your ankles to keep your blood circulating. If you are immobilized for a long period of time, your legs also may be mechanically elevated and placed in plastic sleeves called sequen-tial compression devices (SCDs), which are alter-nately filled with air and deflated. The resulting pumping action keeps the blood flowing normally.

If you are a woman over 35 who smokes and you want to take oral contraceptives, ask your doc-tor for information about quitting smoking (see page 29).

Pulmonary Embolism

Pulmonary embolism usually occurs as a serious complication of deep vein thrombosis (see previ-ous article). A blood clot detaches from the wall of a deep vein and moves into the bloodstream, through the heart, and through the pulmonary artery to the lungs. If the loose clot (called an embo-lus) is large, it can lodge in an artery inside the lungs and block blood flow to the lungs. If most of the pulmonary artery is obstructed, the right ven-tricle of the heart is forced to pump harder, which can lead to heart failure. The obstruction reduces the volume of freshly oxygenated blood returning to the left side of the heart. If the volume of blood is reduced significantly, shock (see page 579) can result. A pulmonary embolism can be fatal.

The condition affects women more frequently than men. People who are confined to bed, espe-cially after pelvic surgery or surgery involving the hip or knee, are at increased risk.

Symptoms

Symptoms of pulmonary embolism depend on the size of the embolus and its location in the lungs. Because the heart and tissues are not getting enough oxygen, the main symptom is usually shortness of breath. The person may also feel faint and have chest pain when inhaling. Other possible symptoms include a cough, bloody phlegm, and cyanosis (a bluish tinge) around the mouth.

Any blockage of blood flow to the lungs can lead to heart failure (see page 570). If a large pul-monary embolism causes the circulatory system to stop functioning, death usually occurs within minutes.

Diagnosis

Anything that predisposes you to deep vein throm-bosis also increases your risk of pulmonary embolism. See your doctor if you have symptoms of either disorder, especially if you have recently been confined to bed. Your doctor will examine you and may order a chest X-ray and an electrocardio-gram (ECG; see page 559) to determine whether your heart, especially the right side, is under strain.

To confirm the diagnosis, the doctor may order a radionuclide scan (see page 114) or CT scan (see page 112) of the lungs. If any doubt remains, he or she may order a pulmonary angiogram to examine arteries in the lungs. A pulmonary angiogram is the same as a coronary angiogram (see page 561), except that it examines the arteries in the lungs instead of in the heart.

Treatment

If you have a pulmonary embolism, you will need to be hospitalized for treatment with anticoagulants (blood thinners) and possibly thrombolytic drugs (clot busters). Heparin, an anticoagulant, helps prevent more blood clots from forming in your lungs and veins. The drug is infused directly into a vein. Occasionally, thrombolytic drugs such as streptokinase or tPA (tissue plasminogen activator) are used to help dissolve blood clots in

Pulmonary Angiogram

A pulmonary angiogram, also called a pulmonary arteriogram, allows doctors to examine the pulmonary arteries on film. A catheter (a thin, flexible tube) is usually inserted into a large vein in the groin area and threaded up through the heart to the pulmonary artery (the main artery in the lungs). A contrast medium (dye) is injected through the catheter into the pulmonary artery, and a series of rapid-sequence X-rays (like a movie) of the artery and its smaller branches is taken. The arteries are clearly visible, allowing the doctor to detect any blood clots in the blood vessels.

the lungs. Because treatment with the combination of thrombolytic and anticoagulant drugs carries a risk of internal bleeding, your doctor will closely

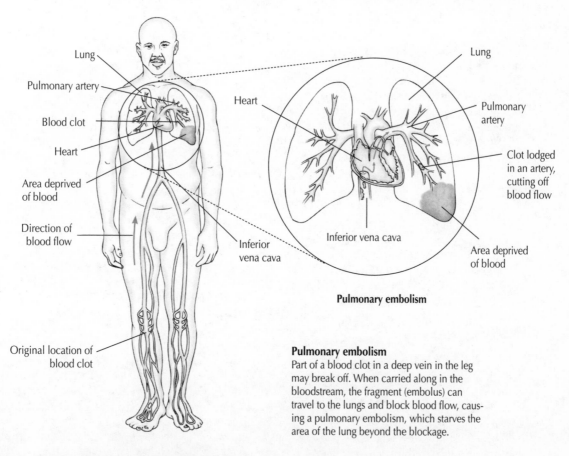

Lung

Pulmonary artery

Blood clot

Heart

Area deprived of blood

Direction of blood flow

Inferior vena cava

Original location of blood clot

Lung

Heart

Pulmonary artery

Clot lodged in an artery, cutting off blood flow

Inferior vena cava

Area deprived of blood

Pulmonary embolism

Pulmonary embolism
Part of a blood clot in a deep vein in the leg may break off. When carried along in the bloodstream, the fragment (embolus) can travel to the lungs and block blood flow, causing a pulmonary embolism, which starves the area of the lung beyond the blockage.

How a pulmonary embolism develops

monitor the ability of your blood to clot normally.

An embolism may damage part of the lung, but a person almost always recovers with treatment that prevents another embolism from forming. The doctor will prescribe an anticoagulant to help prevent the formation of more blood clots, thereby reducing the risk of another embolism.

If an embolism is severe, immediate emergency medical treatment is required. The blockage will probably need to be removed surgically. If a person survives the critical first few days after a massive pulmonary embolism, he or she has a good chance of long-term recovery. The chances of recovery are even better if the source of the embolism, usually deep vein thrombosis (see page 605), is detected and treated successfully.

2

Blood Disorders

Blood has two basic components: blood cells and plasma (the fluid in which blood cells are suspended). Most blood cells are red blood cells, or erythrocytes, which carry oxygen from the lungs to the rest of the body. Red blood cells contain a protein called hemoglobin, which combines with oxygen in the lungs and delivers it to tissues as blood circulates through the body. Red blood cells also return some of the waste product carbon dioxide from the tissues to the lungs, where it is exhaled and eliminated from the body.

Blood also contains several types of white blood cells, which fight infection. Most white blood cells are neutrophils, which attack and surround bacteria and destroy them. Other white blood cells called lymphocytes seek out foreign cells, infectious microorganisms, and other potentially harmful substances in the blood and trigger an immune response in the body. Platelets are cell fragments that enable blood to clot, gathering wherever a blood vessel is injured to begin the blood-clotting process that seals the injury and enables the blood vessel to heal. Proteins in the plasma called coagulation (blood clotting) factors help the platelets to form blood clots.

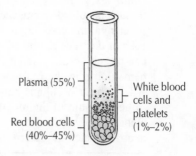

Plasma (55%)

White blood cells and platelets (1%–2%)

Red blood cells (40%–45%)

Basic components of blood
Blood can be broken down easily into its separate parts: plasma, red blood cells, white blood cells, and platelets. Plasma is a yellowish fluid that contains minerals, antibodies (infection-fighting proteins), and blood-clotting factors.

Neutrophil   **Lymphocyte**

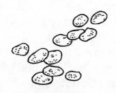

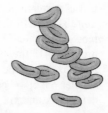

White blood cells
White blood cells protect the body against infection by destroying bacteria and producing antibodies (proteins that fight specific germs recognized by the body). Neutrophils and lymphocytes are two types of white blood cells.

Platelets
Platelets are cell fragments that enable blood to clot, which is essential for wound healing.

Red blood cells
Red blood cells, or erythrocytes, make up about 40 to 45 percent of blood. Red blood cells contain a protein called hemoglobin, which carries oxygen to the tissues.

All blood cells are produced in the bone marrow (a soft tissue inside bone cavities). Lymphocytes are also produced in the lymph glands in the neck, armpits, groin, and other parts of the body. The spleen and lymph glands and the channels and ducts that connect them make up the lymphatic system, which is an important component of the immune system (the body's natural defenses against disease). When red blood cells and platelets are defective, damaged, or old, they are filtered out of the bloodstream and broken down in the spleen and liver.

The different types of blood disorders include lack of hemoglobin (which causes anemia), clotting disorders (which cause bleeding, bruising, or excessive clotting), cancerous changes in white blood cells (which cause leukemia and bone marrow conditions such as multiple myeloma), and lymphatic system disorders such as lymphoma.

Anemia

The main component of red blood cells is an iron-rich protein called hemoglobin, which combines with oxygen in the lungs, carries it through the bloodstream, and delivers it to tissues. In anemia, the body produces too few red blood cells or destroys red blood cells faster than they can be replaced. In some cases, the amount of hemoglobin in the red blood cells is deficient. All of these problems can lead to a shortage of hemoglobin in the blood, which reduces the blood's ability to deliver oxygen from the lungs to nourish tissues and return the waste product carbon dioxide from the tissues to the lungs for disposal.

Anemia is the most common blood disorder in the United States, affecting more than 3 million people. The disorder can be temporary or chronic, and mild or severe. Anemia can result from a deficiency of iron or other nutrients, from loss of blood, or from a chronic or inherited disease or condition. Anemia also may be a complication from taking some medications or from undergoing radiation therapy (see page 23) or chemotherapy (see page 23) to treat cancer.

Iron Deficiency Anemia

Iron is an essential component of hemoglobin, the oxygen-carrying protein in red blood cells. In healthy people, iron from old red blood cells is stored in the body and used to produce hemoglobin in new red blood cells. The small amount of iron that is normally lost from the body is replaced by iron absorbed from iron-rich foods such as lean red meat, green leafy vegetables, and whole-grain products. If the body loses more iron than it absorbs, the bone marrow produces fewer and smaller red blood cells, and anemia develops. Iron deficiency anemia is usually not life-threatening, but it can weaken the body's resistance to the effects of another illness or an injury.

A shortage of iron in the body has a number of possible causes. In most people who have iron deficiency anemia, stored iron has been depleted by excessive blood loss. For example, women who have extremely heavy menstrual periods can deplete their supply of iron and develop anemia. (Women who have normal periods seldom have a problem maintaining an adequate supply of iron.) Blood loss from the intestinal tract can result from digestive system disorders such as gastroesophageal reflux disease (GERD; see page 750), a peptic ulcer (see page 755) or duodenal ulcer (see page 756), polyps (see page 773), or cancer of the colon (see page 775).

Some people may not take in enough iron in their diet to replace the iron they lose each day. This condition occurs mainly in young children, pregnant women, and people who are on a restricted diet. Sometimes a person's digestive system is unable to absorb iron from food, no matter how much iron is in his or her diet. This problem occurs in some disorders of the small intestine that affect absorption of nutrients, such as celiac disease (see page 768), which blocks the absorption of gluten (a protein found in foods that contain wheat, rye, oats, or barley).

Symptoms

Initial symptoms of iron deficiency anemia often are so mild that they go unnoticed. Symptoms can include abnormally pale skin, weakness, fatigue, faintness, or shortness of breath. A person may have palpitations (heartbeats that you're aware of) when his or her heart tries to compensate for decreased blood flow by pumping blood at a faster rate. The person may have a sore, inflamed tongue; headaches; a poor appetite; and an increased susceptibility to infection. Some people with anemia may also experience restless legs syndrome (see page 705), perhaps resulting from impaired blood flow to the legs. They may be unable to keep their legs still, and sometimes may experience a tingling or crawling sensation in their legs.

Diagnosis

If you have symptoms of iron deficiency anemia, your doctor will examine you and order blood tests to evaluate the number, size, and color of the red cells in your blood and the amount of hemoglobin they contain. (Iron-deficient red cells are smaller and paler than normal red cells.) The doctor also will order tests to help determine if an underlying disease is causing the anemia. In most cases, a doctor may order a blood test to measure the level of the protein ferritin. Because ferritin helps the body store iron, a low level of ferritin in the blood indicates a low level of iron. You will probably have tests to measure the amount of iron and vitamin B12 in your blood, and a test to check for blood in your stool. If blood is detected in your stool, you may have additional tests, such as colonoscopy (see page 767), an examination of the rectum and large intestine.

A bone marrow biopsy is sometimes recommended to evaluate the body's iron reserves and to determine the cause of anemia. A bone marrow biopsy is done by passing a hollow needle into a bone—such as the back of the pelvic bone—and removing a small sample of marrow from inside the bone. Local anesthesia is used for the procedure. A bone marrow biopsy can confirm or rule out iron deficiency. It can also help determine other causes of poor red blood cell production, including drug toxicity, lead poisoning, or bone marrow diseases such as multiple myeloma (see page 627), leukemia (see page 621), or aplastic anemia (see page 628).

Treatment

Doctors treat iron deficiency anemia by replacing the lost iron and treating the underlying condition that is causing the shortage of iron in the body. A doctor may prescribe iron supplements to take for several months or longer. (Take the supplements according to your doctor's instructions to avoid indigestion or other gastrointestinal symptoms.) The iron may darken your stool, which is normal. If you have problems taking the supplements, your doctor may inject the iron into a muscle or vein. Iron deficiency anemia usually clears up after a few weeks of treatment with supplemental iron. For severe anemia, a blood transfusion (see page 615) may be necessary.

After your anemia has cleared up, the doctor may recommend that you continue to take iron supplements for a few more months to build up your body's iron reserves. If the cause of the anemia was a poor diet or inadequate absorption of iron, your doctor will recommend changes in your diet to increase your intake of iron. Further treatment will depend on the cause of the iron deficiency.

Preventing Iron Deficiency Anemia

To reduce your risk of iron deficiency anemia, eat plenty of iron-rich foods—such as lean red meat, fish, poultry, eggs, whole grains, dark green leafy vegetables, dried peas and beans, dried fruit, and nuts and seeds—every day. Because vitamin C makes it easier for the body to absorb iron, eat plenty of foods that are rich in vitamin C—such as oranges, grapefruit, strawberries, tomatoes, bell peppers, broccoli, and cauliflower.

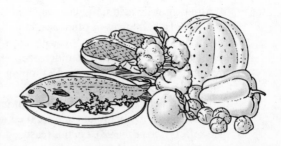

Vitamin Deficiency Anemia

Your body needs an adequate supply of vitamin B12 and folic acid to produce hemoglobin-rich red blood cells, which deliver oxygen throughout the body. A diet lacking these nutrients can lead to vitamin deficiency anemia. Vitamin deficiencies usually develop slowly, over the course of months or years.

Vitamin B12 is vital to maintaining the nervous system and producing red blood cells. The body absorbs vitamin B12 from foods such as lean red meat, poultry, fish, and dairy products. A shortage of vitamin B12 can damage the brain, spinal cord, and peripheral nerves. Vitamin B12 deficiency anemia, also called pernicious anemia, is the most common type of vitamin deficiency anemia. It occurs when the body cannot absorb vitamin B12.

In healthy people, vitamin B12 is stored in the liver. If a person develops an inability to absorb vitamin B12, his or her body will gradually use up the stored vitamin B12, resulting in vitamin B12 deficiency anemia. Surgical removal of a large section of the small intestine (the part of the body where most nutrients are absorbed) and digestive system disorders such as Crohn's disease (see page 764) may impair the body's ability to absorb vitamin B12. Pernicious anemia rarely develops before age 40 and affects men and women in equal numbers. If you have a close relative who has pernicious anemia, you are at increased risk of developing the disorder.

Folic acid deficiency anemia usually results from inadequate intake of the vitamin in the diet. Folic acid is found in foods such as green leafy vegetables, whole grains, nuts, and fortified cereals and grains. Because the body cannot store large amounts of folic acid, folic acid deficiency anemia can develop after only a few weeks of inadequate intake.

Although folic acid deficiency anemia is now rare in the United States, it often occurs in people who drink alcohol heavily, people who may not eat a well-balanced diet (such as older people), and pregnant women (because the developing fetus requires large amounts of folic acid). Folic acid deficiency anemia during pregnancy can lead to birth defects of the brain and spine called neural tube defects (see page 398). For this reason, doctors stress that all women of childbearing age (starting in adolescence) who could become pregnant should get 400 micrograms of folic acid each day. People who have celiac disease (see page 768) are at risk of developing folic acid deficiency anemia because their body cannot absorb enough folic acid, no matter how much of the vitamin they eat in foods.

Some healthy people may have a higher-than-normal biological requirement for folic acid, and need to take in more of the vitamin than other people. Folic acid deficiency anemia also may result from long-term use of some medications, such as some antibiotics, immune-suppressing drugs, anticonvulsants, or potassium-sparing antihypertensive drugs.

Symptoms

The main symptoms of vitamin B12 deficiency anemia and folic acid deficiency anemia are abnormally pale skin, fatigue, shortness of breath, and palpitations (heartbeats that you're aware of), particularly on exertion. In both disorders, a person's mouth or tongue may be sore and his or her skin may appear pale yellow. If the spinal cord is affected by vitamin B12 deficiency anemia, a person may have difficulty walking and maintaining his or her balance. He or she may feel continuous tingling or coldness in the hands and feet, and may experience memory loss, confusion, or depression. See your doctor right away if you have any of these symptoms.

Diagnosis

If you have symptoms of vitamin deficiency anemia, your doctor will examine you and order blood tests to evaluate the level and appearance of your red blood cells. In vitamin deficiency anemia, the level of red blood cells is lower than normal and the red blood cells are larger than normal and underdeveloped. If you have anemia, your doctor will probably order additional tests to determine the underlying cause. Tell the doctor if you have a close relative who has pernicious anemia.

Treatment

Once lost, the digestive tract can never regain the ability to absorb vitamin B12. For this reason, treatment of pernicious anemia and most other types of vitamin B12 deficiency involves taking vitamin B12 injections (which you can administer yourself) for the rest of your life. Initially, you inject vitamin B12 once a day; eventually you inject the vitamin once a month. Problems with walking and balance may take months to improve and, if you had these problems for a long time before beginning treatment, they may not clear up completely. If you stop taking vitamin B12, your symptoms will gradually return.

To treat folic acid deficiency anemia caused by a poor diet, by an inability of the intestines to absorb adequate amounts of the vitamin, or by a greater-than-normal biological need for folic acid, a doctor usually prescribes folic acid supplements. He or she will also recommend changes in the person's diet to take in adequate amounts of folic acid every day.

Preventing Vitamin Deficiency Anemia

The best way to prevent vitamin deficiency anemia is to eat a balanced diet that includes foods rich in vitamin B12 (such as lean red meat, low-fat or fat-free dairy products, and eggs) and folic acid (such as fresh fruits, orange juice, green leafy vegetables, and folic acid–fortified cereals and breads). Talk to your doctor about taking vitamin supplements.

Because smoking interferes with the body's ability to absorb vitamins and increases the risk of vitamin deficiency anemia, quit smoking (see page 29) if you smoke. Cutting back on your intake of alcohol also may improve your body's ability to absorb vital nutrients.

Sickle Cell Disease

Sickle cell disease is a life-threatening inherited form of hemolytic anemia (see page 616) in which hemoglobin (the oxygen-carrying protein in red blood cells) is abnormal. People who inherit a sickle cell gene from both parents develop sickle cell disease. Their red blood cells contain the defective hemoglobin that gives the cells their abnormal, sickle shape. People who inherit a sickle cell gene from only one parent have sickle cell trait. Their red blood cells contain half normal hemoglobin and half defective hemoglobin. Although they will not develop the disease, they can pass the sickle cell gene to their children.

In sickle cell disease, the abnormal, sickle-shaped red blood cells are fragile and have difficulty

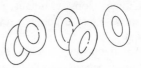

Normal red blood cells

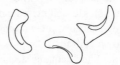

Sickle-shaped red blood cells

Sickle-shaped red blood cells
In sickle cell disease, the body produces abnormal, sickle-shaped red blood cells (bottom). Normal red blood cells are doughnut-shaped (top). Healthy red blood cells flow easily through blood vessels, while sickle-shaped cells tend to block the capillaries (the smallest blood vessels in the body), significantly reducing the amount of oxygen that reaches the tissues.

flowing through the capillaries, the smallest blood vessels in the body. The defective cells tend to clog the capillaries, preventing blood (and oxygen) from reaching tissues and organs, which can lead to severe tissue and organ damage. In addition, the abnormal red blood cells are destroyed faster than they can be replaced; this shortened life of red cells leads to iron deficiency anemia (see page 610).

In the United States, sickle cell disease and sickle cell trait occur most frequently among African Americans and Hispanics of Caribbean ancestry. About 1 in every 10 African Americans carries the gene for sickle cell disease. Each child of a man and woman who both have the sickle cell trait has a 25 percent chance of inheriting the sickle cell gene from each parent and having the disease.

Symptoms

A person who has sickle cell disease has symptoms of anemia, such as weakness, fatigue, shortness of breath, and palpitations (heartbeats that you're aware of). In addition to these symptoms, he or she may have headaches and jaundice (yellowing of the skin and the whites of the eyes). Occasional sickle cell crises occur when the abnormal cells block small blood vessels and cause tissue in the bones, joints, or abdomen to die; a person will have severe pain in the long bones and in the abdomen, sometimes along with nausea and vomiting. The person also may experience fever and shortness of breath.

The frequency of sickle cell crises varies from person to person. Crises are more likely to occur when a person has an infection, has been injured, or has had prolonged exposure to cold weather. Because sickle cell crises can occur during anesthesia and surgery, precautions are taken before surgery to prevent them.

Lack of an adequate blood supply to organs may cause areas of tissue in the organs to die. Poor circulation also can cause sores to develop on the legs and ankles. Damage to the nervous system can lead to stroke (see page 669). Older people with sickle cell disease may develop impaired lung and kidney function. Younger men may develop priapism (see page 840), a condition that causes persistent, often painful, erections.

Diagnosis

For a person who has symptoms of sickle cell disease, a doctor will take a detailed family health history, perform an examination, and order a blood test to check for abnormal hemoglobin and to determine if the person has sickle cell disease or sickle cell trait. Symptoms such as anemia, abdominal and bone pain, and nausea usually indicate sickle cell disease. Sickle cell disease can be diagnosed in a fetus during pregnancy by CVS (chorionic villus sampling; see page 511) between the 10th and 12th weeks of pregnancy or by amniocentesis (see page 510) later in pregnancy. In most states, all newborns are tested for sickle cell disease so that treatment can begin early for a child who is found to have the disease.

Treatment

Because sickle cell disease cannot be cured, treatment focuses on relieving symptoms and preventing sickle cell crises. Sickle cell crises are often treated with analgesics to relieve pain, supplemental oxygen to increase the supply of oxygen to tissues, and both oral and intravenous fluids to help prevent dehydration. For adults with sickle cell disease, a doctor may prescribe a cancer drug called hydroxyurea to increase the amount of hemoglobin F (fetal hemoglobin, which protects against

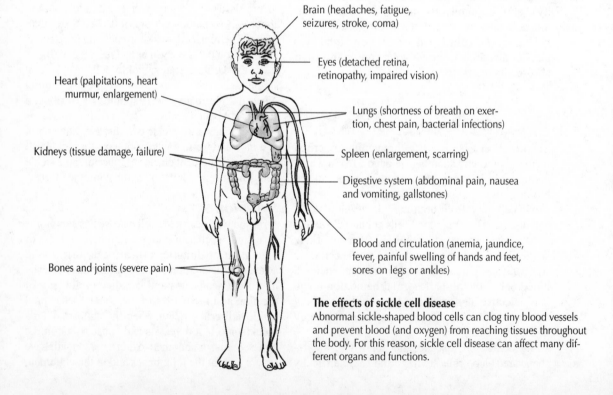

Brain (headaches, fatigue, seizures, stroke, coma)

Eyes (detached retina, retinopathy, impaired vision)

Heart (palpitations, heart murmur, enlargement)

Lungs (shortness of breath on exertion, chest pain, bacterial infections)

Kidneys (tissue damage, failure)

Spleen (enlargement, scarring)

Digestive system (abdominal pain, nausea and vomiting, gallstones)

Bones and joints (severe pain)

Blood and circulation (anemia, jaundice, fever, painful swelling of hands and feet, sores on legs or ankles)

The effects of sickle cell disease
Abnormal sickle-shaped blood cells can clog tiny blood vessels and prevent blood (and oxygen) from reaching tissues throughout the body. For this reason, sickle cell disease can affect many different organs and functions.

sickling) in the blood and decrease the number of sickle-shaped red blood cells. The doctor may prescribe folic acid supplements to increase the body's production of red blood cells to help replace dead and damaged cells. Other treatment options include blood transfusions (see below), antibiotics, and sometimes a stem cell or bone marrow transplant (see page 624), which can have significant risks.

A person who has sickle cell disease needs to do everything possible to maintain good health. He or she should see the doctor regularly for checkups and seek prompt medical treatment for even minor illnesses, such as colds and other viral infections, or minor injuries. As a precaution, a doctor will immunize the person against influenza and pneumonia and will prescribe antibiotics to fight any infection.

Blood Transfusions

If your blood level is low as the result of disease or bleeding (especially from surgery or a severe injury), you may be given a blood transfusion to bring your blood up to a healthy level. A transfusion consists of red blood cells if you have anemia (see page 610) or platelets (which enable blood to clot) if you have bleeding (thrombocytopenia; see page 620).

Blood Donors

Although researchers continue to look for ways to make synthetic blood substitutes, for now people who volunteer to be blood donors are the only sources of blood and blood products. AIDS has highlighted the importance of testing the blood of potential donors for bloodborne infectious organisms such as HIV, hepatitis B and C, malaria, and syphilis.

Before giving blood, all donors are given a blood test to make sure they don't have anemia. If their blood is found to be healthy, about 1 pint of blood is removed from one of their veins with a needle. This procedure takes about 10 to 20 minutes and is painless and safe. Giving blood does not expose a donor to HIV or any other disease-causing organism

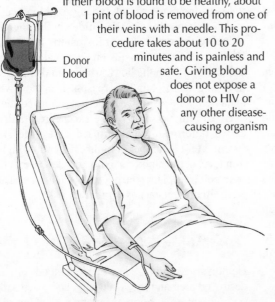

Donor blood

because new, sterile needles are used for each donor.

Self-donation, also called autologous blood donation, is an alternative to using blood from donors. People can donate their own blood in the few weeks before they have a scheduled surgical procedure. During this time, their bone marrow makes new blood to replenish the supply. The donated blood may be stored and used during or after the surgery if needed. An autologous blood donation eliminates the problems of matching blood types and the risk of infections. In directed blood donations, people can select a donor, such as a relative or friend, who gives blood to be used specifically for them.

Blood Groups and Blood Matching

Transfusions are safe and effective if the donor and recipient have compatible blood types. Blood is categorized into four main groups—A, B, AB, and O. In most blood groups, the surfaces of red blood cells are coated with specific proteins called antigens, which are labeled A or B. A person's blood cells have either A or B antigens (A or B blood group), both antigens (AB blood group), or neither antigen (O blood group). In the plasma, a person with A antigens has antibodies against B antigens and a person with B antigens has antibodies against A antigens, which cause a reaction when combined. People with type O blood do not have the A or B antigens to cause a reaction with other blood. For this reason, people with type O blood can donate their blood to people with any other group without causing a reaction. People with AB blood can safely receive A, B, or O blood. Other blood classifications, including Rhesus (Rh) factor (see page 508), are made to ensure a compatible match between donor and recipient.

The blood groups of donor blood are recorded on each unit of blood to make sure that a person having a transfusion gets the right type of blood. Before each transfusion, small quantities of the recipient's and the donor's blood are combined in the laboratory to ensure that they are compatible and that the transfusion is safe.

Having a blood transfusion

Before surgery, people with sickle cell disease are often given a blood transfusion that replaces much of their blood and thereby reduces the risk of sickling. A person who has sickle cell disease should avoid high-altitude activities such as mountain climbing because the decreased amount of oxygen in the air at high altitudes can trigger a sickle cell crisis.

Thalassemia

Thalassemia is a group of blood disorders caused by an inherited genetic defect that blocks the formation of hemoglobin A, the type of hemoglobin in the red blood cells of healthy adults. Hemoglobin is the oxygen-carrying protein in blood. Hemoglobin A is formed by a combination of four proteins—two alpha proteins and two beta proteins—that enable red blood cells to carry oxygen to tissues. Thalassemia is the most common blood disorder in the world, affecting mostly people from the Mediterranean, Middle East, Far East, and Africa. The effects of this recessive genetic disorder can range from mild to severe, depending on the particular genetic defect and whether a person inherits a defective gene from one or both parents.

When thalassemia results from a defect in the production of the alpha protein, it is called alpha thalassemia. Because each parent provides two alpha protein genes, people with this form of thalassemia are usually not severely affected because the healthy two or three copies of the protein override the impact of the deficient ones.

The most serious form of the disorder, called beta thalassemia major, is caused by a deficiency or complete absence of the beta hemoglobin protein. Beta thalassemia major, which occurs when a child inherits a copy of the defective gene from both parents, causes severe anemia. When a person inherits the beta protein defect from only one parent, he or she has what is called thalassemia trait, which rarely causes any serious symptoms or health problems. Thalassemia trait is much more common than beta thalassemia major. The two forms of beta thalassemia can have varying degrees of severity that still allow a person to lead a relatively normal, healthy life.

Symptoms
The form of alpha thalassemia that is most common in the United States, especially among African

Americans and Asians, makes the red blood cells smaller than normal but usually does not produce symptoms. The symptoms that can occur in the various forms include poor growth in an infant, enlargement of the spleen, severe anemia, and jaundice (yellowing of the skin and whites of the eyes). Children with thalassemia may have delayed sexual development and skull deformities. If your child has any of these signs or symptoms, see your doctor right away.

Diagnosis
To diagnose thalassemia, a doctor will order a blood test to detect the abnormal gene. If you have any form of the disease in your family, including thalassemia trait, and are considering having a child, talk to a genetic counselor (see page 952) about your risks of passing the gene on to a child. Thalassemia can be diagnosed in a fetus early in pregnancy with chorionic villus sampling (CVS; see page 511) or later in pregnancy with amniocentesis (see page 510).

Treatment
A child with thalassemia major needs to have regular blood transfusions to provide healthy red blood cells to relieve the symptoms of anemia. These transfusions may use only young red blood cells, which survive longer than older cells, thereby reducing the number of transfusions necessary. However, frequent transfusions eventually lead to a buildup of iron in the body, which can damage the liver and heart. For this reason, a person with thalassemia needs to have the iron removed regularly. To remove some of the excess iron, a drug called deferoxamine is infused under the skin overnight for a number of nights, depending on the iron level in the blood. In extremely severe cases, a stem cell transplant (see page 624) may be considered, although it carries significant risks.

Hemolytic Anemia

Hemolysis is a process in which red blood cells are destroyed prematurely. When hemolysis occurs, the body attempts to compensate by producing new red blood cells. If the destruction of cells exceeds cell production, the resulting disorder is hemolytic anemia. Hemolytic anemia may be inherited and present at birth, or it may be acquired later in life. Inherited hemolytic anemia may occur because the red blood cells do not have enough of a specific enzyme to protect themselves in the presence of some medications or the stress of an infection. Sickle cell disease (see page 613) is an example of inherited hemolytic anemia.

One type of acquired hemolytic anemia occurs when the body mistakenly produces antibodies (proteins that fight specific germs recognized by the body) that destroy the body's own red blood cells. Normally, an immune system organ called the spleen eliminates defective, damaged, or old red blood cells from the body. In hemolytic anemia, the spleen also eliminates healthy red blood cells. Hemolysis may also result when the body produces antibodies against red blood cells received in a blood transfusion (see page 615). Red blood cells can also be destroyed after they are damaged by artificial heart valves, abnormal blood vessel walls, or toxins. Although hemolytic anemia is rarely fatal, some forms of the disease can be difficult to treat.

Symptoms

The main symptoms of hemolytic anemia are fatigue, shortness of breath, and palpitations (heartbeats that you're aware of), especially during physical activity. Your skin may be pale yellow and your urine may contain blood pigment that makes it look darker than usual. If red blood cells are destroyed prematurely over a period of years, gallstones (see page 793) often form from a buildup of bilirubin, a protein by-product of the breakdown of red blood cells.

Diagnosis

Hemolytic anemia is diagnosed with blood tests that look for by-products of red blood cell damage such as bilirubin. Examination of the blood provides valuable information about the shape of the red blood cells, because many types of hemolysis produce abnormally shaped red cells. The spleen may be enlarged from working harder than usual. The blood may be tested for antibodies as well as abnormal types of hemoglobin such as those that occur in sickle cell disease or thalassemia (see previous page).

Treatment

The treatment for some types of hemolytic anemia is a splenectomy, a surgical procedure to remove the spleen. Splenectomy may be used to treat hemolytic anemia caused by an errant immune response and the hereditary form of hemolytic anemia because the spleen produces the antibodies that destroy red blood cells and is the major site of red cell destruction. However, doctors frequently prescribe corticosteroid medications, which may eliminate the need for a splenectomy. Corticosteroids dampen the abnormal immune response that causes the spleen to produce antibodies against red blood cells. Corticosteroids also inhibit the abnormal destruction of red blood cells by the spleen and other parts of the immune system. Doctors may also prescribe immune-suppressing drugs to decrease the immune system's production of antibodies, which can mistakenly attack and destroy red blood cells. If hemolytic anemia is triggered by a medication a person is taking, the doctor will ask him or her to stop taking the drug.

Bleeding and Bruising

Bleeding occurs when a blood vessel is damaged. If an internal blood vessel is injured, blood seeps into surrounding tissue and forms a bruise. When delicate blood vessels are just beneath the surface, such as in the nose, a minor injury or irritation can cause external bleeding. In most people, minor bleeding does not cause problems because three mechanisms in the body quickly act together to stop the bleeding. First, nearby blood vessels contract and restrict the flow of blood to the injured area. Platelets (cell fragments that enable blood to clot) then gather where the blood vessels are damaged and stick to the vessel walls and to each other to form a plug. Interlacing strands of a substance called fibrin form in the damaged area; blood cells become trapped in the fibrin mesh and form a blood clot that seals the wound and stops the bleeding.

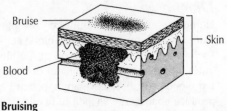

Bruise —

— **Skin**

Blood —

Bruising
If blood from an internal injury seeps into surrounding tissue, it forms a bruise. Once the internal bleeding has stopped, white blood cells called monocytes go to the injured area and help break down the red blood cells, healing the bruise.

In most diseases in which abnormal bleeding occurs (such as hemophilia), one or more of the mechanisms that normally stop bleeding malfunction. Minor injuries can cause persistent or severe bleeding. In a person with hemophilia or another bleeding disorder, bleeding from a cut, which in most people stops within 5 or 10 minutes, may continue for hours or even days. A person with a bleeding disorder may have internal bleeding and bleeding in the joints that can cause severe pain and can damage the joints.

Hemophilia

Hemophilia is an inherited bleeding disorder in which the body does not produce an adequate supply of a protein called antihemophilic globulin (factor VIII), which is essential for proper blood clotting. The disorder usually affects males, but it is passed from one generation to the next by females who carry the gene. In the United States, about 1 in 10,000 males has hemophilia. Nearly 75 percent of people who have hemophilia have a family history of the disease. However, the remaining 25 percent are the first in their family to have the disease, which usually results from a mutation (spontaneous change) in their mother's genes.

Effective treatments have greatly reduced the risk of disability and death from hemophilia. However, care must be taken to avoid serious injuries, which can be life-threatening for a person who has hemophilia.

Symptoms

Although occasionally a male infant with hemophilia will have prolonged bleeding after circumcision, the symptoms of hemophilia usually don't appear until a child becomes active. Bruises form on the knees and elbows when the child crawls, and internal bleeding from falls can produce large, deep bruises that can cause pain and swelling in an arm or leg that last for several days or weeks. Recurring bleeding into joints and the resulting formation of scar tissue stiffen the joints and limit the child's movement and flexibility. The degree of bleeding can vary greatly among people with hemophilia. If you have a son who has symptoms of hemophilia, or if you are an adult male and you notice that you bruise easily, see a doctor as soon as possible.

Diagnosis

If you have symptoms of a bleeding disorder, your doctor may recommend that you see a hematologist (a doctor who specializes in treating diseases of the blood) for an accurate diagnosis. The hematologist will ask about your health history and family health history (to see if any of your close relatives have had bleeding problems) and will perform a physical examination. He or she will order blood tests to measure the amount of blood-clotting factors in your blood and evaluate how well the blood-clotting factors are working.

Because hemophilia is usually inherited, women who have a family history of the disorder and who plan to have children should seek genetic counseling (see page 952) before becoming pregnant. A blood test can confirm whether a woman is carrying the defective gene. During pregnancy, diagnostic tests such as CVS (chorionic villus sampling; see page 511) and amniocentesis (see page 510) can determine if a fetus has hemophilia and enable doctors to plan for possible treatment for the child.

Treatment

If you have hemophilia, unless it is a mild case, your doctor will recommend that you avoid participating in activities that could cause injury, including all contact sports. He or she may recommend moderate exercise such as walking, jogging, or swimming as an alternative. Your doctor will also recommend that you avoid taking aspirin, drugs that contain aspirin, or any nonsteroidal anti-inflammatory drugs because they increase the risk of uncontrolled bleeding. Also, special precautions such as infusions of factor VIII (the deficient clotting substance in hemophilia) to prevent uncontrolled bleeding must be taken before you have any type of surgery, including dental treatment. For people with mild cases, the hormonal drug desmopressin can raise factor VIII levels temporarily.

Preventive treatment for hemophilia involves regular infusions of factor VIII; people can be taught to give themselves these infusions by injection. If you have an injury, any bleeding or bruising that occurs can be stopped with an infusion of factor VIII, which may involve a short hospital stay. These infusions are safe—genetically engineered factor VIII is available that avoids the risk of infection with HIV and other microorganisms, and all blood from donors is screened for HIV, hepatitis, and other disease-causing microbes.

If you or your child has hemophilia, you may be given a card indicating that you have hemophilia. Carry the card with you at all times so that medical personnel will know what treatment you might need in an emergency.

Von Willebrand's Disease

Von Willebrand's disease is the most common inherited bleeding disorder. People who have this disorder have a defect or shortage of a blood protein called von Willebrand factor, which helps platelets (cell fragments that enable blood to clot) function normally. When a person who has von Willebrand's disease is cut or injured, the blood does not clot normally to seal the damaged blood vessels. Severe bleeding can occur during routine dental care, from a sports-related injury, or during surgery or childbirth.

Von Willebrand's disease is more common than hemophilia (see previous article), although hemophilia is the better known blood disorder. Von Willebrand's disease affects about 1 percent of people in the United States. Although its effects are usually mild, about 20 percent of people who have the disorder experience moderate or severe bleeding. The defective gene responsible for the disorder can be inherited from either parent. Unlike hemophilia, which affects mostly males, von Willebrand's disease affects males and females in equal numbers. The disorder poses a bigger health problem for women than it does for men because one of its primary symptoms, heavy menstrual bleeding, can be misdiagnosed as a gynecological problem rather than a bleeding disorder, causing a delay in treatment.

Symptoms

Symptoms of von Willebrand's disease usually appear in childhood, as soon as a child becomes active, and may decrease with age. People who have von Willebrand's disease bruise easily, have recurring nosebleeds, and often bleed heavily from the gums after brushing their teeth or during routine dental care. Rarely, bleeding after an injury also can occur inside the brain, which can be life-threatening.

Women who have the disorder have intense and prolonged menstrual periods that can last for weeks or months without stopping. Such uninterrupted bleeding can cause severe anemia (see page 610) and can interfere with a woman's ability to get pregnant or carry a pregnancy to full term. Women who have the disorder also have an increased risk of potentially severe hemorrhaging immediately after childbirth.

Diagnosis

If you have symptoms of a bleeding disorder, your doctor will probably recommend that you see a hematologist (a doctor who specializes in treating diseases of the blood) to get an accurate diagnosis. After performing a physical examination and obtaining a detailed health history, the hematologist will ask you about any episodes of bleeding in close relatives. He or she will then order blood tests that measure platelet function, clotting factor function, and the levels of certain clotting factors in your blood. These tests are very sensitive and can be made inaccurate by several variables, including the menstrual cycle, the use of aspirin or other nonsteroidal anti-inflammatory drugs that thin the blood, exercise, stress, and a cold environment. For this reason, the tests may need to be repeated before the doctor can confirm the diagnosis.

Treatment

There is no cure for von Willebrand's disease. Mild forms of the disease usually require no treatment other than routine instruction in first aid. For example, you may be shown how to apply pressure with your fingers to help a wound stop bleeding. For moderate or severe bleeding problems, a hematologist may prescribe a hormonal drug called desmopressin, which triggers the body to release the von Willebrand factor. The hormone can be taken by injection or in a nasal spray. People who do not respond to treatment with desmopressin may be given a transfusion of concentrated clotting factors (including von Willebrand factor) called cryoprecipitate.

Women who have heavy bleeding during menstrual periods may benefit from taking birth-control pills. The same hormones that are in birth-control pills can also be rubbed onto the skin or applied as a patch. For unknown reasons, pregnancy often reduces the symptoms of the bleeding disorder; however, immediately after delivery, the risk of bleeding can increase significantly.

Children who have von Willebrand's disease need to reduce their risk of injury by limiting or avoiding contact sports. Children who have the severe form of the disease may have to wear a protective helmet during most forms of physical activity.

If you know that you carry the gene for von Willebrand's disease, or if you already have a child who has the disorder, seek genetic counseling (see page 952).

Thrombocytopenia

Thrombocytopenia results from the destruction or inadequate production of platelets (cell fragments that enable blood to clot). In thrombocytopenia, the blood contains too few platelets, causing prolonged bleeding when a person is injured.

Thrombocytopenia can have different causes. For example, it can result from taking some medications or from having radiation therapy (see page 23) or chemotherapy (see page 23) for cancer (which can inhibit the body's production of platelets). People who have Hodgkin's disease (see page 626) or lupus (see page 920) can develop thrombocytopenia from platelet destruction. Thrombocytopenia also can occur as a result of leukemia (see next page), when cancerous white blood cells crowd out platelet-forming blood cells.

Acute idiopathic thrombocytopenic purpura (ITP) usually occurs when, for unknown reasons, an immune system organ called the spleen forms antibodies (infection-fighting proteins) that mistakenly attack the platelets. In ITP, healthy platelets are damaged and removed from the bloodstream by the spleen at a high rate.

Dilutional thrombocytopenia can develop when a person has many blood transfusions in a short period of time, which can occur during surgery or when abnormal bleeding results from another blood disorder. In dilutional thrombocytopenia, the relative number of platelets in the blood can be reduced significantly.

Symptoms

The main symptom of thrombocytopenia is a rash of tiny bright red and dark red spots caused by bleeding in the skin. The rash can appear on any part of the body, but it often begins on the legs or wherever the skin has been irritated. A person can have frequent nosebleeds and a tendency to bruise easily. If a person's platelet count is very low, prolonged external or internal bleeding can occur after an injury. See your doctor immediately if you develop a dark red rash or if you have any abnormal bleeding.

Diagnosis

If you have symptoms of thrombocytopenia, your doctor will ask about any medications you are taking and will order a blood test to measure the amount of platelets in your blood and to determine if the thrombocytopenia is a symptom of another disease. He or she may order an examination of a sample of your bone marrow under a microscope to evaluate its production of platelets.

Treatment

To treat thrombocytopenia, your doctor will probably ask you to stop taking all medications, because almost any drug can trigger the disease in susceptible people. If abnormal antibody production by the immune system is the cause, your doctor may prescribe a corticosteroid drug to reduce the production of the platelet-destroying antibodies, thereby increasing the number of platelets in your blood. The corticosteroids also reduce the abnormal destruction of platelets by the spleen. In many people, this treatment improves or clears up the disease within several weeks.

If treatment with corticosteroid drugs is not effective, a doctor may recommend a splenectomy, a surgical procedure to remove the spleen. Removing the spleen allows the platelets to circulate in the blood longer. If removing the spleen does not help, the doctor may recommend treatment with high-dose gamma globulin (the pooled antibodies of healthy donors) or immune-suppressing or chemotherapy drugs given intravenously (through a vein) over a few hours. All of these treatments suppress the immune system to keep it from producing the antibodies that destroy the platelets, thereby allowing the platelets to circulate longer.

If you have thrombocytopenia caused by abnormal clotting or by underproduction of platelets by the bone marrow, treatment will depend on the type and severity of the underlying disorder that is causing the problem.

Leukemias

Leukemias are cancers of white blood cells. Normally, the number of white blood cells that the body produces equals the number that die as part of the natural cycle of cell growth and death. This process is designed to keep the total number of white blood cells constant. In leukemia, abnormal white blood cells multiply at an increased rate, and these cancerous cells often tend to live longer than normal—that is, they don't die when they should. As a result, the number of abnormal leukemia cells increases, either gradually or rapidly, accumulating in excess throughout the body and interfering with the functioning of various organs. Also, because leukemia cells are abnormal white blood cells, they usually cannot effectively eliminate infectious agents such as bacteria from the body, as healthy white blood cells can. The two main forms of leukemia affect different types of white blood cells. Myelogenous leukemia is a cancer of the cells from which white blood cells called granulocytes originate. Lymphocytic leukemias are cancers of the white blood cells from which lymphocytes originate. Both forms can be acute (short term and usually severe) or chronic (long-lasting).

Acute Myelogenous Leukemia

Acute myelogenous leukemia (AML) is caused by genetic changes in the cells that produce granulocytes, a type of white blood cell made in the bone marrow (where all the different types of blood cells are made). The resulting abnormal cells (called blasts) fail to mature properly and then multiply and survive longer than normal cells. As their numbers gradually increase, the leukemia cells pack, or fill up, the bone marrow and disrupt the production of normal white and red blood cells and platelets.

As the number of leukemia cells increases, they often spill over into the bloodstream. These cells may invade organs and tissues, especially the spleen and liver, causing the organs to become enlarged. If AML is not treated early, it can be fatal rapidly, sometimes within a few weeks. The major complications of this form of leukemia are severe infections and bleeding. However, as many as 40 to 50 percent of people with AML can be cured, depending on their age and the unique biological characteristics of their leukemia.

Symptoms
The most common symptoms of AML are feelings of fatigue, frequent infections, fever, lip, and mouth sores, and a tendency to bruise and bleed easily. The disease often occurs suddenly, with the symptoms becoming pronounced over a period of 1 to 2 weeks. In some cases, the symptoms develop gradually over about 2 months. If you have any of these symptoms, see your doctor right away.

Diagnosis
If your doctor suspects that you may have AML, he or she will examine you and will probably recommend blood tests and a bone marrow biopsy. For the biopsy, a sample of cells is withdrawn from your bone marrow through a needle and examined under a microscope for the presence of leukemia cells.

Treatment
If you are diagnosed with AML, your doctor will immediately admit you to the hospital. Because the treatment for this type of leukemia is complicated and difficult, it is usually performed by an oncologist (a doctor who specializes in treating cancer) or a hematologist (a doctor who specializes in treating blood disorders). In the hospital, you will be given transfusions of red blood cells and platelets when you need them. Platelet transfusions are usually provided to prevent bleeding. If you develop a fever or other sign of infection, the doctor will identify the infectious agent and give you antibiotics intravenously (through a vein) to fight it.

The first stage of treatment for AML is chemotherapy (see page 23) to try to destroy the cancerous cells. After a few weeks of chemotherapy, your health should return to normal. Chemotherapy produces a remission (disappearance of symptoms) in about 50 to 80 percent of people, depending on their age at diagnosis. However, if treatment is stopped after this first course of chemotherapy, the remission will be brief and the leukemia will recur. A variety of treatment strategies are used during this postremission period, ranging from additional chemotherapy to high-dose chemotherapy followed by a stem cell transplant (see page 624), depending on the person's age and the unique biological characteristics of his or her leukemia. When given at this time, these treatments can prolong survival significantly.

Acute Lymphocytic Leukemia

Acute lymphocytic leukemia (ALL) is characterized by an excess of infection-fighting white blood cells called lymphocytes in the blood and bone marrow. Lymphocytes originate in the bone marrow and other organs of the lymphatic system. In ALL, immature lymphocytes, called lymphoblasts, do not develop into infection-fighting white blood cells as they should. Excessive numbers of these immature lymphocytes collect in the blood, bone marrow, and lymph tissues. If the cancerous cells crowd out other blood cells, including red blood cells (which carry oxygen) and platelets (which enable blood to clot), the bone marrow cannot produce these essential cells in adequate numbers. A deficiency of red blood cells can lead to anemia; a deficiency of platelets can lead to easy bleeding or bruising.

The cancerous lymphocytes can also spread to other organs, including the brain, and to the spinal cord. ALL progresses quickly and affects mostly children and young adults. The prognosis for a person with ALL depends on the person's age and general health, on the characteristics of the leukemia cells seen under a microscope, and on how well the cancer responds to treatment.

Symptoms

The early symptoms of ALL—fever, weakness, fatigue, aching in the bones or joints, and swollen lymph nodes—are similar to those of the flu and other common infections. See your doctor if you have any of these symptoms for more than 2 or 3 weeks.

Diagnosis

Because symptoms in the early stages of ALL can resemble those of the flu, the disease can be difficult to diagnose. If you have persistent symptoms, your doctor may order blood tests to measure the levels of the different kinds of cells in your blood. If the results are abnormal, the doctor may recommend a bone marrow biopsy in which a small sample of your bone marrow is withdrawn through a needle inserted into a bone and the cells are studied under a microscope. The doctor may also recommend a lumbar puncture (see page 693), in which a needle

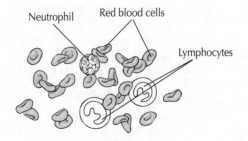

Healthy blood cells

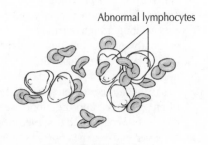

Blood cells in leukemia

Leukemia
In lymphocytic leukemias, white blood cells called lymphocytes have a genetic mutation that makes them abnormal. These abnormal lymphocytes don't function as they should to fight infections and they multiply and stay alive longer than usual, crowding out healthy cells and potentially disrupting the functioning of organs throughout the body.

is inserted through your back into the lower part of the spinal canal to withdraw a sample of cerebrospinal fluid; the fluid is studied under a microscope for the presence of cancerous cells. This information can help the doctor determine the type of leukemia and the best treatment.

Treatment

Chemotherapy (see page 23) is the standard treatment for ALL. Chemotherapy may be given by pill, injected into a vein or muscle, or injected into the cerebrospinal fluid through a needle inserted into the brain or back (to prevent the spread of cancer cells into the spinal fluid). If the cancer cells have spread to the spinal fluid, you will be given additional radiation therapy (see page 23) or chemotherapy in the brain. Once the cancer is in remission and you no longer have any signs of leukemia, you may receive chemotherapy for several years to kill any remaining cancer cells and to keep the cancer from recurring. If the leukemia recurs, you may choose to participate in a clinical trial of a stem cell transplant (see next page). In some cases, a stem cell transplant is recommended as the initial treatment for ALL.

Chronic Myeloid Leukemia

Chronic myeloid leukemia (CML) results from genetic changes in the bone marrow cells that produce granulocytes, a type of infection-fighting white blood cell. As a result of these changes, the number of granulocytes in the blood rises dramatically, often to between 20 and 40 times the normal level. The disease usually responds well to initial treatment. At an early stage of the disease, a stem cell transplant (see next page) can prevent the leukemia from developing into an aggressive, usually fatal form and can result in long-term survival.

Symptoms

People who have CML usually have symptoms at the time the disease is diagnosed. If you have symptoms of CML, you may feel ill, have little appetite, or lose weight. You may have a fever and sweat at night. In addition, if your spleen becomes enlarged from the accumulation of leukemia cells, you will have a feeling of fullness in your upper left abdomen. The excess of granulocytes in your bone marrow limits the ability of the stem cells to

produce the normal amount of red blood cells (which deliver oxygen to tissues) and platelets (which enable blood to clot), which can lead to anemia (see page 610) and easy bleeding.

Diagnosis

If you are having symptoms of a blood disorder, your doctor will recommend blood tests to either rule out CML or to determine if you should have more tests. To make a definite diagnosis of CML, your doctor will probably ask you to have a bone marrow aspiration and biopsy, in which a small sample of your bone marrow is removed through a needle and syringe and examined under a microscope.

Treatment

Most people who have CML can be treated on an outpatient basis unless they are having a transplant. The first treatment consists of anticancer drugs that usually restore bone marrow production to normal and clear up the symptoms. The outlook for people with CML has improved dramatically in recent years with treatment using very high-dose chemotherapy (sometimes with radiation) followed by a stem cell transplant from a compatible donor (usually a sibling). Some people benefit from injections of interferon alfa (a genetically engineered protein that triggers an immune response). A drug called imatinib mesylate is taken by mouth. This medication, called a tyrosine kinase inhibitor, works by blocking the specific enzyme (kinase) in CML that allows the cells to become cancerous and multiply. In many cases, these treatments can induce a complete remission that may increase long-term survival.

Chronic Lymphocytic Leukemia

Chronic lymphocytic leukemia (CLL) is a cancer of lymphocytes (infection-fighting white blood cells). Instead of maturing and dying in the natural way, the cancerous blood cells multiply and stay alive longer than they should. Gradually the leukemia cells crowd out healthy white blood cells in the lymph glands and bone marrow, reducing the immune system's ability to fight infections. The leukemia cells can overflow into the bloodstream and from there into the lymph nodes, spleen, liver, and other parts of the body. As the number of leukemia cells in the bone marrow rises, they increasingly interfere with the ability of the marrow to produce healthy new blood cells. This reduction in the number of healthy blood cells can lead to a variety of problems, including anemia (see page 610), susceptibility to infections, and bleeding.

Symptoms

CLL often produces no symptoms at first and is usually discovered by a blood test done for another reason. The first signs of this form of leukemia may be enlarged lymph glands in the neck, armpits, or groin, or a feeling of fullness in the upper left abdomen caused by an enlarged spleen (an organ of the immune system that contains lymphocytes). Sometimes the first symptoms are those caused by anemia or an infection. Some people with CLL may feel generally ill, have no appetite, lose weight, have a fever, or have night sweats. If you have any of these symptoms, see your doctor right away.

Diagnosis

If your doctor thinks you may have CLL, he or she will examine you and will recommend a blood test. If a blood test shows abnormal cells, you will have further testing, such as a bone marrow aspiration and biopsy, to determine the type of leukemia. In a

Stem Cell and Bone Marrow Transplants

If a closely matched donor is available, a stem cell or bone marrow transplant with very high-dose chemotherapy offers a chance for a cure for some types of cancer and other diseases. Bone marrow is spongy tissue inside the large bones that contains stem cells, which make all the different types of blood cells in the body. The tissue or cells can be taken either from the patient (an autologous transplant) or from a closely matched donor (an allogeneic transplant). A sibling's tissue is usually the best match, but bone marrow registries can often find unrelated donors who may be good matches for transplants.

Stem Cell Transplants

For an allogeneic stem cell transplant, stem cells can be collected from the donor's bloodstream using a procedure called apheresis. In apheresis, blood is drawn from the donor with a needle and syringe and put through a machine that collects stem cells from the blood and infuses the rest of the blood back into the person through another vein. Alternatively, stem cells can be taken directly from the bone marrow while the donor is under general anesthesia.

Before receiving the collected stem cells (either your own or those from a donor), you will be given massive doses of chemotherapy (see page 23), perhaps along with radiation therapy (see page 23), to destroy all the cancerous cells in your body.

Bone Marrow Transplants

A bone marrow transplant is used to replace diseased bone marrow with healthy bone marrow. For an allogeneic bone marrow transplant (which uses bone marrow from a compatible donor), all the bone marrow in your body is first destroyed with high doses of chemotherapy, perhaps along with radiation therapy. Healthy marrow that has been taken from the donor is injected through a needle into one of your veins to replace the bone marrow that was destroyed.

For an autologous bone marrow transplant, some of your bone marrow is taken from you, treated with powerful drugs to kill the cancer cells, and frozen until it is needed. You are then given high-dose chemotherapy (and possibly radiation therapy) to destroy all of your remaining bone marrow. After thawing your frozen, treated bone marrow, the doctor injects it back into your body through a needle into a vein to replace your destroyed, cancerous marrow.

After a Stem Cell or Bone Marrow Transplant

Immediately after the stem cell or bone marrow transplant or intensive chemotherapy, you will have virtually no white blood cells and therefore no ability to fight infections. Because of this, you will be placed in a germ-free environment to avoid the possibility of infection. Once the transplanted stem cells or bone marrow begin to produce white blood cells in adequate numbers, this isolation will no longer be necessary because your immune system will have regained some of its ability to resist infections. You will be given medications derived from human proteins called growth factors to stimulate the growth of healthy blood cells.

Death from infection or severe bleeding can sometimes result after a stem cell or bone marrow transplant or high-dose chemotherapy. A complication of an allogeneic transplant may occur when the donor cells recognize the recipient's tissues as foreign and react against them. To prevent this graft-versus-host response, you will be given immune-suppressing medications for several months or longer after the transplant.

bone marrow aspiration and biopsy, a sample of bone marrow is withdrawn with a needle from one of your large bones (such as the hip) and examined under a microscope.

Treatment

If your leukemia is at an early stage, you do not need any treatment. Your doctor will recommend regular checkups to monitor the progression of the cancer, a flu shot (see page 650) every year, and a vaccination against pneumonia (see page 145) every 5 years. You will need treatment, however, once you start having symptoms, such as a significant increase in the size of your lymph glands, spleen, or liver; anemia; a low platelet count in your blood; fever; and weight loss.

Your doctor will probably first use an anticancer drug that is usually effective in eliminating or reducing most symptoms of this type of cancer. Your enlarged lymph glands and spleen will probably decrease in size, your blood count will improve, and your symptoms will go away. If this drug does not work, or if it stops working after a while, you will probably be treated with a combination of other anticancer drugs and, perhaps, a corticosteroid (to help reduce inflammation). These drugs are often helpful at this stage.

Many people with CLL live for years without needing treatment. When treatment becomes necessary, it usually keeps a person reasonably healthy for several years. Many people with CLL live a normal life span and die of other causes.

Lymphomas

Lymphomas are cancerous tumors of the lymph glands (organs of the immune system) that result from genetic changes in infection-fighting white blood cells called lymphocytes. Occasionally, lymphomas may develop in people who have a weakened immune system, such as people who are infected with HIV or who have AIDS (see page 909) or who are receiving immune-suppressing drugs to avoid organ rejection after a transplant. In these cases, a virus may be the cause.

Non-Hodgkin's Lymphoma

Non-Hodgkin's lymphoma is a very diverse group of cancers. In a slow-growing form, the disease may not require treatment for years and may even go away on its own for a time. In a fast-growing, aggressive form, the disease requires prompt treatment or can quickly be fatal.

Symptoms

The first symptom of non-Hodgkin's lymphoma is usually a swollen gland. Swollen glands can be anywhere in your body, but they generally appear first in the neck, armpit, or groin. Other possible symptoms include feeling generally ill, loss of appetite, unexplained weight loss, fever, or night sweats. If you have a swelling or lump that persists for no obvious reason for more than 2 weeks, see your doctor.

Diagnosis

If the swelling is an enlarged lymph gland and the doctor sees no sign that the swelling has resulted from a common infection such as a cold, he or she may recommend a blood test and a biopsy of the gland (microscopic examination of a sample of tissue from the gland). Information from the blood test and the biopsy usually can help the doctor determine whether a person has lymphoma and, if so, what type.

Treatment

The treatment for non-Hodgkin's lymphoma depends on the type of lymphoma and on how many areas of the body are affected. To enable the doctor to determine how widespread your cancer is, you will have imaging procedures such as X-rays, a CT scan (see page 112), an MRI (see page 113), a gallium scan, or a PET scan (see page 114). You will also probably have a bone marrow aspiration and biopsy to determine if the bone marrow has been affected.

The standard treatment for non-Hodgkin's lymphoma is chemotherapy (see page 23), which is likely to induce a remission (disappearance of symptoms) and can cure a substantial number of people. For people who fail to respond to the standard-dose chemotherapy, high-dose chemotherapy and a stem cell transplant (see page 624) can be lifesaving.

Hodgkin's Disease

Hodgkin's disease is a cancer that arises from white blood cells (lymphocytes). The cancer can develop in a single lymph node, a group of lymph nodes, or in other parts of the lymphatic system, such as the bone marrow or spleen. Hodgkin's disease is most common in adolescents and young adults and in people over age 50.

Symptoms

The main symptom of Hodgkin's disease is persistent swollen glands, usually in the neck, armpit, or groin. Other possible symptoms include fever, sweating, fatigue, weakness, weight loss, and itching. See your doctor immediately if you have any unexplained swellings—Hodgkin's disease responds well to early treatment.

Diagnosis

If you have symptoms of Hodgkin's disease, your doctor will probably take samples of your blood and remove one of your swollen glands for examination. If these evaluations show that you have Hodgkin's disease, you will need to have tests to determine the extent of the cancer. For example, you may have a bone marrow aspiration and biopsy, in which a small amount of bone marrow is removed

through a needle and syringe and examined under a microscope. Other tests may include a chest X-ray, an MRI (see page 113), a CT scan (see page 112), a gallium scan, or a PET scan (see page 114).

Treatment

If you have Hodgkin's disease, your treatment will depend on the results of your diagnostic tests and the form of Hodgkin's you have. Radiation therapy is often used to treat Hodgkin's disease at an early stage. Radiation therapy can have a success rate higher than 90 percent for some forms of Hodgkin's disease in young people. However, many doctors recommend a combination of chemotherapy drugs for most stages of Hodgkin's disease. Occasionally, both chemotherapy and radiation therapy are recommended.

If the cancer is at an advanced stage when it is detected, combination chemotherapy is given. Combination chemotherapy can cure the majority of cases of Hodgkin's disease. Radiation therapy is sometimes given after chemotherapy to eliminate specific areas of disease. The entire course of treatment usually takes about 6 months. High-dose chemotherapy and a stem cell transplant (see page 624) are recommended for people whose Hodgkin's disease returns after treatment or whose disease has not responded completely to other treatments. Once your treatment is completed, you will need to have regular checkups for several years to make sure the cancer has not returned and to watch for any long-term complications of the chemotherapy or radiation therapy, such as heart disease, thyroid disease, lung cancer, or breast cancer.

Disorders of the Bone Marrow

The marrow inside your bones is an active tissue with a rich blood supply. Blood cells inside the bone marrow, called stem cells, make all the different types of blood cells in the body, including red cells (which deliver oxygen to tissues), platelets (which enable blood to clot), and white cells (which fight infection). Blood that flows through the marrow moves the newly produced blood cells into the bloodstream. In adults, active blood-forming marrow is found only in the

bones of the trunk. The marrow inside the bones of the arms and legs is fatty and, in adults, is usually inactive, but it can become active and produce new blood cells when necessary. In young children, all the bones have active, blood-forming marrow. Disorders of the bone marrow such as polycythemia and aplastic anemia can affect all types of blood cells, while disorders such as multiple myeloma and agranulocytosis affect only one type of blood cell.

Multiple Myeloma

Multiple myeloma is a cancer that affects plasma cells, a type of white blood cell in blood and bone marrow. Plasma cells produce proteins called antibodies to fight infections. Normally, plasma cells make up only a small percentage of the cells in the marrow but, if a plasma cell undergoes genetic changes that cause it to multiply excessively, the result is a cancer called multiple myeloma. The overproduction of plasma cells inside the marrow disrupts the production of red blood cells (which deliver oxygen to tissues). This disruption in red blood cell production can lead to anemia (see page 610). The antibodies produced by the cancerous plasma cells can accumulate and injure the kidneys. This accumulation of plasma cells usually overtakes the production of normal infection-fighting antibodies by healthy plasma cells. The excess of plasma cells can cause painful destruction of bone.

Multiple myeloma makes up about 10 percent of all blood cancers but, for unknown reasons, appears to be increasing in the United States. The cancer affects mostly people over 50 and is slightly more common in men than in women and is more common in blacks than in people of other races.

Symptoms

The most common symptom of multiple myeloma is pain in your bones, particularly in the vertebrae (bones in the spine). Other symptoms include weakness, fatigue, increased levels of calcium in the blood (caused by bone loss), and increased susceptibility to infections, which can be serious. You may also have symptoms of kidney failure (see page 817). If you have any of these symptoms, see your doctor, especially if you are over 50 and have bone pain, particularly in the bones in your back. Chronic kidney failure (see page 817) can occur as the disease progresses.

Diagnosis

If your doctor suspects that you have multiple myeloma, he or she will recommend laboratory analysis of samples of your blood and urine and X-rays of your bones.

Treatment

In the early stage of multiple myeloma, no treatment is necessary if you don't have any complications such as anemia. Because your resistance to infections is low, your doctor may prescribe antibiotics if you have any symptoms of infection. If the cancer has become more advanced and is causing symptoms, you will be given chemotherapy (see page 23) or drugs such as corticosteroids or thalidomide or newer derivatives of thalidomide, depending on your age and the stage of the cancer. Multiple myeloma cannot be cured with traditional chemotherapy but, in some cases, a stem cell transplant (see page 624) with cells donated by a sibling can significantly prolong survival and may cure the disease.

If you have had bone destruction, your doctor will prescribe a medication to repair bone tissue and prevent more bone destruction and pain. Fractures can often be prevented with surgery or radiation therapy (see page 23). If you have anemia, you will be given injections of a human protein called erythropoietin to increase your body's production of red blood cells.

Polycythemia

Normally your body regulates the production of blood cells in the bone marrow, balancing the number of blood cells the marrow makes with the number of cells that die during natural body processes. If you have polycythemia, this regulation is faulty and the marrow produces far more blood cells than the body needs.

Polycythemia has two main forms—polycythemia vera and secondary polycythemia. Polycythemia vera, the more serious form, is an overproduction of red blood cells (which deliver oxygen to tissues), granulocytes (white blood cells that fight infections), and platelets (which enable blood to clot). Although polycythemia vera cannot be cured, it can be treated, and many people have relief from their symptoms for years at a time and live for many years. Possible complications of polycythemia vera include heart attack (see page 567), stroke (see page 669), deep vein thrombosis (see page 605), pulmonary embolism (see page 606), peripheral arterial thrombosis, bleeding, gout (see page 1004), and acute myelogenous leukemia (see page 621).

Unlike polycythemia vera, the secondary form of polycythemia is not triggered by a cancerous overproduction of cells. Secondary polycythemia is brought on by an underlying disorder such as severe lung disease or some kinds of congenital heart disease (see page 389), or by living at high altitudes or smoking, all of which can reduce the amount of oxygen supplied to tissues. In response to the signal that the tissues need more oxygen, the bone marrow produces more oxygen-delivering red blood cells. Secondary polycythemia can also develop as a result of noncancerous or cancerous tumors of the kidney, brain, or liver. To treat secondary polycythemia, a doctor diagnoses and treats the underlying disorder.

Symptoms

The most common symptoms of polycythemia vera include recurring headaches, dizziness, visual disturbances, a feeling of fullness in the head, and a ruddy complexion. You also may have severe itching that worsens when you take a hot bath. The condition can also cause enlargement of the spleen (an organ of the immune system that stores red blood cells and platelets), which a doctor can feel during a physical examination. Secondary polycythemia can cause headache, lethargy, and elevated blood pressure.

Diagnosis

To diagnose polycythemia, a doctor performs a physical examination and will probably recommend a blood test that measures the number of red cells in the blood or that compares the relative amounts of red blood cells and plasma (the fluid in which blood cells are suspended). He or she may also recommend measuring the level of erythropoietin (a protein in the blood that enhances the formation of red blood cells). You may need to have a bone marrow aspiration and biopsy (removal of cells from the bone marrow through a needle and syringe for examination under a microscope) to rule out other disorders.

Treatment

If you have polycythemia vera, you may be able to have treatment on an outpatient basis. The first goal of treatment is to lower the number of red cells in your blood, thereby reducing the thickness of your blood and your risk of developing blood clots or sludged blood, which can block blood flow. About a pint of blood is taken regularly from a vein in your arm. The frequency of blood removal (phlebotomy) is based on how long the number of red blood cells stays at a healthy level.

Drugs are sometimes used to control the overproduction of red blood cells. These drugs are usually taken by mouth for months to years, depending on how well they control blood cell production. Rarely, doctors recommend injections of radioactive phosphorus to reduce the number of red blood cells in the blood. Drugs are usually used only for people who cannot have their blood drawn regularly or for whom blood removal alone has not been effective in maintaining a healthy balance of red blood cells.

Aplastic Anemia

If you have aplastic anemia, your bone marrow's production of blood cells decreases, causing a gradual or sudden reduction in the total number of cells in your bloodstream. In most cases of aplastic anemia, the cause cannot be identified. Sometimes it can be traced to exposure to radiation or a toxic substance such as benzene or to taking a particular medication. Many cases are thought to result from an overactive immune system that inhibits the ability of the bone marrow to produce blood cells. The condition may improve spontaneously or with treatment, but progressive failure of the bone marrow can also occur, making the condition worse.

Symptoms

Aplastic anemia has three main groups of symptoms. The decrease in the production of red blood cells causes the symptoms of iron deficiency anemia (see page 610). The decrease in the production of granulocytes, a type of infection-fighting white blood cell, makes you more susceptible to infections. The decrease in the production of platelets (cell fragments that enable blood to clot) causes the bleeding disorder thrombocytopenia (see page 620), which leads to easy bruising, red spots on the skin, and bleeding from the nose, mouth, and other areas. The bleeding may be severe enough to become life-threatening. If you have any of these symptoms, see your doctor right away.

Diagnosis

If you have symptoms of aplastic anemia, your doctor will probably ask you to have a blood test. If the test results show that you may have aplastic anemia, you may need to have a bone marrow aspiration and biopsy, in which a small amount of your bone marrow is removed through a needle and syringe and examined under a microscope. A bone marrow biopsy usually enables a doctor to make a definite diagnosis.

Treatment

If you have aplastic anemia that has resulted from taking a medication for another condition, your doctor will ask you to stop taking the medication and will prescribe a substitute drug. If there is a possibility of continuing exposure to a toxic substance at your workplace or at home, you need to eliminate the toxic substance from your environment; you may need to change jobs or move to another home.

Your doctor will probably treat the anemia and bleeding with blood transfusions and will treat infections with antibiotics, which are usually given intravenously (through a vein). If your condition doesn't improve within a few weeks, your doctor will prescribe medication to stimulate your bone marrow to produce blood cells. Genetically engineered proteins called granulocyte-stimulating factors may also be helpful in stimulating blood cell production. If this treatment does not stimulate normal cell production in your bone marrow, your doctor may recommend drugs such as antithymocyte globulin and cyclosporine, which are effective in improving the levels of blood cells in most people who have aplastic anemia.

Alternatively, your doctor may recommend a stem cell transplant (see page 624) from a sibling if you are otherwise healthy and have a sibling with matching tissue type. The stem cells are injected into one of your veins and make their way to the bone marrow, where they take over the production of blood cells. You may be given granulocyte-stimulating factors after the transplant to enhance the functioning of the donor stem cells within your bone marrow.

Neutropenia and Agranulocytosis

Neutrophils and granulocytes are white blood cells that are the body's first defense against infections. Normally, neutrophils and granulocytes are produced in the bone marrow and released into the bloodstream. In neutropenia, neutrophils are not being produced properly. In agranulocytosis, granulocytes are not being produced at all. The resulting severe reduction in either type of white blood cell significantly decreases the body's ability to fight infections.

Neutropenia is usually a complication of chemotherapy (see page 23). Occasionally, neutropenia results from a medication taken for another disorder. Agranulocytosis can result from a viral infection or from an errant immune response that mistakenly attacks a person's own white blood cells. Neutropenia or agranulocytosis can be the first sign of leukemia (see page 621) or aplastic anemia (see previous page).

Symptoms

The main symptom of both neutropenia and agranulocytosis is susceptibility to infections, especially in the mouth and throat. In some cases of agranulocytosis, infections such as pneumonia progress unusually rapidly and can be extremely severe or fatal. If you have frequent infections, see your doctor, especially if you are taking any prescription or over-the-counter drugs or supplements, because some medications can damage the bone marrow.

Diagnosis

Make sure your doctor knows about all medications you are taking. He or she will probably want you to have a blood test. If the results of the test show that you may have neutropenia or agranulocytosis, your doctor will confirm the diagnosis by performing a bone marrow aspiration and biopsy, in which a small amount of your bone marrow is removed through a needle and syringe and examined under a microscope.

Treatment

The treatment for neutropenia and agranulocytosis involves waiting for the levels of neutrophils and granulocytes to return to normal while dealing with any complications that may occur, including bleeding (which is treated with infusions of red blood cells and platelets) and infections (which are treated with antibiotics). In some cases, drugs called hematopoietic growth factors may be used to stimulate the production of white blood cells. If the cause is a medication you have been taking for another condition, your doctor will ask you to stop taking that drug and will prescribe a substitute.

3

Disorders of the Respiratory System

Respiration is the process by which oxygen reaches the body's cells and is used by them to produce energy. Internal respiration is the exchange of gases between the blood and body tissues. External respiration, which we call breathing, is the exchange of gases between the lungs and the blood.

During breathing, your lungs take in oxygen from the air when you inhale and release carbon dioxide from your blood when you exhale. The channel that carries the air in and out of your lungs is called the respiratory tract and includes the sinuses, nasal cavity, pharynx (throat), larynx (voice box), trachea (windpipe), lungs, and a system of arteries, veins, and smaller vessels that carry blood to and from the lungs.

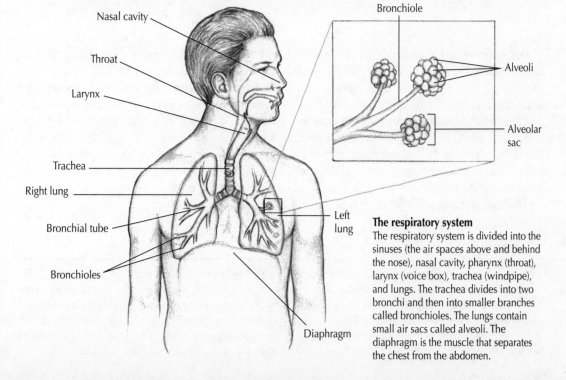

Nasal cavity

Throat

Larynx

Trachea

Right lung

Bronchial tube

Bronchioles

Diaphragm

Bronchiole

Alveoli

Alveolar sac

Left lung

The respiratory system
The respiratory system is divided into the sinuses (the air spaces above and behind the nose), nasal cavity, pharynx (throat), larynx (voice box), trachea (windpipe), and lungs. The trachea divides into two bronchi and then into smaller branches called bronchioles. The lungs contain small air sacs called alveoli. The diaphragm is the muscle that separates the chest from the abdomen.

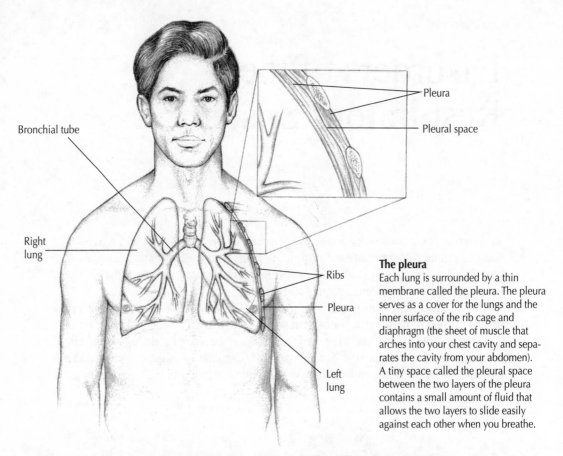

Bronchial tube

Right lung

Pleura

Pleural space

Ribs

Pleura

Left lung

The pleura
Each lung is surrounded by a thin membrane called the pleura. The pleura serves as a cover for the lungs and the inner surface of the rib cage and diaphragm (the sheet of muscle that arches into your chest cavity and separates the cavity from your abdomen). A tiny space called the pleural space between the two layers of the pleura contains a small amount of fluid that allows the two layers to slide easily against each other when you breathe.

Deep in the chest, the trachea divides into two main tubes called bronchi. Each bronchus leads to a lung, where the bronchus divides into smaller air passages called bronchioles. At the tip of each bronchiole are clusters of balloonlike structures called alveoli; the lungs contain about 300 million alveoli. The exchange of oxygen for carbon dioxide occurs through tiny blood vessels in the thin walls of the alveoli.

The body uses several muscles to draw air into the lungs. The diaphragm is a dome-shaped muscle attached to the lower ribs that separates the chest cavity from the abdomen. When the diaphragm contracts (along with other muscles between the ribs), the contraction creates a mild vacuum inside your lungs, causing the lungs to expand and draw air into the respiratory tract. When the muscles that help draw air into the lungs relax, the lungs spring back, forcing the air back out of the lungs.

The Nose

The nose is the uppermost part of the respiratory tract. Protective hairs just inside the nose trap large dust particles and other debris. A mucous membrane that contains many tiny blood vessels lines the nose. This lining cleans, moistens, and warms the air you breathe as it goes through the nasal passage toward your throat and lungs. The nasal passage is winding rather than straight, running along the top of the palate (the roof of the mouth) and turning down toward the throat. In several places, the nasal passage opens into sinuses (air-filled cavities in bones of the skull).

Respiration

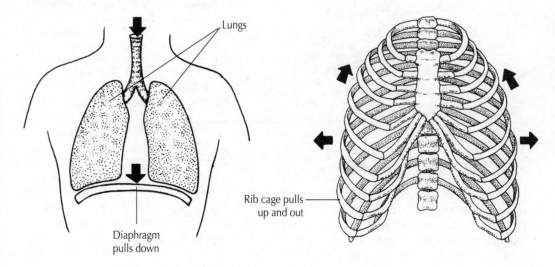

Lungs

Rib cage pulls
up and out

Diaphragm
pulls down

Breathing in

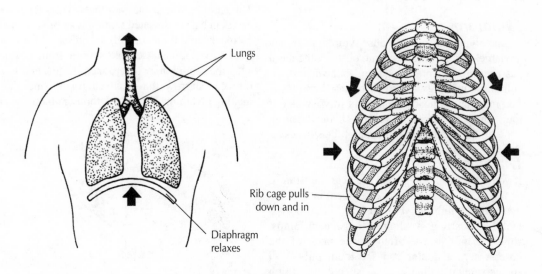

Lungs

Rib cage pulls
down and in

Diaphragm
relaxes

Breathing out

How you breathe

When you breathe in, your diaphragm is pulled down and flattened (top left). The muscles between your ribs may also contract and pull your rib cage upward and outward (top right), expanding and drawing air into your lungs. The stronger this muscle action is, the more air that enters your lungs.

Your breathing rate is determined by the amount of carbon dioxide expelled from your bloodstream. When you breathe out, your chest muscles and diaphragm relax (bottom left), making your rib cage sink (bottom right) and your lungs contract and squeeze out air.

633

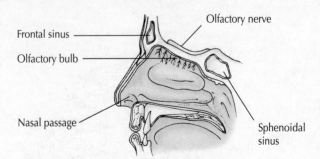

Frontal sinus

Olfactory bulb

Olfactory nerve

Nasal passage

Sphenoidal sinus

Cross section of the nose
The nasal passage is linked to sinuses, which are air-filled cavities in the skull. The sensitive hairlike endings of the olfactory nerves project into the nasal passage. The olfactory nerves detect odors in the air and pass the information to the olfactory bulb, which transmits the information to the brain (which recognizes or perceives the odors).

Nasal Polyps

Nasal polyps are benign (noncancerous) growths of the mucous membrane that lines the nose. They protrude into the nasal cavity. Polyps result from an immune response that triggers fluid buildup and swelling in the lining of the nose. Nasal polyps develop most frequently in people who have chronic conditions such as asthma (see page 640) that cause recurring inflammation in the nasal cavity or in people who are sensitive to aspirin.

Symptoms

Nasal polyps don't always cause symptoms. If they are large or numerous, they can obstruct the nasal passages, making breathing through the nose difficult and impairing your sense of smell and taste. You may have a headache or pain in your face if they cause an infection and block the opening between the nasal cavity and one of the sinuses.

Diagnosis

If you have nasal polyps that are near the front of your nose, you may be able to see them in a mirror by shining a light up your nostrils. Nasal polyps look like pearly gray, slightly translucent lumps. However, polyps are often at the back of the nose, where a doctor can see them only with an instrument called a nasal speculum, which holds the nostrils open. Nasal polyps that haven't caused symptoms are often discovered by a doctor during an examination of a person's nose for other reasons.

Treatment

Nasal polyps sometimes go away in a few years with no treatment. Your doctor may prescribe a corticosteroid nasal spray to help reduce inflammation and shrink the polyps. If your nasal polyps are causing severe symptoms, your doctor may refer you to a specialist who may recommend that you have the polyps removed surgically. To shrink the polyps before surgery, you may need to take oral corticosteroid medication. Polyps have a tendency to recur even after surgery.

Deviated Septum

The nasal septum is the wall that divides the nasal cavity in half. A deviated septum is an off-center or crooked septum that usually has resulted from an injury. Even if the nose looks straight from the outside, the septum may be crooked. A deviated septum can narrow the nasal cavity on one side, making breathing difficult. Although no one has a

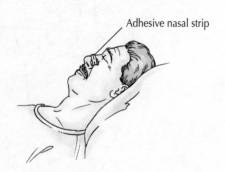

Adhesive nasal strip

Adhesive nasal strips
Adhesive nasal strips consist of two bands of plastic in an adhesive pad. When the strips are placed correctly across the bridge of the nose, they safely lift the sides of the nose and widen the space in the nasal passage, making it easier to breathe through the nose. Many people wear the strips when they sleep to help reduce snoring.

septum that is perfectly straight, it is rare to have a deviation that significantly diminishes air flow through the nose.

Diagnosis

To determine how crooked your septum is, your doctor will examine the inside of your nose using an instrument called a nasal speculum, which holds the nostrils open. He or she will also evaluate how much your breathing is affected by the deviated septum.

Treatment

Your doctor may recommend that you use adhesive nasal strips to widen your nasal passage and make it easier for you to breathe. These strips are especially helpful to wear when you're sleeping and when you're exercising. Your doctor also may prescribe a corticosteroid nasal spray or oral corticosteroid tablets to reduce the inflammation in the nasal passage and improve your breathing. If the spray, tablets, or breathing strips do not improve your breathing, your doctor may recommend surgery.

The Throat

The throat, also called the pharynx, is part of a multipurpose passageway leading from the back of the nose and mouth down to the trachea (windpipe) and esophagus. When you breathe, air passes through your throat into the trachea on its way into and out of the lungs. When you swallow, chewed food lubricated with saliva moves down your throat into the esophagus on its way to the stomach.

The throat splits into two parts at the opening to the larynx (voice box), which is at the top of the trachea. The larynx consists of cartilage, muscle, and connective tissue. At the upper end of the larynx are two paired folds of fibrous tissue. The upper pair are the false vocal cords, which do not produce sound but close along with the epiglottis (the flap of cartilage that lies behind the tongue and in front of the larynx) during swallowing to prevent food from entering the larynx. The lower pair are the vocal cords. Air passing between the vocal cords makes them vibrate to produce the broad range of sounds that your mouth shapes into speech.

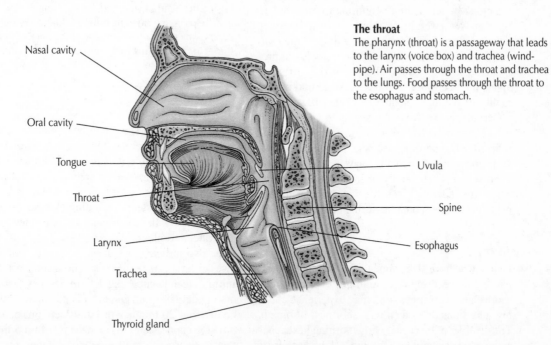

The throat
The pharynx (throat) is a passageway that leads to the larynx (voice box) and trachea (windpipe). Air passes through the throat and trachea to the lungs. Food passes through the throat to the esophagus and stomach.

Nasal cavity

Oral cavity

Tongue

Throat

Larynx

Trachea

Thyroid gland

Uvula

Spine

Esophagus

Sleep Apnea

Sleep apnea is a serious and potentially life-threatening breathing disorder that can cause a person to stop breathing for short periods during sleep. Breathing can cease for 20 seconds or more, sometimes becoming so inadequate that the person's skin turns blue because of the lack of oxygen. As blood oxygen levels drop, the person may stir enough to take some normal breaths (but does not fully wake up). After some normal breathing, the person falls back asleep. This cycle can repeat itself 20 to 30 times an hour each night.

The most common type of sleep apnea, called obstructive sleep apnea, is caused by an overly relaxed or sagging base of the tongue, uvula (the small piece of tissue that hangs from the middle of the back of the throat), or soft palate (roof of the mouth). These sagging tissues obstruct air flow to and from the person's windpipe. Using alcohol or sleeping pills worsens sleep apnea by making the airway tissue more likely to sag during sleep. In the less common type of sleep apnea called central sleep apnea, the brain fails to send the required signals to the breathing muscles to continue regular inhalation and exhalation during sleep.

Sleep apnea occurs in people of all ages, including children, and is more common in men than in women. Overweight people are most likely to develop sleep apnea, although with age the connection between sleep apnea and obesity is less pronounced. Other people who are at risk for sleep apnea include those who have a structural abnormality of the nose or throat or other parts of the upper airway. The disorder seems to run in families. It has been linked to some cases of sudden infant death syndrome (see page 388). People with sleep apnea are often totally unaware that they have the disorder. Their family or friends suspect sleep apnea after hearing excessive snoring or seeing the person struggle to breathe during sleep.

Symptoms

People who have sleep apnea snore loudly between pauses in breathing (although not everyone who snores has sleep apnea) and may experience choking sensations or awaken with shortness of breath. The disorder often causes early morning headaches and daytime sleepiness. Chronic lack of sleep from sleep apnea may cause depression, irritability, learning and memory difficulties, and sexual problems. Sleep deprivation also places a person at risk of vehicle collisions and work-related accidents.

Sleep apnea can cause the heart to beat irregularly. It can contribute to high blood pressure and heart failure because the heart beats harder in the long term trying to make up for the chronically low oxygen levels. In people who already have heart disease (see page 558), sleep apnea can contribute to heart attacks.

Snoring

Snoring occurs when tissue at the back of your throat—the tonsils, adenoids, back of the tongue, or uvula—vibrates as air travels over it while you breathe during sleep. When this tissue becomes enlarged or when it develops poor muscle tone (which often results from excessive, long-term alcohol consumption), snoring is more likely to occur. Swollen and inflamed nasal passages resulting from a cold or allergies can also cause temporary snoring. Most snoring is not serious, but heavy or loud snoring can be a sign of sleep apnea.

If your snoring disrupts your sleep or the sleep of other people, see your doctor. The remedy may be as simple as changing your sleep position or raising the head of your bed. Losing weight may also help. Taking sleeping pills, drinking alcohol, or smoking can cause the tissue at the back of your throat to relax during sleep, increasing the chances that you will snore.

Diagnosis

Because disturbed sleep can have many causes, doctors use two specific tests to diagnose sleep apnea and determine its severity. Both are conducted overnight in a sleep center. The first test, polysomnography, measures a variety of body functions during sleep, including eye movement, muscle activity, the electrical activity of the brain, heart rate, and blood oxygen levels. Polysomnography also indicates when the person enters and leaves different stages of sleep. The second test, the multiple sleep latency test, determines how fast the person falls asleep. In general, people take an average of 10 to 20 minutes to fall asleep, but people with sleep apnea tend to fall asleep within 5 minutes. Because the multiple sleep latency test is conducted periodically over the course of a day, the doctor can also find out the degree of daytime sleepiness of a person with sleep apnea.

Treatment

People whose sleep apnea is mild often benefit from lifestyle changes, such as losing weight and avoiding alcohol and sleeping pills. Some people with mild sleep apnea have breathing pauses only when they lie on their back. Learning to sleep on their side often improves the condition. Devices, fitted by a dentist, help some people with mild to moderate sleep apnea by repositioning the jaw or tongue.

The most effective treatment for people with severe sleep apnea is called nasal continuous positive airway pressure (CPAP). In CPAP, a person with sleep apnea wears a mask over his or her nose during sleep. Pressure from an air blower forces air through the nasal passages, holding the airway open and preventing tissue in the throat from sagging. If it is used properly, CPAP is very effective in reversing sleep apnea (and therefore sleep apnea's detrimental effects on the heart). Possible side effects of CPAP include drying and irritation of the nose, facial discomfort, abdominal bloating, sore eyes, and headaches. These side effects sometimes make CPAP uncomfortable to use, but adjustments in pressure and the use of a humidifier may help lessen the discomfort.

Some people with sleep apnea need to have surgery to increase the size of the airway. In children, the most common corrective surgical procedures include removal of the adenoids (lymph glands at the back of the nose), tonsils (lymph tissue at the back of the throat), or, rarely, nasal polyps (small growths in the lining of the nose). In adults, surgeons perform a surgical procedure called uvulopalatoplasty to remove excess tissue from the tonsils, uvula, or soft palate. People who have sleep apnea resulting from a deformity of the jaw may be helped with reconstructive jaw surgery. In severe, life-threatening cases of sleep apnea, surgeons sometimes perform a tracheostomy, in which they make a small hole in the windpipe and insert a tube in the hole for air. The tube stays closed during waking hours but is opened during sleep to allow air to flow directly into the lungs.

Tumors of the Larynx

Both cancerous (malignant) and noncancerous (benign) growths can develop in the larynx (voice box). Papillomas and vocal cord polyps or nodules are the two most common types of benign tumors that develop in the larynx. Papillomas, which are caused by a virus, are usually multiple and occur more often in children than in adults. Nodules are hard, calluslike growths that frequently develop in pairs on both sides of the larynx. Polyps are softer than nodules and usually develop on only one side of the larynx. Both polyps and nodules usually result from overuse of the voice.

Cancerous tumors of the larynx occur most often in smokers. Cancer of the larynx can almost always be cured if it is diagnosed at an early stage. If cancer is not detected until a later stage, it can spread to other parts of the throat or elsewhere in the body.

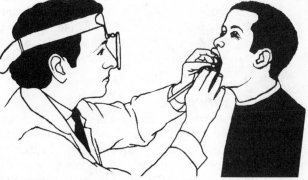

Examining the larynx
To examine your larynx, an otolaryngologist (a doctor who specializes in disorders of the ears, nose, and throat) uses a system of mirrors in a procedure called laryngoscopy. A mirror attached to a band on his or her head reflects light down your throat (the mirror has a hole in it for the otolaryngologist to look through). He or she holds a smaller mirror at the back of your throat to reflect light and enable him or her to view the larynx. If the otolaryngologist cannot see your larynx well using the mirrors, he or she will numb your nose with an anesthetic spray and pass a small, flexible viewing tube down your nose to the larynx.

Symptoms

Because growths on the larynx are painless and develop slowly, they often go undetected during the early stages. Hoarseness is usually the only symptom, although papillomas can also cause difficulty breathing. Hoarseness caused by noncancerous tumors can be intermittent or continuous, while hoarseness caused by a cancerous tumor is always continuous and gets worse over time. If a tumor is cancerous and allowed to grow, it can eventually make swallowing difficult. The cancer may eventually spread to lymph nodes in the neck, producing an obvious lump in the neck. Do not ignore changes in your voice that occur for no obvious reason. If you are hoarse for more than a week or have hoarseness that recurs, see your doctor.

Diagnosis

If, after examining your throat, your doctor rules out inflammation from laryngitis, he or she will refer you to an otolaryngologist (an ear, nose, and throat specialist) for a more thorough examination of your larynx. If the otolaryngologist sees signs of a growth, he or she will probably schedule an outpatient procedure called endoscopy. During the endoscopy, he or she will insert a viewing tube (laryngoscope) through your mouth to the larynx and will take a sample of cells from the larynx for examination under a microscope to determine if the growth is cancerous.

Treatment

Voice-retraining therapy can help relieve pressure on the vocal cords, sometimes causing nodules to shrink enough to stop causing symptoms such as hoarseness. Polyps and nodules can go away on their own, but sometimes a surgeon may need to remove them. If you have surgery, you will be given general anesthesia. The doctor uses an operating microscope to magnify the area, making it easier for him or her to see and remove the abnormal tissue. Papillomas can recur after surgery and may need to be removed several times.

Malignant tumors that are detected early can be successfully treated either with radiation therapy (see page 23) or by removing part of the larynx. With either of these treatments, total loss of voice is rare (the voice is usually preserved at least partially). In advanced cancer, the entire larynx may be removed or the person may be given chemotherapy (see page 23) along with radiation therapy (called chemoradiation) to eliminate the cancerous cells. Even in relatively advanced cases, the chances for a cure are good.

If the surgeon removes your entire larynx, different types of therapies are available to help you regain your speech. With the help of a speech therapist, you may learn how to use your esophagus to speak. Or you may be able to learn to use a special vibrating device that you manipulate with your tongue and teeth to produce the sounds of speech. In some cases, a surgeon implants a valve between the trachea and esophagus (see illustration below) to divert air from the lungs into the esophagus to produce the sounds of speech.

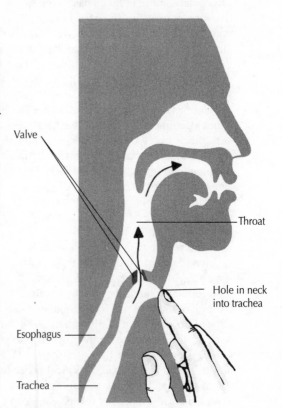

Speaking without your larynx

Surgery can enable you to speak after having your larynx removed by creating a system to produce speech sounds. The surgeon makes a small hole in your neck into your trachea. He or she then implants a valve between the trachea and esophagus. When you want to speak, you place a finger over the hole in the trachea. Blocking the opening in the trachea allows air from your lungs to pass through the new valve, which makes the pharynx vibrate to produce sound.

The Lungs and Chest

Your two lungs lie on either side of the central cavity of the chest. The upper tips of the lungs are slightly above the collarbone. The bottom surfaces of the lungs rest on the diaphragm, a sheet of muscle that arches up into the chest cavity and completely separates the chest cavity from the abdomen.

The bronchi are the main airways that branch into each lung from the trachea. They divide into smaller and smaller airways called bronchioles. Each bronchiole ends in a cluster of tiny air sacs called alveoli. Each lung contains about 150 million alveoli. Each alveolus contains several minute blood vessels called capillaries. The walls of the capillaries are thin enough to allow oxygen and carbon dioxide (a waste product from body processes) to move between the air and the blood. The alveoli transfer oxygen from the air you breathe to your blood, which transports the oxygen to all tissues in your body. Your blood releases carbon dioxide into your lungs and you exhale it. The heart pumps blood that contains mostly carbon dioxide through the pulmonary arteries back to the lungs for a fresh supply of oxygen (to deliver to body tissues) and to release the carbon dioxide.

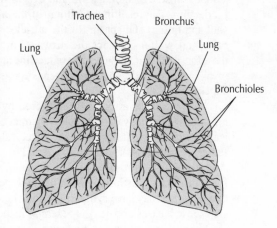

The bronchial tree
The lower end of the trachea (windpipe) divides into the two main airways to the lungs—the right and left main bronchi. The bronchi branch into many tiny airways called bronchioles.

Other Lung Problems

Some of the following terms are specific lung diseases or disorders; others are terms doctors use to describe symptoms of (or symptoms that result from) lung disorders:

- **Adult respiratory distress syndrome** Adult respiratory distress syndrome is a form of pulmonary edema (see right) that results from injury, infection, or, in rare cases, allergies.
- **Alveolitis** Alveolitis is inflammation of the alveoli (the tiny air sacs in the lungs where the exchange of oxygen and carbon dioxide takes place). It is a symptom of some allergies (see page 912) or of autoimmune disorders such as rheumatoid arthritis (see page 918).
- **Chronic obstructive pulmonary disease** Chronic obstructive pulmonary disease (also called chronic obstructive lung disease) is the general term for any progressive disease such as chronic bronchitis (see page 655) or emphysema (see page 656) that is characterized by a persistent obstruction of air flow into or out of the lungs.
- **Interstitial fibrosis** Interstitial fibrosis is thickening and scarring of fibrous tissue caused by an autoimmune disease, idiopathic pulmonary fibrosis (see page 645), occupational lung diseases (see page 645), tuberculosis, or fungal diseases (see page 662).
- **Lung abscess** A lung abscess is a contained infectious area in a lung.
- **Pleural effusion** Pleural effusion is an accumulation of fluid in the space between the pleura (the two membranes that surround the lungs) caused by infection, an autoimmune disease, injury to the chest wall, congestive heart failure, or a tumor (usually one that has spread to the pleura from another site).
- **Pleurisy** Pleurisy (also called pleuritis) is inflammation of the pleura (the two membranes that surround the lungs) usually caused by infection, congestive heart failure, injury to the chest wall, an autoimmune disease, or fluid in the abdomen.
- **Pulmonary edema** Pulmonary edema is a buildup of fluid in the lung tissue.
- **Pulmonary empyema** Pulmonary empyema is the presence of pus (which indicates inflammation and infection) in pleural effusion.

Asthma

Asthma is a chronic disease of the air passages (bronchi and bronchioles) of the lungs, characterized by inflammation and constriction of the smooth muscle of the airways and excess mucus production. The resulting swelling (of the airway wall and lining) and spasm (of the muscles in the bronchial walls) obstruct the airways, increase the effort it takes to breathe, and reduce the amount of oxygen the body can take in, causing asthma attacks.

Asthma attacks are usually triggered by viral infections (especially of the respiratory tract), medications, inhaled irritants (such as tobacco smoke, fumes, or pollutants), vigorous exercise, or stress. Allergies (such as to pets, pollen, mold, or some foods) can cause asthma attacks in some people. Other people may have symptoms only when they are exposed to cats or when they exercise in the cold (and breathe in cold air). The cause of asthma is often unknown.

Approximately 17 million Americans have asthma, including increasing numbers of children. Five to 10 percent of children have some form of asthma, compared with about 5 percent of adults. The disease has a genetic component; children who have a parent with asthma are more likely to develop asthma than children whose parents don't have asthma. Most children eventually outgrow their asthma; however, it may recur after adolescence.

In the United States, about 5,000 deaths a year result from asthma. Blacks and Hispanics are five times more likely to die of asthma than whites. Factors associated with an increased risk of dying of asthma include underestimating the severity of the disease, delaying treatment, and not following the prescribed drug regimen for a severe case. People at increased risk of dying are those who frequently require emergency treatment for severe asthma attacks, who use corticosteroids often or continuously, or who have a history of asthma attacks that require the use of a mechanical ventilator.

Symptoms

The symptoms of asthma vary widely from person to person and in the same person over time. You may have shortness of breath and tightness in your chest, and you may cough up whitish phlegm. You may also wheeze (make a high-pitched sound) when you breathe because you are trying to force air out of narrowed airways. The wheezing may be very loud or may be so low that it can only be heard by a doctor through a stethoscope. During a severe asthma attack, you may sweat profusely, have an increased pulse rate, and be extremely anxious.

Diagnosis

If you think you may have had an asthma attack, write down what you were doing and where you were when the symptoms occurred. Try to give your doctor a clear description of what occurred before and during the attack. He or she will examine you,

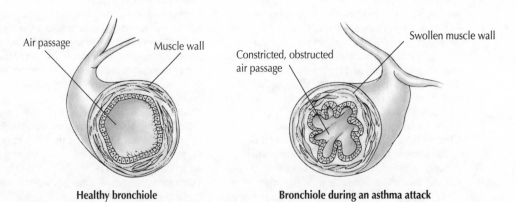

Air passage   Muscle wall   Constricted, obstructed air passage   Swollen muscle wall

Healthy bronchiole   **Bronchiole during an asthma attack**

Asthma attack
An asthma attack results when the smooth muscle wall of the airways is swollen from inflammation and becomes constricted, obstructing the airways. Breathing becomes difficult and the body gets less oxygen.

including listening to your lungs with a stethoscope, and may recommend lung function tests such as peak flow monitoring (see page 647) to measure the breathing capacity of your lungs and to help confirm the diagnosis.

An allergy that may trigger asthma is diagnosed by skin or blood tests. In the skin prick test, small amounts of the possible allergen are placed on your skin, and your skin is pricked. If you are allergic to the substance, your skin will react (usually with itching, redness, and mild swelling). Blood tests measure the levels of antibodies the body produces in response to suspected allergens. Blood tests are recommended for diagnosing asthma in people who are not able to take the skin prick test (either because they cannot stop taking antihistamines or because they have skin rashes—both of which interfere with the results of skin tests) and in people who are at risk of having a severe reaction from a skin test. Your doctor will decide which method is best for you.

In making a diagnosis, doctors classify asthma into the following four general forms:

- **Mild intermittent asthma**   People with mild intermittent asthma have symptoms less often than twice a week, and nighttime symptoms less often than twice a month. Their lung function test results (see page 647) are in the normal range.
- **Mild persistent asthma**   People with mild persistent asthma have symptoms more often than twice a week, and nighttime symptoms more often than twice a month. Their lung function test results are in the normal range.
- **Moderate persistent asthma**   People with moderate persistent asthma have symptoms every day, and nighttime symptoms more often than once a week. Their lung function test results are slightly abnormal, which indicates that their lung function is decreased.
- **Severe persistent asthma**   People with severe

persistent asthma have symptoms continuously throughout the day (even with little physical activity), and frequent nighttime symptoms. Their lung function test results are substantially abnormal, which indicates that their lung function is decreased.

Treatment

Asthma has no cure, but it can be controlled; the obstruction to airflow that occurs in asthma is at least partly reversible. Your first step in treatment is to try to identify the triggers that are causing your asthma. Keep a diary of your symptoms and review it regularly with your doctor. It can help your doctor determine treatment. Once you have identified an allergen or situation that triggers your asthma, the best course is to avoid exposure to that substance or any substance that could irritate your lungs.

Asthma treatment is based on the severity of the disease. Asthma medications are categorized into long-term–control medications (used to achieve and maintain control over time) and quick-relief medications (used to treat acute asthma attacks). These medications are often used in various combinations. Inhalers and nebulizers allow you to breathe the medication directly into your lungs.

Inhalers and Nebulizers

Inhalers and nebulizers are devices that help deliver asthma medication directly to the site of the obstruction in the lungs of people who are having an asthma attack. Some inhalers are breath-activated—they start to work when the person inhales. Devices that attach to inhalers called spacers can help ensure that the medication is delivered to the lungs correctly. Nebulizers use either air or oxygen to disperse the medication in a fine mist, which the person inhales through a face mask. Nebulizers are usually used during acute asthma attacks by people who are not able to use an inhaler correctly (such as young children).

Your doctor may recommend one or more of the following medications for your asthma:

- **Bronchodilators**   Bronchodilators are drugs that relax the smooth muscle of the airways, allowing air to get through. Short-acting bronchodilators, which can be used every 4 to 6 hours as needed,

| MY STORY | **Asthma** |

My son Marcus woke up in the middle of the night gasping for breath. I heard him coughing a couple of times—a dry cough, like he was trying to clear his throat. But then he called me into his room. He said he couldn't breathe and his chest felt tight. I could hear him wheezing. When he started having trouble talking because he was breathing so fast, I got scared and called 911.

I had asthma when I was a kid, but I outgrew it. It was never so bad that it woke me up at night, but I remember how it felt when my chest got tight, so I was pretty sure that's what Marcus had. He gets short of breath from time to time, especially if it's cold outside or if he's around a smoker. But I didn't think it was serious, so I never mentioned it to the doctor. After the paramedics came and took Marcus to the emergency room that night, sure enough, the doctor there said it was asthma.

The emergency room workers gave Marcus a shot of adrenaline to open up his airways and he felt better right away. Then they put some liquid asthma medicine in a machine called a nebulizer—which looks sort of like a vaporizer—and they had him inhale the medicine as a spray through a mask.

I told him to tell the other boy that the doctor said he could play ball and run as much as the other kids as long as he takes his asthma medicine.

Marcus is only 6 years old, and the doctor was afraid he wouldn't be able to press down on an inhaler the right way, so she prescribed a nebulizer for us to use at home and showed Marcus and me how to use it. They gave us a list of things that can trigger asthma and then let us go home.

During the first few nights after the emergency room visit, Marcus was afraid to go to sleep because he thought he would wake up in the middle of the night and not be able to breathe. I had to reassure him over and over that the medicine was making sure that wouldn't happen again. He finally settled down on about the fourth night and he's been fine ever since. One day he said that one of the other kids in his class told him he couldn't play ball because of his asthma. I told him to tell the other boy that the doctor said he could play ball and run as much as the other kids as long as he takes his asthma medicine.

There's a lot of dust and pollution where we live, which is bad for Marcus's asthma, but we can't move right now. We gave our dog to friends because she was making my son's asthma worse. But it was worth it because Marcus is doing so much better now.

provide relief in 5 to 15 minutes. The effects of long-acting bronchodilators last 12 hours. Bronchodilators are usually well tolerated but may increase heart rate. Call your doctor if you need to use a short-acting bronchodilator more often than twice a week; this indicates that your asthma is not under control. Bronchodilators such as salmeterol, albuterol, terbutaline, and ipratropium are inhaled; bronchodilators such as theophylline are taken orally.

● **Mast cell stabilizers**   Mast cell stabilizers such as cromolyn are used in inhalers to help prevent constriction of the bronchi and inhibit the release of inflammatory substances (such as histamine) from mast cells, which play a role in the immune response and in allergic reactions. Mast cell stabilizers are the safest asthma medications

and have few side effects. However, they are not as effective as bronchodilators or inhaled or oral corticosteroids.

● **Inhaled corticosteroids**   People with moderate persistent or severe persistent asthma need to inhale corticosteroids, which decrease inflammation and mucus production. Inhaled corticosteroids must be used daily to be effective. Your doctor can help you find the one that works best for you. Side effects of inhaled corticosteroids, which are usually related to dosage, include oral thrush, sore throat, and hoarseness. Inhaled corticosteroids usually do not cause symptoms in other parts of the body because they are not absorbed into the bloodstream. However, in higher doses, inhaled corticosteroids can cause health probems such as glaucoma, cataracts, and osteoporosis.

- **Oral corticosteroids** Oral corticosteroids may be necessary to treat severe symptoms of asthma. Usually oral corticosteroids are taken for 2 to 3 weeks or less, although longer courses may be necessary. Side effects, which can increase with dosage, include weight gain (from increased appetite and fluid retention) and osteoporosis. If high doses of corticosteroids are necessary, the function of the adrenal glands (the glands on top of each kidney that secrete hormones) may be suppressed. Corticosteroids are generally safe when taken in low to moderate doses for short periods.

- **Leukotriene modulators** The newest drugs prescribed to prevent asthma attacks are leukotriene modulators (also called leukotriene synthesis inhibitors or leukotriene receptor antagonists). Leukotrienes are immune system proteins that trigger asthma attacks by causing inflammation and constriction of the airways. Leukotriene modulators, which are taken by pill, work by interfering with the production or the action of a leukotriene called cysteinyl leukotriene. For unknown reasons, leukotriene modulators are not always effective in every person.

Exercise and asthma

Exercise-induced asthma is asthma that becomes worse when you exercise. You should be able to exercise and play a sport if your asthma is well controlled and you take a few precautions. Nearly 10 percent of Olympic athletes have asthma.

Make sure that your coach, trainer, and others you exercise with know you have asthma. They may need to help you if you have an attack while exercising. Make up a plan of action (with your doctor's input) to follow if you have an attack. Review the plan with your trainer and teammates.

Using your inhaler immediately before exercising will help prevent an asthma attack. Warming up for at least 15 to 20 minutes before more vigorous exercise and cooling down gradually for 15 to 20 minutes afterward can also help decrease your risk of having an attack. Avoid exercising in cold air whenever possible because breathing in cold air can trigger asthma attacks.

Pregnancy and asthma

During your pregnancy, your doctor will monitor your condition carefully. Poorly controlled asthma may decrease the amount of oxygen that gets to the fetus and limit the fetus's growth and chances for survival. Many of the medications used to treat asthma are safe to use during pregnancy, but talk to your doctor about which medications are best for you. If you become pregnant while taking asthma medication, do not stop taking it without talking to your doctor first. Almost all asthma drugs are safe for the fetus.

Preventing Asthma Attacks

Avoiding the substances, situations, or conditions that trigger your asthma is your first line of defense. Here are some steps to take to minimize contact with common asthma triggers:

- Avoid exposure to smoke from cigarettes and cigars. Smoke in the environment at home or work can be a major trigger for asthma. People who have asthma, especially children, should live in smoke-free homes.

- Reduce the amount of dust in your home. Do not sweep (sweeping spreads dust around), and have someone who does not have asthma do the vacuuming. Eliminate rugs or carpets. Use washable window coverings, and wash them frequently. Dust and damp-mop your floors once a week.

- Don't have a pet, especially one with fur or feathers. If you already have a pet, don't allow it in the bedroom. Keep it outdoors if possible.

- Don't use strong chemicals for cleaning; avoid insecticide sprays and perfumed air fresheners.

- Replace feather pillows and comforters with those filled with nonallergenic material. Enclose pillows, mattresses, and box springs in covers that will keep out dust mites.

- Prevent cockroach and other insect infestations. Wash dishes and remove food from drains before going to bed. Store food and garbage inside sealed containers. Don't leave unwrapped food out on tables or counters. Wash your pet's food and water dishes nightly. Clean litter boxes daily.

- Limit the time you spend outdoors on days when the pollen or mold count is high. Use an air conditioner and a clean-air machine to decrease your exposure to irritants in the air.

- In cold weather, wear a scarf around your mouth or an air-warming mask (available at pharmacies) to warm air before you breathe it in. Avoid exercising outdoors in cold weather.

- Vent your furnace to the outside. Avoid wood-burning fireplaces.

- Get a flu shot (see page 650) every year, and get a vaccination against pneumococcal pneumonia (see page 145) as often as your doctor recommends. Avoid contact with anyone who is sick with a cold or the flu.

Pneumothorax

Pneumothorax is partial or total collapse of a lung that occurs when air gets between the two layers of the pleura (the membrane that covers the lungs and lines the chest cavity). The pleura keeps your chest cavity airtight. When a lung collapses, air is squeezed out. The exchange of oxygen and carbon dioxide cannot occur because air cannot move into or out of the collapsed part of the lung. Usually, pneumothorax results from a congenital (present at birth) blister on the surface of the lung or from a blister that develops as a result of a disorder such as emphysema (see page 656). The blister ruptures and lets air seep between the pleural membranes. A small rupture usually is not noticeable and will heal on its own. But sometimes a large amount of air enters the space and causes a large portion of the lung to collapse.

In a potentially fatal condition called tension pneumothorax, air cannot escape from the pleural space and begins to accumulate there. The air squeezes the healthy lung and may squeeze the veins in the chest, preventing blood from returning to the heart. Pneumothorax occurs primarily in otherwise healthy young women for unknown reasons or in older men and women who have damaged lungs from disorders such as emphysema or asthma (see previous article). In people with these respiratory disorders, death from respiratory failure is possible; severe tension pneumothorax can be fatal in anyone.

Symptoms

The major symptoms of pneumothorax are breathlessness, pain in the chest, and sometimes pain at the side of the neck adjacent to the shoulder. The pain occurs suddenly and is usually sharp, or it may only be uncomfortable.

The severity of the symptoms depends on the degree to which the lung has collapsed and on your health. If you are young and in good health, you may have only slight pain and little difficulty breathing, even if a large portion of your lung has collapsed. If you are older and have a lung disorder such as emphysema, even a small, partial lung collapse can be very painful and cause extreme difficulty breathing.

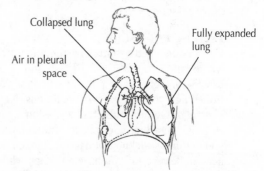

Collapsed lung
Air in pleural space
Fully expanded lung

Collapsed lung
If air is present in the pleural space, it can push into the adjoining lung, reducing the lung's ability to expand as you breathe air in.

Diagnosis

If you have symptoms of pneumothorax, your doctor will examine you to see if the affected side of your chest moves less than the unaffected side when you breathe, and tap your chest with his or her fingers to listen to (and interpret) the sounds produced by the tapping. If your doctor thinks you have pneumothorax, he or she will probably admit you to the hospital for observation. He or she also will recommend diagnostic tests such as a chest X-ray and lung function tests (see page 647).

Atelectasis: Lung Collapse as a Symptom of Other Disorders

In a type of lung collapse called atelectasis, a lung collapses because of an obstruction of the air passages of the lungs. The obstruction is usually a plug of dry mucus or vomit, an inhaled object, or a tumor. In rare cases, the obstruction may be caused by enlarged lymph glands. A doctor will recommend a chest X-ray, CT scan (see page 112), or bronchoscopy (see page 661) to help determine the cause of the obstruction. Treatment may include postural drainage (see page 660) to remove fluid or mucus, bronchoscopy to view and remove a foreign object or diagnose a tumor, antibiotics to treat an infection such as a lung abscess (a pus-filled cavity surrounded by inflamed tissue), or radiation therapy (see page 23) or laser therapy to shrink a tumor. Any object that penetrates the pleura (such as a broken rib) can also cause a collapsed lung.

Treatment

Treatment for pneumothorax depends on the amount of air in the chest, the extent of the lung collapse, and the condition of the lungs. A small pneumothorax often heals on its own. In rare cases, a doctor may recommend hospitalization to treat a collapsed lung. After administering a local anesthetic into the chest, the doctor may use a needle and syringe to suck the air out of the chest cavity, allowing the lung to reinflate. If the collapsed portion of the lung is large, the doctor may remove the air with a flexible tube (catheter) inserted through the chest into the pleural space. Or a doctor may inject a substance into the area of the leak to cause inflammation and make the two pleural membranes fuse, sealing the leak and allowing the membranes to heal.

If the pneumothorax persists, a doctor will recommend surgery to permanently close the leak. The surgeon may scrape the affected area of the lung, producing an effect similar to that of injecting the inflammatory substance, making the membranes stick together as they heal.

Occupational Lung Diseases

You may be exposed to poisonous substances in the form of gases, vapors, fumes, particles, or powders while on the job, whether you work in an office or factory or on a farm. Many of these substances can damage the respiratory tract or cause lung diseases. The sources of some occupational lung diseases (such as inhaling a toxic gas that instantly makes breathing difficult) are obvious. Other causes, such as exposure to asbestos (an insulating building material) or coal dust, can take 10 to 25 years to cause disease. Pneumoconiosis (dust lung) is the name for lung diseases that occur from long-term exposure to metallic or mineral dusts such as asbestos (asbestosis), beryllium (berylliosis), coal (coal miners' lung, also called black lung disease), and silica (silicosis).

If your lungs are repeatedly exposed to harmful substances, the chronic inflammation can lead to permanent scarring of lung tissue and potentially fatal respiratory failure (see right) and congestive heart failure (see page 570). Exposure to some substances increases your risk of lung cancer, especially if you smoke cigarettes.

Symptoms

Breathing in toxic substances can cause the following symptoms in the lungs: fluid buildup, bleeding, inflammation, scarring (fibrosis), and a dry cough or a cough that produces phlegm. The phlegm of coal miners is often black. An affected person may have breathlessness that goes away after a few hours or difficulty breathing that becomes progressively worse. Molecules from inhaled fumes can enter the bloodstream and cause other symptoms, such as fever with chills or a headache.

WARNING!

Respiratory Failure

If you have symptoms of respiratory failure or congestive heart failure (such as swelling of the ankles and legs, bluish skin color, sweating, wheezing, or severe difficulty breathing), get to a hospital emergency department as soon as possible. Treatment includes helping you breathe with the aid of a ventilator, supplemental oxygen, and medication.

Diagnosis

If you are continuously exposed to hazardous substances (or think you may have been) and have symptoms, your doctor will recommend that you have diagnostic tests such as a chest X-ray and lung function tests (see page 647) to see if, and how severely, your lungs are affected.

Treatment

If you have an occupational lung disease, change jobs if possible. If you can't change jobs, try to avoid the toxic material or fumes. Avoid unventilated areas. Wear a canister face mask while working. If you smoke, stop (see page 29). Smoking increases your risk of developing other lung disorders.

Idiopathic Pulmonary Fibrosis

Idiopathic pulmonary fibrosis, also called interstitial pulmonary fibrosis or fibrosing alveolitis, is an inflammatory disorder that results in thickening and scarring of the fibrous tissue of the lungs. Over time, this scarring can accumulate to such an extent that the lungs can no longer provide sufficient oxygen to the body. The disorder affects men and women in equal numbers and is usually diagnosed between ages 40 and 70. Although the cause is unknown, some doctors think that it may result from an autoimmune response (in which the immune system mistakenly attacks its own tissues), a lung infection (usually a viral infection), taking certain medications, or undergoing radiation therapy (see page 23) for breast cancer. In some cases, heredity seems to be a factor. Idiopathic pulmonary fibrosis may lead to other conditions, such as respiratory failure (see previous page) or congestive heart failure (see page 570).

Symptoms

The symptoms of idiopathic pulmonary fibrosis include a dry cough and shortness of breath, especially during exertion. Enlargement or clubbing of the fingertips develops in most people. As the disease progresses, you may have symptoms of respiratory failure or congestive heart failure such as swelling of the ankles and legs, bluish skin color, or wheezing and breathlessness.

Diagnosis

To diagnose idiopathic pulmonary fibrosis and to help determine the type you have, your doctor may recommend diagnostic imaging tests such as a chest X-ray or a CT scan (see page 112). He or she also may recommend a blood test to determine the level of oxygen in your blood. The only sure way to diagnose idiopathic pulmonary fibrosis is by examining tissue or phlegm samples from the lungs, usually obtained in a procedure called bronchoscopy (see page 661) or through an endoscope inserted into the pleural cavity through a skin incision.

Treatment

There is no effective treatment for 90 percent of the cases of idiopathic pulmonary fibrosis. In the remaining 10 percent of cases, a doctor may prescribe the corticosteroid prednisone to reduce inflammation or the immune-suppressing drug cyclophosphamide to reduce the abnormal activity of the immune system. Some people with the disorder may also need supplemental oxygen to boost oxygen levels in their blood, reduce breathlessness, and enable them to become more active. Your doctor may recommend a lung transplant (see page 658) if you are a good candidate for a transplant.

Lung Cancer

Lung cancer is the uncontrolled growth of abnormal cells in the lungs. The abnormal cells crowd out and destroy healthy lung tissue. Lung cancer is the leading cause of cancer deaths in men and women. For every 10 women who die of breast cancer each year, 17 die of lung cancer. Nineteen out of 20 cases of lung cancer result from smoking cigarettes. People who smoke cigars or pipes also have a greater risk of lung cancer than nonsmokers, but not as high a risk as cigarette smokers. Nonsmokers can develop lung cancer from long-term exposure to smoke at home or work. Your chances of developing lung cancer depend on how much you smoke. Only when you stop smoking will your risk start to decrease.

Normal cells in the lungs can also become cancerous when they are exposed to carcinogens other than those in tobacco smoke, such as coal tar and radon (a radioactive gas that can seep into houses from the ground). Exposure to asbestos (an insulating building material) can cause cancer of the pleural membranes that surround the lungs. The risk of developing lung cancer is related to the amount of exposure to the cancer-causing substance. Some carcinogens react together to significantly increase the risk of lung cancer. For example, if you smoke cigarettes and are exposed to asbestos or radon, your risk of lung cancer multiplies. In rare cases, cancer cells from other parts of the body (usually the breasts, bones, thyroid gland, or kidneys) may be carried through the bloodstream or lymphatic system to the lungs, where they form tumors composed of the same type of cancerous cells as that of the original tumor.

Lung cancer that begins in the lungs is classified as one of two types: small cell (also called oat cell) and non–small cell. Non–small cell lung cancer accounts for 80 percent of all cases of lung cancer but usually spreads to distant organs more slowly than small cell lung cancer. Small cell lung cancer is more likely to spread throughout the body quickly, but it is also more likely than non–small cell lung cancer to respond to chemotherapy (see page 23).

Symptoms

An early symptom of lung cancer is a persistent cough, which usually produces bloodstained

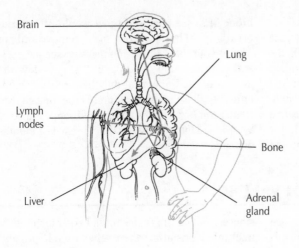

Brain

Lung

Lymph nodes

Bone

Liver

Adrenal gland

If lung cancer spreads
If lung cancer goes undetected, it can spread (metastasize) from the lungs to other areas of the body. The areas to which lung cancer is most likely to spread include the lymph nodes, brain, bones, liver, and adrenal glands. The symptoms of cancer in these sites vary depending on the organs that are affected. For example, a tumor in the brain can cause paralysis.

phlegm. You also may be breathless, wheeze when you breathe, and have chest pains. The chest pains may be dull and persistent, or sharp, intensifying when you take a deep breath.

However, most cancerous tumors in the lungs begin to grow without causing symptoms. Often, people who have lung cancer do not develop symptoms until the cancer is at an advanced stage. It can take 10 to 12 years for a cancerous cell to grow into a tumor that is large enough to cause symptoms or be detected on an X-ray. Sometimes the lung cancer is not detected until it has spread to another organ where it causes symptoms. For this reason, the majority of cancerous tumors in the lungs are diagnosed at a late stage, usually too late for a cure. Only 7 percent of all people with lung cancer are cured. If a person with lung cancer cannot be cured with surgery at the time the cancer is found, death will occur in less than a year in 50 percent of cases.

Diagnosis

If you are having symptoms of lung cancer, your doctor will listen to your chest with a stethoscope and order a chest X-ray. If your doctor suspects you have lung cancer or if the X-ray shows signs of a possible tumor, he or she will probably recommend more diagnostic tests such as a CT scan (see page 112). He or she will also examine phlegm or tissue samples from your lungs to see if they contain cancerous cells. These biopsy samples are obtained by bronchoscopy (see page 661), needle aspiration (in which tissue samples are removed from the lungs using a needle and syringe), or surgery.

The biopsy surgery usually can be done through three small incisions in the side of the chest in a procedure called video-assisted thoracic surgery (VATS). In VATS, a doctor inserts a tube (with a camera and light attached) through one of the incisions into the space between the lungs and the chest wall. The camera sends an image to a monitor that the doctor uses as a guide to take biopsy samples using instruments inserted through the other two incisions.

Lung Function Tests

Lung function tests (also called pulmonary function tests or spirometry) are a series of tests used to diagnose and monitor respiratory problems. These tests, which are administered by technicians, measure the amount of air the lungs hold, how effectively the lungs work, and the maximum air flow in a person's breathing.

- **Forced vital capacity**   Forced vital capacity (FVC) and forced expiratory volume in 1 second (FEV_1) measure the total volume of air exhaled (the FVC test) and the volume of air exhaled in 1 second (the FEV_1 test) using a spirometer. To measure FVC or FEV_1, you inhale and then exhale into the spirometer as hard and as quickly as you can for as long as you can. You repeat each test three times; the highest readings are your FVC or FEV_1 values. Your spirometer readings are compared with values based on age, sex, and body size from a standard table. FEV_1 is normally 75 to 80 percent of FVC.
- **Peak expiratory flow**   Peak expiratory flow (PEF) measures the degree of narrowing of your airways using a handheld device called a peak flow meter. To measure PEF, you inhale and then exhale into the meter as hard as you can. You do this three times; the highest reading is your PEF value. The result is normal if the highest value is 80 percent of the normal predicted value. This test is less accurate than FEV_1.

Treatment

If you have lung cancer, stop smoking now (see page 29). Doing so may help slow or even stop the growth of the tumor. The treatment of lung cancer depends on the type of cancer, the location and size of the tumor, and your age and general health. Surgical removal of the tumor is the most effective treatment if the cancer is not too advanced and if you have no other health problems such as chronic bronchitis (see page 655) that would affect your breathing. The surgeon may remove all or part of your lung. Radiation therapy (see page 23) and chemotherapy (see page 23) may slow the growth of the tumor and may help relieve symptoms, but these treatments rarely cure lung cancer. Remission (a partial or complete disappearance of symptoms) that follows treatment may last months or years.

Infections of the Respiratory Tract

Most infections of the respiratory tract are caused by viruses or bacteria. Upper respiratory tract infections affect the nose, throat, sinuses, and larynx (voice box). Lower respiratory tract infections affect the trachea (windpipe) and lungs.

Colds

Approximately 200 different viruses can cause the common cold. In most cases, the virus that causes a cold is confined to the nose and throat. Sometimes a cold virus travels to other parts of the respiratory tract, such as the larynx (voice box) or lungs, causing other infections, such as laryngitis or acute bronchitis. A cold virus can also lead to a bacterial infection, which can have more severe symptoms. The bacteria can travel to the ears, sinuses, or airways in the lungs and cause infection.

Usually, you catch a cold by touching an infected person or contaminated surface or by inhaling infected droplets coughed or sneezed into the air. A sneeze or a cough from a person with a cold can spread virus-containing droplets up to 10 feet away. Most people have their first cold by the time they are 1 year old. With each cold, you develop lifelong immunity to that particular cold virus. Because most people acquire more immunity as they grow older, they tend to get fewer colds and have less severe symptoms when they do get colds.

Symptoms

To some extent, the symptoms of a cold depend on the cold virus that caused it. Symptoms can include watery eyes, runny and stuffy nose, sneezing, sore throat, hoarseness, and coughing. The nasal discharge from a cold is usually watery and clear or yellow. You may also have a headache or slight fever. A cold will usually clear up in 3 or 4 days, although some colds can last 10 days or more.

Diagnosis

See your doctor if your cold lasts longer than 10 days, if your symptoms are especially severe or persistent, if you have a temperature of 102°F or higher, or if the infection seems to have spread to your ears (causing an earache), lungs (causing wheezing, shortness of breath, or a painful cough), or sinuses (causing pain in the upper cheeks or forehead). Also see your doctor if you have a severe, persistent sore throat, if your fever lasts longer than

Preventing the Spread of a Cold

Stay home if at all possible to keep from spreading the infection. If it is not possible to stay home from work or school, take the following steps to avoid spreading the cold virus:

- Wash your hands frequently. Hand-to-hand and hand-to-surface contact are the most common ways in which cold viruses are transmitted.
- Avoid touching other people or surfaces that other people might touch.
- Cover your mouth and nose with a disposable tissue when you cough or sneeze (and throw the tissues away promptly). If a tissue is not available, use the crook of your elbow or your shoulder (not your hand) to block your cough or sneeze.

3 or 4 days, or if the nasal discharge has changed from thin and clear or yellow to thick and green. A very high temperature and body aches are more likely to be symptoms of the flu.

Treatment

There is no cure for the common cold, but you can take measures to help relieve the symptoms. Breathing steam from a hot shower or boiling water can help to temporarily break up congestion. Drink plenty of water to help prevent dehydration. An

Q & A

Colds

Q. *My 3-year-old son, who is in day care, frequently has colds. His doctor never prescribes antibiotics for his colds. How can I convince his doctor that he needs them?*

A. Your doctor doesn't prescribe antibiotics for your child's colds because colds are caused by viruses. Antibiotics are used to fight infections caused by bacteria, not viruses. If antibiotics are taken unnecessarily, a stronger strain of bacteria could develop that is resistant to the effects of the antibiotic. This resistance makes a true bacterial infection more difficult to treat, and stronger antibiotics may need to be used. In addition, antibiotics can destroy some of the body's helpful bacteria along with those that cause illnesses, potentially causing stomach upset and, in girls, frequent vaginal infections.

Q. *I would like to strengthen my immune system before the cold season starts. Will echinacea or other herbal remedies keep me from catching a cold or lessen the severity of one?*

A. There is no scientific proof that herbal remedies such as echinacea or zinc lozenges can prevent or cure a cold. Talk to your doctor before using any herbal remedies, especially if you are taking a prescription medication. Mixing some herbal remedies with prescription medications can cause potentially serious health problems.

Q. *My mother always told me that I would catch a cold if I went outdoors in cold weather without a jacket. Was she right?*

A. Colds are caused by viruses, not exposure to cold weather. While you should always dress warmly when going outdoors on cold days, there is no evidence that being outside without being properly dressed will cause a cold. Colds are more common when the weather is cold because people tend to spend more time indoors, giving cold viruses a better chance to spread from person to person.

over-the-counter pain reliever such as acetaminophen or ibuprofen can ease aches and pains and help you sleep. Using a saline nasal spray and elevating the head of your bed may improve your breathing if you have a stuffy nose.

For infants and very young children who cannot blow their nose, use a bulb syringe (available at most pharmacies) to suck the mucus out of their nose. This will help them breathe easier and keep mucus from dripping down their throat, which can cause coughing and stomachaches (from swallowed mucus).

Nasal decongestants (available as tablets, sprays, or drops) shrink and dry out the swollen, mucus-producing tissue inside the nose and sinuses, making it easier to blow the mucus out of your nose. An over-the-counter cold medication called pleconaril begins to ease cold symptoms in a day and clears up a runny nose up to a day earlier than usual. Unlike other cold medications, pleconaril attacks the virus itself rather than just relieving cold symptoms.

Because antibiotics are effective only against bacteria, don't ask your doctor to prescribe an antibiotic for a cold. Your doctor will prescribe an antibiotic only if you have symptoms of a bacterial infection such as an earache, sinusitis, shortness of breath, or a painful cough.

Influenza

Influenza, usually called the flu, is a viral infection of the respiratory tract. The flu can spread from the nose or mouth to the rest of the respiratory system, including the lungs. It is usually spread by touching an infected person or contaminated surface or by inhaling infected droplets coughed or sneezed into the air. If a bacterial infection develops in addition to the viral infection and travels from the upper respiratory tract to the lungs, it can cause more serious disorders, such as acute bronchitis (see page 655) or pneumonia (see page 660). Influenza kills about 20,000 people a year in the United States.

There are three main types of influenza virus—A, B, and C. If you have had the flu caused by a type C virus (a relatively mild type of flu with symptoms similar to those of a cold), you are immune to it for life. If you have been infected with a particular strain of a type A or B influenza virus, you have immunity to that strain only. Although both

A and B influenza viruses can produce new strains that can overcome a person's immunity, the type B virus seldom alters itself sufficiently to do so. But the type A virus constantly changes, and the changes are significant enough to make it look like a new virus to the immune system. For this reason, most flu epidemics and severe outbreaks are caused by type A viruses. These strains are usually named after their place of origin (such as the Hong Kong flu).

Influenza usually occurs in small outbreaks, often in the winter. Every few years, in unpredictable intervals, it occurs in epidemics. Two or three epidemics caused by different strains of the virus can occur at the same time. Epidemics die out when everyone who has been infected by a particular strain of a flu virus becomes immune to that strain.

Symptoms

Symptoms of the flu vary widely. You may have a fever with shaking and chills, sneezing, headache, muscle aches, and a sore throat. You may then develop a dry, hacking cough and chest pain. You will probably feel very weak. Some children have abdominal pain and seizures. If you have no complications, you should recover in 1 to 2 weeks, although you may still feel weak for a few weeks. If you seem to be the only person who has the flu,

you may have some other viral illness such as mononucleosis (see page 935).

See your doctor if your symptoms are severe, last longer than 10 days, or seem to have spread to your lungs (causing wheezing, shortness of breath, or a painful cough), or if you have a chronic disease (especially a lung disorder or an immune system disorder). You should also see your doctor if your fever lasts longer than 3 or 4 days.

Q & A

Influenza

Q. *My company is offering free flu shots. My sister said that she got sick after getting a flu shot last year. Can getting a flu shot make you get the flu?*

A. No. The virus used to make the flu vaccine is inactivated and therefore cannot cause an actual flu infection. However, you can get the flu if you are exposed to the virus within a week or two after getting vaccinated (before the vaccine's protection takes effect) or if a prevalent strain of the virus that year was not included in the vaccine. After getting the shot, you may feel sore at the site of the injection, but you will not get the flu from the shot.

Diagnosis

Doctors can usually diagnose the flu by the symptoms, especially when they occur during flu season in fall or winter. If you have symptoms that persist, your doctor will examine you to see if they could be caused by another disease.

Treatment

There is no cure for influenza, but you can take measures to relieve the symptoms. Rest, stay comfortably warm (but not hot), and drink plenty of water to help prevent dehydration. Take an over-the-counter pain reliever such as acetaminophen or ibuprofen to ease aches and pains and help you sleep. Check with your doctor before you use a cough suppressant or any other medication advertised to relieve flu symptoms.

For infants and very young children who cannot blow their nose, use a bulb syringe (available at most pharmacies) to suck the mucus out of their nose. This will help them breathe more easily and keep mucus from dripping down their throat, which can cause coughing and stomachaches (from swallowed mucus).

Flu Shots

Because a flu infection can be debilitating or life-threatening, most doctors recommend that even healthy young adults and children get a flu shot every year. The vaccine now also comes in a nasal spray. The flu vaccine protects you for only a year (sometimes less), even against the strain it is meant to resist. Flu shots are usually administered in late fall after scientists have determined which strains are likely to cause the most widespread infections that year. In rare cases, flu shots can cause minor flulike symptoms such as a low fever and aches for a day or two. Because the vaccine is made from eggs, people who are allergic to eggs should not get a flu shot.

Doctors especially recommend flu shots every year for the following people:

- Those over age 65
- People who have a chronic disease (such as diabetes or cancer) or any disease that impairs the immune system (such as AIDS)
- Those who have a chronic lung disorder
- Health care workers
- Healthy children between 6 months and 2 years of age.

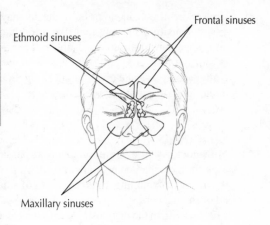

Front view

Antibiotics are not effective against the viruses that cause influenza. Your doctor will prescribe an antibiotic only if your influenza has been complicated by a bacterial infection. If you are older or in poor health, your doctor may prescribe amantadine, oseltamivir, or zanamivir if you have been exposed to the flu virus or if you have flu symptoms. These antiviral drugs can prevent or relieve symptoms caused by an influenza A virus.

Sinusitis

The paranasal sinuses are spaces filled with air in the bones around the nose. Sinusitis is inflammation of the mucous membranes of these sinuses caused by a viral, bacterial, or, in rare cases, a fungal infection. The ethmoid sinuses, the small sinuses behind and between the eyes, are those most frequently affected by sinusitis.

Sinusitis is fairly common; some people who smoke get it every time they have a cold. People who have hay fever are also more likely to develop sinusitis; treating the hay fever can decrease the frequency and severity of sinusitis. Damaging the nasal cavity (such as with a foreign object) or introducing bacteria deep into the sinuses (such as by jumping into water feet first without holding your nose) can cause sinusitis. In some cases, sinusitis of the maxillary sinuses (the sinuses below the eyes and on either side of the nose) is brought on by a tooth abscess (see page 1104). Occasionally, an infection may spread from the roots of a tooth into a sinus after dental work.

In rare cases, sinusitis can spread through the mucous membranes of the sinuses into the eye sockets or bones. If it spreads to the brain, the infection can cause meningitis (see page 692) or an abscess (a pus-filled cavity surrounded by inflamed tissue).

Symptoms

The area over an inflamed sinus may be painful and swollen and you may have a greenish discharge

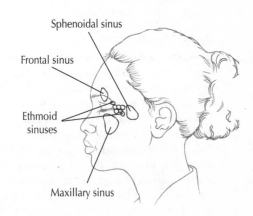

Side view

Sites of sinusitis
Inflammation of the frontal sinuses, and sometimes the sphenoidal sinuses, causes a headache or pain over one or both eyes. Pain in the cheeks on either side of the nose and the sensation of a toothache may indicate an infection in the maxillary sinuses. Pain behind or between the eyes usually points to sinusitis of the ethmoid sinuses.

from your nose. As the sinusitis worsens, the passages between your nose and sinuses may close up, preventing the discharge from flowing out of your nose and making your nose even more stuffed up. You may breathe through your mouth, have bad breath, and feel generally ill.

If the sphenoidal sinuses are affected, you may have a headache over one or both of your eyes that is worse when you lie flat or when your head is lower than the rest of your body. If the maxillary sinuses are affected, one or both cheeks may hurt, or the sinusitis pain may feel like a toothache in your upper jaw. If the ethmoid sinuses are affected, one or both lower eyelids may be swollen, especially when you wake up in the morning. See your doctor if your symptoms persist for more than 3 or 4 days.

Diagnosis

Your doctor will examine your nasal passage to look for a discharge and signs of inflammation of the mucous membrane. In severe cases of sinusitis, he or she may order X-rays or a CT scan (see page 112) to confirm the diagnosis. X-rays may also rule out a tooth abscess. A CT scan can help the doctor determine the extent of the inflammation and the severity of the sinusitis.

Treatment

If you have sinusitis, your doctor may recommend inhaling steam to relieve nasal congestion by promoting the drainage of mucus. Add moisture to the air in your home with a vaporizer or humidifier. Blow your nose gently to avoid damaging your sinuses. You will be more comfortable if you keep your head elevated, especially while you sleep. Use decongestant tablets only if your doctor recommends them; although decongestants shrink the swollen mucous membrane (widening the respiratory airways), when used incorrectly they can cause heart problems such as arrhythmias (see page 580).

If your symptoms persist, your doctor may recommend a corticosteroid nasal spray. He or she will prescribe antibiotics only if your sinusitis is caused by a bacterial infection. In rare, severe cases, surgery may be necessary to enlarge the opening of the affected sinus.

Strep Throat

A sore throat is usually a symptom of a viral infection but sometimes can result from a bacterial infection. Strep throat is caused by a streptococcus bacterium that can be contracted when you inhale infected droplets coughed or sneezed into the air or by touching an infected person or contaminated surface. Strep throat is more common in children than in adults.

Symptoms

Symptoms of strep throat vary from person to person. Usually the throat is very red and the tonsils are swollen and have white patches of pus. The throat may be so sore that it is difficult to swallow, although some people have no throat pain. Other symptoms include fever (often higher than 101°F), headache, swollen lymph nodes in the neck, and general body aches. Children may lose their appetite and have abdominal pain and nausea. If you have strep throat, you usually do not have a runny or stuffy nose or a cough.

In rare cases, strep throat infections can lead to infections in the ears, bloodstream, kidneys, or lungs, or to scarlet fever (see page 443) or rheumatic fever (see page 432). Call your doctor immediately if you develop any of the following symptoms: rash; extreme fatigue; bloody nasal discharge; painful, swollen joints; cough; shortness of breath; chest pain; recurring fever; earache; or seizures.

Diagnosis

The only way for your doctor to definitively diagnose strep throat is to take a sample of secretions from your throat, grow the sample (culture) in a laboratory for 2 to 3 days, and examine it under a microscope for the presence of strep bacteria or other microorganisms. Your doctor may give you a so-called rapid strep test, which can usually produce results in about 10 to 30 minutes. However, the results are not as accurate as those from a throat culture, and the test can only detect one type of strep bacteria and no other microorganisms. If the results of the rapid strep test show a strep infection, no further testing is necessary. If the results are negative, your doctor will send a sample to a laboratory for a culture to verify the results.

Treatment

Strep throat is usually treated with an oral antibiotic. Although your symptoms may subside in a few days, you need to complete the full course of the antibiotic to be sure all the bacteria have been killed and to avoid creating a stronger strain of bacteria that is resistant to antibiotics.

To relieve the symptoms of strep throat, gargle with warm salted water every few hours to help soothe the throat pain and help eliminate pus from the infected area. Drink plenty of water. Take an over-the-counter pain reliever to ease pain and reduce your fever.

For people who have severe, frequent strep throat infections (more than twice a year for an adult and more than four times a year for a child), your doctor may recommend removing the tonsils (tonsillectomy; see below right).

Tonsillitis

Tonsillitis is acute inflammation of the tonsils, usually resulting from a bacterial or viral infection, including strep throat (see previous article). The tonsils are two masses of tissue at the back of the throat that are part of the lymphatic system, which plays an important role in the immune system. Normally, the tonsils are very small at birth, gradually increase in size until age 6 or 7, and then shrink (although they usually do not disappear entirely). In young children, the tonsils help control infections in the nose and throat and protect against upper respiratory tract infections. This function is taken over by other lymphatic tissues if the tonsils are removed or when the tonsils shrink normally with age. Tonsillitis occurs most often in children but can occur occasionally in adults.

Symptoms
If you have tonsillitis, your throat may be red and swollen and may hurt when you swallow. Your tonsils may have white patches of pus. You may also have ear pain, a headache, swollen lymph nodes, and fever with chills. A child with tonsillitis may

also have stomach pain or seizures. A single episode of what seems to be tonsillitis could be mononucleosis (see page 935), especially if the symptoms last longer than 2 weeks.

Diagnosis
If you have symptoms of tonsillitis, your doctor may take a sample of secretions from your throat to test it for the presence of bacteria or other microorganisms to rule out a strep throat infection. The sample (culture) is grown in a laboratory and examined under a microscope. Growing bacteria in a culture can take up to 2 days.

Treatment
If, after examination of a throat culture, your doctor determines that the tonsillitis is caused by a bacterial infection, he or she will prescribe an antibiotic. To relieve your sore throat, take an over-the-counter pain reliever. Gargle with warm salted water to help soothe your sore throat and remove pus from your tonsils if they are infected.

If you have recurring, severe throat infections that have caused significant problems such as excessive time off from school or work, your doctor might recommend a tonsillectomy (see below).

Tonsillectomy
Tonsillectomy is surgical removal of the tonsils. Before the widespread use of antibiotics, it was a common procedure in childhood. Tonsillectomies are performed in people who have frequent, recurring tonsillitis (more than four times a year for a child and more than twice a year for an adult). They are also recommended when a tonsil develops an abscess (a pus-filled cavity surrounded by inflamed tissue) or cancerous tumor, or when the tonsils obstruct breathing during sleep (sleep apnea; see page 636), especially in young children. Teenagers and adults have more postoperative bleeding and seem to have more pain after surgery than children do.

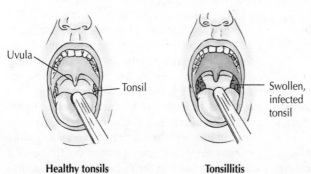

Healthy tonsils   **Tonsillitis**

Tonsillitis
Tonsillitis is inflammation of the tonsils, usually caused by a bacterial or viral infection. The tonsils are two masses of tissue at the back of the throat, on either side of the uvula (the fleshy lobe of tissue that hangs down the middle of the back of the throat).

Pharyngitis

Pharyngitis is acute inflammation of the throat (pharynx). It is similar to tonsillitis (see previous article) and caused by the same bacteria and viruses but tends to be less severe. Pharyngitis is a common symptom of a cold or the flu and is often the first symptom of mononucleosis (see page 935). Pharyngitis can also be caused by substances (such as alcohol, tobacco, or hot beverages) that irritate or burn the lining of the throat. People who have gastroesophageal reflux disease (GERD; see page 750) often have chronic pharyngitis.

Symptoms

If you have pharyngitis, your throat is red and very sore, and swallowing is painful. You may have white patches of pus on your throat, a fever, swollen lymph nodes, or an earache. In rare cases, a person may have difficulty breathing. See your doctor if your sore throat lasts longer than a few days or if the pain is severe.

Diagnosis

Your doctor may take a sample of secretions from your throat to test it for the presence of bacteria or other microorganisms to rule out strep throat. The sample (culture) is grown in a laboratory and examined under a microscope. Growing bacteria in a culture can take up to 2 days.

Treatment

Pharyngitis usually clears up on its own. Gargling with warm salted water, sucking on mild throat lozenges, and taking an over-the-counter pain reliever can temporarily ease the pain in your throat. Don't smoke, and don't eat or drink anything that could irritate your throat. If the pharyngitis is caused by a bacterial infection, your doctor will prescribe an antibiotic.

Laryngitis

Laryngitis is inflammation of the larynx (voice box). The larynx is the organ at the top of the trachea (windpipe) that contains the vocal cords. Laryngitis is usually caused by a virus (such as a cold), but it also can result from exposure to an allergen (an allergy-causing substance) or irritants such as tobacco smoke or alcohol, from overusing the voice, or from violently clearing the throat or coughing. Occasional, uncomplicated bouts of laryngitis are not serious, but recurring episodes can lead to persistent hoarseness or abnormal growths on the vocal cords (see page 637).

Symptoms

The main symptom of laryngitis is a distorted or cracking voice or a complete loss of voice. The inflammation causes the vocal cords to swell, distorting their normal sound, usually for no more than 2 or 3 days. Speaking may be painful, and sometimes a person with laryngitis has a fever. In children, the opening of the larynx is narrow, and inflammation can cause difficulty breathing. See your doctor if symptoms persist for more than 4 or 5 days or if you cough up phlegm.

Diagnosis

If, after examining your larynx, your doctor finds no sign of inflammation, he or she will recommend that you have more tests; you could have a polyp, nodule, or tumor on your larynx.

Treatment

If you have laryngitis, rest your voice as much as you can and drink plenty of water. Don't drink alcohol or smoke cigarettes, because alcohol and smoke can irritate the larynx. Do not whisper; whispering strains the larynx and vocal cords. Use a humidifier or vaporizer to add moisture to the air.

Respiratory Syncytial Virus

The respiratory syncytial virus (RSV) is one of the most common causes of respiratory infections in both children and adults and is the leading cause of lower respiratory tract infections such as pneumonia (see page 660) and bronchiolitis (see page 421) in infants and young children.

Most children contract an RSV infection by the time they are 2 years old and have no problems. However, children who were born prematurely, are younger than 6 months old, or have chronic lung, heart, or immune system disorders are at increased risk of complications from an RSV infection. They also are more likely to later develop long-term respiratory problems such as asthma (see page 640) or other chronic lung diseases after an RSV infection.

Outbreaks of RSV occur throughout the year but are most common in the fall and winter. The virus is highly contagious and can be contracted when a person inhales infected droplets coughed or sneezed into the air or by touching an infected person or contaminated surface (the virus can live from 4 to 7 hours on inanimate surfaces).

Symptoms

The symptoms of an RSV infection resemble those of a cold, such as a runny and stuffy nose, sore throat, and a slight fever. In children who are at high risk, symptoms may be severe and include a high fever, coughing, wheezing, and difficulty breathing or rapid breathing. Severe cases can cause respiratory failure. The infection usually lasts about 5 days. A person can become infected with RSV more than once, but subsequent infections tend to be milder.

Diagnosis

It is especially important to identify an RSV infection early in children who are at increased risk. To diagnose an RSV infection, a doctor will listen to the lungs with a stethoscope to detect any unusual sounds. He or she may then recommend a chest X-ray and test samples of blood and phlegm to determine if the infection is caused by RSV.

Treatment

No vaccine exists for RSV. Treatment of mild RSV infections in older children and adults is similar to the treatment for colds—drinking water to prevent dehydration, inhaling steam to break up congestion, taking an over-the-counter pain reliever to reduce fever and ease pain, and using a saline nasal spray to relieve a stuffy nose.

To treat a severe RSV infection, a doctor may prescribe an antiviral drug called ribavirin, which is administered through an aerosol spray. In children who are at increased risk, a severe RSV infection may require hospitalization.

Prevention

To help prevent the spread of RSV, wash your hands frequently and avoid contact with people who seem to have a cold. When possible, keep at-risk children away from people who are sick. To prevent RSV infections in at-risk children, doctors may recommend giving them antibodies (immune proteins) to fight RSV. This medication, called palivizumab, is given in a shot once a month during RSV season (usually from November to April).

Acute Bronchitis

Acute bronchitis is inflammation of the airways of the lungs (the bronchi and bronchioles) that is usually caused by a viral infection such as a cold or the flu, although it may also be caused by a bacterial infection. Most cases occur in the winter. Acute bronchitis usually affects people who are very young or very old, have a lung disorder or congestive heart failure (see page 570), or smoke or continuously breathe polluted air.

Symptoms

The symptoms of acute bronchitis include a cough that may produce phlegm, a mild fever, and sometimes slight wheezing. You may also have pain in your upper chest that worsens when you cough. Acute bronchitis usually clears up on its own in a few days. See your doctor if you have a fever over 101°F, if your wheezing is severe, or if you cough up blood.

Diagnosis

If you have symptoms of acute bronchitis, your doctor will listen to your chest with a stethoscope and may recommend an X-ray to rule out pneumonia. He or she also may take a sample of secretions to test it for the presence of bacteria or other microorganisms. The sample (culture) is grown in a laboratory and examined under a microscope.

Treatment

For acute bronchitis, your doctor may recommend an over-the-counter pain reliever (to ease discomfort and reduce a fever) and a cough medication. If the phlegm produced by your coughing is green, which usually indicates a bacterial infection, he or she will prescribe an antibiotic. If you are having trouble breathing or are coughing, your doctor may recommend using an inhaler with a bronchodilator drug to open your airways.

Chronic Bronchitis

Chronic bronchitis is recurring inflammation of the airways of the lungs (the bronchi and bronchioles) brought on by prolonged exposure to inhaled irritants. Cigarette smoke, including secondhand smoke, is usually the cause of chronic bronchitis. Nonsmokers who are exposed to secondhand smoke at home or at work have lung damage equal to that of people who smoke 1 to 10 cigarettes a day. People who live near or in industrial or polluted areas also can develop chronic bronchitis. Chronic bronchitis is sometimes a complication of a disease such as cystic fibrosis (see page 958) that affects the lungs.

Irritation of the airway lining increases the production of mucus. With persistent irritation, the mucus glands and cells multiply and grow larger, thickening the lining of the airways. As the lining thickens, the airways narrow. Irritants such as cigarette smoke also damage the tiny hairlike projections called cilia that help move mucus along the airways. When the cilia can no longer move the mucus, it stays in the airways, where it can become infected with bacteria. Over time, the chronic inflammation can damage the lining of the airways and destroy the cilia.

If the infection spreads into the alveoli (the air sacs at the ends of the bronchioles in the lungs), it can cause pneumonia (see page 660). Chronic bronchitis may also lead to heart or circulation problems such as pulmonary hypertension (see page 594) or congestive heart failure (see page 570).

Symptoms

The first symptom of chronic bronchitis is a persistent cough (especially in the morning), usually from smoking, that brings up phlegm from the lungs. The person coughs and wheezes throughout the day. People with chronic bronchitis become progressively more breathless and experience a gradual decline in their ability to tolerate exercise. Some people who have severe chronic bronchitis may look blue in the face, especially around the lips, because they are not getting enough oxygen. They may eventually experience respiratory failure (see page 645) because their lungs cannot supply their body with enough oxygen.

Diagnosis

If you have symptoms of chronic bronchitis, especially a chronic cough, your doctor will ask you if

---

Q & A

Chronic Bronchitis

Q. I have chronic bronchitis and my coughing keeps me up at night. Why did my doctor ask me not to take cough suppressants?

A. Although cough-suppressing medications may relieve your cough, most contain derivatives of opium (such as codeine) that keep you from coughing up phlegm. The phlegm can dry and plug up your lungs and airways, making your bronchitis worse.

---

you smoke (and how much) and where you live and work. He or she also will recommend diagnostic tests such as a chest X-ray and lung function tests (see page 647).

Treatment

The treatment for chronic bronchitis depends on how far it has progressed before it is diagnosed. If you are having difficulty breathing, your doctor probably will prescribe a bronchodilator (see page 641) administered through an aerosol inhaler to open the airways and make your breathing easier. You will probably use the bronchodilator three or four times a day, every 4 to 6 hours. Your doctor may prescribe a small dose of an antibiotic to take for several weeks or months to help prevent bacterial infections. Alternatively, he or she may prescribe a full course of antibiotics only for flare-ups or obvious infections.

If you smoke, the best thing you can do for your chronic bronchitis is to quit smoking (see page 29) and avoid smoky environments. If you work or live in a polluted environment, consider changing jobs or moving. If you move, try to choose not only a cleaner environment but also a warmer, drier one. Warm, dry air is easier to breathe than cold, humid air. Avoid contact with people who have a cold or the flu because illnesses that affect the respiratory system can bring on an episode of bronchitis. Get a vaccination against pneumococcal pneumonia (see page 145) every 5 to 7 years and a flu shot (see page 650) every year.

Emphysema

Emphysema is a disease that causes a permanent change in the structure of the alveoli (the tiny air sacs in the lungs where the exchange of oxygen and carbon dioxide takes place). Cigarette smoking is almost always the cause of emphysema. The smoke from cigarettes causes inflammation in lung tissues and inactivates a beneficial enzyme called alpha$_1$-antitrypsin, which normally protects the alveoli. In response to chronic inflammation in the alveoli caused by cigarette smoke, infection-fighting white blood cells go to the site of the inflammation and release a different enzyme to eliminate it. However, because alpha$_1$-antitrypsin no longer protects the alveoli, the enzyme released by the white blood cells damages the walls of the alveoli, causing emphysema.

Other factors that can cause the airways of the lungs to narrow and contribute to the development of emphysema include pollution, recurring respiratory tract infections, and allergies that affect the respiratory tract. In rare cases, emphysema also may develop in people who have an inherited disorder called alpha$_1$-antitrypsin deficiency and lack the protective enzyme.

Healthy lungs are elastic, and contract and expand fully. When the alveoli of the lungs are stretched out, as occurs in emphysema, the alveoli rupture and merge to make fewer and larger air spaces. The increased pressure caused by labored breathing and spasms of coughing weakens the walls of the alveoli even more. Emphysema can make you more susceptible to chest infections such as pneumonia (see page 660) and can lead to respiratory failure (see page 645) or congestive heart failure (see page 570).

Symptoms

The main symptom of emphysema is shortness of breath. At first, the shortness of breath occurs only during exercise or strenuous activity. But over time, the shortness of breath worsens and occurs during everyday activities. The person's chest may become barrel-shaped because, as the lungs lose their elasticity, air becomes trapped in the lungs. If you also have chronic bronchitis (see page 655), as most people with emphysema do, you may cough up phlegm.

Diagnosis

To confirm a diagnosis of emphysema, your doctor probably will tap your chest with his or her fingers and listen to and interpret the sounds produced by the tapping. He or she will also listen to your lungs with a stethoscope and will probably recommend diagnostic tests such as a chest X-ray and lung function tests (see page 647).

Treatment

Emphysema cannot be cured, but the symptoms can be treated and the progression of the disease can be slowed if you stop smoking. Treatment can improve the quality and length of your life. Quitting smoking (see page 29) is the single most important step you can take. Avoid places with polluted air and people who have a cold or the flu. Exercise regularly but avoid breathing in cold, humid air. Get a vaccination against pneumococcal pneumonia

every 5 to 7 years (see page 145) and a flu shot (see page 650) every year.

To relax the muscles of your bronchial tubes and reduce inflammation (and make your breathing easier), your doctor may prescribe a bronchodilator (see page 641), taken through an aerosol inhaler or in tablets. He or she may also prescribe a corticosteroid to help reduce inflammation and relieve shortness of breath. If you develop a bacterial infection such as pneumonia, your doctor will prescribe an antibiotic.

For some people with emphysema, physical therapy and breathing exercises can be helpful. Your doctor may suggest joining a pulmonary rehabilitation program to improve your physical conditioning, which can help reduce your breathing needs during ordinary activities. If you have severe emphysema, your doctor may prescribe supplemental oxygen. You can have oxygen tanks delivered to your home or use an oxygen concentrator, which extracts oxygen from the air. You breathe the

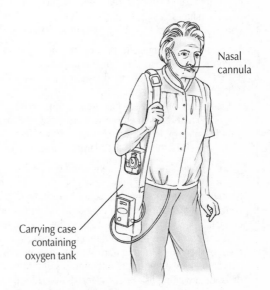

Nasal cannula

Carrying case containing oxygen tank

Using a portable oxygen tank
People whose lungs have lost the ability to absorb sufficient amounts of oxygen may need to use supplemental oxygen from either a portable oxygen supply that they can take with them wherever they go, or from a larger, stationary tank at home. A plastic tube called a cannula attached to the tank delivers the oxygen through the person's nasal passages to his or her lungs. Although somewhat cumbersome, portable oxygen provides mobility to a person who would otherwise be confined to his or her home.

oxygen through one or two plastic tubes called cannulas inserted into your nostrils. The treatment does not interfere with your ability to talk, eat, or drink.

In rare, severe cases of emphysema, a lung transplant (see below) may be the only option. The heart is frequently transplanted along with the lung (also below).

Bronchiectasis

Bronchiectasis is a disorder that causes permanent damage to and enlargement of one or more bronchi (the main air passages of the lungs). The condition takes years to develop and is usually the result of frequent infections during childhood. The damage to the airways prevents fluid in the airway from draining. Bacteria can multiply in the stagnant fluid and cause infections. If you have bronchiectasis, you are more susceptible to developing lung infections.

Symptoms

The main symptom of bronchiectasis is a frequent cough that brings up large quantities of unpleasant-

---

Lung Transplants and Heart-Lung Transplants

Lung Transplants

Doctors recommend a lung transplant when a person has irreversible lung failure that cannot be corrected with other medical or surgical treatments. Surgeons may transplant two lungs, a single lung, or part of a lung. The most common causes of lung failure requiring a transplant are:

- Emphysema (damage to the tiny air sacs in the lungs)
- Pulmonary fibrosis (scarring of lung tissue)
- Cystic fibrosis (an inherited disease that affects the lungs and digestive system)
- Deficiency of a liver protein (alpha$_1$-antitrypsin deficiency) that leads to emphysema (see page 656)
- Pulmonary hypertension (elevated blood pressure in the vessels of the lungs that damages the heart)

Lung transplants can be performed on people ranging in age from infancy to 60 years, but the person must be in otherwise good health. Conditions that can prevent someone from getting a lung transplant include cancer, an untreatable infection, or serious heart, liver, or kidney problems that could make a transplant risky. A team of specialists in lung transplantation evaluates each person seeking a transplant and places suitable candidates on a waiting list. Because the demand for donor lungs far exceeds the supply, a person could wait several years for a suitable donor organ. When an organ becomes available, it goes to the person who has been on the waiting list longest and whose blood type and body size most closely match those of the donor.

Surgeons must transfer a donor lung to the recipient within 4 to 6 hours of the donor's death. During surgery, the recipient is placed on an artificial breathing machine called a ventilator, which takes over his or her breathing. The surgeons remove the diseased lung along with the blood vessels that attach the lung to the heart and a bronchus (large airway) and replace them with those from the donor. If both lungs are being replaced, the second diseased lung will then be removed and replaced with the donor lung. After transplant surgery, the recipient may stay on the ventilator for up to 12 hours while recovering in the intensive care unit. After 7 to 10 days, he or she can go home.

As with any organ transplant, the major risk is possible rejection of the transplanted organ by the body. The immune system treats the new lung as an invading organism and tries to destroy it. To reduce the risk of rejection of the donated lung, the person must take drugs to suppress his or her immune system. However, in addition to reducing the risk of organ rejection, drugs that suppress the immune system increase the person's risk of severe infections such as pneumonia. For this reason, the person will also need to take antibiotics and other infection-fighting medications. Drugs that suppress the immune system have to be taken for life.

Complications that can occur after lung transplant surgery include severe bleeding or blood clots, pneumonia that can be life-threatening, and pulmonary edema (fluid buildup in the donated lung). Survival rates for organ transplantation in general and lung transplants in particular continue to improve. About 75 percent of all lung transplant recipients are alive 1 year after surgery, and 45 percent are alive after 5 years.

Heart-Lung Transplants

A heart-lung transplant is the transfer of a heart and two lungs (in rare cases, one lung) from an organ donor to a recipient. Doctors recommend a heart-lung transplant when a person has advanced lung disease that has also affected the heart and when all other medical and surgical options have been unsuccessful. The leading smelling phlegm that may contain small amounts of blood. The coughing and the amount of phlegm usually increase when you change position, such as when you lie down.

Diagnosis

If you are coughing up large amounts of phlegm, your doctor will listen to your lungs with a stethoscope and will probably recommend diagnostic tests such as a chest X-ray and lung function tests (see page 647) to confirm the diagnosis.

Treatment

If you have bronchiectasis, your doctor will probably recommend that you learn some body postures called postural drainage (see next page) to help airway secretions drain from your lungs. If you smoke, stop (see page 29). Avoid breathing in smoky or polluted air. Try to avoid getting colds and other respiratory infections. Your doctor will prescribe an antibiotic at the first sign of an infection. In severe, frequently recurring cases of bronchiectasis, a doctor may recommend surgery to remove the affected part of the lung.

condition for which heart-lung transplants are performed is severe pulmonary hypertension (elevated blood pressure in the vessels of the lungs that limits blood flow; see page 594) caused by a birth defect of the heart such as cystic fibrosis (see page 958). People under age 45 are the best candidates for the procedure, although it can be performed up to age 60.

Organ availability is an obstacle to successful heart-lung transplantation. There is a scarcity of potential donors who have normally functioning lungs because lung infections and changes in lung function begin to occur very soon after death. Like all people with transplants, heart-lung recipients must take antirejection drugs for life. The outlook for heart-lung transplant recipients depends on the person's age and general health but, overall, about 70 percent of people who receive combined heart-lung transplants in the United States survive for 1 year.

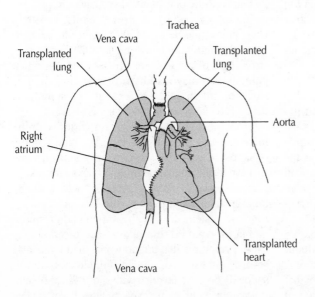

Heart-lung transplant

The donor's heart and lungs may be transplanted directly from the donor at the time of surgery or removed from the donor a few hours before transplantation and kept cool in a special solution. The heart and lungs are removed by severing the trachea, aorta, and the point at which the heart connects to the venae cavae (the two major veins that drain oxygenated blood from the body into the right side of the heart). Blood vessels linking the donor heart and lungs are left intact.

To transplant the donor's organs (shaded areas) into the recipient, a surgeon makes an incision in the breastbone of the recipient and opens the chest. The recipient is connected to a heart-lung machine, which removes carbon dioxide and replaces it with oxygen, and allows blood flow to bypass the heart and lungs. The recipient's diseased heart and lungs are removed separately. The new lungs are attached first, then the heart, followed by the blood vessels. The main reconnections are between the recipient's and the donor's tracheas and aortas and between the right atrium of the donor's heart and the recipient's venae cavae.

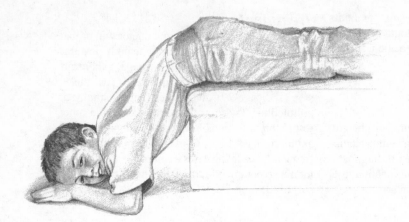

Postural drainage
Postural drainage techniques help you drain phlegm from your lungs. In one position, you lie facedown on a bed with your head and chest hanging over the edge of the bed for 5 to 10 minutes twice a day to help your lungs drain. Have someone gently clap your back and the sides of your chest at the same time to help loosen phlegm (learn how to do this properly from a respiratory therapist).

Pneumonia

Pneumonia is a general term for inflammation of the lungs. It is usually caused by a bacterial or viral infection but can also result from damage to the lungs from toxic substances (such as poisonous gases) or from injury. Less frequently, pneumonia is caused by fungi, yeasts, or other microscopic organisms. Pneumonia is a common complication of a variety of disorders, including upper respiratory tract infections such as the flu (see page 649) or acute bronchitis (see page 655). Pneumonia can also be a complication of a chronic disease such as congestive heart failure, cancer, stroke, or emphysema. In people who have these diseases, pneumonia is often given as the cause of death.

Pneumonia is very common in people who smoke or who have chronic lung infections and in people who cannot cough up phlegm forcefully enough to clear their lungs (such as people who are very sick or weak). It is especially common in people who are taking drugs that suppress the immune system (such as after an organ transplant to prevent rejection) or whose immune system is impaired because of an illness such as AIDS (see page 909).

Pneumonia has many different medical names, usually depending on the location of the inflammation in the lung (such as interstitial pneumonia or lobar pneumonia), on the virus or bacterium that caused the pneumonia (such as pneumococcal pneumonia), or on how the pneumonia was contracted (aspiration pneumonia or hospital-acquired pneumonia). Atypical pneumonia is pneumonia caused by microorganisms other than bacteria (bacterial pneumonias are more common). Walking pneumonia usually refers to milder forms of pneumonia that do not require hospitalization.

Symptoms

The symptoms of pneumonia depend on the cause of the infection and on a person's general health. No single symptom is characteristic of all types of pneumonia. In general, you should consider the possibility that you have pneumonia if you have a respiratory illness with coughing, fever with chills, sweating, chest pains, muscle aches, fatigue, headache, nausea and vomiting, a bluish tinge to the lips or skin (from lack of oxygen), or green or blood-stained phlegm. You may also have mental confusion or shortness of breath. The severity of symptoms depends on how much of the lung is affected.

How quickly symptoms begin varies with the infection. Some symptoms can start within hours of exposure to the disease-causing organism, some in a few days, and some up to 10 days after exposure. An especially strong strain of bacteria can be quickly fatal for a person who has an impaired immune system. In a healthy young adult, pneumonia from a mild respiratory tract infection may cause symptoms that are no worse than those of a severe cold. See your doctor immediately if you suddenly become feverish with shortness of breath, if your chest hurts when you breathe, if you have a temperature over 101°F with chills, or if you cough up blood-stained phlegm.

Diagnosis

If you have symptoms of pneumonia, your doctor will examine you, listen to your lungs with a stethoscope, and tap your chest with his or her fingers to listen to (and interpret) the sounds produced by the tapping. Your doctor may recommend that you have a chest X-ray and may take blood and phlegm samples to examine them for the presence of microorganisms that could cause pneumonia. He or she may need to take a tissue sample from your lungs for examination and evaluation (biopsy) using a procedure called bronchoscopy (see below).

Treatment

The treatment of pneumonia depends on a number of factors, including the type of bacterium or other microorganism that is causing it and the person's general health. For example, pneumonia caused by a virus does not respond to antibiotics, which are effective only against bacteria. However, even in cases of viral pneumonia, a doctor may prescribe antibiotics to help prevent a bacterial infection from developing and causing more severe symptoms.

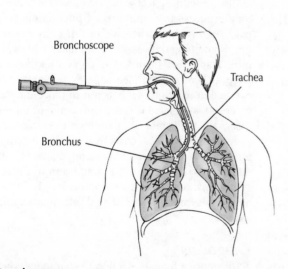

Bronchoscope

Trachea

Bronchus

Bronchoscopy
Bronchoscopy is a procedure that allows a doctor to see inside the lungs. A bronchoscope is a thin, hollow tube that can be passed down the nose or throat. It is primarily used to view or take pictures of the inside of the lungs, but a doctor can also pass instruments down the hollow tube to collect phlegm or tissue samples for a biopsy or to remove tumors or foreign objects.

If laboratory tests confirm that you have a bacterial infection, your doctor will prescribe an antibiotic; the type of antibiotic will depend on the bacterium that is causing the infection. If your doctor thinks that the pneumonia you have could become life-threatening, he or she will admit you to a hospital. If you are very short of breath and your skin and lips look blue (from lack of oxygen), you will probably be given oxygen through a mask or tube. If your symptoms persist, your doctor may perform a bronchoscopy to determine if a tumor or a foreign object in a lung is the cause.

Inhalation Anthrax

Anthrax is a rare, noncontagious disease caused by the bacterium Bacillus anthracis. Inhalation anthrax is particularly rare, developing after a person inhales microscopic particles (spores), usually from contaminated soil. Although there seems to be a wide variation in individual susceptibility to anthrax infection, a person usually has to inhale at least 2,500 of the microscopic spores (which have no smell or taste) to become infected. Anthrax has been used in bioterrorist attacks (see page 30), although most cases of inhalation anthrax in the United States are the result of occupational exposure to contaminated animal hides.

Symptoms of inhalation anthrax usually develop about 7 to 10 days after exposure to the spores, but the bacterial spores can linger in the lungs for 60 days or longer before they mature and cause symptoms. An infected person may have symptoms that include fever with chills, fatigue, coughing, muscle pain, chest pain, or shortness of breath.

A respiratory anthrax infection is usually treated with antibiotics such as ciprofloxacin, doxycycline, or penicillin. To prevent people from becoming infected and to treat those who have symptoms, doctors usually prescribe antibiotics for at least 40 to 60 days to people who have been or might have been exposed to anthrax spores. A vaccination is also available for anthrax and is offered, in addition to the course of antibiotics, to people who have been exposed to anthrax. If treatment is not begun early, a person may die, usually from respiratory failure resulting from tissue damage caused by toxins produced by the bacteria.

If you are young and healthy, you should recover from pneumonia within 2 to 3 weeks, although you may tire easily and cough for a month or two after the infection is cleared up. If you smoke or have a chronic illness, your recovery may take longer.

Severe Acute Respiratory Syndrome

Severe acute respiratory syndrome (SARS) is a form of pneumonia that appears to have originated in China in 2003. The infection is caused by a virus of the coronavirus family, to which the common cold virus belongs. The SARS virus seems to spread through close person-to-person contact, usually in infected droplets from coughs or sneezes. Those most at risk include household members and health care workers who come in close contact with an infected person. The virus may be able to live on inanimate surfaces for 24 hours, unlike the common cold virus, which can live only up to 3 hours on inanimate surfaces. Most people recover from SARS but, in some people, the infection is fatal.

Symptoms and Diagnosis
Symptoms of SARS usually develop within 10 days of exposure to the virus and include a fever higher than 100.4°F accompanied by coughing or difficulty breathing. Some people have only mild symptoms, while others have severe, life-threatening respiratory symptoms. There is no specific diagnostic test for SARS.

Treatment
There is no effective treatment or cure for SARS. If SARS is suspected, the person is hospitalized and put in isolation to prevent the virus from spreading. Treatment is given based on the person's symptoms and may include an antiviral medication such as ribavirin (usually given intravenously) along with corticosteroids (to reduce inflammation in the lungs) and antibiotics (if the person also has a bacterial infection). The person may also be given fluids intravenously. If a person has severe breathing problems, he or she may need a ventilator to assist with breathing. Up to 90 percent of people start to recover within 6 to 7 days of developing symptoms.

Fungal Diseases of the Lungs

Several diseases that infect the lungs can result from breathing in fungal spores. These fungal infections are contracted primarily by inhaling the spores (usually found in soil) from bird or bat droppings or from decaying plant matter such as old wood or dead leaves. The diseases are named for the fungus that causes them. For example, aspergillosis is caused by a species of the fungus Aspergillus, blastomycosis by Blastomyces dermatitidis, coccidioidomycosis by Coccidioides immitis, cryptococcosis by Cryptococcus neoformans, and histoplasmosis by Histoplasma capsulatum. In healthy people, the immune system destroys the spores. However, in some people (usually people who have an impaired immune system or who are very old or very young), the fungal infection can spread throughout the body in the bloodstream and become life-threatening.

Symptoms
Many fungal diseases of the lungs begin with mild, chronic, flulike symptoms such as fever with chills, coughing, chest pain, and muscle aches, but may progress to symptoms of pneumonia (see page 660) such as wheezing or difficulty breathing. Some fungal diseases of the lungs can cause other respiratory disorders, such as allergies (see page 912) or asthma (see page 640). Some may cause skin reactions such as a rash (coccidioidomycosis), skin lesions (blastomycosis), or mouth ulcers (histoplasmosis) in addition to respiratory symptoms. Cryptococcosis may not cause symptoms or may cause weight loss, night sweats, and meningitis (see page 692) in addition to flulike symptoms. See your doctor immediately if you have any symptoms of a fungal infection in your lungs.

Diagnosis
To diagnose a fungal infection in your lungs, your doctor will examine you and listen to your lungs with a stethoscope. In addition, he or she may order blood tests and test samples of your phlegm, urine, or spinal fluid to determine if you have a fungal infection. For a definite diagnosis, you may have a bronchoscopy (see previous page).

Treatment

Fungal diseases sometimes clear up on their own without treatment. If your symptoms are mild, your doctor may prescribe an oral antifungal medication. However, if your symptoms are severe or if you are susceptible to infection because your immune system is weakened, your doctor will probably administer an antifungal medication intravenously (through a vein).

Legionnaires' Disease

Legionnaires' disease is a potentially serious form of pneumonia (see page 660) caused by a bacterium that breeds in warm, moist environments, usually water and air-conditioning systems. Infection can occur when a person inhales droplets of contaminated water. Older people, smokers, people who have lung disorders, and people with an impaired immune system are most susceptible to infection, and some can die of the infection. Young, healthy people generally recover fully.

Symptoms

The symptoms of Legionnaires' disease develop about a week after exposure to the bacterium and include fever with chills, headache, muscle aches, chest pain, coughing, abdominal pain, nausea and vomiting, and diarrhea.

Diagnosis

Your doctor can determine if you have Legionnaires' disease by testing samples of phlegm and urine for the presence of the disease-causing bacterium.

Treatment

Usually a person with Legionnaires' disease is given antibiotics intravenously (through a vein) in a hospital. Young, healthy people may be treated on an outpatient basis.

Tuberculosis

Tuberculosis (TB) is a contagious disease caused by a bacterium that can be contracted when a person inhales infected droplets coughed or sneezed into the air. A healthy immune system can fight most TB infections. However, some people (such as those who are malnourished or who have a chronic disease or an impaired immune system) are susceptible to developing the disease. TB primarily affects the lungs but can also spread to other parts of the body such as the brain, kidneys, and bones. As the bacteria multiply, they create an area of inflammation that slowly destroys the surrounding tissue.

The first stage of TB may last several months. A person's immune system will often stop the infection from spreading at this point by killing the bacteria or enclosing the bacteria in a small fibrous capsule, leaving scar tissue in about one third of cases. The infection may never develop beyond this phase. Sometimes the primary infection is not stopped and it spreads beyond the lymph nodes, which can carry it to other parts of the body. In secondary TB, the bacteria can lie dormant for years and be reactivated if a person's immune system becomes impaired by another disease or by malnutrition. However, in many cases, no triggering factor can be identified.

Symptoms

Usually, TB does not cause symptoms. You may not know you have been exposed to the TB bacterium until you have a chest X-ray for other reasons or a tuberculin skin test (see below). If a person becomes infected, the symptoms may include slight fever, muscle aches, night sweats, weight loss, fatigue, shortness of breath, chest pain, and a cough that produces blood-stained phlegm.

Tuberculin Skin Test

A tuberculin skin test is used to determine if you have ever been exposed to the TB bacterium. After cleaning a small area of skin with an alcohol-soaked pad, a health care worker injects a small dose of tuberculin (a purified protein extract of TB bacteria) into the skin of your forearm. If you don't have a skin reaction at the site of the injection in 2 days, it indicates that you have never been exposed to the bacterium and you have no immunity against it. If a small area of the skin around the site becomes red, hard, and slightly swollen, it indicates that you have been infected with TB, either through exposure to the bacterium or from a previous immunization.

Diagnosis

If you have any symptoms of TB or if you have been exposed to someone who has it, your doctor will examine you, take chest X-rays, and perform a tuberculin skin test. If the X-ray shows signs of infection, he or she will take samples of phlegm to test for the presence of the TB bacterium. If you have ever had TB, the chest X-ray may show shadows that indicate scarred, healed areas of TB.

Treatment

If you have TB, your doctor will prescribe both antibacterial and antibiotic medications, sometimes as many as three or four different drugs, which must be taken exactly as prescribed to be effective. The treatment is prolonged, lasting 6 to 9 months, but it can cure the disease. Try to eat a well-balanced diet and get as much rest as possible during treatment.

4

Disorders of the Brain and Nervous System

The nervous system is made up of two parts—the central nervous system and the peripheral nervous system. The brain and spinal cord comprise the central nervous system, which coordinates all the body's interactions with the environment. The human brain is a highly complex organ that regulates most of the body's functions and changes in response to stimulation from the environment. The brain uses the outside world to build itself after birth and goes through critical periods in childhood during which brain cells need to have specific kinds of stimulation to develop such powers as language, smell, vision, muscle control, and reasoning. Not only does the brain have the ability to change in response to stimulation, such as learning new information, it also continues to make new brain cells throughout life.

The peripheral nervous system is a vast network of nerves that runs from the spinal cord to the rest of the body. The peripheral nerves connect at different levels with the spinal cord, through which information flows back and forth between the nerves and the brain. This system controls your conscious movements and automatically maintains your posture and muscle tone with a system of reflexes. Peripheral nerves called the cranial nerves connect directly to the brain through openings in the skull. The cranial nerves serve functions such as vision, eye movement, hearing, and facial movement and feeling.

All the biochemical processes inside your body and the actions of your internal organs are involuntary—that is, you are not aware of them and you have no control over them. A system of nerves called the autonomic system regulates vital functions such as heartbeat, blood pressure, and body temperature.

Disorders of Blood Vessels in the Brain

Four major arteries deliver blood to the brain: two carotid arteries in the front of the neck and two vertebral arteries in the back of the neck. At the base of the brain, the four arteries join together to form a circle of connections from which smaller arteries branch out to supply blood to all parts of the brain.

Vascular disorders such as a stroke occur when an artery ruptures or becomes blocked, cutting off the blood supply to part of the brain. Areas of the brain that receive blood from a single artery are especially vulnerable to damage from an obstruction of blood flow.

The Nervous System and the Brain

The Nervous System

The central nervous system, which includes the brain and spinal cord, is an intricate communications network that controls the inner workings of our body and allows us to respond to our environment. The peripheral nervous system is made up of the peripheral nerves, which run from the spinal cord to all other parts of the body. The central nervous system and the peripheral nervous system work together as a unit: the peripheral nerves gather information from the environment through the senses (such as touch and smell), transmit the sensory information to the central nervous system, and carry signals from the central nervous system to the skin, muscles, bones, joints, and internal organs (including the heart).

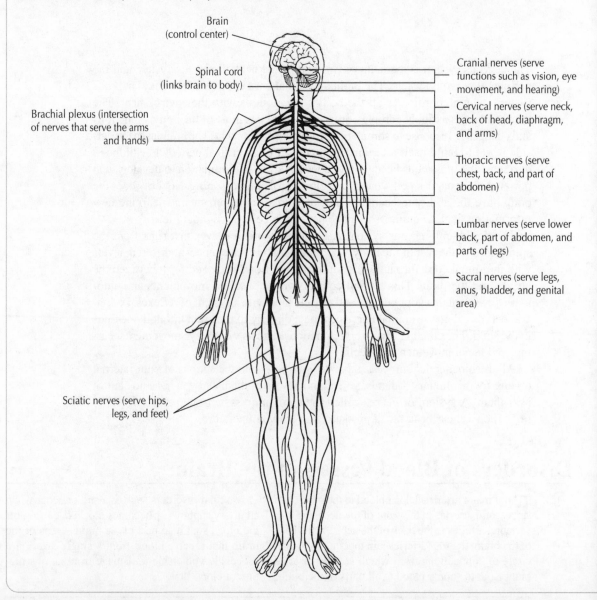

Brain (control center)

Spinal cord (links brain to body)

Brachial plexus (intersection of nerves that serve the arms and hands)

Cranial nerves (serve functions such as vision, eye movement, and hearing)

Cervical nerves (serve neck, back of head, diaphragm, and arms)

Thoracic nerves (serve chest, back, and part of abdomen)

Lumbar nerves (serve lower back, part of abdomen, and parts of legs)

Sacral nerves (serve legs, anus, bladder, and genital area)

Sciatic nerves (serve hips, legs, and feet)

The Brain

The brain lies well protected within the rigid, bony case of the skull. The cerebrum, the largest part of the brain, is responsible for the processes involved in movement and thinking. The cerebellum, located under the cerebrum at the top of the spinal cord, controls functions such as balance and coordination. The brain stem, which merges into the top of the spinal cord, contains nerve centers for the cranial nerves and fibers that connect the brain to the rest of the body. The brain stem controls vital functions such as breathing, heart rate, and circulation.

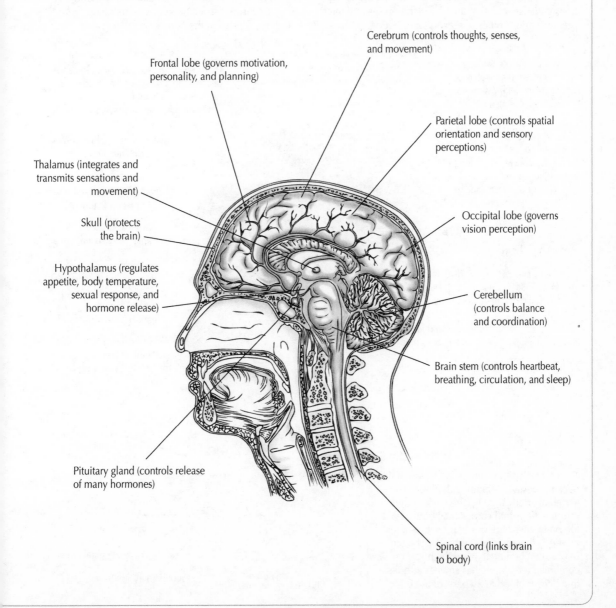

Cerebrum (controls thoughts, senses, and movement)

Frontal lobe (governs motivation, personality, and planning)

Parietal lobe (controls spatial orientation and sensory perceptions)

Thalamus (integrates and transmits sensations and movement)

Skull (protects the brain)

Occipital lobe (governs vision perception)

Hypothalamus (regulates appetite, body temperature, sexual response, and hormone release)

Cerebellum (controls balance and coordination)

Brain stem (controls heartbeat, breathing, circulation, and sleep)

Pituitary gland (controls release of many hormones)

Spinal cord (links brain to body)

The Cerebral Cortex

The cerebral cortex processes and interprets information coming in from the environment and is responsible for voluntary movement, sensations (such as hearing, vision, taste, and smell), and such higher functions as speech, memory, and intelligence. Some of these functions are localized in specific areas—for example, the primary auditory cortex detects qualities of sounds such as degrees of loudness. Adjacent to the areas of known function, called primary areas, are sections called association areas, which process and interpret the various types of sensory information (such as sound) received by the primary areas and relay the sensory information to other regions for voluntary and involuntary motor responses. For example, while the primary auditory cortex detects simple qualities of sound such as volume, the auditory association cortex analyzes the information to allow us to recognize whole sounds such as spoken words or musical melodies. These association areas—the auditory association cortex, the visual association cortex, and the somatic sensory association cortex—make up more than three fourths of the cortex.

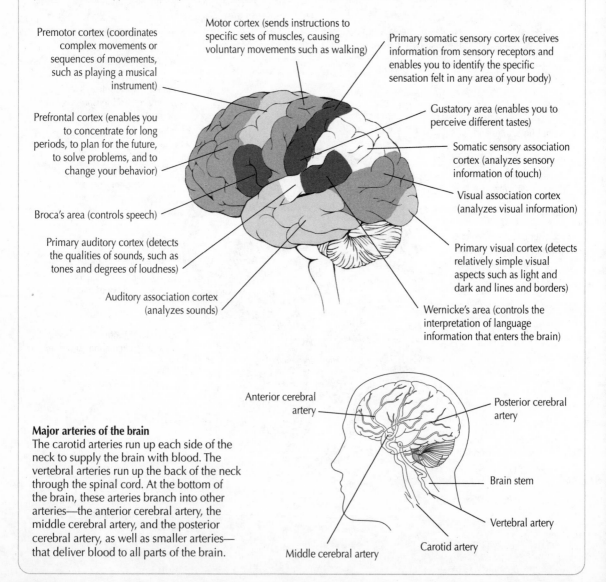

Premotor cortex (coordinates complex movements or sequences of movements, such as playing a musical instrument)

Motor cortex (sends instructions to specific sets of muscles, causing voluntary movements such as walking)

Primary somatic sensory cortex (receives information from sensory receptors and enables you to identify the specific sensation felt in any area of your body)

Prefrontal cortex (enables you to concentrate for long periods, to plan for the future, to solve problems, and to change your behavior)

Gustatory area (enables you to perceive different tastes)

Somatic sensory association cortex (analyzes sensory information of touch)

Visual association cortex (analyzes visual information)

Broca's area (controls speech)

Primary auditory cortex (detects the qualities of sounds, such as tones and degrees of loudness)

Primary visual cortex (detects relatively simple visual aspects such as light and dark and lines and borders)

Auditory association cortex (analyzes sounds)

Wernicke's area (controls the interpretation of language information that enters the brain)

Major arteries of the brain

The carotid arteries run up each side of the neck to supply the brain with blood. The vertebral arteries run up the back of the neck through the spinal cord. At the bottom of the brain, these arteries branch into other arteries—the anterior cerebral artery, the middle cerebral artery, and the posterior cerebral artery, as well as smaller arteries—that deliver blood to all parts of the brain.

Anterior cerebral artery

Posterior cerebral artery

Brain stem

Vertebral artery

Middle cerebral artery

Carotid artery

Stroke

A stroke occurs when blood flow to part of the brain is obstructed, cutting off the supply of oxygen and nutrients and damaging brain tissue, affecting the physical or mental functions that are controlled by the damaged area of the brain. The effects of a stroke may be temporary or permanent, mild or severe. Most strokes, called ischemic strokes, result from a blocked artery. Hemorrhagic strokes result from a ruptured or leaking artery.

Cerebral thrombosis, cerebral embolism, and cerebral hemorrhage are three possible causes of stroke. Cerebral thrombosis occurs when an artery that supplies blood to the brain becomes narrowed, usually as a result of atherosclerosis (see page 557). In atherosclerosis, fatty deposits called plaque build up in artery walls, narrowing the artery. Over time, the surface of a plaque may become roughened or cracked, providing an ideal site for blood cells to clump together and form a clot (thrombus) inside the blood vessel. The clot may continue to grow until it partially or completely blocks blood flow through the artery.

Cerebral embolism occurs when an artery that supplies blood to the brain is blocked by an embolus. An embolus is usually a bit of debris (such as a fragment of plaque) or a blood clot that has traveled through the bloodstream from another part of the body. The embolus becomes wedged in an artery and obstructs blood flow to part of the brain.

Cerebral hemorrhage occurs when an artery ruptures or leaks, and blood seeps into surrounding brain tissue. An artery may leak or rupture as a result of an aneurysm (a weakened area of a blood vessel wall), damage to the artery caused by uncontrolled high blood pressure or diabetes, or an arteriovenous malformation (an abnormal connection between an artery and a vein, which can rupture). Although the initial effects of a hemorrhagic stroke may be more severe than those of an ischemic stroke, the long-term effects of both types of stroke depend on the part of the brain affected and the extent of the lasting damage.

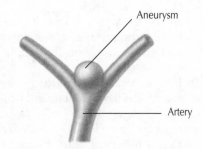

Berry aneurysm
A berry aneurysm results from a congenital (present at birth) defect in an artery wall. It forms at the base of the brain, where an artery branches. When a berry aneurysm ruptures, blood can spurt into surrounding brain tissue and cause brain damage.

Strokes are a leading cause of death and long-term disability in the United States. The effects of a stroke can differ widely from person to person. About one out of three younger people who have a stroke has long-term impairment, while three out of four older people have permanent disability.

Risk Factors

The following factors can increase your risk of stroke. However, most of these factors can be controlled or eliminated through lifestyle changes.

- **Heart disease**   Heart failure (see page 570) and irregular heart rhythms (see page 580) promote blood clot formation.

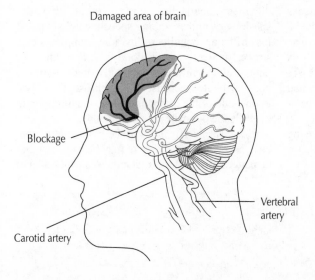

Stroke
When an artery in the brain is blocked, the blood supply to part of the brain is cut off. The lack of blood can damage the area of the brain normally supplied by the artery. An interruption in blood flow to one side of the brain can cause symptoms such as numbness, weakness, or paralysis on the opposite side of the body.

- **High blood pressure**   Uncontrolled high blood pressure damages blood vessels and promotes atherosclerosis.
- **Undesirable cholesterol profile**   An undesirable cholesterol profile (see page 146) promotes atherosclerosis.
- **Lack of exercise**   Being inactive can lead to weight gain and an undesirable cholesterol profile.
- **Being overweight**   Weighing more than your ideal body weight (see page 11) increases your risk of having an undesirable cholesterol profile, high blood pressure, and type 2 diabetes—all risk factors for stroke.
- **Diabetes**   Uncontrolled diabetes increases blood levels of LDL (bad) cholesterol and promotes atherosclerosis.
- **Smoking**   Smoking (including secondhand smoke) increases blood pressure, damages the lining of blood vessels, and increases the risk of blood clot formation.
- **Heavy drinking**   Too much alcohol can raise blood pressure and increase the amount of triglycerides (a potentially harmful type of fat) in the blood.
- **Previous strokes or transient ischemic attacks**   People who have had transient ischemic attacks (TIAs; see page 675) or who have already had a stroke have a significantly increased risk of stroke.
- **Family history of heart disease or stroke**   A family history of heart disease or stroke increases your risk, especially if your father or brother had heart disease before age 55, or your mother or sister had heart disease before age 65.
- **Race**   Blacks have an increased risk of having high blood pressure, which is a strong risk factor for stroke.

- **Stress**   Long-term stress can contribute to high blood pressure.
- **High C-reactive protein levels**   Inflammation (which contributes to atherosclerosis) leaves a chemical by-product in the blood called C-reactive protein (CRP); the higher a person's CRP level, the greater his or her risk of a stroke or heart attack.
- **High homocysteine level**   Too much of a chemical called homocysteine (see page 559) in the blood can damage artery walls and promote formation of blood clots.

Symptoms

Symptoms of a stroke can occur suddenly and without warning. For example, you may wake up and be unable to speak or to move part of your body. You may suddenly feel numbness or weakness in your face or in an arm or leg. In some cases, a stroke begins with sudden loss of consciousness. Sometimes, however, a stroke is preceded by temporary warning signs called transient ischemic attacks. It is important to see your doctor immediately if this occurs so that you can begin treatment to prevent a stroke.

Other possible symptoms of a stroke include dizziness, headache, blurred vision, difficulty speaking or understanding speech, confusion, and loss of balance and coordination. Symptoms of a stroke frequently occur along with drowsiness or nausea and vomiting. Often only one side of the body is affected, because damage is usually limited to one side of the brain, and each side of the brain controls the opposite side of the body.

Because specific areas of the brain control specific parts of the body, there may be a characteristic pattern of symptoms that indicates which area of

WARNING!

Signs of a Stroke

A stroke is a medical emergency. If you have the following symptoms of a stroke, call 911 or your local emergency number immediately. Rapid treatment is vital to limit the extent of brain damage and to improve your chances of recovery. Even a mild stroke is a danger signal; it may be the first in a series of more serious strokes. When caused by stroke, various combinations of the following symptoms occur suddenly. They may be accompanied by drowsiness or nausea and vomiting, especially if there is bleeding in the brain.

- Numbness or weakness in the face, an arm or leg, or on one side of the body
- Severe headache
- Confusion
- Difficulty speaking or understanding speech
- Vision problems (such as dimness or blurred vision) in one or both eyes
- Difficulty walking or loss of balance or coordination

MY STORY   Stroke

I'm 52 and have been overweight most of my life. A few years ago I started a new job and was sent to a doctor for a complete physical. She asked a lot of questions about my health and my habits and then examined me. My blood pressure was high and she said she wanted to check it again in a few days. About a week later, my blood pressure was even higher, and a blood test showed that I had too much bad cholesterol in my blood.

The doctor wrote a couple of prescriptions and told me I needed to quit smoking. She also told me that losing weight and exercising would help lower my blood pressure. She gave me a couple of pamphlets about exercise, healthy eating, and losing weight. I took my medication every day, started eating healthier foods, like fresh fruits and vegetables and whole grains, and tried to cut back on salt, fat, and cholesterol. I started taking walks after dinner. After a couple of weeks, I started to feel pretty good and the weight started coming off—3 pounds that first week. After a couple of months, I had lost about 10 pounds and I was feeling really good. In fact, I felt so good that I stopped taking the medication. Eventually I stopped taking walks and fell back into my old eating habits. And I was still smoking.

One day when I woke up, the right side of my face was numb and I couldn't see too well out of my right eye. I had a really bad headache and was dizzy. I tried to tell my wife, but the words came out slurred. She ran to the phone and called 911 for an ambulance.

In the emergency room, some doctors and nurses gathered around and asked me a few questions, but I couldn't talk. My wife told them what had happened. A couple of the doctors examined me and hooked me up to a machine that showed my heartbeat on a monitor, which looked like little blips on a screen. Then a nurse gave me an injection and told me it was medication that would dissolve the blood clot that was causing my problem. One of the doctors told me that he was putting me in the intensive care unit for a few days so they could monitor my symptoms. A day or so later I started to get the feeling back in my face and could see OK, but I still couldn't talk right. A speech therapist said that the stroke might have permanently damaged the part of my brain that controls speech. She said if my speech didn't get better in a couple of days, she would start to work with me. I couldn't help thinking that I might have prevented this stroke if I had followed a healthier lifestyle.

I now feel lucky. It's been a couple of months since my stroke and I have totally recovered. I am talking normally again and I'm taking much better care of my health. My wife is very supportive and we both eat lots of fruits and vegetables and other healthy foods and take long walks together every day. My wife and I have both lost weight and we feel better than ever.

> *I couldn't help thinking that I might have prevented this stroke if I had followed a healthier lifestyle.*

---

the brain has been damaged. For example, damage to the cerebrum can affect vision or speech, while damage to the cerebellum can impair balance and coordination. A stroke that affects the brain stem (the area where the brain and spine connect) may impair swallowing, breathing, strength, balance, or sensation in various combinations. The symptoms of a stroke usually persist for at least 24 hours. A person who has had a stroke may be partially paralyzed or otherwise affected for a number of weeks before his or her condition begins to improve with consistent physical therapy (see next page).

Diagnosis

The diagnosis of a stroke is based on the symptoms, a physical examination, and the results of tests. Your doctor will probably order a CT scan (see page 112) or MRI (see page 113) of your brain to determine the type of stroke and location and the extent of the damage. The doctor will also order blood tests to evaluate blood clotting. In addition to these tests, he or she may order a cerebral angiogram, an X-ray examination of the arteries in the brain. A cerebral angiogram enables the doctor to detect blocked or narrowed arteries and to evaluate blood

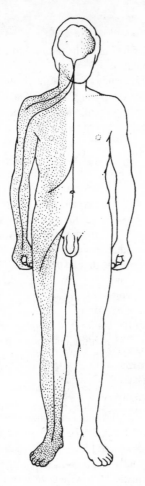

Effects of a stroke
Each side of the brain controls the opposite side of the body. For this reason, damage to the left side of the brain may result in paralysis and loss of sensation in the right side of the body.

flow in the arteries. Your doctor may also order an echocardiogram (an ultrasound examination of the heart; see page 561) to check for blood clots and to determine if your heart is pumping effectively.

If the stroke was caused by a blood clot and treatment is early enough, the doctor will administer thrombolytic drugs to dissolve the clot and restore blood flow to the affected part of the brain. These drugs are safest and most effective when given within 3 hours of the onset of symptoms. The doctor will also order a Doppler ultrasound scan (see page 111) of the neck or an MRA (magnetic resonance angiogram) to evaluate blood flow in arteries in the brain. The doctor will order an electrocardiogram (ECG; see page 559), a recording of

the electrical activity of the heart. Some people may need to wear a portable ECG device called a Holter monitor for 24 hours or more to check for abnormal heart rhythms. While you go about your daily routine, the monitor records your heart's electrical activity on a cassette tape. After 24 hours, the doctor reviews the recorded heart information and any symptoms you describe to help make a diagnosis.

Treatment

If you have had an ischemic stroke (caused by a blockage in an artery), your doctor may prescribe aspirin or other drugs that prevent blood clotting (anticoagulants). He or she may recommend that you take anticoagulant drugs for the rest of your life. If one of your carotid arteries is severely narrowed, your doctor may recommend a surgical procedure called carotid endarterectomy (see page 674) to clear plaque from the artery walls, improve blood flow to the brain, and reduce the risk of another stroke. He or she will also treat any abnormal heart rhythms (see page 580), which may be promoting the formation of blood clots. For some hemorrhagic strokes, doctors may perform surgery to clip an aneurysm, remove a clot or a blood vessel malformation, or relieve pressure on the brain. If you have high blood pressure, you will be given medication to lower it.

Rehabilitation After a Stroke or Other Brain Injury

For many people who have had a stroke or other brain injury, rehabilitation is essential for recovery. The goal of rehabilitation is to improve strength and coordination and help the person remain as independent as possible. The speed and extent of recovery from a stroke or brain injury vary from person to person, depending on factors such as the severity of the stroke and the person's general health and attitude. The sooner rehabilitation begins, the more likely a person will recover some or all of the function in the impaired area and return to a productive life.

Rehabilitation usually begins in the hospital as soon as the person's condition is stable. The therapy may continue in a hospital rehabilitation unit, a rehabilitation facility, or a skilled nursing facility. Rehabilitation may also be provided at an outpatient clinic or at home, with assistance from a home

Aphasia

Aphasia is a speech disorder that usually results from damage (such as from a stroke) to the major language centers of the brain, but it is sometimes a symptom of a partial seizure, a migraine, or a mental disorder. The symptoms of aphasia include partial or total loss of the ability to speak or to understand words and, depending on the extent of brain damage, impairment of specific language functions. For example, a person who has aphasia may be unable to speak but may still be able to write, or may have trouble remembering particular categories of words such as names. Sometimes, although the person's own speech is impaired, his or her comprehension of the speech of others remains unaffected. People who have aphasia are often able to repeat words they cannot recall on their own.

Aphasia differs from a speech disorder called dysarthria, which results from lack of control of the muscles of the lips, tongue, and face. Injection of dental anesthetics may sometimes produce temporary dysarthria, but the disorder can also result from injury to either the nerves or the area of the brain that controls the muscles used in speech. People who have dysarthria are able to understand what they hear, can read and write, and can correctly choose the words they want to speak, but their speech is unintelligible to others.

Aphasia is treated by diagnosing and treating the underlying cause of the disorder. When aphasia results from a stroke, recovery depends on the extent of the damage to the speech center of the brain. A person's language skills usually improve spontaneously (to some extent) in the weeks and months following a stroke. Speech therapy may help the person adapt to the problem or recover his or her communication skills.

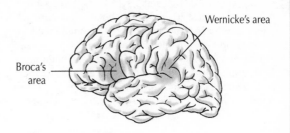

Damage to the brain's language centers
Broca's area and Wernicke's area are the brain's language centers. Broca's area controls speech; Wernicke's area controls language comprehension. Damage to these areas can impair a person's ability to speak or to understand spoken language.

---

health care provider (such as a therapist) or caregivers (family members who have been trained by a nurse or therapist).

Therapy usually begins slowly, with less difficult activities such as changing positions in bed and performing range-of-motion exercises (see page 190); these activities help keep the blood flowing, maintain muscle tone and joint flexibility, and prevent pressure sores (see page 184). Gradually, you can be helped to sit up in bed and move from the bed. You will stand and walk with assistance until you are strong enough to stand and walk on your own. Eventually you will be encouraged to do more complex tasks such as bathing, dressing, and using the toilet.

Rehabilitation is more likely to be successful if the caregivers know what to expect and what to do. If you are caring for someone who is recovering from a stroke, ask the doctor or nurse what the person can do alone, what he or she needs help doing, and what he or she cannot do. If you do not understand something, ask questions. As much as possible, encourage the person to practice doing things for himself or herself.

Classes for stroke survivors and their families and friends are available in many communities. Support groups are also good sources of information and guidance. Ask your doctor to recommend classes or a support group in your area.

A rehabilitation team of health care professionals and others works closely with a stroke survivor and his or her caregivers. A rehabilitation team may include the following:

- **Doctors** Doctors—such as a neurologist (a doctor who specializes in treating disorders of the nervous system), a physiatrist (a doctor who specializes in physical medicine and rehabilitation), and an internist, family doctor, or geriatrician (a doctor who specializes in treating health problems in older people)—provide acute care, supervise the rehabilitation process, and coordinate long-term care.

- **Nurses** Nurses who specialize in rehabilitation teach stroke survivors and their caregivers about

Carotid Endarterectomy

Carotid endarterectomy is a surgical procedure to remove fatty deposits (called plaque) caused by atherosclerosis (see page 557) from affected sections of the walls of one of the carotid arteries (the main arteries in the neck) to restore blood flow to the brain and prevent blood clots from forming and causing a stroke.

Doctors usually recommend carotid endarterectomy for people who have had warning signs of a stroke called transient ischemic attacks (TIAs; see next page) or a mild stroke, especially if an imaging examination called a cerebral angiogram shows significant narrowing (at least 70 percent) of the affected carotid artery. Carotid endarterectomy is not recommended when an artery is completely blocked.

The procedure usually takes less than an hour. During surgery, you are under general anesthesia. The surgeon makes a vertical incision in the side of your neck to reveal the carotid artery and clamps the artery at both sides of the obstruction to temporarily stop blood flow through the artery. He or she then makes a vertical incision in the artery wall at the obstructed area, exposing the plaque. The surgeon scrapes the fatty material away from the artery wall, removes it from the artery, and stitches closed the incisions in the artery and in the neck. In some cases, a damaged section of the artery is replaced with a graft.

After surgery, you will need to remain in the hospital while your condition is monitored. Before you leave the hospital, your doctor will probably talk to you about making positive lifestyle changes—such as exercising regularly, maintaining a healthy weight, and controlling your cholesterol—to help you avoid another stroke. He or she may also prescribe medication to improve your cholesterol profile (see page 146) and anticoagulant medication to help prevent new blood clots from forming.

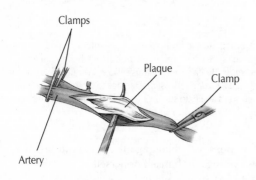

Separating plaque from the artery wall

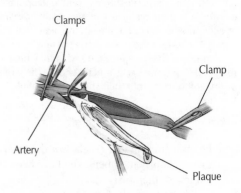

Removing plaque from the artery

eating, exercising, taking medication, preventing pressure sores, and other aspects of home health care.

- **Physical therapists** Physical therapists evaluate a person's physical abilities and develop and carry out a treatment program designed to help him or her regain muscle strength, mobility, flexibility, and coordination. The program may include exercise, massage, and other therapies. Physical therapists can teach people how to use equipment such as walkers, canes, and wheelchairs.

- **Occupational therapists** Occupational therapists help the person regain muscle control and coordination and adjust to and compensate for physical limitations. They help the person relearn the basic activities of daily living (such as eating, bathing, and dressing). Occupational therapists teach people how to use equipment such as canes, walkers, and wheelchairs. They also show people how to change their home environment to make it safer and more user-friendly.

- **Speech therapists** Speech therapists help people regain the ability to speak, or teach them (and their families) other methods of effective communication. Speech therapists also help people learn to deal with swallowing problems.

- **Social workers** Social workers can provide counseling, guidance, support, and direct assistance. They can evaluate the person's needs for assistance and make arrangements or referrals for needed services such as transportation, financial assistance, legal assistance, home health care, and housing.

- **Mental health professionals** A psychiatrist, psychologist, or other mental health professional can help the person deal with depression (see page 709) or other psychological problems that frequently occur after a stroke (see box below).
- **Vocational therapists** Vocational therapists can help people return to work by helping them develop résumés, assisting in job searches and retraining programs, and providing referrals to vocational rehabilitation agencies.

Stroke and Mental Health

After a stroke, many people experience depression. They may feel isolated or frustrated, especially if their recovery is progressing slowly or if they are having problems communicating. Symptoms of depression include sleeplessness, indifference, and withdrawal. For most people, the depression is temporary, and they may benefit from joining a support group or talking to a psychiatrist or other mental health professional. If the depression persists, a doctor may prescribe antidepressant medications (see page 712) such as tricyclics, selective serotonin reuptake inhibitors (SSRIs), monoamine oxidase inhibitors (MAOIs), or bupropion.

Some people who have had a stroke may have difficulty controlling their emotions. For example, they may experience mood swings or they may laugh or cry more easily than usual. These emotional changes result from injury to the brain, so it is important for family and friends to understand that this is not deliberate behavior.

Preventing Strokes

If you have had a stroke, you are at risk of having another one. You can reduce your chances of having a stroke by doing the following:

- **Exercise regularly.** Regular, moderate exercise—such as brisk walking or swimming—lowers your blood pressure, helps you maintain a healthy weight, reduces stress, improves your cholesterol profile, and reduces your risk of diabetes.
- **Eat a healthy diet.** Eating a wide variety of nutritious foods—especially fruits, vegetables, and whole grains—that are low in salt, fat, and cholesterol improves your cholesterol profile, lowers your blood pressure, and helps you control your weight.

- **Control your cholesterol.** You can improve your cholesterol profile by eating a nutritious, low-fat, high-fiber diet; exercising regularly; losing weight if you are overweight; and quitting smoking if you smoke. If necessary, your doctor can prescribe medications to lower your cholesterol.
- **Control your blood pressure.** Have your blood pressure checked regularly, and work with your doctor to keep your blood pressure at a healthy level.
- **Take in at least 400 micrograms of folic acid every day.** Consuming enough of the B vitamins folic acid and vitamins B6 and B12 (in food or in vitamin supplements) lowers your homocysteine level (see page 559), which may decrease your risk of stroke. For foods that are rich in B vitamins, see page 4.
- **Keep diabetes under control.** If you have diabetes, work with your doctor to control your blood sugar and avoid possible complications.
- **Don't smoke.** Ask your doctor for information about how to quit smoking (see page 29).
- **Take anticlotting medication according to your doctor's instructions.** If your doctor has prescribed anticlotting medication, take it exactly as prescribed, and do not take other medications without checking with your doctor first.
- **Have regular checkups.** See your doctor as often as he or she recommends to help detect and treat health problems in their early stages.
- **Manage your stress.** Find positive ways to cope with or reduce the stress in your life, such as by exercising regularly and getting enough sleep.

Transient Ischemic Attacks

A transient ischemic attack (TIA) is a significant warning sign that a person is at risk of having a stroke. In a TIA, some brain tissue does not receive sufficient oxygen because the artery that supplies that area of the brain with blood is temporarily blocked. The symptoms of a TIA are temporary, usually lasting from 2 to 15 minutes (although they can last longer, but rarely more than an hour).

A TIA usually occurs when a small blood clot or a fragment of plaque (a buildup of fatty deposits) breaks away from the wall of an artery or a heart valve and is carried through the bloodstream to the brain. As the fragment passes through blood vessels in the brain, it temporarily obstructs blood flow to an area of brain tissue and causes strokelike symptoms. Symptoms vary, depending on the area of the brain that is affected. As the clot dissolves, blood flow is gradually restored and the affected tissues recover. Although the blockage is temporary, the problem is likely to recur and the risk of permanent damage from a stroke increases.

Factors that increase the risk of a TIA are the same as those for a stroke (see page 669), including uncontrolled high blood pressure, uncontrolled diabetes, an unfavorable cholesterol profile, obesity, and lack of exercise. Recurring TIAs are often warning signs of an impending stroke. Nearly half of all people who have TIAs have a stroke within 5 years of their first TIA.

Symptoms

The symptoms of a TIA resemble those of a stroke and can include dizziness, tingling, numbness, blurred vision, confusion, difficulty speaking, and paralysis on one side of the body. If an artery that delivers blood to an eye is blocked, you may have temporary blindness in that eye. If you have sudden, temporary strokelike symptoms, see your doctor right away.

Diagnosis

To diagnose a TIA, your doctor will examine you and may refer you to a neurologist (a doctor who specializes in treating disorders of the nervous system). The doctor will try to identify the location of a possible blood clot, such as in one of the two carotid arteries in your neck. To detect signs of narrowing of the carotid arteries, a doctor may listen through a stethoscope placed in various locations on your neck. He or she may also place the stethoscope on your chest to listen for abnormal heart valve sounds or for an irregular heart rhythm (see page 580). The doctor may order an electrocardiogram (ECG; see page 559), an examination of the electrical activity of the heart. You may be asked to wear a portable ECG device called a Holter monitor for 24 hours or longer. The doctor may also order an ultrasound examination (see page 111) of your carotid arteries and heart.

If these tests indicate that one of your carotid arteries is narrowed or blocked, your doctor may recommend surgery. In addition, your doctor may order an angiogram (see page 110) to evaluate blood flow and the condition of the blood vessels that may be causing the problem. A CT scan or MRI may be done to look for previous, undetected strokes. An MRA (magnetic resonance angiogram) may be done to help evaluate blood flow through the arteries in the brain.

Treatment

The treatment of a TIA focuses on preventing additional TIAs and a possible stroke. The preventive measures that a doctor may recommend depend on a person's age and general health. You may be asked to take an aspirin once a day every day for the rest of your life. Aspirin helps prevent TIAs and stroke by reducing the risk of blood clots. Doctors sometimes prescribe other anticoagulant drugs instead of or in addition to aspirin. More powerful anticoagulants can help reduce the risk of stroke in people with abnormal heart rhythms. In some cases, a doctor may recommend a surgical procedure called carotid endarterectomy (see page 674) to remove the fatty deposits that have narrowed the arteries.

Transient ischemic attack
A transient ischemic attack is often caused by a clump of blood cells (a clot) flowing with the blood until it blocks a small artery in the brain. The effects of a transient ischemic attack are temporary; the clump quickly breaks up and is swept away in the bloodstream, restoring blood flow.

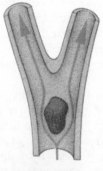

Blood clot in an artery

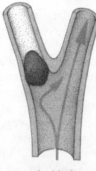

Clot blocks artery

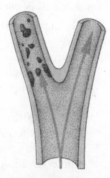

Clot breaks up; blood vessel reopens

Subarachnoid Hemorrhage

The surface of the brain is covered by three membranes called meninges. The thick, outermost membrane, the dura mater, adheres to the skull, while the thin, innermost membrane, the pia mater, adheres to the brain. The middle membrane, the arachnoid, is closer to the dura mater than to the pia mater because the space between the arachnoid and the pia mater (called the subarachnoid space) is filled with cerebrospinal fluid. A subarachnoid hemorrhage occurs when blood leaks into the subarachnoid space, usually as the result of a ruptured aneurysm (see page 599). The blood may remain in the cerebrospinal fluid or it may burst through the pia mater into brain tissue when the aneurysm ruptures.

A major hemorrhage (one that causes loss of consciousness) can cause permanent brain damage or death. One third of people who survive a major hemorrhage have additional hemorrhages. The permanent damage that can result from a hemorrhage varies according to which areas of the brain are affected. A person can have partial paralysis, weakness, numbness, or vision and speech problems that can linger or be permanent. Subarachnoid hemorrhage most often occurs in people between ages 40 and 60 and is slightly more common in women than in men. People who have high blood pressure (see page 574) or diabetes (see page 889) are at increased risk.

Symptoms

The main symptom of a subarachnoid hemorrhage is a sudden, severe headache. A person also may have a stiff neck, be extremely sensitive to bright light (photophobia), or have strokelike symptoms including faintness, dizziness, confusion, drowsiness, nausea, and vomiting. A major hemorrhage can cause sudden loss of consciousness.

Diagnosis

For a person who is unconscious, the doctor will take steps to restore and maintain circulation and breathing. He or she will order a CT scan (see page 112) to determine if there is bleeding in the brain or if some other condition is causing the loss of consciousness. If the scan is normal, the doctor may recommend a lumbar puncture (see page 693), a procedure in which a hollow needle is inserted into the lower part of the spine to withdraw a sample of cerebrospinal fluid for microscopic examination to look for blood or inflammation.

Treatment

If blood is found in the cerebrospinal fluid, the treatment of a subarachnoid hemorrhage will concentrate on preventing further bleeding. The doctor will order an angiogram (see page 110), an X-ray examination of the arteries that supply blood to the brain, to locate the source of the bleeding and to look for an aneurysm. If an aneurysm is detected, surgery will be performed in which the doctor places a tiny clip across the neck of the aneurysm, blocking blood flow to that part of the artery. In some cases, an aneurysm can be sealed from the inside by passing a small coil or balloon through the arteries to the site of the aneurysm. The coil or balloon is released from the tip of the catheter to obstruct the opening of the aneurysm, blocking

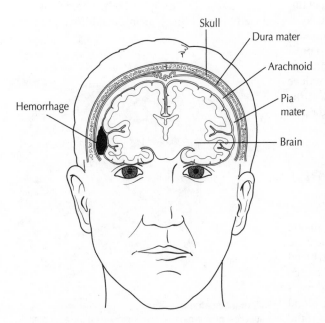

Subarachnoid hemorrhage
In a subarachnoid hemorrhage, a ruptured blood vessel causes blood to leak into the space between the arachnoid and the pia mater, the middle and inner membranes of the three membranes that cover the brain. If enough blood puts pressure on brain tissue, it can cause permanent brain damage and be life-threatening.

blood flow to the area and reducing pressure on the damaged artery wall. The person may be given medication orally or intravenously (through a vein) to prevent spasms of the blood vessels.

If an aneurysm is not detected and a person survives after a subarachnoid hemorrhage without further problems, chances for a full recovery are good. Until the person is out of danger, the doctor will recommend complete bed rest to keep blood pressure down. He or she may prescribe medication to promote relaxation, prevent seizures, and reduce narrowing or spasms of the blood vessels. If the person's blood pressure is very high, the doctor may prescribe antihypertensive medication.

Subdural Hemorrhage and Hematoma

In subdural hemorrhage, blood leaks from blood vessels in the dura mater, the outermost of the three membranes that cover the brain. The ruptured blood vessels are usually small veins that break on the underside of the dura mater. Because blood pressure in veins is less than that in arteries, blood tends to seep slowly into the space between the dura mater and the arachnoid (the middle of the three membranes) and causes a hematoma (a collection of clotted blood). Subdural hemorrhage usually results from a head injury (see page 680), most often in older people who have fallen or bumped their head; the veins stretch and tear upon impact.

Symptoms

The symptoms of subdural hemorrhage develop gradually over a period of hours or, sometimes, days. Symptoms can include drowsiness, confusion, weakness or numbness on one side of the body, loss of balance and coordination, or persistent or recurring headaches and nausea. Initially the symptoms may come and go, but eventually they become persistent.

Diagnosis

A diagnosis of subdural hemorrhage and hematoma is made from the symptoms, a physical examination, and the results of a CT scan (see page 112) or MRI (see page 113).

Treatment

The treatment of subdural hemorrhage depends on the size of the hematoma and may include surgery to remove the clot. If the clot is small, surgery may not be necessary because the blood clot will gradually be reabsorbed by the body. The doctor will closely monitor the person's condition, and may

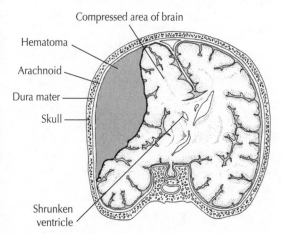

Compressed area of brain

Hematoma

Arachnoid

Dura mater

Skull

Shrunken ventricle

Subdural hematoma
A subdural hemorrhage is bleeding between the dura mater and the arachnoid, two of the three membranes covering the brain. A subdural hematoma results when the blood collects there and clots. In addition to compressing brain tissue, the hematoma can cause shrinkage of the ventricle (one of four cavities in the brain that produce cerebrospinal fluid) on that side of the brain. The symptoms of a subdural hematoma are similar to those of a stroke but can take days or weeks to develop.

recommend rehabilitation therapy (see page 672) to help him or her recover any lost function.

Epidural Hemorrhage

Epidural hemorrhage occurs when blood vessels rupture outside or in the dura mater (the outermost of the three membranes that cover the brain) and blood leaks into the space between the dura mater and the skull. The condition usually results from a head injury that causes some of the blood vessels in the outer surface of the dura mater to rupture. Because these vessels are usually arteries, a significant amount of blood can leak into the space.

Symptoms
The symptoms of an epidural hemorrhage may develop up to a few hours after a head injury. These symptoms can include a headache that increases in severity, nausea and vomiting, and increasing drowsiness and weakness, which eventually can lead to unconsciousness, coma, and death.

WARNING!

Brain Hemorrhage
If you or someone you know has symptoms of an epidural hemorrhage, call 911 or your local emergency number immediately, or take the person to the nearest hospital emergency department without delay, especially after a blow to the head within the past 24 hours. Without prompt treatment, bleeding in the brain can cause permanent brain damage or death.

Diagnosis
A person who reports to a hospital emergency department with symptoms of a head injury will be evaluated immediately with diagnostic tests to determine the severity of the injury and its effects.

Treatment
If the injury has caused an epidural hemorrhage, the doctor will perform surgery immediately to stop the bleeding and relieve pressure on the brain. With prompt surgical treatment, most people recover completely from an epidural hemorrhage.

Structural Disorders of the Brain and Spinal Cord

A structural disorder of the central nervous system occurs when part of the brain or spinal cord is distorted, malformed, or damaged. These problems can result from an injury, a tumor, or a disorder that affects the tissues, membranes, or adjacent bones. Some people are born with malformed blood vessels in the brain that may not cause any symptoms until later in life.

Arteriovenous Malformations

Arteriovenous malformations are congenital (present at birth) abnormalities of blood vessels that can occur in any part of the brain or spinal cord. The blood vessels are tangled, and there may be abnormal connections between arteries and veins, with fewer capillary connections than normal. Pressure can build up in these blood vessels and cause blood to leak into the brain. An arteriovenous malformation that causes a subarachnoid hemorrhage (see page 677) or bleeding into the brain or spinal cord can cause permanent damage or be fatal.

Symptoms
Although people are born with arteriovenous malformations, most do not cause symptoms for years. Symptoms such as recurring headaches and seizures develop when the malformation starts leaking blood into the brain or spinal cord or the subarachnoid space (the space between the middle and inner layers of membranes covering the brain and spinal cord). The damage that causes the seizures may be limited to only one part of the brain. These seizures may not always cause unconsciousness but can cause intermittent symptoms such as uncontrollable twitching in a part of the body controlled by the area of the brain in which the malformation is located.

Diagnosis
If you have symptoms of an arteriovenous malformation, your doctor may recommend that you have a CT scan (see page 112) or MRI (see page 113) and possibly an MRA (magnetic resonance angiogram) to look for abnormal blood vessels.

Treatment

Doctors usually use a combination of treatments for arteriovenous malformations. Leaking blood vessels in a malformation can sometimes be removed surgically or closed to cut off their blood supply. For some malformations, doctors inject an acrylic material through the arteries in the brain into the malformation to destroy all of it or, in some cases, to eliminate the most fragile parts of the malformation that are at risk of leaking. For malformations that are not easy to reach surgically, radiation therapy (see page 23) may be recommended. In this procedure, doctors use angiography (see page 110) and a CT scan or MRI to find the exact location of the malformation. High-energy radiation is then directed into the center of the malformation to form scar tissue and close the abnormal blood vessels while minimizing injury to the surrounding brain tissue.

Brain Injury

A minor head injury usually results in little or no damage to the brain and it heals rapidly and completely. However, a more forceful blow to the head can damage the brain even if the skull is not fractured. In these closed head injuries, the brain can strike the inside surface of the skull, resulting in damage. After a severe head injury, the brain may swell and press against the skull, causing more brain damage. In a small percentage of cases, brain damage is severe enough to cause permanent mental and physical disability or death. A severe head injury may also cause a cerebral hemorrhage (bleeding into the brain), which can lead to brain damage with symptoms resembling those of a stroke (see page 669). If the skull is fractured, bacteria or other microorganisms can enter the brain through the fracture and infect brain tissue, causing meningitis (see page 692). Severe brain injuries are most often caused by motor-vehicle collisions (especially those involving motorcycles), industrial work-related injuries, falls, fights, explosions, or gunshot wounds.

Symptoms

The symptoms of a brain injury may not appear immediately and depend on how badly the brain is damaged. A minor injury may cause a headache or dizziness that lasts for only a few days. Moderate injuries can progress over hours or days as the brain swells from the injury or from irritation from bleeding. A severe injury can cause immediate unconsciousness, which can last hours, days, or weeks. A person who loses consciousness may be confused and dizzy when he or she regains consciousness. He or she also may have headaches, fatigue, muscle weakness, difficulty speaking, dilated pupils, and memory loss (especially of what happened immediately before the injury). A person may vomit or have a seizure in addition to the above symptoms. The injury can also cause bleeding in the membranes surrounding the brain or inside the brain. Symptoms of bleeding in the brain or a stroke—such as headache, weakness, confusion, and loss of consciousness—may develop hours or days after the injury.

The symptoms from a brain injury usually improve gradually as the injury heals. However, in severe cases, a person has permanent brain damage that causes lasting physical symptoms (such as paralysis) and decreased mental function. In some

Coma, Concussion, and Contusion

The following terms referring to brain injury or unconsciousness are frequently used and often confused:

- **Coma**   A coma is a state of unconsciousness in which a person does not respond to stimulation. Coma results from a disturbance in or damage to areas of the brain involved in consciousness caused by disease, injury, or drugs.

- **Concussion**   A concussion is an injury to the brain as the result of a blow to the head. A person may have loss of consciousness caused by a disturbance of the electrical activity in the brain. A mild concussion is a brief period of feeling stunned, sometimes with momentary loss of consciousness; the person may not remember the injury or what happened immediately before or after it. A severe concussion can cause prolonged unconsciousness, impairment of brain functions (including breathing, muscle strength, and coordination), dilated pupils, and a weak pulse.

- **Contusion**   A contusion is a bruise of the brain as the result of an injury to the head. It may or may not be associated with a fractured skull. There may be bruising and scattered bleeding in the brain near the point of impact.

cases, a head injury can cause emotional problems such as depression that can develop long after the injury. Permanent brain damage after a severe head injury may also cause seizures as a result of scarring. The risk of seizures is increased if the skull has been penetrated and the brain has been injured directly.

WARNING!

Never Shake or Toss a Baby

Activities such as shaking or tossing a baby—or jogging with a baby in a carrier or backpack—can tear the fragile veins around the child's brain or make the brain bang against the hard bone of the skull, injuring the brain. These brain injuries can cause loss of vision; severe, permanent brain damage; or death.

Diagnosis

If you have had a recent head injury (even within the past few months) and are having symptoms, your doctor will probably recommend a CT scan (see page 112) or MRI (see page 113) to see if you have any brain damage and, if so, to determine the extent of the damage.

Treatment

If you have had a minor head injury, rest for 2 to 3 days; don't take any medication that hasn't been prescribed by your doctor. Make sure family and friends know about the injury so they can watch for any problems. If you develop symptoms, they should call the doctor right away. If you have had a severe head injury, have someone call 911 or take you to the nearest hospital emergency department. You will be admitted to the hospital and may be given medications such as mannitol or corticosteroids to reduce the swelling in your brain. A surgeon may place a monitoring device in your brain to measure the amount of pressure and to remove cerebrospinal fluid to relieve some of the pressure. If your skull is fractured, the surgeon will remove any bone fragments from your brain and may replace the damaged area of the skull with a metal plate. Recovery from a severe brain injury may take many months and you may need rehabilitation therapy (see page 672) and counseling.

Spinal Cord Injury

The nerves that make up the spinal cord transmit impulses between the brain and the rest of the body, allowing you to control your movements and detect sensations such as pain. If the spinal cord is injured, parts of the body below the point of injury may be affected; the closer to the head, the more areas will be affected. Most spinal cord injuries result from motor-vehicle collisions, diving injuries, sports injuries, falls, or knife or gunshot wounds.

Spinal cord injuries can be permanent and can cause severe disability. If the injury causes numbness, you can hurt the numbed area because your nerves are not transmitting pain messages to your brain. Injury to part of the spinal cord in the neck can be fatal if the injury damages the nerves that control the muscles necessary for breathing.

Symptoms

The symptoms of a spinal cord injury are almost always immediate but can worsen gradually over a few hours to days as the affected area becomes inflamed and swells. Symptoms depend on the location of the damage and include numbness and muscle weakness or paralysis below the level of the injury (including the muscles that control the intestines and bladder). Sometimes the injury affects muscles on only one side of the body. If nearby bones and nerves are injured, you may have severe pain, although pain is not always a symptom of a spinal cord injury.

Diagnosis

To diagnose a spinal cord injury, after immobilizing your spinal cord (to prevent further damage), your doctor will test different parts of your body and may ask you to try to move them. He or she will order X-rays, a CT scan (see page 112), or an MRI (see page 113) to verify the location of the injury and determine the extent of the damage. Your doctor may perform a procedure called myelography. In this procedure, he or she injects a contrast medium (dye) into the cerebrospinal fluid (the liquid that surrounds the brain and spinal cord); the contrast medium, which can be seen on an X-ray or CT scan, will highlight the damaged areas of the spinal cord.

Treatment

Treatment of a spinal cord injury starts immediately. You will be immobilized because any movement could cause more damage to your spinal cord. Your doctor will immediately give you high doses of a corticosteroid medication to quickly reduce inflammation and swelling in the spinal cord. If the muscles that assist breathing have been weakened or paralyzed, you will be placed on a ventilator. A surgeon will remove any bone fragments and repair any damaged vertebrae that press on your spinal cord. If you have lost the ability to control your bladder, a catheter (a thin, flexible tube) will be inserted into your urethra to drain urine. After your doctor has determined the extent of your injury and your condition is stable, he or she may recommend occupational and physical therapy and counseling.

Most spinal cord injuries result in permanent damage. Research is currently being done on ways to stimulate muscles to restore some degree of function. Drugs are being tested to try to improve the conduction of impulses through the damaged surviving nerve fibers.

Brain Tumor

A brain tumor is an abnormal growth in the brain that can be either benign (noncancerous) or malignant (cancerous). Whether cancerous or not cancerous, a brain tumor is always dangerous because the skull makes it impossible for a growing tumor to expand anywhere but inward, into the brain. If untreated, a brain tumor can grow and cause permanent brain damage or death.

Cancerous brain tumors that originate in the brain (called primary brain cancer) are less common than cancerous tumors that have spread to the brain from another part of the body such as the breasts or lungs (called secondary, or metastatic, brain cancer). Primary brain tumors, which may be congenital (present at birth) or acquired later in life, seldom spread to other parts of the body. Secondary brain tumors, like most cancers, are more common later in life.

Symptoms

As a brain tumor enlarges, it may cause headaches that are worse in the morning or when you lie down. Over time, the headaches may become more severe and may be accompanied by nausea and vomiting. Other symptoms—such as blurred or double vision, dizziness, muscle weakness or loss of sensation (such as in the face or on one side of the body), hearing or memory loss, seizures, or a change in behavior—may develop, depending on the location of the brain tumor.

Diagnosis

If you have symptoms of a brain tumor, your doctor will refer you to a neurologist (a doctor who specializes in disorders of the nervous system). The neurologist will order a CT scan (see page 112) or MRI (see page 113) to determine if you have a brain tumor. If a tumor is found, the neurologist will order X-rays of other parts of your body, such as your chest, because of the possibility that the brain tumor originated elsewhere. He or she may recommend an angiogram (see page 110) to help identify the type of tumor, and to see if it is pressing on blood vessels. The neurologist may order an electroencephalogram (EEG; see page 687) to determine if the tumor is causing seizures.

Treatment

Corticosteroids to reduce swelling and surgery are usually the initial treatments for a primary brain tumor. A sample of tissue (biopsy) taken during the surgery can help determine the type of brain tumor and the best course of treatment. Surgery to remove a noncancerous tumor is most successful if the tumor is detected at an early stage. It is usually not possible to successfully remove multiple secondary brain tumors. However, a single metastatic tumor can sometimes be removed. If removing a tumor could cause permanent brain damage, a surgeon may be able to remove part of the tumor to reduce pressure on the brain and relieve the symptoms.

Instead of surgery, or if a cancerous tumor cannot be removed completely by surgery, your doctor may use radiation therapy (see page 23) or chemotherapy (see page 23) to destroy the tumor cells. Some tumors that cannot be reached using conventional surgery can be treated by implanting radioactive seeds into the tumor or by using a device called a gamma knife, which directs focused radiation at the tumor.

Your doctor may prescribe antiseizure medications to control seizures, strong pain relievers to relieve the pain of severe headaches, and corticosteroids to reduce inflammation and swelling and relieve pressure around the tumor.

Spinal Cord Tumor

The spinal cord may be compressed by bone tumors or tumors of the nerve coverings (sheaths). Tumors of the spinal cord itself are rare growths that may be

DISORDERS OF BRAIN FUNCTION 683

benign (noncancerous) or malignant (cancerous). Spinal cord tumors must be treated immediately because an expanding tumor can press on the nerves in the spinal cord and cause severe, sometimes incapacitating, symptoms.

Symptoms

The symptoms of a spinal cord tumor depend on which part of the spinal cord and which nerves are damaged by the tumor. Persistent, worsening back pain is the most common symptom. Other symptoms include numbness, tingling, and loss of the sensations of hot and cold below the level of the tumor; muscle weakness (especially in the legs); difficulty urinating; or loss of bladder or bowel control.

Diagnosis

To diagnose a spinal cord tumor, your doctor will perform a thorough physical examination and may refer you to a neurologist (a doctor who specializes in disorders of the nervous system). The neurologist will order an MRI (see page 113) and may perform a procedure called myelography, in which a contrast medium (dye) that can be seen on X-rays is injected into the cerebrospinal fluid (the liquid that surrounds the brain and spinal cord) to highlight the areas of obstruction, such as a tumor, in the spinal cord. While performing the myelograph, the neurologist may take a sample of cerebrospinal fluid from your spine to look for cancer cells.

Treatment

Surgery is the most common treatment for a tumor that is pressing on the spinal cord, although tumors inside the spinal cord usually cannot be removed completely. Corticosteroids are given to reduce swelling. Removing all or part of the tumor can help relieve pressure on the spinal nerves and reduce pain and other symptoms. For tumors that have spread from elsewhere in the body (secondary tumors) to the bones of the spine, or for tumors inside the spinal cord that cannot be removed surgically, a doctor may use radiation therapy (see page 23) to destroy the tumor cells. Depending on the type of tumor, chemotherapy (see page 23) may also be recommended.

Disorders of Brain Function

Although some brain disorders have an identifiable underlying cause, such as an infection, a tumor or other growth, or a blocked artery, the causes of other brain disorders, such as migraine and epilepsy, are less well understood and are often difficult to diagnose. Most of these disorders result from problems with how the brain and its blood vessels function.

Tension Headaches

A tension headache (also called a muscle contraction headache) is the most common type of headache. Tension headaches usually result from strain on muscles in the face, neck, or scalp, and can be triggered by factors such as anxiety, stress, eyestrain, a noisy environment, or too little sleep. They can also result from overeating, drinking too much alcohol, or heavy smoking. Prolonged coughing or sneezing, a head or neck injury, or poor posture can bring on a tension headache. Tension headaches that occur nearly every day are called chronic daily headaches.

Symptoms

The pain of a tension headache is usually aching and can be mild to moderate and widespread or limited to a specific area. Chronic daily headaches can cause fatigue, depression, or difficulty sleeping.

Diagnosis

A tension headache is diagnosed by a person's symptoms and by a neurological examination that rules out other, more serious, possible causes. A doctor may perform diagnostic tests to rule out other possible causes of headaches.

Treatment

The pain of a tension headache can usually be relieved with over-the-counter pain relievers such as aspirin, acetaminophen, ibuprofen, or naproxen. These medications are most effective when taken at the onset of symptoms. For some people, relaxation techniques (see page 59) such as deep breathing, meditation, or yoga may help. Getting a good night's sleep (see page 57) may also be helpful. Doctors sometimes prescribe antidepressants (see page 712) or muscle relaxants to treat chronic daily headaches.

Migraines

A migraine is a severe, persistent headache that usually starts on one side of the head and spreads to the other side as it gradually increases in intensity. For many people, migraines can be disabling. Because migraines tend to run in families, doctors think that there may be a genetic component.

During a migraine, the arteries leading to the brain first become narrowed and then become dilated (widened) by nerve impulses inside the brain. Doctors believe that these changes in the diameter of the arteries produce the pain of a migraine. Narrowing of the arteries reduces blood flow to various parts of the brain, which may help explain some of the sensory disturbances—such as increased sensitivity to light, noise, or odors—that can accompany a migraine.

In many cases, specific substances, conditions, or circumstances trigger a migraine. Common triggers include consuming alcohol, chocolate, caffeine, monosodium glutamate (MSG) in processed foods, nitrates or nitrites in processed meats, and tyramine in cheese or red wine. Other possible triggers include exposure to fluorescent light, glaring light, high altitudes, strong odors, or sudden changes in environmental temperature or barometric pressure. For some women, migraines are associated with menstrual periods. Other people may develop migraines during or immediately following times of emotional stress.

Migraines seldom occur before puberty, but most people who have migraines usually have their

Headache Diary

Keeping a headache diary can help you determine what triggers your headaches so you can take steps to prevent them in the future. Bring your headache diary with you when you visit your doctor. The information it contains will help your doctor identify the cause of your headaches and plan appropriate treatment. Whenever you have a headache, write down the following information:

- Date
- Time the headache began
- Time the headache ended
- Intensity of pain (such as mild, moderate, or severe)
- Type of pain (such as aching, throbbing, or stabbing)
- Location of the pain
- Other symptoms (such as nausea, vomiting, or sensitivity to light)
- Medication taken for headache (type and amount) and results

- Self-treatment for headache (such as sleep, cold compresses, or relaxation techniques) and results
- Activity you were engaged in when headache began (such as working or exercising)
- Where you were when the headache began (such as indoors or outdoors)
- Potential allergens nearby when the headache began (such as pollen, tobacco smoke, dust, or pets)
- Other environmental factors (such as noises, odors, or room temperature)
- Food or drink you consumed before the headache began
- Your emotional state (such as angry, stressed, or tired) before the headache began
- Medication you are taking for other reasons (both prescription and over the counter)

first one before age 40. Migraines are more common in women than in men.

Symptoms

The main symptom of a migraine is intense, throbbing pain that gets worse. The headache is usually accompanied by other symptoms—such as nausea, vomiting, diarrhea, aches, sweating, or extreme sensitivity to light or noise—that can vary from one person to another. Your eyes may be bloodshot and your skin may appear abnormally pale. Other symptoms may include numbness or tingling around your mouth or in one arm or down one side of your body, dizziness, ringing in your ears, or, rarely, temporary confusion.

Some people experience a warning sign called an aura just before the onset of a migraine, during which they feel uncomfortable and fatigued and may experience some sort of visual disturbance, such as a zigzag distortion. An aura can last from several minutes to several hours, but once the headache begins, the warning symptoms usually fade.

The duration of a migraine and its timing can vary, but you may be able to learn from experience to predict the nature and duration of your headaches. Migraines usually last several hours—severe migraines can last a few days. Episodes may occur several times over the course of a week or once every few years. If you have recurring, severe headaches that you cannot control with over-the-counter pain relievers, see your doctor as soon as possible.

Diagnosis

A migraine is diagnosed by the symptoms and by a neurological examination that rules out more serious possible causes. In some cases, doctors perform specific diagnostic tests to rule out other possible underlying causes of the headaches.

Treatment

Your doctor will probably recommend that you keep a headache diary (see previous page) to help identify symptoms, triggers, and patterns associated with your migraines. This detailed record will help you and your doctor plan an effective course of treatment. Although there is no cure for migraines, their symptoms can be relieved, often dramatically.

The doctor may recommend taking over-the-counter pain relievers such as aspirin, acetaminophen, ibuprofen, or naproxen. If these drugs are not effective, he or she may prescribe vasoconstrictors (drugs that narrow the blood vessels) such as sumatriptan, ergot alkaloids, or serotonin agonists. For severe migraines, these drugs may be injected into a vein or muscle as soon as the symptoms start. To control nausea and vomiting, the doctor may prescribe antihistamines or phenothiazines.

It may take several months of trying different medications—such as beta blockers, calcium channel blockers, antiseizure medications, or antidepressants used in combination with nonsteroidal anti-inflammatory drugs—before you and your doctor find the drug or drug combination that works best for you. Taking medication at the onset of your symptoms can help reduce the severity and duration of a migraine. To avoid side effects, take your medication exactly as prescribed.

Because oral contraceptives (see page 470) can trigger migraines in some women, a doctor may prescribe a different contraceptive or recommend changing birth-control methods to eliminate the headaches. Because tobacco smoke can irritate blood vessels, your doctor may recommend that you stop smoking if you smoke. For some people, relaxation techniques such as meditation, yoga, or biofeedback help prevent migraines.

Cluster Headaches

Cluster headaches are severe, recurring headaches that affect one side of the head. The headaches often occur during the night or early in the morning and can last from 15 minutes to several hours. Cluster headaches go away but often return within a few hours or at the same time the next day. After several days or weeks of recurring headaches (referred to as the cluster), the headaches disappear and may not return for several months or years. Cluster headaches are more common in men than in women.

Symptoms

The symptoms of cluster headaches include sudden, intense pain that is usually centered in and around one eye or on one side of the face. The eye on the affected side is watery and red, and the eyelid may droop. The person's nose may be either runny or stuffy.

Diagnosis

Cluster headaches are diagnosed by the person's symptoms and by a neurological examination that rules out more serious possible causes. In some cases, doctors perform specific diagnostic tests to rule out other possible underlying causes of the headaches.

Treatment

Cluster headaches are usually treated with over-the-counter pain relievers such as aspirin, acetaminophen, ibuprofen, or naproxen. Doctors may also prescribe antihistamines or corticosteroid drugs to reduce inflammation, triptan drugs (such as sumatriptan) to relieve pain and nausea, or antiemetic drugs to control nausea and vomiting. For some people, inhaling oxygen helps relieve symptoms. Daily preventive treatment with an antihypertensive medication (such as a calcium channel blocker) or an ergot derivative can reduce the frequency and severity of cluster headaches in some people. Less frequently, doctors prescribe the mood stabilizer lithium to treat chronic cluster headaches.

Epilepsy

Epilepsy is abnormal electrical activity in the brain that causes miscommunication among brain cells. In a healthy person, brain cells communicate with one another by sending electrical signals back and forth but, in a person who has epilepsy, the signals from one group of brain cells occasionally become so strong that they temporarily overwhelm nearby parts of the brain. This sudden, excessive electrical activity causes seizures (uncontrolled movements or temporary loss of consciousness or memory).

Generalized seizures—grand mal seizures or petit mal (or absence) seizures—affect the entire brain. Partial seizures affect a specific area of the brain. Partial seizures can be either simple partial seizures (during which the person remains aware) or complex partial seizures (during which the person loses touch with his or her surroundings and, sometimes, loses consciousness).

In most people with epilepsy, the cause is unknown. In some cases, the disorder can result from a problem such as a brain tumor, stroke, severe head injury, a brain infection, or a blood vessel malformation. Pesticide poisoning, withdrawal from alcohol or other drugs, drug overdose, or a chemical imbalance in the body can also trigger epilepsy. Between 1 and 2 percent of Americans have some form of epilepsy. The disease may run in families and affects men and women in equal numbers. Petit mal seizures occur mainly in children. Isolated, nonrecurring seizures (called febrile seizures) can occur in infants and toddlers as a result of a high fever from an infection. A child who has febrile seizures does not have epilepsy, but the seizures may increase his or her risk of developing the disorder later in life.

In people who have epilepsy, seizures can occur spontaneously or, occasionally, can be triggered by flickering or flashing lights, loud noises, or monotonous sounds. The risk of having a seizure increases with stress, lack of sleep, fatigue, or hunger, or when a person does not take his or her antiseizure medication properly.

Symptoms

Many people who have epilepsy experience a warning of an oncoming seizure called an aura, which may occur just before or as much as several hours before a seizure. An aura may be a vague feeling of tension or unease, or it may be a recognizable sensory change such as a specific sound, disturbing odor, physical sensation, or visual disturbance.

Grand mal seizure

During a grand mal seizure, a person experiences loss of balance and coordination, loss of consciousness, and uncontrollable twitching and jerking body movements. Some people may also lose bladder and bowel control. A seizure normally lasts 1 or 2 minutes, after which the person is usually disoriented and exhausted and does not remember the seizure.

Petit mal seizure

During a petit mal seizure, a person (usually a child) suddenly stops whatever he or she is doing and becomes unaware and inattentive, staring blankly for a few seconds to half a minute. Some people may also experience brief confusion, slight muscle twitching, or rapid eye movements. The symptoms are subtle, and the person is not aware of the seizure. Children who have petit mal seizures are sometimes thought to be daydreaming. The seizures can occur hundreds of times throughout the day, interfering with a child's ability to concentrate or to complete simple tasks.

Simple partial seizure

A simple partial seizure does not cause loss of consciousness. It usually begins with sudden, uncontrollable muscle twitching in one part of the body, which gradually spreads to other parts of the body. For example, the thumb of one hand may start twitching, then the entire arm twitches, and then the rest of that side of the body twitches. Other symptoms of a simple partial seizure can include tingling or hallucinations (of smell, taste, or vision). The person is aware of the seizure as it occurs and can recall the seizure afterward.

Complex partial seizure

A person who has a complex partial seizure usually experiences an aura that lasts just a few seconds. He or she appears unaware and performs involuntary behaviors such as laughing for no apparent reason, speaking nonsensically, walking in circles, or smacking his or her lips. He or she may also lose consciousness. The person is not aware of the seizure as it occurs and does not recall it afterward. After a complex partial seizure, the person may sometimes feel detached from reality, be confused, or have memory problems.

Diagnosis

To diagnose epilepsy, a doctor performs a complete neurological examination that includes tests to evaluate the functioning of the nervous system, such as vision, reflexes, hearing, sensation, movement, and balance and coordination. The doctor will identify the type of seizure the person is having, usually by evaluating information provided by people who have witnessed the seizures. Sometimes video monitoring of epileptic seizures can help the doctor diagnose the type of seizure the person is having and determine the best course of treatment.

The doctor will order an electroencephalogram (see below left), an examination of the electrical activity of the brain. He or she may also order a CT scan (see page 112) or an MRI (see page 113) of the brain to help rule out other possible causes of the seizures, such as a brain tumor. To check for an infection, the doctor may order blood tests or, in some cases, a lumbar puncture (see page 693), in

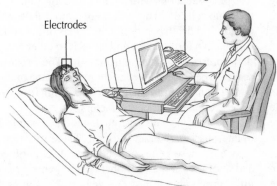

Recording of wave pattern
(electroencephalogram)

Electrodes

Electroencephalogram
In an electroencephalogram (EEG), electrodes are attached to the scalp to record electrical impulses from different areas of the brain using a device called an electroencephalograph, which records the impulses as a wave pattern on a moving strip of paper or on a computer screen. An EEG is used to diagnose brain disorders such as epilepsy.

Helping a Person Who Is Having a Seizure

The most important thing to do for someone who is having a seizure is to make sure that he or she is not injured. During a grand mal seizure, a person will begin to twitch or jerk and may fall to the ground. If a person is having a seizure:

- Do not panic.
- Do not attempt to move the person unless he or she is in immediate danger.
- Do not hold or attempt to restrain the person.
- Do not put your finger or another object in the person's mouth because he or she may bite down on it. (It is not possible for a person to swallow his or her tongue.)
- Move large or sharp objects out of the person's way.
- After the seizure, turn the person on his or her side and turn his or her head to one side to prevent choking on vomit. Loosen the person's collar and try to pull the jaw forward and extend the neck so he or she can breathe easily. Make sure that the person's airway is not blocked by food, chewing gum, dental devices, or vomit.
- Call 911 or your local emergency number if a seizure continues for more than about 5 minutes, if this is the person's first seizure, or if another seizure starts a few minutes after the first seizure ends.
- After the person regains consciousness, call a doctor or take the person to the nearest hospital emergency department.

which a hollow needle is inserted into the spine and a sample of cerebrospinal fluid is withdrawn and examined under a microscope.

Treatment

Epilepsy usually cannot be cured. A doctor prescribes antiseizure drugs such as carbamazepine, phenytoin, or valproic acid to help prevent or control seizures. With the help of medication, most people who have epilepsy can live an active, productive life. Your doctor will tell you how to obtain an identification bracelet, pendant, or card that indicates you have epilepsy. Always carry this identification with you so that emergency medical personnel will know what treatment to provide in case of an emergency.

If medication does not control your seizures, your doctor may recommend surgery to remove tissue in the area of the brain where your seizures originate. For some people, surgery can reduce or eliminate the seizures and improve their quality of life.

If your condition results from an underlying disorder, your doctor will treat that disorder. As the underlying disorder improves, you should have fewer seizures. Some people can control their seizures by following a special diet.

Degenerative Diseases of the Brain

Degenerative diseases of the brain are characterized by the progressive deterioration and death of brain cells. The exact cause of these disorders is not known, but some forms can be inherited. The diseases and their symptoms differ by the type of degenerative changes and by the areas of the brain that are affected. For example, Alzheimer's disease affects the areas of the brain responsible for intellect and memory, Parkinson's disease affects areas involved with movement, and amyotrophic lateral sclerosis (ALS) affects nerve cells that control muscles.

Alzheimer's Disease

Alzheimer's disease is the most common cause of dementia, a brain disorder that results in a progressive and irreversible decline in mental functioning that eventually makes a person unable to perform daily activities. Alzheimer's disease causes severe memory loss, disorientation of space and time, and decline in the ability to think clearly and speak coherently.

The incidence of the disease escalates with age, affecting 1 in 10 people over 65 and 1 in 2 people over 85. An inherited form of Alzheimer's disease can develop in people in their 30s, 40s, and 50s. An estimated 4 million Americans may have Alzheimer's disease, which affects more women than men, perhaps because women tend to live longer than men. People can live with Alzheimer's disease for years, gradually losing more and more function. The average time from diagnosis to death is 4 to 8 years, but some people live with the disease for up to 20 years.

The most characteristic features of Alzheimer's disease are found in and around brain cells. Dense deposits of protein called neuritic plaques form around the brain cells at the same time that twisted strands of fiber called neurofibrillary tangles form inside the brain cells. These plaques and tangles are linked to the degeneration of brain cells and to their loss of connections with other brain cells. Some of the brain cells die. This process of brain cell degeneration and death begins in the regions of the brain responsible for memory and spreads to other areas that control language and thought. The process seems to be amplified by inflammation in the brain, which can be brought on by a combination of genetic and environmental factors.

Scientists have discovered genes that are linked to late-onset Alzheimer's disease. Three variations of one of these genes are called apoE-2, apoE-3, and apoE-4. People can inherit these genes in six different combinations (one gene from each parent): two apoE-2s, two apoE-3s, two apoE-4s, apoE-2 and apoE-3, apoE-3 and apoE-4, and apoE-2 and apoE-4. ApoE-4 confers the greatest risk of Alzheimer's; apoE-2 provides the most protection against the disease. Nearly two thirds of us inherit two copies of apoE-3, giving us an average chance of developing Alzheimer's disease. A person who inherits two copies of the apoE-4 gene is eight times more likely to develop Alzheimer's, while a person who inherits two apoE-2 genes has the lowest risk of all. As researchers learn more about how these genes are linked to Alzheimer's disease, they will be able to develop more effective ways to prevent, diagnose, and treat the disorder.

Symptoms

Doctors believe that the early stages of Alzheimer's disease probably begin decades before symptoms appear, as more and more plaques and tangles form in the brain. When symptoms become evident, they appear slowly. The first sign may be slight forgetfulness, especially of recent events. The person may have no trouble remembering what happened long ago, but may forget what happened 10 minutes ago and can't remember the date and current events. He or she may become disoriented, getting lost in familiar surroundings. Simple math problems become impossible to solve. Such mild symptoms are often mistaken for normal signs of aging.

Usually, personality does not change as a person gets older but, in the early stages of Alzheimer's disease, two key aspects of personality—conscientiousness and the ability to handle stress—may decline. People with the disease eventually display poor judgment and may become angry and belligerent, especially when someone tries to prevent them from doing something inappropriate or tries to help them.

In general, symptoms become more obviously abnormal as the disease progresses. People with Alzheimer's disease have difficulty expressing themselves and understanding what is said to them, and they have trouble reading and writing. They may have problems sleeping and may feel anxious, suspicious, and agitated. They frequently are restless and may pace. These behavior problems often get worse in the evening, a situation doctors call sundowning.

When mentally impaired people live alone, or when they are unsupervised, they are in danger of falling, setting fires, or having other accidents. Impaired hearing or vision can complicate the problem, preventing them from taking their medications as prescribed, crossing the street safely, or eating properly. Some people wander away from home frequently. You can minimize these risks by giving your loved one proper supervision and an identification bracelet to wear at all times or a card to carry, with your address and telephone number on it.

The late stages of Alzheimer's disease bring speech loss as well as the loss of bladder and bowel control. People with the disease lose weight as they lose their appetite or simply forget to eat. They may neglect their personal hygiene and need help using the toilet. They may forget how to perform simple tasks, such as combing their hair or using a can opener, and be unable to recognize family members. Eventually, people with Alzheimer's disease become totally dependent on their caregivers, who are usually family members—primarily spouses or daughters. Caregivers face an immense amount of pressure as they are forced to look after the person 24 hours a day. Many families are forced to make the difficult decision to place their loved one in a nursing care facility.

Diagnosis

No test is available to diagnose Alzheimer's disease in a living person. At present, the only way to make a definite diagnosis is by performing an autopsy to detect the characteristic plaques and tangles in the brain. A doctor can, however, diagnose probable Alzheimer's disease with about 85 percent accuracy using a number of diagnostic tools. He or she will get a detailed personal health history and a family health history, ask for a description of the person's

---

Other Causes of Dementia

Dementia is a term for a progressive loss of memory and other mental functions, such as language. Alzheimer's disease is the most common form of dementia. Vascular dementia, the second most common form of dementia, occurs when small blood clots obstruct tiny blood vessels in the brain, causing multiple strokes that damage brain tissue. The symptoms of vascular dementia can be identical to those of Alzheimer's disease.

Lewy body dementia results from the presence of abnormal structures (Lewy bodies) in multiple areas of the brain. Symptoms often start with hallucinations or impaired thinking and movement difficulties similar to those of Parkinson's disease (see page 691). Less common types of dementia can result from thyroid problems (see page 901), vitamin B deficiencies, hydrocephalus (enlargement of the fluid chambers in the brain), syphilis (see page 483), or AIDS (see page 909).

Creutzfeldt-Jakob disease and a variant of it, bovine spongiform encephalopathy (also called mad cow disease), are degenerative diseases of the brain caused by an infectious protein called a prion.

symptoms, and evaluate the person's emotional status and living environment. Because Alzheimer's disease may be mistaken for depression, a doctor will want to rule out depression. Testing the person's mathematical ability, language skills, and ability to complete tasks that require memory can also provide helpful information in diagnosing Alzheimer's disease. A thorough physical examination, laboratory tests, and a CT scan (see page 112) or MRI (see page 113) can help identify or rule out other possible causes of the dementia such as a stroke or tumor. If the problem turns out to result from another disorder, early diagnosis makes successful treatment more likely.

Treatment

Alzheimer's disease has no cure, but several drugs—including donepezil, rivastigmine, and galanthamine—are available for treatment. These drugs can help improve the early symptoms of Alzheimer's disease in some people, but they do not stop the disease from progressing. They work by slowing the breakdown of the neurotransmitter acetylcholine in the brain, one of the processes that lead to loss of memory and other mental functions. A newer drug called memantine is available for treating people with moderate to severe Alzheimer's disease. The drug slows down the decline of their thinking skills and ability to perform daily activities such as dressing and bathing. Memantine appears to work by regulating the activity of glutamate, a chemical messenger in the brain that plays an essential role in learning and memory. Some doctors also prescribe antianxiety medications to help relieve the sleeplessness and agitation common in people with the disorder.

Treatment focuses primarily on managing the symptoms and supporting the person's ability to function independently for as long as possible. If you are a caregiver, your doctor will help you learn how to provide the best possible care for your loved one. For example, keeping routines and surroundings familiar can be comforting and stabilizing for people with Alzheimer's disease, who have difficulty learning and organizing new information. Explaining each step in a daily task such as dressing can help the person perform the task more easily. Do as much as you can to simplify the tasks by, for example, laying out the person's clothes in the order in which he or she should put them on. Show

> ## Care for the Caregiver
>
> The job of caring for a person with Alzheimer's disease can be overwhelming and exhausting. If you are a caregiver, the stress you are experiencing may make you feel depressed, frustrated, angry, guilty, or isolated. But for you to be able to help your loved one, you need to protect your own health. The most significant step you can take to keep yourself healthy is to share your caregiving responsibilities. Don't be afraid to ask for help or to accept it when it is offered. Seek assistance from siblings and other family members, and take advantage of the time to yourself to get some needed rest and relaxation. Find resources such as home health aides, hired caregivers, or day care centers in your community. You may also be able to arrange for your loved one to be admitted to a nursing care facility for a brief period to allow you to take a break from your responsibilities. Use this time to go on a trip or find things that you enjoy doing.

the person what to do by performing each task so he or she can copy your actions. Use calendars, clocks, and lists to help the person maintain some sense of time and purpose.

Preventing Alzheimer's Disease

Researchers are studying some promising strategies for preventing Alzheimer's disease and improving the quality of life of people with the disease. For example, studies have found a link between Alzheimer's disease and mental stimulation, education levels, and other social and behavioral factors. People who continue to engage in intellectually challenging activities as they grow older seem to be less likely to develop symptoms of Alzheimer's disease than people who do not stay mentally active. Like a muscle, the brain needs stimulation to function at peak performance. Do crossword puzzles, take a class, read books, learn a foreign language—activities such as these may help you avoid or postpone symptoms of Alzheimer's disease.

Studies are under way to determine if herbal therapies such as ginkgo biloba (see page 90) can slow the development of dementia or reduce the rate of cognitive loss from aging. Some doctors prescribe vitamin E supplements (400 IUs daily) to their patients to possibly reduce the risk of Alzheimer's disease. Vitamin E is an antioxidant that can help neutralize the cell damage caused by molecules in the body called free radicals; this cell damage can cause inflammation in the brain, which has been linked to Alzheimer's disease.

Anti-inflammatory drugs such as ibuprofen also may provide some protection against Alzheimer's disease, based on the observation that people who take anti-inflammatory medications for chronic conditions such as arthritis or other immune disorders seem to have lower rates of Alzheimer's disease. Drugs called statins, which are used to lower cholesterol, may also have some benefit; cholesterol in the brain contributes to the formation of waxy buildups called amyloid plaques, which are linked to Alzheimer's disease.

Keep in mind that none of these therapies has yet been scientifically proven to be effective in preventing Alzheimer's disease, and many doctors are waiting for further evidence before recommending them to patients. Always talk to your doctor before you consider taking any kind of drug, including herbal or vitamin supplements.

Parkinson's Disease

Parkinson's disease is a gradual, progressive deterioration of the nerve centers in the brain that coordinate movement. Changes in these nerve centers upset the delicate balance between two chemicals in the brain, dopamine and acetylcholine, which are essential for controlling the transmission of impulses from the brain to the motor nerves in the spinal cord that control muscle movement. This chemical imbalance disrupts the nerve impulses, affecting muscle control and coordination.

In most cases, the cause of Parkinson's disease is unknown. The disease is thought to result from a combination of factors including environmental toxins, genetic predisposition, accelerated aging, and damage from free radicals (molecules in the body that can damage cells). In some cases, Parkinson's disease may result from a brain infection such as encephalitis (see page 694), strokes (see page 669), hydrocephalus (see page 400), a chemical imbalance in the body, or high doses of medications prescribed to treat a mental disorder such as schizophrenia (see page 728). In rare cases, Parkinson's disease may result from carbon monoxide poisoning or high levels of certain metals in body tissues. Parkinson's disease usually develops in late middle age or later and affects men and women in equal numbers.

Symptoms

Early symptoms of Parkinson's disease are subtle and appear gradually. The first symptom may be a slight rhythmic trembling (tremor) of the hands and feet that occurs at rest. Eventually, the arms, legs, and head may also tremble. Gradually, speech may become quiet, slow, and halting, and the person's handwriting may become very small. Movement is slow, and walking becomes increasingly difficult. Falls may become frequent because of impaired balance and coordination. The trembling is worse during times of stress. Other possible symptoms include drooling, abdominal cramps, a flat facial expression, and, later in the disease, problems with memory and thought processes. The person may have difficulty sleeping and may become depressed.

Diagnosis

A diagnosis of Parkinson's disease is usually based on the symptoms and the results of a complete neurological examination that includes tests to evaluate the functioning of the nervous system, such as vision, reflexes, hearing, sensation, movement, and balance and coordination. The doctor may order a CT scan (see page 112) or MRI (see page 113) to rule out conditions that can mimic Parkinson's disease.

Treatment

There is no cure for Parkinson's disease but, in most cases, medication can help relieve symptoms and slow the progression of the disease. Doctors frequently prescribe a combination of levodopa and carbidopa, which the brain uses to make dopamine. Because this treatment becomes less effective after several years, doctors often prescribe drugs that enhance the effects of dopamine (called dopamine agonists) in an attempt to extend the treatment period. Sometimes these drugs are given before the person starts taking levodopa and carbidopa. A doctor also may prescribe an anticholinergic medication (a drug that blocks the effects of acetylcholine) such as benztropine to reduce trembling.

If symptoms become severe and unresponsive to treatment, a doctor may recommend a surgical procedure in which wires are implanted in the brain to stimulate a specific area with a mild electric current to help control the tremors. Less frequently, a surgical procedure called pallidotomy or thalamotomy is done in which the small area of brain tissue that is causing the symptoms is destroyed. A stem cell transplant (see page 624) of cells that can mature to make dopamine is being tried in some people. The stem cells are taken from the person's adrenal glands or from human embryos.

Amyotrophic Lateral Sclerosis

Amyotrophic lateral sclerosis (ALS), also called Lou Gehrig's disease, is a progressive disease of the motor neurons (nerve cells that control muscle movement). In ALS, motor neurons gradually deteriorate, causing muscles to weaken and waste away, which eventually leads to paralysis. ALS usually occurs after age 40 and affects more men than women. Its cause is not known.

Symptoms
In ALS, the affected parts of the body become increasingly weak, with twitching and cramping in the muscles. The person has difficulty swallowing, breathing, and walking. The disease eventually affects all of the body's motor functions. In the final stages of ALS, a person is unable to speak or move, but his or her intellect and awareness are unchanged.

Diagnosis
Diagnosis of ALS is based on the symptoms and the results of diagnostic tests such as an electromyogram (an evaluation of the electrical activity of muscle tissue) and a muscle biopsy (a diagnostic test in which samples of muscle cells are examined under a microscope). An MRI (see page 113) and blood tests may be done to rule out other conditions that can cause similar symptoms.

Treatment
ALS cannot be prevented or cured. Treatment focuses on relieving the discomfort and helping the person remain as mobile and independent as possible for as long as possible. Doctors may prescribe a medication called riluzole to help slow the course of the disease. Specialized ALS treatment centers in many states offer comprehensive support services and treatment to help relieve symptoms; ask your doctor to recommend one. A person may eventually need a ventilator to assist with breathing, and feeding through a tube when he or she can no longer swallow. Most people with ALS die within 5 years of diagnosis.

Infections of the Brain and Nervous System

Infections of the brain and nervous system are less common than infections in other parts of the body because the brain and spinal cord have no direct contact with the environment. However, infections in the nervous system can cause severe symptoms and can be life-threatening. The bacteria, viruses, and other organisms that cause these infections gain entry to the brain and nervous system through the sinuses, the air spaces in the ears, the bloodstream, or fractures in the skull. Early treatment can prevent long-term damage to the nervous system and can be lifesaving.

Meningitis

Meningitis is inflammation of the meninges (the membranes that surround and protect the brain and spinal cord), usually caused by a viral or bacterial infection. The severity of meningitis depends on the infection-causing microorganism. The infection may have traveled to the brain from a localized infection (such as a sinus or ear infection), from the blood as part of a more widespread infection (such as a respiratory infection), or from outside the body through a fracture in the skull. Like many viral or bacterial infections, meningitis can occur in epidemics (usually in winter, when people are in close contact indoors).

The most common cause of meningitis is a virus that is spread when an infected person coughs or sneezes. Viral meningitis (also called aseptic meningitis) is usually relatively mild. Most of the time, a person with viral meningitis will recover in a few days or weeks. Symptoms of viral meningitis may be uncomfortable but usually do not cause permanent damage to the nervous system.

Untreated bacterial meningitis can be fatal or cause permanent brain or nerve damage, including blindness, deafness, or mental deterioration. Infants and young children, older people, or people who have an impaired immune system (such as those who have a chronic illness or who are taking drugs that suppress the immune system) have an increased risk of permanent nerve damage and death.

Vaccination for Meningitis

Widespread immunization of American children has markedly reduced the incidence of Haemophilus influenzae type b (Hib), which used to be the most common cause of bacterial meningitis in children. Because bacterial meningitis can be life-threatening, many doctors recommend that people who are at risk of developing the infection be vaccinated against it. People who are at increased risk include the very young or very old, people who live in close contact (such as in military housing or college dormitories), and people with an impaired immune system (such as those who have a chronic illness or who are taking drugs that suppress the immune system). Vaccines are also available for infections caused by Neisseria meningitidis (which causes meningococcal meningitis) and Streptococcus pneumoniae.

Symptoms

A severe headache, a stiff neck, abnormal sensitivity of the eyes to light (photophobia), nausea and vomiting, and fever usually develop within a few hours of exposure to the bacteria that cause bacterial meningitis. If bacterial meningitis is not treated promptly, you may become sleepy and lose consciousness. You may also develop a deep red or purple rash. Seizures may occur, especially in children, and the soft spot on the top of an infant's head may bulge and be tightly drawn because of swelling over the brain. In viral meningitis, symptoms are milder but still may include headache, a stiff neck, nausea, and photophobia.

The symptoms of meningitis can be less evident in infants and young children, older people, and people with an impaired immune system because they may have a less active immune response. In these cases, a change in responsiveness along with fever or headache may prompt the doctor to check for meningitis.

Diagnosis

If you have symptoms of meningitis (particularly a stiff neck, headache, and photophobia), your doctor may perform a procedure called lumbar puncture (see below) in which a sample of cerebrospinal fluid (the liquid that surrounds the brain and spinal cord) is taken from your spine. If the cerebrospinal fluid is cloudy and contains pus-filled cells, the meninges are likely to be infected with bacteria, and the doctor will prescribe antibiotics immediately. At the same time, he or she will send the fluid to a laboratory to identify the specific bacterium that is causing the infection and to determine which antibiotic is most effective against it.

If the fluid is clear, meningitis still may be present, but it is more likely caused by a virus. A doctor can sometimes determine what virus caused the infection by drawing blood samples immediately and again several weeks later (to see if your immune system has produced antibodies against it). In most cases of viral meningitis, the only treatment needed is pain relief and rest.

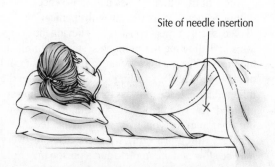

Site of needle insertion

Lumbar puncture

A lumbar puncture (formerly called a spinal tap) is a procedure used mostly to diagnose and treat disorders of the brain and spinal cord. For a diagnosis, a doctor inserts a hollow needle into the lower part of the spinal canal to withdraw a sample of cerebrospinal fluid (the liquid that surrounds the brain and spinal cord) for examination in a laboratory. For imaging examinations such as X-rays or CT scans, a lumbar puncture is used to inject a contrast medium (a dye that can be seen on the film) into the cerebrospinal fluid. The procedure can also be used to deliver medications such as anesthetics or anticancer drugs.

Antiviral medications are prescribed for some types of viruses.

Treatment

Treatment of bacterial meningitis is started immediately. If you have bacterial meningitis, you will probably be hospitalized for 1 to 2 weeks. Your doctor will prescribe a pain reliever and fever-reducing medication, along with large doses of antibiotics and fluids given intravenously (through a vein).

If you have viral meningitis, you will probably recover completely in a few weeks. Rest, drink plenty of water, and take an over-the-counter medication such as acetaminophen or ibuprofen to relieve pain and reduce fever. Antibiotics are not effective against viral meningitis.

Encephalitis

Encephalitis is inflammation of the brain, usually caused by a virus. The most common and severe cases of encephalitis are caused by the herpes simplex virus and are called herpes simplex encephalitis. In many cases, encephalitis results from a generalized viral infection such as mononucleosis (see page 935). West Nile virus (see page 944), which is carried by mosquitoes and can be transmitted to people by mosquito bites, can cause encephalitis. In people who have an impaired immune system (such as people who have AIDS; see page 909), encephalitis may result from viruses such as the cytomegalovirus (see page 508) or the varicella-zoster virus; these organisms generally do not cause illness in healthy people.

Encephalitis can sometimes result from an infection with a bacterium such as the one that causes Lyme disease (see page 942), or another type of microorganism (a protozoan) that causes toxoplasmosis (see page 508).

Life-threatening encephalitis is not common in healthy people; most people recover with no problems. The risk of serious illness or death depends on a person's age (the very young and the very old are more likely to have more severe cases of encephalitis), on his or her general health, and on the particular disease-causing organism. A small percentage of cases (usually those caused by the herpes simplex virus) result in permanent memory impairment or brain damage.

Symptoms

The symptoms of encephalitis can vary widely. In mild cases, symptoms may be limited to fever, headache, and fatigue. Encephalitis is usually accompanied by meningitis (see previous article), and a person may also have a stiff neck. In severe cases, especially if a person has herpes simplex encephalitis, brain function is affected more, causing confusion, odd behavior, irritability, or restlessness. A person may also have muscle weakness in the arms and legs, muscle spasms, loss of coordination and balance, speech or vision impairment, or seizures. The infection can sometimes lead to coma and death.

Diagnosis

If you have symptoms of encephalitis, your doctor will recommend that you have a CT scan (see page 112) or MRI (see page 113) of your brain, and an electroencephalogram (EEG; see page 687) to evaluate the electrical activity of your brain. A lumbar puncture (see previous page) is done to help identify the disease-causing organism. In rare cases, a biopsy of the brain is done to make a diagnosis. Blood tests may be repeated after several weeks to test for antibodies (infection-fighting proteins) to various microorganisms that can cause encephalitis.

Treatment

Life-threatening types of encephalitis (such as those caused by the herpes simplex virus) are treated with antiviral drugs such as acyclovir. In people who have a weakened immune system, an infection caused by the cytomegalovirus or the varicella-zoster virus may respond to treatment with antiviral drugs such as ganciclovir, foscarnet, or cidofovir. Encephalitis associated with toxoplasmosis can be treated effectively with a combination of sulfadiazine (a sulfa drug) and pyrimethamine (an antimalarial drug).

Most of the other viruses that cause encephalitis do not respond to treatment with medication. For these cases, treatment consists of relieving the symptoms and allowing the immune system to eliminate the virus. Your doctor may prescribe corticosteroid drugs to reduce the swelling in your brain from the inflammation. If the muscles that assist breathing are affected, you will be put on a ventilator. If swallowing is impaired, you may need to be fed intravenously (through a vein). In severe cases, recovery may be slow and incomplete and a person may need therapy to relearn basic skills such as speaking.

Polio

Polio (short for poliomyelitis) is a viral infection that affects muscle-controlling nerves in the brain and spinal cord. The virus, which is spread by contact with an infected person or by eating or drinking contaminated food or liquids, usually causes only a mild infection. Widespread, mandatory vaccination (see page 374) of children in developed countries (such as the United States) has almost eliminated the infection in those countries. A person who has had polio may, years later, experience muscle deterioration, pain, or weakness in previously affected muscles; this condition is called postpolio syndrome.

Polio Booster for Foreign Travel

If you or members of your family are going to travel to a country in which polio still occurs—such as many developing countries in Africa, the Middle East, and Asia—ask your doctor if you should have a polio booster before you leave.

Symptoms

The early symptoms of polio include headache, stomachache, sore throat, fever, and diarrhea. The symptoms may begin suddenly and last only a few days. In a small percentage of cases, polio invades the brain and develops into a severe infection, with pain and stiffness in the neck, back, and legs. In severe cases, muscles (including the muscles that control breathing) may become weak and cause paralysis or, sometimes, death.

Diagnosis

If you have recently traveled abroad or have not been vaccinated against polio and have symptoms of polio (such as fever and pain in your muscles, neck, and back), your doctor will take a sample of saliva from your throat or a stool sample to determine if the polio virus is the cause. He or she will also recommend a lumbar puncture (see page 693), in which a sample of cerebrospinal fluid (the liquid that surrounds the brain and spinal cord) is taken from the spinal canal and examined under a microscope to look for inflammation or the presence of infection-fighting white blood cells and proteins.

Treatment

There is no cure for polio. Most infections do not result in permanent damage. In people who are paralyzed from polio, physical therapy can help retain muscle function and limit further muscle damage. If breathing has been affected, a ventilator may be necessary to assist breathing. For people with postpolio syndrome, treatment may involve pain medication, physical therapy, and the use of a brace for parts of the body that are weakened, such as the legs.

Epidural Abscess

An epidural abscess (also called an extradural abscess) is a collection of pus in the space between the skull and the dura mater (the outermost of the three membranes that cover the brain and spinal cord). An epidural abscess is usually caused by a bacterial infection that has spread from a nearby infection such as an ear infection, sinusitis, or an infection in the bones of the skull or spine as the result of an injury or surgery. As the pus collects, it irritates surrounding tissues, causing pain. Inside the spinal cord, the pus can press on the cord and cause symptoms resembling those of a spinal cord tumor (see page 682). In rare cases, the bacteria produce toxins that can damage the dura mater.

Symptoms

The symptoms of an epidural abscess include headache, confusion, fever, chills, muscle weakness, or loss of sensation. Except for fever, symptoms may be similar to those of a stroke (see page 669), including difficulty speaking. In rare cases, an epidural abscess causes seizures.

WARNING!

Weakness or Numbness

If you experience muscle weakness or loss of sensation anywhere in your body, call your doctor immediately. If you can't reach your doctor, call 911 or your local emergency number. These symptoms require immediate medical attention to prevent permanent damage.

Diagnosis

To diagnose an epidural abscess, a doctor will recommend a CT scan (see page 112), an MRI (see page 113), and, in some cases, an X-ray examination of the spinal cord called myelography. He or she will also take blood samples to identify the bacterium that caused the abscess.

Treatment

Antibiotics are usually the initial treatment for an epidural abscess. If an abscess is putting pressure on the brain or spinal cord, surgery may be necessary to relieve the pressure and prevent permanent damage. For the surgical procedure, the doctor makes an opening in the skull or in the spine to remove the pus. After the surgery, treatment with antibiotics is continued to eliminate the bacteria.

Other Brain and Nervous System Disorders

Some disorders of the nervous system do not fit easily into a precise classification. Some neurological disorders, such as carpal tunnel syndrome, develop when nerves are injured. Others, such as Bell's palsy and Guillain-Barré syndrome, may be triggered by an infection. For many of these disorders, the cause is not known, and the symptoms can vary from person to person.

Bell's Palsy

Bell's palsy is a relatively common disorder of the facial nerves that results in weakness of the facial muscles. The facial nerves, located on each side of the face, pass through an opening in the skull just behind each ear. Bell's palsy occurs when a facial nerve swells and presses on the opening in the skull. Some doctors think that a virus such as the herpes simplex virus may be the cause. Bell's palsy is usually a temporary condition that comes on suddenly at any age, occurs on only one side of the face, and does not recur. The major risk is of dryness of and irritation or injury to the eye on the affected side because the eyelid muscles cannot close to protect it.

Symptoms

The recognizable symptom of Bell's palsy is muscle weakness on one side of the face from the forehead to the mouth. This weakness is characterized by a drooping mouth, an inability to close the eye, and distortion of facial expressions. In some cases, taste is impaired because the facial nerve that carries signals from some taste buds of the tongue is affected. Sounds may seem unnaturally loud because a nerve to the stapedius muscle of the ear (which normally dampens sound) is also affected. Sometimes a person has pain near the ear or on one side of the face and a middle ear infection or sore throat.

Diagnosis

A doctor can usually diagnose Bell's palsy by a physical examination and the person's health history. Sometimes it is necessary to rule out other possible causes of the muscle weakness, such as a stroke (see page 669).

Treatment

To treat Bell's palsy, your doctor may prescribe a corticosteroid medication such as prednisone to reduce inflammation and relieve pain. If your Bell's palsy is the result of a herpes simplex virus infection, your doctor may also prescribe the antiviral medication acyclovir. If your eye won't close, he or she will recommend wearing a protective eye patch and applying an eye ointment or eyedrops to protect and lubricate the exposed eye.

If the weakness in your face improves in 2 to 3 weeks, you will probably recover fully. However, if the first signs of returning muscle function do not begin within 2 months, recovery may take longer. In rare cases of permanent disfigurement, surgery may help improve a person's appearance.

Multiple Sclerosis

Multiple sclerosis (MS) is an autoimmune disease in which the body's immune system mistakenly attacks and destroys myelin. Myelin is an insulating material that covers nerve cells throughout the central nervous system and promotes rapid passage of electrical impulses along the nerve pathways. In MS, the myelin in random locations in the brain and spinal cord becomes inflamed, swollen, and damaged, which interferes with normal transmission of electrical impulses. In addition to myelin, nerve fibers and nerve cells also are damaged.

Multiple Sclerosis

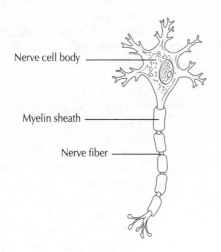

Nerve cell body

Myelin sheath

Nerve fiber

Healthy nerve cell

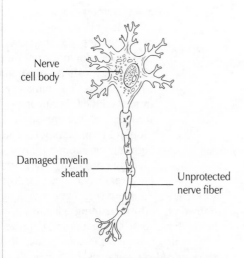

Nerve cell body

Damaged myelin sheath

Unprotected nerve fiber

Nerve cell damaged by multiple sclerosis

Multiple sclerosis
Myelin is an insulating material that covers nerve fibers throughout the nervous system and promotes rapid passage of electrical impulses along the nerve pathways. In multiple sclerosis, the myelin in random locations in the central nervous system becomes inflamed, swollen, and damaged, which interferes with the normal transmission of electrical impulses.

Although the cause of MS is unknown, researchers think it may result from a combination of genetic susceptibility and environmental factors such as a viral infection that occurs early in life. Some evidence suggests that people who spend the first 15 years of life in a temperate climate have an increased risk of developing MS compared with people who live in the tropics. MS can run in families. Whites are twice as likely as blacks to develop MS, and women are twice as likely as men to develop the disease. Most people who have MS live a normal life span.

Symptoms

The symptoms of MS usually appear between ages 15 and 50. Dizziness is an early symptom of the disease. Later symptoms include blurred vision, numbness and tingling, muscle weakness, fatigue, loss of balance and coordination, tremors (trembling), stiffness, and slurred speech. Initially, symptoms may come and go. In the later stages of the disease, symptoms may worsen. As the disease progresses, a person may develop muscle spasms, urinary tract infections, constipation, loss of bowel and bladder control, sexual dysfunction, depression, or mood swings. Many people experience problems with concentration, memory, and judgment, although their language skills do not change. Symptoms may worsen when the person's body temperature rises—such as after exercise or a hot bath, during a fever, or when the environmental temperature is high. Repeated episodes of MS can cause progressive nerve damage that significantly limits activity and movement. This nerve damage can make recovery after later episodes more difficult and may lead to permanent disability.

Diagnosis

If you have symptoms of MS, your doctor will recommend that you see a neurologist (a doctor who specializes in treating disorders of the nervous system). A diagnosis of MS is usually based on a person's neurological history; a neurological examination that includes tests to evaluate the functioning of the nervous system, such as vision, reflexes, hearing, sensation, movement, and balance and coordination; and an MRI (see page 113), which may show damage to the nerve pathways and changes in brain tissue characteristic of MS.

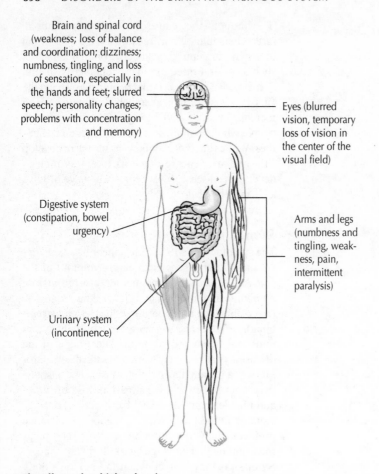

Brain and spinal cord (weakness; loss of balance and coordination; dizziness; numbness, tingling, and loss of sensation, especially in the hands and feet; slurred speech; personality changes; problems with concentration and memory)

Eyes (blurred vision, temporary loss of vision in the center of the visual field)

Digestive system (constipation, bowel urgency)

Arms and legs (numbness and tingling, weakness, pain, intermittent paralysis)

Urinary system (incontinence)

The effects of multiple sclerosis
Because the brain and spinal cord control all parts of the body, damage to the central nervous system from multiple sclerosis can affect many different organs and functions.

The neurologist will order blood tests to help rule out other possible causes of the symptoms, such as vitamin deficiencies, chronic infections, or other inflammatory diseases, such as lupus (see page 920). A neurologist may perform an evoked response test in which electrodes are placed on the person's head and the electrical activity of the brain is recorded while the person is exposed to various sensory stimuli such as sound or light. Another possible diagnostic test is a lumbar puncture (see page 693), in which a hollow needle is inserted into the spine and a sample of cerebrospinal fluid (the liquid that surrounds the brain and spinal cord) is withdrawn and examined under a microscope to look for inflammatory proteins.

Treatment

Although MS has no cure, medications such as interferon beta, glatiramer, and mitoxantrone can reduce the frequency of episodes with symptoms and slow progression of the disease. It is not yet known how effective these treatments will be in preventing progressive impairment over the long term. They seem to be most effective when used early in the course of the disease.

During acute episodes of MS or when a person has difficulty walking or talking, doctors often prescribe corticosteroid drugs to reduce inflammation in the nervous system. Medications are also available that can relieve long-term problems such as muscle spasms and stiffness, help restore bladder control, and alleviate pain, fatigue, depression, and, in some cases, tremors.

To help people whose attacks do not respond to treatment with corticosteroids, doctors sometimes use a procedure called plasmapheresis, which removes inflammatory proteins from the blood. For people who have frequent, severe episodes, immunoglobulin (a preparation of infection-fighting antibodies) is sometimes given intravenously. These treatments, however, may not be effective.

Exercising regularly, eating a nutritious diet, and maintaining a healthy weight can help relieve some symptoms and improve the person's ability to cope with impairments. Doctors also recommend staying cool (such as with air-conditioning in the summer) to help prevent fatigue. Physical therapy can help strengthen muscles and maintain range of motion in joints. Occupational therapy can help the person learn easier, more efficient ways to perform everyday tasks. Equipment such as braces, walkers, canes, and wheelchairs can help some people stay active. Support groups such as those sponsored by local chapters of the National Multiple Sclerosis Society are excellent sources of information, help, and encouragement.

Carpal Tunnel Syndrome

Carpal tunnel syndrome is a disorder caused by compression of the median nerve as it passes through a narrow channel (called the carpal tunnel) in the wrist formed by the wrist bones and a strong ligament (a tough, elastic tissue that holds bones together). Tendons (strong fibrous bands that join muscle to bone) also pass through the channel. The compression usually results from repetitive manual activities that put excessive stress on the surrounding tissues, causing the ligament to thicken and the tendons to swell. The median nerve carries sensations from the thumb, index finger, middle finger, part of the ring finger, and the palm of the hand to the spinal cord. The median nerve also controls the muscles of the hand and forearm that enable the wrist, fingers, and thumb to move and the forearm to rotate.

Carpal tunnel syndrome is fairly common and occurs frequently in pregnant and menopausal women (probably because of fluid retention or hormonal changes) and in people with medical conditions such as acromegaly (a disorder that makes the bones abnormally long and the hands and feet unusually large). People who have diabetes (see page 889) or hypothyroidism (see page 903) or who are obese also seem to be susceptible because of swelling or a buildup of fluid in the carpal ligament, or from thickening of connective tissue. Carpal tunnel syndrome may also result from an inflammatory condition such as rheumatoid arthritis (see page 918) or from an injury such as a bone dislocation or fracture.

Activities that involve repetitive or strenuous use of the hands and wrists—such as working on a keyboard or an assembly line, doing dental work, or knitting or sewing—most often cause carpal tunnel syndrome. People who use jackhammers, chainsaws, or other machines that repeatedly jar the nerves also are at increased risk of carpal tunnel syndrome.

Ulnar tunnel syndrome is similar to carpal tunnel syndrome, but it affects the ulnar nerve, which carries sensations to the ring and little fingers, to the outer part of the palm, and to the elbow. Ulnar tunnel syndrome can occur on its own or along with carpal tunnel syndrome. Ulnar tunnel syndrome is usually caused by damage to the elbow or, occasionally, damage to nerves in the armpit from using crutches.

Symptoms

The symptoms of carpal tunnel syndrome usually appear gradually over weeks or months and include tingling, a burning sensation, and intermittent numbness in part of one or both hands, often accompanied by pain in the fingers that shoots up the forearm from the wrist. The pain is generally worse at night. In severe cases, a person with carpal tunnel syndrome may develop permanent numbness and a weak grip. In ulnar tunnel syndrome, the tingling, burning, and numbness occur along the ulnar nerve.

Diagnosis

To diagnose carpal tunnel syndrome, your doctor will ask you questions about any activities that could be causing the disorder and will perform a thorough physical examination to rule out other medical conditions. He or she may ask you to do some simple maneuvers with your hand and wrist to see if the movements cause symptoms. Although

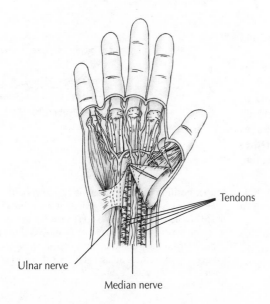

Tendons

Ulnar nerve

Median nerve

Carpal tunnel syndrome
Carpal tunnel syndrome is pain, numbness, or tingling in the thumb, first two fingers, part of the ring finger, and the palm caused by excessive, prolonged pressure on the median nerve as it passes through a narrow passage in the wrist called the carpal tunnel.

X-rays are not useful in diagnosing carpal tunnel syndrome, your doctor may order X-rays to rule out other disorders, such as arthritis or fractured bones. You are likely to have diagnostic tests such as a nerve conduction velocity test (to measure how fast your nerves transmit impulses) and electromyography (to evaluate your muscle activity).

> ## Repetitive Stress Injuries
>
> Chronic upper limb pain syndrome, cumulative trauma disorder, overuse syndrome, repetitive motion disorder, repetitive strain syndrome, and repetitive stress disorder are general terms for injuries to part of the hand or arm caused by repetitive movements of the wrist or hand. These disorders can affect nerves, muscles, tendons, or connective tissue. Carpal tunnel syndrome, ulnar tunnel syndrome, tendinitis (see page 984), and bursitis (see page 1002) are a few examples of repetitive stress injuries.

Treatment

The basic treatment for carpal tunnel syndrome and ulnar tunnel syndrome is to relieve the compression of the affected nerve. Varying your activities and adjusting your workstation may be enough to relieve your symptoms. Rest and limit flexing of your wrist by using a wrist splint or brace (which allows the swollen tissues to shrink and relieves pressure on the median nerve). Use over-the-counter pain relievers such as aspirin or ibuprofen. If they don't ease symptoms, your doctor may inject a corticosteroid or other anti-inflammatory medication into your wrist to reduce inflammation and ease pain. If you still have weakness or pain, a surgeon can relieve pressure on the median nerve by opening the space for the median nerve in a minor surgical procedure.

Preventing Carpal Tunnel Syndrome

Although it is not always possible to prevent a stress injury such as carpal tunnel syndrome, the following steps can help reduce your risk:

- Lose weight if you're overweight (excess fat in the wrist can compress the nerve).

- Get treatment for any disorder, such as arthritis, that may be contributing to your carpal tunnel syndrome.
- Switch hands frequently during tasks.
- Don't rest your wrist on hard surfaces for long periods.
- Adjust your work position to reduce flexing of the wrists.
- Avoid bending, twisting, or extending your hands for long periods; take frequent breaks from repeated hand movements to give your hands and wrists some rest.
- Avoid working with your arms too close to or too far from your body.
- Don't use tools that are too large for your hands.

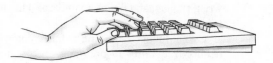

Incorrect position of wrist

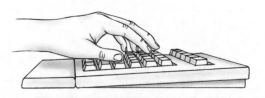

Correct position of wrist

Proper position of wrists when using a keyboard
If you use a keyboard for long periods, position your keyboard at a height at which you don't have to bend your wrists up or down while you type. Your elbows should bend at a 90-degree angle and your forearms should be parallel to the floor. To make these adjustments, try either raising your chair or lowering your keyboard.

Trigeminal Neuralgia

Trigeminal neuralgia, also called tic douloureux, is severe facial pain resulting from a damaged trigeminal nerve, one of the major nerves in the face. The cause of trigeminal neuralgia is unknown. The disorder usually occurs in older people, when a twisted

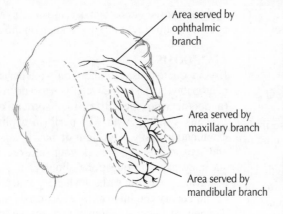

Area served by
ophthalmic
branch

Area served by
maxillary branch

Area served by
mandibular branch

Trigeminal nerve
The trigeminal nerve, which supplies sensation to the scalp,
face, eyes, nose, mouth, teeth, sinuses, tongue, and jaw
muscles, divides into three main branches—the ophthalmic
branch, the maxillary branch, and the mandibular branch.
Damage or disease in one branch of the trigeminal nerve can
cause pain and inflammation in the area of the face or head
served by that nerve branch.

artery presses on the trigeminal nerve. It sometimes
occurs in younger people who have multiple sclerosis (see page 696). Trigeminal neuralgia can be
temporary or chronic.

Symptoms
Trigeminal neuralgia produces severe, shooting
pain on one side of the face, usually in the cheeks,
lips, gums, or chin. The pain can be disabling and
can last from a few seconds to a few minutes. The
pain can occur without warning or, in some people,
can be triggered by touching a sensitive area of the
face. In some cases, the pain recurs every few minutes over a period of several days or weeks.

Diagnosis
Trigeminal neuralgia is diagnosed by the symptoms
and a neurological examination. Your doctor may
refer you to a neurologist (a doctor who specializes
in treating disorders of the nervous system) for
diagnostic tests and treatment.

Treatment
Doctors prescribe pain relievers to treat trigeminal
neuralgia, usually along with anticonvulsant medications or antidepressants, to prevent irritated

nerves from firing pain messages to the brain. In
severe cases, doctors may recommend surgery to
remove a blood vessel that is pressing on the nerve.
Occasionally, doctors will destroy the damaged
nerve. Because destruction of the nerve results in
permanent numbness in the face, doctors usually
recommend this type of surgery only in cases of
extreme, recurring pain.

Myasthenia Gravis

Myasthenia gravis is a rare, chronic autoimmune
disease in which the body's immune system mistakenly produces antibodies that interfere with the
transmission of nerve impulses to muscle tissues,
preventing muscle contraction. The thymus gland,
which is part of the immune system, has a significant role in this faulty immune response that doctors do not fully understand. Although myasthenia
gravis can occur at any age, it usually affects
women under 40, but can also occur later in life,
when it is more likely to be associated with a tumor.

Symptoms
The main symptom of myasthenia gravis is muscle
weakness. Weakness in the eye muscles can cause
drooping eyelids and blurred vision. Because the
muscles that control the mouth are also affected,
some people may have difficulty speaking, chewing,
or swallowing. Weakened muscles in the arms,
hands, and fingers may make it difficult to perform
simple manual tasks. Weakened leg muscles may
make standing or walking difficult. Breathing problems can result from weakened respiratory muscles.
The weakness increases with physical exertion and
decreases with rest. The degree of weakness can vary
throughout the day and from one day to the next.

Diagnosis
To diagnose myasthenia gravis, a doctor takes a
detailed health history and performs a physical
examination. He or she pays special attention to
signs of problems with eye movement and muscle
weakness. The doctor also may order a blood test to
check the blood for antibodies (infection-fighting
proteins), nerve conduction tests to determine if
another condition is causing the symptoms, and an
electromyogram to evaluate the electrical activity of
muscles. A CT scan (see page 112) or an MRI (see
page 113) may be used to look for a growth in the

thymus gland. A lung function test (see page 647) can evaluate the severity of breathing problems resulting from muscle weakness.

Treatment

Myasthenia gravis has no cure, but treatment can relieve the symptoms and enable a person to lead an active, productive life. A doctor may prescribe a long-acting medication such as pyridostigmine to restore transmission of nerve impulses to the affected muscles and increase muscle strength. He or she also may prescribe corticosteroids or immune-suppressing drugs to reduce inflammation and inhibit the errant immune response. Infusions of human immune globulin also can help counteract the body's faulty immune response. A treatment called plasmapheresis, which filters antibodies from the blood, helps some people recover from acute episodes. Doctors often recommend surgery to remove the thymus, which can eliminate the symptoms of myasthenia gravis.

Peripheral Neuropathy

Peripheral neuropathy is damage to the peripheral nerves (the nerves that spread out from the brain and spinal cord). Peripheral neuropathy sometimes occurs as a result of nerve inflammation or as a complication of disorders or conditions such as diabetes, alcoholism, deficiencies of vitamins B or E, AIDS, cancer, kidney disease, or vasculitis (inflammation of blood vessels). Some neuropathies occur as inherited conditions that run in families. Peripheral neuropathy can also be caused by overexposure to some medications (such as the drugs used in chemotherapy; see page 23) and by exposure to toxic chemicals such as insecticides or metals such as lead, arsenic, or mercury.

Symptoms

The symptoms of peripheral neuropathy usually develop gradually over many months and include tingling, numbness, and pain in the feet and later in the hands. The symptoms sometimes spread slowly along the arms and legs to the trunk. In some cases the muscles of the feet, hands, and legs gradually weaken and may atrophy (waste away). When autonomic nerves are affected, impairments in sweating or in bladder, stomach, or bowel function may occur.

Early diagnosis is important because the nerve damage may not be reversible, depending on the cause.

Diagnosis

If your doctor suspects that you have peripheral neuropathy, he or she may refer you to a neurologist (a doctor who specializes in disorders of the nervous system), who will perform a physical examination, test you for signs of muscle weakness and sensory loss, and check your reflexes. He or she may ask you questions about your general health and your family's health history to determine if a hereditary condition may have caused the nerve damage. The neurologist may perform the following tests: blood tests to check vitamin levels and look for evidence of diabetes, thyroid disease, or inflammatory conditions; a nerve conduction velocity test to measure how fast your nerves transmit impulses; and electromyography to evaluate your nerve and muscle activity. The neurologist also may take a biopsy (sample of tissue) from a small nerve in the ankle called the sural nerve to look for the cause of the neuropathy.

Treatment

The treatment of peripheral neuropathy depends on the cause. For example, a doctor will prescribe vitamins to treat a vitamin deficiency, and corticosteroids or drugs that suppress the immune system to treat an inflammatory disorder such as vasculitis. A person with diabetes will be given medication to lower blood sugar, and a person with abnormal thyroid function will be given medication to correct it. In severe cases of irreversible neuropathy, treatment includes physical therapy, the use of assistive equipment (such as canes, walkers, bath rails, and grab bars), and prevention of sores and infections that could result from injuries caused by the person's inability to feel pain.

Guillain-Barré Syndrome

Guillain-Barré syndrome, also called acute inflammatory polyneuropathy or idiopathic polyneuritis, is a potentially severe form of peripheral neuropathy (see previous article) resulting from a faulty immune response that can follow a viral infection such as the flu, a cold, mononucleosis (see page

935), or diarrhea. The condition affects the peripheral nerves (the nerves that spread out from the brain and spinal cord). Infection-fighting antibodies and white blood cells of the immune system confuse the nerves with the virus (because the nerves and the virus have a similar molecular structure) and mistakenly attack the nerves. The nerve damage and muscle weakness caused by Guillain-Barré syndrome usually are temporary—most people recover from even severe cases. Recovery time ranges from a few weeks to a year or more.

Symptoms

Symptoms of Guillain-Barré syndrome usually develop within about 3 to 4 weeks after a viral infection but can develop within a few hours. Symptoms include recurring tingling and numbness and then weakness and paralysis that usually begin in the feet and spread to the legs and later to the trunk and arms. Guillain-Barré syndrome may progress to complete muscle paralysis, affecting the muscles that assist in breathing and swallowing.

Diagnosis

Guillain-Barré syndrome can be difficult to diagnose when the symptoms first begin. Because nerve responses are slow in Guillain-Barré syndrome, a doctor may perform a nerve conduction velocity test, which measures how fast the nerves send messages to the brain. An electromyogram can help determine the severity of the nerve damage. Because the cerebrospinal fluid (the liquid that surrounds the brain and spinal cord) of a person with Guillain-Barré syndrome contains more protein than usual, a doctor may take a sample of the fluid from the person's spine using a procedure called lumbar puncture (see page 693) to test it for excess protein.

Treatment

Treatment of Guillain-Barré syndrome depends on the symptoms and on how far the disorder has progressed. If the muscles that assist breathing are affected, you will be put on a ventilator; if your ability to swallow is impaired, you may need to be fed intravenously (through a vein) until the symptoms subside. If the nerves that control blood pressure and heart rhythm are affected, you will need a pacemaker (see page 584) to regulate your heartbeat. Plasmapheresis (a procedure that removes antibodies from the blood) or immunoglobulin therapy (treatment in which a doctor injects high doses of immune proteins into a vein) removes or blocks the action of the antibodies that are causing the abnormal immune response, reducing the severity and duration of symptoms.

Sleep Disorders

Sleep is as important to good health as a nutritious diet and regular exercise. When you fail to get enough sleep, your body releases higher than normal levels of the stress hormone cortisol, which can have a harmful effect on body tissues, making you more prone to infections and other diseases. Sleep deprivation or fragmented sleep can also interfere with your daily activities by causing daytime sleepiness, poor concentration, performance and memory problems, delayed responses, and difficulty controlling your emotions. Most people occasionally have trouble falling asleep, and many people routinely fail to get enough sleep because of work and family demands or shift work.

Some medical conditions, such as asthma (see page 640) or heart failure (see page 570) and disorders such as arthritis (see page 996) that cause chronic or occasional pain, can interrupt sleep. Other sleep-disrupting medical problems include heartburn or gastroesophageal reflux disease (GERD; see page 750), osteoporosis (see page 989), Alzheimer's disease (see page 688), and chronic lung diseases such as emphysema (see page 656) or chronic bronchitis (see page 655). A number of medications, including those used to treat high blood pressure, heart disease, or asthma, can also adversely affect sleep. Alcohol, caffeine, and nicotine can all make it harder to fall asleep and stay asleep. The time changes produced by air travel, especially when traveling west to east, also can interfere with the body's natural sleep cycle, causing jet lag (see page 705).

Although adults need an average of 8 hours of sleep every day, the amount you require to stay alert during the day may be more or less because the quantity of sleep needed varies from person to person. Additionally, as you age, you may not be able to sleep as long as you once did, although the amount of sleep you need remains the same. Some people have difficulty sleeping because of a medically recognized sleep disorder such as insomnia, restless legs syndrome, or narcolepsy.

Insomnia

People who have insomnia get insufficient sleep or experience poor-quality sleep because they have difficulty falling asleep, wake up often and cannot fall back asleep, or wake up too early in the morning. Insomnia can cause serious problems—including drowsiness, diminished energy, poor concentration, irritability, and a greater risk of accidents—during the day. Work performance and personal relationships often suffer.

Q & A

Sleep

Q. *I read somewhere that many famous people, such as Thomas Edison, got by on very little sleep. There is so much to do and so little time. How can I make a few hours of sleep work for me?*

A. You can't. Cutting down on your sleep will make you less productive, not more. Sleep is necessary to refresh your tired brain, organize the day's experiences, and stimulate hormones that build and repair body tissues. It has been said that Edison slept 6 hours a night, but the untold part of the story is that he was able to fall asleep quickly and took naps frequently throughout the day, possibly up to two 2-hour naps a day—a total of 10 hours a day.

Q. *I'm a 20-year-old college student and I frequently pull all-nighters to study for early-morning tests. My roommate told me that I'm not doing myself any good and, I have to admit, my grades don't reflect the amount of time I spend studying. What am I doing wrong?*

A. Staying awake longer than normal can impair your memory. Essentially, learning is about forming permanent memories. People remember more of what they have learned if they have sufficient sleep right after studying. A few hours won't do. In the last few hours of dream sleep, the brain concentrates on strengthening and reinforcing the connections between nerve cells that make up a new memory. A good night's sleep helps the brain organize and retrieve information.

A number of factors can cause insomnia. Many people experience short-term or intermittent insomnia when they are under increased stress, have jet lag (see next page), or sleep in a noisy environment. The side effects of some medications also can cause insomnia. Certain conditions, such as depression (see page 709) or anxiety (see page 718), seem to make people more susceptible to insomnia. Although the disorder affects people of all age groups, it occurs more often in women (especially after menopause) and older people.

The causes of chronic insomnia are often complicated, involving a number of underlying physical or psychological disorders. Depression is one of the most frequent causes of long-term insomnia. Other disorders, such as arthritis (see page 996), kidney disease, heart failure (see page 570), asthma (see page 640), multiple sclerosis (see page 696), Parkinson's disease (see page 691), and hyperthyroidism (see page 901), also are common causes of insomnia. Other sleep disorders, such as sleep apnea (see page 636) and restless legs syndrome (see next page), can also cause insomnia.

Your risk of having insomnia increases if you smoke (because nicotine is a stimulant that disrupts sleep) or if you consume too much alcohol or caffeine, or use other stimulants before bedtime. Shift work or other activities that promote irregular sleep patterns also can affect your ability to fall asleep and stay asleep. Excessive worrying (including worrying about not being able to sleep) can contribute to insomnia. Making lifestyle changes is often enough to improve your sleep.

Symptoms

The difficulty sleeping that is characteristic of insomnia falls into three main classes—short-term, intermittent, and chronic. Short-term or transient insomnia usually lasts only a few weeks or less. Short-term insomnia that occurs from time to time is said to be intermittent. Chronic or long-term insomnia happens on most nights and persists for a month or longer.

Diagnosis

If you have insomnia, your doctor will take a detailed health history (see page 130), including a sleep history. You may be asked to keep a sleep diary to find out how much sound sleep you get each night. The doctor may also ask your sleep partner about the quality of your sleep and how long you sleep each night.

Treatment

Short-term and intermittent insomnia may need no medical treatment if the doctor thinks the insomnia can be taken care of with lifestyle adjustments, such as reducing caffeine or alcohol consumption. If the problem persists or causes excessive daytime sleepiness and impaired performance, a doctor may prescribe a short-acting sleep medication for a brief period of time. Doctors usually do not recommend using over-the-counter medications to treat insomnia. Some doctors are prescribing the hormone melatonin (which resets the body's sleep cycle) for some people who have insomnia; ask your doctor about it.

To treat chronic insomnia, your doctor will diagnose and treat any medical or psychological problems that may be contributing to the disorder. He or she also will try to identify any behaviors, such as excessive napping, that could be making your insomnia worse and suggest ways to reduce or stop them. Your doctor may prescribe a sleep medication, but may instruct you to take it for only a short time to minimize side effects and to reduce the possibility of your becoming dependent on it. The dosage of some of these sleep medications must be gradually reduced as they are discontinued. To avoid problems, make sure you work with your doctor to gradually stop any sleep medication you are taking.

Many doctors recommend treating insomnia with simple behavioral techniques, such as relaxation therapy, which reduces anxiety and tension and helps you sleep more restfully. Sleep restriction is another behavioral technique that benefits some people by allowing only a few hours of sleep each night at first and then gradually increasing sleep time to a more normal span. A third behavioral treatment is called reconditioning, in which a person learns to associate the bed and bedtime only with sleep by not using the bed for any activity other than sleeping or sex.

Jet Lag

Jet lag is characterized by fatigue, sleep disturbances, irritability, and dehydration that occur after long plane flights. Lengthy plane trips disrupt the natural rhythms of the body by exposing them to abrupt time changes. Jet lag is more likely to occur if you are traveling east through several time zones (for example, from the United States to Europe or from Hawaii to the US mainland) because your body finds it harder to adjust to a shorter day than to a longer one.

The following simple measures can help lower your chances of having jet lag:

- Drink a lot of water during the flight; carry a bottle of water with you, and don't be reluctant to ask flight attendants for water.
- Avoid caffeine because it can keep you awake and cause dehydration.
- Avoid alcohol because it can cause dehydration.
- Try to get a good night's sleep before your flight.
- Begin to think in terms of your destination's time zone and plan your meals and sleep accordingly.

No special diets have been proven effective in reducing the effects of jet lag. Some people take the hormone melatonin to induce sleep either on the plane or before going to bed at night when they reach their destination. Melatonin resets the body's sleep cycle. You can buy melatonin as an over-the-counter supplement. Ask your doctor if he or she recommends taking melatonin to avoid or treat jet lag.

Restless Legs Syndrome

Restless legs syndrome is a neurologic disorder characterized by unpleasant sensations in the legs and, less often, in the arms. Restless legs syndrome is sometimes categorized as a sleep disorder because the symptoms can disrupt normal sleep, making a person feel tired or fatigued during the day. The cause of restless legs syndrome is unknown, although doctors think it may be hereditary. Restless legs syndrome affects people of all ages but is more common and more severe in older people. Younger people with restless legs syndrome are sometimes misdiagnosed with attention deficit hyperactivity disorder (ADHD; see page 730) or incorrectly said to be experiencing "growing pains."

Symptoms

The sensations associated with restless legs syndrome are most often described as creeping, crawling, pulling, tingling, or painful. The symptoms worsen during periods of rest or inactivity, or during the evening or at night. A person with restless legs syndrome may have periodic involuntary jerking in his or her legs or arms while asleep. Involuntary movements of the toes, feet, or legs can make a person with restless legs syndrome appear fidgety.

Diagnosis

There are no tests for diagnosing restless legs syndrome. A diagnosis is usually made from the symptoms and from the information a person gives the doctor. Sometimes an underlying condition such as iron deficiency anemia, diabetes, rheumatoid arthritis, or hormonal changes during pregnancy or menopause produce symptoms of restless legs syndrome. In these cases, the symptoms usually subside once the condition is treated (or after childbirth). Some medications—such as calcium channel blockers (used for treating high blood pressure and heart disease), antinausea drugs, some cold and allergy medications, some tranquilizers (including haloperidol and phenothiazines), the antiseizure medication phenytoin, and antidepressant medications—can worsen the symptoms of restless legs syndrome.

Treatment

Doctors frequently recommend medication for treating restless legs syndrome. The drugs most often prescribed include benzodiazepines (which induce sleep by depressing the central nervous system) or dopaminergic agents (usually used to reduce tremors in people with Parkinson's disease). The effectiveness of a medication depends on the severity of the symptoms.

People who have a less severe form of restless legs syndrome may find relief from the symptoms by walking, stretching, taking hot or cold baths, or practicing relaxation techniques or yoga. Lifestyle changes such as limiting consumption of caffeine and alcohol and eating a healthy, balanced diet also may help lessen the symptoms.

Narcolepsy

Narcolepsy is a chronic sleep disorder in which a person is overcome by such overwhelming sleepiness that he or she falls asleep at inappropriate times (for example, while eating dinner or having a conversation) during the day. These daytime "sleep attacks" are uncontrollable and often occur without warning. The sleep attacks appear to occur when the messages about sleep and waking sent by the brain to other parts of the body deviate from their normal course or arrive at the wrong time. This process causes a disturbance in the normal order and length of sleep stages, so that rapid eye movement (REM) sleep, when dreaming occurs, happens at sleep onset or even during the day. The person usually remains conscious.

Strong emotions such as anger, fear, or laughter, or strenuous physical activity often trigger these episodes. Some attacks can be accompanied by loss of muscle function and total body collapse, a condition called cataplexy.

Narcolepsy often interferes with a person's job and personal life and restricts his or her activities. Roughly 1 in 2,000 people has narcolepsy, which can occur in people of all ages, although symptoms usually begin between ages 15 and 30. Narcolepsy seems to run in families, but it is often misdiagnosed as depression (see page 709), epilepsy (see page 686), or the side effects of medication. The length of time between the appearance of symptoms and a diagnosis of narcolepsy can be up to 15 years.

Symptoms

Overwhelming daytime sleepiness at inappropriate times is usually the first symptom of narcolepsy. People with narcolepsy also may experience sleep paralysis, in which their body becomes temporarily immobile during the time they fall asleep or wake up. A person may have intense, often frightening hallucinations (abnormal perceptions not based on reality) when he or she dozes off or falls asleep. Affected people sometimes display automatic behavior, in which they perform routine tasks repeatedly without full awareness that they are doing so.

Diagnosis

After performing a thorough physical examination and taking a detailed health history, your doctor will probably order two tests to diagnose narcolepsy. The first, called polysomnography, measures brain waves, heart rate, blood oxygen levels, and muscle movements during sleep. The second, the multiple sleep latency test, measures how fast you fall asleep when given a chance to nap every few hours. Both tests can be performed in a sleep laboratory or at home.

Treatment

To treat narcolepsy, your doctor will tailor a treatment plan to your individual needs, depending on the severity of your symptoms. Medications called central nervous system stimulants are the recommended treatment for narcolepsy. These drugs promote wakefulness during the day to reduce the effects of excessive daytime sleepiness.

Antidepressant drugs (see page 712) that suppress REM sleep may also be prescribed to control cataplexy. The doctor may recommend taking 10- to 15-minute naps two or three times a day to help relieve daytime sleepiness. It may take several weeks or months of adjustment before your treatment plan is effective; even then, complete control of your symptoms may not be possible. Joining a support group may help you and your family learn to cope with the emotional effects of narcolepsy and learn ways to avoid situations in which you could be injured if you fell asleep unexpectedly.

5

Behavioral, Emotional, and Mental Disorders

A mental disorder is a condition that adversely affects a person's thoughts, feelings, and behavior. Because they often produce anxiety, mood changes, and disturbances in perception, mental disorders have traditionally been seen as different from physical disorders. However, we now know that, like any other illnesses including heart disease and cancer, mental disorders result from an interaction of biology (such as a chemical imbalance or structural abnormality in the brain), genes, and environment. Mental disorders not only cause psychological symptoms but also can cause a variety of uncomfortable and frightening physical symptoms, including heart palpitations, nausea, and dizziness.

Stressful life events—both positive and negative—can trigger some mental disorders. Others seem to arise spontaneously with no obvious cause. The effects they produce are no less real than the effects of a heart attack or cancer.

Mood Disorders

Mood disorders are mental disorders that affect a person's emotional state. Occasionally feeling sad, dejected, or elated is a normal part of the human experience. But people with a mood disorder feel these emotions more strongly, and the feelings can persist for months or years. Roughly one in seven people experiences some kind of mood disorder each year. Factors that have been implicated in their development include an inherited susceptibility, an imbalance in brain chemicals that regulate mood, a structural abnormality in a part of the brain that controls emotions, and environmental influences. Often, a combination of these factors comes into play. The most common mood disorders are depression, bipolar disorder (formerly known as manic depression), and seasonal affective disorder (SAD). Mood disorders are among the most treatable of all mental disorders.

Depression

Depression is a disorder of mood regulation, caused by an imbalance of brain chemicals called neurotransmitters, which enable brain cells to communicate with each other. People with depression endure overwhelming feelings of despair and hopelessness that last for long periods. It is normal to feel unhappy when you lose your job or when a loved one dies, but such feelings usually subside with the passage of time. Depression can impair your functioning at home and at work and cause you to withdraw from family and friends.

Women are twice as likely as men to have

Psychiatric Terms

Many terms used in this section have clearly defined meanings for medical professionals, but may seem vague to most of us. You may find the following definitions helpful:

Psychiatrist A physician who has completed medical school and residency training and specializes in diagnosing and treating mental problems (with medical and physical causes) and behavioral disorders. Psychiatrists employ treatments such as medication and psychotherapy.

Psychologist A professional who has completed graduate training in human psychology but not in medicine (and, therefore, cannot prescribe medication in most states). Many psychologists conduct psychological testing and statistical analysis. Clinical psychologists practice psychotherapy.

Psychotherapist A psychiatrist, psychologist, or social worker who looks for the cause of a person's problems and helps the person develop coping strategies to deal with them.

Psychotherapy Also called talk therapy, a term that covers several types of treatment—including suggestion, analysis, and persuasion—for mental disorders. Frequently used forms of psychotherapy include:

- Cognitive-behavioral therapy, which teaches you how to change inappropriate or negative patterns of thought and behavior.

- Psychoeducation, which shows you how to recognize signs of relapse so you can get help early. Social rhythm therapy is a form of psychoeducation that teaches a person with a disorder such as bipolar disorder how to regulate his or her daily routine to help prevent manic episodes.

- Family therapy, which evaluates the interactions of family members to help lower the level of family stress that might be worsening your disorder or that might result from it.

- Interpersonal therapy, which helps you improve your relationships with other people.

Neurosis Now an outdated, nonmedical term for an emotional disorder that is not as severe as a psychosis. People with neuroses have symptoms, such as anxieties or fears, that they recognize as being irrational but cannot control.

Psychosis A mental disorder in which a person has difficulty distinguishing reality from fantasy. Hallucinations (abnormal perceptions not based on reality), delusions (false, irrational beliefs), and distorted speech patterns are hallmark symptoms.

Psychosomatic Physical symptoms thought to be caused by a mental or emotional problem. The symptoms can often be treated by addressing the associated psychological problem.

---

depression. The disorder can occur at any age, but usually first appears between ages 18 and 44. Depression in childhood and adolescence has been linked to an increased risk of teen suicide. Depression among older people is extremely common and can be worsened by the death of friends and recognition of the physical limitations of aging.

Structural abnormalities in the brain such as from a moderate to severe head injury can contribute to the development of depression. Biological factors, such as blockage of the arteries to the brain (stroke; see page 669) and age-related brain chemical or structural changes, can also trigger depression. Genes play a role, too; if you have a close relative who has had depression, you are more likely than other people to develop it. Stressful life events, such as the death of a family member, may trigger depression in susceptible people. This vulnerability to depression probably involves a combination of genetic, biological, psychological, and environmental factors.

Recreational or prescription drug abuse, alcohol use, or exposure to a poison or toxin can produce symptoms of depression. Depression can also be a symptom of a number of medical conditions, including Cushing's disease (see page 898), stroke, hypothyroidism (see page 903), or cancer of the pancreas (see page 800). People who have a serious physical illness, such as heart disease, cancer, or diabetes, also are at risk of developing depression.

Depression can deter a person who has a serious medical condition from seeking or complying with treatment—for both the physical illness and the depression. Depression caused by a medical condition often goes unrecognized and, therefore, untreated. But early diagnosis of depression can improve overall health. About 70 to 80 percent of people with depression experience relief of their symptoms after receiving treatment.

Symptoms

Depression usually occurs in episodes that last at least 2 weeks. During this time, the primary symptoms are overriding melancholy, despair, and hopelessness. The person becomes apathetic and loses interest in enjoyable activities, including sex. It is also common for a person with depression to have difficulty concentrating. He or she may show signs of agitation, such as pacing or hand wringing, along with slowed speech and response time. Fatigue can be so great that even the smallest everyday tasks, such as dressing, seem to require enormous effort.

Depressed people often feel a diminished sense of self-worth—so much so that they may unreasonably feel responsible for unfavorable events that are beyond their control. For example, a salesman may blame himself for failing to make sales even when the general economy is bad and most other salespeople are also missing their sales targets. The intensity of symptoms often varies with the time of day. Often, a depressed person wakes up early with almost no energy but improves as the day goes on, although some people experience worse symptoms at night. As the disorder progresses, depression may deepen until it becomes chronic and the person may become totally withdrawn.

Characteristic symptoms of depression can change with age. Depressed children may express vague physical discomforts (such as a stomachache), be irritable, cry a lot, express a fear of death, or withdraw socially. They may also be extremely sensitive to rejection or failure. Adolescents who have depression often sleep excessively, display disruptive or reckless behavior, are frequently absent from school or perform poorly in school, and abuse alcohol or drugs. They may also have a concurrent anxiety disorder (see page 718).

The most serious risk of depression is suicide. If you think that you or someone you know may be depressed, talk to your doctor immediately. Untreated, depression often persists and can worsen, with episodes occurring more frequently and becoming more severe over time. This is why it is so important to seek treatment early.

The Risks and Warning Signs of Suicide

Recognizing and treating depression and other mental disorders as early as possible can be lifesaving. About 70 percent of people who commit suicide or attempt it are depressed. Always take a suicide attempt—even just talking about suicide—very seriously. Attempted suicide is always a plea for help from someone who is combating a mental disorder or a substance abuse problem. If someone you know threatens to commit suicide, listen to him or her without judgment, try to get him or her to see a doctor or call a suicide hot line, or call a suicide hot line yourself.

Women attempt suicide more often than do men, but men are four times as likely to be successful. More than 20 percent of adolescents seriously consider suicide each year, and the risk increases with age. The highest suicide rate occurs in white males over age 85. The following factors put a person at risk of committing suicide:

- Having previously attempted suicide
- Having a mental disorder
- Having a family history of a mental disorder, substance abuse, suicide, or physical or sexual abuse
- Keeping a firearm in the home
- Being imprisoned

- Being exposed to the suicidal behavior of others, including media exposure

A suicide attempt often follows clearly visible warning signs such as the following:

- Talking about suicide or death, even jokingly
- Having problems coping with an adverse life event (such as job loss or the death of a loved one)
- Withdrawing from friends and activities
- Hoarding pills or purchasing a gun
- Abusing alcohol or other drugs
- Giving away prized possessions
- Showing a lack of interest in the future
- Writing notes or poems about death
- Changing eating or sleep habits
- Neglecting personal appearance
- Behaving impulsively

The best way to prevent someone from attempting suicide is to get professional help for him or her immediately. Limiting access to firearms also helps; nearly 60 percent of suicides in the United States are committed with a firearm. If someone you know is in immediate danger, call 911 or your local emergency number.

Diagnosis

If you have symptoms of depression, your doctor will perform a thorough physical and psychological evaluation. You will probably receive a neurological examination that assesses the functioning of your brain and nervous system by testing your coordination, reflexes, and balance. The doctor may also order blood and other laboratory tests to rule out any medical conditions that could be causing your symptoms. He or she will interview you to find out if any of your close relatives have ever had a mood disorder or if you abuse any substances, including alcohol, that could be contributing to your condition. After making a preliminary diagnosis of depression, your doctor will recommend treatment or refer you to a psychiatrist (see page 710) or other mental health professional for treatment.

Medications for Mental Disorders

Medications cannot cure a mental disorder, but they can help control and alleviate its symptoms. The length of time a person needs to take a given medication depends on the disorder. In addition, medications prescribed for mental disorders do not produce the same effect in every person. You may need to try more than one drug before you and your doctor find the one that is right for you. Sometimes a combination of medications works best.

Medications for Mood Disorders

The two most common classes of drugs prescribed for mood disorders are antidepressants, which are used to treat depression (see page 709), and mood stabilizers, which are used to treat bipolar disorder (see page 715).

Antidepressants

Doctors prescribe antidepressants for severe depression, although antidepressants also can be used to treat certain anxiety disorders (see page 718) and phobias (see page 721). It takes about 1 to 3 weeks before an antidepressant begins to improve symptoms. How long a person needs to take an antidepressant depends on the severity of the illness, but treatment usually lasts for several months and may continue up to a year or more. Up to 70 percent of people who have depression will get better if they regularly take the appropriate antidepressant medication.

Selective Serotonin Reuptake Inhibitors   Selective serotonin reuptake inhibitors (SSRIs) have become the treatment of choice for depression. They work by altering the activity of serotonin, a neurotransmitter (chemical messenger) in the brain. SSRIs have fewer side effects than the older antidepressant medications.

The most common SSRIs are fluoxetine, sertraline, citalopram, fluvoxamine, and paroxetine.

Serotonin Norepinephrine Reuptake Inhibitors
Serotonin norepinephrine reuptake inhibitors (SNRIs) are newer antidepressants that work by altering the activity of serotonin and norepinephrine, two important neurotransmitters (chemical messengers) in the brain. Like SSRIs, they have fewer side effects than the older antidepressants. The most common SNRIs are venlafaxine and milnacipran.

Tricyclic Antidepressants   Once the first-line treatment for depression, tricyclic antidepressants have a number of side effects, including blurred vision, constipation, weight gain, and drowsiness, although not every person experiences every side effect. They alleviate the symptoms of depression in a way similar to that of SSRIs and SNRIs. Examples of tricyclic antidepressants include imipramine, doxepin, amitriptyline, nortriptyline, and desipramine.

Monoamine Oxidase Inhibitors   Monoamine oxidase inhibitors (MAOIs) work by obstructing a protein that breaks down certain neurotransmitters needed for feelings of well-being. MAOIs can interact adversely with many prescription and over-the-counter drugs and also with red wine and some foods, such as aged cheese, causing life-threatening symptoms, including dangerously high blood pressure. Common MAOIs include phenelzine, tranylcypromine, and isocarboxazid.

Other Antidepressants   Newer drugs have been developed that work on neurotransmitters other than, or in combination with, serotonin. They seem to have fewer side effects than the older drugs. Examples

Treatment

Treatment of depression usually is a combination of medication and some form of psychotherapy. The form of therapy most frequently used to treat depression is cognitive-behavioral therapy, which can help you learn the underlying cause of your depression, develop skills to cope, and teach you how to transform your negative ways of thinking and behaving into more positive ones. Some depressed people also benefit from interpersonal therapy, which helps them learn how to interact more effectively with other people.

Antidepressant medications (see previous page) such as tricyclic antidepressants and monoamine oxidase inhibitors (MAOIs) work by evening out the balance of the brain chemicals serotonin, norepinephrine, and dopamine. These medications can have unpleasant side effects such as dry mouth,

include mirtazapine, nefazodone, trazodone, and bupropion.

Mood Stabilizers

Doctors prescribe mood stabilizers to even out the manic highs and depressive lows of bipolar disorder. The drug most commonly used to treat bipolar disorder is the mineral lithium. The exact way lithium works is not known, but it lessens symptoms in about 5 to 14 days. Some people with bipolar disorder respond better to anticonvulsant drugs, which are used to treat epileptic seizures (see page 686). In addition to lithium, common mood stabilizers include divalproex, carbamazepine, lamotrigine, gabapentin, and olanzapine.

Medications for Anxiety Disorders

Antianxiety medications have a calming and relaxing effect on people with anxiety disorders. Most antianxiety drugs fall into two classes—benzodiazepines and azaspirones. Many doctors also prescribe antidepressants for people who have panic attacks.

Benzodiazepines

Benzodiazepines produce a calming effect by depressing the central nervous system. They can be habit-forming, so doctors usually prescribe them for only brief periods or intermittently. Other than drowsiness, side effects are few, but withdrawal can occur if the person suddenly stops taking the drug. Commonly prescribed benzodiazepines include chlordiazepoxide, alprazolam, clonazepam, diazepam, lorazepam, and clorazepate.

Azaspirones

Azaspirones are a class of drugs that is usually prescribed for generalized anxiety disorder. Buspirone is the most frequently prescribed medication of this type.

Medications for Psychosis

Antipsychotic medications are used to treat the symptoms of psychosis, principally schizophrenia. Doctors consider a number of factors—including age, weight, and the severity of the condition—when deciding which antipsychotic drug to prescribe because each one has its own level of potency and side effects.

Antipsychotics

People vary in how they respond to antipsychotic drugs and in how fast their symptoms improve. It is not clear how these medications work, but they have tranquilizing properties; they may work by interfering with the activity of dopamine (a chemical messenger in the brain). Sometimes these drugs completely reverse the psychosis after treatment. In other cases, medications have to be taken indefinitely. Weight gain is a common side effect of antipsychotic medications, but a potentially long-term effect is the appearance of involuntary movements. Examples of antipsychotic medications include chlorpromazine, thioridazine, molindone, trifluoperazine, fluphenazine, perphenazine, and haloperidol.

Newer Antipsychotics

Although the exact way in which the newer, atypical antipsychotic medications work is not fully understood, they seem to have an effect on dopamine and serotonin, two neurotransmitters (chemical messengers) in the brain. Examples include clozapine, olanzapine, risperidone, and ziprasidone.

drowsiness, constipation, headaches, nausea, or insomnia, but these side effects subside as your body adjusts to the medication. Newer antidepressants, called selective serotonin reuptake inhibitors (SSRIs) and serotonin norepinephrine reuptake inhibitors (SNRIs), are as effective as the older drugs but with fewer side effects. You will have to take an antidepressant for a few weeks before you see an improvement in your mood.

You may have to try more than one drug before you and your doctor find the one that works best for you. Some people respond better to one drug or a combination of drugs than to others. Doctors prescribe antidepressant medications for a fixed period—usually 6 to 18 months—but the beneficial effects usually last long after you stop taking the drug. Many people experience anxiety along with their depression, so doctors sometimes also prescribe antianxiety medications (see previous page) for people who have depression.

In severe cases, depression may require hospitalization, especially if a person has contemplated or attempted suicide. In the hospital, the doctor will monitor the person's condition carefully and begin treatment with drugs and psychotherapy. Temporary care in a day hospital may make it easier for a person to make the transition from the hospital to home. In a day hospital, you receive

MY STORY   Depression

My husband died 3 years ago and I felt horrible for months. I found myself crying all the time, wanting to stay in bed all day, and avoiding my friends and even my children. Life didn't seem worth living. I used to love spending time with my grandchildren, taking them to movies and museums, but even that no longer seemed fun. My old friends kept calling me and inviting me to dinner or out to lunch and I always made up excuses not to go. I felt that no one wanted to spend time with me anyway because I was such a mope—they were just trying to be nice.

Then one day my daughter came over to the house and sat down with me and told me how worried she was about me. She said that the children kept asking her what was wrong with Grandma and why didn't I like to be with them anymore. She said that they all missed our big family dinners together and talked about the fun we used to have whenever we got together. She suggested that I talk to my doctor about how sad I felt all the time, but I dismissed her, saying, "There's nothing that can be done about the way I feel, so why bother?" She told me that a friend of hers had had a severe bout of depression after her second child was born and she was able to get help from her doctor and is now feeling much better.

I'm grateful that my daughter pushed me to do something about my depression—I was beginning to think I would never enjoy life again.

Even though I had no energy and little interest in doing anything for myself, my daughter seemed so upset that I finally agreed to talk to my doctor at my next appointment. I told the doctor about how sad I was all the time and how I didn't want to do anything but sleep. He asked me questions about my life and how I felt about different things and said that he thought I might be suffering from depression. He explained that depression is common, especially in older people who have lost a spouse, and that it can be treated successfully. He prescribed a medication called paroxetine to take every day and told me that I should start feeling better after a few weeks.

The doctor also referred me to a psychiatrist for further treatment. I saw the psychiatrist regularly for about 6 months. I was able to talk openly about my feelings for the first time, and the doctor helped me learn how to cope with the death of my husband and take steps toward making a happy life for myself. I started feeling better after a couple of weeks and I stopped taking the medication after about a year. I'm enjoying my family and friends again, taking a class at a community college, and taking up some of my old hobbies. I'm grateful that my daughter pushed me to do something about my depression—I was beginning to think I would never enjoy life again.

treatment at a care facility during the day and return home at night.

For some severe cases of depression, psychiatrists may use electroconvulsive therapy (ECT), formerly known as electroshock therapy, in which electrical stimulation is applied to the brain (while the person is under general anesthesia) to produce a seizure (abnormal electrical activity in the brain). The effects of ECT are similar to those of medications used to treat depression, but ECT is more intense. ECT is one of the most effective treatments for severe depression, benefiting 80 to 90 percent of affected people. Memory loss is a common side effect of ECT, but memory usually is restored within about 4 to 6 weeks. Advances in the way doctors apply the technique have lowered its side effects significantly.

A promising newer treatment for depression is the use of magnetic fields applied to the skull to stimulate electrical impulses in the brain. This technique has a success rate almost as high as that of ECT but does not trigger seizures, causes no pain, and does not require anesthesia.

Bipolar Disorder

People with bipolar disorder experience episodes of intense euphoria or mania that can, at times, alternate with periods of severe depression. The intensity of the disorder's dramatic mood swings is different from the normal ups and downs that most people experience. Bipolar disorder tends to be cyclical, with the episodes of mania and depression interrupted by periods of normal mood. Manic states can occur suddenly or gradually and can last for days, weeks, or months. The first episode of mania usually occurs between ages 15 and 25. Stressful life events can trigger the onset of bipolar disorder in people who are genetically susceptible to developing the disorder.

Bipolar disorder affects about 1 percent of the population, striking men and women in equal numbers. The condition results from a combination of genetic and environmental factors. Almost 90 percent of affected people have a close relative with either bipolar disorder or depression. Additionally, an imbalance in brain chemicals and a deficiency in the production of some hormones (substances in the body that control key functions) may contribute

Dysthymic Disorder

People who experience low-level symptoms of depression—either most of the time or intermittently—for 2 or more years have dysthymic disorder (also called dysthymia), a mild but persistent form of depression. Such people may not realize they are depressed, believing that they simply have a gloomy temperament. To others, people with dysthymic disorder may appear pessimistic, passive, introverted, and self-critical. They may have difficulty enjoying themselves and often are preoccupied with feelings of inadequacy and fear of failure. Other symptoms of dysthymic disorder include either poor appetite or overeating, sleep problems, low energy levels, poor concentration, and low self-esteem.

The cause of dysthymic disorder is not known, although it seems to carry the same inherited risk as major depression. Women are more frequently affected than men. The disorder may begin in childhood or adolescence, usually starting earlier than depression. People with dysthymic disorder may have difficulties in their relationships and usually have a negative perception of themselves. The principal danger of dysthymic disorder is that it can develop into major depression.

Dysthymic disorder often goes undiagnosed and untreated. Many people with dysthymic disorder fail to seek treatment because they think that feeling gloomy is normal. It is common for a person seeking help for the disorder to state that he or she has felt mildly depressed for years. If you or someone you know feels this way, discuss it with your doctor because a number of effective treatments can help you feel better.

Doctors frequently prescribe antidepressants (see page 712) to treat dysthymic disorder. Along with medication, doctors usually recommend psychotherapy (see page 710), including interpersonal therapy, to help affected people learn more effective ways to interact with others, and cognitive-behavioral therapy, to learn how to recognize and change negative thought patterns and behaviors into more positive ones. People with dysthymic disorder can often benefit from vocational counseling—they seem to be especially good at jobs that require concentration and attention to detail.

to bipolar disorder. The sudden and intense mood swings that characterize bipolar disorder can seriously disrupt a person's life by damaging relationships and negatively affecting job attendance and performance. Alcohol and drug abuse are common among people with bipolar disorder. Anxiety disorders, especially posttraumatic stress disorder (see page 720) and obsessive-compulsive disorder (see page 720), also commonly coexist in people with bipolar disorder.

Effective treatment for bipolar disorder is available but, during the manic phase, many people with the disorder feel so elated that they may fail to seek treatment or refuse to follow the doctor's treatment recommendations. A mild level of mania, known as hypomania, may even improve a person's productivity and performance. However, when the upbeat mood inevitably subsides, the person is left feeling lower than normal and may be more responsive to medical help. Family members and friends should strongly encourage the person to seek treatment, taking him or her to the doctor or to a hospital emergency department for evaluation if necessary.

Symptoms

During the manic phase of bipolar disorder, a person has an elevated mood, unrealistically inflated self-esteem, a decreased need for sleep, rapid speech, racing thoughts, and poor impulse control. He or she can be easily distracted, may have exaggerated beliefs about his or her abilities, and may say or do things simply to shock others. Mania also can compel people to go on unrestrained spending sprees, to have impulsive and promiscuous sexual encounters to fulfill an increased sex drive, or to enthusiastically start (but rarely finish) new projects. Extreme mania can progress to delirium (profound mental confusion) or paranoia (extreme or irrational suspicion).

The depressed phase produces the characteristic symptoms of depression (see page 709), including persistent sadness, anxiety, and feelings of emptiness and despair. The person may feel hopeless, helpless, pessimistic, guilty, and worthless. Loss of interest in activities that were once enjoyable, including sex, is common. Decreased energy and difficulty concentrating are accompanied by irritability and restlessness. When depressed, a person may sleep too much or be unable to sleep enough.

He or she may have chronic pain or other uncomfortable sensations that are not caused by physical illness or injury. He or she may think about death or suicide.

Some people with bipolar disorder have a mixed state in which symptoms of mania and depression occur at the same time. In this state, a person may feel sad and hopeless while at the same time feeling full of energy. In a state called rapid cycling (see next page), a person can experience four or more episodes of mania or depression in a year.

Diagnosis

Like other mental disorders, bipolar disorder cannot be diagnosed by a specific medical test. But your doctor will perform a physical examination to rule out any physical disorder that could be causing the symptoms. If no physical conditions are detected, the doctor will probably refer you to a psychiatrist or other mental health professional, who can diagnose bipolar disorder based on your health history and a description of your feelings and behavior.

Treatment

Although bipolar disorder is a condition that occurs in episodes, treatment must be continuous to prevent the severe mood swings that are characteristic of the disorder. A regimen that combines medication and psychotherapy (see page 710) is usually the most effective. Affected people who are experiencing a severe episode of mania or depression may need to be hospitalized for treatment. If they are a danger to themselves or others or if they are unable to care for themselves, they may need to be hospitalized against their will.

Doctors usually prescribe drugs called mood stabilizers (see page 713) to treat bipolar disorder. The drugs may need to be taken indefinitely to control a person's mood. The most common mood stabilizer prescribed for bipolar disorder is lithium, a naturally occurring mineral, which seems to act on the central nervous system to dampen the manic and depressive phases of the disorder. The dosage of lithium needs to be carefully controlled because a toxic dose is very close to the dose needed to control symptoms. For this reason, if you are taking lithium, you will need to have regular checkups and blood tests to measure the levels of lithium in your blood. Too much lithium can cause weight gain,

Rapid Cycling and Cyclothymia

Rapid cycling is a form of bipolar disorder in which the episodes of mania and depression occur at least four times a year. In serious cases (called ultrarapid cycling), the episodes can occur several times a day. Up to 20 percent of all people with bipolar disorder develop rapid cycling at some point in their lives, and 90 percent of those who do are women. Rapid cycling is more common in people with bipolar disorder who have a thyroid abnormality.

Lithium is less effective in treating rapid cycling than other forms of bipolar disorder, and antidepressant medications sometimes induce rapid cycling. For these reasons, an antiseizure medication called divalproex is usually used instead; divalproex works by stabilizing the limbic system (the areas of the brain responsible for emotions). Thyroid hormone also may be helpful in treating rapid cycling in people with mood disorders who have thyroid abnormalities.

Cyclothymia is a disorder marked by less severe episodes of mania and depression than bipolar disorder, and the episodes last only a few days. The instability produced by these milder episodes of mania can cause such erratic behavior as frequent changes of residence, irregular work attendance, repeated romantic breakups, and an intermittent pattern of alcohol and drug abuse. A rare form, called chronic hypomania, causes predominantly manic episodes and produces a personality that is overly cheerful, impulsive, and excessively energetic.

People with cyclothymia have a greater risk of developing bipolar disorder than the general population, but only a third actually go on to develop it. Treatment may not be required for cyclothymia if the person can learn to live within the extremes of his or her temperament. Otherwise, a doctor will prescribe mood stabilizers (see page 713).

severe trembling, dizziness, confusion, nausea, vomiting, diarrhea, and heart palpitations. Lithium also can affect the functioning of the thyroid gland. As an alternative to lithium, antiseizure drugs such as divalproex are sometimes prescribed to stabilize mood. For maximum effect, doctors sometimes combine lithium with an anticonvulsant drug.

To help treat your bipolar disorder, your doctor will recommend one or more types of psychotherapy to give you support and guidance in coping with the disorder. You and family members may also benefit from joining a support group to share experiences with other people who are going through the same difficulties.

Seasonal Affective Disorder

Seasonal affective disorder (SAD) is a form of depression that occurs in the fall or winter in response to shorter days with less sunlight. The disorder subsides in the spring or summer as daylight increases. The exact cause of SAD is unclear. The deficiency of light during fall and winter is thought to decrease the level in the brain of the chemical messenger serotonin. Serotonin affects emotions, behavior, and thought. People with SAD may also have altered circadian rhythms, or internal biological clocks, that cause a shift in the signals that indicate when to fall asleep and when to wake up.

Normally, the light-sensing pineal gland in the brain responds to the lessening light of day by secreting the hormone melatonin, which promotes relaxation and sleep. Daylight signals the pineal gland to shut off the production of melatonin to allow us to wake up. Melatonin levels should be low in the morning and high at bedtime, but melatonin is produced in increased quantities throughout the day in winter, when the days are shorter and darker. Maintaining this cycle becomes more difficult in the fall and winter because the body is no longer responding to stark contrasts in day and night or light and darkness.

The short daylight hours and lack of sunlight during winter can also cause a chemical imbalance in an area of the brain called the hypothalamus, which plays a role in regulating the body's biological clock. Cold weather adds to the chemical imbalances caused by low light levels by encouraging people to spend more time indoors. Some doctors think that SAD may be the human counterpart to the seasonal cycles of animals that influence activities such as hibernation. SAD affects more women than men and is most common in people in their 20s and 30s.

Symptoms

The symptoms of SAD are severe and usually appear around September or October and continue until March or April. They are similar to the symptoms of depression (see page 709), including decreased energy, excessive sleepiness, or fatigue. In some cases, a person has feelings of sadness and a decreased interest in sex or physical contact. He or she may withdraw from family and friends. Many people with SAD gain weight, perhaps because of an increased appetite and a craving for carbohydrate-rich or sugary foods.

The symptoms subside in the spring and summer, either gradually with increasing sunlight or suddenly. Some people experience bursts of energy or creativity or elevated moods during this time, similar to the manic episodes that occur in bipolar disorder (see previous article).

Diagnosis

A diagnosis of SAD can usually be made after two or more consecutive winters of symptoms of depression that go away when the weather turns warmer and daylight increases. People with SAD may notice that their symptoms recur or worsen if the amount of indoor light they are exposed to decreases or if the weather is overcast at any time of year. A doctor may recommend a thorough physical examination and laboratory tests to rule out other possible conditions. If your doctor thinks you may have SAD or another type of depression, he or she will refer you to a mental health professional who has experience treating the various forms of depression, including SAD.

Treatment

Light therapy (phototherapy) provided by a fluorescent light box or by wearing a visor with a fluorescent light attached is commonly used to treat SAD. The amount of light needed to provide effective therapy varies from one person to another. Phototherapy usually is done in the morning or early evening to extend the feeling of daylight. Your doctor will monitor the therapy carefully because of possible side effects such as eyestrain, headache, and insomnia.

If you have SAD, try to expose yourself to daylight as much as possible. Outdoor light, even on a cloudy day, is brighter and can provide more light than a light box. Daily exercise can be helpful in treating SAD and is especially beneficial when done outdoors. Eating a balanced diet can help to offset cravings for carbohydrates and sweets.

Antidepressant medications (see page 712) may be effective in eliminating or at least reducing the symptoms of SAD. Psychotherapy (see page 710) can often help people with SAD deal with their depression. Some people benefit from a combination of light therapy, medication, and psychotherapy.

Other Types of SAD

Many people gain weight and lack energy at times in the fall and winter. This mild form of SAD, called winter depression or winter "blues," is a more moderate reaction to seasonal variations in light than SAD and often occurs around the time of the winter solstice (December 21). Some people who think they have the winter blues may simply be coming down with the holiday blues, a time when they are likely to eat more.

A reverse form of SAD, called summer depression, is characterized by irritability, insomnia, and decreased appetite with accompanying weight loss. Symptoms of reverse SAD may be related to the excessive heat of summer rather than to a reaction to light.

Anxiety Disorders

The human body evolved a rapid hormonal response system to deal with danger and to ensure survival. Our physical reactions to dangerous or stressful situations—increased heart rate, rapid breathing, tensed muscles—help us survive and succeed. A genuine threat, such as a speeding car heading right for you, provokes this survival response. But people who have an anxiety disorder respond in this way even when they are not faced with a threat or when a threat is only minor. They experience almost constant fear or dread that disrupts their family life and job performance and prevents them from enjoying a full life.

People with anxiety disorders seem to have a biological vulnerability that makes them easily aroused by stress. Factors that contribute to an increased risk for anxiety disorders include an inherited tendency, family behavior that may be learned, abnormalities in brain chemistry, and a chemical hypersensitivity to such substances as high levels of carbon dioxide. Traumatic events in childhood, such as physical or sexual abuse, also can bring about an anxiety disorder in childhood or later in life.

Anxiety disorders represent the most common form of psychological illness in the United States—

more than 19 million Americans are affected by an anxiety disorder each year. Depression (see page 709) often accompanies an anxiety disorder, which can lead a person who has an anxiety disorder to contemplate suicide (see page 711) at some time in his or her life. The most common anxiety disorders are panic disorder, obsessive-compulsive disorder, posttraumatic stress disorder, phobias, acute stress disorder, and generalized anxiety disorder.

Panic Disorder

Panic disorder is an anxiety disorder that produces sudden, unexpected episodes of overwhelming fear accompanied by alarming physical symptoms, such as a rapid heartbeat or a choking sensation. Initial episodes often occur when the person is experiencing severe stress such as from overworking or going through a dramatic life event such as getting married. After having the first panic attack, a person often lives in fear of having another attack. This anticipatory fear causes some affected people to limit their activities to avoid situations that could trigger another attack.

Panic disorder can progress to a higher level, known as agoraphobia, in which the person fears being in a place where escaping or finding help might be difficult. Such people avoid being in a crowd, standing in line, going to the store, or riding in cars or on public transportation. In severe cases, people are afraid to leave their home.

Panic attacks appear to occur when the brain's usual way of reacting to a threat, called the flight or fight response, is activated inappropriately. The disorder is twice as common in women as in men. Initial attacks can appear anytime between late adolescence and middle age. Other psychological conditions, including specific phobias (see page 721), social phobia, and depression (see page 709), often coexist with panic disorder.

Symptoms

Panic disorder causes episodes of extreme terror and dread, accompanied by physical symptoms such as heart palpitations, light-headedness, difficulty breathing, chest pains, hot flashes or cold chills, and tingling or numbness in the hands. The physical symptoms may appear first, making you afraid that you suddenly have a life-threatening condition, such as a heart attack, and are going to die. You may feel that you can't get enough air and you begin breathing rapidly, triggering light-headedness. Some people report feeling waves of energy flowing down their body.

These episodes of panic accompanied by uncomfortable physical sensations occur unpredictably and take you completely by surprise, triggering the urge to flee or escape. The physical symptoms usually last from a few minutes to an hour, and can recur at any time. Some people experience periods of remission (when they have no panic attacks) that can sometimes last for months or even years.

Diagnosis

Panic disorder can convincingly mimic some serious medical conditions, such as a heart attack, so it is important to get an accurate diagnosis. To diagnose panic disorder, your doctor will give you a thorough medical examination, including blood tests and an electrocardiogram (ECG; see page 559), to rule out other disorders, such as elevated thyroid hormone levels or abnormal heart rhythms (arrhythmias; see page 580), that can cause similar symptoms. Only then can the doctor make a diagnosis of panic disorder based on your description of your symptoms.

Treatment

Without treatment, repeated panic attacks can occur for years, disrupting your relationships and interfering with your ability to do your job. You could start to avoid situations that you fear will trigger a panic attack and become severely depressed. Treatment of panic disorder usually includes antidepressants (see page 712) or antianxiety medication (see page 713) and cognitive-behavioral therapy (which changes the thought patterns that can trigger symptoms and attempts to change the person's behavior). Seventy to 90 percent of people can expect near total relief of their symptoms with treatment.

Obsessive-Compulsive Disorder

Obsessive-compulsive disorder is marked by persistent, intense, and inappropriate thoughts or images known as obsessions, which a person tries to compensate for with repetitive behavior, called compulsions, that he or she feels driven to perform. Examples of common obsessions include recurring doubts (about having turned off the stove or locked the door, for example), thoughts about contamination (such as from touching a doorknob or shaking hands), requiring things in a certain order, violent or shocking impulses (such as to hurt someone or laugh out loud at a funeral), and intrusive sexual images. Compulsive behaviors performed to lessen the anxiety produced by such obsessive thoughts range from repeated hand washing or checking, to praying or counting. In the extreme, ritual compulsions can consume hours every day, disrupting a person's life.

Obsessive-compulsive disorder is thought to result from abnormal activation of specific areas of the brain. In children with obsessive-compulsive disorder, infections with streptococcal bacteria (such as strep throat; see page 652) have been implicated in either triggering the disease or making it worse.

Symptoms

The obsessive thoughts characteristic of obsessive-compulsive disorder produce a great deal of anxiety and distress. The affected person may attempt to ignore or suppress such thoughts but inevitably feels compelled to perform the ritualistic action to get rid of the uncomfortable anxiety. The thoughts keep returning, prompting the compulsion, and the cycle repeats indefinitely. The person usually recognizes that this behavior is unreasonable but can't keep from doing it. If he or she resists the compulsion, an overwhelming feeling of physical tension occurs, which can be relieved only by giving in to the compulsion. Some people with obsessive-compulsive disorder also have tics, which are repeated, purposeless actions or muscle contractions; examples include blinking, throat clearing, and mouth twitching.

Diagnosis

A doctor can make a diagnosis of obsessive-compulsive disorder from a person's description of his or her feelings, physical symptoms, and behavior.

Treatment

Antidepressant drugs (see page 712) called selective serotonin reuptake inhibitors (SSRIs) are the first line of treatment for obsessive-compulsive disorder because they increase the availability of the brain chemical serotonin, which helps regulate mood and behavior. Half of all affected people benefit from these medications. Most doctors also prescribe a type of cognitive-behavioral therapy called desensitization, which exposes the person to a compulsion-producing situation (such as using a public bathroom) while attempting to reduce the compulsive response (such as repeated hand washing).

Posttraumatic Stress Disorder

Posttraumatic stress disorder is a condition that occurs after a terrifying experience, such as a violent personal attack, child abuse, a severe injury, a natural disaster, or military combat. The traumatizing event can be something that the person has either experienced or witnessed. After the incident, the person continues to relive the event through nightmares or intrusive daytime memories called flashbacks. Any traumatizing experience can trigger posttraumatic stress disorder, although not all people who experience a horrifying event develop the disorder. The condition affects millions of Americans. Because some people who have posttraumatic stress disorder are at increased risk of suicide (see page 711), getting prompt treatment can be lifesaving.

Symptoms

During the traumatic event, you may have felt profound fear, helplessness, and horror. Flashbacks cause you to feel that you are reliving the incident, recalling the sounds, odors, and feelings related to the event to the exclusion of physical reality. Even when you are not reliving the event, you may feel numb and detached from your surroundings and be easily startled. You may also have difficulty returning affection and engaging in activities you previously enjoyed. Irritability, aggression or violence, and sleep problems are common. People with posttraumatic stress disorder are highly susceptible to depression (see page 709) and substance abuse (see page 732).

Diagnosis

Your doctor can diagnose posttraumatic stress disorder after listening to a description of your experiences and symptoms. The diagnosis is confirmed if you have had symptoms for more than a month.

Treatment

Antidepressant and antianxiety medications (see page 709) can reduce the symptoms of depression and help with sleep problems in people with post-traumatic stress disorder. Psychotherapy (see page 710), especially cognitive-behavioral therapy, which helps to change negative patterns of thought and behavior into more positive ones, can also be helpful. Many people with the disorder find group therapy beneficial because they can share their feelings with others who have had similar experiences.

Phobias

For people with phobias, certain objects or situations provoke irrational fear so overwhelming that it interferes with normal life. The two main types of phobias are specific phobias and social anxiety disorder. When fear is connected to a particular object, such as bridges, snakes, or water, a person is said to have a specific phobia. Specific phobias can arise at any age. In children, specific phobias are learned, either by experiencing a traumatic event, such as being bitten by a vicious dog, or by observing a parent who is afraid of some object. Adults typically develop specific phobias as a learned response after experiencing intense anxiety in a particular situation, such as being confined in a stalled elevator.

Social anxiety disorder can involve fear of being humiliated in front of other people. A person may experience a social phobia in most social situations or only at certain times, such as when speaking in public or performing onstage. Social anxiety disorder usually first appears between ages 15 and 20 and occurs equally in men and women. Doctors believe that people who have social anxiety disorder have an inborn tendency to have exaggerated physical responses, such as blushing or increased heart rate, in social situations.

Both types of phobias run in families. People with phobias may be genetically programmed to easily learn to be fearful, or they may acquire their fear from watching the fearful behavior of others.

Symptoms

In both specific phobias and social anxiety disorder, the anxiety produced by the feared object or situation is so great that it produces physical symptoms, including a pounding heart, sweating, and rapid breathing. Anticipation of a situation in which the person might have to face the object of fear can cause loss of sleep and loss of appetite. People with social anxiety disorder have difficulty talking to other people in everyday social situations, both in person and on the telephone. They may blush or shake in front of other people, believing that others are watching them closely and waiting for them to make a mistake. Their anxiety may become so extreme that they begin to have panic attacks (see page 719) and may take extreme measures to avoid situations that could trigger attacks. People with phobias are especially susceptible to substance abuse (see page 732).

If you think you may have a specific or social phobia, tell your doctor, especially if your fears are keeping you from functioning fully in your everyday life. It is difficult to change the way you feel without help from a professional.

Diagnosis

If your doctor thinks you may have a phobia, he or she will perform a physical examination and ask you to describe your symptoms. Doctors can usually diagnose phobias based on a person's explanation of the way he or she feels.

Treatment

To treat a specific phobia, your doctor will recommend a type of cognitive-behavioral therapy known as desensitization or exposure therapy, which gradually and in increasing stages exposes you to the object or situation that frightens you until your fear diminishes. For example, if you are afraid of flying, you may first be taught relaxation exercises (see page 59), shown pictures of airplanes, and asked to imagine flying in an airplane. The next step would be to go to an airport and then, eventually, fly in an airplane. About 75 percent of people with specific phobias find relief from their symptoms with this type of therapy. No drugs are available for treating specific phobias, although your doctor may prescribe an antianxiety medication (see page 713) for a limited time to help reduce your symptoms.

Exposure therapy also can benefit people with social phobia because it allows them to gradually become more comfortable in social situations and helps them learn how to handle disapproval or criticism. However, for people with social phobia, most doctors recommend exposure therapy in combination with antidepressant medications (see page 712) called selective serotonin reuptake inhibitors (SSRIs) or monoamine oxidase inhibitors (MAOIs). People who have public-speaking anxiety sometimes benefit from drugs called beta blockers (medications used for lowering blood pressure), which they take before participating in the event they are anxious about.

Generalized Anxiety Disorder

Feelings of anxiety that arise before an important event, such as a wedding or the first day of a new job, are normal and experienced by most people. But people with generalized anxiety disorder feel worried and tense constantly, worrying excessively about everyday events as well as special occasions. People who have the disorder always seem to expect the worst, are unable to relax, and are easily irritated.

Generalized anxiety disorder affects about 4 million people in the United States every year. More women than men are affected. The disorder most often begins in childhood or adolescence but also can first appear in adulthood. It does not seem to run in families but may coexist with other psychological disorders, including depression (see page 709), substance abuse (see page 732), or another anxiety disorder. Some physical conditions, such as irritable bowel syndrome (see page 765), also can accompany generalized anxiety disorder.

Symptoms

The hallmark symptom of generalized anxiety disorder is constant, excessive, and often unrealistic worrying about family, finances, work, or other routine aspects of life. Physical symptoms—including fatigue, headaches, muscle tension and pain, trembling, sweating, hot flashes, poor concentration, nausea, or insomnia—often accompany the worry. A person also can be irritable, have trouble concentrating, and develop insomnia.

Diagnosis

If you think you may have generalized anxiety disorder, tell your doctor about your excessive worrying and any physical symptoms you may have. He or she will want to know if any family member has had an anxiety disorder or depression, if you consume a lot of caffeine or alcohol, or if you have experienced any stressful events recently. The doctor may ask you to take a test that can evaluate your anxiety levels to help diagnose generalized anxiety disorder.

Treatment

Treatment of generalized anxiety disorder usually combines antianxiety medications (see page 713) called benzodiazepines (which can become addictive) or azaspirones with some form of psychotherapy (see page 710). Doctors usually also recommend stress management techniques to enable the person to cope better with the routine demands of life. It may take a few weeks before the prescribed medication begins to work and you start feeling better.

Personality Disorders

A personality disorder is a long-lasting pattern of maladaptive behavior that adversely affects a person's ability to interact with others. The disorder usually first appears in adolescence or early adulthood. The person's behavior is noticeably different from expected behavior. Psychiatrists classify personality disorders into three different clusters. Cluster A personality disorders (paranoid, schizoid, and schizotypal) are characterized by odd or eccentric behavior. Cluster B personality disor-

ders (antisocial, borderline, histrionic, and narcissistic) are marked by dramatic and highly emotional behavior. Cluster C personality disorders (avoidant, dependent, and obsessive-compulsive) are typified by anxious, fearful behaviors.

Personality disorders affect up to 3 percent of the general population. A personality disorder can affect both men and women, but some, such as antisocial personality disorder and paranoid personality disorder, are more prevalent in men.

Symptoms

The symptoms of a personality disorder depend on the type. It is possible to have a personality disorder that displays traits of more than one type. The disorders described here are the most common medically recognized personality disorders.

Paranoid personality disorder

People with paranoid personality disorder are so distrustful and suspicious of other people's motives that, without any evidence, they may assume that others intend to harm, exploit, or deceive them. They bear grudges, do not forgive perceived injustices, and react with anger when they think they are being attacked.

Schizoid personality disorder

People with schizoid personality disorder are not interested in forming close relationships and seem cold and indifferent. They prefer to be alone and do not express much emotion, including anger. This type of personality disorder is thought to be a limited form of schizophrenia (see page 728) and sometimes eventually becomes schizophrenia.

Schizotypal personality disorder

People with a schizotypal personality disorder are uncomfortable in close relationships, seem eccentric, and are preoccupied with superstitions or the paranormal. They may believe they have special powers, such as clairvoyance, or that they have magical control over others. This type of personality disorder is also thought to be a limited form of schizophrenia (see page 728).

Antisocial personality disorder

The essential feature of antisocial personality disorder is callous disregard for other people's rights or suffering. A person with this disorder may be contemptuous, deceitful, and manipulative and often break the law by destroying property, stealing, or conning other people.

Borderline personality disorder

People with borderline personality disorder have a lifelong history of mood instability and fear real or imagined abandonment. They try to counteract it by impulsively entering and ending relationships, engaging in spending sprees, having promiscuous sex, driving recklessly, or abusing drugs or alcohol. They lead tempestuous lives and may engage in self-mutilation or attempt suicide. Borderline personality disorder may be related to bipolar disorder (see page 715).

Histrionic personality disorder

Attention-seeking and shallow, exaggerated emotionality characterize histrionic personality disorder. Affected people demand to be the center of attention, are sexually seductive, and are easily influenced by others.

Narcissistic personality disorder

People with narcissistic personality disorder have an exaggerated sense of self-importance. They assume they are superior to others and feel slighted when their superiority is not recognized. They require excessive admiration, have a sense of entitlement, and exploit others to realize their own ambitions. Doctors think this personality disorder is a limited form of bipolar disorder (see page 715).

Avoidant personality disorder

A person with avoidant personality disorder has a lifelong fear of rejection, is preoccupied with feelings of inadequacy, and harbors fears of criticism. He or she longs to have a social life but avoids social gatherings, intimate relationships, and new activities because they may prove embarrassing. This type of personality disorder is thought to be related to social anxiety disorder (see page 721).

Dependent personality disorder

The distinguishing feature of dependent personality disorder is a strong need to be taken care of. This need creates submissive and clinging behavior in relationships. People with this personality disorder always depend on other people to make decisions and assume responsibility.

Obsessive-compulsive personality disorder

Not to be confused with obsessive-compulsive disorder (see page 720), obsessive-compulsive personality disorder produces a preoccupation with orderliness, perfectionism, and control over both thoughts and other people. People with this disorder are inflexible and often inefficient because they adhere excessively to rules, schedules, lists, and trivial details.

Diagnosis

When diagnosing a personality disorder, a psychiatrist or other mental health professional interviews the person and his or her family to find out what kind of behavior the person displays and the nature of his or her relationships with other people. The doctor must take care not to mistake the person's cultural habits, ethnic customs, or religious beliefs for a personality disorder. For example, people from countries in which food and other necessities are scarce may exhibit disregard for others by cutting in front of people who are waiting in line. This behavior does not mean that they have an antisocial personality disorder, which requires evidence that the person also had a conduct disorder (aggressive behavior that disregards the rights of others) before the age of 15 years. When diagnosing a personality disorder, the doctor also carefully rules out the presence of another mental disorder or evidence of substance abuse or a medical condition, such as a severe head injury, when making a diagnosis.

Treatment

Psychiatrists treat personality disorders with psychotherapy and, at times, with a combination of medication and psychotherapy, depending on the disorder. Each of the three clusters calls for a specific type of medication. Cluster A personality disorders (paranoid, schizoid, and schizotypal) may respond to antipsychotic medication (see page 713). People with Cluster B disorders (antisocial, borderline, histrionic, and narcissistic), which typically cause mood instability, usually benefit from drugs called mood stabilizers (see page 713), which are also prescribed for bipolar disorder. No medication works very effectively for antisocial personality disorder, however. Doctors treat cluster C personality disorders (avoidant, dependent, and obsessive-compulsive) with antianxiety medications (see page 713) or antidepressants (see page 712). Cognitive-behavioral therapy also helps people with personality disorders change their ineffective thought and behavior patterns to enable them to improve their relationships.

Eating Disorders

Few people are genetically programmed to be thin, but this image is the ideal in our society. The unrealistic desire to be slim has made many people, especially women, feel uncomfortable, awkward, or ashamed of their body shape. People who have a negative body image are more likely to be depressed, have low self-esteem, and struggle with weight loss. At any given time, 45 percent of American women and 25 percent of American men are on a diet. For some people, simple dieting crosses the line into an eating disorder. People at increased risk for an eating disorder often engage in sports (such as gymnastics or figure skating) or have careers (such as modeling or acting) that depend on their being thin or having an attractive physical appearance.

Most people who have an eating disorder also have depression (see page 709) or an anxiety disorder (see page 718). About 40 percent have obsessive-compulsive disorder (see page 720). Eating disorders can severely and irreversibly harm the body and can be fatal. They can also cause serious psychological problems. In addition to placing tremendous pressure on a person's relationships with family and friends, eating disorders can lead to the following health problems:

- Irregular heartbeat or cardiac arrest
- Heart failure
- Kidney damage
- Liver damage
- A weakened immune system
- Permanent loss of bone mass, leading to bone fractures and osteoporosis
- Infertility (from interruption of the menstrual cycle)
- Anemia
- Malnutrition
- Loss of muscle mass
- Depression
- Imbalances of electrolytes (sodium, potassium, and other minerals)

Binge eating also increases the risk of obesity, heart disease, diabetes, and colon cancer. The most common types of eating disorders are binge eating, anorexia, and bulimia.

Binge Eating Disorder

Overeating is common in the United States, where the food supply is abundant and meals are a time to socialize with family and friends. But some people overeat compulsively, frequently consuming huge amounts of food in secret. These people have a binge eating disorder. Binge eating also occurs in another eating disorder called bulimia (see next article), but people with bulimia typically purge their body of food—usually by self-induced vomiting—after they eat. Purging is not a part of binge eating disorder. Binge eating is probably the most common of all the eating disorders. An estimated 2 percent of the adult American population—about 4 million people—may have a binge eating disorder, which affects more women than men.

The causes of binge eating are unclear, although about half of all people with the disorder also struggle with depression (see page 709). Many people who binge eat report feeling angry, bored, unhappy, or anxious right before an episode of bingeing. Doctors think that affected people may have more difficulty controlling their impulses than other people. Inherited tendencies or brain chemical interactions also seem to contribute to the development of binge eating.

Binge eaters face a number of health risks, especially if they are obese. These risks include diabetes, high blood pressure, elevated cholesterol levels, gallbladder problems, heart disease, and some types of cancer.

Symptoms

People with a binge eating disorder are typically overweight, although their weight may fluctuate. They engage in regular episodes of overeating in which they consume unusually large amounts of food in a short period of time. They eat quickly, even after feeling full, until they feel uncomfortable. They tend to prefer junk foods that are high in carbohydrates and fat. Binge eaters usually eat alone because they don't want anyone to see how much food they are consuming. Afterward, they often feel guilty, depressed, and angry with themselves for having eaten so much food. They may periodically try to diet to lose the excess weight, but either the diet fails or they soon gain the weight back.

Some people are so obsessed with binge eating that they miss work, school, or social events so they can overeat at home alone. They may reach a point at which they avoid social situations completely because they are so ashamed of their overeating. Many binge eaters have depression.

Diagnosis

A doctor can diagnose binge eating by listening to a person's description of his or her feelings and behavior and eating habits.

Treatment

Binge eaters think that losing weight will help them feel better about themselves, but the treatment for binge eating focuses on the binge eating rather than weight loss. Some psychotherapeutic methods have proven successful in treating this disorder. Cognitive-behavioral therapy can help a person learn to change his or her negative thoughts and abnormal eating patterns into more positive, healthy thoughts and behaviors.

Interpersonal psychotherapy can help binge eaters look at their relationships with family members and friends to find ways to improve their social interactions and relationships. Self-help groups offer a source of encouragement and allow people to share useful information and their experiences and ways of overcoming their problem. Some people with a binge eating disorder may also benefit from antidepressant medications (see page 712) if depression is a factor. Working with a registered dietitian, binge eaters can develop a sensible eating plan that emphasizes healthy foods, along with a program of regular exercise to help them lose weight gradually and keep it off.

Anorexia and Bulimia

Anorexia nervosa is a life-threatening eating disorder whose distinguishing features are self-starvation and excessive weight loss. People with anorexia have an irrational fear of gaining weight and a distorted perception of their appearance, believing that they are fat when, in reality, they are extremely thin. They are at a much lower weight than the healthy weight for their height, body type, and level of activity. They consider being thin a unique achievement that gives them some control over at least one part of their lives. Anorexia can cause permanent physical and psychological problems, including the bone-thinning disorder osteoporosis, infertility, heart attack, and depression.

Anorexia most often starts between the ages of 12 and 25 years and affects women and girls more frequently than men and boys. About 10 percent of people with anorexia are male. Doctors think that this gender disparity reflects the intense pressure society places on women to be thin. Roughly 1 percent of adolescent girls have anorexia.

Bulimia nervosa also is a serious disorder that can be life-threatening. Bulimia is characterized by a secretive cycle of binge eating and then purging the body of the food, usually by self-induced vomiting. People with bulimia consume massive quantities of food in a short period of time, ignoring feelings of fullness. During binges, they often feel that their eating is out of control. Such binges make the person worry about gaining weight and trigger the need to compensate by eliminating the food from the body through vomiting or using laxatives (drugs that eliminate solid wastes from the body) or diuretics (drugs that eliminate water from the body). They may often fast, exercise excessively, or use diet pills. Like people with anorexia, people who have bulimia are acutely aware of their body weight and shape. Four percent of all college-age women have bulimia, and half of all people who have anorexia also develop bulimia.

A combination of factors is responsible for the development of anorexia or bulimia, and any given factor may be more or less important for a particular person. The following are the most significant contributing factors:

● **Biological** Eating disorders sometimes run in families, and family members of people with eating disorders have a high risk of developing one themselves. For example, a person whose mother or sister has anorexia is 12 times more likely than average to have the disorder. Over time, the disordered eating pattern changes the person's brain chemistry, producing euphoric feelings that reinforce the eating disorder.

● **Psychological** Some personality types, such as perfectionists, are more prone to having anorexia. People with anorexia have certain shared characteristics. They tend to be conscientious and hardworking. They are good students or employees who try to please, seek approval, and avoid conflict.

In spite of this, they often feel inadequate and powerless, and try to take control of their lives by controlling what they eat. Affected adolescents sometimes fear growing up and taking on adult responsibilities.

● **Family-related** The families of some people with anorexia or bulimia may be overprotective and inflexible. Some families may overvalue physical appearance or make disparaging remarks about their children's looks. Girls seem especially sensitive to critical comments from their father.

● **Social** Dieting is the No. 1 activity that puts a person at risk for anorexia. Media messages that equate success and popularity with thinness encourage excessive dieting and weight loss, especially in women and girls.

● **Environmental** Anorexia or bulimia may begin when a vulnerable person responds to a difficult transition—such as enrolling in a new school, starting a new job, getting married or divorced, or breaking up with a boyfriend or girlfriend—by losing an excessive amount of weight or bingeing and purging.

Treatment of eating disorders can save a person's life. Untreated, anorexia can be fatal. The earlier anorexia and bulimia are treated, the more successful the treatment is likely to be. The recovery rate for people with bulimia is 80 percent when treatment begins within the first 5 years of illness. When treatment is delayed more than 15 years, the recovery rate falls to 20 percent.

Symptoms
Both anorexia and bulimia are characterized by a distorted body image and abnormal eating habits. Many of the symptoms of these disorders are distinct, although many are common to both.

Anorexia
People with anorexia display strange eating habits, including eating in ritualistic ways, chewing food and spitting it out, and shopping and cooking for others while refraining from eating. They may mentally divide foods into good and bad groups, eating only the foods they consider good and eliminating whole categories of foods, such as fat, red meat, or sugar. They often feel superior to people who don't eat the "right" foods. They may also be depressed, irritable, argumentative, or withdrawn.

They may spend a significant amount of time inspecting their body in a mirror. Some people with anorexia exercise compulsively and excessively. They may engage in irrational thinking ("If I don't eat this, I'll feel better."). As their weight drops, women stop menstruating; adolescent girls may not begin to menstruate, a sign of delayed puberty (see page 448). Hormonal changes may produce downy hair growth on their face, arms, and body.

Bulimia

In contrast to people with anorexia, people who have bulimia have problems with impulse control. In addition to binge eating and then purging the food, people with bulimia may engage in risky behavior. For example, they may shoplift or binge-shop, be sexually promiscuous, or abuse drugs or alcohol. Their weight may be normal or even above normal. Many have underlying feelings of depression, loneliness, shame, or emptiness, although, on the surface, they appear confident and are often fun to be with. Like people with anorexia, many people with bulimia tend to be overly dependent on their families.

Repeated vomiting can rupture the esophagus (the muscular tube that connects the throat to the stomach) and make the salivary glands swollen, which make the cheeks puffy. The backs of the front teeth may be damaged by frequent exposure to regurgitated stomach acid. Some people with bulimia have scars or calluses on the backs of their hands from rubbing them against their teeth when they induce vomiting.

Diagnosis

Getting a person to recognize that he or she has an eating disorder can be extremely difficult. Many affected people deny that they have a problem. If you know someone who has anorexia or bulimia, or if you think you may have one of these disorders, get help right away. The earlier treatment begins, the more successful it can be.

After performing a thorough physical examination to rule out another illness and taking a health history (see page 130), including a family health history, a doctor can usually diagnose an eating disorder by listening to the person's description of his or her symptoms and evaluating his or her weight and body fat.

Treatment

Once anorexia or bulimia is diagnosed, the doctor must determine whether the person is so ill that he or she needs to be hospitalized. Conditions that justify hospitalization include excessive and rapid weight loss, severe dehydration that could affect the heart or kidneys, or depression (especially if the person talks about suicide). Whether the person is in the hospital or in outpatient care, a team of specialists will work together to help him or her overcome any emotional problems. If the person is underweight, they will try to bring his or her weight up to normal. Treatment usually combines some form of psychotherapy (usually cognitive-behavioral therapy; see page 710) with antidepressant medication (see page 712). A registered dietitian may provide nutritional counseling.

Psychotic Disorders

P sychotic disorders are mental disorders in which a person loses touch with reality, experiences unusual perceptions (hallucinations), and holds false beliefs called delusions. Psychotic disorders alter a person's thought patterns and reactions to others so severely that he or she undergoes a dramatic change in personality and begins behaving irrationally. These disorders are characterized by the presence of two prominent symptoms: delusions and hallucinations. In most cases, the person does not realize that the hallucinations are not real.

Different types of medical conditions—including brain tumors (see page 682), stroke (see page 669), Huntington disease (see page 969), multiple sclerosis (see page 696), epilepsy (see page 686), migraine (see page 684), thyroid disorders (see page 901), and low blood sugar—can cause psychotic symptoms. Sometimes, psychotic symptoms result from drug abuse or exposure to a poison, or are side effects of a prescribed medication.

Schizophrenia

Schizophrenia is a disorder of the brain that causes alterations in a person's perceptions (hallucinations) and fixed, false beliefs formed with no proof (delusions). A person with schizophrenia may have disorganized speech, catatonia (abnormal movements and posture or lack of movement), and limited emotional expressiveness. Schizophrenia is responsible for severe disruptions in personal relationships, work or school performance, and self-care. Symptoms usually appear between late adolescence and age 25 for men and between ages 25 and 35 for women. The disorder may be lifelong, but episodes tend to recur at times of emotional stress.

Doctors think that schizophrenia may to some extent be inherited. It also may result from brain damage that occurs during fetal development or in early childhood. An increased risk for schizophrenia has been linked to such factors as malnutrition or exposure to an infection such as influenza before birth, complications of birth, or a brain infection (such as encephalitis; see page 694) or neurological disorder early in life. For unknown reasons, schizophrenia is more common among people who live in the inner city than in people who live in rural areas.

Symptoms

For most people with schizophrenia, an episode begins with a gradual or, occasionally, sudden withdrawal from daily activities. The content of the person's speech may become increasingly vague, and he or she may seem unable to follow a simple conversation. An acute episode can occur unexpectedly, but often the onset is so gradual that it is difficult to know exactly when psychotic symptoms appear. Initial symptoms may include disconnected remarks accompanied by blank looks. In early phases of schizophrenia, a person may have symptoms that mimic bipolar disorder (see page 715). However, as schizophrenia progresses, the person becomes unusually detached from other people.

People who have schizophrenia often believe that others can hear and "steal" their thoughts. They frequently have delusions, ranging from a single idea (such as believing that a family member is an impostor) to complex systems of related beliefs (such as believing that the CIA and FBI have been taken over by extraterrestrials, who are controlling everyone). Sometimes they fear they have lost control of their body movements and thoughts, as if they were puppets. They frequently hear voices, often hostile ones. Less often, they have hallucinations of unusual physical sensations, such as feeling that they have been poisoned or otherwise attacked by someone. They may express exaggerated feelings of happiness, bewilderment, or despair, or inappropriately laugh at sad moments or cry for no reason. Other common symptoms include unpredictable agitation, inappropriate sexual behavior, a neglected appearance, and difficulty performing the activities of daily life.

Diagnosis

If you suspect that someone in your family has schizophrenia, try to get him or her to see a doctor, although this may not be easy. If your loved one seems to go out of control, try to stay with him or her to prevent self-destructive behavior until help arrives. People who exhibit the symptoms of schizophrenia may be admitted to a hospital for a preliminary period of observation. In the hospital or at the doctor's office, a doctor will perform a physical examination, order relevant tests, and ask you questions about the person's behavior to rule out any physical disorders that might be contributing to the person's behavior. For a diagnosis of schizophrenia to be confirmed, the person must show signs of the disorder for at least 6 months and have at least one display of delusions, hallucinations, or significant abnormalities in thinking.

Treatment

Treatment of schizophrenia usually involves the use of medications, psychotherapy (see page 710), and rehabilitation. Severe cases are treated in a hospital. The person is given antipsychotic medication (see page 713) to reduce the hallucinations and delusions. As the symptoms gradually subside, doses of the medication are usually reduced, although some people need long-term medication therapy. They may take medication by mouth daily or be given an injection every 2 to 4 weeks to ensure that they are getting the medication. Injections are usually given to people with schizophrenia who fail to take their medication consistently and correctly.

As soon as the person's symptoms are controlled by medication, he or she starts psychotherapy. Techniques of psychotherapy vary, but the goal is the same—to help the person and his or her family understand the emotional factors that can worsen the effects of schizophrenia.

The final stage of treatment is rehabilitation, which helps recovering people regain their normal behavior patterns. In the early stages of hospital treatment, people with schizophrenia are generally given increasingly complex tasks that eventually approximate the routine demands of life. People with schizophrenia often benefit from assistance from community care centers once they are released from the hospital. Many people recover from an episode of schizophrenia enough to return to relative independence. But further episodes may occur, especially if the person does not take the medication as prescribed. In some people, schizophrenia becomes long term. However, most people with schizophrenia do well if they take their prescribed medication regularly and if their family is involved and supportive.

Delusional Disorder

Delusional disorder is a form of mental illness in which a person develops a persistent belief that seems very real to him or her but is not shared by others. The delusion usually is about a situation in the person's life, such as being deceived by a spouse. Apart from the delusion, the person functions normally; a person with delusional disorder does not have the incoherent speech, altered mood, or auditory hallucinations (such as hearing voices) that are characteristic of schizophrenia. Delusional disorder affects men and women equally and tends to appear in midlife, although it can occur at a younger age. The disorder is more common in people who have a family history of schizophrenia and in those diagnosed with a personality disorder (see page 722). For unknown reasons, the incidence of delusional disorder also is higher among people with impaired hearing or sight and among refugee populations and minorities. In vulnerable people, the disorder can be triggered by stress or alcohol or drug abuse.

Symptoms

The prominent symptom of delusional disorder is a false belief about some aspect of a person's personal life. Such delusions usually fall into specific categories, including:

- Being persecuted
- Having a serious medical condition or physical defect

- Believing that a spouse or sex partner is unfaithful
- Believing that a celebrity or person of higher status loves him or her
- Having a special, undiscovered talent, power, or knowledge

Some people have more than one type of delusion. In all other aspects of their life, people with delusional disorder seem relatively normal, although they are often described as cold and aloof. They easily become argumentative and uncompromising, especially when confronted with their erroneous beliefs. Problems may arise when the person decides to act on his or her belief—for example, by stalking an imagined lover or suing someone the person thinks is ruining his or her reputation. People with delusional disorder are only rarely violent or dangerous, but may be perceived as such because they are often angry.

Diagnosis

No test is available that can diagnose delusional disorder. Doctors diagnose the disorder when a person has had the delusional beliefs for at least 3 months and does not have any psychotic symptoms such as hallucinations or other thought abnormalities that would indicate schizophrenia.

Treatment

It can be very difficult to bring a person with delusional disorder in for treatment because he or she will vigorously deny any need for help. The best way to persuade an affected person to seek treatment is to suggest that he or she get help for depression or anxiety instead of for the delusion. Hospitalization usually is not necessary—in fact, it may increase the person's distrust and feelings of persecution. Antipsychotic drugs are the primary treatment for delusional disorder and usually are taken indefinitely. Psychotherapy may be helpful, especially with a supportive therapist who can help the person see how his or her delusional beliefs create problems in his or her life. Group therapy is not recommended for people with delusional disorder because other people usually don't share their beliefs. With treatment, some people with delusional disorder recover fully, and others experience episodes of delusions alternating with periods of normalcy. Others remain delusional even with treatment.

Developmental Disorders

Attention deficit and other developmental disorders are not as well understood as many other diseases. These disorders are thought to be caused by a combination of factors that can affect the development of the brain—including genes, exposure during fetal development to drugs taken by the mother, abnormal development of the brain, or brain injuries at birth or during early childhood.

Attention Deficit Disorders

Attention deficit disorder (ADD) and attention deficit hyperactivity disorder (ADHD) are developmental brain disorders characterized by distinctive and consistent behaviors, including inattentiveness, distractibility, impulsiveness, and, in the case of ADHD, hyperactivity (excessive movement or restlessness). The official diagnosis of the condition is ADHD, but three subtypes are medically recognized—predominantly inattentive, predominantly hyperactive/impulsive, and a combined type. Boys and men more frequently have the hyperactive type of attention deficit disorder; girls and women more often have the inattentive form.

About 4 to 6 percent of the US population have an attention deficit disorder. Although the popular conception is that the condition affects only children, an attention deficit disorder can extend into adulthood. One half to two thirds of affected children continue to have problems as adults. The characteristic behaviors usually appear before age 7 and are much stronger than the normal distractibility and impulsiveness that are common in childhood.

Attention deficit is not a new disorder—its characteristic behaviors have been recognized since the early 1900s. In the past, many people with the condition were diagnosed with minimal brain damage. Although the underlying causes of the neurologic problem remain unknown, doctors now think that abnormal brain development or an imbalance in brain chemicals causes an attention deficit disorder. This means that the inattention, impulsiveness, and hyperactivity that are characteristic of an attention deficit disorder have a physical cause in the brain. The common beliefs that ADD and, especially, hyperactivity result from such lifestyle habits as consuming too much sugar or watching too much TV, or from food allergies are not supported by scientific evidence. The disorder seems to run in families, which indicates a genetic component.

Symptoms

People with the inattentive form of ADHD most often have the following symptoms:

- Making careless mistakes and paying little attention to detail
- Not listening when spoken to directly
- Failing to follow instructions
- Trouble finishing tasks
- Being disorganized
- Absentmindedness and forgetfulness; losing or misplacing things
- Becoming distracted by noise

People with the hyperactive form of ADHD exhibit the following symptoms:

- Fidgeting or squirming
- Difficulty engaging in quiet activities, such as reading
- Constant, driven activity
- Excessive talking
- Difficulty waiting their turn
- Making blunt comments or blurting out answers
- Interrupting

If you think you or your child has an attention deficit disorder, see a doctor for a thorough evaluation. For effective treatment, it is essential to get an accurate diagnosis, which is not always easy.

Diagnosis

To make an accurate diagnosis of ADHD, a doctor will try to gather as much information as possible to rule out other possible causes of the problem behavior. He or she will evaluate the person's health history and perform a physical and neurological examination. Laboratory tests also may be done to rule out other disorders that can mimic ADHD, such as hyperthyroidism (see page 901), pinworms (see page 444), a brain tumor (see page 682), or a sleep disorder such as restless legs syndrome (see page 705). In making a diagnosis for a child, the doctor probably will interview the parents, the child, and the child's teachers and may want to examine school records to put together a profile of the child's behavior. The doctor will then compare the child's behavior to the classic symptoms of ADHD to reach a diagnosis.

Treatment

The most common treatment for an attention deficit disorder is the drug methylphenidate, a central nervous system stimulant. It may not seem logical to prescribe a stimulant for a disorder whose distinguishing feature is hyperactivity, but the drug is effective in calming agitated behavior in children who have an attention deficit disorder. The exact way the drug works is unknown, but the medication seems to affect the chemical dopamine in the brain, which helps in the regulation of attention and concentration. Appetite loss and insomnia are the two most prominent side effects of the medication. Methylphenidate is safe for children over age 6, but it can be addictive when taken in higher-than-prescribed doses.

Another commonly prescribed drug for ADHD is a combination of two different stimulant drugs—dextroamphetamine and amphetamine. This combined drug has a longer duration of action than methylphenidate. However, the drug has a high risk of abuse and addiction. Side effects are similar to those of methylphenidate.

Antidepressants such as bupropion and atomoxetine have also been found to be an effective treatment for some people with ADHD. It is not known exactly how these drugs work, but they seem to influence the absorption of chemical messengers in the brain (especially serotonin and norepinephrine) that help regulate attention, impulsivity, and activity. Because these medications are not stimulants and are not addictive, doctors can prescribe them for longer periods.

Drug therapy works best when combined with other types of treatment. Behavior modification teaches an affected person how to change his or her behavior to better control such tendencies as impulsiveness and disorganization. The person receives praise and rewards each time he or she performs in the desired way. Social-skills training can also help change socially inappropriate behaviors, such as not waiting for a turn or expressing anger or impatience. In psychotherapy, people with ADHD can explore, with their therapist, ineffective patterns of behavior and learn how to change them. Parents of

children with ADHD also may benefit from training that teaches them how to manage their child's behavior more effectively. The family can also join a support group to learn coping skills.

Most people do not outgrow an attention deficit disorder, but can learn to adapt by developing their natural strengths and abilities and transforming their behaviors into more socially acceptable ones. For example, physical exercise and sports are good outlets for a person with hyperactivity, and working on more than one project at a time enables a person with a short attention span to focus on a number of subjects or tasks.

Autism

Autism is a developmental disorder of the brain and nervous system that usually appears during the first 3 years of life and causes lifelong emotional and behavior problems. Autism affects 1 in every 500 people in the United States and, for unknown reasons, the incidence is increasing. Boys seem to be affected about four times as often as girls.

Living with a child who has autism presents daunting challenges to the family. These challenges are further complicated by the fact that children with autism can have multiple mental or emotional disorders—such as impulse-control disorders, psychosis, obsessive-compulsive disorder (see page 720), anxiety disorders (see page 718), or mental retardation—at the same time. Affected children sometimes also have a seizure disorder (see page 686).

Medical researchers are working hard to find the cause of autism. The biological differences in the brain structures of affected people and the fact that autism and related disorders seem to run in families point to a possible genetic influence. No specific gene for the disorder has yet been discovered, but scientists believe that a number of genes may be involved. Other research is examining the possibility of an environmental cause. Doctors do know that autism is not caused by bad parenting or bad choices made by the child about how to behave. There is no scientific evidence to support the theory that autism is linked to a vaccine.

Symptoms

Although children may be affected by the disorder from birth, they often have only subtle symptoms in the first year. Some children with autism seem to develop normally for the first 2 years of their life, acquiring language and other skills at the normal time, only to lose the acquired skill suddenly. Children who have autism usually have an impaired ability to interact socially. They appear indifferent and remote, often avoiding eye contact and not responding to their name. They give the impression that they are completely unaware of how their difficult behavior affects other people, a feature often described by parents as being "walled off."

Autistic children have trouble interpreting other people's tone of voice and facial expressions, so they cannot respond appropriately to verbal and nonverbal cues. Most children with autism start talking later than usual, and tend to express themselves in a singsong manner. Their conversation is on a limited range of topics, and they seldom interact with their listener. Children with autism often respond abnormally to sounds they hear and to being touched. They sometimes resist being held or cuddled. Changes in routine can be extremely upsetting to them.

In the most severe cases of autism, children engage in unusual, repetitive behavior, such as rocking or hair twisting. They may injure themselves by biting themselves or banging their heads repeatedly. They can also become extremely aggressive toward other people. Some children with autism have normal intelligence, while others appear to have below-average intelligence, including mental retardation.

Diagnosis

Autism is often not diagnosed until after the child's second birthday because parents may not notice any developmental impairment until then. To make a diagnosis of autism, doctors usually rely on interviews with the child and parents, careful observation of the child for the characteristic symptoms of the disorder, and a review of the results of the child's previous physical and neurological examinations. There are no medical tests for diagnosing autism, although doctors may order tests to rule out other disorders. The child may have tests that evaluate his or her brain, such as an electroencephalogram (EEG; see page 687), a CT scan (see page 112), or an MRI (see page 113). Genetic tests are also sometimes done to rule out other disorders.

Treatment

There is no cure for autism and no single treatment is effective for all autistic children, but a combination of early intervention programs, special education, family support, and medication can improve the behavior and functioning of affected children and adults. Educational programs for the affected child stress the development of communication and social skills. To help an autistic child reach his or her full potential, parents and siblings are taught behavior training, how to maintain structure in the home, and how to cope with the stresses and challenges of having an autistic child.

Doctors may prescribe some medications for specific symptoms. For example, drugs used to treat anxiety, depression, and psychosis sometimes have a calming effect on a child with autism. Stimulant drugs used to treat hyperactivity may help reduce the frenzied activity sometimes displayed by autistic children.

Addictions and Abuses

Substance abuse poses a threat to both the user and to society. Drug abuse decreases productivity in school and on the job and impairs judgment, increasing the risk of injury. Substance abuse also raises the risk of illness and death from overdose or from serious medical conditions, such as liver damage and some cancers.

This section covers the abuse of and dependence on alcohol and other drugs—both prescription and illegal. It also discusses the abuse of such substances as common household products used as inhalants, often by grade-school children. Although the nicotine found in tobacco products is also highly addictive, it is discussed in another section (see page 27). While not a true addiction, compulsive gambling is a serious and growing problem in the United States and, for this reason, is included in this section.

Alcohol Abuse and Alcohol Dependence

Alcohol abuse is the most serious and most common form of substance abuse in the United States. Regular social drinking can quickly turn into problem drinking and, even if the drinking causes no difficulties at home or at work, it can seriously harm a person's health. Alcoholism, also called alcohol dependence, is a chronic (long-term) disease characterized by a strong craving for and physical dependence on alcohol.

Alcohol dependence is not the only type of alcohol problem. Alcohol abuse can be just as damaging. A person who abuses alcohol may not be dependent on it, but may still drink enough to adversely affect his or her health. Binge drinking—defined as having more than five drinks in a row (for males) or four drinks in a row (for females)—engaged in by many college students, is an example of alcohol abuse that can occur with or without dependence.

The risk of developing alcoholism is inherited, but lifestyle factors also play a role. Peer pressure, the ready availability of alcohol, whether your spouse or partner drinks, and your stress level all contribute to your risk for alcoholism. However, having an inherited tendency to become dependent on alcohol doesn't necessarily mean you will develop a drinking problem. Conversely, not having a family history of alcoholism does not guarantee that you will not develop a problem.

Alcohol abuse and dependence occur in people of every race, gender, and nationality. About 1 in 13 adults—nearly 14 million people nationwide—either abuses alcohol or is dependent on alcohol. Alcohol problems affect men more often than women, but alcohol's intoxicating effects occur more quickly in women, and alcohol damages a woman's health more quickly. Alcohol's harmful effects on the liver also occur earlier in women than in men. Young adults ages 18 to 29 have problems with alcohol at higher rates than do people over 65. However, some older people begin drinking out of loneliness or after losing a loved one. People who also take medications that can interact with alcohol can develop serious health problems.

Heavy drinking (the consumption of more than two drinks a day for men and more than one drink a day for women) can cause the following health problems:

- **Cardiomyopathy** Damage to the heart that can lead to congestive heart failure (see page 570).
- **Liver disease** Scarring of the liver (cirrhosis; see page 790) and alcoholic hepatitis, which is inflammation of the liver.
- **Pancreatitis** Inflammation of the pancreas (see page 799).
- **Cancer of the mouth, throat, and voice box** The risk of developing these cancers rises significantly in people who also smoke.
- **Vitamin deficiencies** Not eating a nutritious diet can cause vitamin deficiencies, which can damage the brain, heart, and nerves.
- **Nerve damage** This damage occurs primarily in the nerves of the arms and legs.
- **Brain damage** Excessive alcohol intake is toxic to brain cells; the death of brain cells can lead to dementia.

WARNING!

Some People Should Never Drink

For most adults, drinking moderate amounts of alcohol (two drinks a day for men and one drink a day for women) poses little health risk and, doctors believe, may even be beneficial. But some people should never drink alcohol. Do not drink if you:

- Are pregnant or are trying to become pregnant (alcohol can seriously harm a developing fetus).
- Plan to drive or use high-speed machinery (alcohol can impair your judgment and slow your reactions).
- Take certain over-the-counter or prescription drugs such as some antianxiety medications (see page 713),

antidepressants (see page 712), or antiseizure drugs, which can interact with alcohol and cause problems.

- Have health problems (such as liver disease) that could be made worse by drinking. Ask your doctor if you have a condition that could be worsened by drinking.
- Are a recovering alcoholic (which puts you at risk of a relapse).
- Are under age 21 (because your brain and nervous system are still developing and could be harmed by excessive alcohol intake).

Heavy drinking also increases a woman's risk of the bone-thinning disorder osteoporosis (see page 989) and possibly breast cancer (see page 857). Alcohol's tendency to loosen inhibitions can make you more likely to engage in risky behaviors such as driving while intoxicated or having unprotected sex. Women who drink even small amounts of alcohol during pregnancy risk harming their fetus; fetal alcohol syndrome (see page 409) is the most common preventable cause of mental retardation in the United States.

Symptoms

People who are dependent on or addicted to alcohol have a strong need or compulsion to drink that cannot be overcome by willpower. If they do not have access to alcohol, they experience severe withdrawal symptoms, including nausea, sweating, tremors, and anxiety. They often feel that they are not able to limit or control their drinking once they start. In addition, their tolerance for alcohol increases and they need to drink increasing amounts of alcohol to feel intoxicated.

Denial is a significant psychological trait of people who are dependent on alcohol. They seldom acknowledge that they have a problem. They also may become depressed, jealous, resentful, or paranoid (unreasonably fearing that other people are hostile or plotting against them). Eventually, they can experience loss of memory and concentration, along with an inability to meet the demands of their job. Physically, alcohol dependence can produce a flushed, veiny face; bruises on the body; a husky voice; trembling hands; and chronic gastritis (inflammation of the stomach; see page 781).

People who abuse alcohol, on the other hand, do not crave alcohol or have withdrawal symptoms when they stop drinking, but they have problems similar to those of people who are dependent on alcohol. They often develop a pattern of drinking that gets them into trouble at work, with their families, or while driving. They may fail to fulfill responsibilities at work, school, or home. They may drive or operate dangerous machinery while intoxicated and may be arrested for driving or assaulting someone while under the influence of alcohol. Problem drinkers also may have blackouts, periods in which they have no memory of what happened during a drinking episode.

Diagnosis

How do you know if you are drinking too much? Your answers to the following four questions can help you find out:

- Have you ever felt you should cut down on your drinking?
- Has anyone ever annoyed you by criticizing your drinking?
- Do you ever feel bad or guilty about your drinking?
- Have you ever had a drink the first thing in the morning to steady your nerves or to get rid of a hangover?

One "yes" answer may indicate that you have a drinking problem. More than one positive response suggests that it is highly likely that you have a problem. If you think that you may have an alcohol abuse or addiction problem, see your doctor right away. He or she will ask you to describe how often and how much you drink and will perform a physical examination to determine the extent to which your drinking has caused any health problems. If necessary, he or she will refer you to an alcohol treatment program.

Q & A

Alcohol and Heart Disease

Q. Is it true that drinking alcohol helps protect against heart disease?

A. Moderate alcohol consumption (two drinks a day for men; one drink a day for women) has been found to lower the risk of heart disease by decreasing the buildup of fatty deposits in the arteries that supply blood to the heart. This buildup of fat in the arteries is a major risk factor for heart disease and stroke (major killers of both men and women). However, in spite of this potentially beneficial effect, you should not start drinking alcohol to prevent heart disease. Alcohol is an addictive substance, and long-term, heavy drinking can contribute to the development of serious health problems, including liver cirrhosis. Overall, the health risks of alcohol consumption outweigh its beneficial effects. You are better off keeping your heart healthy by exercising regularly; eating a nutritious low-fat, high-fiber diet; losing weight if you need to; and quitting smoking if you smoke.

Treatment

Alcoholism cannot be cured, but it can be treated. The type of treatment you receive depends on how serious your alcohol problem is and what treatment programs are available in your community. You may be treated as an outpatient or in a hospital, or a combination of both. You will probably undergo some form of individual or group counseling to help you identify the situations and emotions that trigger your desire to drink so you can learn to avoid them and find other ways of handling stress. Family therapy enlists the support of your family members to encourage you in your recovery.

If you are motivated to stop drinking and are unable to, or if you keep having relapses, your doctor may prescribe a medication, such as disulfiram, that makes you feel ill when you drink alcohol. Some doctors may prescribe a drug called naltrexone to reduce the risk of relapse in some people. If you experience withdrawal symptoms, you will have to undergo detoxification (the process of desensitizing your nervous system to the effects of alcohol). Detoxification is usually done over a period of a week to 10 days in a hospital or treatment center, where your condition can be carefully monitored.

The cornerstone of any treatment regimen is long-term involvement in an alcohol recovery program such as Alcoholics Anonymous. This type of program brings people who are struggling with a drinking problem together where they can give support to and encourage each other to stay sober. But even people who have successfully completed an alcohol recovery program are vulnerable to relapses of drinking. Relapses are common; having a relapse does not mean that you have failed, only that recovery is difficult. To protect your future health and the interests of your family, seek help as many times as you need to, to stop drinking for good.

Drug Abuse and Addiction

Using any drug for a purpose other than that recommended on the label or prescribed by a doctor, or using any drug for nonmedical use, is considered drug abuse. Drug dependence (or addiction) is an uncontrollable physical craving for a drug. Drug abuse and addiction are difficult and serious problems worldwide, and many dangerous drugs that carry the potential for abuse are available both legally and illegally in the United States. Not everyone who takes an addictive drug becomes dependent on it. Some people are more susceptible to drug addiction than others for reasons that include both inherited and environmental factors.

Numerous drugs can cause physical dependence, or addiction, which means that your body gets so used to the substance that it needs the drug just to feel normal. When the drug is not available, you develop severe withdrawal symptoms. Your body eventually builds up a tolerance to a drug that causes dependence, so you must take gradually increasing doses to maintain the enjoyable effects of the drug or to prevent the unpleasant withdrawal symptoms that can develop when you stop using the drug. Most sleeping pills, for example, alter the sleep rhythm so much that, without the drug, a person's sleep becomes disturbed and restless. Withdrawal symptoms from some drugs can be harmful, or even fatal, and withdrawal should be carefully supervised by a doctor.

Many drugs also cause psychological dependence, meaning that they produce such enjoyable sensations that the user feels unable to live without them and is driven to take the drug again and again. The most dangerous drugs have traditionally been alcohol, heroin, and cocaine, but many newer drugs (such as the club drug ecstasy and the prescription pain relievers oxycodone and hydrocodone) can be just as harmful.

People gain access to addictive drugs in a number of ways. Drugs may be prescribed by a doctor to treat a physical or mental disorder, or they may be purchased illegally to provide a high or to avoid or diminish unpleasant feelings or sensations such as pain. Other substances—including household cleaning products, glue, and some substances in aerosol containers—can be used inappropriately to produce a high, especially among preadolescent and adolescent boys (see page 459). Nicotine, found in cigarettes and other tobacco products, is a highly addictive, although legal, drug.

Apart from the obvious risks from the effects of the drugs themselves, abuse carries other serious risks. Users of injected drugs often share needles or fail to sterilize them before use, placing themselves at risk for hepatitis (see page 786), HIV infection (see page 909), and other bloodborne

Prescription Drug Abuse and Addiction

The abuse of prescription drugs is expanding nationwide. An estimated 2 percent of the US population use prescription drugs for nonmedical purposes. The most commonly abused prescription drugs are pain relievers such as oxycodone and hydrocodone, sedatives and tranquilizers such as benzodiazepines and diazepam, and stimulants such as methylphenidate. Many of these drugs are highly addictive, and the longer they are taken—especially at high doses—the more damaging their effects and the more prolonged and difficult the withdrawal.

Some groups of people have a substantially higher risk of abusing or becoming addicted to prescription drugs than others. Doctors prescribe drugs for older people three times as frequently as for the general population. An older person can sometimes receive an inappropriately high dose of a prescription medication (because the body's ability to process medications declines with age), or may mistakenly take higher doses of a drug than prescribed. Commonly prescribed sedatives such as benzodiazepines can increase the risk of falls and vehicle accidents in older people and cause physical dependence after about 4 months.

Adolescents are the No. 1 population group to abuse prescription drugs, especially pain relievers, stimulants, barbiturates, and tranquilizers. Recreational use of the drug methylphenidate, prescribed for attention deficit hyperactivity disorder (ADHD; see page 730), also is on the rise among adolescents and young adults. Oxycodone, often prescribed as a pain reliever for cancer patients, has become a desirable street drug because it produces a long-lasting high. These drugs are usually either bought from a person for whom they were prescribed or stolen and then sold illegally.

Women are far more likely to be prescribed a narcotic or addictive antianxiety drug than are men, although men and women have similar rates of recreational prescription drug use. Also, people who work in the health professions may have an increased risk of prescription drug abuse and addiction because they have easy access to the drugs.

If your doctor gives you a prescription for a drug that can become addictive, ask the doctor if he or she can substitute a medication with a lower potential for dependence. Carefully follow your doctor's instructions to make sure you are taking the correct dose. If you think you may be becoming dependent on a prescription drug, tell your doctor right away so he or she can work with you to gradually stop using the drug and avoid or minimize unpleasant withdrawal symptoms.

---

diseases. The high cost of illegal drugs may lead addicts into crime or prostitution, which poses a high risk for acquiring sexually transmitted diseases (STDs; see page 477). Also, no official agency regulates the purity or strength of illegal drugs. They may be too pure, making them too strong, or they may be combined with toxic substances to increase the quantity. Many people abuse or become addicted to both alcohol and drugs at the same time. No reliable statistics exist on the total number of people who are dependent on drugs in the United States because many addicts obtain their drugs illegally and many never seek treatment.

Symptoms

Each drug produces its own characteristic mental and physical symptoms (see next page). But addiction to any drug is likely to cause a gradual deterioration of a person's work or school performance and attendance, personal relationships, or both. The behavior of drug abusers or addicts is often erratic and their moods may change rapidly, with periods of restlessness and irritability alternating with extreme drowsiness. They also may have loss of appetite and extreme fatigue.

If someone close to you displays some of these symptoms, it does not necessarily mean that he or she is dependent on drugs. But if the person also spends more and more time away from home and always seems to be out of money, the likelihood of drug abuse or dependence is high. People who are addicted to a drug need help, but they are unlikely to seek help themselves unless they are desperate. If you are concerned that you or someone you know has a drug problem, talk to your doctor or a professional at a drug counseling center.

Diagnosis

A doctor can often diagnose a drug problem by listening to a person's description of his or her drug use and its effects on his or her behavior, relationships, and other aspects of his or her life. Laboratory tests to detect drug use include urine drug screens, blood tests, and hair analysis.

Commonly Abused Drugs

The following chart describes the symptoms, effects, and long-term risks of some commonly abused drugs:

Type of Drug	Symptoms	Effects	Risks
Amphetamines Speed or uppers. Prescribed for weight loss, narcolepsy, and attention deficit disorders.	Weight loss, dilated pupils, insomnia, and trembling.	Speed up physical and mental processes.	Psychosis and violent behavior.
Barbiturates Downers. Prescribed as sleeping pills and anticonvulsants.	Slurred speech, confusion, lack of coordination and balance, extreme lethargy, and drowsiness.	Slow down physical and mental processes.	Fatal (from overdose), especially when used with alcohol.
Benzodiazepines Prescribed as tranquilizers or sleeping pills or to reduce anxiety.	Calmness, lethargy, and drowsiness.	Sedate the mind and relax the muscles.	Confusion, coma, and fatal (from overdose).
Cannabis Marijuana and hashish.	Red eyes, dilated pupils, lack of coordination, lethargy, hunger, and mood swings.	Relaxes the mind and body and heightens perception.	Damage to brain, heart, lungs, and reproductive system.
Cocaine Can be snorted, injected, or smoked.	Dilated pupils, trembling, apparent intoxication, agitation, rapid breathing, and elevated blood pressure.	Stimulates the nervous system and produces heightened sensations and sometimes hallucinations.	Ulceration and perforation of nasal passages if drug is snorted, itching (which can lead to open sores), seizures, and abnormal heart rhythms.
Opiates Opium, morphine, heroin, methadone, and synthetic pain relievers such as oxycodone.	Weight loss, lethargy, mood swings, excessive sweating, slurred speech, sore eyes, and drowsiness.	Relieve pain and produce temporary euphoria.	Constipation, infection if drug is injected, absence of periods in women, and fatal (from overdose).
Hallucinogens LSD, mescaline, and psilocybin mushrooms.	Dilated pupils, excessive sweating, trembling, and fever and chills.	Unpredictable. Produce pleasant or frightening hallucinations.	Long-term psychological problems and flashbacks.
Inhalants Fumes from glue, cleaning fluids, or aerosol cans.	Confusion, dilated pupils, flushed face, and unconsciousness.	Produce hallucinations, giddiness, and euphoria.	Damage to brain, liver, or kidneys; and fatal (from suffocation).
Club drugs Ecstasy, GHB (gamma hydroxybutyrate), flunitrazepam, ketamine, and nitrous oxide. GHB, flunitrazepam, and ketamine are known as date rape drugs.	Ecstasy causes confusion, depression, sleep problems, anxiety, paranoia, blurred vision, and fainting. GHB causes lethargy, coma, and seizures. Flunitrazepam causes sleepiness and amnesia. Ketamine impairs motor function and causes delirium and amnesia. Nitrous oxide causes slurred speech and lack of coordination and balance.	Ecstasy stimulates the nervous system and produces hallucinations. GHB depresses the central nervous system. Flunitrazepam has sedative effects. Ketamine produces a dreamlike state and hallucinations. Nitrous oxide dulls the senses and interferes with the absorption of folic acid and vitamin B12.	Ecstasy increases heart rate and blood pressure and causes brain damage. GHB causes coma and seizures. Flunitrazepam is fatal (when mixed with alcohol). Ketamine is fatal (from respiratory failure). Nitrous oxide causes unconsciousness from a depressed nervous system.

Treatment

The treatment for drug addiction usually combines physical detoxification (the process of desensitizing the nervous system to the effects of the drug) with a rehabilitation program. Detoxification is usually done over a period of a week to 10 days in a hospital or treatment center, where your condition can be carefully monitored. At times, a less damaging drug such as methadone is substituted for a more dangerous drug such as heroin. During and possibly after your rehabilitation program, you will participate in group therapy to help you deal with the psychological and social consequences of your past drug use and to show you how to make more positive life choices. To help you stay drug-free over the long term, get involved in an addiction-recovery program such as Narcotics Anonymous.

Pathological Gambling

Legal gambling has become one of the fastest-growing industries in the United States and is more widely accepted than ever before. The proliferation of casinos and state lotteries has generated a steady rise in problem gambling nationwide. Pathological gambling—irresponsible, uncontrolled betting—sometimes is referred to as a gambling addiction but, although it shares some symptoms with alcoholism and substance abuse (see previous article), doctors categorize it as a disorder of impulse control.

Estimates of the number of pathological gamblers in the United States range from 3 million to 10 million. Up to 8 percent of adolescents may be affected. Most problem gamblers are men, but about one third are women. The problem usually begins in adolescence in males and somewhat later in females. Gambling problems affect people in all segments of society but are more prevalent among the poor and the uneducated, perhaps because they see no other way of achieving the affluence they are exposed to around them and in media images.

Problem gambling seems to result from a combination of genetic and environmental factors. Some psychiatrists believe that compulsive gambling is learned behavior that is reinforced by intermittent, random winning, a form of reinforcement known as operant conditioning. This type of conditioning is very difficult to overcome, even when the reward (winning) is removed by losing.

Compulsive gamblers often have other, concurrent mental disorders, including depression (see page 709), panic disorder (see page 719), and substance abuse. Up to 20 percent have attempted suicide. About half of all people who gamble heavily also have an alcohol problem.

Symptoms

The most common characteristics of pathological gambling are:

- A preoccupation with gambling that includes reliving past gambling activities, planning the next bet, or finding ways to obtain money for gambling
- Needing larger bets and more frequent betting to maintain interest, and not being able to quit while ahead
- Lying to family members and friends to conceal problem gambling
- Repeated failed attempts at stopping
- Intolerance of losing, leading to attempts to win back losses
- Restlessness, irritability, and physical symptoms when gambling is unavailable
- Selling personal property or committing illegal acts to finance gambling

Men who have a gambling problem share some personality traits. They are usually highly competitive, energetic, easily bored, easily angered, and seek the approval of others. They also have problems delaying gratification, tend to bend the rules, and rebel against authority. Some pathological gamblers say that they feel secure only when they are gambling, and many construct a dream world in which they fantasize about providing themselves and their friends and family with a luxurious lifestyle as an escape from the difficulties of real life. Women, on the other hand, tend to gamble to escape feelings of depression.

Financial, marital, employment, and legal problems are common among people who gamble heavily. During the periods between gambling sprees, pathological gamblers often experience nervousness, irritability, insomnia, frustration, and indecision, symptoms resembling those of withdrawal from alcohol or drugs.

Diagnosis

Your doctor will ask you about your gambling behavior. If he or she identifies at least four of the characteristics described above, your gambling is likely to be a problem.

Treatment

The recommended treatment for most pathological gamblers is similar to that of alcohol and drug addiction—group therapy in a structured rehabilitation program such as Gamblers Anonymous. Such programs view the gambling problem as a progressive disease and seek to help the gambler face reality in an atmosphere of fellowship and shared experience.

Cognitive-behavioral therapy (see page 710) also has been used with some success to treat pathological gambling by teaching the affected person how to change deeply ingrained patterns of learned behavior and unproductive ways of thinking.

For people who gamble largely to escape their problems—mainly women—the rehabilitation program approach is less successful. Women tend to need more supportive therapy and often require treatment for depression, including antidepressant drugs.

Disorders of the Digestive System

6

Your body needs a regular supply of nutrients to grow, make proteins, replace worn-out or damaged tissue, and supply energy for the thousands of chemical reactions that occur constantly in the body. As it passes through the digestive system, the food you eat is broken down so the bloodstream can absorb nutrients from it. The digestive system consists of the digestive tract (the tube that runs from the mouth to the anus and includes the throat, esophagus, stomach, and intestines) and the digestive glands (which include the liver, gallbladder, and pancreas).

Digestion begins in the mouth, where the teeth tear and chew food into small pieces. The salivary glands produce saliva, which lubricates the food and contains an enzyme (a protein that regulates chemical reactions) that aids digestion by breaking down the starch in food. As you chew your food, the tongue moves it around your mouth and forms it into a ball called a bolus. When you swallow, the bolus enters the esophagus, the section of the digestive tract between the throat and the stomach. Rhythmic contractions of the muscles of the esophagus move the food down the esophagus to the stomach.

After the food enters the stomach, muscles in the stomach wall churn it and mix it with digestive juices (produced in the stomach wall), breaking the food down even more. From the stomach, the food passes through another ring of muscles into the short tube called the duodenum, which makes up the first part of the small intestine.

Waves of contractions from muscles in the walls of the small intestine push the food along. Nearly all nutrients are absorbed in the first part of the small intestine except for vitamin B12, which is absorbed at the very end of the small intestine. Inside the small intestine, the food is broken down by a fluid called bile (which helps make fats easier to digest) and by digestive enzymes. The bile flows from the gallbladder into the small intestine through an opening called the bile duct. The gallbladder contracts, and expels the bile into the small intestine when it is needed. Although the gallbladder stores and concentrates the bile, it does not manufacture it. The liver makes bile, trickling it into the gallbladder through a network of tiny tubes. The enzymes that help bile with digestion in the small intestine come from the pancreas and from the lining of the small intestine itself. The bile and the digestive enzymes reduce the food into microscopic pieces that enable nutrients in the food to get through the lining of the wall of the small intestine and be absorbed into the bloodstream.

The Digestive Process

The digestive system is divided into several sections. Each section has a specific role in the breakdown and absorption of food or in the expulsion of stool. Food moves through the esophagus, stomach, small intestine, large intestine, and rectum by waves of muscular contractions called peristalsis. Digestive enzymes (proteins that speed up chemical reactions) help break down food into pieces small enough to pass through the wall of the small intestine and into the bloodstream.

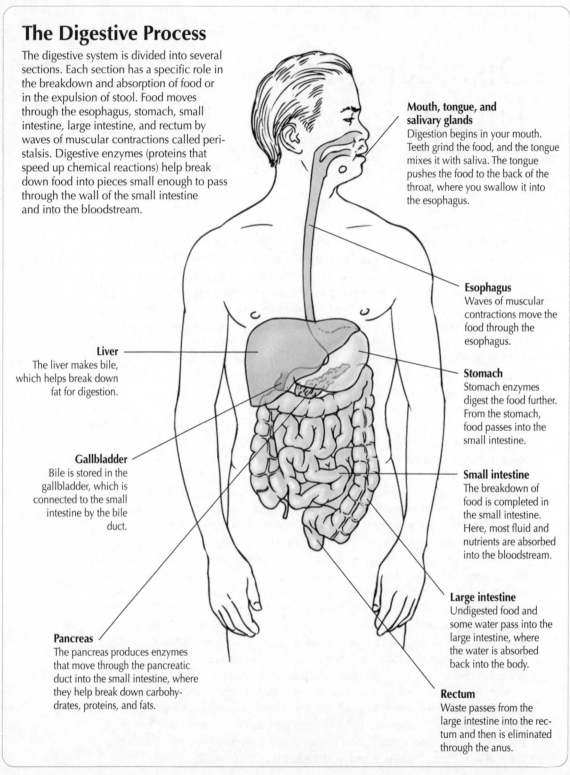

Mouth, tongue, and salivary glands
Digestion begins in your mouth. Teeth grind the food, and the tongue mixes it with saliva. The tongue pushes the food to the back of the throat, where you swallow it into the esophagus.

Esophagus
Waves of muscular contractions move the food through the esophagus.

Stomach
Stomach enzymes digest the food further. From the stomach, food passes into the small intestine.

Small intestine
The breakdown of food is completed in the small intestine. Here, most fluid and nutrients are absorbed into the bloodstream.

Large intestine
Undigested food and some water pass into the large intestine, where the water is absorbed back into the body.

Rectum
Waste passes from the large intestine into the rectum and then is eliminated through the anus.

Liver
The liver makes bile, which helps break down fat for digestion.

Gallbladder
Bile is stored in the gallbladder, which is connected to the small intestine by the bile duct.

Pancreas
The pancreas produces enzymes that move through the pancreatic duct into the small intestine, where they help break down carbohydrates, proteins, and fats.

Once in the bloodstream, nutrients travel to the liver, where some are stored, some are assembled into more complex substances, and some are transported to other parts of the body. The nutrients ultimately are stored in the liquid that surrounds each cell. The cells use the nutrients as needed, pulling them inside their membranes. Once the nutrients are inside a cell, the body sorts them and breaks them down, using some for energy and others to make new tissues and body chemicals such as enzymes.

The remaining food that has not been digested then moves into the colon (the longest section of the large intestine), which absorbs water and a small amount of calcium from the undigested food. Bacteria that are normally present in the colon produce important nutrients for the body; other bacteria digest carbohydrates and starches not absorbed by the small intestine. The rectum, which forms the end of the large intestine, collects the partly solid waste (stool) before it is eliminated from the body through the anus.

Disorders of the Mouth and Tongue

The inside of your mouth is covered with a delicate lining of mucous membrane that is kept moist and lubricated by saliva. Saliva is produced in small glands lining the entire mouth and throat and in three pairs of salivary glands—in the floor of the mouth (the sublingual glands), on each side of the neck below the jaw (the submandibular glands), and above each angle of the jaw (the parotid glands). Your tongue has a complex system of muscles that enables it to move food around as you chew and to mold the food into a ball called a bolus that is small enough to be swallowed. The surface of the tongue is covered with hairlike projections called papillae (known as taste buds). All tongues have creases, but some tongues are more deeply fissured than others. Disorders of the mouth include problems with the lining of the mouth, lips, tongue, and gums.

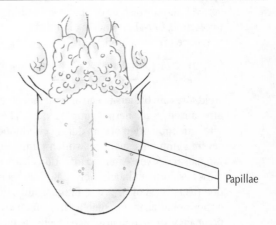

Papillae

The surface of the tongue
The tongue is muscular and flexible and is covered by many projections called papillae (taste buds).

Canker Sores

Canker sores (also called aphthous ulcers or recurrent aphthous stomatitis) are common, noncontagious sores that can develop in the lining of the mouth (and sometimes on the tongue and gums), exposing the sensitive tissue underneath. Canker sores tend to occur when stress, fatigue, or illness has weakened the immune system. The sores occur most frequently in adolescents and young adults and in women just before a menstrual period. Sores can also occur in the mouth as a result of injuries from a toothbrush, a poorly fitting denture, or a jagged tooth, or from biting the inside of the cheek.

Symptoms
You may not know you have a canker sore until you eat something spicy or acidic, which makes the sore sting. Most canker sores are small (up to ¼ inch in diameter), pale yellow spots surrounded by red borders (see page 126). They usually occur singly but may develop in clusters. (Ulcers from an injury are usually large, single sores.) See your doctor about any sore or swelling in your mouth that recurs or that doesn't heal within 2 weeks.

Diagnosis

A doctor usually can diagnose canker sores by the symptoms and their appearance. If the sores persist for more than 10 days, he or she may recommend blood tests and a biopsy (in which samples of cells are taken from the sore and examined under a microscope). It is important to make sure that the sores are canker sores and not a sign of a more serious disease such as inflammatory bowel disease (see page 764) or cancer.

Treatment

Canker sores usually heal without treatment. Over-the-counter medications in the form of gels or lozenges are available that relieve pain and protect the exposed tissue until it heals. Avoid very hot, spicy, or acidic food or drinks. Your doctor may prescribe a mouthwash or ointment containing a corticosteroid, or a short course of oral corticosteroids to reduce inflammation.

Cold Sores

Cold sores are blisters in and around the mouth usually caused by the herpes simplex virus. The initial viral infection often occurs during childhood, with severe symptoms such as swollen gums, extreme fatigue, and fever. After the infection clears up, the virus lies dormant indefinitely. Later, another infection (usually a cold), stress, fatigue, sun exposure, or hormonal changes (such as from menstruation, pregnancy, or menopause) can reactivate the virus. Cold sores are common. The infection is very contagious when blisters are present. Although rare, it is possible to transfer the virus to other parts of your body, such as the genitals (genital herpes, see page 482) or eyes (corneal ulcers, see page 1037).

Symptoms

Some people have a slight tingling sensation of the skin around the mouth before they get a cold sore. The gums may become swollen and red. Once the cold sore appears, the blisters burst and develop into painful sores (see page 126). See your doctor about any sore or swelling in your mouth that recurs or that doesn't heal in 2 weeks.

Diagnosis and Treatment

Doctors diagnose cold sores by their appearance. Mild cases of cold sores usually need no treatment. Applying an ice pack to cold sores for a few minutes at a time often relieves pain. Your doctor may prescribe an antiviral medication such as acyclovir, valacyclovir, or famciclovir for you to take by mouth before the blisters are fully formed. These drugs reduce the rate at which the herpes virus multiplies. For people who have frequent outbreaks, a doctor may prescribe small doses of these medications to take daily to prevent or reduce the frequency of outbreaks.

Oral Thrush

Oral thrush is infection of the mouth with a yeast called Candida albicans. The yeast is one of many microbes that are normally present in the mouth but that are usually kept in check by the helpful bacteria in the mouth. The yeast can multiply to above-normal levels if you have a weakened immune system, if you are taking antibiotics (which kill beneficial bacteria as well as harmful bacteria), or if you are taking inhaled corticosteroids (which can suppress the immune system) for an inflammatory respiratory disorder such as asthma. If a woman has a vaginal yeast infection, her newborn can be exposed during birth and develop oral thrush within a week after birth. Some women who are nursing develop thrush in their nipples (see page 539) and can transmit it to their baby during breastfeeding.

Symptoms

The main symptom of oral thrush is sore, creamy, yellow-white, slightly raised patches in the mouth (and sometimes in the throat). If the patches are rubbed, they become raw and painful. Thrush can also cause denture problems. See your doctor about any sore in your mouth that recurs or that doesn't heal within 2 weeks.

Diagnosis and Treatment

Doctors can diagnose oral thrush by its appearance. Oral thrush is usually treated with a topical antifungal medication or an oral medication such as fluconazole. Your doctor will recommend maintaining good oral hygiene with regular brushing, flossing, and using antiseptic mouth rinses, which may help prevent another infection.

Leukoplakia

Leukoplakia is a disorder in which a portion of the normally soft lining of the mouth thickens, hardens, and turns white, usually over a few weeks. The thickening may be a protective response to repeated injury to the area caused by a rough tooth or a poorly fitting denture or by irritation from tobacco smoke or smokeless tobacco. Some leukoplakia patches can eventually become cancerous. About 5 percent of what are thought to be patches of leukoplakia are actually cancerous tumors (tumors of the mouth and tongue; see page 747). Leukoplakia is especially common in older men who smoke.

Symptoms

A leukoplakia patch can be any size, can be white or gray (see page 126), and is usually painless at first. Later it may become rough and stiff. In advanced stages, the rough patches may develop sores that eventually crack. The open cracks can be sensitive to hot, spicy, or acidic foods. See your doctor about any sore in your mouth that recurs or that doesn't heal within 2 weeks.

Diagnosis

If you have symptoms of leukoplakia, your doctor will first recommend that you stop using tobacco and may recommend that you have a biopsy (in which samples of cells are taken from the affected area and examined under a microscope). He or she may also recommend that you see a dentist to take care of any dental problem that may be causing the irritated patches.

Treatment

The treatment of leukoplakia depends on the cause. If leukoplakia is the result of smoking or using tobacco, your doctor will recommend that you stop immediately. He or she may remove the patches with a laser (a highly concentrated beam of light). If the leukoplakia is the result of a dental problem, your dentist can smooth the tooth or adjust the denture that is causing the irritation.

Oral Lichen Planus

Lichen planus is a skin disorder that can affect the lining of the mouth. Half of all people who have oral lichen planus also have lichen planus of the skin (see page 1071). The cause of lichen planus is unknown, but it seems to be triggered by a weakened immune system. An outbreak usually lasts about 9 months; in rare cases, it can last several years. The disorder occurs most often in middle-aged and older women but can also develop in young people. Less than 5 percent of cases of oral lichen planus develop into cancerous tumors (tumors of the mouth and tongue; see page 747).

Symptoms

The symptoms of oral lichen planus are often unnoticeable and may include only thickening and hardening of the lining of the mouth. In rare cases, symptoms can include small, pale pimples that gradually join to form either a thin, white, lacy network or shiny, red patches of slightly raised tissue (usually on the inside of the cheeks and the sides of the tongue). You may also have a sore mouth and a dry, metallic taste in your mouth. Symptoms can develop suddenly. See your doctor about any sore or swelling in your mouth that recurs or that doesn't heal within 2 weeks.

Diagnosis and Treatment

Doctors usually can diagnose oral lichen planus by its appearance. The doctor may take a sample of tissue from the affected area for examination under a microscope (biopsy) to confirm the diagnosis and to rule out other disorders.

The treatment of oral lichen planus depends on the cause. The symptoms of the disorder can usually be relieved, but the condition itself cannot be cured. Your doctor may prescribe a topical or oral corticosteroid to reduce inflammation or a pain reliever. If the disorder is caused or worsened by a dental problem such as a jagged tooth or a poorly fitting denture, the doctor will recommend that you see your dentist.

Infections of the Salivary Glands

The most common cause of a salivary gland infection is the viral infection mumps (see page 440), but a salivary gland infection can also be caused by bacteria. A persistent salivary gland infection can cause extensive scarring in the affected gland and prevent the gland from producing saliva.

Symptoms

Symptoms of a salivary gland infection include swelling and pain on each side of the neck below the jaw, or above the angle of the jaw. You may have

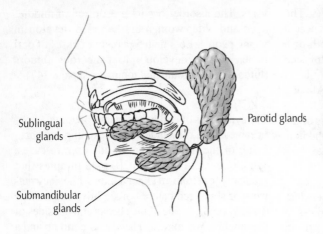

The salivary glands
The mouth contains three pairs of salivary glands: the parotid glands, the submandibular glands, and the sublingual glands. All of the salivary glands secrete saliva, which contains a digestive enzyme that helps break down carbohydrates. Saliva also keeps the mouth moist and lubricates food for swallowing. The parotid glands, the largest salivary glands, are just below and in front of the ears. The sublingual glands lie just beneath the tongue toward the front of the mouth. The submandibular glands lie deeper than the sublingual glands at the back of the mouth and can be felt beneath the jaw.

a bad taste in your mouth from pus discharged by the infected gland. Eating spicy foods or citrus fruits increases the flow of saliva, which can cause swelling if the gland is completely or partially blocked. See your doctor about any swelling in your mouth that recurs or that doesn't heal within 2 weeks.

Diagnosis
If you have symptoms of a salivary gland infection, your doctor will look for swelling, tenderness, and redness in the glands and pus flowing from your salivary ducts. (He or she will massage the glands to see if pus comes out.) If the infection has persisted for a long time, your doctor may recommend a CT scan (see page 112) or order a sialogram, an X-ray of the salivary gland taken after injection of a contrast medium (dye). A sialogram will show the areas of obstruction on X-ray film.

Treatment
Unless the gland is completely blocked, the doctor will probably use lemon juice to stimulate the flow of saliva in the infected gland to flush out the bacteria. He or she will prescribe an antibiotic to treat

the infection and may use probes to try to widen the ducts of the salivary gland to increase the flow of saliva and prevent further infection. If the salivary gland has been irreversibly damaged, your doctor may recommend surgery to remove it.

Stones in the Salivary Ducts or Glands

Salivary duct stones are tiny particles that form when chemicals and salts in saliva collect around a tiny amount of solid material or mucus in the duct of a salivary gland. Stones inside the salivary gland itself are more rare. The stone blocks the duct, preventing saliva from getting through and causing the gland to swell. A persistently obstructed salivary gland duct can cause extensive scarring that reduces the gland's ability to produce saliva. The submandibular glands (on each side of the neck below the jaw) are the most susceptible to blockage. Salivary duct stones most frequently affect middle-aged or older people.

Symptoms and Diagnosis
The main symptoms of a stone in the salivary duct are pain and swelling on each side of the neck below the jaw, above the angle of each jaw, or under the chin, particularly while eating.

To check for a stone in a salivary duct or gland, your doctor may recommend X-rays. If the cause is still not clear, he or she may order a sialogram, an X-ray of the salivary gland and ducts taken after injection of a contrast medium (dye). A sialogram will show the areas of obstruction on X-ray film. In addition, the doctor may recommend a CT scan (see page 112) or ultrasound (see page 111) to help confirm the diagnosis.

Treatment
Salivary duct stones can be removed by a doctor. He or she will try to dislodge the stone by massaging your jaw to widen the salivary duct or by making a superficial cut in the floor of the mouth to allow the stone to pop out. To treat recurring stones, a surgeon can make a permanent opening along the duct to allow saliva to drain into your mouth. Having a permanent opening may help prevent other stones from blocking the duct and can reduce the risk of scarring. If a stone forms inside the salivary gland itself or at the beginning of the duct and causes frequent

infections, your doctor may recommend surgery to remove the entire gland. A procedure called extracorporeal lithotripsy (see page 816) can also be used to direct shock waves at the stones to break them up.

Salivary Gland Tumors

Most tumors in the salivary glands form in the parotid glands (located above the angle of each jaw), although they can form in other salivary glands as well. These tumors usually develop slowly over several years. In some cases, salivary gland tumors become cancerous, especially in the parotid glands.

Symptoms

The main symptom of salivary gland tumors is swelling on either side of the face above the jaw. These tumors seldom cause pain. See your doctor about any swelling in or below your jaw that recurs or that doesn't heal within 2 weeks.

Diagnosis

If you have symptoms of a salivary gland tumor, your doctor may perform an aspiration biopsy to help reach a diagnosis. During an aspiration biopsy, the doctor inserts a small needle into the tumor and uses a syringe to withdraw a small amount of tissue and fluid for examination in the laboratory. A doctor may also order a CT scan (see page 112) or MRI (see page 113) to get a clear image of the tumor.

Treatment

If you have a salivary gland tumor, your doctor will recommend surgery to remove the entire gland, or most of it. If a tumor is cancerous, doctors sometimes recommend radiation therapy (see page 23) to kill any remaining cancer cells. When a submandibular gland is removed, a nerve that controls the lower lip may be injured. During removal of a parotid gland, branches of the facial nerve may be cut, potentially affecting movement on one side of the face and interfering with closing of the eye. However, surgery can often repair any nerve damage.

Tumors of the Mouth or Tongue

Tumors of the mouth or tongue are rare, usually slow-growing, single lumps that may be either benign (noncancerous) or malignant (cancerous; see page 126). A tumor can grow undetected for months and, in rare cases, years. Cancerous tumors of the mouth are rare in people under age 40, except for people who smoke. Oral cancer is most common in people over 60, especially those who smoke cigarettes, pipes, or cigars or who use smokeless tobacco, or who drink alcohol excessively. The risk increases even more when a person both uses tobacco and drinks alcohol excessively.

Symptoms

Both noncancerous and cancerous tumors of the mouth usually start as small, pale, painless lumps. Depending on their size and location, tumors of the mouth may rupture easily and bleed extensively, distort the face, cause fitting problems with dentures and other dental appliances, and make eating, swallowing, and speaking difficult. At first, cancerous tumors of the tongue can make the tongue muscles stiff and difficult to move. A cancerous tumor usually turns into a sore with a hard, raised rim and a fragile center that bleeds easily. The tumor grows and erodes the surrounding area. If a tumor gets very large or is in an awkward location, it can cause pain. See your doctor about any sore or swelling in your mouth that recurs or that doesn't heal within 2 weeks.

Diagnosis

If you have symptoms of a tumor of the mouth or tongue, your doctor will recommend a biopsy (in which samples of cells taken from the tumor are examined under a microscope) to determine if the tumor is cancerous.

Treatment

The treatment of a tumor in the mouth depends on its cause and location. A noncancerous tumor that is not disfiguring or causing problems is usually not treated, although your doctor will check it every 6 months or at least once a year. Any growth or change in a tumor may indicate cancer.

Successful treatment of cancerous tumors depends on the stage of the cancer. Cases that are diagnosed and treated in an early stage are usually cured. If the tumor is in an early stage and the cancer has not spread, a surgeon can remove it. If the tumor is large or has spread, your doctor will order radiation therapy (see page 23), with or without surgery, in combination with chemotherapy (see page 23).

Early diagnosis is more likely to result in treatment that is less disfiguring and less likely to cause speech or swallowing problems. A surgeon can remove disfiguring tumors. If the tumor is on the lips, he or she can reconstruct them. If the tumor is on the gums, special dentures can restore the gums' natural appearance.

Glossitis and Geographic Tongue

Glossitis refers to general inflammation of the tongue. Geographic tongue is a specific inflammatory disorder of the tongue in which the papillae (tiny hairlike projections known as taste buds) are deformed and cover only part of the tongue. Glossitis can result from an infection, an injury, a vitamin deficiency (especially a vitamin B12 deficiency), or an allergic reaction. The cause of geographic tongue is unknown.

Symptoms

In both glossitis and geographic tongue, the tongue is dark red, smooth (a healthy tongue is pink and bumpy) and sore (especially after eating spicy food). Geographic tongue produces a maplike appearance on the tongue, and the pattern changes from day to day. Geographic tongue usually affects smaller areas of the tongue than glossitis, and the symptoms come and go.

Diagnosis and Treatment

A doctor can diagnose geographic tongue by its appearance, but there is no known treatment for the condition. Treating the underlying cause of glossitis, such as an infection or vitamin deficiency, may clear it up. To help relieve soreness, avoid eating hot or spicy food, drinking alcohol, smoking cigarettes, or chewing tobacco.

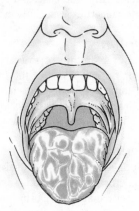

Geographic tongue
In geographic tongue, patches of the surface cells that coat the tongue break down, producing a maplike pattern.

Disorders of the Esophagus

The esophagus is the muscular tube, about 10 inches long, that runs from the back of your throat to your stomach. As you swallow food, the back of your tongue pushes it into the esophagus, the soft palate closes off the passage to the nose, and the flap of tissue (the epiglottis) at the top of the windpipe shuts to prevent food from entering the windpipe and lungs. Contractions of the esophageal muscles move the food down to the base of the esophagus. Muscles at the entrance to the stomach relax to let the food pass through. The lower esophageal sphincter muscle then tightens to prevent food, stomach acid, and digestive enzymes from going back up into the esophagus.

Pharyngeal Pouch

A pharyngeal pouch, also called an esophageal diverticulum, is a rare disorder in which a bulge or sac develops at the back of the throat (pharynx). It usually develops when the upper esophageal sphincter muscle fails to relax. The bundles of muscles spread apart and the muscle lining pushes through, creating an area where food settles during swallowing. As it fills with food, this area stretches and forms a baglike pouch. For unknown reasons, pharyngeal pouches occur most often in middle-aged men. In some cases, a person can inhale fluid and undigested food that has settled in the pouch (especially while sleeping), leading to pneumonia (see page 660).

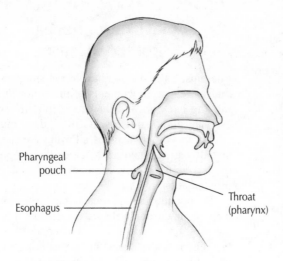

Pharyngeal pouch
A pharyngeal pouch is an abnormal sac that bulges down from the back of the throat.

Symptoms

The symptoms of a pharyngeal pouch include difficulty swallowing and a feeling of swelling in the throat. A person may also cough and have bad breath and a metallic taste in the mouth from regurgitated liquid or undigested food. Some people lose weight because very little food gets into the stomach.

Diagnosis

Your doctor may be able to diagnose a pharyngeal pouch from your symptoms and a physical examination. He or she may recommend a barium X-ray (see page 767) of your throat and esophagus.

Treatment

Some people who have a pharyngeal pouch learn how to empty the pouch into their esophagus by manipulating it with their fingers, by getting into specific positions, or by coughing. If the pouch continues to expand or if you lose weight, your doctor may recommend surgery to remove the pouch.

Indigestion

Indigestion (often called heartburn) is a term used to describe discomfort in the upper abdomen. Some people get indigestion after consuming caffeine or high-fat or acidic foods. Drinking carbonated beverages or wine, beer, or liquor can cause indigestion in some people. Eating too fast or having an exceptionally large meal can also cause indigestion. Some people get indigestion when they are depressed, anxious, or nervous. Pregnant women, heavy smokers, and people who are overweight seem to be most susceptible.

Symptoms

Symptoms of indigestion include a dull, burning, gnawing, or sharp pain in the chest; an uncomfortable or bloated sensation in the abdomen; a sour taste in the mouth; belching; a sensation of butterflies in the stomach; and nausea. If you frequently or repeatedly get indigestion; if symptoms occur suddenly, seem more severe, or do not seem to have an apparent cause; or if you lose your appetite or lose weight for no obvious reason, see your doctor. The symptoms of indigestion can mimic a number of disorders, including a peptic ulcer (see page 755), stomach cancer (see page 757), angina (see page 19), or a heart attack (see page 567).

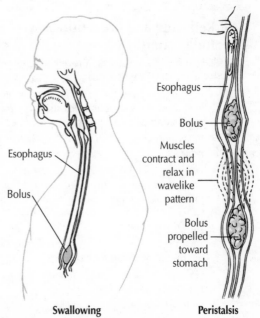

Swallowing   **Peristalsis**

Swallowing
When you swallow, the muscles at the back of your throat push the partially digested food into the esophagus. A circular muscle at the top of the esophagus (the upper esophageal sphincter) relaxes, and the muscles of the throat grasp the bolus of food and push it into the esophagus. With powerful contractions called peristalsis, muscles in the esophagus propel the food down the rest of the esophagus toward your stomach.

Diagnosis

To make sure you don't have anything more serious than indigestion, your doctor will rule out other digestive disorders. He or she may perform a procedure called endoscopy (see page 766) to examine your esophagus and recommend a barium X-ray (see page 767) of your throat and esophagus if you are having trouble swallowing. Other tests may include an ultrasound (see page 111) of the gallbladder and blood tests.

Treatment

The treatment of indigestion depends on the cause. If a doctor has ruled out other disorders, he or she will recommend the measures in the box below. The doctor may also recommend an over-the-counter antacid. If preventive measures or over-the-counter antacids do not relieve your symptoms, your doctor may prescribe a medication to help stop or prevent symptoms.

Relieving and Preventing Indigestion

Take the following steps to prevent indigestion or to help relieve it when it occurs:

- Keep a food diary. Avoid the foods or drinks that seem to cause your indigestion. Different foods affect people differently.
- Relax during a meal and for at least half an hour afterward. Stress can cause indigestion.
- When you eat, breathe through your nose, chew with your mouth closed, and eat slowly to avoid swallowing air along with your food, which can cause bloating and contribute to your discomfort.
- Take small bites and chew your food thoroughly. Good digestion begins in the mouth.
- Stay upright for at least 60 minutes after eating. Avoid late-night eating.
- Don't use aspirin or other over-the-counter pain relievers or caffeine. They can irritate the stomach lining.
- Sleep with your head and shoulders propped up at a 30° angle. Acid production is greatest at night, and gravity helps prevent acid from flowing into the esophagus from the stomach.
- Don't smoke. Smoking encourages the production of stomach acid.

Gastroesophageal Reflux Disease

The muscles at the entrance to the stomach normally prevent the contents of the stomach from moving back up into the esophagus. In gastroesophageal reflux disease (GERD), these muscles relax at inappropriate times, allowing stomach acid and digestive enzymes to enter the esophagus (called acid reflux). Stomach acid can cause inflammation in the esophagus.

The opening to the stomach is controlled by the diaphragm, the dome-shaped muscle that separates the chest from the abdomen. In a condition called hiatal hernia, a weakness in the diaphragm allows part of the upper part of the stomach to protrude into the chest, which can sometimes contribute to the symptoms of GERD. However, a person can have a hiatal hernia and not have any symptoms of GERD (and someone can have severe symptoms of GERD but not have a hiatal hernia).

The chronic inflammation of GERD can lead to ulcers in the esophagus. The chronic inflammation can also cause scarring and narrowing of the esophagus (see page 752). GERD is a common condition, especially in older people, people who are overweight or who smoke, and pregnant women. The chronic inflammation can eventually lead to esophageal cancer (see page 754).

Symptoms

The main symptoms of GERD are increasing pain in the lower part of the breastbone and a burning sensation in the upper abdomen that can extend into the mouth (indigestion; see previous page). The discomfort occurs regularly when your stomach is full or when you change position (such as when you bend over or lie flat). Other symptoms of GERD include belching and an acidic taste in your mouth. Some people may have difficulty swallowing.

Diagnosis

To diagnose GERD, your doctor will probably perform a procedure called endoscopy (see page 766) to examine your esophagus. He or she may also recommend manometry (see next page) to measure changes in pressure in the esophagus that occur during swallowing, and tests to measure the amount of acid in the stomach over 24 hours.

Hiatal hernia

Normally the stomach lies below the diaphragm, the sheet of muscle that separates the chest from the abdomen (right). A hiatal hernia (far right) occurs when part of the stomach protrudes up into the chest through an opening (hiatus) in the diaphragm.

Esophagus

Esophagus

Diaphragm

Stomach

Hiatal hernia

Diaphragm

Stomach

Healthy diaphragm and stomach

Hiatal hernia

Treatment

The treatment of GERD depends on the symptoms. Your doctor may recommend an over-the-counter antacid or prescribe one to neutralize the stomach acid or reduce the amount of acid in your stomach. He or she may also prescribe a medication that increases the speed at which food passes through the stomach and into the intestines. If a hiatal hernia is causing GERD, your doctor may recommend surgery to repair the hernia. Untreated GERD can lead to a rare condition called Barrett's esophagus (a change in the lining of the lower esophagus), which increases the risk of cancer of the esophagus.

Manometry

Manometry is a measurement of pressure. Esophageal manometry measures contractions of the muscular wall of the esophagus to evaluate the functioning of the esophagus. The contractions of the esophagus propel food to the stomach during digestion. In esophageal manometry, a thin, flexible tube that contains pressure sensors is inserted into the nose or mouth, and down the throat into the esophagus. Pressure measurements of the esophagus and of the upper and lower esophageal sphincters are taken while the person swallows water.

Anorectal manometry is used to measure contractions of the rectum and the anal sphincter. In this procedure, a $1/4$-inch flexible tube is inserted 3 to 4 inches into the rectum. Pressure measurements are taken while the rectum and anus are stimulated in various ways such as by moving the tube around in the rectum, inflating a balloon attached to the tube with air or water, or withdrawing the tube.

Preventing Acid Reflux

In addition to the steps recommended on the previous page to prevent indigestion, the following measures can help control GERD or prevent acid reflux:

- Lose weight if you are overweight, which can help reduce abdominal pressure.

- Eat small meals several times a day. When less food is in the stomach, less acid is produced.

- Don't eat late at night or up to 2 hours before going to bed. The stomach produces more acid at night.

- Avoid caffeine and tobacco, which relax the muscle at the bottom of the esophagus.

- In bed, keep your head, neck, and shoulders propped up at a 30° angle. Gravity helps acid flow down and out of the esophagus.

- Don't wear constricting clothing or belts. They can increase pressure inside the abdomen.

- Avoid positions such as lying down or activities such as jogging (especially right after a meal), which can cause acid reflux.

In severe cases, a doctor may recommend a surgical procedure called fundoplication. During this procedure, a section of the upper part of the stomach is pulled up and wrapped around the lower part of the esophagus to make it tighter, limiting the amount of acid that can flow back up into the esophagus.

Esophageal Stricture

Stricture (narrowing) of the esophagus is a common disorder that usually results from an accumulation of scar tissue in the esophagus. A stricture may be both the result and the cause of gastroesophageal reflux disease (GERD; see page 750). Even after treatment, an esophageal stricture caused by GERD can recur.

Symptoms and Diagnosis

Usually the only symptom of an esophageal stricture is difficulty swallowing. To diagnose a stricture of the esophagus, a doctor will order a barium X-ray (see page 767).

Treatment

To treat an esophageal stricture, your doctor will probably refer you to a gastroenterologist (a doctor who specializes in disorders of the digestive system). A gastroenterologist will most likely widen the channel of your esophagus with one of two techniques. In one technique, the doctor inserts a rigid, tapered instrument called a dilator through the stricture and, over a period of days or weeks, widens the channel of the esophagus with a series of increasingly wider dilators. Using an alternate method, the gastroenterologist inserts a lighted viewing instrument called an endoscope (see page 766) into the esophagus and passes a deflated bag or balloon that can be filled with air or water

WARNING!

Food Caught in the Esophagus

In severe cases, food can get stuck in a narrowed esophagus. Because you could inhale it into your lungs, which can be fatal, the food must be removed. If you are choking or you think you may have food stuck in your esophagus, call 911 or your local emergency number or have someone call for you or take you to the nearest hospital emergency department.

through the endoscope. When the bag is inflated, it stretches the tissue at the bottom of the esophagus, opening up the passageway enough to allow food to pass into the stomach more easily. These procedures may require multiple sessions and sometimes must be repeated every 6 months or every year if the symptoms recur. If enlarging the passageway becomes too difficult, surgery may be necessary to remove the scar tissue.

Achalasia

Achalasia is a rare disorder of unknown cause in which the muscle segment between the esophagus and stomach fails to relax after swallowing to permit food to enter the stomach. As a result, food accumulates in the lower part of the esophagus. Eventually other sections of the esophagus muscle are also affected, and the contractions that move food through the esophagus become irregular and uncoordinated. In some cases, as achalasia worsens, a person may inhale food particles (especially while sleeping), which can lead to pneumonia (see page 660).

Symptoms

The main symptom of achalasia is regurgitating food a day or two after eating it. As food accumulates in your esophagus, you may feel discomfort or pain in your chest and have an unpleasant taste in your mouth along with bad breath. At first you will only have difficulty swallowing food, but eventually you will also have trouble swallowing liquids. Because food does not pass into your intestines to be absorbed, you may lose weight and have symptoms of vitamin or mineral deficiencies.

Diagnosis

If you have symptoms of achalasia, your doctor will probably perform a procedure called endoscopy (see page 766) to examine your esophagus to rule out a tumor. Your doctor may also recommend a barium X-ray (see page 767) of your esophagus. Achalasia can be confirmed with a procedure called manometry (see previous page), which measures pressure inside the esophagus to evaluate its contractions. If manometry shows that the muscle at the bottom of your esophagus fails to relax, you have achalasia.

Treatment

To treat achalasia, your doctor will probably refer you to a gastroenterologist (a doctor who specializes in disorders of the digestive system). The gastroenterologist will insert a flexible viewing tube (endoscope) into the esophagus and pass a deflated bag or balloon that can be filled with air or water through the endoscope. When the bag is inflated, it stretches the muscles at the bottom of the esophagus, expanding the opening enough to allow food to pass into the stomach more easily. This procedure carries a risk of perforating the esophagus and usually must be repeated. In some cases, a surgeon will cut some of the muscles at the stomach entrance to open a passageway for food. Although this surgery is sometimes effective, it can increase the risk of gastroesophageal reflux disease (GERD; see page 750).

Esophageal Varices

Esophageal varices are bulging (varicose) veins in the lower part of the esophagus (and sometimes the upper part of the stomach) that usually result from elevated blood pressure in the portal vein, the vein that carries blood from the stomach and intestines to the liver. The increased pressure in the portal vein usually is caused by scarring of the liver from cirrhosis (see page 790). People who have liver damage from uncontrolled hereditary hemochromatosis (see page 961) or a disease such as Wilson's disease (see page 792) are also at increased risk of developing esophageal varices. The veins can widen to the point of rupture, causing bleeding into the esophagus or stomach, which can be fatal.

Symptoms

Symptoms of bleeding from esophageal varices include vomiting blood and passing dark-colored or black stool. The stool is dark from partially digested blood. Some people who have esophageal varices may have other symptoms of liver disease, such as jaundice (yellowing of the skin or whites of the eyes; see page 785). Bleeding can cause a sudden drop in blood pressure, which can lead to shock.

Diagnosis and Treatment

To diagnose esophageal varices, a doctor will perform a procedure called endoscopy (see page

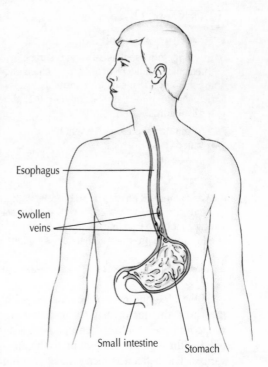

Esophageal varices

Esophageal varices are bulging veins in the walls of the lower part of the esophagus that occur as a result of increased blood pressure in the portal vein, which carries blood from the stomach and intestines to the liver. The condition, which results from liver damage, can be life-threatening if the veins burst and bleed.

766) to examine the veins at the lower end of the esophagus.

If you have esophageal varices, your doctor will prescribe a blood pressure medication such as a beta blocker to lower the pressure in the portal vein. If the varices rupture, you will immediately be admitted to the intensive care unit of the hospital and given a synthetic hormone called octreotide intravenously (through a vein). The hormone decreases pressure in the portal vein and helps reduce the bleeding.

To evaluate the problem, a doctor will pass an endoscope (viewing tube) through your esophagus to the varices. To stop the bleeding, he or she will then either inject a chemical agent through the endoscope into the ruptured vein to cause it to scar or place a rubber band around the vein to seal it off.

If the bleeding cannot be stopped with these measures, the doctor may try inserting an endoscope into the esophagus and passing a deflated balloon through the endoscope to the site of the varices. The balloon is then inflated, putting pressure on the veins in the esophagus and stopping the bleeding. Often, a procedure called transjugular intrahepatic portosystemic shunt (TIPSS) is performed to reroute the portal vein to connect directly to the hepatic vein (which drains blood from the liver), relieving some of the pressure inside the esophagus.

Cancer of the Esophagus

Cancer of the esophagus is rare. But when cancer develops in the lining of the esophagus, the cancer cells multiply rapidly and are likely to spread to other parts of the body. The tumor eventually blocks the passageway to the stomach. Esophageal cancer can be divided into two main types—squamous cell carcinoma and adenocarcinoma. Squamous cell carcinoma develops in the cells that line the esophagus. Because the entire esophagus is lined with squamous cells, squamous cell carcinoma can occur anywhere in the esophagus. Squamous cell carcinoma used to be responsible for 90 percent of all esophageal cancers but now makes up only 50 percent.

Adenocarcinomas usually develop in glandular tissue in the lining of the lower part of the esophagus. Adenocarcinoma can result from tissue changes in the esophagus caused by chronic inflammation from gastroesophageal reflux disease (GERD; see page 750).

Cancer of the esophagus has been linked to long-term exposure to irritants such as tobacco smoke and alcohol. A person's risk of cancer of the esophagus increases even more when he or she both smokes and drinks. The cancer is more common in men than in women and usually develops after age 60. Esophageal cancer is almost always fatal. However, it can be successfully treated if it is diagnosed at an early stage.

Symptoms

The main symptom of esophageal cancer is difficulty swallowing, or pain that becomes progressively worse when swallowing. At first only solids, but eventually liquids, are difficult to swallow. Other symptoms may include weight loss and, occasionally, regurgitating bloody mucus.

Diagnosis

If you have symptoms of esophageal cancer such as difficulty swallowing, your doctor will probably recommend a barium X-ray (see page 767) of your esophagus. He or she may also perform a procedure called endoscopy (see page 766) to examine your esophagus. If an abnormality is found on the X-ray or endoscopy, your doctor may also recommend a biopsy (in which samples of cells are taken from the esophagus and examined under a microscope).

Treatment

Surgery is the usual treatment for cancer of the esophagus. Radiation therapy (see page 23) and chemotherapy (see page 23) may be used alone or in combination to destroy cancer cells. Laser therapy (see page 22) is sometimes used to destroy the part of the tumor that is blocking the esophagus, temporarily relieving symptoms such as difficulty swallowing.

Disorders of the Stomach and Duodenum

After you chew and swallow food, powerful contractions of your stomach wall repeatedly crush and pulverize it. Stomach acid and enzymes break the food down into a pulp. The processed food trickles out of the stomach (through a ring of muscles called the pyloric sphincter) into the duodenum (the upper section of the small intestine at the entrance to the stomach). The duodenum secretes bile and more enzymes, which digest the pulp further before it passes into the rest of the small intestine. It takes from 3 to 5 hours for the contents of a meal to completely empty out of the stomach and duodenum and reach the lower part of the small intestine.

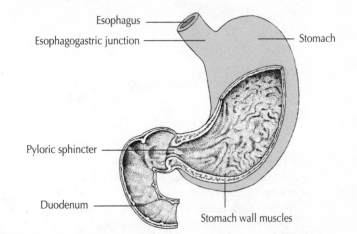

The stomach and duodenum
Food enters the stomach at the esophagogastric junction, where it is stored and partially digested. Muscles of the stomach wall crush the food and move it through the pyloric sphincter and eventually into the duodenum. The food is digested further in the duodenum and then passes into the rest of the small intestine.

Peptic Ulcers

A peptic ulcer is a hole or break in the lining of the stomach or duodenum (the beginning of the small intestine). The digestive juices secreted by the stomach are very acidic. Normally, the lining of the stomach and intestine is protected from this acid by a layer of mucus and a substance called bicarbonate, which is secreted by glands in the stomach wall. When this protective barrier is broken down, the digestive juices can come into contact with cells of the lining, damaging them.

Peptic ulcers that form in the duodenum are called duodenal ulcers. Peptic ulcers that form in the stomach are called gastric ulcers. In rare cases, an ulcer can develop on the lower esophagus and in the lower part of the small intestine. A peptic ulcer can break through the stomach lining completely, causing severe bleeding that can be fatal if not treated immediately.

A number of factors can contribute to the development of peptic ulcers. Infection with the bacterium Helicobacter pylori can cause peptic ulcers in some people by attaching to the protective lining and weakening it. Long-term use of pain relievers such as aspirin, ibuprofen, and naproxen also contribute to the development of peptic ulcers because these drugs can irritate the stomach lining when taken in large doses for long periods. Smoking is also a risk factor. Rarely, peptic ulcers are caused by tumors in the stomach or pancreas. Emotional stress, drinking alcohol, and eating spicy foods do not contribute to the development of peptic ulcers.

Symptoms

The main symptom of a peptic ulcer is burning, gnawing pain in the upper abdomen, lower chest, and, in rare cases, the upper back (between the shoulders). The pain is often worse about 2 hours after a meal and at night and can usually be relieved by eating something or taking an antacid. Other possible symptoms include nausea, vomiting (the vomit may be tinged with blood), and black, tarry stool (from bleeding). A rare condition called pyloric stenosis

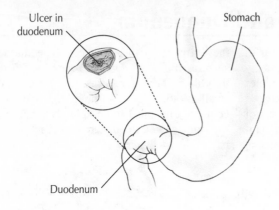

Duodenal ulcer
A duodenal ulcer is a sore in the wall of the first part of the small intestine (the duodenum) caused by erosion of the lining of the duodenum.

can result if scarring from a peptic ulcer blocks the pylorus (the outlet from the stomach to the duodenum), preventing the stomach from emptying normally and sometimes causing projectile vomiting (forceful vomiting immediately after eating).

Diagnosis
If you have symptoms of a peptic ulcer, your doctor will perform a procedure called endoscopy (see page 766) to examine your esophagus and stomach and possibly to take a sample of tissue for examination under a microscope (biopsy). Your doctor may order tests to look for blood in the stool, or blood tests to check for H. pylori or an iron deficiency (anemia; see page 610). Anemia can be a sign of internal bleeding.

Treatment
Reducing the amount of acid in the stomach is the usual treatment for peptic ulcers. Your doctor may recommend an over-the-counter antacid or may prescribe one. He or she may also prescribe a medication that coats the ulcer to protect it from stomach acid and allow it to heal. If your doctor detects H. pylori in the biopsy, he or she will prescribe antibiotics. Don't take over-the-counter antacids unless your doctor has diagnosed a peptic ulcer and has recommended them. Taking antacids can mask symptoms of more serious disorders such as stomach cancer. Stop smoking, because smoking can irritate the stomach lining and slow healing.

In rare cases, surgery is necessary to treat a peptic ulcer. A surgeon may close a severely bleeding perforated duodenal ulcer with stitches. In a procedure called vagotomy, the surgeon may cut the nerves responsible for controlling the production of stomach acid. Usually the stomach outlet is widened (in a procedure called pyloroplasty) at the same time to prevent tightening of the pyloric muscles that would normally follow vagotomy. For duodenal ulcers, a surgical procedure called gastrojejunostomy (see next page) is sometimes performed to create an opening from the stomach to the middle section of the small intestine (jejunum) and close the opening into the duodenum.

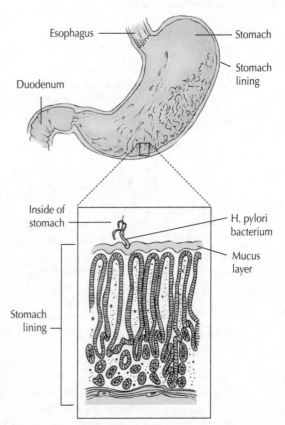

Helicobacter pylori in stomach lining
Helicobacter pylori is a spiral-shaped bacterium that attaches itself to the surface of mucus-secreting cells of the stomach lining. About 50 percent of people over age 60 are infected with H. pylori, and most of them have no symptoms. But about 15 to 20 percent of people who have the bacterium develop a peptic ulcer.

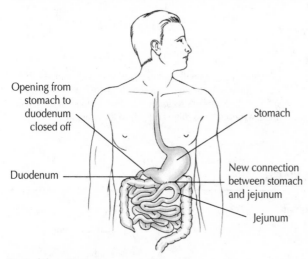

Opening from stomach to duodenum closed off

Stomach

Duodenum

New connection between stomach and jejunum

Jejunum

Gastrojejunostomy
A gastrojejunostomy is a surgically created connection between the stomach and the jejunum (the middle section of the small intestine) sometimes used for treating duodenal ulcers. The doctor seals the duodenum at the opening to the stomach, allowing gastric acid to enter the jejunum rather than the duodenum, where it could irritate the ulcer and cause it to bleed.

Cancer of the Stomach

Cancerous cells can develop anywhere in the stomach and are likely to spread to other parts of the body. Because the symptoms of stomach cancer are similar to those of other, less serious, digestive problems, it is difficult to detect stomach cancer early. It is thought that eating foods that are dried, smoked, heavily salted, or pickled is a risk factor for stomach cancer. Having peptic ulcers (see page 755) of the stomach does not seem to increase the risk of stomach cancer. However, the presence of the bacterium Helicobacter pylori in the stomach (which has been linked to gastric ulcers) may be linked to stomach cancer. Stomach cancer is much less common in the United States than it was in 1940. It is twice as common in men as in women, and the risk increases with age. Smoking also increases the risk of stomach cancer.

Symptoms

The initial symptoms of stomach cancer are easy to ignore and include indigestion (especially right after eating) and loss of appetite. Later symptoms include severe pain in the upper abdomen, weight loss, frequent vomiting (the vomit is usually tinged with blood), and red or dark blood in the stool. A rare condition called pyloric stenosis can result if a tumor blocks the pylorus (the outlet from the stomach to the small intestine), preventing the stomach from emptying normally, and sometimes causing projectile vomiting (forceful vomiting immediately after eating).

Diagnosis

If you have symptoms of stomach cancer (especially if the symptoms are different from your usual indigestion), your doctor will perform a procedure called endoscopy (see page 766) to examine your esophagus and stomach and, possibly, take samples of cells from the stomach for examination under a microscope for cancer (biopsy). He or she may also recommend a barium X-ray (see page 767) of your stomach.

Treatment

The treatment of stomach cancer depends on the stage of the disease. Removing only the part of the stomach affected by cancer (called a partial gastrectomy) is the most common treatment. However, it may be necessary to remove all of the stomach (total gastrectomy). Cases that are diagnosed and treated at the earliest stage have the best chances for a cure. Your doctor will order radiation therapy (see page 23) in combination with chemotherapy (see page 23) to keep the cancer from spreading or returning.

Gastrectomy

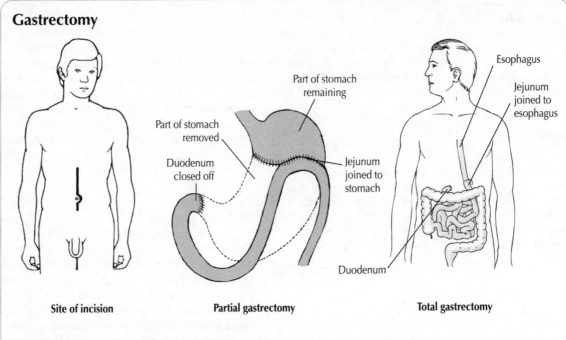

Site of incision   Partial gastrectomy   Total gastrectomy

Part of stomach remaining

Part of stomach removed

Duodenum closed off

Jejunum joined to stomach

Esophagus

Jejunum joined to esophagus

Duodenum

Gastrectomy

A gastrectomy is the surgical removal of a portion of the stomach (partial gastrectomy; above center) or the entire stomach (total gastrectomy; above right). In a partial gastrectomy, the remaining part of the stomach is joined to the jejunum (the middle part of the small intestine), and the duodenum (the first part of the small intestine) is closed off where it used to join the stomach. In a total gastrectomy, the whole stomach is removed and the esophagus is joined directly to the jejunum.

General Abdominal Disorders

The other sections of this chapter cover disorders specific to a particular part of the digestive system (such as the small intestine). However, sometimes a disorder can affect more than one digestive organ in the abdomen (such as the stomach and the intestines). This section discusses the disorders that affect multiple organs, including the stomach, the small intestine, the large intestine, and the peritoneum (the membrane that lines the entire abdominal cavity and encloses many organs). These disorders often involve signs and symptoms such as inflammation, blockage, and paralysis.

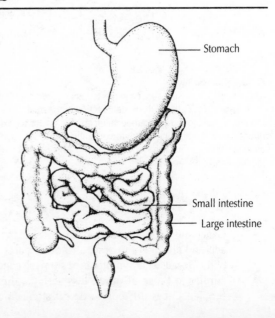

Stomach

Small intestine

Large intestine

The stomach, small intestine, and large intestine

Sometimes a disorder of the digestive system can affect more than one organ, such as the stomach, small intestine, and large intestine.

Peritonitis

Peritonitis is inflammation of the peritoneum, the two-layered membrane that lines the abdominal cavity and covers the stomach, intestines, and other abdominal organs. Peritonitis almost always results from an underlying untreated inflammatory disorder. For example, it may occur as a complication of a disorder of the digestive tract such as a peptic ulcer (see page 755), diverticulitis (see page 772), appendicitis (see page 771), or Crohn's disease (see page 764). In women, peritonitis can be a complication of some disorders of the fallopian tubes such as a ruptured ectopic pregnancy (see page 523). Peritonitis also can be caused by an infection that results from an injury that pierces the abdominal wall.

Full recovery from peritonitis is possible if treatment is started promptly. If untreated, peritonitis can lead to severe dehydration or a chemical imbalance (from repeated vomiting), paralysis of the intestines (ileus; see page 761), or shock (see page 579). Although peritonitis can be fatal, few people die of it because antibiotics can usually clear up the infection.

Symptoms

The main symptom of peritonitis is severe pain in the abdomen. The pain is most severe near the site of the initial disorder and increases when you move. For example, the pain from a ruptured peptic ulcer is worse in the upper midright side of the abdomen. A person usually has a fever. Other symptoms depend on the source of the inflammation or infection and can include nausea and vomiting. After a few hours the stomach becomes bloated and the pain more generalized.

Diagnosis

If you have symptoms of peritonitis, go to the nearest hospital emergency department immediately. The doctor will ask you about your symptoms and feel your abdomen to find the most painful area and identify the source of the inflammation. He or she will also order blood tests and a CT scan (see page 112). If fluid is present in the abdominal cavity, the doctor may perform a procedure called paracentesis, in which he or she inserts a needle into the cavity and withdraws a sample of fluid for evaluation. If the doctor is unsure of the diagnosis, he or she may recommend a surgical procedure

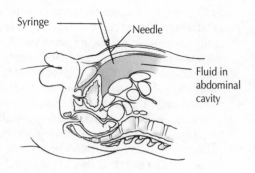

Paracentesis
In abdominal paracentesis, a doctor uses a needle and syringe to draw fluid out of the abdominal cavity for analysis in a laboratory.

called exploratory laparotomy, in which the abdominal cavity is opened to look for the cause of the disorder.

Treatment

If you have peritonitis, surgery must be done immediately to correct the underlying cause. For example, a surgeon may remove a damaged segment of intestine or repair a perforated ulcer. Before surgery you will be given antibiotics intravenously (through a vein) to treat the infection, and fluids if you are dehydrated. The surgeon will place soft rubber tubes in your abdominal cavity to drain the accumulated fluid.

Intestinal Obstruction

An intestinal obstruction is a partial or complete blockage of the intestines. The most common cause of an obstruction is a band of scar tissue (adhesion) that develops as a result of abdominal surgery. The band of scar tissue can wrap around the intestine, or the intestine can wrap around the scar tissue, squeezing the intestine. An intestinal blockage can also result from inflammation from an inflammatory bowel disease (see page 764), a cancerous tumor in the colon (see page 775), a strangulated hernia (see page 762), or an indigestible mass such as hardened bulk laxative. Sometimes an intestine is obstructed because it is knotted or twisted (a condition called volvulus). In rare cases, an intestinal obstruction is caused by intussusception (see page 406), in which the intestine folds back on itself like a telescope. Intussusception occurs more frequently in infants and young children than it does in adults.

Intestinal obstructions are common. If a complete obstruction occurs, the blood supply to the intestine can be cut off, causing the tissue to die. If the blockage is not relieved, the intestine can rupture and cause peritonitis (see previous page). An untreated intestinal obstruction can eventually lead to severe dehydration or a chemical imbalance (from repeated vomiting), paralysis of the intestines (ileus; see next page), or shock (see page 579), or it can be fatal.

Symptoms

Symptoms of intestinal obstruction depend on the location of the obstruction and on whether the obstruction is complete or partial. An obstruction in the small intestine causes cramping pain in the

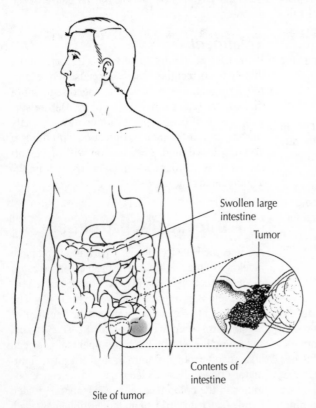

Intestinal obstruction

An intestinal obstruction is a blockage of the small or large intestine. An obstruction such as a tumor may block the flow of food or stool out of the intestine, causing the contents of the intestine to back up, which can cause the intestine to swell.

(labels on diagram)
Swollen large intestine
Tumor
Contents of intestine
Site of tumor

> **WARNING!**
>
> ## Intestinal Obstruction
>
> An intestinal obstruction can be life-threatening. Call 911 or your local emergency number or go to the nearest hospital emergency department immediately if you have the following symptoms:
>
> - Abdominal pain followed by swelling of the abdomen, especially in the lower part of the abdomen
> - Constipation
> - Inability to pass gas
> - Nausea and vomiting

middle of the abdomen and increasingly frequent vomiting; if vomiting temporarily relieves the cramping, the obstruction in the small intestine is probably partial. If the blockage is in the large intestine, you may not vomit or vomit very little; if the obstruction in the large intestine is partial, you will be able to pass gas and very loose stool, which will temporarily relieve the intense cramping. Partial or complete blockage of an intestine prevents gas or stool from passing.

Diagnosis

If you have symptoms of an intestinal obstruction, the doctor will take an X-ray of the abdomen (while you are standing, if possible). If the doctor is unsure of what is causing the blockage, he or she may recommend a barium X-ray (see page 767) or CT scan (see page 112). If the results are still unclear, he or she will recommend a surgical procedure called exploratory laparotomy in which the abdominal cavity is opened to look for the cause of the obstruction.

Treatment

If you have symptoms of an intestinal obstruction, the doctor will pass a long tube down your nose or mouth and into your stomach and intestines to remove fluid and air, which relieves pain by relieving pressure. You may be given fluids intravenously (through a vein) if you are dehydrated. You won't be given any food for 24 to 72 hours to see if the obstruction passes on its own.

If the obstruction does not pass through the intestines in 72 hours, your doctor will perform surgery to locate the blockage and treat it. The surgery will be done sooner if the intestine becomes completely blocked (which could cut off the blood supply to the intestine).

If the cause is a volvulus, the surgeon will try to untwist the intestine and prevent the volvulus from recurring by inserting a tube past the twisted segment. Alternatively, a surgeon may remove the twisted segment of intestine and rejoin the severed ends.

Ileus

Ileus is a serious disorder in which the intestines are paralyzed, disrupting digestion. The paralysis is caused by abnormal electrical activity of the intestinal muscles. The contractions that move food through the intestines slow down or stop entirely, causing gas, fluid, and stool to collect in the intestines. Ileus is usually the result of abdominal surgery, severe infections, or some medications. It can also result from digestive disorders such as an intestinal obstruction (see page 759), peritonitis (see page 759), pancreatitis (see page 799), or a perforated peptic ulcer (see page 755). People with some nervous system disorders such as multiple sclerosis (see page 696) or Parkinson's disease (see page 691) are at increased risk. Ileus can be fatal if the underlying disorder is not treated.

Symptoms

The symptoms of ileus include pain and swelling in the abdomen, constipation, failure to pass gas, and vomiting. If you have these symptoms, see your doctor to determine the underlying cause. If you have these symptoms along with a fever, you could have a life-threatening infection that requires emergency medical attention.

WARNING!

Ileus

Paralysis of the intestine can be life-threatening if it causes an infection. If you have a fever with any of the following symptoms, call 911 or your local emergency number or go to the nearest hospital emergency department immediately:

- Abdominal pain and swelling
- Constipation
- Inability to pass gas
- Vomiting

Diagnosis

If you have symptoms of ileus, the doctor will examine you and will order an X-ray of your abdomen. To rule out other disorders, he or she will take a detailed health history and order blood tests to check the level of calcium and electrolytes (such as sodium, potassium, and magnesium) and evaluate the functioning of your thyroid gland. Abnormalities in any of these can slow the electrical activity of the intestines.

Treatment

If you have symptoms of ileus, a doctor will pass a long tube down your nose or mouth into your stomach and intestines to remove fluid and air, which relieves pain by relieving the pressure the blocked intestine is putting on adjacent tissues and organs. Further treatment of ileus depends on the cause. Because some degree of intestinal paralysis is common after abdominal surgery, doctors try to avoid or minimize the use of narcotics for pain relief because the drugs can slow the movement of the intestines.

Carcinoid Tumors

Carcinoid tumors are cancerous tumors that are most often found in the appendix but can also develop in the wall of the intestines or stomach. Although they are cancerous tumors, they develop so slowly that 50 percent of people who have them never have symptoms and the tumors are found during tests or surgery for another disorder. However, if the carcinoid tumor grows large enough, it can cause symptoms of an intestinal obstruction (see page 759). In 10 percent of cases, cells from the tumor spread through the bloodstream to the liver, where the cells multiply and form hormone-producing tumors. The hormones released by these tumors produce symptoms that are collectively called carcinoid syndrome.

Symptoms

The main symptom in carcinoid syndrome is flushing of the head and neck that lasts several hours and is usually triggered by exercise or drinking alcohol. If the cancer spreads to the liver, signs can include abdominal cramping, sudden episodes of watery diarrhea, symptoms of asthma (see page 640) such as wheezing, and symptoms of heart failure (see page 570) such as breathlessness.

Diagnosis

Carcinoid tumors can be difficult to diagnose. If you have symptoms of carcinoid syndrome, your doctor may order blood and urine tests to identify the hormone that the carcinoid tumor is secreting. He or she may also recommend a CT scan (see page 134), colonoscopy (see page 767), or endoscopy (see page 766) to examine your stomach and intestines. You may also have capsule video endoscopy (see page 767), in which you swallow a small pill containing a camera that takes a video of your small intestine.

Treatment

Surgery is the usual treatment for carcinoid tumors. However, all the tumors must be removed to eliminate the symptoms of carcinoid syndrome, which can be difficult. Your doctor may prescribe a medication called somatostatin to reduce the frequency and length of the attacks of flushing, antidiarrheals to control episodes of diarrhea, bronchodilators to relieve symptoms of asthma, and chemotherapy (see page 23) to slow the growth of the tumors.

Hernia

A hernia is a bulge of soft tissue that forces its way through or between a weak area in the muscle wall that usually contains it. Normally, body muscles are tight and firm and hold tissues and organs in position. The abdominal wall is made up of flat sheets of muscle that cover and protect the abdominal organs such as the stomach, intestines, liver, kidneys, and reproductive organs. In a hernia, muscles in the abdominal cavity that become weak and slack because of a strain, congenital (present at birth) weakness, or abdominal surgery push through a

---

WARNING!

Strangulated Hernia

A strangulated hernia can cut off the blood supply to the intestine, causing the tissue to die, which can be life-threatening. Call 911 or your local emergency number or go to the nearest hospital emergency department immediately if you have any of the following symptoms of a strangulated hernia:

- A hernia that is very painful
- A hernia that you cannot push back into place
- A hernia that is very warm, red, and swollen

Incisional Hernia

An incisional hernia can result from abdominal surgery if the cut abdominal wall muscles and fibrous layers do not heal properly, if the incision becomes infected, or if broken stitches cause defects in the abdominal muscle wall. Incisional hernias can range from small to large areas of weakness in the abdominal wall. You are more likely to develop an incisional hernia after abdominal surgery if you are inactive after the surgery, older, overweight, extremely underweight, or weak.

---

weak point in the muscle wall. A hernia usually occurs when the abdominal wall is put under pressure, such as when you cough, lift a heavy object, or strain to pass urine or have a bowel movement. An umbilical hernia (see next page) is a soft bulge of tissue around the navel of a newborn whose abdominal wall is not fully developed.

Hernias develop in many parts of the body but are most common in the abdominal wall. If a significant portion of an intestine has squeezed through the weak part of the abdominal wall, the contents of the intestine may be prevented from moving through the intestine, causing an intestinal obstruction (see page 759). If the blood supply to the intestine is cut off, the result is a condition called a strangulated hernia.

Symptoms

Usually the only symptom of a hernia is a bulge or swelling. The bulge usually forms slowly over several weeks, but it can also appear suddenly. Other symptoms include a feeling of heaviness, tenderness, or aching at the site of the hernia. If the hernia has caused an intestinal obstruction, you will have symptoms such as nausea, vomiting, or increasing abdominal pain.

Diagnosis and Treatment

A doctor can usually diagnose a hernia through a physical examination. Most hernias can be treated temporarily by pushing the organ or soft tissue back through the weak point in the muscle wall and wearing a supportive device called a truss to keep the organ in place. However, surgery is usually necessary to treat a hernia permanently. A strangulated hernia or a hernia that causes an intestinal obstruction is a medical emergency and must be treated

Types of Hernias

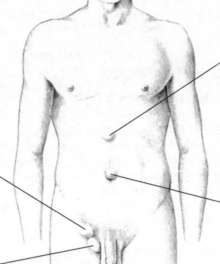

Inguinal hernia
An inguinal hernia appears as a bulge in the groin. It can develop when abdominal organs push aside weak abdominal wall muscles that cover the groin; this is called a direct inguinal hernia. In men, a loop of intestine can pass through a weakness in the inguinal canal (the passage through which the testicles descend) and become trapped; this is called an indirect inguinal hernia.

Femoral hernia
A femoral hernia occurs in a slightly lower position in the groin than an inguinal hernia. This type of hernia is most common in overweight women and in women who have had several children.

Epigastric hernia
An epigastric hernia occurs between the navel and the breastbone when a small piece of the fatty apron that covers the intestine protrudes through a weak point in the fibrous tissue that joins the central abdominal muscles. Epigastric hernias are more common in men than in women.

Umbilical hernia
An umbilical hernia occurs when a weakness develops in the abdominal wall muscles around the navel. It occurs most often in infants, and more often in women than in men.

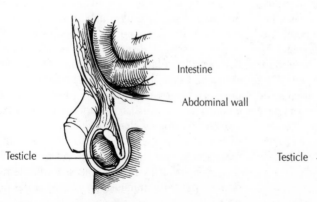

Intestine

Abdominal wall

Testicle

Normal inguinal canal

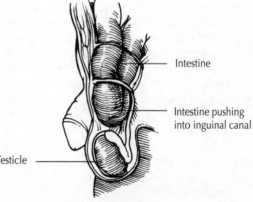

Intestine

Intestine pushing into inguinal canal

Testicle

Inguinal hernia

Inguinal hernia
In males, the inguinal canal is the opening through which the spermatic cord passes and eventually through which the testicles descend into the scrotum. Normally, it closes completely before birth. In an inguinal hernia, the opening does not close, causing part of the intestine to protrude into the canal.

immediately. A surgeon will push the protruding muscle or tissue back into place and tighten the loose muscles (usually by sewing them together). A thin, meshlike piece of plastic is sometimes used to reinforce a weak muscle or a muscle that has been replaced by scar tissue from previous hernia surgery.

Inflammatory Bowel Disease

Inflammatory bowel disease refers to disorders that cause recurring inflammation of the intestines. Crohn's disease and ulcerative colitis are examples of inflammatory bowel disease. Crohn's disease can occur in any part of the digestive tract but usually occurs in the intestines. Ulcerative colitis usually affects the large intestine and the rectum (but sometimes just the rectum). The cause of inflammatory bowel disease is unknown, but doctors think the inflammation may be an immune system response to a viral or bacterial infection. Neither disorder results from stress or from eating specific foods, although these factors can trigger symptoms in some people who have the disorder.

Inflammatory bowel disease tends to run in families and affects men and women in equal numbers. The inflammation may produce ulcers in the intestine and colon and scar tissue that thickens and narrows the intestinal wall, possibly causing an intestinal obstruction (see page 759). In ulcerative colitis, sores form where inflammation has killed cells in the intestinal lining. About 20 percent of people who have Crohn's disease develop anal fistulas (abnormal channels from the intestine to the surface of the skin or other organs; see page 779). Fistulas can leak to the skin or other organs and cause peritonitis (see page 759). People who have inflammatory bowel disease, especially ulcerative colitis, have an increased risk of developing cancer of the intestine (see page 775).

Symptoms

The symptoms of inflammatory bowel disease can include diarrhea (that may contain blood or pus), abdominal pain, fatigue, fever, and, in children, failure to grow. In ulcerative colitis, or Crohn's disease that involves the colon, the stool may be especially bloody because of bleeding ulcers in the intestine. If inflammatory bowel disease persists for years, it can cause a gradual deterioration in bowel function.

If you have fistulas that prevent digested food from being absorbed, you may lose weight. If a fistula connects to your skin, the contents of your intestines may leak out of your body. Inflammatory bowel disease can also cause symptoms such as red eyes, rashes, joint pain, or liver abnormalities in areas of the body other than the intestines.

Diagnosis

If you have symptoms of inflammatory bowel disease, your doctor will perform a physical examination. He or she may perform a procedure called colonoscopy (see page 767) to examine your colon. If just the lower third of the colon is examined, the procedure is called sigmoidoscopy (see page 144). He or she may also order a barium X-ray (see page 767) of your intestines. You may also have capsule video endoscopy (see page 767), in which you swallow a small pill containing a camera that takes a video of your small intestine. Your doctor may also order blood tests and tests to look for blood, bacteria, or viruses in your stool to rule out cancer or a viral or bacterial infection. He or she will probably take samples of cells from your intestine for examination under a microscope (biopsy) to confirm the diagnosis.

Treatment

To treat Crohn's disease, a doctor may prescribe anti-inflammatory medications such as sulfasalazine or mesalamine, corticosteroids such as prednisone or budesonide, or drugs such as azathioprine or methotrexate that suppress the body's abnormal immune response. He or she may prescribe the corticosteroids in large doses for an initial, severe attack and then in gradually decreasing doses to prevent a recurrence. If Crohn's disease affects the colon, a doctor will also prescribe antibiotics such as metronidazole or ciprofloxacin.

For ulcerative colitis, the usual treatment is mesalamine taken both by mouth and by enemas or rectal suppositories. In some cases, corticosteroids or more powerful immune-suppressing drugs may be necessary.

Surgical removal of part of the colon in a procedure called partial or total colectomy (see page 776) is sometimes necessary to treat Crohn's disease that does not respond to medication or to treat complications such as fistulas or scarring. A total colectomy may be done for ulcerative colitis that has not responded to other treatments.

Irritable Bowel Syndrome

Irritable bowel syndrome (also called spastic or irritable colon) is a common disorder that can cause a number of symptoms in any organ in the gastrointestinal tract, including the esophagus, stomach, and small and large intestines. The cause of the disorder is unknown, but it may result from a dysfunction of the involuntary nerves or muscles in these organs. In irritable bowel syndrome, the waves of muscular contractions that normally move stool through the intestines become uncoordinated. The condition is twice as common in women as in men, and is more common in young adults. The symptoms can be triggered or worsened by stress or a poor diet.

Symptoms

The symptoms of irritable bowel syndrome vary from person to person and resemble the symptoms of other gastrointestinal disorders. Symptoms include abdominal discomfort anywhere in the colon, nausea, digestive noises such as rumbling and gurgling, and gas. People often have constipation, diarrhea, or a feeling that the rectum is not completely empty. Sometimes diarrhea alternates with bouts of constipation.

Diagnosis

To diagnose irritable bowel syndrome, a doctor performs a physical examination and rules out other possible disorders such as inflammatory bowel disease (see previous page) or colon cancer (see page 775) by ordering a series of tests. He or she may order blood tests and stool tests to rule out cancer or an infection. You may have a CT scan (see page 112) or an ultrasound (see page 111). In rare cases, a doctor will recommend a biopsy, in which samples of cells are taken from the intestine and examined under a microscope, or capsule video endoscopy (see page 767), in which you swallow a small pill containing a camera that takes a video of your small intestine. The doctor may perform a procedure called colonoscopy (see page 767) to examine the colon. If just the lower third of the colon is examined, the procedure is called sigmoidoscopy (see page 144). He or she also may recommend a barium X-ray (see page 767) of your intestines.

Treatment

Irritable bowel syndrome can be difficult to treat because the cause is not clear. Several factors can make the condition worse. Try to identify and avoid substances and situations (including psychological or emotional ones) that you think may be causing your symptoms. Taking steps to avoid indigestion (see page 750) and gastrointestinal reflux disease (GERD; see page 750) may help alleviate some of your symptoms. If you are constipated or have alternating bouts of diarrhea and constipation, your doctor may recommend a high-fiber diet with insoluble fiber (fiber that cannot be broken down by the digestive tract) such as wheat bran. People who have diarrhea or excessive gas may benefit by following a bland diet. In rare cases, a doctor may prescribe antispasmodic medications to help decrease intestinal contractions. If stress is triggering your attacks, your doctor may prescribe antidepressants (see page 712) or antianxiety medications (see page 713) to help reduce symptoms of stress. Do not take any over-the-counter medication unless your doctor has recommended it.

Disorders of the Small Intestine

The small intestine is a tube about 1½ inches in diameter and 14 to 20 feet long. It runs from the stomach to the colon (the longest section of the large intestine). The process of breaking down food into small particles that begins in the stomach continues in the small intestine, aided by the secretion of additional enzymes and digestive juices from the pancreas, the gallbladder, and the wall of the small intestine. When food particles dissolve into their smallest units, they pass through the thin lining of the small intestine into the bloodstream. (Fats pass into the lymphatic vessels in the small intestine before they enter the bloodstream.) The inside surface of the wall of the small intestine is covered with tiny fingerlike projections called villi. These projections make the digestive surface area larger, so that more of the tiny particles can be absorbed.

Common Diagnostic Procedures

Doctors can choose from a number of imaging procedures to diagnose disorders of the digestive tract. Some of these procedures are also used for treating gastrointestinal disorders. Following are descriptions of some of the most common diagnostic procedures.

Endoscopic Procedures

Endoscopes are viewing tubes that doctors use to examine a body cavity. Endoscopes are usually flexible, but some (such as the laparoscope) are rigid. Endoscopes contain small cameras, instruments with which to take tissue samples or perform medical procedures, and lights or light sources. During an endoscopic procedure, a camera or video recorder can take pictures or transmit images to a monitor. Air may be passed into the digestive tract at the time of the procedure to open up the cavity and provide a clearer image.

Here are some of the endoscopic procedures that are used to diagnose or treat disorders of the gastrointestinal tract:

ENDOSCOPIC PROCEDURES		
Procedure	**Part of Body Examined**	**Where Endoscope Is Inserted**
Esophagoscopy	Esophagus	Into the nose or mouth
Gastroscopy	Stomach	Into the nose or mouth
Laparoscopy	Abdominal cavity	Through small incision in abdomen
Colonoscopy	Colon	Into the rectum
Sigmoidoscopy	Lower third of the colon	Into the rectum
Anoscopy, proctoscopy, rectoscopy	Anus and rectum	Into the rectum
Capsule video endoscopy	Small intestine	Swallowed

Upper endoscopy
A number of endoscopic procedures can be used to view structures in the upper part of the gastrointestinal tract. A doctor passes the endoscope down the esophagus until it reaches the part of the digestive tract to be examined or treated.

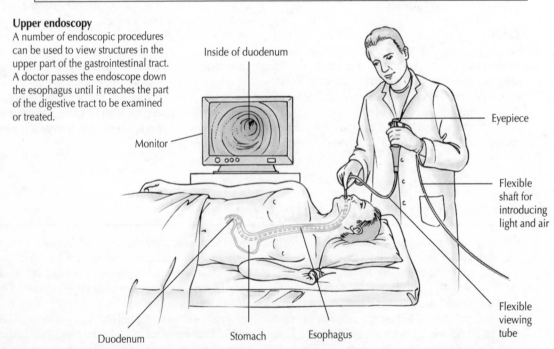

Inside of duodenum

Monitor

Eyepiece

Flexible shaft for introducing light and air

Flexible viewing tube

Duodenum   Stomach   Esophagus

Colonoscopy

In colonoscopy, a narrow, flexible tube (colonoscope) is inserted through the anus and rectum and threaded up through the colon. As the colonoscope is slowly withdrawn, the doctor examines the lining of the colon for abnormalities such as inflammation, polyps, or tumors. A tiny camera at the end of the colonoscope displays images of the inside of the colon on a video monitor. The procedure is painless but can be uncomfortable, so a person is given a sedative to relax him or her and to reduce any discomfort. Growths such as polyps can be shaved and removed through the endoscope. Bleeding blood vessels or ulcers can also be treated through the endoscope.

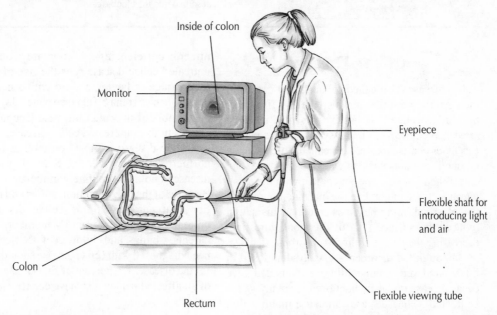

Inside of colon

Monitor

Eyepiece

Flexible shaft for introducing light and air

Colon

Flexible viewing tube

Rectum

Capsule Video Endoscopy

Capsule video endoscopy is a diagnostic imaging test that uses a miniature color video camera placed inside a pill-shaped capsule that a person swallows with a sip of water. The so-called edible camera travels through the intestinal tract by way of peristalsis, the natural contractions of the intestines. Along the way, the camera captures video images of the inside of the intestinal tract and transmits the images to sensors on a belt worn around the person's abdomen. The sensors store the images on a recorder. The process takes about 8 hours. The person then returns the belt and recorder to the doctor's office, where the doctor can download the images and view them on a computer screen to check for any abnormalities in the intestinal tract. The disposable (flushable) camera passes out of the body naturally during a bowel movement, usually within 24 hours.

Barium X-Ray Examinations

Tests using a contrast medium (dye) called barium are performed to detect abnormalities in the digestive tract. Barium is a metallic chemical that X-rays cannot pass through. When barium is mixed with water and passed into an area of the body to be examined, it allows an image of the area to show up on X-ray film. Sometimes air is introduced into the digestive tract to get a clearer image of less-visible abnormalities.

- Before an examination of the esophagus, stomach, and duodenum, barium is swallowed in a drink or ingested in a cookie or tablet.

- For an examination of the small intestine, barium is usually swallowed in a drink or ingested in a cookie or tablet. Sometimes the barium is passed into the small intestine through a tube inserted through the rectum.

- For an examination of the large intestine, barium is passed into the large intestine through a tube inserted through the rectum.

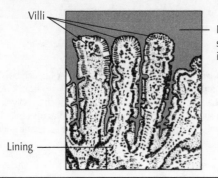

Small intestine
The inner wall of the small intestine is lined with tiny fingerlike projections called villi, which increase the surface area of the intestinal lining for digestion. The villi secrete enzymes to break down fats, proteins, and carbohydrates and enable the resulting particles to be absorbed into the bloodstream.

Celiac Disease

Celiac disease (also called celiac sprue) is a common inherited disorder in which the tiny fingerlike projections called villi that line the small intestine are damaged by the immune system after a person eats foods containing a protein called gluten. Gluten is found in grains such as wheat, barley, rye, and oats. When gluten comes in contact with the small intestine, the villi that line the intestine flatten, and the intestinal lining becomes smooth. This action reduces the surface area of the small intestine, decreasing the body's ability to absorb nutrients.

Although the disorder is usually diagnosed in infants and very young children, adults can have celiac disease that is undiagnosed for many years. Untreated, celiac disease can cause malnutrition and other malabsorption or deficiency disorders such as anemia (from an iron deficiency; see page 610), osteoporosis (from poor calcium absorption; see page 989), seizures (see page 686), or abnormally short stature (from general vitamin and

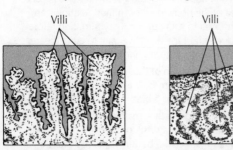

Villi in celiac disease
Villi (left) are tiny fingerlike projections that line the inner wall of the small intestine and help break down and absorb nutrients from food. In people with some intestinal disorders such as celiac disease, the villi flatten out (right), reducing the body's ability to absorb nutrients.

mineral deficiencies). A pregnant woman with untreated celiac disease runs the risk of having a miscarriage or having a child with a neural tube defect such as spina bifida (see page 398). Cancerous tumors of the small intestine (see next page) can result from untreated celiac disease.

Celiac disease is most common in people of northern European descent. Screening for celiac disease is not done routinely in the United States. Because of the risk of complications and malnutrition that can develop if celiac disease goes untreated, first-degree family members (such as parents, siblings, and children) of people who have been diagnosed with celiac disease should be tested for the disease. Ten percent of first-degree relatives of an affected person also have celiac disease.

Symptoms

Gastrointestinal symptoms of celiac disease depend on the amount of gluten ingested. Symptoms may include a swollen abdomen, excess gas, abdominal pain, chronic diarrhea, or pale, foul-smelling stool. Other symptoms (of malnutrition) can include canker sores (see page 743), tooth discoloration, pain in the bones and joints, muscle cramps, tingling and numbness in the legs, rash (dermatitis; see page 1062), weight loss, or fatigue. In addition to the above symptoms, celiac disease can cause failure to thrive in infants and delayed growth in children. In women, celiac disease can cause missed menstrual periods (amenorrhea; see page 846) and bone loss leading to osteoporosis and fractures.

Diagnosis

If you have symptoms of celiac disease, your doctor will perform a physical examination and may order blood tests to determine the levels of antibodies (proteins the body has produced to defend itself against gluten). He or she will try to rule out cancer or a viral or bacterial infection by testing stool samples for blood, viruses, or bacteria. A diagnosis of celiac disease can be confirmed with a biopsy (in which samples of cells are taken from the intestine and examined under a microscope) to check for damage to the villi.

Treatment

The usual treatment for celiac disease is to eliminate all gluten-containing foods from the diet. Your doctor will advise you to avoid baked goods, cereals, pasta, and any other foods (or drinks such as beer, ale, vodka, gin, or whiskey) that contain wheat, barley, rye, or oats. Although oats may not cause symptoms in all people who have celiac disease, they should be avoided because gluten in oats can damage the villi without causing symptoms. Gluten can also be found in medications, mouthwashes, and some additives, preservatives, and stabilizers. Within a few days of following a gluten-free diet, most symptoms improve and the intestinal lining starts to heal. In rare cases, some people with celiac disease don't respond to a gluten-free diet and may need to take corticosteroids or other medications to reduce inflammation. Some people have to be fed intravenously (through a vein) to get adequate nutrition.

Tumors of the Small Intestine

Like tumors elsewhere in the body, tumors of the small intestine can be malignant (cancerous) or benign (noncancerous). Most are benign (only 1 of 10 cases is malignant). Tumors of the small intestine may cause no symptoms and are often diagnosed by tests performed for another reason. In rare cases, they may be carcinoid tumors (see page 761).

Symptoms

Tumors in the small intestine can cause symptoms of anemia (see page 610) such as paleness, fatigue, or palpitations (heartbeats that you are aware of). You may have traces of blood in your stool or very dark, bloody stool. If a tumor is very large, it may cause abdominal pain and an intestinal obstruction (see page 759). If the cancer spreads to other parts of the body, it may cause symptoms such as weight loss or fatigue.

Diagnosis and Treatment

If you have symptoms of an intestinal tumor, your doctor will perform a barium X-ray (see page 767) of your intestines or capsule video endoscopy (see page 767). Surgery is the usual treatment for both cancerous and noncancerous tumors of the small intestine. Radiation therapy (see page 23) and

---

Constipation and Diarrhea

Constipation is generally defined as having hard, dry, difficult-to-pass stools and infrequent bowel movements. Usually constipation is the result of not drinking enough water, not eating enough fiber-containing food, lack of exercise, stress, or delaying bowel movements. Some medications (such as cough suppressants and antianxiety medications) can cause constipation. Overusing laxatives can lead to constipation by overemptying the bowel and making a person dependent on them to have a bowel movement. (Also, the effect of laxatives diminishes when used repeatedly.) A number of conditions, such as hypothyroidism (see page 903) or a high level of calcium in the blood, can cause constipation. If constipation persists for more than 2 weeks, see your doctor.

Diarrhea is usually considered to be an abnormal increase in the looseness and amount of stool and very frequent bowel movements. In general, the more frequent the bowel movements, the looser the stool. Sometimes diarrhea can be brought on by stress or as a side effect of some medications (such as antacids or antibiotics), but it is usually the result of a viral or bacterial infection or food poisoning. Some foods (such as some fruits and dairy products) can cause diarrhea. If diarrhea persists for more than 3 days or if you see blood in your stool, see your doctor. Also call your doctor if you have diarrhea and your stool is bloody or contains pus or if you are extremely thirsty or weak, have a fever, or have pain in your abdomen.

People differ markedly in the pattern and consistency of their bowel movements. See your doctor about any change in your normal pattern; you could have a serious disorder.

chemotherapy (see page 23) may be used alone or in combination to destroy cancer cells.

Lactose Intolerance

Lactose intolerance results from the body's inability to digest lactose, a sugar found in milk and other dairy products. In lactose intolerance, the body produces little or no lactase, an enzyme in the small intestine needed to break down lactose. Lactose intolerance can cause gastrointestinal disturbances such as bloating, cramping, and diarrhea.

Many of the world's people—especially those of African, Asian, Middle Eastern, Jewish, Hispanic, and Native American descent—are susceptible to developing lactose intolerance. The condition develops over time, usually after age 2. Some people who have lactose intolerance are able to consume small amounts of milk products with no problem. In rare cases, lactose intolerance is congenital (present at birth) and causes bloating and persistent diarrhea immediately, resulting in a child's inability to gain weight.

Symptoms

Symptoms of lactose intolerance include abdominal bloating, cramping, nausea, gas, and diarrhea after consuming a food that contains lactose. The symptoms usually begin within 30 minutes to 2 hours. The severity and duration of the symptoms depend on the amount of lactose a person can tolerate.

Diagnosis

To diagnose lactose intolerance, a doctor will take a detailed health history. He or she may also recommend three tests—the lactose tolerance test (a blood test), hydrogen breath test, and stool acidity test—that measure the amount of lactose your body is digesting. The tests are performed after you fast for a specified length of time and then drink a liquid that contains lactose. The breath and blood tests can be given to older children and adults but not to infants and very young children because excessive amounts of lactose can cause diarrhea, which can lead to dehydration.

Treatment

There is no treatment to increase the amount of lactase your body produces. To prevent symptoms of lactose intolerance, your doctor will recommend limiting or avoiding foods that contain lactose. When shopping, read all product labels to see if foods contain lactose. Your doctor may also recommend taking an over-the-counter lactase enzyme, which will aid in the digestion of lactose. The enzyme comes in tablets or liquid, and you take it before eating or drinking products that contain lactose.

If you need to avoid milk and other dairy products (which are major sources of calcium), a doctor will recommend taking a calcium supplement and eating other calcium-rich foods (see page 5), including green vegetables and fish with bones (such as sardines). Hard cheeses are OK because they contain minimal amounts of whey. (Most lactose is in the whey portion of cheese.) Lactose-reduced milk and other products are available in most grocery stores. If an infant or young child has symptoms of lactose intolerance, a doctor may recommend giving the child soy milk instead of cow's milk.

Disorders of the Large Intestine

The large intestine is a tube about 2 inches in diameter and 5 feet long consisting of the colon (the longest section) and the rectum. The first part of the colon is a pouchlike chamber called the cecum. The appendix (a thin, wormlike pouch that is part of the immune system) hangs from the cecum. The rest of the colon runs up the right side of the abdomen (ascending colon), across and under the rib cage (transverse colon), and down the left side of the abdomen (descending colon and sigmoid colon). The rectum is a short tube about 5 inches long that points down from the end of the colon to the anus. Fluid and mineral salts from the contents of the intestine are absorbed through the colon wall into the bloodstream. The large intestine compacts indigestible solids and moves them toward the rectum. Waste is released from the rectum through the anus in the form of stool.

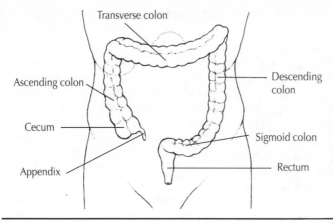

The large intestine
The large intestine is made up of two parts—the colon and the rectum. Undigested food (in liquid form) flows from the small intestine into the large intestine, where most of the water is absorbed back into the body. The partly solid waste (stool) that remains moves down into the rectum. The appendix is a thin sac that hangs from the first part of the large intestine called the cecum.

Appendicitis

Appendicitis is inflammation of the appendix (a small, narrow sac that branches out from the large intestine). If a piece of stool or food plugs up the appendix, it can become swollen and inflamed. Appendicitis is rare in children younger than 2. If appendicitis is not treated, the swollen appendix may burst, releasing the contents of the intestine into the abdomen and causing peritonitis (inflammation of the membrane that lines the abdominal cavity; see page 759). The apron of tissue that covers the intestines also covers the appendix and may prevent an infection from spreading.

Symptoms
The main symptom of appendicitis is abdominal pain that grows more severe over several hours. Usually the pain begins around the navel and then moves to a small area in the lower right abdomen. Slight pressure on the area will increase the pain. Other symptoms can include fever, nausea, vomiting, and loss of appetite. Some people notice that they have not had a bowel movement for a day or two before the attack, while others have bouts of diarrhea. Do not take a laxative if you have symptoms of appendicitis; it can cause an inflamed appendix to rupture.

Diagnosis
Appendicitis is sometimes difficult to diagnose because other disorders have similar symptoms. If you have symptoms of appendicitis, your doctor will perform a physical examination and press on your abdomen to locate the site of the pain. If your doctor thinks you have appendicitis, he or she will admit you to a hospital and order a number of tests, such as blood tests, a CT scan (see page 112), and ultrasound (see page 111), to rule out other disorders. If a diagnosis of appendicitis is uncertain, your doctor will recommend a surgical procedure called exploratory laparotomy in which the abdominal cavity is opened to look for the cause of the disorder.

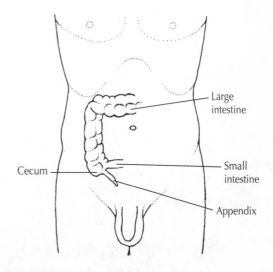

Appendix
The appendix projects from the cecum (the first part of the large intestine) in the lower right side of the abdomen, where the small intestine and the large intestine meet. The appendix is part of the immune system.

Treatment

To treat appendicitis, doctors remove the appendix immediately in a surgical procedure called appendectomy. If ultrasound shows that the appendix is severely abscessed (filled with pus), the appendectomy may be delayed for a few days or weeks until the infection has cleared up with antibiotics and the abscess drained with surgery or by inserting a tube. Because appendicitis is likely to flare up again, the appendix is removed as soon as tests show that the infection has cleared up. Even if the appendix looks normal, the surgeon still removes it because, if the appendix were not removed and the person later develops appendicitis and comes into an emergency department, doctors would recognize the characteristic appendectomy scar and would incorrectly rule out appendicitis as the cause.

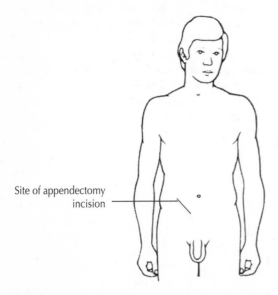

Site of appendectomy incision

Appendectomy

A surgeon can remove an inflamed appendix in a procedure called appendectomy. While the person is under a general anesthetic, the surgeon makes a diagonal incision in the lower right side of the abdomen. He or she clamps the appendix at its base, cuts it off, and sews up the remaining stump.

Diverticulosis and Diverticulitis

Diverticulosis is a common disorder in which small, saclike swellings (called diverticula) develop in the walls of the lowest part of the colon (the longest section of the large intestine). In rare cases, diverticula can develop in other parts of the digestive tract such as the esophagus (pharyngeal pouch; see page 748), stomach, or small intestine. The cause of diverticulosis is unknown. Some doctors think that the condition may result from chronic constipation. Straining during bowel movements increases pressure on the wall of the colon, possibly causing a weak point in the wall to swell. Diverticulosis usually causes no symptoms and is often diagnosed by chance during tests done for another reason.

When one or more of the diverticula become inflamed, the condition is called diverticulitis. Only 10 percent of people with diverticulosis develop diverticulitis. If untreated, diverticulitis can cause an abscess (pus-filled cavity) to form in the intestine. The abscess can rupture, causing inflammation of the membrane that lines the abdominal cavity (peritonitis; see page 759).

Symptoms

Diverticulosis usually causes no symptoms. However, you may have mild abdominal tenderness, cramping in the lower left side of the abdomen (that is relieved after you pass gas or have a bowel movement), constipation, or occasional attacks of diarrhea. The diverticula may bleed, producing blood in the stool or significant bleeding from the rectum.

If you have diverticulitis, you will probably have severe abdominal pain and tenderness in the lower left side of your abdomen that gets worse when you press on the area, although diverticula can sometimes develop on the right side. In some people, the pain becomes disabling within a few hours; in others, the pain is tolerable for a few days before it becomes severe. Other symptoms include nausea and fever. If peritonitis has developed, you will also have a swollen abdomen.

Diagnosis

If you have symptoms of diverticulosis or diverticulitis, your doctor will perform a physical examination and will order a CT scan (see page 112) of your intestines to rule out diverticulitis. He or she may also order blood tests and test your stool for blood.

Treatment

Diverticulosis usually requires no treatment. Your doctor may recommend that you eat more high-fiber foods and drink more liquids to produce softer

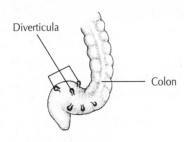

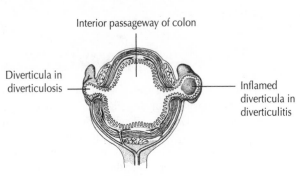

Diverticulosis and diverticulitis
Small pouches called diverticula (top) can form in the outer wall of the colon and project into the abdominal cavity. If these pouches don't cause pain or other symptoms, the condition is called diverticulosis. If the pouches become inflamed, however, they can cause pain; this condition is called diverticulitis (bottom).

stools, which will help prevent straining during bowel movements.

To treat diverticulitis, your doctor will probably prescribe oral antibiotics to take for 7 to 10 days. He or she may recommend a liquid diet to give your colon time to heal. If the abdominal pain continues, your doctor will admit you to a hospital and you will be given antibiotics intravenously (through a vein). Immediate surgery usually is not necessary unless the diverticula continue to bleed or if peritonitis or an intestinal obstruction (see page 759) develops. To treat bleeding diverticula, your doctor may recommend a procedure using angiography (see page 110) to inject a substance into the artery to make the blood clot. In some cases, surgery is necessary to stop the bleeding.

If you are not passing gas or stool, the contents of your stomach and intestine will be sucked out through a long tube and you will be given fluids intravenously. If the swelling in your abdomen doesn't subside, you may have an intestinal obstruction. In rare cases, doctors perform a temporary

colostomy (see page 776). After the inflammation has subsided (usually within a few weeks), the colostomy will be closed and the affected section of the colon removed (colectomy; see page 776). Diverticulosis and diverticulitis usually recur unless the entire colon has been removed.

Intestinal Polyps

Polyps are mushroomlike growths that can develop in the large intestine, either singly or in groups. Most polyps are benign (noncancerous). Two types of polyps occur in the large intestine—adenomatous polyps and hyperplastic polyps. Adenomatous polyps are the most likely to grow large (bigger than $1/2$ inch) and become cancerous. In rare cases, people can have hundreds of polyps in their colon (familial polyposis; see next page). The cause of polyps in the intestine is unknown, but the incidence increases with age. If the polyps are large, they can cause an intestinal obstruction (see page 759).

Symptoms

Intestinal polyps seldom cause symptoms, but they may cause slight bleeding from the rectum or blood in the stool. You may be pale and tired or have other symptoms of anemia (see page 610) if the polyps cause excessive bleeding. In rare cases, if the polyps have caused an intestinal obstruction, symptoms can include abdominal pain and vomiting.

Polyps and Colon Cancer

Because some types of polyps can become cancerous if they are not removed, doctors recommend testing in people who are at risk of having polyps. You should have a diagnostic procedure called colonoscopy (see page 767) on the following schedule:

- Every 5 years if you have been diagnosed with adenomatous intestinal polyps.

- Every 10 years starting at age 40, or 10 years younger than the age at which colon cancer in a first-degree relative (parent, sibling, or child) was diagnosed.

- Every 10 years starting at age 50 if you have no history of polyps or colon cancer.

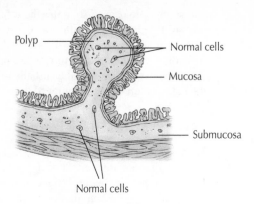

Polyp
Normal cells
Mucosa
Submucosa
Normal cells

Noncancerous polyp

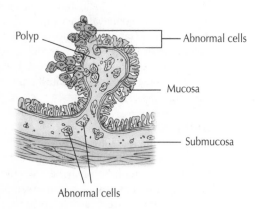

Polyp
Abnormal cells
Mucosa
Submucosa
Abnormal cells

Cancerous polyp

Noncancerous and cancerous polyps
Polyps are growths in the inner lining (mucosa) of the wall of the colon and are usually made up of normal cells. When a polyp becomes cancerous, its cells grow and multiply abnormally. The abnormal cells may grow into the next layer of the wall of the colon (the submucosa). If the cancerous cells continue to multiply unchecked, the cells may invade blood vessels and metastasize (spread) throughout the body.

Diagnosis

Because intestinal polyps usually cause no symptoms, they are often diagnosed by chance from tests performed for another reason. To diagnose intestinal polyps, a doctor performs a procedure called colonoscopy (see page 767) to examine the colon. If just the lower third of the colon is examined, the procedure is called sigmoidoscopy (see page 144). A doctor may also order a barium X-ray (see page 767) of the colon.

Treatment

Intestinal polyps are usually removed through the colonoscope during a colonoscopy. If the polyp is very large, your doctor may be able to remove part of it at that time or may refer you to a surgeon. If the polyp is an adenoma, the larger it is, the greater the risk that it is cancerous. However, sometimes the cancer cells are contained entirely within the polyp, and removal of the polyp is the only procedure necessary.

Familial Polyposis

Familial polyposis (also called familial adenomatous polyposis or polyposis coli) is a relatively rare genetic disorder in which hundreds or thousands of growths—polyps or cysts—form in the colon (the longest part of the large intestine) and sometimes in the stomach or duodenum (the first part of the small intestine). The polyps usually begin to form during puberty; 95 percent of people with familial polyposis have polyps by age 35.

Most people with familial polyposis inherit the disorder from an affected parent. About 30 percent of cases result from a spontaneous change (mutation) in a gene that occurs during conception, which causes the disease to appear for the first time in a family. Because the abnormal gene is dominant (which means that it takes only one copy of the gene to cause the disease), each child of an affected person will have a 50 percent chance of inheriting the abnormal gene and having the disorder. Familial polyposis affects males and females equally and occurs in all racial and ethnic groups.

The polyps eventually become cancerous if they are not removed. However, familial polyposis is responsible for only 1 percent of cases of colon cancer (see next page). The average age at which colon cancer develops in people with untreated familial polyposis is 39 years. If you have familial polyposis, a genetic counselor (see page 952) can help you understand the disorder and evaluate your risk of passing it on to your children.

Symptoms

Although the polyps begin to grow at puberty, most adolescents with familial polyposis have no symptoms. As the disease progresses, symptoms may include blood and mucus in the stool, bleeding from the rectum, a change in bowel habits, diarrhea, abdominal pain, or weight loss. People with some types of familial polyposis tend to produce extra tissue in the form of cysts or bony growths in other parts of the body, including the skin, bones, eyes, thyroid gland, and abdomen.

Diagnosis

To diagnose familial polyposis, your doctor will ask you if anyone in your family has ever been diagnosed with intestinal polyps or colon cancer. He or she will recommend a genetic test that detects the gene mutation that causes familial polyposis. Your doctor will probably perform a procedure called colonoscopy (see page 767) to examine the inside of your colon. He or she may also order a barium X-ray (see page 767) of your colon.

Treatment

Removing the entire colon is the only treatment for familial polyposis because the polyps are too numerous to be removed individually. In some cases, the rectum is also removed. The surgeon may create a temporary or permanent opening on the outside of the abdomen called an ileostomy (see next page) to replace the rectum and through which stool can pass.

Colon Cancer

Cancer of the large intestine is usually called colon cancer or colorectal cancer. It occurs most often in the lowest part of the large intestine. Colon cancer is the third most common cancer (after lung cancer and breast cancer). The cause of colon cancer is unknown, but researchers think that a diet high in animal fat (especially from red meat) and low in fiber may play a role. Smoking cigarettes has been linked to colon cancer. Genes also have an influence—having a family history of colon cancer increases your risk. Having ulcerative colitis (see page 764) also increases your risk—about 1 of 20 people who have had ulcerative colitis for more than 10 years eventually develops colon cancer. Having adenomatous intestinal polyps (see page 773) that are not detected and removed also increases the risk of colon cancer. Men and women are equally susceptible. Colon cancer is most prevalent in people over 40, and the incidence increases with age.

As the cancerous cells multiply, the normally smooth intestinal lining roughens, enlarges, and hardens. If a tumor grows large enough, it can cause an intestinal obstruction (see page 759), blocking the passage of stool. If untreated, colon cancer can spread through the intestinal wall to other abdominal organs or through the bloodstream to other parts of the body. If you have a relative who has had colon cancer, talk to your doctor about having a screening test called colonoscopy (see page 767), which is the most effective way to detect colon cancer.

Symptoms

The symptoms of colon cancer depend on the site of the cancer and on its stage (see page 777). Because the inside of the intestine does not have pain sensors, you won't feel pain in the early stages of colon cancer. The first symptom is usually a change in normal bowel movements, such as constipation, diarrhea, narrow stool, or a feeling that the rectum is not completely empty. Other symptoms can include abdominal discomfort, a bloated feeling, nausea, digestive noises such as rumbling or gurgling, weight loss, blood in the stool, or bleeding from the rectum. In rare cases, a person has no symptoms at all until the cancer causes an intestinal obstruction or until the intestine ruptures and causes peritonitis.

Screening Tests to Detect Colon Cancer

Colonoscopy is the most effective screening test for colon cancer. For people who have a family history of colon cancer, the test is recommended at regular intervals beginning when they are 10 years younger than the age at which a first-degree relative (parent, sibling, or child) was diagnosed. For other people, colonoscopy is recommended every 10 years beginning at age 50, together with annual fecal occult blood tests (see page 142).

Diagnosis

If you have symptoms of colon cancer, your doctor will perform a physical examination, including a digital rectal examination (see page 144). During the digital examination, your doctor will take a sample of stool to test it for blood. He or she will recommend that you have a diagnostic test called colonoscopy to examine your large

Colectomy, Colostomy, and Ileostomy

To treat intestinal disorders such as diverticulitis, ulcerative colitis, and cancer of the large intestine (colon), it may be necessary to remove all or part of an intestine in a procedure called colectomy. If possible, the two severed ends of the colon are sewn or stapled together to maintain a passageway for stool. When it is not possible to maintain this passageway, an opening called a stoma is made in the abdominal wall, through which stool can pass into a bag. The procedure is called a colostomy when the colon opens through the stoma and an ileostomy when the small intestine opens through the stoma.

A colectomy is surgical removal of part or all of the colon. In a partial colectomy, the diseased part of the colon is removed and the two severed ends of the colon are joined together. The surgeon makes a temporary or permanent opening called a colostomy to allow stool to pass directly outside the body through an artificial opening in the abdominal wall (instead of the normal route through the large intestine and rectum). If the colostomy is temporary, the stoma will be closed after the surgically severed ends of the colon heal and fuse together.

In a total colectomy, which is sometimes done for inflammatory bowel disease (see page 764), the entire colon is removed. The rectum may or may not be removed. If the rectum is removed, the doctor may perform an ileostomy.

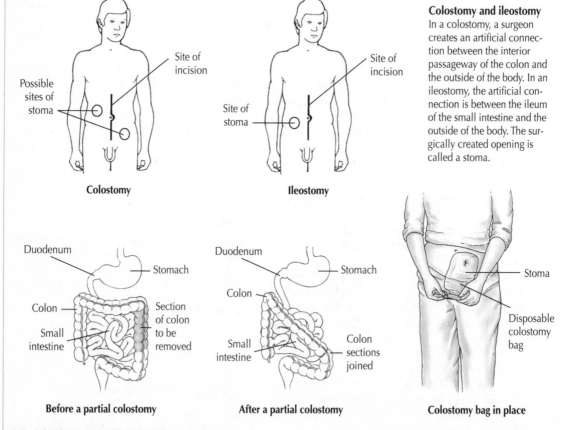

Colostomy

Ileostomy

Colostomy and ileostomy
In a colostomy, a surgeon creates an artificial connection between the interior passageway of the colon and the outside of the body. In an ileostomy, the artificial connection is between the ileum of the small intestine and the outside of the body. The surgically created opening is called a stoma.

Before a partial colostomy

After a partial colostomy

Colostomy bag in place

Partial colectomy with a colostomy

In a partial colectomy, a surgeon removes the damaged section of the colon and joins the two severed ends. He or she then creates an artificial opening called a stoma, through which stool can be eliminated. He or she makes an incision in the abdomen and brings part of the colon through the incision in a procedure called a colostomy. The severed edges of the colon are then stitched to the skin at the edge of the incision to make the stoma. A bag to collect stool can be attached to the skin around the stoma with an adhesive. The bag is replaced after each bowel movement.

Stages of Colon Cancer

In most types of cancer, staging is used to determine how far the cancer has progressed. The cancer is described in terms of how large the primary tumor is, the degree to which the tumor has invaded surrounding tissue, and the extent to which it has spread to lymph glands or other areas of the body. Staging helps a doctor determine the most appropriate treatment. Doctors stage colon cancer in the following way:

- **Stage 0**   The cancer is limited to the innermost lining of the colon or rectum.
- **Stage I**   The cancer has spread to the outer part of the lining of the colon or rectum.
- **Stage II**   The cancer has spread from the intestine to nearby organs or tissues but not to the lymph nodes.
- **Stage III**   The cancer has spread to nearby lymph nodes.
- **Stage IV**   The cancer has spread to other parts of the body, such as the liver or lungs.

intestine. If just the lower third of the large intestine is examined, the procedure is called sigmoidoscopy (see page 144). Your doctor also may order a barium X-ray (see page 767) of your large intestine.

Treatment

For colon cancer that has not spread to other organs, surgery is the most effective treatment. If the cancer is confined to the colon, the surgeon will remove the growth and the surrounding areas of the colon on either side of the tumor in a procedure called colectomy (see previous page); the remaining healthy sections of the colon are stitched together to maintain a passageway for stool. If the cancer is very low in the intestine, you may need to have a colostomy (see previous page). Your doctor may recommend chemotherapy (see page 23) after surgery. Radiation therapy (see page 23) is used in combination with chemotherapy either before or after surgery to treat cancerous tumors that develop in the rectum.

Disorders of the Anus

The anus is the opening at the end of the digestive tract through which stool passes out of the body. It is a 1½-inch-long canal that leads from the rectum through a ring of muscles (the anal sphincter) to the anal opening. Normally an adult can easily control the anal sphincter, regulating when he or she wants to have a bowel movement. Because the function and structure of the anus are relatively simple, only a few disorders affect the anus.

Hemorrhoids

Hemorrhoids are swollen veins (varicose veins; see page 602) that protrude from the lining of the anus. The affected veins lie just under the mucous membrane that lines the lowest part of the rectum and anus. Hemorrhoids can occur anywhere in the anal canal. They may be hidden at the beginning of the canal or visible at the opening.

Hemorrhoids are a common disorder. Straining to pass stool puts pressure on the sphincter muscles and pressure on the veins of the anus, causing them to swell. Some people are more susceptible than others to developing hemorrhoids. Pregnant women and people who are obese can develop hemorrhoids from the extra pressure that increased weight can put on the abdomen and the veins of the anus. Often

people who have advanced cirrhosis (see page 790) have hemorrhoids because blood flow to their liver is obstructed, which can increase blood pressure in the veins of the intestine and anus.

Symptoms

The primary symptom of hemorrhoids is bleeding from the rectum, which is often noticeable only on toilet paper or in toilet water. Blood may also be around, but not mixed in, the stool. The walls of the swollen, twisted veins are thin and rupture easily during bowel movements. External hemorrhoids may be visible at all times, or they may protrude outside the anus only during a bowel movement. The ruptured veins produce sore areas that can cause pain during bowel movements. Anticipating pain during a bowel movement can make a person delay passing stool, which, in turn, can lead to harder, drier stool. Although not life-threatening, a blood clot that develops inside a swollen vein can cause considerable pain. A hemorrhoid that protrudes outside the anus prevents the anus from closing fully, allowing a discharge of mucus to seep out and irritate the surrounding area (see box at right).

Diagnosis

If you have symptoms of hemorrhoids, your doctor will perform a digital rectal examination (see page 144). He or she may also perform a procedure called anoscopy (see page 766) to examine the anus and rectum. To make sure that the bleeding from the rectum is not the result of colon cancer, he or she may recommend that you have a colonoscopy (see page 767) or sigmoidoscopy (see page 144).

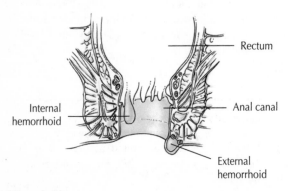

Rectum

Internal hemorrhoid

Anal canal

External hemorrhoid

Hemorrhoids
Hemorrhoids are swollen veins in the lining of the anus that can develop near the opening of the anal canal (internal hemorrhoids) or at the anal opening (external hemorrhoids). Some may protrude outside the anus.

Treatment

To soothe inflamed hemorrhoids, your doctor may prescribe rectal suppositories or ointments that contain hydrocortisone and pain relievers. If a blood clot has developed in a hemorrhoid and is causing extreme pain, your doctor may remove the clot. If a hemorrhoid does not heal, the doctor may wrap a rubber band around its base to cut off its blood supply; without a supply of blood, the hemorrhoid withers and falls off. Other techniques used to remove hemorrhoids include destroying tissue by freezing

Self-Help for Anal Itching

Anal itching (also called pruritus ani) is a common problem, usually caused by hemorrhoids or irritation. In children, the itching may be caused by pinworms (see page 444), especially if the itching is worse at night. Anal itching is more prevalent in older people because the skin becomes drier and less elastic with age.

If you have anal itching, your doctor may recommend the following tips to help heal irritated tissue and relieve the itching:

- Soak in a warm bath once or twice a day.
- Cleanse the anal area with mild soap and water (or just water) and dry the area gently but thoroughly.
- Use unscented soaps, lotions, and toilet paper to avoid irritation.
- When you are away from home, carry with you prepackaged pads that contain soothing lotions or oils to clean the anal area.
- Don't scratch or rub the inflamed area.
- Wear cotton underwear to keep the area dry.

Self-Help for Hemorrhoids

If you have hemorrhoids:

- Don't delay having a bowel movement, or strain or sit too long on the toilet.
- Eat plenty of high-fiber foods (such as fruits, vegetables, and whole-grain or bran cereals or breads) and drink lots of fluids (especially water) to make your stool soft and easy to pass.
- To increase the water content of your stool, which makes it softer and easier to pass, take a psyllium-based fiber supplement (not a laxative) with a large glass of water.

- Exercise regularly to stimulate bowel movements to help relieve constipation.
- If you have protruding hemorrhoids, push them back in with your finger after every bowel movement.
- Apply an ice compress to the anal area to help relieve swelling.
- Sit on a doughnut-shaped pillow to ease pressure on sore areas.
- If you are having a painful attack, rest in bed.
- To relieve anal itching and irritation, use the self-help tips in the box above.

(cryosurgery), injecting a chemical to shrink the hemorrhoid, or using heat (infrared coagulation) to seal the hemorrhoid and prevent it from bleeding. Only in rare cases are hemorrhoids removed surgically (called a hemorrhoidectomy). In this procedure, a surgeon stretches the hemorrhoid, ties it off at the base, and slices it off using a scalpel or laser. The laser seals the blood vessels as it cuts.

Rectal Abscesses

Rectal abscesses are pus-filled cavities surrounded by inflamed tissue that can develop in the tissue surrounding the anus, deeper in the rectum (between the muscles of the anal sphincter), or in tissues higher up in the rectum. People who have an inflammatory bowel disease (see page 764), leukemia (see page 621), or diabetes (see page 889), or who engage in anal sex are at increased risk of developing rectal abscesses. If a rectal abscess is untreated, it can lead to an anal fistula (an abnormal channel from the anal canal to the skin's surface; see right).

Symptoms
The symptoms of rectal abscesses include intense pain in the rectal area (especially during a bowel movement), and bleeding and a discharge of pus-filled mucus from the rectum. A rectal abscess outside the body may be swollen and feel warm. You also may have a fever with chills.

Diagnosis and Treatment
To diagnose a rectal abscess, a doctor performs a digital rectal examination (see page 144) to feel for the abscess. He or she may also perform a procedure called anoscopy (see page 766) to examine the anus and rectum to look for an abscess. Ultrasound (see page 111) may also be used to help detect an abscess in the rectum. An abscess in the rectum is usually drained surgically. If the abscess is deep, general anesthesia may be necessary. The doctor will prescribe antibiotics to kill the bacteria.

Anal Fissures

An anal fissure is an elongated ulcer (sore) that extends upward into the anal canal from the anal opening. The cause is not known, but it may result from passing a large, hard stool. An anal fissure can also occur from injury to the delicate tissues of the anal canal during anal sex.

Symptoms
An anal fissure is easily irritated during a bowel movement. The fissure may also cause bleeding from the rectum. Sometimes the area is so painful that the anal sphincter tightens (spasms), causing more pain.

Diagnosis and Treatment
A doctor can diagnose an anal fissure by looking inside the anal canal. Most fissures heal on their own. For an anal fissure caused by constipation, a doctor will recommend eating high-fiber foods, drinking lots of water, exercising, and not delaying bowel movements or straining or sitting too long on the toilet. Sit on a doughnut-shaped pillow or rest in bed if you are having a painful attack. Your doctor may also recommend the self-help tips for anal itching to help heal irritated tissue and the self-help tips for hemorrhoids on the previous page because these tips also would help an anal fissure. If the fissure does not heal or if it recurs, your doctor may recommend surgery to widen the anal sphincter muscle and close the fissure.

Anal Fistulas

An anal fistula is a rare condition in which a tiny tubelike opening starts in the anal canal and ends in a small hole in the skin near the anal opening. The fistula is caused by the erosion of tissue from a spreading rectal abscess (see left). Anal fistulas are often a complication of Crohn's disease (see page 764) or colon cancer (see page 775).

Symptoms and Diagnosis
A continuous discharge of watery pus through the fistula irritates the skin and causes pain and itching. The abscess itself may be painful. To diagnose an anal fistula, your doctor will order a barium enema (see page 767) or a CT scan (see page 112) with a contrast medium (dye). He or she will also perform a procedure called sigmoidoscopy (see page 144) to examine the anus and rectum.

Treatment
The treatment of an anal fistula depends on its cause. Fistulas caused by Crohn's disease often heal when the inflammatory disorder is brought under control. To treat an anal fistula caused by a rectal abscess, a doctor will remove the fistula and drain the abscess.

Rectal Prolapse

Rectal prolapse is the displacement of the rectum from its normal position. In complete rectal prolapse, the membrane that lines the rectum and the muscle wall of the rectum protrude out of the anus. The disorder usually results from straining during bowel movements. Rectal prolapse is most common in older people because the tissues that support the perineum (the area between the genital organs and the anus) can weaken with age. In some women, the ligaments of the rectal area are weakened during childbirth, putting them at increased risk for rectal prolapse.

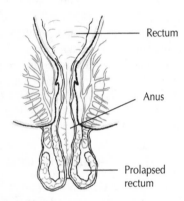

Rectum

Anus

Prolapsed rectum

Rectal prolapse
In a rectal prolapse, the lining of the rectum protrudes outside the anus.

Symptoms and Diagnosis

In its earliest stages, rectal prolapse may not be evident outside the body. The first symptoms may be fecal incontinence (see right) and a discharge of mucus or blood from the rectum. You may have some discomfort, but rectal prolapse rarely causes pain. The most obvious symptom is the protrusion of the rectum from the anus, especially when straining during a bowel movement.

A rectal prolapse is diagnosed with a procedure called a defecogram, in which an X-ray video is taken of the rectum while a person has a bowel movement.

Treatment

Treatment of a rectal prolapse depends on the person's age and general physical condition and on the severity of the prolapse. Rectal prolapse in children usually corrects itself with a high-fiber diet. In adults, a surgeon may implant a band of elastic, wire, or nylon around the muscle of the anus to enable it to support the rectum and keep it in place. Rectal surgery also may involve raising and repositioning the rectum or removing tissue from the rectum. More extensive surgery involves opening the abdomen and removing the displaced segment of the rectum. Surgery is not always successful, and rectal prolapse frequently recurs.

Fecal Incontinence

Fecal incontinence is the inability to retain stool (feces) in the rectum. Fecal incontinence may be caused by damage to the muscles or nerves of the anal sphincter or rectum, diarrhea, lack of elasticity of the walls of the rectum, or dysfunction of the pelvic floor. Damage to the muscles or nerves can occur during childbirth, especially if the doctor uses forceps or does an episiotomy (see page 533). Surgery of the anus or rectum (such as to treat hemorrhoids; see page 778) can also damage the sphincter. Straining during a bowel movement or having a stroke (see page 669) or another disorder that affects the nerves, such as diabetes (see page 889) or multiple sclerosis (see page 696), can also cause fecal incontinence. Having rectal surgery, radiation therapy (see page 23), or an inflammatory bowel disease (see page 764) can cause scarring that makes the walls of the rectum stiff—the rectum can't stretch and hold the usual amount of stool. Fecal incontinence can also be a consequence of rectal prolapse (see left).

Diagnosis

If you have fecal incontinence, your doctor will perform a physical examination. He or she may also order a series of tests such as manometry (see page 751) to check the tightness of your anal sphincter and the function of your rectum, an ultrasound (see page 111) to evaluate the structure of the anal sphincter, and electromyography to test for nerve damage. The doctor may perform a procedure that measures how much stool your rectum can hold and how well it holds and eliminates stool. During a procedure called sigmoidoscopy (see page 144), the doctor will examine your lower intestine and rectum to look for signs of disease such as inflammation, growths, or scarring.

Treatment

The treatment of fecal incontinence depends on the cause. Your doctor may recommend changes in your diet and eating habits such as avoiding particular foods (for example, caffeine relaxes the anal sphincter muscle), eating small meals more frequently, eating foods with more fiber, and drinking lots of water to avoid dehydration. Your doctor also may prescribe medications such as vitamin supplements and antidiarrheals. Exercises to strengthen the pelvic muscles (Kegel exercises; see page 874)

or training the bowels to empty at a particular time of day can be helpful. Because constant contact with stool can cause anal skin inflammation, use the tips on page 778 to soothe irritated anal tissue. If fecal incontinence is the result of injury to the pelvic floor, rectum, or anal sphincter, surgery may be necessary to repair the damage. Some people who have chronic fecal incontinence decide, after discussing it with their doctor, to have a colostomy (see page 776).

Infections of the Digestive Tract

The intestines normally contain harmless bacteria; some bacteria that inhabit the intestines have beneficial functions such as manufacturing vitamins. An infection of the digestive tract occurs when infectious agents, such as viruses or bacteria, multiply rapidly in the stomach or intestines. The presence of microorganisms in the digestive tract is not considered an infection unless the microorganisms exist in large numbers and cause symptoms.

Gastroenteritis

Gastroenteritis is a general term that refers to irritation and inflammation of the digestive tract, especially the stomach and intestines. It is most often caused by a viral infection that spreads easily from person to person—even without having direct contact or consuming contaminated food or water. Viral infections are the most common cause of the 24- to 48-hour attacks of vomiting and diarrhea that are commonly called stomach or intestinal flu.

Eating or drinking contaminated food or water (food poisoning; see page 783) can also cause gastroenteritis. Gastroenteritis that occurs after eating something that contains a toxic substance, such as a nonedible mushroom or a rhubarb leaf, is not actually food poisoning but can cause a severe attack. Eggs, milk products, and shellfish can cause allergic reactions in people who are sensitive to those foods (see page 915).

Another possible cause of gastroenteritis is a change in the population of bacteria that normally live in the digestive tract. If you have an illness that weakens your immune system, or if you suddenly make changes in your diet (such as when visiting another country), the balance of bacteria in your digestive tract can become disturbed. When some strains of bacteria become stronger and multiply at the expense of others, the result can be an upset stomach and irritated intestines. Antibiotic drugs also can disturb the bacterial equilibrium in the intestines, permitting unchecked growth of bacteria that can lead to infections such as the common yeast infection candidiasis (see page 880).

The severity of an attack of gastroenteritis depends on the type of infectious agent, the number of infectious microbes, the amount of contaminated food substances you have eaten, and your age and general health. The risk of serious illness is greatest for newborns, children younger than 18 months, and older people who are chronically ill or who have a weakened immune system. In a healthy person, an episode of vomiting and diarrhea is rarely serious. But persistent diarrhea can cause dehydration and loss of essential body salts, which upsets body chemistry and, if not treated, can lead to shock (see page 579). Severe and persistent pain in the abdomen (not just an occasional cramp) can be a sign of a more serious abdominal disorder.

Symptoms

The symptoms of gastroenteritis range from a mild attack of nausea followed by diarrhea to a severe illness. You may have only one or two bouts of vomiting and soft stool, or you may vomit repeatedly and have recurring attacks of watery diarrhea with abdominal pain and cramps, fever, and extreme weakness. Occasionally, a severe case of gastroenteritis lasts so long that it is disabling. In most cases, however, the symptoms go away within 24 to 48 hours. If your symptoms last for 5 days or more, if you notice any blood in your stool, or if you have symptoms of dehydration (such as lightheadedness, a rapid pulse, and little urine output), see your doctor right away.

Diagnosis

If you have symptoms of gastroenteritis, your doctor will perform a physical examination and may take a stool sample for laboratory evaluation. The doctor will ask you questions about what you have eaten and whether any family members or other people you have come into contact with are also ill. He or she may know about a local epidemic of gastroenteritis and its cause, which will help determine treatment.

Treatment

Because most attacks of gastroenteritis clear up on their own, you can perform self-help measures at home to keep you from getting dehydrated. If you have been vomiting, once you can keep liquids down, drink an oral rehydration solution (a mixture of water, salts, and glucose that helps your body absorb water and get it into cells), which will significantly reduce your risk of dehydration. Rehydration solutions are available over the counter in most pharmacies.

If you have diarrhea, drink the rehydration fluid at half-hour intervals until your urine becomes pale yellow again, a sign that you are no longer dehydrated. An adult with severe diarrhea may need to drink a few quarts of the solution per day before his or her urine returns to its normal color. Once the diarrhea begins to ease, start drinking other kinds of fluids such as tea and clear broth or bouillon; gradually add flavored gelatin, cooked cereal, and other bland, soft foods. After about 2 or 3 days, you should be able to resume your normal diet.

Over-the-counter antidiarrhea medications may help relieve symptoms, but they are not an alternative to the fluid replacement that is essential for treating diarrhea. However, you should not take antidiarrhea medication if there is blood in your stool. Also, do not take antibiotics without talking to your doctor. Antibiotics can make it more difficult to identify the cause of diarrhea, and some antibiotics can upset the bacterial balance in the intestine and cause an inflammatory form of diarrhea called Clostridium difficile colitis.

There is no specific treatment for viral gastroenteritis. If the diagnosis is definite and your nausea and diarrhea are relatively mild, your doctor will probably recommend continuing the self-help measures described above. If your vomiting is severe, your doctor may prescribe an antiemetic drug in suppository form or by injection. Diarrhea caused by a virus is sometimes treated with medications such as narcotic-type drugs or antispasmodic drugs that slow intestinal activity and may help relieve cramping. Treatment is usually stopped as soon as the intestines begin to function normally again.

If your vomiting and diarrhea are so severe that you become dehydrated, or if you have a chronic disease such as diabetes (see page 889) or kidney problems, your doctor may admit you to the hospital to give you fluids intravenously (through a vein) and restore the balance of your body chemistry.

Gastrointestinal Anthrax

Anthrax is a very rare, noncontagious disease caused by the bacterium Bacillus anthracis. Gastrointestinal anthrax (also called intestinal or ingestion anthrax) results from eating the meat of contaminated animals, usually beef. The disorder is rare in humans in the United States because livestock is vaccinated routinely for anthrax in areas where the anthrax bacterium can be found in the soil. (Other forms of anthrax have been used in bioterrorism; see page 30.)

Anthrax bacteria settle in the lining of the intestines, where they multiply and produce a toxin. The symptoms of gastrointestinal anthrax occur 1 to 7 days after a person eats raw or undercooked meat containing the bacteria. Symptoms initially resemble those of gastroenteritis (see previous page), including nausea, vomiting, diarrhea, fever with chills, and abdominal pain. Later symptoms include headaches, back pain, pain in the arms and legs, bloody diarrhea, and bleeding of the mucous membranes. Gastrointestinal anthrax can be treated easily with antibiotics. If untreated, it can be fatal.

Food Poisoning

Food poisoning, also known as foodborne illness, refers to a group of disorders caused by the ingestion of food or beverages contaminated with infectious microorganisms such as viruses or bacteria. Food, such as some mushrooms, also can contain toxins that produce illness, and some microorganisms produce toxins as they grow inside food. Infants, children, older people, pregnant women, and people with a compromised immune system from illness or cancer treatment are most vulnerable to the more serious effects of food poisoning.

More than 250 different foodborne illnesses are known to exist, and up to 80 million cases of food poisoning occur in the United States every year. The most common types of food poisoning include botulism, cryptosporidiosis, shigellosis, mushroom poisoning, traveler's diarrhea; and campylobacter, cyclospora, E. coli, salmonella, and staphylococcus infections. Infection by the parasite that causes trichinosis from eating undercooked pork is now relatively rare, but it can be contracted from eating undercooked game meat such as bear, wolf, fox, or squirrel.

Symptoms

Many types of food poisoning cause nausea, vomiting, abdominal cramps, and diarrhea, but the different types also produce various characteristic symptoms. The chart below describes the sources

Type of Food Poisoning	Common sources	Symptoms
Botulism	Contaminated home-canned food	Muscle weakness, blurred vision, dilated pupils, difficulty breathing, paralysis
Campylobacteriosis	Raw or undercooked chicken	Abdominal cramps and pain, fever, bloody diarrhea
Cryptosporidiosis	Contaminated water, unpasteurized apple cider, raw vegetables and fruits	Watery diarrhea, fever, chills, headache, body aches, abdominal cramps, nausea, vomiting
Cyclosporiasis	Contaminated food	Diarrhea
E. coli infection (or colibacillosis)	Undercooked ground beef, alfalfa sprouts, unpasteurized apple cider	Watery diarrhea, abdominal pain; can cause hemolytic uremic syndrome (see page 429) in children and older people
Giardiasis	Contaminated water	Diarrhea, nausea, vomiting, abdominal pain
Infant botulism	Contaminated honey	Muscle weakness, a weak cry, poor sucking, increased heart rate, constipation
Listeriosis	Contaminated soft cheeses, unpasteurized milk, vegetables grown in soil fertilized with manure	Fever, body aches, vomiting; can cause meningitis in people who have a weakened immune system
Mushroom poisoning	Poisonous wild mushrooms	Abdominal pain, diarrhea, vomiting, difficulty breathing, sweating, dizziness, seizures, hallucinations, liver or kidney damage
Norwalk and Norwalk-like viruses	Uncooked food contaminated with the feces of infected food handlers; contaminated drinking water and ice made from contaminated water	Nausea, vomiting, diarrhea, abdominal pain, muscle aches, headache, fatigue, fever
Salmonellosis	Undercooked poultry and eggs	Abdominal pain, diarrhea, nausea, headache, fever, severe dehydration
Shigellosis	Food or water contaminated with the feces of infected food handlers	Bloody diarrhea, fever, nausea, vomiting, abdominal cramps
Staphylococcosis	Contaminated, hand-prepared food, such as sandwich spreads	Nausea, vomiting, diarrhea
Traveler's diarrhea	Food or beverages contaminated with bacteria, viruses, or parasites	Watery diarrhea, abdominal cramps, fever, nausea, vomiting
Vibriosis	Contaminated fish or shellfish	Diarrhea, abdominal cramps, vomiting, headache, fever

of the most common types of food poisoning and their hallmark symptoms.

Diagnosis

Most cases of food poisoning improve on their own within 2 or 3 days. Call your doctor if your fever is higher than 102°F, if blood appears in your stool, if you are dehydrated, or if the diarrhea lasts longer than 3 days. To diagnose the source of the food poisoning, your doctor will take a sample of your stool and send it to a laboratory for testing.

Treatment

There are many different kinds of food poisoning and they may require different treatments, depending on the cause. Most cases cause vomiting and diarrhea, which can cause dehydration. You should replace lost fluids by drinking plenty of liquids or an oral rehydration solution. You can help relieve diarrhea by taking the over-the-counter drug bismuth subsalicylate. Your doctor will prescribe antibiotics only if the food poisoning was caused by bacteria such as shigella, salmonella, or campylobacter.

Handling Food Safely

Bacteria and other microorganisms that cause food poisoning can quickly contaminate the food in your kitchen if you don't handle it carefully. Poultry, especially, is a major source of contamination with salmonella bacteria, which can also be harbored by raw eggs. Most cases of food poisoning are caused by the following:

- Contamination of food by other foods (for example, when raw meat, poultry, or eggs touch cooked foods)
- Not cooking meat, poultry, or eggs sufficiently
- Insufficient hand washing
- Leaving foods out at room temperature when they should be refrigerated, frozen, or kept hot

You can protect your family's health at mealtimes by following these simple guidelines:

- Always wash your hands thoroughly before handling food and after handling raw meat, poultry, or eggs.
- Wash the knives and cutting boards you use for meat or poultry in hot, soapy water.
- Never reuse a plate or cutting board that held raw meat or poultry for cooked foods or for preparing other foods.
- Rinse meat, fish, and poultry before cooking.

- Never eat raw or undercooked beef, poultry, fish, or eggs. Cook these foods at a temperature above 140°F to kill infectious microorganisms.
- Use or freeze raw meat within 3 days, and poultry within 2 days. Separate raw meat and poultry from other foods when storing them in the refrigerator.
- Always defrost food in the refrigerator for 12 to 24 hours (not at room temperature) or in the microwave.
- Never refreeze foods that you have thawed (bread is an exception).
- Don't leave cooked or raw foods at room temperature for more than 2 hours.
- Make sure the temperature in your refrigerator is below 40°F and your freezer is set at 0° or lower.
- Refrigerate leftovers right away. You don't have to wait for hot foods to cool down first.
- Eat leftovers within 2 or 3 days or freeze them.
- Throw away a can or jar if it hisses or food spurts out when you open it—the food may contain the bacterium that causes botulism, a life-threatening form of food poisoning. (Some vacuum-packed cans do hiss slightly when opened, which is normal.) Avoid buying dented or swollen cans of food.

Disorders of the Liver, Gallbladder, and Pancreas

The liver, gallbladder, and pancreas are not actually part of the digestive system, but they play a vital role in digestion and the body's use of nutrients from food. The liver is the heaviest organ in the body, spreading across the upper right part of the abdomen behind the lower ribs. The liver is the body's chemical factory, performing vital functions such as converting food into nutrients the body can use; storing nutrients including fats, vitamins, sugars, and iron until the body needs them; producing proteins necessary for blood clotting; and removing or neutralizing potentially harmful substances such as alcohol. Most of the cholesterol in your body is made by your liver from saturated fats in foods that you eat (such as whole-milk dairy products and red meat).

To aid digestion, the liver secretes a fluid called bile, which helps neutralize stomach acid and break down fat. Bile trickles through tiny tubes (called bile ducts) into the gallbladder, a baglike collecting organ that rests against the lower back of the liver to absorb water and store bile. During digestion, the duodenum (the first part of the small intestine, from the stomach) releases a hormone that stimulates the gallbladder to contract and release bile into the duodenum through the common bile duct.

The pancreas lies just behind the lower part of the stomach. The pancreas makes insulin, a hormone that controls the body's use of sugar for energy and regulates the body's use of fat and amino acids, which are essential for storing energy and building proteins. The pancreas also makes enzymes, digestive juices that flow down the pancreatic duct into the duodenum, where they break food down into particles small enough to be absorbed and used by the body.

Liver, gallbladder, and pancreas

Although the liver, gallbladder, and pancreas are not actually considered organs of the digestive system, each plays an important role in digestion and in enabling the body to use nutrients for energy. The liver spreads across the upper right abdomen behind the lower ribs. The gallbladder rests against the lower back of the liver. The pancreas lies just behind the lower part of the stomach. The pancreas is connected to the duodenum (the upper part of the small intestine at the exit from the stomach) by the common bile duct. The bile duct transports the digestive fluid bile from the gallbladder to the intestines to help in the digestion of fats.

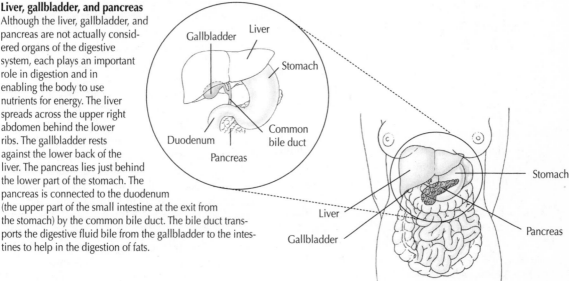

Jaundice

Jaundice is a condition that results from excess bilirubin in the blood; bilirubin is a yellow pigment by-product of the breakdown of aging red blood cells. An excess of the yellow pigment discolors the skin and the whites of the eyes (see pages 118 and 127). Normally, the liver filters bilirubin from the bloodstream and excretes it into the bile ducts, which carry it to the gallbladder. From the gallbladder, bilirubin eventually flows into the small intestine, where most of it is broken down by bacteria that are normally present in the intestine. Bilirubin is eliminated from the body as pigmented compounds in stool.

Jaundice usually occurs as a result of liver diseases, including the viral infection hepatitis (see next page), cirrhosis (see page 790), cancers that spread to the liver, or blockage of a bile duct, or as a reaction to a medication.

Jaundice can also result from an obstruction of the bile ducts—such as gallstones (see page 793) or pancreatic tumors (see page 800)—which can prevent bilirubin from entering the intestines, causing it to build up in the blood. Jaundice can occur in hemolytic anemia (see page 616), in which red blood cells are destroyed at an excessive rate, releasing bilirubin into the blood. In hemolytic anemia, the liver functions normally but is unable to remove bilirubin from the blood rapidly enough.

If you notice that the whites of your eyes are yellow and your skin tone is yellowish, see your doctor right away. He or she will examine you and may order various diagnostic tests to find the underlying cause of your symptoms. Treatment will depend on the underlying disorder. Once that disorder is treated or cured, the jaundice should clear up.

Hepatitis

Hepatitis is inflammation of the liver caused by one of several hepatitis viruses—A, B, C, D, or E. The diseases caused by the hepatitis viruses share many of the same symptoms, but the way in which they are transmitted and the progression of the diseases and their outlook differ. Hepatitis A, B, and C are the most common in the United States. Hepatitis D occurs only along with hepatitis B. Hepatitis E is much more common in developing countries than in the United States.

Hepatitis A

Hepatitis A is found in the feces of people who are infected and is spread from person to person by close contact or by consuming food or water contaminated with infected feces. From 90,000 to 180,000 people in the United States are infected with hepatitis A each year, but the disease is especially widespread in developing countries with inadequate sanitation systems. If you are planning to travel to a developing country, talk to your doctor about having a vaccination against hepatitis A (see next page).

Children, especially those under age 6, who are infected with hepatitis A often have no symptoms. Adults usually develop flulike symptoms such as fever, headache, aching joints, and weakness. Other symptoms include lack of appetite, nausea, abdominal pain, dark urine, and light-colored stool. Jaundice (yellowing of the skin and whites of the eyes; see previous page) usually develops after a few days. In nearly all cases, the symptoms gradually subside on their own in a few weeks or months. In rare cases, the infection eventually leads to liver failure, and a liver transplant (see page 790) is recommended. In very rare cases, the infection can be fatal.

Hepatitis A is diagnosed with a blood test that checks for antibodies (proteins the body produces to fight the virus), which are detectable 5 to 10 days before symptoms develop and can persist for up to 6 months. No treatment is available for hepatitis A. Once a person has been infected, he or she is immune to the disease for life.

Hepatitis B

Hepatitis B virus causes inflammation of the liver that, in some people, can damage liver cells and lead to scarring of the liver (cirrhosis; see page 790) and an increased risk of liver cancer (see page 792). The hepatitis B virus is spread by contact with the blood, semen, or vaginal secretions of an infected person. Thousands of people in the United States become infected with hepatitis B each year. The virus can be transmitted through sexual activity with an infected person, sharing contaminated intravenous needles, or using unsterilized needles for tattoos or body piercing. Health care workers who come into frequent contact with blood are also at increased risk.

An infected pregnant woman can transmit the hepatitis B virus to her baby during a vaginal delivery. Giving the baby an injection of antibodies to fight the virus and a vaccination within 24 hours of birth can help to prevent infection; this treatment is effective in 95 percent of cases. Like all newborns in the United States, the babies of infected women also receive the required series of three hepatitis B vaccinations during the first 6 months of life. A few months after they receive the last dose of the vaccine, they are tested to determine if their body is making antibodies against the virus, which will protect them from hepatitis B for life. Infected mothers can safely breastfeed their babies because the hepatitis B virus is not transmitted in breast milk.

When first infected with hepatitis B, a person may not have any symptoms or may have mild flulike symptoms, including loss of appetite, fatigue, muscle aches, fever, and possibly jaundice. The virus can be in the body for an incubation period of 45 to 180 days or more before symptoms develop. During this time, however, a person is highly infectious and can spread the virus to other people. A person continues to be infectious even after the symptoms have cleared up.

Most people who are infected with hepatitis B develop antibodies against the virus and recover with no treatment within 6 months. They become immune to the virus for life and can no longer spread it to others. However, in about 5 to 10 percent of infected adults, the virus stays in the body, often without causing any noticeable symptoms, and can infect other people. This percentage is much higher in infected children and in people who have a weakened immune system. A person who continues to harbor the virus is called a carrier. Carriers are at increased risk of eventually developing cirrhosis, liver cancer, and liver failure. The only way to know if you are infected or if you carry the virus is to have a blood test that looks specifically for hepatitis B. (The hepatitis B virus may not show up on the test during the incubation period, so you will need to repeat the test.)

> ## WARNING!
>
> ## Don't Combine Alcohol and Acetaminophen
>
> Using the over-the-counter pain reliever acetaminophen with alcohol on a regular basis can cause severe liver damage and liver failure. If you have hepatitis, your doctor will recommend that you avoid alcohol altogether. But even people without liver disease should avoid taking acetaminophen if they drink alcohol regularly (especially if they consume more than two or three drinks a day).

Hepatitis C

Hepatitis C is inflammation of the liver caused by the hepatitis C virus, which is more likely than the other hepatitis viruses to become chronic. The disease can progress slowly for 10 to 40 years, eventually causing liver damage in some people. The infection is transmitted through contact with an infected person's blood. Those most at risk of contracting hepatitis C are intravenous drug users who share needles with an infected person, or people who have unsanitary tattooings or body piercings. Less commonly, the infection can be transmitted sexually.

The virus used to be spread primarily through blood transfusions, but all donor blood in the United States is now screened for the virus. However, you could have hepatitis C if you received a blood transfusion or organ transplant before 1992 or blood products (such as clotting factors used for treating hemophilia; see page 618) before 1987. Nearly 4 million Americans are infected with hepatitis C and, because it seldom causes symptoms, most do not know they have it. Some doctors recommend being tested for the virus even if you don't have symptoms. If the test shows that you are infected, you can take antiviral medications such as interferon and ribavirin to slow progression of the disease and prevent liver damage. Ask your doctor about being tested for hepatitis C.

Hepatitis C is diagnosed with a simple blood test that detects antibodies that the body produces to fight the virus. The antibodies can be detected as early as 5 weeks or up to 16 weeks after exposure to the virus. If the test result is positive, the test is repeated to confirm the diagnosis.

Diagnosis

If your doctor thinks you may have viral hepatitis, he or she will ask you about your risk factors, perform a physical examination, and order a blood test to look for one of the viruses. He or she will want to determine which hepatitis virus you are infected with and whether you have any liver damage or liver function problems, and evaluate the severity of the illness. Blood tests may be repeated at regular intervals to monitor the health of your liver and to watch for any signs of liver damage.

Treatment

If you have hepatitis and your symptoms are mild, your doctor will probably recommend that you stay home and rest for a week or two, avoid spreading the infection to others, eat a nutritious diet, and avoid alcohol (which can promote liver damage). If your symptoms are more severe or if laboratory tests indicate that you have liver damage, you may be admitted to the hospital for evaluation and treatment. You may have a liver biopsy (in which a sample of tissue is withdrawn from your liver through a needle for study under a microscope). If you have hepatitis C, you will probably be given antiviral

> ### Hepatitis Vaccinations
>
> Hepatitis B vaccinations are required for all American children and recommended for adults who are at risk of exposure to the virus, such as people who have several sex partners, health care workers, college students who live in dormitories, or people who live with an infected person. Ask your doctor about having a hepatitis B vaccination.
>
> If you are planning a trip to a developing country, where hepatitis A is often widespread, ask your doctor about having a vaccination for hepatitis A. An injection of immune globulin (infection-fighting proteins) can provide immunity to the virus for 2 to 3 months. The two-shot vaccination against hepatitis A provides even more protection after the second shot, although exactly how long the protection lasts is unknown.

medications such as interferon and ribavirin; for hepatitis B, you will be given lamivudine.

Preventing Hepatitis B and C

You can avoid becoming infected with hepatitis B or C or transmitting the virus to other people if you are already infected by taking the following steps:

- If you have hepatitis B, have everyone in your household get tested for the virus. If the test shows that someone is not immune to the virus (and does not already have it), he or she should be vaccinated against hepatitis B.
- Practice safer sex (see page 477) because hepatitis B is a common sexually transmitted disease.
- Tell your sex partners that you have hepatitis B. They should have a blood test to see if they are immune to the virus and, if not, they should be vaccinated against it. Until a blood test shows that they are immune to the virus, always use a condom during sex.
- To prevent spreading the virus, avoid touching your sores and keep them covered with a bandage.
- Don't share any personal items that could have infected blood on them, including toothbrushes, razors, nail clippers, pierced earrings, or body-piercing instruments.
- Clean up all blood spills with a 10 percent solution of bleach (10 parts water to one part bleach). Dispose of tampons and sanitary napkins in a plastic bag.
- If you are infected, don't chew food before giving it to your baby.
- If you are exposed to hepatitis B and have not been vaccinated, get an injection of immune globulin and start the vaccination process as soon as possible.
- If you are exposed to hepatitis B and have been vaccinated, see your doctor for a blood test to detect hepatitis B antibodies, which indicate infection.

Chronic Hepatitis

The risk of developing progressive, chronic hepatitis is greater with the hepatitis B and C viruses than with the others. Up to half of all people who are infected with hepatitis C go on to develop

---

Hepatitis

Q. My friend told me that you can get hepatitis B or C from donating blood or having a blood transfusion. Is this true?

A. No. You cannot get hepatitis or any other infectious disease from donating blood; a new, sterilized needle is used to draw blood from each donor. You are very unlikely to get hepatitis B or C from a blood transfusion with donated blood because all donor blood in the United States is screened for the viruses.

Q. Can any of the hepatitis viruses be transmitted sexually?

A. Yes. Hepatitis B is more likely to be transmitted through sexual activity than hepatitis C or hepatitis A. Hepatitis B—which is found in blood, semen, and vaginal fluids—is a common sexually transmitted disease and is much more infectious than HIV (the virus that causes AIDS). If you or your partner is infected with hepatitis B, always practice safe sex. The partner who is not infected should have a hepatitis B vaccination. Once a follow-up blood test shows that his or her body has produced antibodies to fight the hepatitis B virus, he or she is protected from the infection for life. Hepatitis C is rarely transmitted sexually. Hepatitis A, which is present in an infected person's feces, can be spread through anal-oral sexual contact.

Q. Is there a hepatitis E? I never heard of it before.

A. Yes, but it is extremely rare in the United States. Nearly all cases in the United States occur in people who have traveled to countries in which the virus is widespread, especially developing countries that have inadequate sanitation systems. Like hepatitis A, the hepatitis E virus is spread in feces, often in contaminated drinking water, and it causes similar symptoms. However, unlike hepatitis A, hepatitis E is not transmitted easily from person to person. There is no vaccination for hepatitis E. If you travel to a developing country, drink bottled water, don't put ice in your drinks, and avoid uncooked shellfish and uncooked fruits or vegetables that are peeled or prepared by someone else. During pregnancy, especially in the second or third trimester, a hepatitis E infection can be severe and is more likely to lead to liver failure in the woman.

chronic hepatitis C and are more likely to have liver disease eventually. Hepatitis C is the leading cause of chronic hepatitis and cirrhosis worldwide, and the leading reason for a liver transplant in the United States.

Many people, however, develop chronic hepatitis without being infected with the virus. For example, autoimmune hepatitis is triggered in some people when their immune system mistakenly attacks the liver. In other people, hepatitis results from a severe reaction to a medication.

Chronic hepatitis is classified into two main types—chronic persistent hepatitis and chronic active hepatitis. In both diseases, the body responds with a faulty immune response that can damage cells in the liver. Chronic persistent hepatitis progresses slowly over a period of 10 to 40 years, but is unlikely to progress to cirrhosis (see next page).

Chronic active hepatitis is less predictable—in many cases, a steady, progressive destruction of liver cells leads to cirrhosis. The severity of chronic active hepatitis can vary from person to person. Some people have no symptoms for long periods but occasionally have episodes of jaundice (yellowing of the skin and whites of the eyes; see page 785), pain in the joints, nausea, fever, and loss of appetite. In some people, the disease comes and goes and does not respond to treatment. In others, the disease responds well to treatment and the symptoms clear up.

In rare cases, people with chronic hepatitis B have flare-ups of illness caused by hepatitis D, also called the Delta virus, which affects only people who are already infected with hepatitis B. Having a hepatitis B vaccination prevents hepatitis D.

Diagnosis

Blood tests can indicate whether you are infected with hepatitis B or C. Your doctor will diagnose a form of chronic hepatitis if your health does not return to normal after an acute attack of jaundice and if liver function tests continue to be abnormal. If you are diagnosed with chronic hepatitis C, the doctor will test the levels of two liver enzymes—alanine aminotransferase (ALT) and aspartate aminotransferase (AST)—that are released when liver cells are injured or die. These levels can fluctuate from elevated to normal during the illness. If your liver enzyme levels are normal, your doctor will test them regularly over a 6- to 12-month period. If your enzyme levels continue to be normal

during this time, he or she may recommend blood tests less frequently, such as once a year. Your doctor may order a liver biopsy (examination of a small sample of tissue taken from the liver for examination under a microscope) to help evaluate your condition and determine appropriate treatment.

Treatment

Depending on your general health and the results of the liver biopsy, your doctor may be able to determine if the disease is likely to clear up without treatment. If the results of blood tests and a liver biopsy show that the disease could progress to cirrhosis, your doctor will recommend treatment based on whether you have hepatitis B or C. In either case, the doctor will recommend that you have a vaccination against pneumonia (see page 660), hepatitis A, and hepatitis B (if you have hepatitis C) to prevent further strain on your liver. (There is no vaccination for hepatitis C.)

To treat chronic active hepatitis B, a doctor will prescribe an antiviral medication such as interferon alfa-2b or lamivudine. Injections of interferon are usually given for 4 to 6 months. Interferon can cause a number of side effects including fatigue, headache, nausea and vomiting, loss of appetite, depression, and thinning hair. Because interferon can depress the blood cell–producing bone marrow, you will have regular blood tests to measure your blood cell levels. Lamivudine is taken by mouth for at least a year. Lamivudine is not quite as effective in eliminating hepatitis B as interferon and, in some cases, the virus becomes resistant to lamivudine.

To treat chronic hepatitis C, a doctor may prescribe an antiviral medication such as interferon or ribavirin, often in combination. Interferon is given by injection; ribavirin is taken by mouth. The side effects of ribavirin include sudden, severe anemia (see page 610) and birth defects; for this reason you should not get pregnant or get anyone pregnant while you are taking ribavirin and for 6 months after your treatment ends.

Many people with chronic hepatitis C respond to treatment at least temporarily, and some of them become virus-free after 6 months of therapy. In others, however, the disease progresses over a period of 30 to 40 years to cirrhosis and eventually liver failure. A liver transplant (see next page) is frequently recommended for people who have end-stage hepatitis C.

Liver Transplants

In liver transplantation, a diseased liver is removed and replaced with a healthy liver (or part of a liver) from a donor. About 80 to 90 percent of people survive liver transplant surgery. Survival rates have improved over the past several years thanks to drugs such as cyclosporine and tacrolimus, which suppress the immune system to prevent it from attacking and damaging the donor liver.

Transplants are usually recommended for people whose liver has been severely damaged by chronic cirrhosis or for children who have congenital (present at birth) abnormalities of the bile ducts. Transplants can be successful in people who stop drinking alcohol permanently. However, a transplant is not recommended for people who have advanced cirrhosis caused by drinking alcohol if alcohol has already damaged other organs, such as the heart.

The procedure

For a liver transplant, a person receiving the transplant is given general anesthesia, and the transplant surgeon makes an incision in the upper part of the abdomen. The surgeon then cuts the major blood vessels—the vena cava, the hepatic artery, and the portal vein—and the bile duct to remove the diseased liver. The donor liver is put in place and connected to the blood vessels and bile duct. In some cases, a small tube is inserted into the bile duct to allow bile to drain out of the body into a small bag.

The transplant recipient is connected to a ventilator

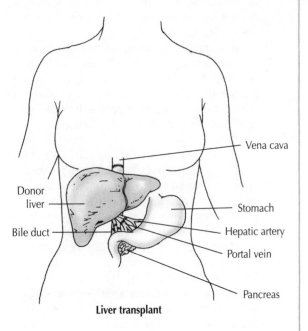

Liver transplant

to assist with breathing until his or her condition stabilizes. The new liver starts to function immediately. The bile-collecting bag may remain attached to the tube for a week or more. Once the bag is removed, the tube may be capped but will remain in place for several months to enable the doctor to perform tests to monitor the transplant. Most people who receive a liver transplant are able to lead active lives.

Cirrhosis of the Liver

Cirrhosis of the liver is a chronic condition in which scar tissue replaces healthy liver tissue, reducing the liver's ability to perform its many vital functions. Cirrhosis has many causes; alcohol dependence (see page 733) and chronic hepatitis C (see page 787) are the most common causes in the United States. The disease can also result from other liver diseases, such as hepatitis B (see page 786), hemochromatosis (see page 961), or autoimmune hepatitis. Although liver damage from cirrhosis cannot be reversed, treatment can stop or slow progression of the disease and reduce the risk of complications.

Symptoms

In the early stages, many people with cirrhosis have no noticeable symptoms because the liver can continue functioning with fewer than normal healthy cells. As the disease progresses, a person may lose his or her appetite, lose weight, and experience general weakness and fatigue.

Eventually, a number of complications can develop. For example, if the liver loses its ability to make the proteins necessary for blood to clot, a person may bleed and bruise easily; small, red, weblike marks called spider nevi may appear on the face, arms, and upper part of the trunk. If the liver can no longer make the protein albumin, fluid can build up in the legs (edema) or abdomen (ascites). A

WARNING!

Herbal Remedies and Liver Disease

Herbal remedies and dietary supplements contain many ingredients and, because dietary supplements are not regulated by the federal government, the contents are not standardized and can vary from one brand to another. In addition, the contents listed on the label can differ from what's actually inside. Doctors believe that many cases of sudden, severe hepatitis not related to a hepatitis virus are caused by repeated use of some herbal products. Use of these herbs causes many cases of nonviral hepatitis and unexplained cirrhosis. Herbal remedies that are thought to be potentially harmful to the liver include chaparral, a Chinese herbal product called jin bu huan, kava kava, germander, comfrey, mistletoe, skullcap, margosa oil, maté tea, gordolobo tea, and pennyroyal (squawmint oil). Always talk to your doctor about any supplement you are taking.

person can develop jaundice (yellowing of the skin and whites of the eyes; see page 785) when the liver does not absorb the yellow pigment bilirubin, causing it to build up in the blood.

If blood cannot be delivered to the liver from the digestive system, blood pressure can build up in the veins around the junction of the esophagus and stomach, a condition called portal hypertension. The increased pressure in these veins causes them to bulge, making them susceptible to bursting, which can cause life-threatening bleeding (esophageal varices; see page 753). If the damaged liver can no longer remove toxins from the blood, they can build up in the brain (a condition called encephalopathy), causing mental confusion, reduced intellectual functioning, and sometimes personality changes. Cirrhosis can also affect the immune system and kidneys, causing frequent infections, kidney dysfunction, and kidney failure (see page 816).

See your doctor if you have any symptoms of cirrhosis, especially if you consume an excessive amount of alcohol or if you have chronic hepatitis (see page 788).

Diagnosis

A doctor can often diagnose cirrhosis from the symptoms, a health history, and a physical examination. He or she will press on your abdomen to feel your liver and, if it feels harder or larger than normal, the doctor will order blood tests to see if you have liver damage. The doctor may also want to examine your liver on an image such as a CT scan (see page 112), an ultrasound (see page 111), or a radioisotope scan (which highlights the liver using a harmless radioactive substance). In some cases, a doctor will want to look at the liver directly using laparoscopy, in which a viewing tube (laparoscope) is inserted through a small incision in the abdomen to transmit pictures to a computer screen. To confirm a diagnosis of cirrhosis, a liver biopsy may be done. During a liver biopsy, a doctor inserts a needle through the abdomen into the liver to remove a small sample of tissue to examine for signs of scarring or disease.

Treatment

The treatment of cirrhosis depends on the underlying cause. For example, if it is caused by alcohol dependence, your doctor will ask you to avoid drinking alcohol. Abstaining from alcohol can help prevent cirrhosis from getting worse and should enable you to lead a relatively active life. If the cirrhosis arose from hepatitis (see page 786), your doctor will prescribe medications such as interferon to treat a hepatitis infection or corticosteroids to suppress the abnormal immune response in autoimmune hepatitis.

If you have nausea, your doctor can prescribe medication to relieve it. He or she will recommend that you eat frequent small meals or snacks during the day rather than three large meals. Don't take any over-the-counter medications, including vitamin supplements and herbal remedies, without talking to your doctor, because your liver cannot filter substances normally.

Any complications of cirrhosis will also be treated. For example, if you have fluid buildup, your doctor will recommend a low-sodium diet and diuretics (drugs that remove fluid from the body). He or she may recommend removing fluid from your abdomen through a needle in a procedure called paracentesis (see page 759). For portal hypertension, your doctor may prescribe a blood pressure medication such as a beta blocker. A low-protein diet can help decrease the buildup of toxins in the blood and brain that can occur when the liver is not filtering normally. If complications cannot be controlled, or if the liver is so damaged that it stops functioning, a liver transplant (see previous page) can be lifesaving.

Tumors of the Liver

Liver tumors can be benign (noncancerous) or malignant (cancerous). Benign tumors in the liver are extremely rare; if they are detected, they can usually be removed safely and completely.

Two types of cancerous tumors develop in the liver—those that have spread there from another part of the body (metastases) and those that originate in the liver (primary cancers). About one third of all cancers in the body eventually spread to the liver. Once a cancer has spread to the liver, the outlook is poor. Cancers that originate in the liver are rare. These tumors often result from infection with the hepatitis B or C virus or from cirrhosis (see page 790).

Liver cancer is twice as common in men as in women and usually is diagnosed after age 60. People who have a family history of this cancer are at increased risk.

Symptoms

If a person has liver cancer that has spread from elsewhere in the body, he or she may first experience symptoms from the primary cancer, most frequently the breast (see page 857), lung (see page 646), or gastrointestinal tract (see page 775). As liver cancer develops, it causes loss of weight and appetite, feelings of fullness, pain in the upper abdomen on the right side (possibly extending to the back and shoulder), bloating, weakness, fatigue, and nausea and vomiting. A person may eventually develop jaundice (yellowing of the skin and whites of the eyes; see page 785) as the liver is damaged.

Diagnosis

If your doctor thinks that you may have liver cancer, he or she will perform a physical examination and feel your abdomen for lumps in the liver or nearby organs or changes in the shape or size of organs. He or she also will feel your abdomen for an abnormal buildup of fluid and will examine your skin and eyes to look for jaundice. You may have blood tests to detect any problems and to evaluate liver function.

Your doctor may examine your liver using an imaging procedure such as a CT scan (see page 112), ultrasound (see page 111), MRI (see page 113), or angiogram (see page 110). In some cases, doctors remove a sample of tissue from the liver for examination under a microscope to look for cancer cells (biopsy). Depending on the size of the sample required for examination, a liver biopsy can be done using a small needle (aspiration biopsy), a thicker needle (core biopsy), or a laparoscope (a viewing tube that is inserted into a small incision in the abdomen). In rare cases, a biopsy is done through a large incision in the abdomen.

Treatment

Treatment of liver cancer usually depends on the condition of the liver, the number of tumors and their size and location, and whether the cancer has spread outside the liver. A doctor also considers the person's age and general health. Doctors usually recommend surgery to remove tumors that originate in the liver or a single tumor that has spread to the liver from elsewhere. (Liver transplants are recommended only for tumors that originate in the liver, not for metastases.)

If a tumor cannot be removed surgically—usually because a person has a liver disease such as cirrhosis, the tumor is not easily accessible, or a person has other health problems—a number of treatment options may be considered to help control the cancer and extend the person's life. Treatment options include applying heat to the tumors to destroy them with radiofrequency waves, lasers, or microwaves; injecting ethanol (a type of alcohol) into the liver tumor to kill cancer cells; freezing the cancer cells (cryosurgery) to destroy them; or injecting or infusing anticancer drugs directly into the tumor.

For tumors that are found in both lobes of the liver, that have spread to the liver from the colon and are confined to the liver, or that have spread to other parts of the body, chemotherapy (see page 23) may help slow the growth of the tumors.

Wilson's Disease

Wilson's disease is an inherited disorder in which excessive amounts of copper accumulate in the liver or brain. Copper, a mineral present in most foods, is essential to the body in small amounts. In healthy people the unneeded copper is excreted but, in people who have Wilson's disease, the liver cannot release copper as it normally does, causing copper to accumulate in the liver and damage liver tissue. Over time, the damage to the liver causes it to release the copper directly into the bloodstream, which carries the mineral throughout the body. The excess copper can eventually damage the kidneys, brain, and eyes. If not treated, Wilson's disease can cause severe brain damage, liver failure, and death. Although a person is born with the disorder and copper begins to accumulate immediately after birth, the symptoms usually don't appear until late adolescence.

Because the gene for the disorder is recessive, to be affected, a person needs to inherit a copy of the defective gene from both parents. If you or your partner has a family member with Wilson's disease, you may want to talk to a genetic counselor (see page 952) about being tested before you have children to see if you are at risk of passing the disease to your children. The test would look for the precise genetic mutation that runs in your family. There is no test yet available for widespread screening for the gene or for prenatal diagnosis. When detected and treated early, people who have Wilson's disease can lead a normal, healthy life.

Symptoms

When excess copper attacks the liver, a person can develop symptoms of hepatitis (see page 786), including jaundice (yellowing of the skin and whites of the eyes; see page 785), abdominal swelling and pain, and vomiting blood. Excess copper in the brain produces tremors in the arms and hands, rigid muscles, and speech and language problems. Women who have Wilson's disease may have irregular menstrual periods or no periods, infertility, or multiple miscarriages.

Diagnosis

A diagnosis of Wilson's disease can be made relatively easily even in people who don't have symptoms. The doctor will feel your abdomen for signs of swelling of the liver or spleen or fluid buildup in the lining of the abdomen. He or she will also order tests to measure the level of copper in your blood, urine, and liver. An eye examination may be done to look for a rusty-brown ring around the cornea (called the Kayser-Fleischer ring) that is characteristic of Wilson's disease. The earlier the diagnosis is made, the less damage to the liver and brain and the better the outcome.

Treatment

Wilson's disease is treated with zinc (which blocks the absorption of copper) or penicillamine or trientine (which help remove copper from tissues). You will need to take the medication throughout your life. You will also need to avoid eating copper-rich foods such as mushrooms, nuts, chocolate, dried fruit, liver, and shellfish. Ask your doctor if you should take a zinc supplement to help prevent your intestines from absorbing copper.

Gallstones

Stones of varying composition sometimes form in the gallbladder, the reservoir in which the digestive substance bile collects. Bile flows from the liver to the gallbladder, which excretes bile into the intestines to help neutralize stomach acid and aid in the digestion of fat. Bile is rich in cholesterol (a fat that is manufactured and excreted by the liver) and bilirubin (a substance formed from the breakdown of old red blood cells). Sometimes, if the balance of the cholesterol and bilirubin in the bile is upset, a tiny solid particle can form in the gallbladder. The particle may grow to become a gallstone as more cholesterol or, less often, bilirubin builds up around it. Some people may have only one gallstone, while others have several.

An estimated 20 million people in the United States have gallstones, with 1 million new cases diagnosed each year. Autopsy studies have shown that 80 percent of all people who reach 90 years of age have gallstones when they die.

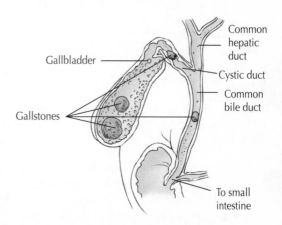

Common sites of gallstones
Gallstones may remain in the gallbladder or pass easily through the bile duct into the upper part of the small intestine (the duodenum) without causing symptoms. However, problems can develop if a gallstone gets trapped in the cystic duct or in a bile duct.

Symptoms

Between one third and one half of people with gallstones do not have any symptoms. However, some gallstones flow out of the liver in bile and get stuck in the common bile duct. A stone in the bile duct causes severe pain in the right side or in the center of the upper abdomen, which can radiate around the ribs or through to the back; this pain is called biliary colic. Biliary colic results when the gallbladder and the muscle of the bile duct clamp down and try to empty the stone into the intestines. If the stone falls back into the gallbladder, or is forced along the bile duct into the intestines, the blockage goes away and the pain quickly subsides. For this reason, the pain tends to build to a peak over a period of a few hours and then fade. A person usually has nausea and vomiting. If you have severe pain on your right side or in your upper abdomen, call your doctor immediately or go to the nearest hospital emergency department.

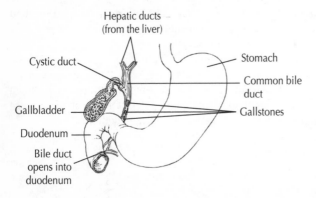

Biliary colic
A gallstone can sometimes get stuck in the common bile duct, causing pain in the right side or in the center of the upper abdomen. If the stone falls back into the gallbladder or into the duodenum (the upper part of the small intestine), the pain subsides.

A more common problem develops when a stone blocks the cystic duct (the tube that carries bile to and from the gallbladder) and causes inflammation in the gallbladder. Having gallstones also increases the risk of acute pancreatitis (see page 798) if a gallstone gets stuck in the pancreatic duct, which drains into the bile duct.

Diagnosis

If you have severe pain resembling biliary colic, your doctor will examine you and question you

about the pain. If the doctor suspects that you may have gallstones, he or she will probably order an ultrasound scan (see page 111) of the abdominal area to detect and locate any stones. You will have blood tests to measure liver proteins to help evaluate the functioning of your liver. You may also have a hepatobiliary (HIDA) scan, a test that can detect a gallbladder obstruction by tracking a radioactive dye through your liver and gallbladder. In HIDA, a nuclear scanner takes multiple pictures of your abdominal area, and a radiologist (a doctor who specializes in the use of radiation for medical diagnosis or treatment) interprets the pictures.

Treatment

If you are having severe pain from a gallstone, your doctor may give you an injection of a strong pain reliever to reduce the pain immediately. If tests show that you have gallstones in your bile duct, the doctor will recommend that you have them removed. One of several procedures will be performed, depending on your condition and the location of the stones. Gallstones are frequently removed in a procedure called laparoscopic cholecystectomy (see next page), which is performed through small incisions in the abdomen. In rare cases (for people who are very ill), more extensive surgery that opens the abdomen is performed in which an incision is made in the bile duct and the stone is removed directly from the duct. In both of these procedures, the gallbladder is also removed to avoid the risk of more stones forming.

Primary Sclerosing Cholangitis

Primary sclerosing cholangitis is inflammation and scarring of the bile ducts inside and outside the liver. The bile ducts carry bile out of the liver into the small intestine, where it helps break down fats from food. As the scarring builds up in the bile ducts, it can block the ducts, causing bile to accumulate in the liver, damaging liver cells. Over time, the condition can cause liver failure.

The cause of primary sclerosing cholangitis is unknown, but doctors think it involves a faulty immune response triggered by an infection. Between 70 and 80 percent of people who have primary sclerosing cholangitis also have an underlying inflammatory bowel disease (usually ulcerative

Laparoscopic Cholecystectomy

Laparoscopic cholecystectomy is a common procedure used to remove the gallbladder. It can usually be done through four small incisions in the abdomen using a laparoscope (viewing tube). After determining the number of gallstones and their location using an imaging procedure such as ultrasound, the surgeon inserts the laparoscope through one of the incisions. The laparoscope's fiberoptic viewing system transmits a clear image of the abdominal cavity onto a video monitor. The surgeon then passes tiny precision instruments through the laparoscope or through the abdominal incisions to remove any gallstones.

The surgeon puts clips on the cystic artery and the cystic duct to close them off and takes an X-ray to look for any hidden stones in the common bile duct. He or she then uses tiny scissors to free the gallbladder from the artery and duct, and removes the gallbladder through a tiny incision below the navel.

During the cholecystectomy, which is commonly done on an outpatient basis, the person is under general anesthesia. The procedure usually takes less than an hour, recovery is relatively quick, and the incisions rarely leave noticeable scars. A person may have nausea and vomiting after the surgery. In about 5 to 10 percent of cases, the gallbladder cannot be removed safely with laparoscopy, and open abdominal surgery is immediately done instead.

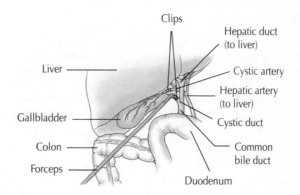

Tying off the cystic artery and cystic duct

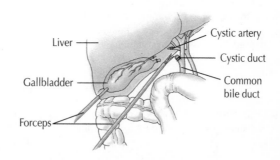

Removing the gallbladder

Laparoscopic cholecystectomy
Before disconnecting the gallbladder from the cystic artery (which supplies the gallbladder with blood) and the cystic duct (which connects the gallbladder to the liver), a surgeon puts clips on the artery and duct to close them off. After the artery and duct to the gallbladder are closed off, the surgeon uses tiny scissors to cut the artery and duct to free the gallbladder. He or she then removes the gallbladder through a small incision below the navel.

colitis; see page 764). Primary sclerosing cholangitis usually begins between ages 30 and 60 and is more common in men than in women.

Symptoms and Diagnosis

A person can have primary sclerosing cholangitis for years before symptoms develop. When symptoms appear, they can include itching (caused by a buildup of bile salts in the skin), fatigue, and jaundice (yellowing of the skin and whites of the eyes; see page 785). If the bile ducts become infected, a person also can have a fever and chills.

Primary sclerosing cholangitis is diagnosed using an imaging procedure called cholangiography, in which a dye is injected into the bile ducts and an X-ray is taken to obtain a picture of the bile ducts.

Treatment

The treatment of primary sclerosing cholangitis includes medication to relieve itching, antibiotics to treat infections, and vitamin supplements (because the disease can reduce the body's ability to absorb some vitamins, particularly A, D, and K). In

ERCP

To diagnose and treat various problems in the bile ducts including tumors, cysts, and narrowing, doctors use a procedure called endoscopic retrograde cholangiopancreatography (ERCP). It is also used to help evaluate jaundice (yellowing of the skin and whites of the eyes; see page 785). In ERCP, an endoscope (a flexible viewing tube) is passed down the esophagus, through the stomach, and into the duodenum. After introducing a dye into the bile and pancreatic ducts, the doctor can see any stones or other abnormalities in the duct on an X-ray image. If a stone is found, a tiny device can be passed through the endoscope to grab the stone (or stones) and pull it out or to dislodge it and allow it to pass through the newly enlarged opening to the duodenum.

The procedure takes from 30 minutes to 2 hours. If the procedure is done for diagnosis only, you will be able to leave the hospital after the sedative wears off, probably after about 1 to 2 hours. If a gallstone was removed or other treatment given, you may need to stay overnight in the hospital. Possible complications of ERCP, which are rare, include pancreatitis (inflammation of the pancreas; see page 798), infection, bleeding, and perforation of the duodenum.

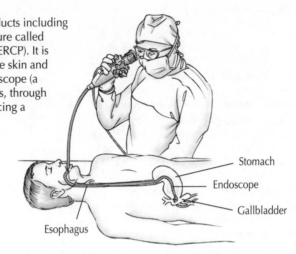

Stomach

Endoscope

Gallbladder

Esophagus

ERCP

In ERCP, a flexible viewing tube (endoscope) is passed into a person's mouth and esophagus through the stomach into the first part of the small intestine (duodenum). After locating the stone on an X-ray image, the doctor inserts an instrument through the endoscope into the bile duct to grab the stone and pull it out or to dislodge it and allow it to pass on its own into the duodenum.

---

some cases, a blockage in the common bile duct is opened using ERCP (see above), in which a wire coil (stent) is inserted into the blockage and expanded; the stent remains in place to keep the duct open. If the liver starts to fail, the doctor may recommend a liver transplant (see page 790).

Cholangiocarcinoma

A cholangiocarcinoma is a relatively rare cancerous growth in one of the bile ducts, which carry the digestive fluid bile from the liver to the small intestine. Cholangiocarcinomas, which can develop anywhere along a bile duct, are usually slow-growing and don't cause symptoms until they block the duct. The tumors occur in people of both sexes equally and are usually diagnosed after age 65. People who have primary sclerosing cholangitis (see page 794) or another disorder that causes chronic inflammation in the bile ducts have an increased risk of developing cholangiocarcinomas.

Symptoms

The symptoms of a cholangiocarcinoma include clay-colored stool, jaundice (yellowing of the skin and the whites of the eyes; see page 785), itching of the skin, pain in the right upper abdomen that may radiate to the back, loss of appetite, weight loss, and fever and chills.

Diagnosis

If you have symptoms of a cholangiocarcinoma, your doctor will order tests to look for a tumor or obstruction in a bile duct. You may have an imaging procedure such as a CT scan (see page 112) or ultrasound (see page 111) of your abdomen, or ERCP (see above). In ERCP, the doctor passes a flexible viewing tube (called an endoscope) down your esophagus, through the stomach, and into the small intestine, and introduces a dye into the bile duct. Another diagnostic imaging test is a percutaneous transhepatic cholangiogram (PTCA), in which a thin, flexible needle is inserted through the skin of the upper right side of your abdomen into the liver. An X-ray machine called a fluoroscope transmits images onto a monitor, guiding the doctor as he or she inserts the needle into the bile duct and injects a dye that will show up on the monitor and reveal any abnormalities in the bile duct. If a tumor shows up on an image, the doctor will take a sample of cells during the ERCP or PTCA for examination in the laboratory to look for cancer cells and to confirm the diagnosis.

Treatment

The treatment for cholangiocarcinoma is to surgically remove the tumor, if possible, which can result in a cure if the cancer is found early and has not spread from the bile duct. Sometimes chemotherapy (see page 23) or radiation therapy (see page 23) is given after surgery to reduce the risk of a recurrence. If the tumor cannot be removed surgically, treatment to clear the obstruction in the bile duct and relieve symptoms may be done through an endoscope. Radiation therapy, sometimes combined with chemotherapy, may follow.

Cholecystitis

In cholecystitis, the gallbladder becomes inflamed and swollen, usually because a gallstone has become lodged in the cystic duct, blocking the flow of bile from the gallbladder into the intestine and causing severe pain (called biliary colic). In rare cases, the inflammation results from an infection that has spread from the intestine to the gallbladder. Three out of four people who have cholecystitis have had previous gallbladder problems.

Symptoms

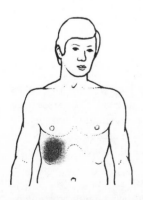

Site of pain in cholecystitis

If a gallstone becomes lodged in the cystic duct, a person will have severe pain in the upper right area of the abdomen that can spread around to the back and to the right shoulder blade. As cholecystitis develops, a person's temperature rises and he or she will probably have nausea and vomiting. If the condition is not treated, jaundice (yellowing of the skin and whites of the eyes; see page 785) can develop.

Diagnosis and Treatment

To diagnose cholecystitis, a doctor may recommend tests such as a hepatobiliary (HIDA) scan, a test that can detect an obstruction in the cystic duct by tracking a radioactive dye through the liver and gallbladder. In HIDA, a nuclear scanner takes multiple pictures of the abdominal area, and a radiologist (a doctor who specializes in the use of radiation for diagnosis or treatment) interprets the pictures.

If you have cholecystitis, you probably will be admitted to the hospital and given fluids intravenously (through a vein) to provide you with nutrients and fluid. You will not be allowed to eat or drink for a few days, and you will be given a pain reliever and antibiotics by injection or intravenously. If you have cholecystitis, the doctor will recommend that you have your gallbladder removed. In severe cases, removal is done within a day or two after a person is admitted to the hospital. However, some doctors prefer to wait until the inflammation has subsided.

Laparoscopic cholecystectomy (see page 795) is the procedure used most often to treat cholecystitis. In an alternative treatment, gallstones may be dissolved by long-term treatment with drugs. However, this treatment has several disadvantages. For example, you may need to take the drugs for 1 to 2 years before the stones disappear completely. The drugs work for only 50 percent of people who use them, and after the stones are gone, the risk is high that they will recur when the medication is stopped. In addition, the drugs can cause side effects such as diarrhea in some people.

Cancer of the Gallbladder

Cancer of the gallbladder is an uncommon cancer that occurs more frequently in women than in men and in people who have gallstones (see page 793) or chronic inflammation of the gallbladder. The cancer has also been linked to obesity and to cigarette smoking. Because gallbladder cancer often does not cause symptoms in the early stages, it frequently is found by chance during laparoscopic cholecystectomy (see page 795).

Symptoms

The symptoms of gallbladder cancer are similar to the symptoms of gallstones, including pain in the right side or in the upper abdomen. Frequently, gallbladder cancer causes no symptoms in the early stages. When symptoms develop, they can include persistent pain above the stomach, loss of weight, fever, or jaundice (yellowing of the skin and whites of the eyes; see page 785).

Diagnosis

If you have symptoms of gallbladder cancer, your doctor may order an imaging procedure such as ultrasound (see page 111), a CT scan (see page 112), or MRI (see page 113) to look for signs of cancer in the gallbladder and to help determine if it has spread to the common bile duct, nearby lymph nodes, or liver. You may also have angiography (see page 110), cholangiography, or ERCP (see page 796) to see if a tumor is blocking a blood vessel, the bile duct, or the pancreatic duct. However, because the gallbladder is hidden behind other organs, it can sometimes be difficult to make a diagnosis with imaging alone. A doctor may recommend laparoscopic surgery (see page 795) to remove tissue samples from the gallbladder and nearby organs for examination under a microscope for cancer cells (biopsy). The gallbladder may be removed at this time if a person has gallstones or another obvious gallbladder problem.

Treatment

The treatment for gallbladder cancer depends on the extent of the cancer, whether it has spread from the gallbladder, and the person's general health. If gallbladder cancer has been found on a biopsy or during a laparoscopic cholecystectomy, the gallbladder will be removed through a larger incision in the abdomen to avoid releasing cancer cells into the abdominal cavity while removing the gallbladder. Part of the liver near the gallbladder and lymph nodes in the abdomen may also be removed.

Radiation therapy (see page 23) may be used alone or before or after surgery. Chemotherapy (see page 23) may be given in combination with radiation therapy to make cancer cells more sensitive to the radiation. These therapies are sometimes used to help shrink a tumor before surgery.

If your cancer is detected at a later stage, or if it recurs after treatment, your doctor may talk to you about participating in a clinical trial that evaluates experimental treatments for gallbladder cancer.

Acute Pancreatitis

Acute pancreatitis is a condition characterized by sudden, severe inflammation of the pancreas. Worldwide, about half of people who develop acute pancreatitis have gallstones. Most cases of acute pancreatitis in the United States are caused by alcohol abuse. Other possible causes include reactions to medications such as acetaminophen, sulfa drugs, thiazide diuretics, some antibiotics, zidovudine (an AIDS drug), or mercaptopurine (an immune-suppressing drug); a penetrating duodenal ulcer (see page 755); hyperparathyroidism (see page 904); or an abdominal injury. The condition can also result from pancreatic cancer (see page 800), elevated levels of triglycerides or calcium in the blood, or anatomical abnormalities.

Most people recover completely after their first attack of pancreatitis. The major danger is shock (see page 579), which can result from internal bleeding around the pancreas and can be fatal. Acute pancreatitis can sometimes lead to chronic, recurring attacks.

Symptoms

The primary symptom of acute pancreatitis is severe pain in the center of the upper abdomen. It often begins 12 to 24 hours after eating a large meal or drinking an excessive amount of alcohol. The pain seems to bore through to the back and is accompanied by vomiting. In severe cases, a person can become extremely ill and feverish and have bruise marks on his or her abdomen from internal bleeding around the pancreas. Cystlike blisters (pseudocysts) sometimes form on the pancreas after an attack. If they cause symptoms such as pain, they may need to be removed surgically or drained.

Diagnosis

If you have symptoms of acute pancreatitis, your doctor will admit you to the hospital. To make a diagnosis, the doctor will order a CT scan (see page 112) to examine the pancreas and blood tests to measure levels of some pancreatic enzymes and other proteins that are linked to acute pancreatitis.

Treatment

If you have acute pancreatitis, you will probably be given a pain reliever and should not eat or drink (fasting reduces the levels of pancreatic juices). Shock is treated with fluids given intravenously (through a vein). If you have a bacterial infection, you will be given antibiotics. As you recover, you can gradually start eating and drinking again. Your doctor will tell you to avoid alcohol to prevent chronic pancreatitis (see below). After you have recovered from the attack of acute pancreatitis, your doctor will recommend an ultrasound scan (see page 111) to look for gallstones to determine if they were the cause of the attack. If you have gallstones, the doctor may recommend having them removed (see page 795). If pancreatitis is severe, debridement (removal) of part of the inflamed tissue of the pancreas may be required.

Chronic Pancreatitis

Chronic pancreatitis is a disease of the pancreas that develops gradually, usually after several years of alcohol abuse (see page 733). Chronic pancreatitis occurs when digestive enzymes attack and destroy the pancreas and nearby tissues, causing scarring. As the disease progresses, the pancreas eventually loses its ability to supply digestive juices and hormones (such as insulin). The resulting lack of digestive fluids can reduce the body's ability to absorb nutrients from food. If insulin is not available to push glucose into cells, glucose can build up in the blood, causing diabetes (see page 894).

Alcohol-related chronic pancreatitis is more common in men than in women and usually develops between ages 30 and 40. The condition can sometimes be triggered by one attack of acute pancreatitis (see previous page), especially if the pancreatic ducts are damaged; this damage can cause inflammation in the pancreas that can kill pancreatic cells and lead to scarring. The pancreatic ducts can be damaged or blocked by an injury or by pseudocysts (cystlike accumulations of pancreatic fluid) that form in the duct.

People with the inherited genetic disorder cystic fibrosis (see page 958) are at risk of developing chronic pancreatitis because the defective gene that causes cystic fibrosis makes a protein that plugs up the pancreatic ducts (which normally deliver digestive enzymes to the intestine). The buildup and activation of digestive enzymes in the pancreas cause the pancreas to digest itself, damaging tissue and causing severe pain. An inherited form of pancreatitis has the same progression as the noninherited forms, but people with inherited pancreatitis have a 50-fold increased risk of eventually developing pancreatic cancer (see next page). In many cases, the cause of chronic pancreatitis cannot be determined.

Symptoms

Pain is the major symptom of chronic pancreatitis, although 10 percent of affected people do not have any pain. The pain, which occurs primarily in the abdomen and back, is dull and cramping, usually worsens when you drink alcohol or eat, and is relieved when you sit up and lean forward. As the disease progresses, the pain becomes constant.

People often lose weight, even when eating normally, because their body is not absorbing nutrients from food. As a result, fat, protein, and sugar are excreted in stool, producing yellow, foul-smelling diarrhea. If the insulin-secreting cells in the pancreas are destroyed, a person develops the symptoms of diabetes. See your doctor immediately if you have any of these symptoms.

Diagnosis

Chronic pancreatitis is sometimes difficult to diagnose. Your doctor may recommend a test to determine if your pancreas is making sufficient amounts of digestive enzymes. You may also have an imaging procedure such as ultrasound (see page 111), ERCP (see page 796), or a CT scan (see page 112) to look for signs of chronic pancreatitis, such as calcification of the pancreas. In more advanced stages, after a person has developed problems such as diabetes or malabsorption (inability to absorb nutrients from food), a doctor will use blood, urine, and stool tests to diagnose chronic pancreatitis or to monitor its progression.

Treatment

The first step in treating chronic pancreatitis is to relieve the pain. Your doctor will tell you that to avoid painful attacks, you must avoid alcohol and closely follow a special diet high in carbohydrates and low in fat. He or she will give you detailed dietary guidelines. If your pancreas is not producing enough digestive enzymes, your doctor may prescribe pancreatic enzymes to take with meals to help your body digest food. If you have diabetes, your doctor will prescribe insulin or a glucose-lowering medication to control your blood sugar level. If you stop drinking alcohol permanently, follow your prescribed diet, and take the pancreatic enzymes, your chances of long-term improvement are good.

In some cases, as the disease progresses and the pain becomes even more severe, surgery may be recommended to relieve the pain by, for example, draining an enlarged pancreatic duct, removing damaged tissue from the pancreas, or cutting the nerves that transmit pain signals from the pancreas to the brain.

Cancer of the Pancreas

Pancreatic cancer is the second most common gastrointestinal cancer after colon cancer and the fourth leading cause of cancer death in the United States. The exact cause of cancer of the pancreas is not known. As with most cancers, the risk of developing pancreatic cancer increases with age. People who smoke are two to three times more likely than nonsmokers to develop pancreatic cancer. People who have diabetes (see page 889) and people who have a family history of pancreatic cancer are also at increased risk. The cancer is more common in men than in women and is more prevalent in African Americans than in other people.

Symptoms

Pancreatic cancer is often called a silent disease because it seldom causes symptoms in the early stages. As the cancer progresses, symptoms can include loss of appetite, weight loss, nausea and vomiting, and jaundice (yellowing of the skin and whites of the eyes; see page 785). If the cancer affects the body and tail of the pancreas, a person will experience pain in the upper abdomen that may spread to the back. Cancer in the head of the pancreas often causes no symptoms until the tumor has become incurable.

Diagnosis

If you have symptoms of pancreatic cancer, your doctor will want to rule out other possible causes, such as gallstones (see page 793). He or she will perform a physical examination to look for jaundice and feel your abdomen for any changes in the pancreas or surrounding organs and for a buildup of fluid. You will probably have blood, urine, and stool tests to look for abnormalities in substances such as the liver protein bilirubin, which can build up in the blood, urine, or stool if the common bile duct is blocked by a tumor.

To examine the pancreas, your doctor may also recommend an imaging procedure such as a CT scan (see page 112), an endoscopic ultrasound or MRI (see page 113), or ERCP (see page 796). In ERCP, the doctor can examine the pancreas, liver, and gallbladder ducts to look for narrowing or blockage of the ducts, which can be a sign of pancreatic cancer in some people. A doctor may take a sample of tissue from the pancreas during ERCP for examination under a microscope to look for cancer cells (biopsy).

Treatment

Pancreatic cancer is difficult to control with available treatments. If pancreatic cancer is detected at an early stage, surgery to remove part or all of the pancreas may provide a cure. In one surgical procedure, part of the pancreas and part of the small intestine and some of the tissue around the small intestine are removed. Enough of the pancreas remains to produce insulin and aid in digestion.

After surgery for pancreatic cancer, chemotherapy (see page 23) and radiation therapy (see page 23) may be used alone or together, but they are generally not very effective for this type of cancer. When pancreatic cancer is detected at an advanced stage, the outlook is poor and treatment focuses on reducing the person's discomfort and the risk of complications. For example, if a tumor blocks the bile duct or duodenum (upper part of the small intestine), a doctor can create a bypass to allow fluids to flow through the digestive tract. Alternatively, a stent (a mesh tube) may be inserted into the duct or intestine to relieve the blockage and reduce the discomfort. Your doctor may talk with you about participating in a clinical trial of an experimental new treatment for pancreatic cancer.

7

Disorders of the Urinary Tract

As your body uses up the nutrients from the food you eat, it produces toxic waste products that the blood carries to the kidneys and liver for removal. The kidneys filter the waste products from the blood, combine them with water, and excrete them from the body as urine. The production and excretion of urine are essential to maintain life.

The kidneys are bean-shaped organs, each about the size of a fist, at the back of the abdominal cavity, just above the waist and on each side of the spine. The functions of the kidneys include regulating blood pressure, maintaining the balance of body fluids and electrolytes (essential minerals that help regulate various body processes), eliminating waste products, and stimulating bone marrow to produce red blood cells.

Each kidney contains more than 1 million tiny filtering units called nephrons, which allow amino acids, glucose, mineral salts, and waste products to pass from the blood into a series of microscopic tubes (tubules). The tubules reabsorb the essential nutrients (such as glucose, sodium, and potassium) and secrete waste products and excess water as urine. A steady stream of urine flows from the kidneys down to the bladder (a hollow, muscular organ in the pelvis that serves as a reservoir for urine) through a pair of narrow muscular tubes called ureters.

During urination, the bladder contracts and expels urine through a larger muscular tube called the urethra. In males, the opening of the urethra is in the tip of the head of the penis; in females, the opening is directly in front of the vagina. The system that runs from the kidneys to the urethra is called the urinary tract.

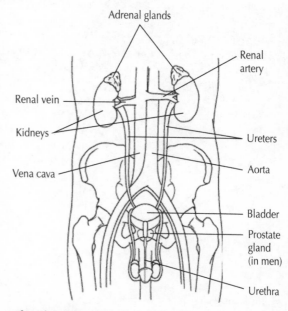

The urinary tract
The kidneys are at the back of the abdominal cavity, just above the waist and on each side of the spine. The ureters carry a steady stream of urine from the kidneys to the bladder, which is in the pelvis just behind the pubic bone. The bladder expels urine from the body through the urethra.

The urinary tract is susceptible to a number of disorders. For example, infection or inflammation of the kidneys or fat buildup (atherosclerosis; see page 557) in the small arteries inside the kidneys can cause scarring of the filtering tissue. This scarring may ultimately lead to kidney failure. Mineral deposits called kidney stones can form, obstructing the flow of urine and causing severe pain. Stones may also form in the bladder, especially when the bladder does not empty properly. Tumors can form anywhere along the urinary tract.

How the Urinary Tract Functions

The urinary tract consists of the kidneys, ureters, bladder, prostate gland (in men), and urethra. The kidneys filter the blood and excrete waste products and excess water as urine. The ureters carry urine from the kidneys to the bladder, which serves as a reservoir. The urethra carries urine from the bladder out of the body during urination.

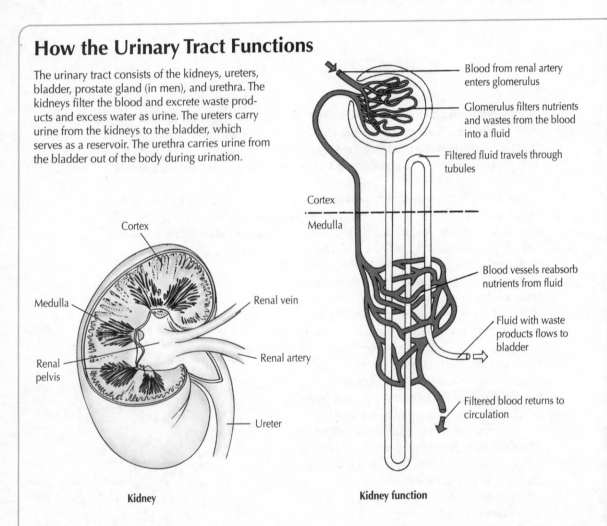

Kidney

Kidney function

The kidneys

Each day, the kidneys filter more than 200 quarts of blood. Blood from the renal artery first passes through the glomeruli. These tiny, globelike tangles of blood vessels in the outer part of the kidney (the cortex) filter a fluid containing nutrients and wastes from the blood. The fluid then flows into the center of the kidney (the medulla) through long, thin tubes called tubules. The tubules are surrounded by blood vessels that reabsorb the nutrients from the fluid. The filtered blood passes through a cavity called the renal pelvis, leaves the kidneys through the renal vein, and returns to the circulation. The filtered fluid, which contains waste products from the blood, continues down through the tubules, which form collecting ducts that lead into the ureters.

Infections, Inflammation, and Injury

In a healthy person, there are usually no micro-organisms in the urinary tract and urine is sterile. However, infectious agents, especially bacteria, can enter the urinary tract from outside the body by moving up the urethra into the bladder. Microorganisms can also travel through the bloodstream to the urinary tract from other parts of the body. Once the infectious agents enter the urinary tract, they can multiply and spread, causing inflammation and disrupting normal functioning. Infections of the urinary tract can be acute (short term, usually severe) or chronic (long-lasting).

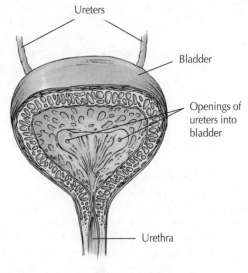

Ureters

Bladder

Openings of ureters into bladder

Urethra

The bladder
The bladder is a hollow, muscular organ that can store about 1 pint of urine. Urine flows down the ureters from the kidneys to the bladder. As the bladder fills with urine, its elastic, flexible walls expand. Nerves in the bladder signal the brain when the bladder is full. When you urinate, the bladder walls contract to expel urine through the urethra. The muscle layers within the bladder walls and the sloping angle at which the ureters enter the bladder combine to act as a valve to prevent urine from flowing backward through the ureters into the kidneys.

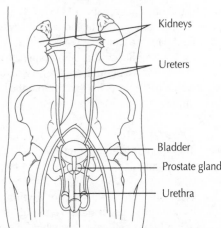

Kidneys

Ureters

Bladder
Prostate gland

Urethra

Kidneys

Ureters

Bladder

Urethra

The male urinary tract

The female urinary tract

Male and female urinary tracts
The structure of the male urinary tract differs slightly from the structure of the female urinary tract. The male urethra is about 10 inches long and provides an outlet for semen as well as urine. The female urethra is about 1½ inches long and lies, with the bladder, just in front of the reproductive organs.

Infection of the kidney is called pyelonephritis. Infection of the bladder is called cystitis. Kidney inflammation (nephritis) can occur without an infection, such as when it is caused by medication. Glomerulonephritis, inflammation of the glomeruli (the network of tiny blood vessels inside the nephrons, the basic filtering units of the kidneys), can also occur without infection.

Direct injury to the kidneys from a blow is rare because the kidneys are located at the back of the abdominal cavity and are protected by the rib cage and the fat and muscles of the back. The bladder is also well protected inside the pelvis. Direct injury to the urinary tract usually occurs along with severe injuries that require hospitalization, such as from a motor vehicle collision or a bullet wound.

Acute Pyelonephritis

Acute pyelonephritis is an infection of the kidneys that develops suddenly. The infection and the inflammation it causes affect mainly the tissue in the kidneys that contains tiny filtering units (nephrons). In most cases, the bacteria causing the infection come from the tissues surrounding the opening of the urethra (the tube that carries urine from the bladder out of the body). If the bacteria multiply, they can enter the urethra and move up through the bladder and ureter to the kidneys. Acute pyelonephritis occurs more frequently in women than in men because the rectum is closer to the urethra in women and the urethra is shorter in women, increasing the likelihood that bacteria will enter the urinary tract.

Acute pyelonephritis is more likely to occur when the normal flow of urine is partially blocked as a result of a condition such as pregnancy, kidney stones (see page 814), a tumor of the bladder (see page 813), or an enlarged prostate gland (see page 832). In these conditions, urine can collect and become stagnant, encouraging bacteria to multiply; the reduced urine flow prevents the bacteria from being easily eliminated from the urinary tract.

Acute pyelonephritis can also develop when bacteria from an infection in another part of the body are carried through the bloodstream to the kidneys. The condition also sometimes occurs for unknown reasons in otherwise healthy people.

Symptoms

Often the first symptom of acute pyelonephritis is sudden, intense pain in the back just above the waist. Although both kidneys may be affected, the pain is usually worse on one side of the body and spreads around that side and down into the groin. A person with acute pyelonephritis quickly develops a fever (often reaching 102°F to 104°F), which may produce chills or trembling and may be accompanied by nausea and vomiting. He or she may also experience difficult or painful urination and is likely to feel a constant urge to urinate, even when the bladder is empty. The urine is often cloudy and may appear reddish if blood has leaked into it. Rarely, this condition can lead to blood poisoning (see page 937) or shock (see page 579), or can be fatal.

Diagnosis

The diagnosis of acute pyelonephritis is based on the symptoms. Your doctor will probably order blood tests or urine tests to determine the type of bacteria causing the infection. To check for conditions that may be obstructing the flow of urine through the urinary tract, your doctor may order an ultrasound (see page 111) or CT scan (see page 112) to evaluate your kidneys, or cystoscopy (see next page) to examine your bladder. He or she may order a voiding cystourethrogram (see next page) to check for vesicoureteral reflux, a condition in which urine flows backward from the bladder to the kidneys.

Treatment

Treatment for acute pyelonephritis usually includes rest, plenty of fluids (at least eight large glasses of water every day), and antibiotics given intravenously (through a vein) or in pills. People who have a fever, nausea and vomiting, or an elevated white blood cell count, or who are very young or very frail may need to be hospitalized for treatment with intravenous antibiotics. The antibiotics usually bring the infection under control within 24 to 48 hours, although, in some cases, treatment may need to continue for 14 days or longer. The doctor will also treat any underlying condition

Diagnostic Tests for Disorders of the Bladder or Urethra

Doctors frequently perform the following diagnostic tests to evaluate the condition of the bladder and the urethra and to determine how well the bladder functions.

Cystoscopy

Cystoscopy is a diagnostic imaging technique that allows a doctor to look directly inside the urethra and bladder to examine the bladder, look for any stones or tumors, and check for other abnormalities. Cystoscopy is often done using local anesthesia, but spinal or general anesthesia is sometimes used. The procedure is usually performed on an outpatient basis.

As you lie on your back, the doctor inserts a narrow viewing tube (called a cystoscope) through your urethra and into the bladder. The cystoscope has a tiny light and camera at its tip that enables the doctor to view the urethra and bladder directly or on a video monitor. He or she may also insert a small instrument through the cystoscope to remove a tiny sample of tissue for examination under a microscope (biopsy). In some cases, a doctor may pass water into the bladder to see how much it can hold.

Although most cystoscopic examinations do not cause problems, there is a small risk of bladder infection or injury to the urethra or bladder. After the test, you probably will experience a temporary burning sensation or pain in the urethra, especially when urinating. You may also notice a small amount of blood in your urine during the first day or two after the procedure; this is normal. However, contact your doctor if these symptoms persist, if you have difficulty urinating, or if you have a fever. These symptoms can indicate an injury or a bladder infection.

Voiding Cystourethrogram

A voiding cystourethrogram is an X-ray procedure that allows a doctor to evaluate bladder function during urination. This test is usually performed to diagnose anatomical problems that may be the underlying cause of conditions such as vesicoureteral reflux, in which urine in the bladder is forced back up through the ureters toward the kidneys instead of down through the urethra and out of the body. The procedure is usually performed on an outpatient basis.

As you lie on your back, a catheter (a thin, flexible tube) is inserted through your urethra and into the bladder. After the catheter is in place, the doctor injects fluid containing a contrast medium (dye) into your bladder through the catheter. Several X-rays are taken while your bladder is being filled with the fluid. After the catheter has been removed, the doctor will ask you to urinate into a handheld urinal or bedpan. Additional X-rays are taken as you empty your bladder.

Although most voiding cystourethrograms do not cause problems, there is a small risk of infection or an allergic reaction to the contrast medium. Also, for a few hours after the catheter has been removed, some people experience temporary irritation of the urethra that causes a slight burning sensation while urinating. If you have persistent burning or pain when urinating, tell your doctor; these could be symptoms of a bladder infection.

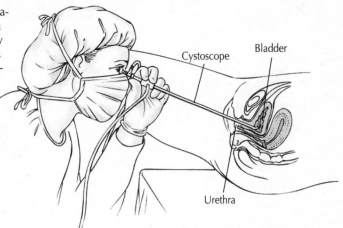

Cystoscopy

In cystoscopy, a doctor inserts a viewing tube called a cystoscope through the urethra and into the bladder. A tiny light and camera at the tip of the cystoscope allow the doctor to view the bladder directly or on a video monitor.

causing the infection. With prompt treatment, long-term complications are unlikely. People who have repeated episodes of acute pyelonephritis may have an anatomical problem in the urinary tract that requires surgery.

Chronic Pyelonephritis

Chronic pyelonephritis is a recurring kidney infection that causes progressive scarring of kidney tissue over a period of several years. Doctors think the condition begins in childhood and persists undetected into adulthood. After years of scarring, symptoms of kidney disease, including chronic kidney failure (see page 817), may develop.

The bacteria that cause chronic pyelonephritis probably enter the urinary tract through the urethra (the tube that carries urine from the bladder out of the body). The infection is usually limited to the lower parts of the urinary tract, because the outflow of urine and the valvelike openings between the ureters and the bladder normally keep the bacteria from spreading upward. When a healthy person urinates, the bladder contracts and forces urine out of the body through the urethra. At the same time, the openings between the ureters and the bladder close like valves, preventing urine from flowing back into the kidneys. However, in some cases, this valvelike action does not work properly and, when the bladder contracts, urine is forced up through the ureters and back into the kidneys. This backward flow is called vesicoureteral reflux.

Doctors think that a combination of recurring infections and reflux probably causes chronic pyelonephritis in most people who develop the condition. Kidney stones (see page 814) also may cause the disorder by blocking the normal flow of urine and providing a reservoir for bacteria. In some people, chronic pyelonephritis may be preceded by repeated episodes of other urinary tract infections, such as acute pyelonephritis (see

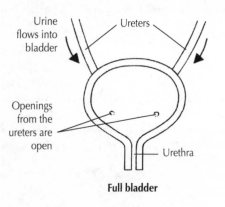

Urine flows into bladder

Ureters

Openings from the ureters are open

Urethra

Full bladder

The flow of urine
A possible cause of kidney infection is ineffective closing of the valvelike openings between the ureters and the bladder. If the openings between the ureters and the bladder do not close properly when you urinate, urine may be squeezed back up the ureters and into the kidneys. Microorganisms in the urine can then enter the kidneys.

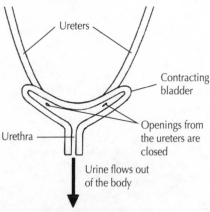

Ureters

Contracting bladder

Openings from the ureters are closed

Urethra

Urine flows out of the body

Normal flow of urine

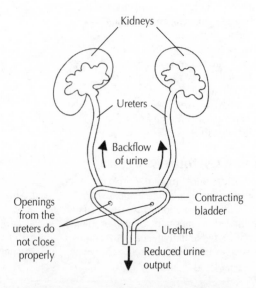

Kidneys

Ureters

Backflow of urine

Openings from the ureters do not close properly

Contracting bladder

Urethra

Reduced urine output

Abnormal flow of urine in vesicoureteral reflux

page 804) or cystitis (see next page). However, doctors do not think that these infections cause chronic pyelonephritis.

Symptoms

Chronic pyelonephritis often does not produce symptoms until years after the condition develops. Eventually, early symptoms of kidney failure may develop, including fatigue, nausea, and itching skin. If you have recurring mild urinary tract infections, or any symptom of chronic kidney failure, see your doctor.

Diagnosis

If you have recurring urinary tract infections, your doctor will examine you and will probably order blood and urine tests to determine the type of bacteria that is causing the infection. He or she may also order an ultrasound (see page 111) or CT scan (see page 112) to evaluate your kidneys, cystoscopy (see page 805) to examine your bladder, or a voiding cystourethrogram (see page 805) to find out how your bladder functions during urination. In many cases, the condition is detected at an earlier stage by a blood or urine test performed for another purpose.

Treatment

If you have chronic pyelonephritis but no symptoms, your doctor may recommend that you drink plenty of fluids (at least eight large glasses of water every day) and limit your intake of foods high in protein and sodium to avoid overworking your kidneys. Your doctor may also recommend that you have blood tests every 6 to 12 months to monitor your condition and watch for infections.

Treatment for chronic pyelonephritis depends on how advanced the condition is when it is diagnosed. Surgery to repair the faulty valvelike action at the openings of the ureters into the bladder may be performed on a child, but the procedure is usually not performed on adults. Your doctor will treat any underlying cause of the chronic infections, such as kidney stones. He or she will probably prescribe an antibiotic to take for a specified amount of time whenever you have a urinary tract infection. Alternatively, a doctor may prescribe a low dose of an antibiotic to take for 3 to 6 months to try to keep the urine free of bacteria.

Because chronic pyelonephritis progresses slowly, your doctor may recommend that you watch

for symptoms of kidney disease (such as frequent urination, abnormal-looking urine, pain in your side or back between the rib cage and hip, or puffiness in your face) and have regular checkups.

Glomerulonephritis

Glomerulonephritis refers to several related diseases that damage the kidneys. Some types of glomerulonephritis are linked to disorders in which the immune system mistakenly attacks the glomeruli (the network of tiny blood vessels inside the nephrons, the basic filtering units of the kidneys).

In a healthy kidney, blood passes through the glomeruli, which filter out chemicals including waste products. Most of the water and essential chemicals (such as glucose, sodium, and potassium) are reabsorbed into the bloodstream. The remaining waste materials collect as urine and pass down the ureters to the bladder for storage until you urinate.

If the glomeruli are damaged, red blood cells can leak through them into the urine, and protein can pass from the blood into the urine. If the loss of protein is excessive, it can cause a condition called nephrotic syndrome (see page 429). As more of the glomeruli are damaged, the kidneys become less efficient as filters and regulators of the chemical content of the blood. Waste products accumulate in the blood and can damage the kidneys.

Glomerulonephritis can be mild or severe, and it may be acute, flaring up over a few days, or chronic, taking months or years to develop. The condition is not common, but approximately 60 percent of people who have end-stage kidney failure (see page 819) first have signs and symptoms of chronic glomerulonephritis. Acute glomerulonephritis can result from infections such as HIV (see page 909), hepatitis (see page 786), or endocarditis (see page 593). It also can occur as a result of inflammation or cancer anywhere in the body. Because the kidneys have a major role in regulating blood pressure, glomerulonephritis can eventually lead to high blood pressure (see page 574). Glomerulonephritis also may lead to chronic kidney failure (see page 817).

Symptoms

Mild, chronic glomerulonephritis produces no symptoms. In many cases, a doctor detects the condition with blood or urine tests performed for another purpose. In some cases, small amounts of blood in the urine may cause it to look smoky; larger amounts of blood make the urine look bright red.

In severe, acute glomerulonephritis, you may feel generally ill, with drowsiness, nausea, and vomiting—all symptoms of impending kidney failure. You will probably be producing very small amounts of urine. You may urinate less frequently during the day and wake up at night to urinate. Fluid may accumulate in your body tissues, causing a condition called edema, which makes your skin, particularly around the ankles, look puffy. You may notice swelling around your eyes in the morning. If fluid accumulates in your chest, you may become short of breath.

Diagnosis

If you have symptoms of glomerulonephritis, your doctor will order a urine test to check for protein and red blood cells. If the test results indicate that you could have glomerulonephritis, the doctor will probably order additional tests, such as blood tests, an ultrasound (see page 111) or a CT scan (see page 112), or a kidney biopsy, in which a small sample of kidney cells is removed through a hollow needle and examined under a microscope.

Treatment

Many forms of glomerulonephritis require no treatment other than rest. Other forms of the disease can be treated with corticosteroids or immune-suppressing drugs to relieve inflammation or dampen the errant immune response. If an underlying condition is causing the problem, you will receive treatment for the condition.

If you have edema, your doctor may prescribe diuretics to reduce the amount of fluid your body retains. To treat high blood pressure, your doctor may prescribe antihypertensive medication to help control your blood pressure. If you have developed iron deficiency anemia (see page 610) as a result of the disorder, your doctor may prescribe iron and vitamin supplements. If glomerulonephritis leads to end-stage kidney failure, a doctor will treat the kidney failure.

Cystitis

Cystitis is inflammation of the bladder, usually caused by a urinary tract infection. The bladder functions as a temporary storage site for urine, and expels urine from the body through a muscular tube called the urethra. Cystitis occurs more frequently in women than in men because a woman's urethra is shorter, providing bacteria and other germs from outside the body easier access to the bladder. Cystitis in men usually results from an inflamed or enlarged prostate gland or another abnormality of the lower urinary tract.

Symptoms

The main symptom of cystitis is a frequent urge to urinate that produces only a small amount of urine, which is sometimes strong-smelling or bloody. Because the urethra often also becomes inflamed in cystitis, you are likely to experience a burning or stinging sensation when you urinate. You may wake up during the night with a strong urge to urinate, and you may have a feeling of discomfort below your navel, where your bladder is. Cystitis can also cause a fever.

Diagnosis

If you have symptoms of cystitis, your doctor may order a urine test to check for bacteria and white blood cells, which are signs of infection. The urine sample is grown in a laboratory to confirm the presence of an infection, identify the microorganism that is causing the infection, and determine the best treatment.

Treatment

To help relieve your symptoms, your doctor will recommend drinking large quantities of water (at least eight large glasses every day). If there are bacteria in your urine, your doctor will prescribe antibiotics. The medication should clear up the infection within a few days, but you should continue taking the drugs until your doctor tells you to stop. If the symptoms recur after you have completed treatment, see your doctor.

Injury to the Kidneys or the Ureters

Injury to the kidneys or the ureters (the muscular tubes that carry urine from the kidneys to the bladder) usually results from a direct blow to the side of the body or a crushing force (such as from a motor vehicle collision). Another possible cause of injury is penetration by a sharp object (such as a knife) or a bullet. In any injury, a kidney may be bruised or its tissue torn or fractured. The ureters also may be bruised, obstructed, or torn. Sometimes a large blood clot forms under the fibrous capsule that surrounds the kidney and produces a lump over the kidney. It is also possible for blood or urine to leak into the abdomen through a tear in a kidney or a ureter.

Symptoms and Diagnosis

A slight injury to a kidney or a ureter may cause pain and tenderness in the lower part of your back. You may have a fever and notice occasional traces of blood in your urine (you may not see any blood until a day or two after the injury). If you have severe pain or large amounts of blood in your urine, you may have a serious injury to one or both kidneys and possibly the ureters.

If you have a kidney or bladder injury, your doctor will probably order diagnostic tests such as an ultrasound (see page 111) or a CT scan (see page 112) to evaluate the severity of the injury and determine the best course of treatment.

Treatment

Because the kidneys are often able to heal themselves, even major tears and injuries usually require no treatment other than 7 to 10 days of bed rest. Your doctor will probably recommend that you stay in the hospital for several days to allow him or her to monitor your pulse, blood pressure, and blood count, and to check your urine frequently for signs of severe internal bleeding.

Surgery to repair a damaged ureter is usually performed immediately. If your kidney does not heal on its own after a period of bed rest, the doctor may perform surgery to remove it. The remaining healthy kidney may increase in size and level of function and do the work of both kidneys.

Injury to the Bladder or the Urethra

Because the bladder is low inside the pelvis, it is usually protected from injury. When an injury does occur, it generally results from a direct blow to the pelvis that fractures a pelvic bone and causes a sharp fragment of the bone to pierce the bladder wall, or from a direct, forceful blow to a full bladder that causes the bladder to rupture. The bladder

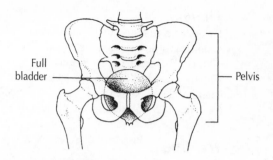

Location of the bladder
The bladder is a hollow organ that serves as the temporary storage site for urine. It lies behind the pubic bone and is protected by the circle of bones that form the pelvis.

can occasionally be damaged during abdominal surgical procedures such as a cesarean section (see page 534) or laparoscopy. These injuries can be serious if urine leaks from the bladder into the abdominal cavity.

Because the male urethra (the tube that carries urine from the bladder out of the body) is longer than the female urethra, rupture of the urethra occurs more frequently in men than in women. A ruptured urethra can result from a fall or any other kind of serious injury to the pelvis. This type of injury usually occurs in a motor vehicle collision that fractures the pelvis.

Rupture of the bladder is dangerous because urine can leak into the abdominal cavity and cause peritonitis (see page 759). This condition requires prompt treatment in a hospital. Damage to the urethra, however, usually does not lead to peritonitis. For a man, the major risks of damage to the urethra are narrowing of the urethra from scarring or inflammation (urethral stricture; see page 837) and erection problems (see page 486).

Symptoms

A ruptured bladder causes severe abdominal pain. The condition also may produce symptoms of peritonitis—such as fever, bloating, or nausea and vomiting—and of shock (see page 579)—such as sweating, faintness, shallow breathing, rapid pulse, or pale, cold, clammy skin. A ruptured bladder usually results in the inability to urinate. An injury to the urethra causes extreme pain and an inability to urinate. In some cases, a person has a bloody discharge from the urethra.

Diagnosis

If you have an injury to the bladder, urethra, lower abdomen, or urinary tract, see your doctor immediately. He or she may order X-rays of your abdomen and bladder, a CT scan (see page 112) to examine the abdomen and pelvis, and cystoscopy (see page 805) to examine the bladder.

Treatment

If you have an injury to your bladder or urethra, you will be hospitalized and probably given antibiotics to prevent infection. If your bladder is ruptured but urine does not leak into the abdominal cavity, you may need to have a catheter (a thin, flexible tube) placed inside the bladder to allow urine to drain from your body and to prevent urine from leaking into your abdomen. Use of the catheter allows the rupture to heal while preventing the bladder from filling with urine and stretching. If urine leaks from the bladder into the abdominal cavity, the doctor will perform surgery to drain the leaking urine and, if possible, repair the injured bladder. If the urethra is damaged, the doctor will probably insert a catheter into the bladder through

the abdominal wall for several days to drain urine. Although the urethra usually heals on its own, surgery is performed occasionally to repair an injured urethra that has not healed within 3 to 6 months.

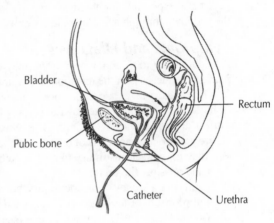

Urinary catheter
A urinary catheter is a long, flexible tube that is inserted through the urethra into the bladder to allow urine to drain from the body.

Cysts, Tumors, and Stones

The urinary tract can be affected by two kinds of growths—cysts and tumors. Cysts are usually soft, fluid-filled sacs and are usually, but not always, benign (noncancerous). Solid tumors are usually cancerous. Other types of growths, such as kidney stones or bladder stones, occur more frequently. Stones are hardened accumulations of particles (usually mineral salts) that form in the urine. Although stones can cause great discomfort, they are usually not life-threatening.

Simple Kidney Cysts and Acquired Kidney Cysts

There are three major types of kidney cysts—simple cysts, acquired cysts that result from kidney failure (see page 816), and cysts that develop in polycystic kidney disease (see next page). Simple cysts, which are the most common type, are soft, fluid-filled pouches lined with cells called renal epithelial cells. Simple cysts can be single or multiple and can occur in both kidneys. They usually cause no symptoms and are often detected by tests performed for another purpose. It is estimated that

about one of four people over age 50 has simple kidney cysts.

Acquired cysts occur only in kidney failure. They develop in the nephrons (the basic filtering units of the kidneys) and increase in number and size as the kidney failure progresses. More than 75 percent of people who receive dialysis (see page 818) develop acquired cysts after 5 years of treatment. Doctors monitor these cysts closely because they can develop into adenomas (noncancerous tumors that could become cancerous) or adenocarcinomas (cancerous tumors). Cysts that develop on the kidneys of people who are on dialysis are often cancerous.

Symptoms

Simple kidney cysts usually do not cause symptoms; many people who have simple kidney cysts don't know it. Rarely, a simple cyst grows large enough to cause pain in the back or in the abdomen. Blood in the urine is another possible symptom. Acquired cysts rarely cause symptoms.

Diagnosis

Simple kidney cysts are usually detected during an ultrasound (see page 111), CT scan (see page 112), or MRI (see page 113) performed for another purpose. Because of the slight possibility that cancer cells are present in the cyst, your doctor may order an aspiration biopsy of the cyst, in which a small sample of fluid and cells is withdrawn through a hollow needle (guided by ultrasound, CT, or MRI) and examined under a microscope. Aspiration of a kidney cyst is usually painless with the use of a local anesthetic.

Treatment

No treatment is required for a painless, noncancerous kidney cyst. If it grows large enough to press on other organs or is causing discomfort or pain in the back or abdomen, the cyst may be drained by inserting a hollow needle into it (guided by ultrasound, CT, or MRI) and withdrawing the fluid. If it becomes large enough to be painful, fluid can be removed with a needle (aspirated) periodically, or the cyst can be drained with laparoscopy. If the cells in the fluid are found to be normal, no treatment is needed. If a cyst recurs after being drained, a doctor may perform laparoscopic surgery to remove it permanently. If a cyst is found to be cancerous, surgery is performed to remove part or all of the affected kidney. The healthy kidney will increase in size and level of function and do the work of both kidneys.

Polycystic Kidney Disease

Polycystic kidney disease is an inherited disease characterized by the growth of numerous fluid-filled cysts in the kidneys. The cysts grow out of the tiny filters (called nephrons) inside the kidneys. The cysts enlarge and eventually separate from the nephrons, and the kidneys begin to enlarge as the cysts multiply. The number of cysts can reach into the thousands. Over time, the cysts may make up the bulk of the kidneys, affecting kidney function and eventually causing kidney failure.

There are two types of inherited polycystic kidney disease—autosomal dominant (the most common type) and autosomal recessive. Autosomal dominant polycystic kidney disease, which primarily affects adults, occurs when a person inherits a copy of the defective dominant gene from only one parent, who also has the disease. Typically, the family has a long history of kidney problems. But in about one fourth of all cases, a mutation of a gene in a parent's egg or sperm produces the disease for the first time in a family. This form of the disease is the most common life-threatening inherited disorder in the United States, affecting roughly half a million people. The disorder affects men and women in equal numbers.

The autosomal recessive form, which is rare and affects only infants and children, occurs when a copy of the defective recessive gene is inherited from both parents. A third form of polycystic kidney disease, which is not inherited, is called acquired cystic kidney disease and occurs mainly in people who have another long-term kidney disease and are on kidney dialysis (see page 818).

Symptoms

In autosomal dominant polycystic kidney disease, cysts may begin to develop early in life without causing any symptoms. The age at which symptoms first appear varies from person to person, but most people begin to notice signs of the disease between ages 30 and 40. Common symptoms include pain in the back and in the sides between the ribs and hips, headaches, blood in the urine, urinary tract infections, kidney stones, and an enlarged abdomen. High blood pressure is common.

The disorder can affect the entire body, causing liver, pancreas, and intestinal problems. It can also weaken blood vessels, producing an aneurysm (a balloonlike swelling) that can rupture in a blood vessel of the abdomen or brain. Blood vessels in the walls of the intestine or abdomen can also be affected, producing a hernia (see page 762). One quarter of people with polycystic kidney disease have an abnormality in a heart valve, called mitral valve prolapse (see page 591), that causes a fluttering feeling or pounding in the chest, along with possible chest pain. Cysts can also form in the ovaries, testicles, pancreas, spleen, central nervous system, and liver. By age 60 the disease advances to kidney failure in more than half of all affected people. The risk of kidney failure increases in people who have high blood pressure or blood or protein in their urine.

Infants and children who have the rare recessive form of polycystic kidney disease have the above symptoms along with high blood pressure and frequent urinary tract infections. They usually develop kidney failure within a few years of birth; in rare, severe cases, a baby dies within a few hours or days of birth. Children who live into adolescence or early adulthood are small for their age because the abnormal kidney function inhibits growth.

Diagnosis

Doctors use ultrasound imaging (see page 111), along with a family health history (see page 130), to diagnose both forms of inherited polycystic kidney disease. Kidney cysts are usually clearly visible on an ultrasound. Sometimes doctors detect the first signs of the disorder when an affected adult discovers blood in his or her urine or during a routine examination when high blood pressure is detected. Scientists are working on developing a genetic test (see page 953) that can screen for polycystic kidney disease before cysts begin to develop.

Treatment

Currently there is no cure for polycystic kidney disease, but treatment of the symptoms can relieve pain and prolong life. Over-the-counter pain medication may help reduce back or headache pain. Severe pain may require surgery to drain and remove the cysts that are causing the pain, but surgery cannot prevent the disease from getting worse. Doctors prescribe antibiotics to treat the frequent urinary tract infections that develop. High blood pressure can be controlled with medication, diet, and exercise. Eventually, if the kidneys fail, the person must begin dialysis or have a kidney transplant (see page 820).

Kidney transplantation is a relatively common and successful treatment for kidney failure caused by polycystic kidney disease. Healthy transplanted kidneys do not develop cysts, and donor kidneys are slightly more available than other organs because a person can donate one of his or her kidneys to an affected person and still function normally with the remaining kidney.

Kidney Tumors

A tumor is an abnormal mass of tissue that forms when cells reproduce at an increased rate. There are two major types of kidney tumors, both of which are cancerous. One type, called renal cell carcinoma, occurs only in adults. The other type, called Wilm's tumor (see page 430), affects mainly children.

Renal cell carcinoma occurs most often in men over age 40. Renal cell carcinomas are highly malignant tumors whose cells can enter the bloodstream and spread to other parts of the body, particularly the lungs or bones. Because these tumors can grow for years without causing symptoms, they may go undetected until they are at an advanced stage. As the tumor enlarges, it can grow into healthy kidney tissue, gradually diminishing the ability of the kidney to filter blood.

Symptoms

A kidney tumor often causes symptoms such as pain in the side, loss of appetite, weight loss, anemia (see page 610), or blood in the urine, and can cause a variety of symptoms throughout the body.

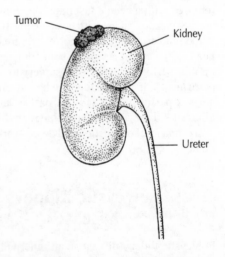

Kidney tumor
A kidney tumor can grow for many years without causing symptoms. Doctors use diagnostic imaging techniques such as X-rays, ultrasound, CT, or MRI to detect kidney tumors that are too small to be felt during a physical examination.

For example, symptoms such as bone pain or a cough can develop if the tumor spreads to other organs, such as the bones or lungs. Your urine may appear reddish or cloudy because of bleeding from the tumor.

Diagnosis

If your urine looks reddish or cloudy, or if you have pain in your side, your doctor will order urine tests. If your doctor thinks you may have a kidney tumor, he or she will probably also recommend other diagnostic tests such as an ultrasound (see page 111), a CT scan (see page 112), or an MRI (see page 113) of the abdomen and pelvis, including the kidneys.

Treatment

If the diagnostic tests indicate that you have renal cell carcinoma, your doctor will perform tests to determine if the tumor has spread to other organs. Part or all of the affected kidney will be removed surgically in a procedure called nephrectomy. The remaining, healthy kidney will increase in size and level of function and do the work of both kidneys.

If cancerous cells have spread to other parts of the body (metastasized), your doctor may recommend treatment such as radiation therapy (see page 23), which uses high-energy radiation to kill the cancer cells, or immunotherapy, which uses drugs such as interferon or interleukin to boost the body's natural ability to fight cancer. Your doctor will perform regular checkups to monitor your condition.

Bladder Tumors

Bladder tumors are usually malignant and tend to recur, but are not likely to spread. The tumors originate from cells that line the bladder and most of the urinary tract, and they tend to produce a growth or growths that project inward, into the space inside the bladder where urine is stored. The tumors may also invade the muscle of the bladder. Any tumor in the urethra or near where a ureter (the muscular tube that carries urine from the kidney to the bladder) enters the bladder can block the flow of urine. Urine can then build up in a kidney, causing it to expand (a condition called hydronephrosis). Bladder tumors occur more frequently in men than in women. Cigarette smoking increases the risk of bladder cancer.

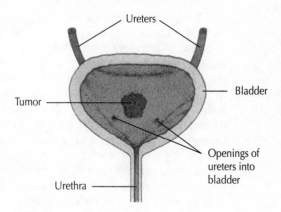

Bladder tumor
Most bladder tumors project inward from the bladder's inside wall. If the tumor develops near the openings to the ureters, it can block the flow of urine from the kidneys to the bladder. If it develops near the urethra, the tumor can block urine flow from the bladder out of the body.

Symptoms

The main symptom of a bladder tumor is a frequent, urgent need to urinate. Urination is usually not painful, but you may have pain after you finish urinating. You may also have a burning sensation and a tendency to urinate small amounts at frequent intervals. There may be blood in the urine. If hydronephrosis has developed, you may also have pain in your back or side.

Diagnosis

To help diagnose a bladder tumor, your doctor will order a urine test to check for blood in the urine. He or she may also order other diagnostic tests, including cystoscopy (see page 805), or an ultrasound scan (see page 111), CT scan (see page 112), or MRI (see page 113) of the bladder. If the doctor detects a tumor that has not penetrated the wall of the bladder, he or she will probably remove it using instruments inserted through a cystoscope (viewing tube). Cells from the tumor are then examined under a microscope to see if they are cancerous.

Treatment

Treatment of bladder tumors depends on their location. Tumors in the lining of the bladder are often removed with instruments passed through a cystoscope. At some stages of bladder cancer, a doctor may insert a catheter through the urethra into the bladder to deliver a solution containing anticancer medications or an immune system stimulator, such as tuberculosis vaccine. You will be asked to hold the solution in the bladder for 1 or 2 hours before urinating. The medication causes the bladder to shed its lining, which is then replaced by healthy cells. Although these treatments may effectively destroy the tumor and prevent its recurrence, the doctor will recommend regular checkups to monitor the condition.

If a tumor has affected a large area of the bladder, or if it has grown into nearby tissue, the doctor may recommend surgical removal of part, or all, of the bladder. After removing the bladder, the surgeon may connect the ureters to a portion of the intestine that he or she has formed into a pouch. The surgeon then attaches the pouch to the urethra, creating a new bladder, which allows you to urinate normally. Alternatively, the surgeon may attach the ureters to a disconnected section of the small intestine, the end of which is sewn to an opening in the skin; urine flows through the opening into a removable external pouch, which you must empty from time to time. After surgery, the doctor may prescribe chemotherapy to destroy any remaining abnormal cells.

Kidney Stones

A kidney stone usually begins as a tiny speck of solid material deposited in the renal pelvis, the tissues in the kidney where urine collects before flowing into the ureter (the tube that connects the kidney and the bladder). As additional material adheres to the first speck, it gradually increases in size. This process can occur in one or both kidneys. Over time, a stone that is 1 inch or more in diameter can develop. Most kidney stones contain calcium. Other substances, such as uric acid or amino acids, can crystallize in the urine and form a stone.

Tiny stones seldom cause problems because they are easily carried in the ureters and urethra and passed in urine. Any stone with a diameter of about $\frac{1}{5}$ inch or more, however, can cause severe pain if it enters the ureter. Passage of a kidney stone is a frequent cause of brief hospital admissions for pain control and administration of fluids.

Kidney stones run in families. Men are more susceptible to developing kidney stones than women, and the risk increases after age 30. Kidney stones

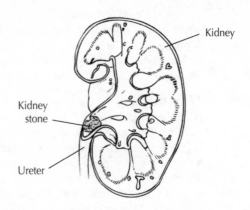

Kidney stone
A kidney stone is a hardened accumulation of mineral salts or other substances that forms in a kidney. A stone that is smaller than $\frac{1}{5}$ inch in diameter can usually pass through a ureter and urethra without difficulty. However, a larger stone can become lodged in the ureter, blocking the flow of urine and causing severe pain.

occur more frequently in people who live in hot climates because of increased loss of body water in very warm weather. Also, unless their fluid intake is substantial, people in hot climates produce a smaller, more concentrated volume of urine, which contains a higher proportion of stone-forming material. In rare cases, children develop a type of kidney stone caused by a chemical abnormality in the blood.

Most kidney stones are eventually passed in the urine. An occasional stone may get stuck in a ureter and block the flow of urine on one side; surgery may be required to remove the stone because of the risk of severe kidney infection and kidney damage.

Symptoms

If a kidney stone is too large to pass from the kidney into the ureter, it may not cause any symptoms or may cause only occasional pain as small pieces break off and are carried down the ureter. The most common symptom of a kidney stone is renal colic, a severe, stabbing pain that tends to come in waves, often a few minutes apart. Renal colic can develop when a stone passes from a kidney down one of the ureters, blocking the flow of urine. The pain will subside if the stone moves into the bladder. The pain usually occurs on one side of the body, but if you have stones in both kidneys, a subsequent attack of pain can occur on the other side.

Pain from a kidney stone usually occurs first in the back, just below the ribs on one side of the spinal column. Over the next few hours or days, the pain may follow the course of the stone as it travels through the ureter—from the back around to the front of the body and down toward the groin. In men, the pain may radiate to the testicles; in women, the pain may radiate to the labia. You may feel nauseated, and notice traces of blood in your urine. After the stone reaches the bladder, it usually passes more easily through the remainder of the urinary tract.

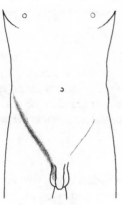

Site of kidney stone pain

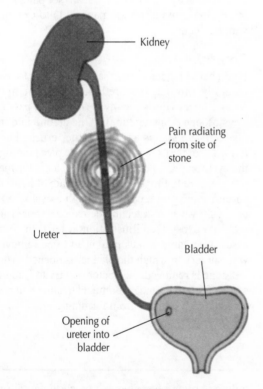

Kidney

Pain radiating from site of stone

Ureter

Bladder

Opening of ureter into bladder

Path of a kidney stone

Pain from kidney stones
A kidney stone can cause severe pain as it travels from the kidney to the bladder. This process can take several days. The location of the pain often indicates the position of the stone.

Diagnosis

If you have renal colic, your doctor will probably order blood and urine tests and a CT scan (see page 112) or ultrasound (see page 111) to find the cause of your symptoms, locate any stones, and help determine if treatment is necessary.

A 24-hour urine test can determine if your body excretes too much of a specific mineral salt or other stone-forming substance or if your urine does not contain enough of a specific body chemical that inhibits stone formation. Half of all people who develop a kidney stone will develop a second stone within 10 years.

Treatment

If you have symptoms of a kidney stone, your doctor will recommend drinking large quantities of water (at least eight large glasses of water every day) to help flush any stones through your urinary tract and to help prevent more stones from forming by keeping your urine diluted. Your doctor will prescribe pain relievers if you are having pain. Your doctor also will ask you to try to collect the stone when you pass it so he or she can examine it to determine the type of stone and possibly plan additional treatment.

There is no effective treatment for most kidney stones that have already formed. However, if your body forms stones made of uric acid, your doctor may prescribe drugs that can prevent more stones from forming or, sometimes, dissolve existing stones. Doctors prescribe thiazide diuretics for people whose stones are caused by excessive excretion of calcium in the urine. If a stone causes a blockage in the lower third of the ureter, it can sometimes be removed during a procedure called cystoscopy (see page 805), in which a doctor passes tiny instruments through a cystoscope (viewing tube) into the bladder and up into the ureter, where the stone is trapped. When the doctor withdraws the instrument, the stone often comes out with it. The doctor can also pass a smaller viewing tube called a ureteroscope into the ureter to remove the stone or crush it with a laser (a highly concentrated beam of light) or ultrasonic probe passed through the ureteroscope.

Stones in the upper part of the ureter or in the kidney may be crushed using a technique called extracorporeal lithotripsy, in which a machine called a lithotriptor produces shock waves that pulverize the stones into a powder that can pass out of the body in urine. Lithotripsy has made surgery for kidney stones unnecessary in most cases.

In rare cases, stones severely damage one of the kidneys, and the entire kidney may need to be removed. The healthy remaining kidney increases in size and level of function and does the work of both kidneys.

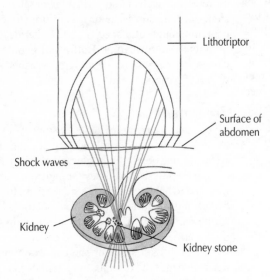

Lithotriptor

Surface of abdomen

Shock waves

Kidney

Kidney stone

Extracorporeal lithotripsy
Extracorporeal lithotripsy is a procedure used to destroy kidney stones. A machine called a lithotriptor, which is placed against the abdomen, generates a shock wave that passes through the body to the stone, causing it to disintegrate into a powder that passes from the body in urine.

Bladder Stones

A kidney stone (see page 814) that has traveled through one of the ureters (the tubes that connect the kidney and the bladder) into the bladder is usually relatively small and will pass easily out of the body through the urethra. Stones that form inside

the bladder, however, tend to be larger than kidney stones and may remain in the bladder. These stones form when the bladder does not empty properly, such as when the opening into the urethra is obstructed by an enlarged prostate gland (see page 832).

Symptoms
A bladder stone may cause symptoms such as a frequent urge to urinate, pain when you pass urine, an intermittent stream of urine, or blood in the urine. Often the blood seems to be squeezed out in the last few drops of urine.

Diagnosis
If you have symptoms of a bladder stone, your doctor will examine you and order a urine test to check for bacteria and white blood cells, which are signs of infection. He or she may also order an abdominal X-ray (see page 109), a CT scan (see page 112), or an ultrasound scan (see page 111) to examine your bladder.

Treatment
If you have bladder stones that are too large to pass naturally through the urethra, the doctor must remove them. This is usually performed by passing a cystoscope (viewing tube) up the urethra into the bladder. The stones are then either crushed and removed, or they are removed in one piece through the cystoscope. To crush the stones, a doctor may use a laser (a highly concentrated beam of light) or an ultrasonic probe passed through a cystoscope, or shock waves in a technique called extracorporeal lithotripsy (see illustration at left). In some cases, very large stones may need to be removed with surgery in which the bladder is opened. After the stone is removed, the doctor will try to find the cause of the stone and recommend treatment to prevent additional stones from forming.

Kidney Failure

K idney failure, also called renal failure, occurs in one of three forms: acute, chronic, or end stage. Acute kidney failure is a condition in which the kidneys suddenly stop functioning, sometimes within a few days or even hours. Acute kidney

failure is often reversible. Chronic kidney failure develops undetected over many years and can ultimately lead to end-stage kidney failure. In end-stage kidney failure, the kidneys are severely damaged and can no longer function properly.

Acute Kidney Failure

If a person's kidneys suddenly stop functioning, it is usually for one of three reasons: exposure to toxic agents, an immune reaction to a drug, or the result of an infection or disease that affects the kidneys, such as acute glomerulonephritis (see page 807). A sudden drop in blood pressure from a serious burn, severe bleeding, or a major heart attack can deprive the kidneys of an adequate supply of oxygen-rich blood, damaging them. The flow of urine may be suddenly and completely obstructed by a blockage in the urinary tract, such as in the urethra from an enlarged prostate gland (see page 832) or from a crushing injury in which myoglobin (the oxygen-carrying pigment of muscle) filters through the network of tiny blood vessels inside the kidneys and blocks the kidney's microscopic filtering tubes.

If the kidneys cannot produce urine, waste products build up in the bloodstream, and water accumulates in the body. A dangerous imbalance of essential body chemicals that are normally regulated by the kidneys may develop.

Symptoms

In acute kidney failure, you may pass significantly less urine than usual, possibly less than a cup a day. Almost immediately, you will lose your appetite, feel increasingly nauseated, and begin to vomit. Delaying treatment can lead to drowsiness, confusion, seizures, coma, and death.

Diagnosis

Acute kidney failure is a medical emergency that requires immediate treatment in a hospital. If the cause of kidney failure cannot be determined easily, you will probably undergo an intensive series of diagnostic tests, including blood and urine tests; an ultrasound (see page 111), CT scan (see page 112), or MRI (see page 113) of the kidneys; and possibly an aspiration biopsy. In an aspiration biopsy, a small sample of kidney cells is removed through a hollow needle and examined under a microscope.

Treatment

If the cause of acute kidney failure is heavy bleeding or a heart attack, the person must be treated for shock (see page 579). If the cause of acute kidney failure is a urinary tract obstruction, surgery will be performed to eliminate the blockage. If the underlying cause of acute kidney failure is kidney disease, or if the kidneys remain severely affected after the cause of the failure has been treated successfully, additional treatment will be determined by the doctor.

If shock or severe fluid loss (from hemorrhaging, vomiting, or diarrhea) has led to acute kidney failure, the doctor will administer an intravenous saline (salt) solution, plasma (the fluid in which blood cells are suspended), or blood, sometimes with an adrenalinelike substance, to restore blood pressure to a more normal level and improve blood flow to the kidneys.

Diuretics (drugs that help remove excess water from the body by increasing the amount of water in urine) occasionally can help reestablish urine flow, but only after fluid loss is restored to the bloodstream by fluids given intravenously (through a vein). Kidneys can recover most or all of their lost function within a few days to several weeks. In some cases, such as in acute glomerulonephritis, treatment with medication may be effective. But when little or no urine is being formed and kidney damage is severe, a doctor will recommend kidney dialysis (see next page), a treatment that takes over the function of the kidneys until they recover.

While you are being treated, you may need to follow a special diet that is high in calories and low in protein and includes no more than 1 liter of fluid per day. This diet will provide the energy you need without overtaxing your kidneys.

Chronic Kidney Failure

Chronic kidney failure ultimately leads to end-stage kidney failure (see page 819), in which dialysis (see next page) or kidney transplantation (see page 820) becomes necessary to sustain life. Diabetes (see page 889) is the most frequent cause of kidney failure, but it also can result from other conditions that affect the blood vessels, such as glomerulonephritis (see page 807), or from conditions that cause kidney inflammation, such as chronic pyelonephritis (see page 806). Infections such as HIV (see page 909), hepatitis (see page 786), or endocarditis (see page 593) can lead to kidney failure. Overuse of drugs containing

Dialysis

If your kidneys are temporarily unable to function, or if they have been badly damaged by chronic inflammation, you will probably receive a treatment called dialysis. In dialysis, the functions of the kidneys, which include removing waste products from the body and regulating the body's chemical and water balance, are performed by a machine called a dialysis unit or by infusing a special fluid into the abdomen.

There are two forms of dialysis—hemodialysis (usually called, simply, dialysis) and peritoneal dialysis. Hemodialysis filters waste products from the blood. To do this, blood from an arm or leg artery is passed through a thin tube to the dialysis unit, through its filter, and back through another tube into an adjacent vein. A special solution in the filter draws out waste, and suction draws out excess fluid. A standard hemodialysis treatment lasts 4 hours and is repeated two or three times a week, which is enough to control the levels of waste products and excess water in the body.

Before beginning dialysis treatment, you must first have a minor surgical procedure in which an artery and a vein in your arm are connected to enlarge the vein and provide permanent access to your bloodstream for hemodialysis. If your veins are too small for this procedure, a synthetic blood vessel is placed under your skin to connect an artery and a vein. Temporary dialysis is performed using a thin, flexible tube (catheter) placed in a large blood vessel.

People on dialysis learn how to insert their own needles and run the machine themselves. Small portable dialysis units are available that allow people on home dialysis to travel and take their machine with them. People who receive a kidney transplant (see page 820) no longer need dialysis.

In peritoneal dialysis, the doctor makes a small incision in your abdominal wall and threads a thin plastic tube into your abdomen. A special fluid flows slowly through the tube and fills the peritoneal space (the space between the inner and outer layers of the lining of the abdomen). The fluid draws in waste products from the blood vessels that line the abdomen, and drains from the abdomen along with excess water. The process takes several hours. Peritoneal dialysis is a painless procedure.

If you have acute kidney failure, you will gradually be weaned off of dialysis as your kidneys recover. If the damage to your kidneys is permanent, you may be taught to perform peritoneal dialysis yourself. This procedure (called continuous ambulatory peritoneal dialysis, or CAPD) is performed at home, during the day or overnight, and allows you to carry out your normal daily activities.

Dialysis unit — Pump — Tube from dialysis unit to vein — Tube from artery to dialysis unit

How hemodialysis is done

In hemodialysis, blood from an artery in your arm or leg flows through a tube and into a machine called a dialysis unit. Inside the dialysis unit, a membrane filter that works as an artificial kidney cleanses the blood, which then flows out of the machine and back into your body through another tube, which has been inserted into a vein in the same arm or leg.

phenacetin or poisoning from heavy metals (such as lead or mercury) may also lead to chronic kidney failure.

In chronic kidney failure, body chemicals gradually build up in the blood, and the kidneys gradually lose their ability to filter and excrete waste products and excess water. Because the kidneys also help regulate blood pressure, chronic kidney failure can cause high blood pressure (see page 574). The kidneys can become scarred and continue to lose function, which eventually leads to end-stage kidney failure (see next page).

Symptoms and Diagnosis

Symptoms of chronic kidney failure develop gradually. At first you may notice that you are urinating less often than usual, because your kidneys are not functioning efficiently. If you are urinating less often during the day, you may awaken at night to urinate. You may also feel increasingly tired and lethargic. If chronic kidney failure continues to get worse, it will produce symptoms of end-stage kidney failure (see right).

If your doctor suspects that you have chronic kidney failure, he or she may order blood and urine tests to measure the levels of electrolytes (essential minerals that help regulate various body processes) and to evaluate kidney function.

Treatment

If you have chronic kidney failure, your doctor will probably recommend eating a low-protein diet to avoid overworking the kidneys. If you develop high blood pressure, the doctor may ask you to exercise regularly and cut back on salt to help lower your blood pressure. You may also be asked to monitor your fluid intake and urine output. Your doctor will probably recommend that you exercise regularly. Do not take any over-the-counter or prescription medications unless your doctor has prescribed them, to avoid potentially dangerous side effects.

Your doctor may prescribe medications to control your blood pressure and prevent bone damage. He or she may also prescribe medications to lower the pressure inside the filters of the kidneys, or to

treat anemia (see page 610) or an underlying disease. With regular checkups, a carefully planned diet, and medication, most people with chronic kidney failure can lead active, productive lives.

End-Stage Kidney Failure

End-stage kidney failure is the most advanced form of kidney failure, usually occurring when chronic kidney failure (see page 817) or acute kidney failure (see page 817) progresses to a point at which the kidneys can no longer function. An infection such as pneumonia, which places added stress on the already limited filtering capacity of the kidneys, can tip the balance from chronic kidney failure to end-stage kidney failure.

Symptoms

A variety of symptoms can occur in end-stage kidney failure, including lethargy, weakness, headache, confusion, delirium, and seizures. A person may also have fluid buildup around the heart, an irregular heartbeat, or fluid buildup in the lungs (producing shortness of breath) or just under the skin (producing generalized swelling). The condition can also cause oral thrush (see page 744); nausea, vomiting, and diarrhea; pain in the chest or bones; or intensely itchy skin. Severe anemia (see page 610) results from kidney failure, because the kidneys stop producing erythropoietin, a hormone that stimulates the bone marrow to produce red blood cells (which deliver oxygen to other cells throughout the body). In both men and women, the sex hormones and sexual function are affected. A woman with end-stage kidney failure may stop menstruating.

Diagnosis

Doctors diagnose end-stage kidney failure by the symptoms and the results of urine and blood tests. Your doctor will probably ask you to immediately report any illness or any change in your condition.

Treatment

Most people who develop end-stage kidney failure are already receiving treatment for acute or chronic kidney failure. Treatment for end-stage kidney failure is a complex team effort to tailor the various aspects of the treatment program to each patient's needs.

Because the kidney damage is irreversible, the only effective treatment for most people is either dialysis (see page 818) or a kidney transplant (see below). However, some people with end-stage kidney failure may be too ill for either treatment. Doctors treat anemia with regular injections of erythropoietin and prescribe other medications as needed to relieve specific symptoms.

Dialysis and kidney transplantation have significantly improved the chances of survival for people who have end-stage kidney failure. More than half of the people with end-stage kidney failure who are treated with dialysis or a kidney transplant continue to lead active, productive lives 10 to 15 years after the initial diagnosis.

Kidney transplants

A kidney transplant is relatively straightforward and less risky than many other organ transplants. While rejection of a transplanted heart, liver, or lung can be fatal, rejection of a kidney is not necessarily life-threatening because a person whose body rejects a transplanted kidney can be kept alive with dialysis. In some cases, a kidney transplant may be performed primarily to improve a person's quality of life rather than as a lifesaving measure. Of people who have a kidney transplant, more than two thirds are alive 2 years after surgery, with the transplanted kidney functioning normally. In about one sixth of recipients, the transplanted kidney is rejected, but they are able to go back on dialysis until another kidney becomes available for transplantation.

Transplants

Organ transplantation is the surgical removal of an organ, such as a kidney, liver, or heart, from one person to transfer to another. An organ is transplanted when a person's own organ has failed because of a serious medical condition or injury. Doctors recommend transplantation only after all other measures have been tried or considered; replacing the organ may be the only way doctors can save a critically ill person's life. Organs that can be transplanted include the kidney, liver, heart, lungs, pancreas, and intestine. Kidney transplants are the most commonly performed procedures, followed by liver transplants. Sometimes surgeons transplant two organs at once, such as the heart and lungs, or a kidney and the pancreas. Surgeons can transplant not only organs but also body tissues such as the cornea (the transparent outer covering of the eyeball), bone or cartilage, skin, heart valves, and veins in the leg.

Surgery to replace damaged body organs with healthy ones has become routine, and several thousand transplants are performed every year around the world. Most replacement organs come from the bodies of people who have died. The donor's surviving relatives must consent to the medical use of the organs after death, or the donor must have agreed in advance,

while still alive, to donate his or her organs (see page 544). (Many state and national organizations provide organ donor cards for people who are willing to donate their vital organs.) Organs such as the kidneys or parts of the liver or lungs can be obtained from living donors, who are usually family members of the person who needs the transplant.

Quick action is of critical importance in organ donation. For instance, a kidney must be removed within 30 minutes of a donor's death and can be kept in storage for only 15 to 18 hours before transplantation. Hearts must be transplanted from donor to recipient within 4 to 5 hours.

More than 50 organ-procurement organizations in geographic regions across the country coordinate the retrieval of donated organs. People who are candidates for a transplant are placed on a waiting list, and the waiting time can be several years, depending on the demand for a particular organ and the availability of donor organs. Strict government regulations determine which person on the list has the highest priority. The rules vary by type of organ but, in general, when an organ becomes available, it goes to the person on the local waiting list who has the most urgent need and can benefit most from transplantation.

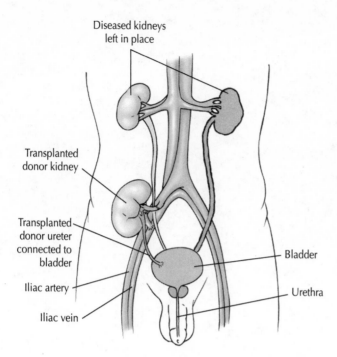

Diseased kidneys
left in place

Transplanted
donor kidney

Transplanted
donor ureter
connected to
bladder

Iliac artery

Iliac vein

Bladder

Urethra

Kidney transplant

A kidney transplant can be an effective treatment for kidney failure. The
donor kidney is usually placed in the
right lower abdomen and connected
to the iliac artery and the iliac vein.
The ureter (the tube that carries urine
from the kidney to the bladder) of the
donor kidney is connected to the
bladder. The diseased kidneys are
usually left in place because they are
usually harmless, they may have
some hormonal function, and removing them requires additional surgery.
The transplant procedure takes 3 to 6
hours and is followed by up to 2
weeks of recovery in the hospital.
The donor kidney may begin producing urine right away, or it may take
several weeks to begin working.

Risks of Organ Rejection

The primary risk of organ transplantation is potential
rejection by the body. The immune system treats a
transplanted organ as if it were an invading organism
and tries to destroy it. For this reason, for most transplants (except for heart and lung transplants; see page
658), doctors try to find a donor whose blood and tissue types are as close to those of the recipient as possible. (Because the heart and lungs can be kept alive for
only a brief time outside the body, there is not enough
time for tissue matching.) A parent or sibling is the
person most likely to be a compatible donor. Corneal
transplants do not require tissue matching because the
cornea has no blood supply and does not trigger
rejection.

To prevent rejection of a transplanted organ, doctors
have to suppress the recipient's immune system with
drugs. Older immune-suppressing drugs had serious
side effects and were not always effective. With the
availability of better immune-suppressing drugs such as
cyclosporine, tacrolimus, and mycophenolate, survival
rates have improved dramatically. Immune-suppressing
drugs have to be taken for life to avoid organ rejection.
Side effects from the drugs can include high blood
pressure, fluid retention, shakiness, excessive hair

growth, and, rarely, kidney damage. To offset these
side effects, a person may need to take additional
medications.

Because the person's immune system is weakened
from the antirejection drugs, he or she is at increased
risk of developing severe infections such as pneumonia.
For this reason, doctors also prescribe antibiotics and
other infection-fighting medications for people having
transplants. The risk of cancer, especially skin cancer, is
also higher for transplant recipients than for the general
population. Some types of cancer develop in transplant
recipients as side effects of the immune-suppressing
medications; others occur as a consequence of the
person's weakened immune system. Other side effects
that occur depend on the type of organ transplanted.

Outlook

The survival outlook for organ transplant recipients is
bright and continues to improve each year. Nationwide, 98 percent of people who receive a donated
organ of any type are alive after 1 year, and 91 percent
survive at least 3 years (except for heart-lung transplant
recipients). Most people who have had a transplant
find that the procedure has improved the quality of
their life.

8

Disorders of the Male Reproductive System

The male reproductive system is made up of the penis, testicles, prostate gland, Cowper's glands, seminal vesicles, and vas deferens. Each of the two testicles is suspended by a spermatic cord inside a pouch of skin and muscle called the scrotum. The spermatic cord is made up of the vas deferens, nerves, and blood vessels. The testicles produce sperm and the male sex hormone testosterone. Sperm are collected and stored in a long, tightly coiled tube called the epididymis, which lies above and behind each testicle. Sperm mature over a period of about 3 weeks inside the epididymis before they pass into the vas deferens, a long duct that acts as a storage and transport system. Sperm travel from the vas deferens, past the prostate gland, into a pair of sacs called the seminal vesicles.

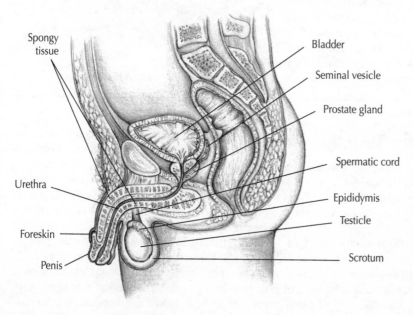

Spongy tissue

Bladder

Seminal vesicle

Prostate gland

Spermatic cord

Urethra

Epididymis

Testicle

Foreskin

Scrotum

Penis

The male reproductive system
The visible parts of the male reproductive system are the penis and scrotum, the pouch of skin and muscle that protects the two testicles. When a male is sexually aroused, spongy tissue inside the penis fills with blood. The testicles produce sperm and the male sex hormone testosterone. From the testicles, sperm travel through a duct called the vas deferens into a pair of sacs called the seminal vesicles. The prostate gland, Cowper's glands (not shown), and seminal vesicles produce fluids that are added to sperm to create semen, which is ejaculated during orgasm.

The prostate gland, Cowper's glands, and seminal vesicles produce fluids that support sperm and make up about 98 percent of semen. When a male is sexually aroused, spongy tissue inside the penis fills with blood, causing the penis to become erect. During an orgasm, semen is ejaculated through the urethra (a muscular tube inside the penis that carries urine and semen out of the body). The muscular action of ejaculation automatically closes the neck of the bladder, temporarily preventing urine from entering the urethra and preventing semen from entering the bladder.

Infections of the reproductive and urinary tracts are rare in men because the length of the urethra usually provides an effective barrier against infectious agents. However, because the organs of the reproductive system are connected to the organs of the urinary tract, a disorder in one system can cause symptoms in the other.

Disorders of the Testicles and Scrotum

The testicles develop inside the abdomen of a male fetus. By the time the baby is born, the testicles have usually descended through the abdominal wall and are suspended inside a pouch of skin and muscle called the scrotum. Each testicle is connected to the body by a single spermatic cord, which is composed of the vas deferens (sperm duct), nerves, and blood vessels.

Sperm are collected and stored in the epididymis (a tightly coiled tube that lies above and behind each testicle) until they mature (which takes about 3 weeks). Fully developed sperm pass into the vas deferens, where they are stored. During orgasm, sperm travel from the vas deferens to the seminal vesicles, where they mix with fluids produced by the prostate gland, Cowper's glands, and seminal vesicles to form semen. Semen is ejaculated from the body through the urethra. Sperm that are not ejaculated in semen during orgasm gradually break down and are reabsorbed by the body.

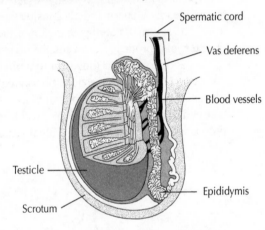

Cross section of a testicle and scrotum

Cancer of the Testicle

Cancer of the testicle (or testicular cancer) is a growth of malignant cells inside a testicle. Although testicular cancer accounts for only about 1 percent of all cancers in men, it is the most common form of cancer in men between ages 18 and 35. In the United States, 6,000 to 8,000 cases of testicular cancer are diagnosed each year. Cancer of the testicle occurs more often in whites than in people of other races. Advances in the development of new drugs and diagnostic tests have significantly increased the survival rates of people with testicular cancer. With early diagnosis and treatment, cancer of the testicle is frequently curable.

The two different types of testicular cancer are seminomas (which account for about 35 to 40 percent of cases) and nonseminomas (which account for about 60 percent of cases). Seminomas consist of a single type of immature germ cell that probably arises from the cells that produce sperm. Because seminomas tend to grow slowly, they are usually detected before they spread to other parts of the body. Nonseminomas consist of a mix of different types of cells. Because nonseminomas tend to grow more rapidly, they often spread to other parts of the body before they are detected. An estimated 60 to 70 percent of men who are diagnosed with nonseminomas have cancer that has spread to nearby lymph nodes.

The risk of developing testicular cancer is increased in men who were born with undescended testicles—a condition called cryptorchidism (see page 431). That risk rises if cryptorchidism is not corrected surgically before a boy reaches puberty. Other factors that can increase the risk of testicular cancer include previous testicular cancer and a family history of testicular cancer. Additional risk factors include low birthweight, fetal alcohol syndrome (see page 409), and the chromosomal disorder Klinefelter syndrome (see page 957).

Symptoms

In some men, testicular cancer causes no symptoms. However, in most cases, there is a lump or swelling in a testicle. Other possible symptoms include enlargement of a testicle, a feeling of heaviness in the scrotum, a sudden collection of fluid in the scrotum, or enlargement or tenderness of the breasts. Although testicular cancer usually does not cause pain, some men may experience soreness or discomfort in a testicle or in the scrotum or a dull ache in the back, lower abdomen, or groin. If you have any of these symptoms, see your doctor right away. Although not all lumps are cancerous, any lump in a testicle must be evaluated by a doctor to rule out cancer.

Diagnosis

Most testicular cancers are detected by men themselves, either by chance or while performing a testicle self-examination (see page 139). If your doctor suspects that you may have cancer of the testicle, he or she will perform a complete physical examination, including a careful examination of the testicles. The doctor will also order blood and urine tests to rule out other possible causes of your symptoms, such as an infection. If the examination and tests do not detect an infection or other disorder, the doctor will order additional tests to detect or rule out testicular cancer. You will probably have an ultrasound scan (see page 111) of the testicles, which uses high-frequency sound waves to create images of the testicles.

The only sure way to determine if a testicular tumor is cancerous is for the doctor to perform a biopsy to examine cells in the testicle for cancer. For this biopsy, the entire affected testicle is removed through a small incision in the groin in a surgical procedure called a radical inguinal orchiectomy.

Removing just a portion of the testicle is usually not an option because cutting through the outer layer of the testicle can cause any cancer to spread. Removing the testicle also helps prevent the cancer from spreading to other parts of the body. Removal of one testicle usually does not interfere with a man's fertility or ability to have an erection.

Cancer staging

Once cancer has been diagnosed, a doctor determines how far the cancer has spread by performing tests—such as blood tests, imaging tests, and biopsies—to categorize, or stage, the disease. Staging helps a doctor determine the most appropriate treatment for each case. The three stages of testicular cancer are:

- Stage I—the cancer has not spread beyond the testicle
- Stage II—the cancer has spread to lymph nodes in the back of the abdomen
- Stage III—the cancer has spread beyond the lymph nodes to sites away from the abdomen

The doctor uses blood tests to check for tumor-associated markers, which are substances that are often present in abnormal amounts in people who have cancer. By comparing the levels of these markers before and after surgery, the doctor can determine if a cancer has spread beyond the testicles. Measuring marker levels before and after a person undergoes chemotherapy (see page 23) helps determine how well the chemotherapy is working.

Treatment

Treatment of testicular cancer depends on the type of tumor (seminoma or nonseminoma), how far the cancer has spread, and the person's age and general health. Because seminomas tend to grow slowly and usually do not spread, they usually are diagnosed in stage I or II. If performed early enough, removal of the entire affected testicle may be the only treatment necessary for a seminoma. However, treatment for seminomas usually combines testicle removal, radiation therapy (see page 23), and chemotherapy. Surgical removal of lymph nodes usually is not necessary for men who have seminomas because this type of tumor responds well to radiation treatment. Doctors usually treat stage III seminomas with multidrug chemotherapy and radiation.

Although nonseminomas grow more rapidly than seminomas and often spread before they are detected, the cure rate is high. Because nonseminomas do not respond as well to radiation therapy, surgical removal of the lymph nodes is often necessary after the cancer has spread beyond the testicle. Treatment of nonseminomas also can include multidrug chemotherapy. Men who have a stage II nonseminoma who have had surgery to remove the affected testicle and lymph nodes may need no further treatment. However, some doctors recommend a short course of multidrug chemotherapy to reduce the risk of recurrence. Most stage III nonseminomas can be treated effectively with chemotherapy.

The condition of men who have been treated for cancer of the testicle is carefully monitored for at least 2 years after treatment to make sure the cancer has not recurred. The disease recurs in about 10 to 15 percent of men who have been treated for stage I testicular cancer. If the cancer recurs, it is treated with chemotherapy.

After a man has been cancer-free for 3 years, cancer of the testicle seldom recurs. Men who have been treated for cancer in one testicle have about a 1 percent chance of developing cancer in the remaining testicle. If cancer develops in the second testicle, it is usually a new tumor rather than the result of cancer cells that have spread from the first tumor. After treatment for testicular cancer, men should continue to perform monthly testicle self-examinations.

Torsion of the Testicle

Each testicle is suspended in the scrotum by a spermatic cord that consists of the vas deferens, nerves, and blood vessels. In torsion of the testicle, one of the testicles becomes twisted on the spermatic cord, cutting off blood flow to and from the testicle. The condition is rare, and the cause is usually unknown. Although testicular torsion develops most often during adolescence, it can occur at any age.

In some cases of testicular torsion, the testicle untwists by itself. However, if the testicle does not return to its usual position naturally, and the condition is not treated within 4 to 8 hours, the sperm-producing parts of the testicle or the entire testicle can be permanently damaged, and the tissue may die (gangrene; see page 601). For this reason, torsion of the testicle is a medical emergency.

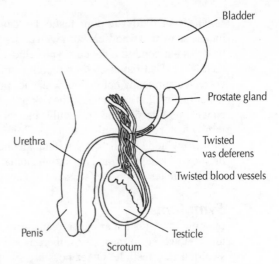

Torsion of the testicle
Each testicle is suspended in the scrotum by a spermatic cord. In torsion of the testicle, a testicle becomes twisted on the spermatic cord, cutting off blood flow to and from the testicle.

Pain from an injury, inflammation, or testicular cancer can sometimes resemble torsion of the testicle. Even if the problem seems to have cleared up on its own, it is important to see your doctor right away to rule out other possible problems.

Symptoms and Diagnosis

The main symptom of testicular torsion is sudden, severe pain in the groin area. One side of the scrotum is swollen and can be red and tender, and the affected testicle may rest higher than usual or may lie horizontally in the scrotum. Other possible symptoms include fever, light-headedness, fainting, and nausea and vomiting. A diagnosis of testicular torsion is based on the symptoms and a physical examination, including an examination of the testicles.

WARNING!

Testicle Strangulation

If the spermatic cord becomes twisted, blood flow to and from the testicle can be blocked. The lack of blood can permanently damage the testicle. If you have sudden, severe pain in your groin, along with other symptoms of testicular torsion, see your doctor immediately or go directly to the nearest hospital emergency department. Prompt medical treatment can help prevent permanent damage to the testicle.

Injury to the Testicles

Because the testicles are suspended outside the body in the scrotum, they are vulnerable to injury. A direct blow to the testicles can cause extreme pain that spreads from the testicles to the lower abdomen and may be accompanied by dizziness, sweating, and nausea. The pain results when the testicle swells and presses on surrounding nerves. The pain of testicular injury is deep, intense, and widespread, resembling the pain of injury to an internal organ.

Although the pain may be severe and cause you to double over, it usually subsides quickly without damage to the testicles. Applying an ice pack to your scrotum and taking over-the-counter anti-inflammatory drugs such as aspirin or ibuprofen will usually relieve the pain and swelling.

If the pain and swelling persist for more than an hour or if your scrotum is bruised, see your doctor immediately or go directly to the nearest hospital emergency department. The testicle may have ruptured, or it may have twisted on the spermatic cord. Also, the sperm-producing tubes inside the testicle may have pushed out through a tear in the membrane that covers the testicle. If these problems are not treated promptly, the testicle can be damaged permanently. Surgery may be necessary to stop any bleeding and to prevent blood clots, infertility, or loss of the testicle.

WARNING!

Don't Give Aspirin to Children or Adolescents

Do not give aspirin to children or adolescents who have a fever; use of aspirin in children has been linked to Reye's syndrome (see page 411)—a rare but potentially fatal childhood disorder. Carefully check the label before giving any over-the-counter medication to your child.

Treatment

If you have torsion of the testicle, your doctor may try to untwist the testicle with gentle manipulation. If he or she cannot untwist the testicle, or if the testicle does not stay untwisted, prompt surgery to prevent testicular strangulation is required. During the procedure, the surgeon untwists the testicle and fixes it in a position that will help prevent the problem from recurring. He or she will also secure the other testicle in place to prevent torsion. Surgery to remove the affected testicle may be necessary if it has been damaged severely and permanently.

Epididymitis

Epididymitis is inflammation of the epididymis (the coiled tube that lies above and behind each testicle) or the top of the testicle. The condition can result from a bacterial or viral infection that spreads from the urinary tract into the vas deferens (sperm duct) or by the backward flow (reflux) of infected urine from the urethra. In younger men, epididymitis usually results from the sexually transmitted diseases nongonococcal urethritis (see page 481), chlamydia (see page 477), and gonorrhea (see page 480).

Symptoms

Epididymitis often produces severe pain and swelling on the affected side of the scrotum. The swelling develops over the course of a few hours, and the swollen area may feel hot and tender. The affected testicle may feel painful or heavy. You may have a slight fever and chills. You may also have discomfort in your lower abdomen or in the groin area, and pain or burning during urination. In some cases, there may be a discharge from the penis, pain during ejaculation, or blood in the semen. If you have any of these symptoms, see your doctor right away.

Diagnosis

To diagnose epididymitis, a doctor examines the testicle and may order tests of your blood, urine, and prostate fluid to help identify the cause of the infection. To obtain a sample of prostate fluid, a doctor inserts a gloved, lubricated finger into the rectum and massages the prostate, which then releases the fluid through the urethra.

Treatment

If epididymitis results from a bacterial infection, the doctor will prescribe antibiotics. He or she may also recommend bed rest, ice packs applied to the scrotum, elevation and support of the scrotum, and nonsteroidal anti-inflammatory drugs such as aspirin, ibuprofen, or naproxen to relieve pain and inflammation. Rarely, in severe or chronic cases, a doctor may recommend surgery to remove the infected epididymis.

If your epididymitis was caused by a sexually transmitted disease, it may also be necessary to treat your sex partner to avoid reinfection and reduce the risk of pelvic inflammatory disease (see page 871) in your female partner.

Orchitis

Orchitis is inflammation of one or both testicles that usually results from the viral infection mumps (see page 440) but also can result from an injury or a bacterial infection in the prostate gland or epididymis. This rare condition can permanently damage one or both testicles and, in some cases, can result in infertility.

Symptoms and Diagnosis

Orchitis causes pain, swelling, and a feeling of heaviness in the scrotum. You also may have a fever and nausea. In some cases, symptoms include discharge from the penis, pain during urination, pain during sexual intercourse or ejaculation, or blood in the semen.

To diagnose orchitis, a doctor will perform a manual examination of the affected testicle and will probably recommend an ultrasound scan (see page 111) of the scrotum. He or she will order blood and urine tests to help determine the cause of the infection.

Treatment

In many cases, orchitis can be treated successfully by limiting activity, placing an ice pack on the affected testicle, and wearing an athletic supporter. For pain, doctors usually recommend over-the-counter pain relievers. If orchitis results from a bacterial infection, a doctor will prescribe an antibiotic or an antibacterial drug.

Hypogonadism

Hypogonadism, or testosterone deficiency, is a disorder in which the testicles fail to produce the male sex hormone testosterone, which stimulates

sexual development. There are two main types of hypogonadism: primary and secondary. Primary hypogonadism, also known as primary testicular failure, arises from an abnormality in the testicles. Secondary hypogonadism signals a defect in the pituitary gland, a small structure at the base of the brain that secretes a variety of different hormones, which regulate many processes in the body.

When the pituitary gland does not send hormones to the testicles, the testicles cannot produce testosterone. Hypogonadism affects about 1 in 500 men and boys.

Primary hypogonadism can be caused by a number of factors, including:

- A genetic disorder such as Klinefelter syndrome (see page 957), in which an extra X chromosome causes abnormal testicle development
- Absence of testicles at birth
- Undescended testicles
- Hemochromatosis (see page 961), an inherited disorder that causes iron to build up in the blood
- Injury to the testicles
- Hernia surgery
- Chemotherapy or radiation therapy for cancer
- Inflammatory diseases such as sarcoidosis (see page 929)
- Mumps contracted during adolescence or in adulthood
- Normal aging

The possible causes of secondary hypogonadism include disorders that affect the functioning of the pituitary gland, severe head injury, or taking some medications.

Symptoms

The symptoms produced by hypogonadism vary depending on the age at which the disorder occurs. If it occurs during fetal development, too little testosterone is produced, resulting in a condition in which the infant's genitals are not fully developed and his or her gender cannot be determined. During puberty, hypogonadism can cause such symptoms as slowed growth, underdeveloped muscle mass, small penis and testicles, and scant growth of body hair. Other signs during puberty include breast enlargement, disproportionately long arms and legs, and failure of the voice to deepen.

Men who develop hypogonadism can have scant

beard and body hair growth, testicles that are smaller or less firm than normal, and enlarged breasts. They may also have increased body fat and decreased muscle mass and bone density, erection problems, and infertility from an inability to produce sperm. The lowered testosterone levels can also produce symptoms similar to those of menopause in women, including hot flashes, a reduced sex drive, and mood swings.

Diagnosis

If your son has signs of hypogonadism, take him to a doctor for an evaluation because early detection can prevent delayed puberty (see page 449). Early diagnosis and treatment in adulthood can help prevent osteoporosis.

If you have signs of hypogonadism, your doctor will ask about your physical symptoms, your mood, and your sex drive. He or she will perform a physical examination to check for delayed or reduced male sexual development. Blood tests can measure the level of testosterone in your blood, and other tests can determine if the problem is caused by a disorder of the testicles or of the pituitary gland. You may have hormone tests, a semen analysis, an MRI (see page 113) or a CT scan (see page 112) of the pituitary gland, genetic studies, or a biopsy (microscopic examination of a tissue sample) or ultrasound scan (see page 111) of the testicles.

Treatment

The treatment for hypogonadism depends on its cause. Disorders of the testicles are treated with testosterone injected into a muscle, delivered in a skin patch, or rubbed onto the abdomen in a gel. For pituitary disorders, doctors give pituitary hormones to stimulate sperm production. A growth or tumor in the pituitary gland may require medication or surgical removal. If you are interested in restoring your fertility, your doctor may refer you to a doctor who specializes in treating infertility.

Fluid Accumulation in the Scrotum

For a number of reasons, various types of fluid can accumulate in the scrotum. A hydrocele is an accumulation of the watery lubricating fluid that is normally found in the membrane that covers the testicles. This condition develops when the membrane produces excess fluid or when the body does not reabsorb fluid normally. A hematocele is a collection of blood around the testicle that may result after injury to or rupture of a testicle. A spermatocele is a cyst filled with dead sperm cells that develops next to the epididymis. A varicocele is a mass of varicose (swollen) veins in the spermatic cord that can develop when the valves in the veins are not working properly, causing the veins to stretch and bulge. An untreated varicocele can sometimes cause infertility. Although any of these accumulations of fluid can increase in size, they are usually harmless and do not necessarily require treatment. However, any mass or persistent swelling in the scrotum needs to be evaluated by a doctor.

Symptoms

Fluid accumulations in the scrotum usually produce a mass on one side of the scrotum. The mass may be soft or firm and may or may not be painful. Some men experience a heavy, dragging feeling in the scrotum. Although a large mass can cause pressure and discomfort in the scrotum, it does not affect a man's ability to achieve and maintain an erection.

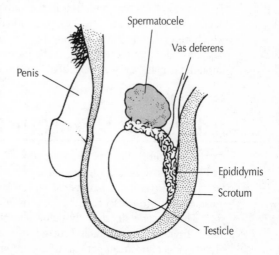

Spermatocele

A spermatocele is a cyst filled with dead sperm cells that arises from the epididymis and usually causes a painless swelling in the upper back portion of one or both testicles. Although spermatoceles may grow large enough to cause pressure and discomfort in the scrotum, they are usually harmless.

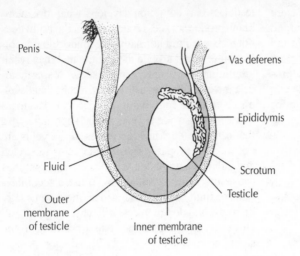

Hydrocele
A hydrocele is usually a soft, painless swelling around a testicle that develops when excess fluid accumulates between the testicle and its membrane covering. If a large hydrocele is causing discomfort, a doctor will probably recommend outpatient surgery to open the membrane around the testicle to prevent fluid from reaccumulating. Alternatively, the doctor may administer a local anesthetic and drain the fluid from the scrotum with a needle and syringe.

Diagnosis
To diagnose fluid accumulation in the scrotum, a doctor will perform a physical examination during which he or she may use a strong light source to pass light through the scrotum. If the light passes through the mass, the mass is probably a hydrocele.

If the light does not pass through the mass, it could be a hematocele or a varicocele. A spermatocele may light up under a strong light source in a darkened room. To confirm the diagnosis, the doctor will order an ultrasound scan (see page 111) of the scrotum or a biopsy (in which a sample of cells is removed from the mass and examined under a microscope).

Treatment
If an accumulation of fluid in the scrotum is not growing and is not causing discomfort, treatment may not be necessary. However, your doctor may ask you to watch for any increased swelling. If the condition results from a bacterial infection, the doctor will prescribe antibiotics. To relieve pain and inflammation, he or she may prescribe nonsteroidal anti-inflammatory drugs such as aspirin, ibuprofen, or naproxen, and may recommend wearing supporting briefs or an athletic supporter. If a hydrocele becomes very large or painful, your doctor may recommend surgery to open the membrane covering the testicle and turn it inside out to prevent fluid from reaccumulating.

If a hematocele, spermatocele, or varicocele continues to grow and is causing discomfort, your doctor will probably recommend surgery to remove it. If you have a varicocele and are having problems with fertility, your doctor will perform surgery to remove the varicose veins from the spermatic cord. All types of fluid accumulation in the scrotum can recur after surgery.

Disorders of the Prostate Gland

The prostate gland is a collection of small glands; it weighs about an ounce and is about the size of a walnut. It is covered with a layer of muscle and fibrous tissue called the prostatic capsule. The prostate sits directly below the bladder and in front of the rectum, and surrounds the neck of the bladder and the upper part of the urethra (the muscular tube that carries urine from the bladder out of the body).

The main function of the prostate gland is to produce part of the seminal fluid, the fluid that supports sperm in the semen. During orgasm, fluid from the prostate is squeezed into the urethra as sperm and other substances enter the urethra from

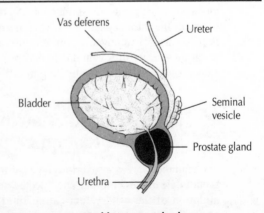

Healthy prostate gland

the seminal vesicles and vas deferens. When combined, these substances form semen, which carries sperm through the urethra and out of the penis during ejaculation.

After age 40, men are more prone to two types of prostate disorders—an enlarged prostate and cancer. Because the prostate gland surrounds the urethra, nearly all disorders of the prostate gland cause symptoms related to urination, such as a weak or interrupted urinary stream or a frequent or urgent need to urinate. The three most common prostate problems are inflammation (prostatitis), enlargement (benign prostatic hyperplasia), and prostate cancer.

Prostatitis

Prostatitis is inflammation of the prostate gland. The three basic forms of prostatitis are bacterial prostatitis, nonbacterial prostatitis (also called chronic pelvic pain syndrome), and asymptomatic inflammatory prostatitis. Prostatitis can occur with or without an infection.

The two types of bacterial prostatitis (also called infectious prostatitis) are acute bacterial prostatitis and chronic bacterial prostatitis. Acute bacterial prostatitis is a rare but serious disease caused by bacteria in the prostate gland. The bacteria may have come from an infection elsewhere in the body. Chronic bacterial prostatitis occurs primarily in older men who have an enlarged prostate (see next page). It is a recurring infection of the prostate gland that usually results from previous bacterial infections that were not eliminated completely.

Nonbacterial prostatitis is the most common but least understood form of the condition. It may be inflammatory or noninflammatory. In the inflammatory form, there is no evidence of an infecting microorganism but infection-fighting cells are present. In the noninflammatory form, there is no evidence of either infection or infection-fighting cells.

In asymptomatic inflammatory prostatitis, a man has infection-fighting cells in his semen but has no symptoms. Asymptomatic inflammatory prostatitis is usually diagnosed when a doctor is testing the prostate for other disorders.

Symptoms

The initial symptom of both bacterial and nonbacterial prostatitis is often pain in and around the base of the penis and behind the scrotum. Your rectum may feel full, and you may have an urge to have a bowel movement. Later, you may experience a strong, frequent urge to urinate but find it difficult and painful to urinate. You may pass only a small amount of urine and have blood in your urine. Other possible symptoms include pain at the tip of the penis, pain in the testicles, and lower back pain. In bacterial prostatitis, symptoms can include fever, chills, or nausea. If you have any symptoms of prostatitis, see your doctor right away.

Diagnosis

Diagnosis of prostatitis is usually based on the symptoms, a physical examination, and the results of urine tests. A doctor may perform a digital rectal examination, in which he or she inserts a gloved, lubricated finger into the rectum to feel the prostate gland. If you have symptoms of an acute bacterial infection, your doctor probably will not perform a digital rectal examination because manipulation of the prostate gland can release bacteria into the bloodstream.

Your doctor may perform a test called prostatic localization to diagnose chronic bacterial prostatitis. In this test, the doctor asks you first to urinate and collect the first few drops of urine. You then will collect a midstream sample of urine (in which you urinate for several seconds before collecting the sample of urine). The doctor then performs a digital rectal examination and massages the prostate gland to release prostatic fluid, which is collected. Finally, another urine sample, which also contains some of the prostatic fluid, is taken. The doctor compares all of the samples to confirm the presence of an infection, identify the microorganisms that are causing it, and determine the best treatment. The samples are grown in a laboratory and examined to determine if the infection is in the urethra, the bladder, or the prostate.

In some cases, a doctor may also examine the prostate gland with a cystoscope (a flexible, lighted, viewing tube) inserted through the urethra. An accurate diagnosis is important because different types of prostatitis require different treatments.

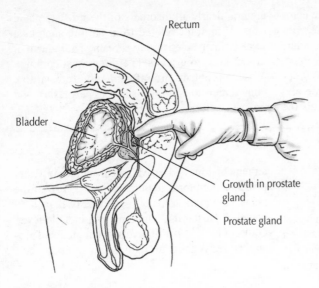

Digital rectal examination
For a digital rectal examination, your doctor will probably ask you to stand and bend forward at the waist. He or she will insert a gloved, lubricated finger into your rectum to feel for any abnormalities in the prostate gland. The examination may also be performed while you lie on your side with your knees bent toward your chest.

Treatment

To treat bacterial prostatitis, doctors prescribe antibiotics. If your symptoms are severe, your doctor may recommend bed rest and nonsteroidal anti-inflammatory drugs to relieve pain and inflammation. You may be admitted to the hospital for treatment if your urethra becomes blocked, if you have a high fever that leads to dehydration, or if the bacteria spread to other parts of your body. Because it is difficult to eliminate bacteria from the prostate gland, your doctor may prescribe antibiotics to take for 4 to 6 weeks. For chronic infections, antibiotics are taken for several months. Doctors rarely perform surgery for chronic bacterial prostatitis and only as a last resort—usually when the condition makes you unable to urinate (causing urinary retention) or causes kidney problems.

Nonbacterial prostatitis is not treated with antibiotics. To help relieve the symptoms of nonbacterial prostatitis, your doctor may recommend the following:

- Take over-the-counter nonsteroidal anti-inflammatory drugs such as aspirin, ibuprofen, or naproxen to relieve pain and inflammation.
- Soak in a warm bath.
- Avoid caffeine, alcohol, and spicy foods, which can irritate the prostate gland.
- Exercise regularly and practice relaxation techniques such as deep breathing and meditation to help relieve stress-related pain.

Benign Prostatic Hyperplasia

Benign prostatic hyperplasia (BPH) is noncancerous enlargement of the periurethral glandular tissue of the prostate (the portion of the prostate gland immediately surrounding the urethra). As the prostate becomes larger, it can tighten around the urethra and block the flow of urine. Starting urination is difficult, and the urine stream is weak. The blockage may cause the bladder muscles to enlarge and the bladder to become irritable, causing contractions of the bladder that result in a frequent urge to urinate. Eventually the muscles are no longer able to force urine past the blockage, causing the urine to back up. This backup of urine can result in damage to the bladder muscles, frequent urinary tract infections, and urinary retention (the inability to urinate). BPH usually does not affect sexual function, although the flow of semen may be blocked. Without treatment, late stages of BPH can lead to kidney damage or kidney failure.

By age 50, more than half of all American men have signs of prostate enlargement. Although doctors are not sure what causes BPH, they know that it is linked to the male sex hormone testosterone and aging. (BPH does not occur in men whose testicles were surgically removed before puberty or in men whose testicles cannot produce testosterone.)

A diet high in fat and cholesterol may be a risk factor for BPH. Obesity is also a risk factor—men who have a waist size larger than 43 inches are twice as likely to develop BPH than are men who have a waist size of 35 inches or smaller. The risk increases with age.

Symptoms

The symptoms of BPH can result from either irritation or obstruction in the urinary tract. Symptoms of irritation are related to the bladder muscle and include a frequent need to urinate, numerous trips to the bathroom at night, and urgency (a strong urge to urinate). These symptoms are usually the first

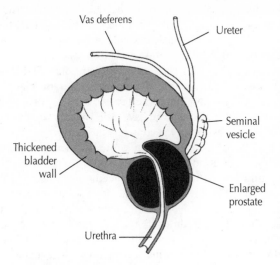

Vas deferens

Ureter

Seminal
vesicle

Thickened
bladder
wall

Enlarged
prostate

Urethra

Enlarged prostate gland
An enlarged prostate can obstruct the urethra (the tube that
carries urine from the bladder out of the body), reducing the
flow of urine and causing the muscular wall of the bladder to
thicken as it works harder to force urine out of the body.

signs of a prostate problem, although they are often
not noticeable until years after the prostate has
begun to enlarge; they can also be a sign of other
urinary tract disorders.

Bladder outlet obstruction is a group of symptoms associated with BPH and related to problems
with urine flow. These symptoms include decreased
force and diameter of the urinary stream, inability
to urinate, trouble starting the flow of urine, a weak
flow of urine, double voiding (a person urinates and
is able to urinate again in 5 to 10 minutes), dribbling after urination, and overflow urinary incontinence (leaking of urine from an overfull bladder).
Frequent urinary tract infections, characterized by
a burning sensation during urination, strong-
smelling urine, and some blood in the urine, may
also result from BPH. Bladder outlet obstruction
tends to come and go.

Diagnosis

To diagnose BPH, a doctor takes a health history
and performs a physical examination, including a
urinalysis, to rule out infection. He or she may
try to feel the bladder (which normally cannot be
felt) by pressing down on the abdomen above the
pelvic bone. The doctor also performs a digital rectal examination (by inserting a gloved, lubricated

finger in the rectum) to feel the prostate and determine if and how much it is enlarged. He or she may
recommend a test that uses a device called a
uroflometer that measures the rate at which urine
flows, to determine if the flow of urine from the
bladder is obstructed. He or she may also perform
an ultrasonic postvoid residual (PVR) urine test, a
noninvasive test that measures the amount of urine
left in the bladder after urination.

Blood tests may be recommended to rule out
kidney disease or to screen for prostate cancer (see
page 835). A procedure called cystoscopy (examination of the urinary tract with a viewing tube) may
be done to evaluate the urinary tract and determine
the extent of obstruction.

Treatment

BPH is a normal effect of aging, and therefore cannot be cured. However, the symptoms can be
relieved with medication or surgery. If your
symptoms are mild, your doctor may recommend a
period of watchful waiting. During this time, he or
she will carefully monitor your symptoms and try
to determine whether external factors—such as
consumption of alcohol or caffeine, exercise, or
stress—are triggering your symptoms. The doctor
will also perform tests regularly to check for signs
of damage to your kidneys or bladder.

If your symptoms begin to worsen, your doctor
may recommend treatment with medications called
alpha blockers, which relax the prostate and lower
blood pressure. Alpha blockers are effective in
about 75 percent of men who have bladder outlet
obstruction. These medications, such as tamsulosin
and terazosin, work by relaxing the muscle of the
prostate, allowing urine to flow more freely. However, alpha blockers can cause unpleasant side
effects, including low blood pressure and dizziness
on standing. Tamsulosin is less likely to cause these
side effects, which usually lessen or disappear with
continued use of either drug. Less frequently, a doctor may prescribe other medications to shrink the
prostate. Because your symptoms usually will
return when you stop any of these medications, you
may need to take them indefinitely.

All of the surgical procedures for treating BPH
involve eliminating excess prostate tissue. A prostatectomy is the removal of the overgrown portion of
the prostate gland. A prostatectomy can be either
closed or open. In a closed prostatectomy, the gland

or the excess tissue is removed through a resectoscope (viewing tube) that is inserted up the urethra. In an open prostatectomy, the gland or the excess tissue is removed through an incision in the lower abdomen. Although closed prostatectomies have mostly replaced open prostatectomies, open procedures are still performed if the prostate gland is very large or if the surgeon plans to perform other procedures at the same time.

Transurethral resection of the prostate (TURP) is a closed procedure. TURP involves passing a resectoscope into the urethra and inserting a tiny wire loop or cutting edge through the scope to shave away excess prostate tissue from around the urethra. A major benefit of this procedure is the relief of many of the urinary symptoms associated with BPH. However, a relatively common effect of TURP is retrograde ejaculation, in which a man ejaculates backward into the bladder. Also, up to 1 percent of men who have this procedure experience subsequent problems with urinary incontinence. The procedure may need to be repeated if the tissue that was removed grows back.

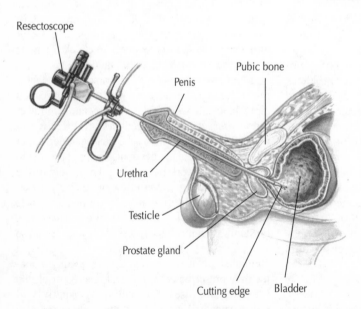

Transurethral resection of the prostate
Transurethral resection of the prostate (TURP) is a closed surgical procedure in which the surgeon passes a viewing tube called a resectoscope through the urethra to the prostate gland. He or she then guides a tiny wire loop or scalpel through the resectoscope to shave away and remove excess prostate tissue from around the urethra.

Another closed procedure is called transurethral incision of the prostate (TUIP). In TUIP, the surgeon makes deep single or double cuts completely through the prostate to loosen its grip on the urethra. TUIP is a bit less effective than TURP but has a lower risk of causing retrograde ejaculation. Because it is less effective, TUIP is not appropriate for all men who have BPH. In some cases, the procedure may need to be repeated.

Other treatments for BPH include microwave thermotherapy, intraurethral stents, laser therapy, and transurethral needle ablation (TUNA). Microwave thermotherapy uses heat generated by microwaves to eliminate excess prostate tissue. Intraurethral stents are small tubelike devices inserted into the urethra to enlarge it and provide relief from urinary symptoms. Laser therapy uses a highly concentrated beam of light to vaporize excess prostate tissue. TUNA uses microwave technology to cut away obstructing tissue. Doctors are still evaluating the long-term effectiveness of these techniques. Discussing with your doctor the risks and benefits of any treatment you are considering can help you make an informed decision.

If you find that some foods and medications increase the intensity of your symptoms, try the following lifestyle tips and keep track of your symptoms to see if they improve:

- Eat a low-fat, low-cholesterol diet (see page 38). Men who follow such a diet have a lower risk of BPH.
- Eat more fruits and vegetables. Men who do so have a lower rate of BPH than those who do not.
- Ask your doctor if you should limit your fluid intake, particularly at bedtime. It may reduce the number of times you have to get up to urinate during the night.
- Avoid caffeine, alcohol, and spicy foods. They can irritate the prostate and increase the need for nighttime urination.
- Monitor your medications. Some drugs—including oral bronchodilators, diuretics, tranquilizers, antidepressants, and over-the-counter medications such as antihistamines and decongestants—can worsen urinary problems. Check with your pharmacist.

Prostate Cancer

Prostate cancer is a common form of cancer in American men. Each year in the United States, doctors diagnose about 200,000 new cases of prostate cancer and more than 30,000 men die of the disease. Prostate cancer is the third leading cause of cancer death in American men, after lung cancer and colon cancer. The risk of prostate cancer increases significantly after age 50, especially in African American men. Your risk of developing prostate cancer is increased if a close relative (such as your father or brother) has the disease, which indicates a genetic component.

Some prostate cancers grow slowly, and are not detected for several years. Some prostate cancers never threaten health because they develop later in life; many older men who have prostate cancer die of another cause. However, in a significant number of cases, the cancer is more aggressive and grows and spreads rapidly.

Symptoms

Prostate cancer usually causes no noticeable symptoms in the early stages. In some men, the cancer grows so slowly that it never causes symptoms. Rarely, in the late stages of the disease, symptoms can develop, including weight loss, weakness, decreased appetite, a weak or interrupted flow of urine, inability to urinate, difficulty starting the flow of urine, and frequent urination (especially at night). Other possible symptoms include blood in the urine, pain or burning during urination, or persistent pain in the lower back, pelvis, or upper thighs.

Diagnosis

Doctors usually detect prostate cancer in one of three ways—during a digital rectal examination, from a prostate-specific antigen (PSA) blood test (see right), or during a surgical procedure called transurethral resection of the prostate (TURP; see previous page), performed to treat an enlarged prostate. Annual digital rectal examinations are recommended starting at age 50 for white men who have no family history of prostate cancer, and at age 45 for all African American men and for white men who have a family history of prostate cancer. If you have any symptoms of prostate cancer, see your doctor right away.

The PSA Test

The prostate-specific antigen (PSA) test measures the amount of prostate-specific antigen, a protein that circulates in your bloodstream and is produced mainly by the prostate gland. Normally, very little PSA is in the blood. Elevated PSA levels can be a sign of prostate cancer, but usually indicate other, less serious, prostate problems, such as benign prostatic hypertrophy (see page 832), infection or inflammation of the prostate, or a minor injury, such as bruising caused by a long bike ride. For this reason, additional tests, such as a biopsy (in which a doctor removes a small sample of tissue from the prostate gland for examination under a microscope), are performed to rule out prostate cancer.

Doctors disagree about whether all men should have routine PSA testing after age 50. The PSA test is not designed to diagnose prostate cancer, so some men who have low PSA levels may still have prostate cancer. Conversely, most men who have elevated PSA levels do not have prostate cancer. Uncertain test results can cause anxiety and may lead to unnecessary procedures, such as a biopsy or surgery. Any kind of prostate cancer surgery poses the risk of problems such as urinary incontinence (leaking of urine) or erection problems (see page 486). However, although the PSA test is imperfect, when combined with a digital rectal examination, many doctors consider it to be dependable for detecting prostate cancer in the early stages, when it is more likely to be curable.

The American Cancer Society recommends an annual PSA test along with an annual digital rectal examination for all men over age 50, and at age 45 for younger men who have an increased risk of developing the disease—such as African Americans and men whose father or brother has prostate cancer. Talk to your doctor about the PSA test so you can make an informed decision about having the test.

Treatment

Treatments for prostate cancer include surgery, radiation therapy, hormone therapy, chemotherapy, cryotherapy, or combinations of these. Your doctor will work with you to develop an appropriate treatment plan based on the benefits, possible side effects, and risks of each treatment; your age; your overall health; your preferences; the likelihood of your living at least 10 more years; and the stage of your cancer. Doctors may recommend watchful waiting for older men whose cancer is at an early stage and is growing slowly. Watchful waiting involves regular digital rectal examinations, a PSA test every 3 to 6 months, and, in some cases, an annual prostate biopsy.

Radical prostatectomy is the most common surgical procedure for prostate cancer. Doctors perform this procedure to treat cancer that has not spread beyond the prostate. In a radical prostatectomy, the surgeon removes the entire prostate and the seminal vesicles, along with surrounding tissue and pelvic lymph nodes. In rare cases, doctors perform TURP to relieve symptoms before using other treatments. TURP is usually used to treat benign prostatic hyperplasia (see page 832). To treat cancer that has not spread beyond the prostate gland, surgeons occasionally perform a procedure called cryosurgery, in which cancerous cells are destroyed by freezing them with a metal probe. Cryosurgery is not used routinely for treating prostate cancer.

A doctor may use one or two types of radiation therapy—external radiation therapy or internal radiation therapy (also called brachytherapy)—to treat prostate cancer. In external radiation therapy, the doctor uses a machine to aim high-power rays (gamma rays or X-rays) or particles (electrons, protons, or neutrons) directly at the tumor and sometimes at surrounding lymph nodes. In brachytherapy, the doctor permanently inserts low-level radioactive pellets (each about the size of a grain of rice) into the prostate gland using ultrasound (see page 111) or CT scanning (see page 112) to guide the procedure. The pellets release radiation for a number of weeks or months.

Doctors usually use hormone therapy alone to treat prostate cancer that has spread to other parts of the body or that has recurred after treatment. The goal of hormone therapy is to lower the levels of androgens (male sex hormones such as testosterone, which can stimulate growth of cancer cells in the prostate gland), thereby shrinking the cancer or slowing its growth. The two most commonly used methods for lowering androgen levels are a surgical procedure called orchiectomy (removal of the testicles, the source of androgens) or regular injections of testosterone-lowering drugs.

Because the adrenal glands produce small amounts of androgens, drugs called antiandrogens are sometimes used to curb production of the hormones by these glands. Antiandrogens are usually taken in pills one to three times a day and are most effective when used along with hormone therapy.

If hormone therapy is not effective in treating prostate cancer that has spread beyond the prostate gland, doctors may recommend chemotherapy, which uses high doses of powerful anticancer drugs to destroy cancer cells. The goal of chemotherapy is to slow tumor growth and relieve pain. Because chemotherapy does not kill all of the cancer cells in the prostate, it is not used to treat early stages of the disease.

Possible side effects of the various treatments for prostate cancer include:

- Sexual problems such as erection problems (see page 486)
- Urinary problems such as frequent urination, urinary incontinence (leaking of urine), obstruction of the flow of urine, blood in the urine, or a burning sensation during urination
- Intestinal problems such as diarrhea, blood in the stool, or irritation
- Swelling of the penis, scrotum, or prostate gland
- Bruising of, pain in, or damage to the treated area or nearby tissues
- Breast enlargement or tenderness or hot flashes
- Loss of muscle mass or thinning bones (osteoporosis; see page 989)
- Fatigue, infection, heart disease, hair loss, or sores in the mouth

Disorders of the Bladder, Urethra, and Penis

The bladder is a hollow, elastic organ in the pelvis that acts as a reservoir for urine. The urethra is a narrow, muscular tube that carries urine from the bladder out of the body. In men, the urethra also carries semen out of the body during ejaculation. Ducts leading from the testicles, the seminal vesicles, and the prostate gland join the urethra just below the point where it leaves the bladder.

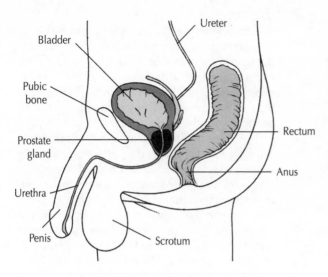

Bladder

Pubic
bone

Prostate
gland

Urethra

Penis

Ureter

Rectum

Anus

Scrotum

Location of the bladder, urethra, and penis

Most of the urethra lies inside the penis, which consists of three cylinders. The two cylinders on the upper surface of the penis are made up of spongy tissue that is filled with blood when the penis is erect and empty when the penis is relaxed. The third cylinder surrounds the urethra and does not fill with blood during an erection.

In uncircumcised men, the head of the penis (called the glans) is covered by a loose flap of skin called the foreskin. In the United States, the foreskin is frequently removed at birth in a surgical procedure called circumcision (see page 375).

Disorders of the bladder and urethra that affect both men and women are discussed in the chapter on disorders of the urinary tract (see page 801). Those included here affect men exclusively or affect men differently than women.

Cystitis in Men

Cystitis is inflammation of the bladder. Cystitis is rare in men and usually results from a more serious underlying disorder, such as a blockage or tumor in the urinary tract or an infection that has spread from elsewhere in the urinary tract, such as the urethra or the prostate gland.

Symptoms

The symptoms of cystitis include pressure or pain in the lower abdomen, an itching or burning sensation when urinating, an urgent need to urinate, increased frequency of urination, and reddish or brownish or strong-smelling urine. Other possible symptoms include fatigue, fever, chills, vomiting, pain in the side, or pain in the penis.

Diagnosis

A preliminary diagnosis of cystitis is based on the symptoms. A doctor will order a urine test to check for bacteria or blood in the urine. The urine sample is grown in the laboratory to confirm the presence of an infection, identify the microorganism that is causing the infection, and determine the best treatment. If there is no infection, the doctor will probably recommend tests—such as cystoscopy (see page 805), an ultrasound (see page 111), or a CT scan (see page 112)—to determine if an underlying disorder is causing the problem.

Treatment

If the cystitis is caused by a urinary tract infection, your doctor may prescribe antibiotics or antibacterial drugs, depending on the cause of the infection. He or she will also treat any underlying disorder that is causing the problem. Your doctor will probably recommend that you increase your intake of fluids (to at least eight glasses of water every day), while avoiding fluids (such as alcohol, citrus juices such as orange juice, and beverages that contain caffeine) that could irritate your bladder.

Urethral Stricture

Urethral stricture is a condition in which the urethra gradually narrows because of contracting scar tissue in the walls of the urethra. The scarring may result from long-term use of a catheter, from surgery, or from chronic inflammation of the urethra caused by an injury or an infection such as gonorrhea (see page 480).

Urethral stricture can interfere with urination and ejaculation. In rare cases, the condition results in kidney damage if urine builds up in the urinary tract and flows backward into the kidneys. Urethral

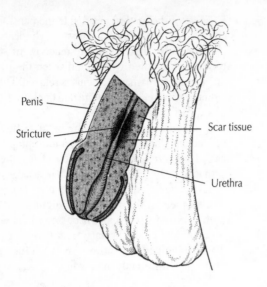

Urethral stricture
Injury or chronic inflammation can cause scar tissue (dark areas) to form in the walls of the urethra and narrow the channel inside the urethra. Narrowing of the channel can block the flow of urine, causing problems in the urinary tract.

stricture can sometimes be a factor in urinary tract infections.

Symptoms

Urethral stricture may make it increasingly difficult and painful to urinate. Other possible symptoms include a frequent urge to urinate with a small output of urine, dribbling urine after urination, pain in the lower abdomen or pelvis, blood in the urine, blood in semen, and a discharge from the penis. Urethral stricture can lead to recurring urinary tract infections.

Diagnosis

A diagnosis of urethral stricture is based on the symptoms and a physical examination. A doctor may also order urine tests to check for infection. If the urethral stricture continues to narrow the urethra, the doctor may refer you to a urologist (a doctor who specializes in treating disorders of the urinary tract). The urologist may perform a postvoid residual (PVR) urine test, which measures the amount of urine left in the bladder after urination. To confirm the diagnosis, he or she may perform cystoscopy (see page 805), an examination of the urethra with a cystoscope (viewing tube).

Treatment

To treat a urethral stricture, a urologist may first try to widen the urethra with a long, thin, flexible instrument called a dilator. In this procedure, the penis is numbed with a local anesthetic and the dilator is inserted through the urethral opening in the tip of the penis. You may need follow-up treatments to keep the channel open.

If treatment with a dilator is not effective, the urologist may recommend surgery using a cystoscope. The scar tissue may be removed through the cystoscope using tiny surgical instruments or a laser (a highly concentrated beam of light). In some cases, surgery is performed through an incision to remove the tissue that contains the stricture and replace it with tissue taken from another part of the body. After surgery, a urethral stent (a small plastic tube) is sometimes placed in the channel to keep it open.

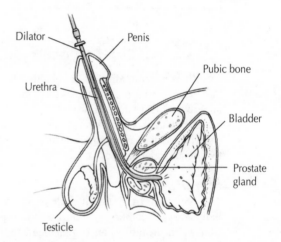

Urethral dilation
To stretch the urethra, the doctor numbs the penis with a local anesthetic and inserts a long, thin, flexible instrument called a dilator through the urethral opening in the tip of the penis. You may need follow-up treatments to keep the channel open.

Balanitis

Balanitis (also called balanoposthitis) refers to several common types of inflammation of the foreskin and the head of the penis (glans). The inflammation can result from infection, poor hygiene under the foreskin, friction from damp clothing, or irritation from chemicals in soap, clothing, condoms, or spermicides. Balanitis occurs more frequently in uncircumcised men than in men who are circumcised.

Symptoms

Balanitis causes redness, soreness, and swelling in the foreskin and head of the penis that make the foreskin difficult to retract (pull back). If it is painful or difficult to pull back your foreskin, see your doctor right away.

Diagnosis

A diagnosis of balanitis is based on the symptoms and a physical examination. In some cases, a doctor may recommend blood and urine tests to determine if a yeast infection or a sexually transmitted disease such as gonorrhea (see page 480), genital herpes (see page 482), or syphilis (see page 483) is causing the problem.

Treatment

Balanitis usually clears up on its own after successful treatment of the underlying cause. If the condition is caused by poor hygiene, your doctor will recommend keeping the area clean to prevent recurrences. You should also avoid using strong soaps, detergents, or shampoos, which could irritate the skin. If the condition results from an infection, your doctor will prescribe an antifungal or antibiotic lotion or an oral medication to clear up the infection and help relieve inflammation. For persistent cases of balanitis, a doctor may recommend circumcision (surgical removal of the foreskin).

Phimosis

Phimosis refers to tightening of the foreskin around the head of the penis (glans). The condition is normal before about age 5, but the foreskin naturally loosens by adolescence. In older men, phimosis can result from persistent irritation and inflammation of the head of the penis, and it can interfere with urination and sexual activity. Doctors think that phimosis may be a factor in cancer of the penis.

A diagnosis of phimosis is based on the symptoms and a physical examination. The condition is usually detected during puberty, when erections cause pain in the penis. If you have phimosis, your doctor will probably recommend circumcision (surgical removal of the foreskin).

WARNING!

Paraphimosis

Paraphimosis is the inability to pull a retracted foreskin back over the head of the penis. This condition often results from phimosis. The symptoms include pain and swelling, especially in the head of the penis. Paraphimosis can also cause loss of blood flow to the head of the penis, which is a medical emergency that requires immediate medical treatment. If you cannot pull your foreskin back over the head of your penis, call your doctor right away or go directly to the nearest hospital emergency department. Paraphimosis is usually treated with circumcision (surgical removal of the foreskin).

Peyronie's Disease

In Peyronie's disease, the penis bends or curves during an erection. In this noncancerous, progressive condition, a scar called a plaque develops in the erectile tissue inside the penis after an infection or injury, or for no obvious reason. The scar usually forms in the upper or lower part of the penis, but can form in both. If the plaque does not clear up within a few months, it can develop into permanent scar tissue or calcium deposits that do not allow the spongy tissue of the penis to expand, causing it to bend during an erection.

Symptoms

In Peyronie's disease, the penis bends at an angle during an erection, making intercourse painful and sometimes impossible. The curvature may develop slowly or rapidly and can be mild or severe. The condition is usually painful, but the pain sometimes decreases over time. In some men, Peyronie's disease causes erection problems (see page 486).

Diagnosis

A doctor can diagnose Peyronie's disease by the symptoms and by a physical examination. The doctor may inject medication into the penis to induce an erection so he or she can evaluate the curvature. Ultrasound (see page 111) of the penis is sometimes performed to locate the plaque that is causing the problem.

Treatment

The treatment of Peyronie's disease depends on how severe the curvature is and on how long the person has had it. Some treatments can reduce the pain but cannot correct the bend in the penis. Because surgery can cause complications and make the condition worse, doctors usually try other measures first. For example, most doctors recommend treatment with vitamin E supplements to help prevent the plaque from growing. Other treatments include injecting corticosteroids, calcium channel blockers, or other medications into the scar tissue to keep the scar from growing; using an electric current to deliver a drug to the scar tissue to keep the scar from growing; or directing high-energy radiation (using ultrasound guidance) to the affected site to break up the scar.

In most cases, surgery to correct Peyronie's disease is successful. In one procedure, the surgeon removes the plaque and grafts a patch of skin or other material onto the treated area. In another procedure, tissue on the unaffected side of the penis is removed, which straightens the curve but makes the penis shorter when it is erect. In some cases, inserting an implant into the penis can straighten it. Although these procedures can cure Peyronie's disease, they can also cause further scarring that could make the condition worse or cause erection problems (see page 486).

Priapism

Priapism is a painful, persistent erection that occurs without sexual stimulation. This rare condition can occur when an underlying condition leads to blood vessel or nerve abnormalities that cause blood to become trapped in the penis. Possible underlying conditions include medications, blood clots, urinary tract infections, sickle cell disease, leukemia, or a tumor.

WARNING!

Persistent Erection

Priapism is a medical emergency that requires immediate medical treatment. If you have an erection that persists for no reason, call your doctor right away, or go directly to the nearest hospital emergency department.

If priapism is not treated promptly, the spongy tissues of the penis can be permanently damaged, preventing future erections. The tissue can also die (gangrene; see page 601).

Diagnosis and Treatment

A diagnosis of priapism is based on the symptoms and a physical examination. The doctor will take a detailed health history to help find the possible underlying cause of the condition.

Emergency treatment of priapism involves draining excess blood from the penis with a needle and syringe and irrigating the spongy tissue of the penis with an antihistamine fluid to relax the erection and wash out old blood or blood clots. Priapism may be treated with surgery to bypass the blockage or drugs that relax the muscle in the penis, allowing blood to flow out of the penis. For people who have sickle cell disease (see page 613), blood transfusions to reduce the number of abnormal (sickled) blood cells can be effective. If priapism is treated promptly, the erection will subside and the person will eventually be able to have normal erections again.

Cancer of the Penis

Cancer of the penis is the growth of cancerous cells on the skin and in the tissues of the penis. Although the exact cause of penile cancer is not known, it seems to be associated with chronic irritation and inflammation of the head of the penis. There is a link between penile cancer and the human papillomavirus (HPV; see page 480), the virus that causes cervical cancer in women. Cancer of the penis occurs most frequently in men over age 55 and in blacks. Penile cancer rarely occurs in circumcised men, and is rare in the United States.

Although cancer can occur anywhere on the penis, it usually develops on the head (glans) or foreskin. Because this type of cancer is usually slow-growing, early detection and treatment will save the penis in most cases. If left untreated, cancer of the penis can spread to other parts of the body, usually through the lymphatic system (see page 908) or the bloodstream.

Symptoms

The main symptom of penile cancer is a sore or wartlike lump on the penis. Other possible symptoms include pain in the groin, a lump or swelling in the groin, a discharge from the penis, or bleeding during an erection.

Diagnosis

If you have symptoms of penile cancer, your doctor will examine your penis and may recommend a biopsy. For a biopsy, a small sample of tissue from the penis is removed for examination under a microscope for cancer cells. The biopsy will help the doctor distinguish cancer of the penis from syphilis (see page 483) or genital warts (see page 480), both of which can resemble a cancerous growth.

If cancer is detected, the doctor will order an imaging test such as ultrasound (see page 111), a CT scan (see page 112), or MRI (see page 113) of the pelvis to see if the cancer has spread. He or she also may perform an aspiration biopsy, in which a sample of cells is withdrawn through a hollow needle from a lymph node in the groin area. The cells are then examined under a microscope to determine if the cancer has spread to the lymph nodes. A test called lymph node dissection, in which lymph nodes in the groin area are removed and examined for the presence of cancer cells, may also be done.

Treatment

If you have cancer of the penis, your doctor probably will recommend surgery. Possible methods of surgery include wide local excision (in which the surgeon removes the cancer and some surrounding healthy tissue) or microsurgery (in which the surgeon removes the cancer and a very small amount of the surrounding healthy tissue while looking through a microscope). In laser surgery, the surgeon uses a concentrated beam of light to destroy the cancerous cells. Penectomy, a surgical procedure in which the penis is partially or totally removed, is the most common effective treatment for penile cancer. The surgeon may also remove some lymph nodes during a penectomy.

Surgery for cancer of the penis may be followed by radiation therapy (see page 23), in which X-rays or other forms of radiation are used to destroy or slow the growth of cancer cells, or chemotherapy (see page 23), in which powerful drugs are used to destroy cancer cells throughout the body. In biological therapy, a relatively new, experimental cancer treatment, a doctor administers injections of the protein interferon to boost the natural ability of the body's immune system to fight cancer.

Disorders of the Female Reproductive System

Most women will experience problems with their reproductive system at some time in their life. By recognizing the most common symptoms and talking about them with your doctor, you can often detect these problems in their early stages, when they are easiest to treat. The more information you have, the better you can protect or improve your reproductive health.

Your reproductive system is partly hidden and partly exposed. Your external genitals include the clitoris; the outer and inner labia, or lips; and the opening to your vagina. Together these external genitals are called the vulva. Your internal reproductive organs—the vagina, cervix, uterus, fallopian tubes, and ovaries—lie inside your body so the processes of conception and pregnancy can be protected. All of the sexual and reproductive functions that these organs fulfill are directed by a system of hormones coordinated by the brain.

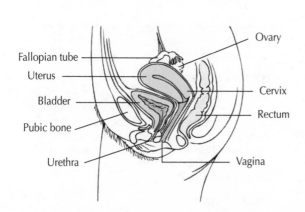

Side view of reproductive organs

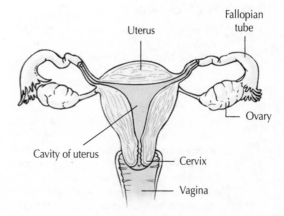

Front view of reproductive organs

The internal female reproductive organs

Your reproductive organs are inside your lower abdomen, where the processes of conception and pregnancy can take place in a protected environment. Each month, one of your ovaries releases an egg, which travels through a fallopian tube toward your uterus. If the egg is fertilized by a sperm, it will implant in the lining of the uterus. If unfertilized, it will be shed during menstruation.

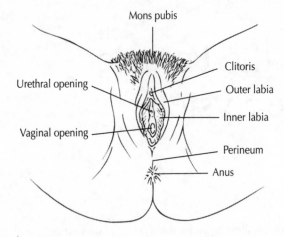

Mons pubis

Clitoris

Urethral opening

Outer labia

Inner labia

Vaginal opening

Perineum

Anus

The external genitals
Your genitals are on the outside of your body
near the openings to your vagina and urethra.
Vulva is the medical term for the external female
genitals.

Inside your outer and inner labia lies the clitoris, the organ of sexual arousal in women. Just below is the opening to the urethra, from which urine passes out of your body. The vaginal opening is behind the urethral opening and is partially covered by a membrane called the hymen until the first time you have intercourse. The perineum is the skin and underlying muscle between the vagina and the anus.

The vagina is the entrance to your internal reproductive organs. After intercourse, sperm travel up the vagina, past the cervix, and into the uterus. From the uterus, the sperm make their way up through the fallopian tubes, possibly to fertilize an egg produced by one of your ovaries. Usually, one ovary releases an egg each month. If a sperm fertilizes an egg, the fertilized egg implants in the uterus, beginning the process of pregnancy. An unfertilized egg is shed during menstruation (see next page).

Sex Hormones

The delicately balanced and precisely timed release of the sex hormones controls the female reproductive system. The sex hormones include the following:

Estrogen

Produced mainly in the ovaries, estrogen is the most important female sex hormone. Estrogen is responsible for triggering puberty in girls, including development of secondary sex characteristics such as breasts and pubic hair. The hormone maintains the healthy functioning of the reproductive system throughout life. Estrogen is also produced in small amounts in the testicles in men and in the brain in both men and women.

Follicle-Stimulating Hormone (FSH) and Luteinizing Hormone (LH)

FSH and LH are manufactured by the pituitary gland in both men and women. In women, the hormones regulate menstruation by stimulating the

release of an egg (ovulation) every month. In men, these hormones coordinate the production of sperm in the testicles.

Progesterone

After ovulation, the ovaries produce progesterone, which stimulates the lining of the uterus to thicken with blood in preparation for the implantation of a fertilized egg. During pregnancy, the placenta (the organ that links the woman's blood supply to that of the fetus) produces progesterone to maintain a healthy pregnancy.

Testosterone

Testosterone is the primary male sex hormone, responsible for the development of the secondary sex characteristics in boys at puberty. The hormone also has a role in maintaining sex drive in both men and women. Testosterone is produced in a man's testicles and, in small amounts, in a woman's ovaries.

Menstruation

Your body gets ready for the possibility of pregnancy each month during the years between the time you enter puberty and the time you reach menopause. Every 28 days or so, one of your two ovaries releases an egg, a tiny single cell that is invisible to the naked eye but that contains half of your genetic material. This process is called ovulation. The egg travels down a fallopian tube to the uterus, taking about 5 days to complete its journey. If you have intercourse shortly before or after the egg is released, your egg may be fertilized by your partner's sperm inside the fallopian tube. Sperm can live for as long as 6 days, so if you have intercourse 5 days before the release of your egg or 24 hours after, a sperm will still be able to fertilize the egg.

A few days before ovulation, the lining (endometrium) of your uterus gradually thickens. This process prepares your body for the possibility of fertilization and pregnancy. The thickened lining will become the first food supply for your fetus. By the time a fertilized egg reaches the uterus, the lining is ready for the egg. Once the egg attaches itself to the lining, it starts developing into an embryo, and you are officially pregnant.

If the egg is not fertilized, the thickened, blood-filled lining of the uterus will begin to shed, along with the unfertilized egg, about 14 days after ovulation. The bloody fluid passes out of the cervix (the lower opening of the uterus) into the vagina and out of the body. This process, called menstruation, lasts

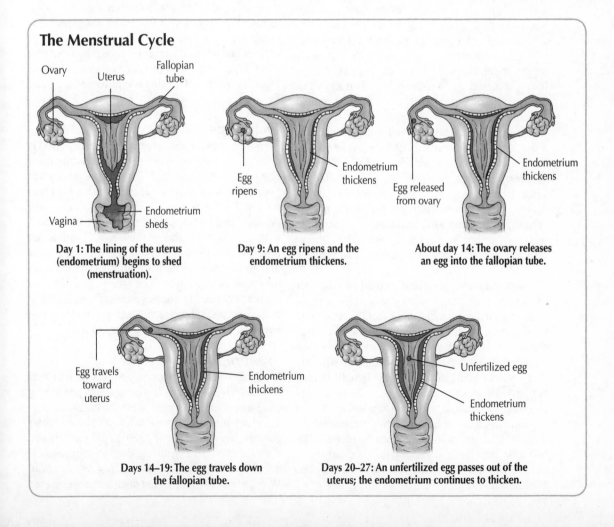

The Menstrual Cycle

Ovary
Uterus
Fallopian tube
Vagina
Endometrium sheds

Day 1: The lining of the uterus (endometrium) begins to shed (menstruation).

Egg ripens
Endometrium thickens

Day 9: An egg ripens and the endometrium thickens.

Egg released from ovary
Endometrium thickens

About day 14: The ovary releases an egg into the fallopian tube.

Egg travels toward uterus
Endometrium thickens

Days 14–19: The egg travels down the fallopian tube.

Unfertilized egg
Endometrium thickens

Days 20–27: An unfertilized egg passes out of the uterus; the endometrium continues to thicken.

an average of 5 days. During the next 9 days, another egg matures and grows in an ovary, starting the process of ovulation again.

The entire menstrual cycle lasts an average of 28 days, although in most women it fluctuates by 1 or 2 days and sometimes more. Each stage of the menstrual cycle is controlled by a cascade of inter-related hormones produced by the hypothalamus and pituitary gland in the brain and by the ovaries.

Periods usually start between ages 11 and 14. The first period is called menarche. Periods may be irregular for the first couple of years because ovulation often does not occur regularly at first. Periods can also become irregular after about age 45 because of fluctuating hormone levels and variable ovulation. Periods finally stop permanently at menopause (see page 851), at the average age of 51.

Absence of Periods

The temporary or permanent absence of periods is known medically as amenorrhea. In some girls, periods fail to start at the normal age, usually between ages 11 and 14. This is called primary amenorrhea, which usually results from a normal but late onset of puberty but can also be caused by a hormonal imbalance or an abnormality in the reproductive system. Usually doctors do not look for abnormalities until a girl reaches age 16 without having a period, or 14 if she has not had any signs of sexual development, such as breast enlargement or pubic hair.

It is common to miss a period once in a while. In a woman who has normally had regular periods, a delay in or absence of periods is called secondary amenorrhea. One obvious cause of secondary amenorrhea is pregnancy. But, like primary amen-orrhea, secondary amenorrhea can result from a change in the balance of hormones that control the release of an egg from an ovary. Secondary amen-orrhea occurs much more frequently than primary amenorrhea.

Hormone activity can be disrupted by a number of factors, including severe stress, rapid weight loss, or a medical condition, or from taking some medications. Women who stop taking oral contra-ceptives may experience secondary amenorrhea for a few months. Sometimes secondary amenor-rhea results when a disorder of the hypothalamus, pituitary gland, or ovaries disrupts the hormone-signaling system that triggers ovulation.

Normally, a balance exists between estrogen and progesterone (the major female sex hormones). If a hormone imbalance is causing the amenorrhea, a woman can have hormone-related problems. For example, failure to have periods for a number of

months can indicate a lack of estrogen, which can lead to bone loss (osteoporosis; see page 989). In some cases, a hormone imbalance results from obe-sity, a condition called polycystic ovarian syndrome (see page 865), high blood pressure, or diabetes, any of which can block the body's production of progesterone. Without progesterone, increased estrogen levels can raise the risk of a precancerous condition called endometrial hyperplasia (see page 868) or endometrial cancer (see page 869). In rare cases, amenorrhea can be a sign of a more serious disorder, such as Cushing's syndrome (see page 898).

Diagnosis

If your periods are fairly regular and your period is delayed 2 weeks or more, pregnancy is the most likely cause. A doctor will first do a pregnancy test to determine if that is the cause. If you are not preg-nant and are otherwise healthy, your doctor will probably tell you to wait for a few months to see if your periods start again on their own. If you do not have a period for 6 months, your doctor may order diagnostic tests to check for an underlying disor-der, such as hypothyroidism (see page 903). The doctor may need to check your hormone levels to make sure you are producing estrogen and that you have not gone into premature menopause.

Treatment

If you are not having periods, your doctor will treat the underlying cause. If you are not producing estrogen, your doctor may prescribe hormone ther-apy (see page 853). Women who don't have regular periods may have difficulty getting pregnant. If you want to become pregnant, the doctor may prescribe a fertility drug (see page 499) to restart ovulation. Women who have the eating disorder anorexia (see

The Female Athlete Triad

The benefits of physical activity almost always outweigh the risks. But some women who train intensively for athletic competition and do not consume enough calories to compensate for their increased activity level risk developing a condition known as the female athlete triad. This disorder is a cluster of three conditions—eating disorders (see page 724), lack of periods, and the bone-thinning disorder osteoporosis (see page 989)—that can occur together in women who engage in intense athletic exercise or training.

The prevalence of the female athlete triad is difficult to assess because many women with an eating disorder are secretive about their eating habits. Among the contributing factors are pressure by coaches and parents to win at all costs, frequent weigh-ins that penalize athletes for weight gain, and society's preference for a thin body. The girls and women most at risk of developing the condition are those in activities such as gymnastics, figure skating, distance running, ballet, and swimming.

The female athlete triad can place you at risk for some potentially serious health problems. The lack of periods indicates inadequate production of the female sex hormone estrogen, which is essential for maintaining bone strength. If you miss your period for more than 4 months, you will begin to lose bone mass, which can lead to frequent stress fractures and osteoporosis. Failing to keep your body weight at a normal level can have adverse effects on your heart, hormone system, and digestive system.

In addition to the lack of periods, common symptoms of the female athlete triad include:

- Fatigue
- Anemia
- Depression and other psychological problems
- Stress fractures
- Inability to concentrate
- Intolerance to cold; having cold hands and feet
- Constipation
- Dry skin
- Light-headedness
- Slow pulse
- Low blood pressure
- Downy hair growth on the face and body

Having your periods stop is not a normal consequence of intense training. It is a sign that your body is not getting enough nourishment and, to help protect you from starving, your body has shut down your reproductive system. If you exercise vigorously on a regular basis and your periods have stopped, see your doctor so you can prevent further bone loss. He or she will encourage you to gradually gain some weight and cut back on your training, enough to restart your periods. Your doctor may also prescribe estrogen replacement therapy (possibly in the form of birth-control pills; see page 470), which may help forestall bone loss until your body weight returns to normal.

---

page 726), who are very thin, or who exercise excessively or do vigorous athletic training on a regular basis can have either a delayed onset of menstruation or cessation of their periods (see above). This condition usually indicates that they are not consuming enough calories to maintain a normal weight or proportion of body fat, which reduces estrogen production.

If you have amenorrhea, remember that an egg can be released from an ovary at any time, so if you want to prevent pregnancy, you must still use some form of contraception throughout your menstrual cycle.

Irregular Periods

A woman's periods are considered irregular when 35 or more days (at least 7 more than the usual 28)

pass from the first day of one cycle to the first day of the next. Variations in the regularity of menstruation can result from stress, a change in contraceptive method, or taking medications such as corticosteroids. Menstruation depends on a balance of estrogen and progesterone (the two main female sex hormones). When this balance is disturbed, irregular periods can result. Menstrual periods and ovulation (release of an egg) are sometimes irregular after menstruation begins in puberty and for several years before menopause (see page 851).

Vaginal bleeding between periods sometimes indicates an unrecognized pregnancy or an early miscarriage. Abnormal tissue in the lining of the uterus can also cause bleeding between periods. Sometimes underlying disorders of the uterus, ovaries, or pelvic cavity can produce irregular or painful periods.

Diagnosis

Keeping track of your periods on a calendar can help you become aware of any variations in your cycle. If your periods are irregular only occasionally, such as once or twice a year, the irregularity is probably caused by stress. If your periods are frequently irregular, your doctor will give you a physical examination and may order diagnostic tests to find out if an underlying disorder, such as endometriosis (see page 870), might be causing the problem.

Treatment

Your doctor will treat any underlying disorder that is causing your irregular periods. If he or she does not find any physical problem, stress may be the cause. Try to eliminate stress as much as possible from your daily life and see if that helps regulate your periods.

Painful Periods

Many women experience cramping pain in the lower abdomen during their periods, and some women have painful menstrual cramps just about every month. This type of pain is known as primary dysmenorrhea and is thought to result from the normal hormonal changes that occur during menstruation. Primary dysmenorrhea can persist for years until menopause. Painful periods that are a symptom of another disorder—such as endometriosis (see page 870), pelvic inflammatory disease (see page 871), or fibroids (see page 867)—are called secondary dysmenorrhea.

Symptoms

Menstrual pain varies considerably. Some women have dull pain in the lower abdomen or lower back; others have severe, cramping pelvic pain. The pain is usually worse at the beginning of the period and may begin 12 to 24 hours before the onset of bleeding. Sometimes the pain is accompanied by nausea, vomiting, and leg cramps.

Diagnosis and Treatment

Your doctor can diagnose dysmenorrhea from your description of the symptoms. Painful periods are very common, but most cases are mild and do not require treatment. Over-the-counter nonsteroidal anti-inflammatory drugs (NSAIDs) such as ibuprofen can be effective in relieving menstrual pain. Your doctor may prescribe a stronger NSAID if the over-the-counter medications do not provide relief. Applying a heating pad to your pelvic area may also help. Oral contraceptives can help reduce menstrual cramps.

See your doctor if you develop severe menstrual pain that is not relieved by over-the-counter medications. He or she will examine you to find out what is causing the pain. Sometimes a surgical procedure called laparoscopy is needed to discover the cause of severe pelvic pain.

Heavy Periods

Unusually heavy or prolonged periods are known medically as menorrhagia or hypermenorrhea. Heavy periods are defined as periods that last longer than 7 days or that soak a large sanitary pad in less than 2 hours. A spontaneous disturbance of the hormones that control the menstrual cycle may cause heavy periods. Heavy periods can also result from fibroids (see page 867), small growths in the lining of the uterus called endometrial polyps, or a precancerous buildup of the endometrium, the tissue that lines the uterus (endometrial hyperplasia; see page 868). Endometrial hyperplasia is easily treated but, if not treated, can progress to cancer of the uterus (see page 869). Uterine cancer usually must be treated with a hysterectomy (surgical removal of the uterus; see page 870). Some kinds of IUDs (see page 472) can also cause heavier periods in a small percentage of women.

Some women regularly have heavy periods; others have them only occasionally. The condition frequently occurs in young women who have not yet established a regular ovulation cycle, and is especially common in women approaching menopause. If you regularly have heavy periods and do not consume enough iron-rich foods, you can develop iron deficiency anemia (see page 610).

Diagnosis

If you have a single, unusually heavy period and the bleeding does not diminish within 24 hours, or if you have been having heavy periods for some time, call your doctor. If your period is late as well as heavy, you may be having an early miscarriage. In this case, see your doctor immediately. Your doctor will ask you questions and examine you to find out the extent of bleeding and to see whether there could be an abnormality in your uterus. The doctor may do a Pap smear (see page 140) to check for cancer of the cervix, and an endometrial biopsy (see below) to screen for cancer of the uterus. A blood test will help determine if the heavy bleeding has caused anemia and will identify any other blood or hormone problems that could be contributing to your heavy periods.

Treatment

If you have a single heavy period and do not think you are pregnant, reduce your activity, drink extra fluids, and take an iron supplement. If you have consistently heavy periods and tests do not find the cause, your doctor may prescribe a medication that contains the hormone progesterone (or estrogen combined with progesterone) to reduce the bleeding. These are the same hormones contained in oral contraceptives. Nonsteroidal anti-inflammatory drugs sometimes help reduce the bleeding. If you are using a copper-containing IUD, your doctor may recommend that you consider another method of contraception. If blood tests indicate that you are anemic, you will need to take iron supplements.

If these measures do not limit the bleeding after a few months, your doctor may evaluate your pelvic organs using an ultrasound scan called a sonohysterogram. Even if no abnormality is found, the doctor may consider doing a hysteroscopy (see below) to examine the inside of your uterus. If a problem is found, the doctor will perform a procedure called endometrial ablation. In endometrial ablation, the doctor removes all or most of the lining of the uterus (endometrium) using a controlled delivery of heat from a balloonlike device inserted through the hysteroscope into the cavity of the uterus. Because endometrial ablation destroys the lining of the uterus, a woman's fertility is affected. The procedure is performed mainly on women who want

Hysteroscopy

To diagnose some gynecologic conditions, such as heavy or prolonged periods or bleeding between periods, a doctor needs to examine the inside of the uterus. In a procedure called hysteroscopy, the doctor can view the uterus directly to diagnose, evaluate, and treat disorders such as uterine fibroids, endometrial polyps, hyperplasia (thickening of the lining of the uterus), or benign or malignant tumors. Hysteroscopy can be performed in a hospital outpatient clinic or in a doctor's office using a local anesthetic with sedation.

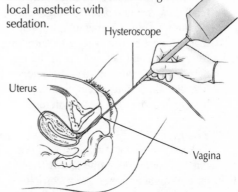

Hysteroscopy
During a hysteroscopy, the doctor inserts a flexible, lighted viewing instrument called a hysteroscope through the vagina into the uterus. He or she introduces a small amount of liquid or gas through the hysteroscope to expand the uterus. The doctor can also pass medical instruments through the hysteroscope to remove growths from the uterus or to perform procedures such as biopsies.

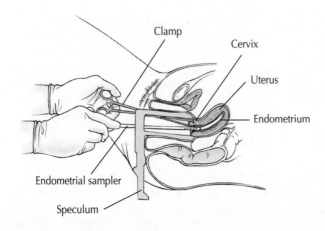

Endometrial biopsy
For an endometrial biopsy, the doctor takes a sample of tissue from the endometrium (lining of the uterus) for analysis in the laboratory for signs of cancer. Using an instrument called a speculum to open the vagina, the doctor stabilizes the cervix with a clamp and then inserts a very thin, flexible tube (endometrial sampler) into the uterus to take the tissue sample.

to avoid the major surgery of a hysterectomy. In some circumstances, however, a hysterectomy is the best treatment.

Premenstrual Syndrome

The combination of physical and emotional changes that sometimes occur in the week or so before your period is called premenstrual syndrome (PMS). Doctors believe that PMS results from hormonal fluctuations during the menstrual cycle. A number of other factors may also contribute— such as changes in the levels of a chemical messenger in the brain called serotonin (which helps regulate mood), stress, inadequate levels of some vitamins and minerals, eating salty or caffeine-containing foods, or drinking excessive amounts of alcohol.

Up to 75 percent of women who menstruate experience some uncomfortable premenstrual symptoms, and 30 to 40 percent have symptoms serious enough to disrupt their daily activities. PMS occurs most commonly in a woman's 20s or 30s and in the years preceding menopause; for each woman, the symptoms tend to follow a predictable pattern.

Symptoms

Common symptoms of PMS include mood swings, tender and swollen breasts, weight gain from fluid retention, a bloated abdomen, fatigue, food cravings, headaches, difficulty concentrating, irritability, anxiety, and depression in the days before a period. Some women also experience joint and muscle pain or nausea and vomiting. Most women have only some of these symptoms.

Diagnosis

Talk to your doctor if symptoms of PMS are affecting your normal routine and if lifestyle changes have brought no relief. No specific tests are available to diagnose PMS with certainty, but your doctor will be able to make a diagnosis based on your description of your symptoms and on their pattern. He or she may suggest that you keep track of your symptoms on a calendar every month to help you recognize the pattern.

Treatment

You may need to try different treatments for your PMS to find the ones that are most effective. Some women find that their symptoms are relieved by over-the-counter pain relievers such as ibuprofen or naproxen. The combined oral contraceptive pill, which evens out the normal fluctuations in the female hormones estrogen and progesterone, can ease PMS symptoms by blocking ovulation. Some women obtain relief by taking diuretics (drugs that remove excess water from the body); eating a diet that minimizes consumption of caffeine (including from chocolate), sugar, alcohol, red meat, and salt (which can increase water retention and bloating); and taking calcium, magnesium, vitamin B complex, and vitamin E supplements. Regular exercise and adequate rest also can help diminish PMS symptoms. Antidepressant drugs called selective serotonin reuptake inhibitors (see page 712), which modify levels of the brain chemical serotonin, reduce PMS symptoms in many women and can be taken at lower doses and for shorter periods than those prescribed for depression.

If your symptoms are not relieved with these measures, your doctor may prescribe mild pain relievers or tranquilizers to take on the days when your symptoms are most severe. If you have persistent depression that occurs at other times (not only before your periods), your doctor may refer you to a psychologist or psychiatrist.

Abnormalities in Sex Hormone Production

Several hormones regulate the menstrual cycle. Each month, the hypothalamus, deep in the brain, produces chemicals called releasing hormones. Releasing hormones pass into the pituitary gland at the base of the brain and stimulate the production of pituitary hormones, which in turn cause the ovaries to release an egg. These hormones also stimulate the production of the female sex hormones estrogen and progesterone in the ovaries.

A number of factors can throw this hormonal cycle out of balance. For example, stress, extreme weight changes, excessive exercise, drug abuse, or a severe illness can affect the hypothalamus, altering the production of releasing hormones. In rare cases, some brain disorders such as a brain tumor can affect the hypothalamus. Rare disorders of the pituitary gland and ovaries also can affect hormone production.

Symptoms

The main symptom of abnormal sex hormone production is infrequent or absent menstrual periods (see page 846). If the problem resides in the pituitary gland, other symptoms—such as the abnormal production of breast milk, irregularities in growth, thyroid problems, or underactivity of the adrenal gland—also may occur.

Some disorders of the ovaries or adrenal glands cause an overproduction of the male sex hormone testosterone, which is also naturally produced in women. Excess testosterone can cause hair growth on the face and body, deepening of the voice, acne, and weight gain.

Diagnosis

If your periods have become irregular or have stopped completely, your doctor will perform a pregnancy test. If the test shows that you are not pregnant and you have missed fewer than three periods, the doctor may recommend returning after you have missed three periods, especially if you want to become pregnant. He or she will then perform a thorough physical examination to determine if an underlying disorder is causing the problem. If your doctor suspects an underlying disorder, you may need to have blood and urine tests to evaluate your hormone levels, and a CT scan (see page 112) or MRI (see page 113) of your pituitary gland.

Treatment

The treatment for abnormal sex hormone production depends on the underlying cause. Treatment may include some type of hormone therapy, such as oral contraceptives or progesterone medication.

Menopause

Menopause is the period in a woman's life when menstrual cycles and ovulation stop permanently. The term perimenopause is often used to describe the transition phase that occurs during the 3 to 5 years before menopause. After menopause, your body makes much less of the female sex hormones, especially estrogen. In the years leading up to menopause, your menstrual cycle changes and your periods may become irregular as your hormone levels rise and fall. Eventually your periods stop altogether. Doctors consider menopause to be complete when a woman has not had a period for 1 year. The average age of menopause in the United States is 51 years, but it can occur earlier or later and varies from woman to woman. Cigarette smokers tend to reach menopause earlier than nonsmokers; toxins in cigarette smoke damage the ovaries, decreasing their normal span of activity. With an average life expectancy of 81 years, a woman can expect to live more than one third of her life after she has gone through menopause.

Women of childbearing age who have had both of their ovaries removed during a hysterectomy (see page 870) experience an abrupt menopause called surgical menopause. Because their hormone production ends so quickly, these women may experience the symptoms of menopause more severely than women who go through menopause naturally.

If you are sexually active, remember that you may still be fertile as you start menopause. Continue to use contraceptives for 12 to 24 months after the date of your last period.

Symptoms

Most women experience some symptoms during menopause. Only about 10 percent of women aren't aware of any changes at menopause other than an end to their periods. You may begin to notice some signs during perimenopause that come and go before your periods stop completely. Hot flashes are the most common symptom of menopause, affecting more than 60 percent of menopausal women in the United States.

See your doctor right away if you bleed between periods, have prolonged or excessive menstrual bleeding, or have any bleeding 6 months or more after what appeared to be your last period. These symptoms could signal a number of disorders, including a precancerous condition or cancer of the uterus (see page 869).

Hot flashes

A hot flash is a sudden physical sensation of intense heat that usually affects the upper part of the body but can affect the whole body. Your face and neck may become flushed, and red blotches may appear on your chest, back, and arms. Hot flashes, which can last from a few minutes to half an hour, cause profuse sweating, sometimes followed by chills as your body struggles to readjust its temperature. Hot flashes happen unexpectedly—more often at night—and usually start several years before other symptoms of menopause. They should gradually decline in frequency and intensity as you get older.

Most women who have hot flashes experience them for no more than 2 years. Hot flashes seem to be the body's response to a falling estrogen level, which affects the body's temperature regulator in the brain. They usually occur without warning, but some women find that alcohol, stress, or caffeine can trigger hot flashes or make them worse.

Hormone therapy (see next page) relieves the discomfort of hot flashes for most women. Some women find that taking vitamin E provides minor relief. Taking a herb called black cohosh (sold as a vitamin supplement) and eating foods containing soy seem to help reduce the intensity and frequency of hot flashes in some women. To better cope with hot flashes, dress in layers so you can take off a layer when you feel a hot flash coming on. Drink a glass of cold water at the first sign of a hot flash, and keep a pitcher of ice water or an ice pack next to your bed.

Changes in the vagina and urinary tract

As you age, the walls of your vagina become thinner, dryer, and less elastic, sometimes causing pain during intercourse. You may find it helpful to lubricate your vagina before intercourse with a water-soluble lubricant to help reduce the risk of infection. Don't use petroleum jelly; it can damage latex condoms and cause allergic reactions in some women.

The tissue in your urinary tract also changes at menopause, making you more vulnerable to stress incontinence (the involuntary leaking of urine; see page 877). Activities such as jogging or heavy lifting—or even sneezing, coughing, or laughing—can put enough pressure on your bladder to release a small amount of urine. Doing Kegel exercises (see page 874) regularly can help alleviate or reverse mild stress incontinence in menopausal women.

After menopause, your vagina and urinary tract may also become more susceptible to infection. To prevent urinary infections, drink lots of water, keep your genitals clean, and wash your genitals before and after intercourse. Ask your partner to wash his genitals before intercourse.

Changes in mood

While some women going through menopause may experience depression, anxiety, irritability, difficulty concentrating, lack of confidence, or sleep disturbances, most do not. For many women, menopause does not cause unpredictable mood swings or depression. In some women, menopause even seems to improve mental health. Many cases of depression in middle-aged women develop in response to life stresses as they struggle to cope with children who are leaving home or aging parents who require extended care. Lower estrogen levels may bring about a decline in sexual interest. However, sexual activity may increase in some women who are relieved that pregnancy is no longer a concern.

For many women, engaging in regular moderate aerobic exercise such as walking at least 5 days a week helps improve their mood by enabling them to sleep better. Better sleep can enhance concentration and memory. If you experience emotional problems related to menopause or other life changes, see your doctor, who may prescribe an antidepressant (see page 712) or refer you for counseling.

Bone loss

One of the most serious health issues for menopausal women is the bone-thinning condition osteoporosis (see page 989). Directly connected to declining estrogen levels in women, osteoporosis causes loss of bone tissue, especially in the first several years after menopause, which can result in thin, brittle bones that are highly susceptible to fracture. Roughly 300,000 women in the United States fracture a hip each year, often becoming unable to walk and requiring extended care.

The best strategy to combat osteoporosis is prevention, which requires building strong bones in adolescence and young adulthood (see page 452). However, it's never too late to adopt health-promoting practices that can keep you healthy in general and help you maintain the density and strength of your bones after menopause. Get in the habit of exercising at least 5 days a week—even moderate exercise such as walking and light weight lifting are helpful. Fit exercise into your daily routine by trying to take the stairs instead of the elevator whenever possible, or parking farther away from your destination. Eat a balanced diet rich in calcium; you should take in 1,500 milligrams of calcium each day if you are not taking a bone-preserving medication (see page 993). Quit smoking (see page 29) if you smoke, and limit your intake of alcohol—smoking and excess drinking increase the rate of bone loss.

The most effective medications for women who have osteoporosis are estrogen or estrogenlike drugs. For women who cannot or choose not to take estrogen, other effective bone-preserving medications are also available, such as raloxifene, alendronate, and calcitonin.

Menopause and heart disease

Heart disease is the No.1 killer of American women, causing half of all deaths in women over age 50. After menopause, the incidence of heart disease increases in women until it reaches that of men. Menopause brings changes in the levels of fats in a woman's blood. The level of HDL (good cholesterol) tends to decline, while the level of LDL (bad cholesterol) rises. These changes are thought to be caused by the drop in estrogen. An unhealthy cholesterol level profile (that is, low HDL, high LDL) can boost your risk of stroke and heart disease.

Taking estrogen in hormone therapy was once thought to reduce the risk of some types of heart disease in women after menopause. However, a combination of estrogen and a specific progestin called medroxyprogesterone acetate (MPA) in hormone therapy has been found to increase the risk of heart attack, stroke, or blood clots in some women. Research is continuing on the link between heart disease and other combinations of estrogens and progestins and on estrogen alone (without a progestin). (Women who do not have a uterus because they have had a hysterectomy can take estrogen without a progestin.) Women who have a high risk of developing blood clots or a family history of blood clots should not take estrogen, especially if they smoke. Women who smoke are more likely to develop heart disease at any time of life but, after menopause, their risk increases dramatically.

Hormone Therapy

To prevent the symptoms produced by falling estrogen levels during menopause, doctors have traditionally turned to hormone therapy. In addition to having the potential to prevent osteoporosis after menopause, hormone therapy may help reduce the risk of colon cancer. However, hormone therapy seems to increase the risk of breast cancer, heart attack, stroke, and blood clots in some women. Studies are being done to understand the link between reduced estrogen production and tooth loss and age-related macular degeneration (the most frequent cause of loss of vision in people over 50; see page 1046).

If you are considering hormone therapy, talk with your doctor about what the benefits and risks might be for you. Hormone therapy is available in the form of pills, skin patches, and vaginal creams. Most women take estrogen along with a progestin. Doctors recommend this hormone combination because estrogen given alone may slightly increase the risk of cancer of the uterus. (Because women who have had their uterus surgically removed cannot develop uterine cancer, there is no need for them to take progestin with the estrogen to reduce the risk of uterine cancer.)

Menopausal women taking the hormone combination sometimes temporarily resume monthly bleeding or have spotting. Bleeding usually stops within 6 to 12 months. Sometimes all it takes is a different dose of hormones to stop the bleeding. Some women experience breast tenderness, bloating, abdominal cramps, anxiety, irritability, or depression from hormone therapy.

There are medications other than hormone therapy that can help alleviate some menopausal symptoms. For example, water-based vaginal lubricants and estrogen-containing vaginal creams can help relieve vaginal dryness and reduce discomfort during sexual intercourse. Many effective drugs also are available that help maintain a woman's bone density and prevent and treat osteoporosis without increasing the risk of uterine cancer, breast cancer, heart attack, or blood clots.

Breast Disorders

The primary function of the female breasts is to produce milk to feed an infant. The breasts also play a role in a woman's sexuality. Breast sensitivity and sexual response vary among women, but most women's breasts undergo a number of physiologic changes in response to sexual stimulation.

In some women, hormonal fluctuations during the menstrual cycle make the breasts a little larger and tender before periods.

The size and shape of a woman's breasts are determined primarily by genes. Most of the breast consists of fat, which is layered around milk glands,

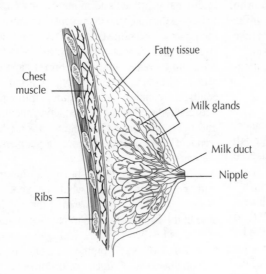

The breast
A woman's breasts consist mostly of fatty tissue surrounding a system of milk glands (called lobules), milk ducts, and connective tissue. The milk glands and ducts radiate out from the nipple. During pregnancy, the milk-producing glands become active. At about the time of childbirth, the milk glands secrete milk into the ducts, where it is stored until an infant needs it. A layer of muscle lies behind each breast.

milk ducts, and supporting fibers. The nipple contains 15 to 20 tiny openings, which are the outlets of milk ducts or sebaceous (oil) glands. The sebaceous glands secrete an oily substance that lubricates and protects the skin. Around the nipple is a pigmented area called the areola, which can vary greatly in size, shape, and color from one woman to another. Small muscles behind the areola make the nipple erect when stimulated. The system of milk glands and ducts radiates out from the nipple.

Infection-fighting lymph nodes drain lymph fluids from the breast to three major areas—the armpit, the area just above the collarbone, and the area under the breastbone. The breasts can develop abnormal growths such as cysts or tumors, or conditions that can result from infections. Breast cancer is the most common cancer in women and the second most common cause of cancer death in women (after lung cancer). To detect signs of breast cancer at an early, more curable stage, every woman should do a monthly breast self-examination, have regular manual examinations by her doctor, and have regular mammograms, usually starting at age 40.

Nipple Discharge

A whitish or gray-green discharge just before or after childbirth is likely to be breast milk, especially if it comes from both nipples. If you have a milky discharge at any other time, it is called galactorrhea (see next page), and can be a sign of an underlying disorder. You need not worry if you have nipple discharge only when the nipple is manipulated, such as during foreplay; this is a normal physiologic response.

Any spontaneous nipple discharge, however, should be evaluated by a doctor. Note whether the discharge comes from one nipple duct (one of the tiny holes in the nipples) or from many. If the discharge is dark (usually dark red or black), especially if it comes from only one breast, see your doctor. The dark coloring is usually caused by blood in the discharge, often from a tiny benign growth in the milk duct called a duct papilloma. In rare cases, however, a dark discharge from the nipple could also be a sign of breast cancer.

Your doctor will examine your breasts and may analyze a sample of the discharge. He or she may also recommend other diagnostic tests, including a mammogram (see page 141) and an ultrasound (see page 111). If anything suspicious is found on the mammogram or ultrasound, the doctor will recommend a biopsy, in which a small sample of tissue is removed from the breast for examination under a microscope. If you have a duct papilloma, it can be removed in a simple surgical procedure.

Inverted Nipples

Some women's nipples are naturally inverted, which is normal for them. The only possible disadvantage of inverted nipples is that they can make breastfeeding more difficult. However, if your nipples are not normally inverted and you notice, especially on only one breast, that a nipple (or any part of your breast) is pulled in, see your doctor. He or she will examine the breast and may order diagnostic tests to rule out breast cancer.

Paget's Disease of the Nipple

Paget's disease of the nipple is an uncommon form of breast cancer that starts in the milk ducts of the nipple. Without treatment, the cancer can gradually spread deeper into breast tissues. The disease resembles the skin condition eczema (see page 1062) and usually affects only one nipple. The nipple itches and burns and may have a sore that doesn't heal.

If you have symptoms of Paget's disease, your doctor will probably recommend removing a small piece of tissue from the affected breast for examination under a microscope for cancer cells (biopsy). Early detection and treatment are your best chances for a cure. The treatment for Paget's disease of the nipple is similar to that for breast cancer (see page 857), depending on the extent of the cancer when it is diagnosed.

Breast Abscess

An abscess is an infected, pus-filled area of tissue. A breast abscess forms when bacteria enter the breast through the nipple and infect the milk ducts and glands. Breast abscesses are not common. They can affect any woman, but occur mostly in women who are just beginning to breastfeed (see page 539). During the first week of breastfeeding, the nipples may become dry and develop cracks, making it easier for bacteria from the baby's mouth to enter the breast.

Symptoms and Diagnosis

An abscess usually develops in the skin around the nipple. As the bacteria multiply, they produce a red, firm, painful swelling or lump in the breast. The glands in the armpit next to the affected breast may be tender, and you may have a fever. Even if you are not breastfeeding, see your doctor right away if you develop any symptoms of a possible abscess. Doctors can usually diagnose a breast abscess from the symptoms.

Treatment

If you have a breast abscess, your doctor will prescribe antibiotics to fight the infection. He or she may recommend periodically applying a warm, moist washcloth to the inflamed area. You may be asked to stop breastfeeding from that breast until the infection clears up; to maintain your milk production and to prevent your breast from becoming engorged, use a breast pump to express the milk from the infected breast during this time.

Occasionally, antibiotics do not clear up the infection, and the abscess needs to be drained. To drain the abscess, a doctor makes a small incision at the edge of the areola to allow the pus to seep out.

Galactorrhea

The breasts normally produce milk after childbirth and, sometimes, for a few weeks before childbirth. Milk production that occurs at any other time in a woman, or at any time in a man, is called galactorrhea. Galactorrhea is uncommon in women and rare in men. In galactorrhea, milk is usually produced by both breasts and is whitish or gray-green. Although galactorrhea can occur for no apparent reason, excessive production of the hormone prolactin is a possible cause. Prolactin is made by the pituitary gland in the brain to stimulate milk production for breastfeeding.

Galactorrhea also can result from a disorder of the pituitary gland such as a tumor (prolactinoma; see page 885). Some medications—especially those that have an effect on the brain, such as drugs used to treat mental disorders—can cause galactorrhea. Galactorrhea also can be triggered by excessive nipple stimulation (such as during sexual foreplay) or friction (such as from not wearing a bra during jogging). In women, galactorrhea is often associated with an absence of periods (see page 846). If you notice any fluid leaking from your nipples, see your doctor.

Diagnosis

If your doctor suspects that the galactorrhea is caused by a pituitary tumor or another underlying hormonal disorder, he or she probably will order a blood test to measure the level of prolactin and may recommend diagnostic tests such as a CT scan (see page 112) or MRI (see page 113) of the brain.

Treatment

If the diagnostic tests do not find a problem, you probably will not need any treatment. For galactorrhea that results from taking a medication, discontinuing the drug will clear it up. If the condition is caused by a disorder of the pituitary gland, the doctor may prescribe hormone therapy or the drug bromocriptine to block milk production. In rare cases, surgery is necessary to remove a pituitary tumor.

Lumps in the Breast

Women who do regular breast self-examinations (see page 137) may occasionally find an area that feels different from the rest of the breast. These areas are referred to as breast lumps. Breast lumps often do not cause any discomfort, but they can sometimes be tender or painful.

Although breast lumps are usually not a cause for concern, always see your doctor if you notice any changes (including seemingly minor ones) in your breasts. Lumps can have a number of causes. They can be cysts (noncancerous fluid-filled sacs), or they can result from thickening of the milk-producing glandular tissue inside the breasts (called fibrocystic changes). They can also result from infections or from noncancerous growths such as fibroadenomas. All of these kinds of lumps are harmless, but, because lumps can also be cancerous, it's essential to have them checked by a doctor.

Benign Lumps and Cysts

Most lumps that develop in the breasts are harmless, non-cancerous growths. Some women have naturally lumpy breasts that tend to develop numerous cysts or fibrous growths. Fibroadenomas are solid lumps that can range from the size of a pea to the size of a lemon.

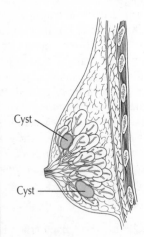

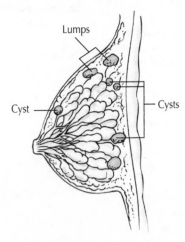

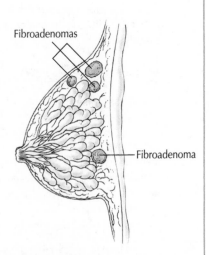

Breast cysts

Cysts are fluid-filled sacs that can develop in the breasts. They are harmless, noncancerous growths that sometimes go away on their own. Some women have several cysts in their breasts, which is normal for them. A doctor may sometimes recommend withdrawing fluid from a lump to confirm that it is indeed a cyst and not a solid mass, which could be cancerous. A lump can also be identified as a cyst using ultrasound.

Fibrocystic breasts

Some women have a condition called fibrocystic breasts, in which they have several small lumps and cysts in one or, usually, both breasts. This is not a disease. However, women who have fibrocystic breasts should become familiar with the location and size of these lumps through regular breast self-examinations so they can recognize any changes and bring them to their doctor's attention.

Fibroadenomas

Fibroadenomas are solid lumps that are firm and rubbery and can be moved around easily. Fibroadenomas seldom cause pain and don't change in response to hormonal fluctuations during the menstrual cycle, although they can sometimes grow larger during pregnancy or breast-feeding. Doctors only remove them when they are unusually large, when they do not appear to be characteristic benign fibroadenomas on an image (such as a mammogram or ultrasound), or if cells taken in a needle biopsy look abnormal. If a needle biopsy confirms that a lump is a benign fibroadenoma, it is not removed but is monitored regularly for changes.

You might want to watch the lump through one menstrual cycle before seeing a doctor because benign lumps sometimes disappear after a menstrual cycle.

Diagnosis

If you still feel the lump after a menstrual cycle, see your doctor, whether or not the lump is painful. You should also see your doctor if a lump you have had for a long time becomes painful or feels different in some way (such as harder or bigger).

Your doctor will examine both breasts and, if the lump feels suspicious, recommend that you have a diagnostic mammogram to evaluate it. The radiologist who studies your mammogram may suggest that you have an ultrasound (see page 111) to determine if the lump is a harmless cyst or a solid mass of tissue that could be cancerous. The radiologist may also recommend taking a sample of tissue from the lump for examination under a microscope for cancer cells (biopsy).

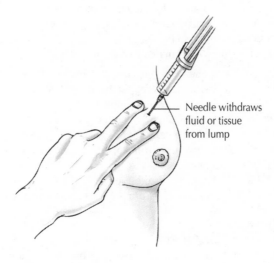

Needle withdraws fluid or tissue from lump

Needle aspiration or biopsy
If you have a lump that looks like a cyst but the doctor is not absolutely sure is a cyst, he or she may recommend withdrawing fluid from the lump with a needle. The doctor locates the lump with his or her fingers and, often guided by ultrasound, inserts the needle into the lump. If fluid comes out, the lump is a cyst, and it will collapse as the fluid is removed. If no fluid comes out, the doctor may then use a larger needle to withdraw tissue from the lump to examine it for cancer cells.

Treatment

The treatment for a breast lump depends on the nature of the lump. If a lump is proven to be a cyst on an ultrasound, it does not need to be aspirated (unless it is causing pain). If a lump does not look like an obvious cyst on a mammogram or ultrasound, the doctor may try to withdraw fluid from the lump through a needle (called needle aspiration; see illustration below left). If it is a cyst, which contains fluid, the cyst usually collapses and disappears when the fluid is withdrawn.

If the cause of a lump (or lumps) is thickening of the glandular tissue in the breasts from fibrocystic changes, treatment is not necessary. However, if the lump feels tender or painful, wearing a bra that provides firm support can help reduce breast tenderness. For some people, limiting their intake of caffeine seems to reduce breast pain. If your breasts are very painful, your doctor may prescribe sex hormones or other medications to reduce the hormone fluctuations that are affecting the lumps.

If a mammogram or ultrasound suggests that the lump could be a cancerous or precancerous tumor, your doctor will recommend a needle biopsy (see illustration), in which a sample of tissue is removed from the tumor through a needle for examination under a microscope for cancer cells. If the cells are found to be cancerous, the lump will need to be removed. The type of surgery depends on the nature of the tumor. If the lump is found on a biopsy to be noncancerous, it does not need to be removed, but the doctor will want to examine it regularly for changes.

Breast Cancer

Cancer of the breast is the most common cancer in women (although lung cancer kills more women each year). The risk of developing breast cancer is actually much lower than that of several other life-threatening diseases, including heart disease (the No. 1 killer of American women), stroke, type 2 diabetes, and osteoporosis. When breast cancer is detected at an early stage and treated, it is cured in 9 out of 10 cases.

Risk Factors

Breast cancer results from changes in the genes of breast cells. The precise cause of these genetic mutations is not fully understood. Breast cancer develops more frequently in whites than in blacks or Asians. The following factors increase a woman's risk of developing breast cancer:

- **Age**   Age is the most significant risk factor for breast cancer. Breast cancer is uncommon in women younger than 35; the risk is higher in women over 50 and especially high in women over 60. Your risk of developing breast cancer at 60 is about 26 times greater than it is at 35.

- **Health history**   If you have breast cancer in one breast, you are at increased risk of developing a cancer in your other breast.

- **Family history**   Although the vast majority of cases of breast cancer occur in women who have no family history of the disease, heredity can play a role. Women who have a close relative (mother, sister, or daughter) with breast cancer (especially if it develops at a young age) are at increased risk of also developing the cancer.

- **Genetic changes**   Alterations in some genes (such as BRCA1 and BRCA2) increase a woman's risk of developing breast cancer. Five to 10 percent of cases occur in women who inherit one of these genes. If several members of your family have had breast cancer, your doctor may talk to you about genetic testing (see page 953) to determine if you have a genetic mutation in one of these genes. You may be able to delay or prevent the cancer or at least have it diagnosed at an early stage.

- **Estrogen**   Exposure to the female hormone estrogen (either made by the body or taken as a drug) appears to play a role in a woman's risk of breast cancer. For example, breast cancer is slightly more common in women who start menstruating early (before age 12) or who go through menopause late (after age 55). Women who have never had a baby or breastfed (and therefore have never had a break in their menstrual cycle) also appear to have a slightly higher risk of breast cancer than women who have had a baby.

- **Late childbearing**   Women who have their first child after age 30 are at greater risk of developing breast cancer than women who have babies at younger ages. The reason for this is not clear, but doctors think it may be that early pregnancy causes breast cells to mature, which makes them less likely to undergo changes that could lead to cancer.

- **Radiation therapy**   Women whose breasts have been exposed to radiation during radiation therapy, such as for Hodgkin's disease (see page 626), are at increased risk of developing breast cancer. The younger the woman when she has the therapy, the higher her risk.

Finding Cancer Early

Because there is no known way to prevent breast cancer, the best chance for successful treatment is to detect it at an early stage. Performing a breast self-examination (see page 138) every month will help you detect a lump early. Have a mammogram (see page 141) as frequently as your doctor recommends, usually starting at about age 40. When a tumor is detected at an early stage and treated before it has spread, you can expect a complete cure or many years of good health.

Symptoms

If you have breast cancer, you may feel a lump or thickening in or near your breast or in the underarm area during a breast self-examination. The lump may or may not be painful; breast pain is usually a sign of a noncancerous condition, although there are exceptions. Although most breast lumps turn out to be benign, see your doctor if you find a lump or notice any of the following:

- A change in the size or shape of a breast
- Spontaneous nipple discharge (especially if it is dark in color) or nipple tenderness
- A nipple that is suddenly pulled back into the breast (inverted)
- Ridges or pitting of the breast resembling an orange peel
- A change in the look or feel of the skin of the breast, areola, or nipple (such as warm, swollen, red, or scaly)

Diagnosis

If you have a lump in your breast or if a lump is detected on a routine mammogram, your doctor will perform a manual breast examination to determine whether more tests are required to rule out cancer. He or she may recommend that you have a diagnostic mammogram to get a close-up view of the area of the lump or an ultrasound of the breast. Your doctor or a breast surgeon may perform a biopsy (take a sample of tissue from the lump for examination under a microscope) or remove fluid or tissue from the lump with a needle (needle aspiration or biopsy; see previous page).

If the lump is found to be cancerous, you will probably have more tests. MRIs (see page 113) and PET scans (see page 114) are being used increasingly to help evaluate breast tumors. A PET scan can help determine if the cancer has spread to the lymph nodes under the arms, but a lymph node biopsy is always done to confirm this. A PET scan can also show whether an advanced cancer has spread to other parts of the body.

Other tests used for diagnosing breast cancer include a hormone receptor test performed on the cancerous tissue to determine if estrogen or progesterone (female sex hormones) stimulates the cancer to grow. Sometimes the tissue is examined to look for a gene called human epidermal growth factor receptor-2 (HER-2), a tumor marker that is associated with an especially aggressive form of breast cancer.

Ductal lavage

A test called ductal lavage is used to evaluate the risk of breast cancer in women who are at high risk, such as those who have a family history of breast cancer. In ductal lavage, an anesthetic cream is applied to the nipple area to reduce discomfort, and a breast pump with gentle suction is applied to the nipple to draw out tiny amounts of fluid from the milk ducts. When fluid is found in a milk duct, the milk duct is washed out with salt water infused through a tiny tube (catheter) inserted into the duct. The collected cells are then examined in the laboratory for precancerous changes or cancer.

Ductoscopy

Ductoscopy is a procedure that uses a thin (smaller than 1 millimeter in diameter), flexible viewing tube (ductoscope) inserted through the nipple into a milk duct to evaluate nipple discharge for abnormalities. The tube is connected to a camera that allows the doctor to examine the ducts directly on a video monitor. Ductoscopy may eventually prove to be useful before a woman has breast-conserving surgery (see next page) to help determine how much tissue to remove, or as a screening test for women who are at high risk of breast cancer.

Treatment

The treatment of breast cancer is complex and depends on many variables, including the characteristics of the tumor (which can sometimes help a doctor determine if it is likely to grow rapidly),

whether the cancer has spread to the lymph nodes or to another part of the body, and the sensitivity of the tumor cells to estrogen (which can stimulate tumor growth in some women). Treatment options for a particular woman also depend on her general health. Surgery is usually the first treatment for breast cancer, which may be followed by radiation therapy, chemotherapy, hormone therapy, or biological therapy, or a combination of these.

After any treatment for breast cancer, doctors recommend frequent checkups, at least twice yearly. If breast cancer recurs, it can usually be controlled for many years with drugs, radiation therapy, and, sometimes, more surgery.

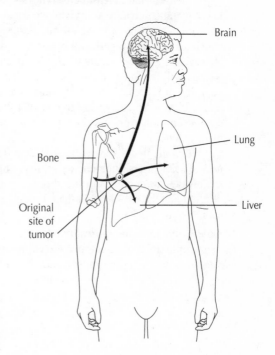

When breast cancer spreads
Groups of lymph nodes under the arms and in the chest are located close to the breasts. Breast cancer cells can enter the lymph nodes and be carried in the lymphatic system and bloodstream throughout the body. The sites to which breast cancer most often spreads (metastasizes) are the lungs, liver, bones, or brain.

Surgery

In most cases of breast cancer, surgery is recommended to remove the tumor. Surgery may involve removing all or part of the breast. The type of surgery performed and the amount of tissue removed depend on the size and location of the tumor and whether the cancer has spread. Occasionally, the entire tumor can be removed during a biopsy.

Breast-conserving surgery

If a breast tumor is small, a woman may be offered the option of having just the lump and a small amount of the surrounding tissue removed (called a lumpectomy or a partial mastectomy), followed by radiation therapy. Some lymph nodes in the armpit are also removed and examined for cancer cells (called a sentinel lymph node biopsy). Radiation therapy after surgery reduces the risk of recurrence of the cancer in the breast and chest wall.

Women who have breast-conserving surgery followed by radiation have a survival rate equal to that of women who have mastectomies (surgery in which all or a major part of a breast is removed). However, if a cancer recurs after a lumpectomy, a woman will later need to have a mastectomy. Ask your doctor if breast-conserving surgery is appropriate for you. You may want to consider getting a second opinion from another doctor before you make a decision.

Studies are under way to evaluate the effectiveness of using lasers (high-energy beams of light) or radiowaves to destroy tumors through a needle inserted into the tumor rather than through a surgical incision.

Simple and modified radical mastectomies

In a simple (total) mastectomy, the entire breast is removed, including the nipple and areola. Chest muscles are not removed. This procedure is sometimes performed to treat precancerous growths in the breast or a tumor that has not spread beyond a limited area of the breast. A simple mastectomy is sometimes performed to prevent breast cancer in women who are at high risk of developing the cancer, usually because of a strong family history.

In a modified radical mastectomy, the entire breast is removed along with many of the lymph nodes under the arm. The lymph nodes are examined to see if the cancer has spread. This surgery may be followed by radiation therapy. The incisions are the same for both the simple mastectomy and the modified radical mastectomy.

Skin-sparing mastectomy with reconstruction

Doctors perform a skin-sparing simple or modified radical mastectomy in women who are having breast reconstruction. In these mastectomies, the nipple and areola are the only areas of skin that are removed, which makes reconstruction easier and limits scarring. An incision is made around the areola and to the side and all the breast tissue is removed through this incision. Breast reconstruction is then performed with muscle taken from the woman's abdomen or back.

Breast reconstruction

Losing a breast is traumatic for every woman. Many women choose to have breast reconstruction surgery (see page 862) after having a mastectomy. Breast reconstruction involves inserting an artificial breast implant into the space or reconstructing

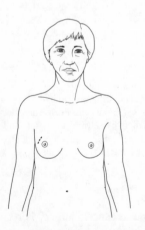

Incision for lumpectomy

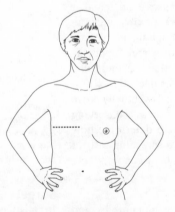

Incision for simple or modified radical mastectomy

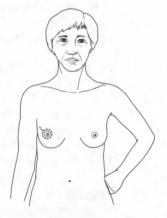

Incision for skin-sparing mastectomy

the breast using skin, fat, and muscle from another part of the woman's body (usually the abdomen or back). The procedure may be performed at the same time as the mastectomy or after a woman recovers from a mastectomy. Reconstruction is always done at the same time as a skin-sparing mastectomy. Another option is to wear a breast prosthesis inside a bra. A prosthesis is matched to the other breast and is nearly undetectable.

After surgery

After surgery for breast cancer, you may have pain and tenderness at the site; if you are in pain, ask your doctor about pain-relief medication. As with any surgery, there is a risk of infection, slow wound healing, bleeding, or an allergic reaction to the anesthetic used for the surgery.

The skin in the area where the breast was removed may be tight, and the muscles in your arm and shoulder may feel stiff. After a mastectomy, some women have some permanent loss of strength in these muscles, but for most women this reduced strength is temporary. Your doctor, nurse, or a physical therapist will recommend exercises you can do to help regain movement and strength in your arm and shoulder.

If nerves were injured or cut during the surgery, you may have numbness and tingling in your chest, underarm, shoulder, or upper arm. These symptoms usually go away within a few weeks or months as the injury heals. Sometimes, when lymph nodes under the arm are removed, fluid can build up in the arm and hand and cause swelling (lymphedema). You will need to take precautions to protect your arm and hand on that side from injury or pressure; let your doctor know right away if an infection develops in your arm or hand.

Radiation therapy

Radiation therapy, the use of high-energy rays to kill cancers in localized areas of the body, is often used in addition to surgery to treat breast cancer. The radiation may be directed at the breast from a machine (called external radiation) or inserted into the breast in thin plastic tubes placed at the site of the cancer (called implant radiation). For external radiation therapy, a person goes to a hospital or clinic, usually 5 days a week for 6 weeks. For implant radiation, a person stays in the hospital with the implants in place for several days. In some cases, especially for small tumors that are removed

in breast-conserving surgery such as lumpectomy, radiation therapy is given after surgery to destroy any breast cancer cells that may remain. For large tumors that cannot be removed easily with surgery, radiation is sometimes given before surgery, alone or with chemotherapy or hormone therapy (see below), to destroy cancer cells and shrink the tumor.

Fatigue is the most common side effect of radiation therapy, especially after several treatments. Although rest is important, your doctor will recommend that you try to stay as active as you can. The skin in the treated area may become red, dry, tender, and itchy, and the treated breast may feel heavy and hard. These symptoms will clear up after the treatments stop. Because the skin in the treated area will be especially tender, you should wear loose-fitting clothing and expose the area to the air as often as possible to help the skin heal. Your doctor will tell you how to care for your skin during this time.

Chemotherapy

For cancer that has spread from the breast, chemotherapy, usually as a combination of drugs, is given to kill cancer cells throughout the body. The drugs are given in pills or by injection at an outpatient clinic, at the doctor's office, or at home.

The side effects of chemotherapy depend on the particular drugs and the dosage. Along with cancer cells, chemotherapy destroys healthy cells, especially those that divide rapidly, such as blood cells and the cells in hair roots and in the lining of the digestive tract. This cell loss can increase your susceptibility to infections and cause easy bruising or bleeding, weakness and fatigue, loss of hair, poor appetite, nausea and vomiting, diarrhea, or mouth and lip sores. Many of these side effects can be controlled with medication and are usually short term. Because the effects of chemotherapy on a fetus are unknown, doctors usually recommend that women avoid getting pregnant during their treatment; discuss birth control (see page 470) with your doctor before your treatment starts.

Hormone therapy for breast cancer

For women whose breast tumors are stimulated by estrogen, hormonal medications such as tamoxifen or raloxifene may be given (usually for 5 years) to block the growth-stimulating effects of the hormone on the tumor. In addition to treating breast cancer, these drugs are also used to prevent breast cancer in high-risk women.

Breast Reconstruction Surgery

Today, just about any woman who loses her breast because of cancer can have a new breast created through reconstructive surgery, although the best candidates are those women whose cancer has been completely eliminated by breast removal. New surgical techniques have given surgeons additional ways to create a breast that closely matches a natural breast. Reconstruction is now possible right after breast removal in many cases. If you have been diagnosed with breast cancer and your doctor has recommended breast removal, discuss your options for surgery with the doctor so you can work together to come up with the best alternative.

Reconstructive breast surgery usually requires more than one operation to insert a breast implant or form a breast using tissue from another part of the body and then to reconstruct the nipple and surrounding areola. Sometimes the surgeon also recommends reducing or enlarging the other breast to create better symmetry. Your surgeon will describe the different reconstructive options, including:

Skin Expansion

After your mastectomy, the surgeon will place a device called a balloon expander under your chest muscle. Over several weeks, he or she will inject a salt solution (saline) into the expander to gradually fill it. As the expander gets larger, the skin over your chest will expand enough to hold a permanent breast implant, which will be inserted in a subsequent operation. Some women do not need skin expansion before getting an implant.

Flap Reconstruction

In flap reconstruction, the surgeon makes a skin flap out of skin, fat, and muscle taken from another part of the body, such as the back, abdomen, or buttocks. The skin flap becomes either the pocket into which the implant is inserted, or the new breast itself. There are two types of skin flap surgery—a pedicle flap and a free flap. For a pedicle flap, the surgeon tunnels the borrowed tissue (usually from the abdomen), which retains its own blood supply, under the skin to the chest. For a free flap, the surgeon removes the tissue from the site of the graft and transplants it to the chest, connecting it to a new source of blood. Flap reconstruction is more complex than skin expansion and requires a longer recovery time.

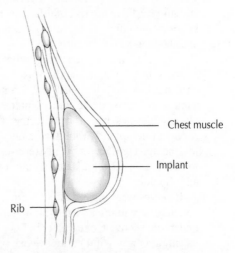

Breast reconstruction using an implant
Following a mastectomy, a saline implant may be inserted under the chest muscle to create a breast or to add bulk to a breast that has been reconstructed with a tissue flap taken from the back or abdomen. The nipple may be reconstructed using tissue from the woman's inner thigh.

The side effects of hormone therapy depend on the particular drug or type of treatment. Tamoxifen may cause hot flashes, vaginal discharge or irritation, nausea, and irregular periods. Women who are still menstruating may become pregnant more easily when taking tamoxifen. Tamoxifen increases the risk of endometrial cancer (see page 869). For this reason, your doctor will recommend regular pelvic exams and, if you are experiencing vaginal bleeding, endometrial biopsies (see page 849) to look for signs of possible cancer. Unlike tamoxifen, raloxifene does not appear to increase the risk of endometrial cancer.

Biological therapy

Newer medications called aromatase inhibitors are starting to replace tamoxifen or be given after the 5-year course of tamoxifen in the treatment of postmenopausal women who have late-stage breast tumors. Aromatase inhibitors such as letrozole, anastrozole, and exemestane block the action of an enzyme that is necessary for the body to produce estrogen. These drugs may also be effective in shrinking tumors before a woman has breast cancer surgery and in preventing breast cancers from recurring. Side effects can include hot flashes and night sweats and an increased risk of osteoporosis.

After Surgery

The risks of reconstructive breast surgery include bleeding, excessive scar tissue formation, and infection. As with any surgery, smokers face a longer healing time and more noticeable scarring. Some women experience capsular contracture, a tightening of the scar tissue around the breast implant, which causes the breast to feel unnaturally hard and may require corrective surgery. For now, out of uncertainty over the safety of silicone gel–filled implants, the Food and Drug Administration approves only saline-filled implants for use in breast reconstruction unless a woman is participating in a medical study.

The usual hospital stay for breast reconstruction is 2 to 5 days. You will probably feel pain and be very tired for the first 2 weeks after surgery. Your doctor will prescribe medication to relieve your discomfort. Stitches are usually removed in about a week to 10 days, and it may take up to 6 weeks to fully recover from the surgery. You probably will not have normal sensation in the reconstructed breast, although some feeling may return over time. By the second year after your surgery, your scars will fade substantially, but they will never disappear completely.

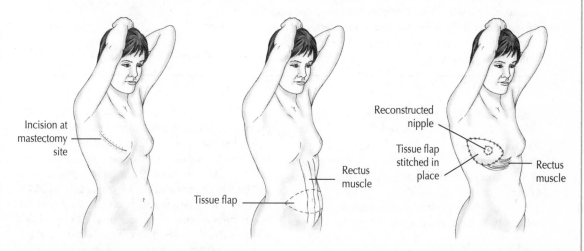

Breast reconstruction using abdominal tissue
For breast reconstruction after a mastectomy, the surgeon cuts out an area from the mastectomy site (left). He or she then cuts out a flap of tissue (including skin, muscle, fat, and attached blood vessels) from the abdomen (center) to use to create the new breast. With the blood vessels still intact, the tissue flap is tunneled up under the skin to the area of the mastectomy, guided out through the incision at the mastectomy site, and stitched in place on the chest (right). The abdominal (rectus) muscle and fat under the skin of the flap produce a natural-looking breast mound. A nipple may be reconstructed in later surgery.

A drug called trastuzumab (Herceptin) is used to treat breast cancer that has spread in women whose tumors produce an excessive amount of the protein associated with the HER2 gene. By blocking HER2, trastuzumab slows or stops the growth of the cancer cells. Trastuzumab is given by injection, either alone or in addition to chemotherapy.

The side effects of biological therapy depend on the substances used and can vary from person to person. Rashes or swelling at the site of the injection and flulike symptoms are common side effects. Trastuzumab can damage the heart, potentially leading to heart failure (see page 570), and can affect the lungs, causing breathing problems that require immediate medical attention. You will be monitored carefully during your treatment.

Experimental treatments

Even when a cancer has spread extensively from the breast, experimental treatments may be helpful for some women. One experimental biological treatment uses antibodies (immune proteins) that block the growth factor receptors on breast cancer cells, which prevents the cells from growing and multiplying. Many of these treatments are available through clinical trials. Ask your doctor about participating in a clinical trial.

Disorders of the Ovaries, Uterus, and Cervix

The two ovaries and the uterus make up the primary female reproductive organs. The ovaries sit on either side of the uterus, just above the pubic bone, and move freely within a small area. Each ovary contains thousands of eggs, which a woman is born with. During your fertile years, one egg (or sometimes more) ripens each month and is released into a fallopian tube. As the egg travels slowly down the tube toward the uterus, it can be fertilized by a sperm. The uterus lies in the pelvis, behind the bladder. The walls of the uterus consist of powerful muscles that contract to push out a baby during delivery. At the lower end of the uterus is a narrow, thick-walled structure called the cervix, which leads into the vagina.

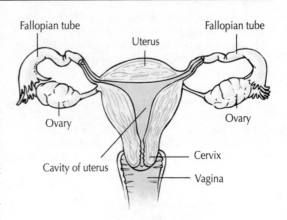

The female reproductive system

Ovarian Cysts

An ovarian cyst is a sac full of fluid that forms on or in an ovary. Most ovarian cysts are harmless and go away on their own within a couple of months. Others can interfere with the ovary's production of sex hormones or become cancerous; for this reason, all cysts should be evaluated by a doctor. Ovarian cysts are common in women of childbearing age and are usually caused by the changing hormone levels that naturally occur during the menstrual cycle. Ovarian cysts can range from the size of a pea to the size of a grapefruit. A woman may develop one cyst at a time or many. Multiple cysts that form repeatedly month after month characterize a disorder called polycystic ovarian syndrome (see next page).

The most common types of ovarian cysts are functional cysts, dermoid cysts, and endometri-omas. Functional cysts form when tissue in the ovary changes during the normal process of ovulation. There are two kinds of functional cysts: follicular and corpus luteum cysts. Follicular cysts develop when the matured follicle containing an egg fails to rupture and release the egg. Instead, the follicle grows larger and becomes a cyst. Functional cysts usually disappear on their own after a few menstrual cycles. The corpus luteum is a normal glandular mass that develops in an ovary every month after the mature follicle releases an egg. The corpus luteum can develop into a cyst if the opening through which the egg is released is sealed off. A corpus luteum cyst usually dissolves on its own within a few months.

Dermoid cysts are composed of different types of tissues—such as skin, hair, fat, and teeth—that are normally found in other parts of the body. Endometriomas are blood-filled cysts that develop when tissue from the endometrium (the lining of the uterus) grows in an ovary. Endometriomas can bleed during menstruation and are signs of endometriosis (see page 870).

Symptoms

Ovarian cysts seldom produce symptoms but may cause a dull ache in the lower abdomen, and pain during intercourse. Some cysts twist, bleed, or rupture, causing sudden sharp pain and internal bleeding, which is life-threatening. When a cyst affects hormone production, symptoms include irregular vaginal bleeding or an increase in body hair.

Common Ovarian Cysts

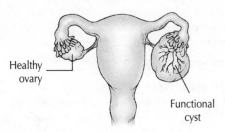

Healthy ovary

Functional cyst

Functional cyst
The most common type of functional cyst occurs when an egg matures but the follicle fails to rupture and release it. The follicle continues to grow, enlarging the entire ovary. This type of cyst usually goes away on its own after one or two menstrual cycles.

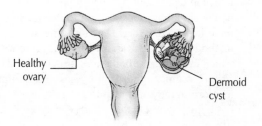

Healthy ovary

Dermoid cyst

Dermoid cyst
A dermoid cyst is made up of tissue—such as skin, hair, fat, and teeth—that is usually found in other parts of the body. Dermoid cysts are usually not cancerous, but doctors remove them for testing to make sure.

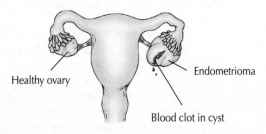

Healthy ovary

Endometrioma

Blood clot in cyst

Endometrioma
Endometriomas are blood-filled cysts that develop when tissue from the endometrium (the lining of the uterus) grows in the ovary. Endometriomas that cause symptoms can be removed surgically.

Diagnosis

Some ovarian cysts are found during a routine pelvic examination. To find out what type of cyst you have, your doctor will probably order a pelvic and vaginal ultrasound to examine your ovaries. If the ultrasound shows an abnormality, the doctor may perform an outpatient surgical procedure called laparoscopy, using a lighted viewing instrument inserted through a tiny incision in your abdomen to examine the pelvic cavity. Depending on your risk factors, the doctor may recommend genetic testing (see page 953) for other diseases, such as ovarian cancer.

Treatment

Most ovarian cysts require no treatment. In many cases, the ultrasound shows a cyst that is obviously benign. You will need only regular follow-up pelvic examinations and ultrasounds until it goes away on its own. If a cyst is large or is causing symptoms, it can be treated with hormone therapy or surgery, depending on the size and type of cyst, your age, and your desire to have children. Doctors sometimes treat functional cysts with oral contraceptives. Large, solid, or persistent cysts are usually removed surgically. Sometimes a cyst can be removed without affecting the ovary, but if the cyst is very large, the only way to ensure complete removal may be to take out the entire ovary and, in some cases, the fallopian tube as well. Women can usually get pregnant with only one ovary and one fallopian tube.

Polycystic Ovarian Syndrome

Polycystic ovarian syndrome is a condition characterized by the presence of multiple small ovarian cysts that do not go away on their own, as do most ovarian cysts. The disorder is relatively common, affecting 5 to 10 percent of all women. Because most women with polycystic ovarian syndrome see their doctor primarily when they are having irregular periods or seeking infertility treatment (see page 498), many doctors consider the syndrome a gynecologic disorder.

However, polycystic ovarian syndrome is recognized as a complication of insulin resistance, a condition in which the body must produce abnormally high amounts of insulin to regulate blood sugar. The high levels of insulin, in turn, stimulate the ovaries to produce too much testosterone and other male sex hormones (androgens), which brings on the disorder's characteristic symptoms (see below). Polycystic ovarian syndrome is thought to be a form of metabolic syndrome (also called prediabetes; see page 53) with a strong link to type 2 diabetes (see page 894) and heart disease (see page 558).

The disorder usually appears in late childhood, around the time of puberty, and lasts throughout an affected woman's life. Although the precise cause is not known, polycystic ovarian syndrome tends to run in families.

Symptoms

In addition to having multiple ovarian cysts, women with polycystic ovarian syndrome have no menstrual periods or irregular periods because they fail to ovulate. The failure to ovulate makes them infertile. Elevated levels of androgens result from the abnormally high amount of insulin circulating in the blood. The excess androgen production can cause acne and excess hair growth on the face and body. Most affected women are overweight and tend to carry their weight around the abdomen.

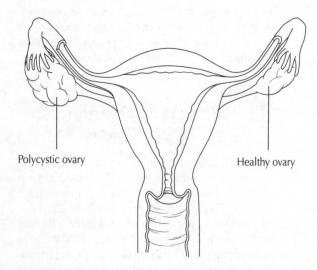

Polycystic ovarian syndrome
The ovaries of women with polycystic ovarian syndrome contain multiple small cysts that never disappear. The cysts are caused by overproduction of male hormones by the ovaries and adrenal glands. This overproduction of male hormones is stimulated by excessively high levels of the hormone insulin.

Diagnosis

Polycystic ovarian syndrome can mimic a number of other disorders, such as adrenal gland problems and thyroid disease, so a doctor will first try to rule these out when making a diagnosis. He or she will diagnose polycystic ovarian syndrome by the presence of its characteristic symptoms, along with a blood test to detect abnormally high levels of testosterone. An ultrasound of the pelvis usually shows enlarged ovaries with many small cysts.

Treatment

Many women who seek treatment for missed periods or infertility caused by polycystic ovarian syndrome receive treatment for these symptoms only. Doctors often prescribe oral contraceptives to regulate a woman's menstrual cycles and suppress the production of testosterone (to reduce symptoms such as excessive hair growth). Other drugs may be prescribed to stimulate ovulation if a woman wants to become pregnant. The best long-term treatment, however, addresses the insulin resistance that underlies the disorder. The most effective drug for treating polycystic ovarian syndrome is metformin, which improves the body's use of insulin and helps restore regular menstrual cycles and ovulation. Metformin may also help lower a woman's risk of developing type 2 diabetes and heart disease later in life.

Ovarian Cancer

Cancer of the ovary is one of the leading causes of death from cancer in women. Although ovarian cancer can occur at any age, it is most common after age 50. The cancer can originate in the ovary or appear as a secondary growth that has spread to the ovary from elsewhere in the body. Mutations in the BRCA1 and BRCA2 genes (see page 858) increase a woman's risk of both breast and ovarian cancer. In women without these genetic mutations, the cause of ovarian cancer is not known.

Several factors can increase a woman's chances of developing ovarian cancer. Risk factors include having a close relative (mother, sister, or daughter) with the disorder, or a personal history of breast cancer or colon cancer. Ovarian cancer seems to be related to the number of times a woman ovulates during her lifetime, with the risk of the disease lower in women who have ovulated less, such as women who have taken birth-control pills. For this reason, women who have never had children (and, therefore, never had a 9-month break from ovulation) and women who have taken fertility drugs (which stimulate ovulation) may be at increased risk. Conversely, women who have taken birth-control pills (and, therefore, have ovulated fewer times) have a significantly lower risk of developing ovarian cancer than other women.

Symptoms

Ovarian cancer often produces no symptoms until late in its development. Eventually, it may cause lower abdominal pain or discomfort, including gas, indigestion, swelling, bloating, or cramps. The first sign may be the feeling that your clothes are getting tighter around your waistline for no obvious reason. Appetite loss, frequent urination, and nausea accompanied by diarrhea or constipation are common. You may also have a feeling of fullness even after light meals.

Diagnosis

Ovarian cancer is difficult to detect in its early stages because the ovaries lie deep inside the pelvis and initial symptoms are vague. If you have any symptoms of ovarian cancer, or if you have a family history of breast cancer or ovarian cancer, your doctor will order an ultrasound to examine your ovaries. If the ultrasound shows multiple cysts on your ovaries, or solid growths containing abnormal tissue (which could indicate cancer), the doctor will do further tests. A blood test that measures the levels of a substance called CA-125 (CA stands for cancer antigen), which is found in high amounts in women with ovarian cancer, can be useful in detecting the disorder in women who are past menopause. In younger women, mildly elevated levels of CA-125 can be present in many noncancerous conditions such as fibroids (see right), endometriosis (see page 870), or pelvic inflammatory disease (see page 871).

Sometimes doctors use a series of X-rays of the colon and rectum (a lower GI series; see page 767) or a CT scan (see page 112) to detect ovarian cancer.

Treatment

If tests detect ovarian cancer, surgery is usually necessary to remove both ovaries, the fallopian tubes, and the uterus (hysterectomy; see page 870). Any cancerous tissue inside the abdomen that may have spread from the ovary and affected lymph glands will also be removed to make sure that no cancer cells remain. Chemotherapy (see page 23) is usually given to kill cancer cells throughout the body and prevent the cancer from recurring or slow its progression (if it has already begun to spread). In rare cases, radiation therapy (see page 23) is used to destroy localized areas of cancer. Blood tests are performed periodically to monitor the effects of the chemotherapy. Any fluid from the tumor that collects in the abdomen can be drained from time to time. The outlook for survival depends on the stage of the disease at the time of diagnosis—generally, the earlier the stage at diagnosis, the better the survival rate. Receiving treatment from a doctor who specializes in gynecologic cancers (called a gynecologic oncologist) can significantly improve a woman's chances of survival.

Some women who are at high risk of ovarian cancer choose to have their ovaries removed before cancer develops. This procedure usually—but not always—protects a woman from ovarian cancer.

Fibroids

A fibroid (also called a myoma) is a benign (noncancerous) tumor in the uterus that can grow large but is unlikely to spread. The tumor develops either inside the muscular wall of the uterus or on the uterine wall, sometimes attached to the wall by a stalk of tissue. Some fibroids take many years to grow to the size of a pea, while others may reach the size of a grapefruit within a few years.

Fibroids are common—up to 30 percent of women over age 30 have them. Fibroids seldom occur before age 20 and are most common between ages 35 and 45. If you have one fibroid, you are likely to develop others. After menopause, the reduction in the level of estrogen often causes fibroids to shrink.

Symptoms and Diagnosis

Most women with fibroids have no symptoms, especially if the fibroids are small. Other women experience heavy bleeding, discomfort or pain in the pelvis, or pressure on nearby organs. Fibroids that lie just under the lining of the uterus can cause excessive blood loss from heavy periods, which can

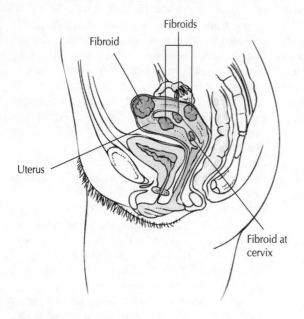

Fibroid
Fibroids
Uterus
Fibroid at cervix

Uterine fibroids
A fibroid is a noncancerous tumor that develops inside the uterus. Uterine fibroids are very common—up to 30 percent of all women have fibroids at some time in their life.

lead to iron deficiency anemia (see page 610). Fibroids under the uterine lining can cause infertility by taking up space that a fertilized egg could use to implant successfully in the uterine wall. Occasionally, a fibroid enlarges rapidly during pregnancy, causing pain, miscarriage, or obstruction during delivery.

A doctor can often detect a fibroid during a routine pelvic examination. He or she can confirm the diagnosis with an ultrasound scan (see page 111), MRI (see page 113), or CT scan (see page 112).

Treatment

Small fibroids that don't cause symptoms do not require treatment. Pain relievers such as ibuprofen can help relieve minor discomfort. If fibroids cause abnormal bleeding, the bleeding can often be controlled with oral contraceptives.

If you have symptoms and you eventually plan to become pregnant, your doctor may recommend a procedure called myomectomy. In myomectomy, the doctor removes the fibroids but leaves the uterus intact. Myomectomy carries a slightly

increased risk of bleeding and, if a woman becomes pregnant after myomectomy, she is more likely to have a cesarean delivery (see page 534).

Women who are no longer planning a pregnancy may choose to have a procedure called endometrial ablation, in which low-voltage heat is applied to the lining of the uterus to permanently block its growth. In cases of severe bleeding or when fibroids grow large enough to cause distortion of the abdomen, a doctor may recommend a hysterectomy (see page 870), in which the uterus is surgically removed.

Endometrial Hyperplasia

Endometrial hyperplasia is a condition in which the lining of the uterus (the endometrium) becomes overly thick and does not shed as it normally does during menstruation. The disorder usually develops when ovulation is not regular, such as in women who are approaching or who are past menopause. Endometrial tissue builds up and can harbor abnormal cells, which can eventually become cancerous. Doctors consider endometrial hyperplasia a precancerous condition caused by the presence of too much estrogen, which can occur in women taking estrogen in hormone therapy (see page 853) without the counterbalancing hormone progesterone.

Endometrial hyperplasia occurs in stages. The mild stages are usually noncancerous, but they need to be treated to prevent them from developing into severe hyperplasia, in which suspicious, abnormal cells can develop into cancer of the uterus (see next page).

Symptoms and Diagnosis

In women of childbearing age, a common sign of endometrial hyperplasia is irregular or heavy periods. The most common symptom after menopause is abnormal vaginal bleeding.

To diagnose endometrial hyperplasia, a doctor takes a sample of endometrial tissue from the uterus for examination under a microscope. This procedure, called endometrial biopsy (see page 849), is done in the doctor's office. Tissue samples can also be taken during a hysteroscopy (see page 849) or a D and C (see next page).

Treatment

If you have missed two consecutive periods and are definitely not pregnant, your doctor will probably recommend inducing a period by prescribing the hormone progesterone to take for 10 days to stimulate the endometrium to shed. If you have endometrial hyperplasia, your doctor will prescribe birth-control pills or progesterone supplements to stimulate shedding of the uterine lining. Surgical removal of the uterus (hysterectomy; see next page) is usually used only for treating severe hyperplasia that recurs after prolonged treatment with progesterone. If your doctor recommends a hysterectomy, you may want to get a second opinion from another doctor.

D and C

In a D and C (dilation and curettage), the lining of the uterus is surgically removed to terminate a pregnancy, treat an incomplete abortion or miscarriage, or determine the cause of frequent or heavy periods. During the procedure, you will probably be sedated and receive some other form of anesthesia. The doctor will gradually widen your cervical opening so he or she can insert instruments to remove the tissue from the uterus with suction or with gentle scraping; the tissue is then examined under a microscope. A D and C is often combined with another procedure called hysteroscopy (see page 849), in which a viewing instrument is inserted through the cervix to enable the doctor to see the exact location of any abnormal tissue. Hysteroscopy can also be used to remove a lost IUD.

A D and C usually takes about 15 minutes. You should be able to go home the same day or the next morning. You will probably have vaginal bleeding for a few days and may have some pelvic and back pain. To reduce the risk of infection, avoid having intercourse or using tampons for 2 weeks (or for as long as your doctor recommends). You can resume most other activities after a few days.

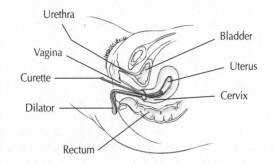

D and C
During a D and C, a doctor inserts instruments called dilators to open up the cervix and inserts an instrument called a curette to gently scrape away the lining of the uterus.

Cancer of the Uterus

Most cancers of the uterus start in the endometrium (the lining of the uterus). After growing in the lining, the cancer can invade the wall of the uterus and, if not treated, spread to the fallopian tubes, ovaries, nearby lymph glands, and other organs. The precise cause of uterine cancer is not known, but it appears to be related to excessive exposure to the hormone estrogen, which can occur in women who have never been pregnant or who have taken the hormone estrogen in hormone therapy (see page 853) for many years without the counterbalancing hormone progesterone. Other risk factors include obesity (because obese women have higher levels of circulating estrogen), diabetes (see page 889), and high blood pressure (see page 574). In a small number of women, cancer of the uterus is caused by a mutation in a gene that also predisposes them to colon, breast, and ovarian cancer.

Cancer of the uterus occurs most often between ages 50 and 70 and is more common in whites than in blacks. Uterine cancer is less likely to be fatal than most other gynecologic cancers because it tends to grow very slowly and it is easier to diagnose at an early stage.

Symptoms

The most common symptom of uterine cancer is abnormal vaginal bleeding. The most obvious symptom of uterine cancer is vaginal bleeding in a woman who has gone through menopause and who has not had periods for some time. Women who are still menstruating may have unusually heavy periods or bleeding between periods. A woman may also have a vaginal discharge that ranges from a watery, pink fluid to a thick, brown, foul-smelling discharge. Uterine cancer may or may not cause intermittent pain similar to menstrual pain.

Diagnosis

If you have any irregular vaginal bleeding, your doctor will perform an endometrial biopsy (see page 849) to take a sample of endometrial tissue from the uterus for examination under a microscope. This procedure is done in the doctor's office, takes only a few minutes, and produces only minor, temporary discomfort. A doctor may also perform a hysteroscopy (see page 849) or a D and C (see left) to diagnose cancer of the uterus.

Treatment

When cancer of the uterus is confirmed, the standard treatment is surgical removal of the uterus, along with the ovaries and fallopian tubes, in a hysterectomy (see below). Radiation therapy (see page 23) and sometimes chemotherapy (see page 23) may be used instead of—or in addition to—surgery. If the cancer is detected at an early stage, your chances for a complete recovery are excellent. About 80 percent of women who are treated in the early stages of uterine cancer are cured.

Hysterectomy

The uterus, sometimes along with the ovaries and fallopian tubes, are removed to treat several different gynecologic disorders, especially in women who are at or near menopause. Because there may be other ways of treating a particular disorder, you may want to get a second opinion from another doctor before deciding to have a hysterectomy.

In the most commonly used method of hysterectomy, the surgeon removes the uterus through an incision in the lower abdomen. Alternatively, the surgeon may make the incision at the top of the vagina and remove the uterus from below. A woman usually is given a general or spinal anesthetic for the surgery, which takes about 1 to 2 hours.

After a hysterectomy, you may experience some vaginal bleeding and discharge for a few days. Your doctor will encourage you to get out of bed and walk around a little the day after the surgery, and you can probably go home in a few days. You should be able to resume your usual activities within 6 to 8 weeks. Removal of the ovaries in a woman who has not yet reached menopause stops estrogen production and brings about early menopause. In this case, the doctor may recommend taking estrogen supplements (hormone therapy; see page 853).

Endometriosis

The lining of the uterus is called the endometrium. During each menstrual cycle, part of the endometrium thickens, becomes engorged with blood, and (if conception does not occur) sheds during menstruation. Endometriosis causes the same kind of tissue to develop in other parts of the pelvic cavity—such as on the ovaries or (less commonly) on the fallopian tubes, vagina, or intestines. The endometrial tissue can also develop on scars that have formed in the abdominal wall after surgery. Each month, these abnormal endometrial tissue fragments bleed like the lining of the uterus does during menstruation. However, because the fragments are embedded in tissue, the blood cannot escape. Instead, the blood collects in sacs (cysts), or the bleeding irritates the surrounding tissue, which responds by forming a fibrous covering around each bleeding area. Over time, scar tissue (adhesions) can develop.

In its mild form, endometriosis is common. Because endometriosis is linked to menstruation, it occurs only during a woman's reproductive years, most often between ages 25 and 50. Endometriosis is most common in women who have not had children. After the onset of menopause, the development of the abnormal endometrial tissue subsides.

Symptoms and Diagnosis

In some cases, endometriosis causes no symptoms or only mild or unnoticeable symptoms. In most cases, symptoms include pain in the lower abdomen or lower back just before periods. Sometimes periods are irregular, with spotting before the flow begins. Intercourse may be painful. Endometriosis can cause infertility if the fallopian tubes become blocked by scarring.

The most common diagnostic procedure used to detect endometriosis is laparoscopy, an outpatient surgical procedure in which the doctor uses a lighted viewing instrument (laparoscope) to see inside the pelvic cavity.

Treatment

Mild cases of endometriosis that don't cause symptoms do not require treatment. If symptoms are severe, doctors frequently remove the abnormal tissue during laparoscopy by cutting it out or destroying it with heat. The doctor may take a sample of tissue at this time for examination under a microscope to look for cancer cells (biopsy). Your doctor may prescribe daily treatment with hormones or hormonelike drugs for several months to suppress the growth of the abnormal tissue.

If endometriosis affects the ovaries, the treatment is the same as that for an ovarian cyst (see page 865) such as hormone therapy or surgery. In severe cases that do not respond to hormone therapy or surgical treatment, a doctor may recommend

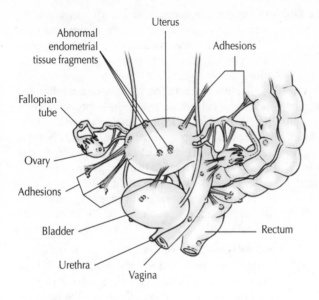

Uterus

Abnormal
endometrial
tissue fragments

Adhesions

Fallopian
tube

Ovary

Adhesions

Bladder

Rectum

Urethra

Vagina

Endometriosis

Endometriosis causes fragments of endometrial tissue to grow on organs such as the bladder, ovaries, and fallopian tubes in the pelvic cavity. These abnormal tissue fragments bleed each month, as does the endometrial lining of the uterus during menstruation. The persistent irritation caused by the repeated bleeding can produce scar tissue called adhesions, which stretch across and bind the organs inside the pelvic cavity, including the intestines. Adhesions can distort and twist the fallopian tubes, causing infertility.

a hysterectomy (see previous page) to remove the uterus, the fallopian tubes, and the ovaries.

Trophoblastic Tumors

Trophoblastic tumors (often called hydatidiform moles) are a rare type of growth in the placenta that may occur during or after pregnancy. (The placenta is the organ that develops in the uterus during pregnancy and links the blood supplies of the pregnant woman and fetus.) Trophoblastic tumors can also develop in placental tissue left in the uterus after childbirth or a miscarriage. Trophoblastic tumors are usually benign (noncancerous). Occasionally, however, they may invade the wall of the uterus or spread to other parts of the body.

Symptoms

The main symptoms of a trophoblastic tumor are irregular vaginal bleeding, nausea, and vomiting during or after a pregnancy or after termination of a

pregnancy. See your doctor right away if you have any of these symptoms.

Diagnosis

If you have symptoms of a trophoblastic tumor, your doctor may order an ultrasound of the uterus. A trophoblastic tumor causes excessive production of the pregnancy hormone human chorionic gonadotropin (HCG), which is normally made by the cells of the placenta during pregnancy. HCG passes into the blood and can easily be detected in the same blood test that is used for confirming a pregnancy (see page 504).

Treatment

If a trophoblastic tumor is present in your uterus, your doctor will remove the growth surgically during a D and C (see page 869). No further treatment is necessary for a benign tumor, other than frequent checkups and blood tests (to check for HCG) for a year to make sure the tumor has not recurred. Your doctor will recommend that you avoid pregnancy during this time; he or she may prescribe oral contraceptives or another reliable form of birth control.

If the tumor is malignant, the doctor may recommend chemotherapy (see page 23), perhaps in addition to a hysterectomy (see previous page). You may have chemotherapy after a hysterectomy to prevent the cancer from spreading and to kill any cancer cells that have spread. After this treatment you will need to have regular checkups. Your chances for a complete cure are good.

Pelvic Inflammatory Disease

Pelvic inflammatory disease (PID) occurs when bacteria or viruses infect the uterus and spread to the fallopian tubes, ovaries, and surrounding tissues. The infection is usually introduced through the vagina during sexual intercourse with an infected person. The sexually transmitted diseases chlamydia (see page 477) and gonorrhea (see page 480) are very common causes of PID. Pelvic infections are most common in young, sexually active women and least common in women who have reached menopause. If the infection is not treated, an abscess (a pus-filled sac) may form in a fallopian tube or ovary, causing scarring and potentially damaging the fallopian tubes. Blockage of the fallopian tubes from the infection can cause infertility (see page 493).

Symptoms

An acute or sudden pelvic infection causes severe pain and tenderness in the lower abdomen and may also cause a high fever. A chronic pelvic infection may cause mild, recurring pain in the lower abdomen and sometimes pain in the back, along with a low-grade fever. In both acute and chronic forms of PID, you may experience pain during intercourse, have irregular periods, and have a heavy, foul-smelling vaginal discharge.

Diagnosis

To diagnose PID, a doctor will perform a pelvic examination and take samples of fluid from inside the cervix. Laboratory analysis of this fluid will help identify the infectious organism that is causing the condition. He or she will also order an ultrasound (see page 111) to look for an abscess around the ovary.

Treatment

Antibiotics are the first treatment for PID; in severe cases, antibiotics are given intravenously (through a vein) in the hospital. If antibiotics do not clear up the infection, or if an abscess shows no signs of shrinking, a doctor may perform a laparoscopic procedure (through a small incision in the abdomen) to remove as much of the infected tissue as possible. Recovery and fertility both depend on the extent of the infection and the surgery required to treat it.

Pelvic Support Problems

The uterus, vagina, and other lower abdominal organs are held in place by strong pelvic muscles and ligaments at the base of the abdomen. If these supporting muscles and ligaments are weakened, they can no longer support organs in the pelvis (such as the bladder, urethra, uterus, vagina, small intestine, and rectum), causing the organs to slip from their original position. Pelvic floor muscles can become stretched and weakened by a number of factors, including injury during vaginal delivery, loss of muscle tone that can accompany aging,

decreased estrogen production after menopause, chronic constipation (which causes straining during bowel movements), a chronic respiratory condition (which can cause persistent coughing), or lifting heavy objects.

The uterus, bladder, rectum, and urethra are especially vulnerable to sagging or prolapse when pelvic floor muscles become weakened. Minor degrees of prolapse are common, especially for a few months after childbirth and later in life. A prolapse can be uncomfortable and inconvenient but poses few risks to your overall health.

Following are some of the most common types of pelvic support problems, which often occur together:

- **Prolapse of the uterus** When the uterus drops from its normal position, it sags downward. This process causes a bulging of the front or back wall of the vagina. Sometimes the uterus may descend so far that the cervix or even the entire uterus bulges out of the body (called a complete prolapse). The displacement of the uterus often brings other pelvic organs, such as the bladder or intestines, down with it.
- **Cystocele** A cystocele occurs when the bottom of the bladder drops into the front of the vagina.
- **Cystourethrocele** A cystourethrocele results from the weakening of the tissues supporting the urethra and bladder.
- **Enterocele** An enterocele forms when a part of the intestine bulges into the top of the vagina.
- **Rectocele** A rectocele is the bulging of the rectum into the vagina.
- **Vaginal vault prolapse** Vaginal vault prolapse occurs when the top part of the vagina (called the vaginal vault) loses its support from the uterus after a hysterectomy (see page 870) and collapses.

Symptoms

The involuntary leaking of urine may be the first sign of a pelvic support problem. A cystourethrocele often causes stress incontinence (see page 877). You may feel a sensation of heaviness and discomfort in your pelvis and an ache in your lower back, especially after lifting or otherwise straining your muscles. If the condition has progressed, and if the back wall of the vagina has descended, bowel movements can be difficult. A large rectocele may

Prolapse of the Uterus

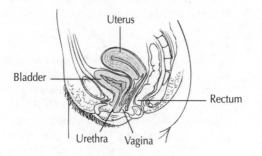

Normal position of uterus

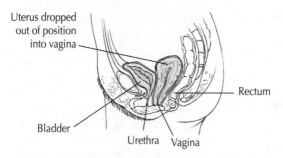

Prolapsed uterus

Prolapsed uterus

One of the most common pelvic support problems is prolapse of the uterus, in which the uterus drops from its normal position into the vagina. The uterus may drop part of the way into the vagina or protrude completely outside the vagina. Prolapse of the uterus can be corrected surgically.

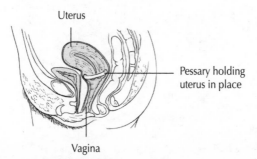

Prolapsed uterus supported by a pessary

A pessary is a rubber or plastic device worn inside the vagina to keep a prolapsed uterus in place. A pessary is a good option for women whose prolapse is not severe and who do not want or cannot have surgery for medical reasons. A pessary is not likely to provide enough support to keep a severely prolapsed uterus in place.

make it difficult to empty the bowels completely. In severe cases, a lump or bulge may protrude outside the vagina. Constipation (see page 769), hemorrhoids (see page 777), and urinary incontinence sometimes accompany pelvic support problems. In severe cases, the pressure from the slipping of the bladder in a cystocele may make urination difficult.

Diagnosis

To diagnose a pelvic support problem, a doctor will perform a thorough pelvic examination. He or she may be able to see or feel one or more of the pelvic organs displaced from their usual position.

Treatment

To treat pelvic support problems, doctors sometimes prescribe a device called a pessary, which is inserted into the vagina to temporarily or permanently hold the uterus in place. Pessaries come in many shapes and sizes and must be fitted for each woman. They have to be cleaned periodically by the doctor and can sometimes cause irritation.

Most pelvic support problems can be corrected with surgery. If uterine prolapse is caused by a large fibroid in your uterus or by supporting tissue that has become severely stretched after multiple vaginal deliveries, your doctor may recommend a hysterectomy (see page 870). During the hysterectomy, your doctor can tighten any sagging of the vaginal walls, bladder, or supporting ligaments. A surgical procedure called an anterior repair can lift and support a sagging bladder. Surgery usually produces excellent results, but prolapse may recur, requiring treatment again.

An alternative treatment to surgery is electrical stimulation of the pelvic floor muscles, which you can give yourself at home over several weeks. A small device inserted into the vagina stimulates the pelvic muscles and causes them to contract, making them stronger.

Exercises called Kegel exercises (see next page) can also help strengthen the pelvic floor muscles after a prolapse. If you are overweight, shedding some pounds may help prevent further prolapse. Eating a high-fiber diet or taking a natural stool softener will help keep you from straining during bowel movements. Avoid heavy lifting. If you smoke, quit, to avoid having a chronic cough, which puts stress on the pelvic floor muscles.

Kegel Exercises

Pelvic floor exercises called Kegel exercises can both prevent and treat pelvic support problems. Doing these simple exercises every day can improve your bladder control and strengthen your vaginal muscles. You can do Kegel exercises at home or at work whenever you have a few free moments.

To do them, alternately contract and relax the muscles around the opening of your vagina as though you were trying to interrupt the flow of urine. Hold each contraction for 3 seconds and gradually work up to 10 seconds. Repeat each contraction 10 times. Try to do a set of 10 contractions 10 times a day for the best results.

Cervical Dysplasia

Cervical dysplasia describes the presence of abnormal, precancerous cells on the surface of the cervix or its canal. Doctors recognize two types of dysplasia: low-grade squamous intraepithelial lesions (LGSIL) and high-grade squamous intraepithelial lesions (HGSIL). The abnormal cells present in LGSIL usually return to normal on their own within 18 to 24 months, but the HGSIL cells, if not treated, can progress to cancer of the cervix (see next page). To detect these changes early, it is essential to have regular Pap smears (see page 140).

Cervical dysplasia can occur at any age after puberty but is most common between ages 25 and 35. The condition has been linked to exposure to specific strains of the human papillomavirus (HPV), which causes genital warts (see page 480). The risk of cervical dysplasia is increased in women who have multiple sex partners, who had unprotected sex at a young age (under 18) or with partners who have had multiple partners, who have a history of sexually transmitted diseases, or who smoke cigarettes.

Symptoms and Diagnosis

Cervical dysplasia often produces no symptoms, but some women have bleeding or spotting after intercourse. Abnormal cells in the cervix are usually found on a routine Pap smear. To confirm the diagnosis after an abnormal Pap smear, a doctor will perform a colposcopy, an examination of the cervix using an instrument with a lighted magnifying lens. Doctors often take a sample of tissue for analysis under a microscope (biopsy) during a colposcopy to determine if dysplasia is present and, if so, to evaluate it and classify it as LGSIL or

HGSIL. Some doctors also take a swab of cells from the cervix to determine if HPV is present and, if so, if it is one of the strains of the virus that are strongly linked to cervical cancer.

Treatment

LGSIL (mild) dysplasia often returns to normal on its own and usually can be managed with frequent follow-up care, including Pap smears every 4 to 6 months. More severe dysplasia (HGSIL), which is more likely to develop into cervical cancer, is usually treated surgically. The procedure doctors use most often to treat dysplasia is called by either of two names—LEEP (loop electrosurgical excision procedure) or LLETZ (large-loop excision of the transformation zone). Both names refer to the removal of the outer layer of cervical cells, which are at highest risk of becoming cancerous. The removed tissue is sent to a laboratory for examination to make sure that all the abnormal cells were removed. Your doctor will advise you not to have intercourse or use tampons for 4 weeks after the procedure. The doctor will recommend a Pap smear every 4 months for the first year after a colposcopy, which has a 95 percent success rate in removing abnormal tissue.

If the area of abnormal tissue extends up into

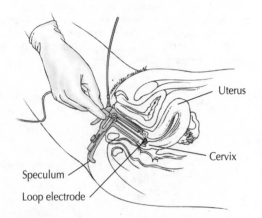

Uterus

Cervix

Speculum

Loop electrode

LEEP/LLETZ
The procedure doctors use most often to treat cervical dysplasia is called by one of two names, LEEP (loop electrosurgical excision procedure) or LLETZ (large-loop excision of the transformation zone). During the procedure, the doctor inserts a rubber-coated, nonconductive speculum to hold open the vagina and then uses a thin-wire, loop electrode to slice off the abnormal tissue with a low-level electric current. LEEP/LLETZ takes less than 30 minutes and requires only a local anesthetic.

the cervical canal, a procedure called a cone biopsy (in which the doctor removes a cone-shaped piece of tissue) may be required. The tissue is sent to a laboratory to look for cancer cells. This procedure is usually performed in an operating room using a local anesthetic during an outpatient visit. Afterward, you may need to rest for a day or so. In very rare cases, a cone biopsy can increase the risk of premature delivery in a future pregnancy, so if you have had a cone biopsy and become pregnant, tell your doctor that you have had the procedure.

Cancer of the Cervix

Cervical cancer occurs when abnormal cells on the outer layer of the cervix (the lower opening of the uterus) spread deep into the tissues of the cervix, or to nearby lymph glands, and up into the uterus. Most cases of cervical cancer develop in women who have either undiagnosed or untreated cervical dysplasia (see previous page) or its more advanced form, called carcinoma in situ. Cervical dysplasia refers to the presence of abnormal, precancerous cells in the lining of the cervix.

Deaths from cervical cancer have declined sharply, thanks to the prevalence of Pap smears (see page 140). Cancer of the cervix is nearly 100 percent preventable if cervical dysplasia is detected by a Pap smear in its early stages. The majority of women who are diagnosed with cervical cancer have not had a Pap smear within the past 3 years. The more advanced the cancer, the more difficult it is to treat—which makes the Pap smear a potential lifesaver.

Some factors increase the chances that cells in the lining of the cervix will become abnormal or cancerous. The most important risk factor is exposure to certain strains of the human papillomavirus (HPV), which can cause the common sexually transmitted disease genital warts (see page 480). Other risk factors include having sex at a young age, having unprotected sex at any age, having multiple sex partners, or having a sex partner who has had multiple partners or who has had a partner with HPV or cervical cancer. Smoking is also a risk factor for cervical cancer. Women whose mothers were given the drug diethylstilbestrol (DES) during pregnancy to prevent miscarriage also have an increased risk of developing cervical or vaginal cancer. Taking drugs, such as cancer drugs, that suppress the immune system, or being HIV-positive (which weakens the immune system)

also raises a woman's risk. Smoking also seems to increase a woman's risk of cervical cancer, but doctors are not sure exactly why.

Symptoms
The main symptom of cervical cancer is abnormal vaginal bleeding that can occur between periods, after intercourse, or after menopause. A watery, bloody discharge, which can be heavy and foul-smelling, is another common symptom. Advanced cases of cervical cancer can cause pelvic pain and back pain.

Diagnosis
If you have an abnormal Pap smear, your doctor may want to do another Pap smear and compare the results or perform some other tests, depending on the degree of abnormality found on the Pap smear. If the doctor can see an abnormality directly, he or she will take a sample of tissue from your cervix for laboratory examination for cancer cells (biopsy).

Doctors often use a procedure called colposcopy, an examination of the cervix using a lighted viewing instrument, to check the cervix for abnormal tissue. Doctors usually take a sample of tissue for analysis under a microscope (biopsy) during a colposcopy to look for cancer cells and to evaluate the stage of the cancer. Another common biopsy procedure is called LEEP/LLETZ (see previous page). If these tests do not clearly show whether abnormal cells have spread beyond the surface of the cervix, the doctor may perform a cone biopsy, in which a cone-shaped sample of tissue is taken from the cervical canal and sent to a laboratory for analysis.

Treatment
Chances are extremely good that cervical cancer can be cured if the cancer has not spread beyond the cervix. In fact, the outlook for cervical cancer is much better than that for most other cancers. Your doctor will discuss the risks and benefits of each form of treatment with you before you choose the best course. Cervical cancer is usually treated with surgery to remove abnormal tissue in or near the cervix. If the cancer is found only on the surface of the cervix or confined to the cervix, a doctor may treat it with a cone biopsy or a hysterectomy (see page 870). Radiation therapy (see page 23) is frequently given along with chemotherapy (see page 23), which helps improve the effectiveness of the radiation.

Even if your reproductive organs are left intact, radiation therapy will probably disrupt your menstrual cycle; you may experience some symptoms of menopause. During radiation treatment and for a few months after radiation therapy, you may have diarrhea and difficulty retaining urine. Long-term radiation therapy may eventually obstruct the ureters (the tubes that connect the kidneys to the bladder), possibly leading to kidney failure. Make sure you have all the follow-up checkups that your doctor recommends to avoid these potential complications.

Cervical Polyps

A cervical polyp is a small, grapelike growth on a stalk that hangs from the lining of the cervix. Polyps usually are single and tiny but can grow to about an inch in length. The exact cause of cervical polyps is unknown, but they are linked to inflammation of the cervix and frequently accompany a chronic infection of the vagina or cervix. They are not contagious, and they rarely recur. The growths are benign (noncancerous) in 99 percent of cases but, in rare cases, can be a sign of early cervical cancer (see previous page).

Symptoms
Cervical polyps can produce a watery, bloody vaginal discharge. Sometimes they can cause bleeding after intercourse or after menopause. Cervical polyps are harmless but, because they produce symptoms similar to those of cervical cancer or

cancer of the uterus (see page 869), it's important to have these symptoms checked out by your doctor.

Diagnosis and Treatment
To determine the cause of your symptoms, your doctor will perform a pelvic examination and a Pap smear (see page 140). If the doctor finds a polyp in your cervix, he or she will probably remove it then in a quick, painless office procedure using biopsy scissors. You may feel slight pain or cramping after the procedure. The doctor will send the removed polyp to a laboratory for examination under a microscope to make sure it is benign.

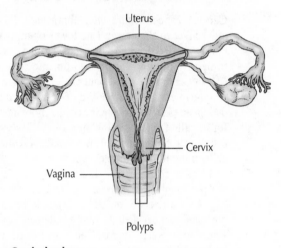

Cervical polyps
Cervical polyps are small, bulbous growths on stalks that protrude into the cervix from the lining of the uterus. Usually they are benign.

Disorders of the Bladder and Urethra

Located in the lower part of your abdomen, the bladder holds urine until you release it from your body during urination. The bladder lies in front of the uterus, just above the pubic bone. Urine drains slowly from your kidneys down two thin tubes called ureters into your bladder, where the urine is stored until you eliminate it through a short passage called the urethra.

Disorders of the bladder and urethra that affect both men and women are discussed in the chapter on disorders of the urinary tract (see page 801). The disorders included here either affect women exclusively or affect women differently than men.

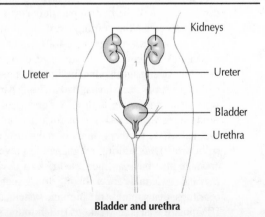

Bladder and urethra

Cystitis in Women

Cystitis is inflammation of the bladder caused by a bacterial infection. The bacteria first infect the urethra and then travel up to infect the bladder. Most women have an episode of cystitis at some time in their life. It is especially common during times of increased sexual activity, such as on a honeymoon. Left untreated, the infection can spread to the kidneys, causing a kidney infection called acute pyelonephritis (see page 804).

To help prevent bladder infections, always wipe from front to back after bowel movements, drink lots of water, keep your genitals clean, wash your genital area before and after intercourse, and empty your bladder after intercourse. Ask your partner to wash his genitals before intercourse.

Symptoms

If you have cystitis, you will feel a frequent, painful urge to urinate, but when you try to urinate, you are able to release only a small amount of urine. The urine may have a strong smell, may contain blood, and you will feel burning or stinging when you urinate. The urge to urinate may be so strong that you cannot control it. You may also have a fever. Other urinary tract problems, such as urethritis (see next page), can produce similar symptoms.

Diagnosis

If you have symptoms of cystitis, your doctor will ask you for a midstream urine specimen in which you collect the urine sample in a sterile container after you have started to urinate. The doctor will test the sample in the office for pus, which indicates an infection, and then send the sample to a laboratory to identify the organism that is causing the infection.

If you have more than two or three episodes of cystitis within 6 to 12 months, your doctor may refer you to a urologist (a doctor who specializes in urinary tract disorders), who can determine whether you have a urinary tract abnormality that is making you susceptible to bladder infections. The urologist will examine you and may ask for additional midstream specimens of urine. Sometimes an ultrasound is performed to detect an abnormality. You may also have a procedure called an intravenous pyelogram (IVP), which is an X-ray of the kidneys and bladder, and an examination of the bladder called a cystoscopy, in which the doctor uses a viewing instrument to see inside your urethra and bladder.

Treatment

If your symptoms are very mild and you do not have a fever, try to flush your urinary tract by drinking lots of fluids—at least eight large glasses a day—to relieve your symptoms. Drinking cranberry juice may help flush out bacteria. If the symptoms persist longer than 24 hours or are severe, see your doctor. He or she will prescribe antibiotics or other drugs to treat the condition.

If you have recurring infections and if diagnostic tests find an abnormality in your urinary tract, the urologist will treat it. If no abnormality is found, the urologist may prescribe low-dose antibiotics or antibacterial drugs for you to take for a month or more, or only around the times you have intercourse.

Stress Incontinence

A sheet of muscles called the pelvic floor muscles lies at the base of the abdomen. These muscles support the bottom of the bladder and help close the top of the urethra, the short channel through which urine passes. When you have stress incontinence, your pelvic floor muscles are so weak that the pressure produced by coughing, sneezing, or laughing can cause an involuntary release of urine.

Stress incontinence is very common—up to 50 percent of women over age 60 experience it to some degree. The pelvic floor muscles can be weakened by vaginal childbirth or obesity. The lack of estrogen after menopause can also weaken these muscles, sometimes producing prolapse of the uterus or vagina (see page 872). Chronic lung conditions, such as emphysema (see page 656), that cause persistent coughing, can also contribute to stress incontinence.

At any age, women can have stress incontinence during exercise, particularly high-impact sports such as running, because repeated jumping can put pressure on the bladder. More than half of all gymnasts and one of every three women who regularly exercise has had stress incontinence.

Diagnosis

To diagnose stress incontinence, the doctor will ask you questions about the activities that tend to cause the leaking of urine. You will probably be asked to provide a midstream urine specimen in which you collect a sample of urine in a sterile container after you have started to urinate. The urine sample is checked for bacteria or other signs of infection. The doctor may ask you to keep a diary of when and how often the leaking occurs.

The doctor may recommend other diagnostic procedures, including a voiding cystogram (an X-ray of your bladder taken while you are urinating), cystoscopy (in which the doctor uses a viewing instrument to see inside your urethra and bladder), and urodynamic testing (which involves filling the bladder with water and then inserting a device that measures the pressure inside the bladder).

Treatment

The treatment for stress incontinence usually includes doing Kegel exercises (see page 874) regularly to strengthen the pelvic floor muscles that support the bladder. If you are overweight, your doctor will recommend that you lose weight because extra weight around the abdomen puts pressure on the pelvic floor muscles. If you are past menopause, the doctor may recommend hormone therapy (see page 853) to help strengthen these muscles. If these measures do not relieve the condition, your doctor may recommend surgery to tighten the pelvic floor muscles.

To relieve stress incontinence that occurs during exercise, try wearing a tampon while you exercise because it will slightly close off the opening to the urethra. Your doctor may be able to prescribe a device called a pessary that, when inserted into the vagina, can help elevate the urethra and block urine leakage.

Urge Incontinence

Urge incontinence, also called irritable bladder, is a condition in which the bladder contracts uncontrollably, causing a sudden urge to urinate. You may pass a small amount of urine before you are able to reach a bathroom. Why certain people develop an irritable bladder is not known, but it sometimes occurs at the same time as a urinary tract infection (see previous page), stress incontinence (see previous page), or a pelvic support problem (see page 872) such as a prolapsed uterus. The condition can also result from damage to the nerves or muscles of the bladder in people who have a neurological dis-

order such as multiple sclerosis (see page 696), Parkinson's disease (see page 691), Alzheimer's disease (see page 688), stroke (see page 669), or a brain tumor (see page 682).

Diagnosis

If you have symptoms of urge incontinence (repeated, sudden urges to urinate), your doctor will ask you to provide a midstream urine specimen, in which you collect a sample of urine after you have started to urinate. The sample is sent to a laboratory, where it is analyzed for bacteria and other signs of infection. Your doctor may also arrange for other diagnostic procedures, including a voiding cystogram (an X-ray of your bladder taken while you are urinating), cystoscopy (in which the doctor uses a viewing instrument to see inside your urethra and bladder), and urodynamic testing (which involves filling the bladder with water and then inserting a device that measures the pressure inside the bladder).

Treatment

You can probably control urge incontinence with a few lifestyle changes if you don't also have stress incontinence or a pelvic support problem. Limit your intake of caffeine-containing drinks such as coffee or cola, which increase fluid loss from the body by increasing the need to urinate. Urinate before leaving the house, and make sure you know where the bathrooms are in malls, restaurants, and other destinations.

If these measures are not effective, your doctor may prescribe a drug that relaxes the contractions of your bladder muscles or reduces the activity of the nerves that control the muscle contractions that affect urination. Another treatment involves inserting an electrode the size of a tampon into the vagina to stimulate the pelvic floor muscles that support the bladder, making the muscles stronger.

Chronic Urethritis

Chronic urethritis is the term used to describe recurring inflammation of the urethra. The symptoms are similar to those of cystitis (see previous page), except that they last for only 1 or 2 days. Infection is the usual cause—often a sexually transmitted disease such as chlamydia (see page 477)—although the microorganism that is responsible cannot always be easily identified. The urethra can also become inflamed during intercourse or from exposure to some spermicides, bath oils, or other chemical irritants.

Symptoms and Diagnosis
Chronic urethritis causes burning and stinging during urination, frequent urination, and a sudden urge to urinate.

If you have symptoms of urethritis, the doctor will ask you for a sample of urine for analysis to find out if an infection is causing the problem. He or she may also take a sample of vaginal discharge to determine if you have a sexually transmitted disease. If these tests do not show signs of infection, the doctor may perform a cystoscopy, in which he

or she uses a viewing instrument to examine the inside of your urethra.

Treatment
If the underlying cause of the inflammation is an infection, it can usually be treated successfully with antibiotics or antibacterial drugs. If no infecting organism is found, the doctor will recommend that you empty your bladder completely after each time you have intercourse or after you engage in any other activities that could irritate your urethra, such as riding a bicycle vigorously or for a long time. Keep your genitals clean by washing them before and after having intercourse. Ask your partner to wash his genitals before intercourse.

Disorders of the Vagina and Vulva

The vulva is the outer area that surrounds the opening to the female urinary and reproductive systems. It consists of two outer folds of tissue called the outer labia, which lie on each side of the openings of the urethra and the vagina. The vulva also includes the inner labia, folds of tissue that enclose several lubricating glands and the clitoris (a small, sensitive organ that swells in response to sexual stimulation). The vagina is the passage that connects the vulva with the uterus. The tissues of the vulva are susceptible to skin problems such as warts or severe itching. The lining of the vagina and glands in the vulva produce fluid that cleanses the vagina, lubricates it during intercourse, and makes it easier for sperm to pass up to the uterus.

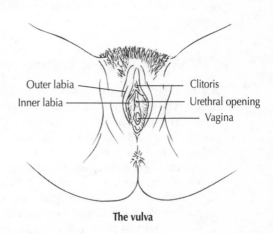

The vulva

Bacterial Vaginosis

Bacterial vaginosis (often referred to as BV) is the most common vaginal infection. It results from an overgrowth of one or more types of bacteria (usually gardnerella bacteria) that are normally present in the vagina in smaller amounts. When these bacteria overgrow, they prevent the protective bacteria from maintaining a healthy balance of microorganisms in the vagina. The infection can affect the vagina, urethra, bladder, and skin in the genital area.

Bacterial vaginosis occurs most often during the reproductive years, although women of all ages are susceptible. The infection is usually not serious, but

if not treated can increase the risk of infection after pelvic or vaginal surgery. In pregnant women, the infection can increase the risk of preterm labor and delivery (see page 529).

Symptoms
In many cases, bacterial vaginosis causes no symptoms and is diagnosed during a routine pelvic examination. If you have symptoms, you may notice that you have more vaginal discharge than usual or that your vaginal discharge is milky with an unpleasant, fishy odor that is worse after sexual intercourse. Other symptoms include itching or burning in or near the vagina.

Diagnosis

Some women mistake bacterial vaginosis for a yeast infection and try to treat it with an over-the-counter product. If you have symptoms of bacterial vaginosis or if you tried to treat a yeast infection with an antifungal vaginal medication and it did not clear up, see your doctor. The doctor will make a diagnosis of bacterial vaginosis based on a number of criteria. Because the doctor needs to test your vaginal secretions to make a diagnosis, do not douche or use vaginal creams or suppositories for a couple of days before you see the doctor.

Treatment

To treat bacterial vaginosis, doctors usually prescribe an antibiotic vaginal gel or cream that a woman inserts for 5 to 7 days. Oral antibiotics such as metronidazole are sometimes prescribed. For severe or recurring cases, a doctor may recommend oral antibiotics for both the woman and her sex partner.

Vaginal Yeast Infection

A yeast infection is the overgrowth of Candida albicans, a type of fungus that is normally present in small amounts in the vagina. If conditions in the vagina change and become more favorable for the fungus, it grows excessively, displacing the harmless bacteria that normally keep the fungus under control.

Using feminine hygiene sprays, douching, or taking antibiotics can kill the helpful bacteria in the vagina and allow the fungus to proliferate. Hormonal changes that occur when you are pregnant or taking oral contraceptives can also change the conditions in the vagina and allow the fungus to overgrow and cause an infection. Women with diabetes are especially susceptible to yeast infections.

Yeast infections are common—three quarters of all women have yeast infections at some time in their life. To prevent yeast infections, wear cotton underpants and avoid exposing your genital area to unnecessary chemicals, such as those in feminine hygiene sprays or powders, bubble baths, or deodorant tampons or sanitary pads. Do not douche.

Symptoms

Vaginal yeast infections cause an unusual thick, white discharge; itching and irritation of the vagina;

and swelling and redness of the vulva. You may experience some mild vaginal tenderness or discomfort during intercourse.

Diagnosis and Treatment

To diagnose a yeast infection, your doctor will take a sample of your vaginal discharge for analysis in the laboratory. The usual treatment for a yeast infec-

Vaginal Hygiene

Most doctors think that washing the area around the vaginal opening (including the minor and major labia, urethra, and clitoris) daily with unscented soap and water is the best way to keep the area clean. Do not use deodorant sprays, which are unnecessary and contain chemicals that can irritate the vaginal lining, the labia, and other areas of the skin.

The vagina cleanses itself by secreting a mucous discharge that flows downward, removing bacteria, old cells, and any menstrual blood that is present. Normal vaginal discharge is minimal, is either clear or white and sticky, and has a mild odor. The discharge dries as a yellowish stain on your underpants. The consistency and volume of the discharge may change when you ovulate, producing mucus from the cervix midway between menstrual periods. Infections of the vagina and cervix can produce more plentiful, thicker vaginal secretions that are often foul-smelling and cause redness, dryness, flaking, itching, and irritation.

Douching is neither necessary nor recommended because it rinses away the beneficial bacteria normally present in the vagina that protect against infection and washes away secretions that can help doctors diagnose infections. Removing the bacteria and secretions, which are part of the vagina's natural self-cleaning system, may actually prolong an infection. (It is also important to understand that douching is not a method of birth control.) Some douching preparations can irritate the mucous membrane that lines the walls of the vagina. In some women, these preparations can cause allergic reactions.

If you have a foul-smelling or unusual vaginal discharge and you think you may have a vaginal infection, see your doctor. He or she will perform a pelvic examination and take a sample of your vaginal discharge for testing. Do not try to treat yourself by douching.

tion is an over-the-counter antifungal drug most often taken in the form of a vaginal suppository or cream. A single-dose antifungal tablet also is effective against yeast infections but can produce adverse reactions when taken with some other drugs. Also, antifungal tablets do not relieve the irritation of the vagina and vulva as quickly as the cream or suppository does. Using the vaginal suppository or cream for about a week usually clears up the problem. If you have repeated yeast infections, your doctor may want to check your blood sugar levels for diabetes and may recommend tests, such as an HIV test (see page 910), to try to determine why your immune system defenses are weakened.

Cancer of the Vulva

Cancer of the vulva—the external, visible part of the female genitals—is a rare cancer. The most common site of cancer of the vulva is the labia majora (outer lips of the vulva). Most women with cancer of the vulva are over age 50, although it is becoming more common in women under 40. Infection with the human papillomavirus (HPV; see page 480) is the most likely cause. Cancer of the vulva tends to grow very slowly and is highly curable when diagnosed at an early stage. If the cancer has not spread to the lymph nodes, the overall survival rate after treatment is 90 percent.

Symptoms and Diagnosis

Cancer of the vulva starts as a small, hard lump in the skin, which gradually breaks down on the surface to form an ulcer (open sore). The ulcer has thickened, raised edges and may ooze or bleed from the center. The ulcer gradually enlarges and, if it is not treated, will eventually spread to other parts of the body.

If you have any lump or ulcer on your vulva, your doctor will perform a pelvic examination and take a small sample of tissue for examination under a microscope (biopsy) for cancer cells.

Treatment

Treatment for cancer of the vulva depends on the stage of the cancer. If the cancer is in its early stages and is present on only the surface of the skin, the doctor will probably remove it surgically. If the tumor has invaded the deeper part of the vulva but has not spread to nearby tissue, the doctor will surgically remove it, along with surrounding skin and nearby lymph nodes. Radiation therapy (see page 23) may be given after the surgery if the cancer has spread to the lymph nodes.

Cancer that has spread to nearby tissues requires surgical removal of the entire vulva (and possibly the lower colon, the rectum, or the bladder), followed by radiation therapy. The doctor may recommend chemotherapy (see page 23) along with the radiation therapy.

Hormonal Disorders

10

Hormones are chemical messengers that are produced by a network of glands called the endocrine system and released directly into the bloodstream, which carries them to organs and tissues throughout the body. A hormone circulating in the bloodstream affects only the target organs or tissues for that hormone. Together with the nervous system (see page 665), the endocrine system coordinates and controls many essential body processes. For this reason, a problem in any part of the endocrine system can affect many body functions.

The endocrine system includes the following glands:

- **Pituitary gland**   The pituitary is a pea-sized gland that is suspended from the base of the brain. The pituitary gland is the most important endocrine gland and is often called the master gland because it produces hormones that control other endocrine glands and many essential body processes.
- **Hypothalamus**   The hypothalamus is a small structure at the base of the brain, below the thalamus (a structure deep inside the brain that processes sensory information) and above the pituitary gland. The hypothalamus coordinates production and release of hormones by the pituitary gland, the thyroid gland, the adrenal glands, the ovaries, and the testicles.
- **Thyroid gland**   The thyroid is a butterfly-shaped gland at the base of the neck, directly below the larynx (voice box) and in front of the trachea (windpipe). The thyroid produces the hormones thyroxine and triiodothyronine, which have an important role in metabolism (the chemical processes that take place in the body), and calcitonin, which helps regulate the calcium level in the blood and enhances bone formation.
- **Parathyroid glands**   The parathyroid glands are two pairs of pea-sized glands next to the thyroid gland. The parathyroid glands produce parathyroid hormone, which helps regulate the calcium level in the blood.
- **Adrenal glands**   The adrenal glands are two small, triangular glands on top of the kidneys. The adrenal glands produce corticosteroid hormones, which have an important role in metabolism; epinephrine, which helps the body respond to stress or danger; aldosterone, which helps regulate blood pressure and the sodium and potassium levels in the blood; and testosterone, which stimulates development of male sexual characteristics.

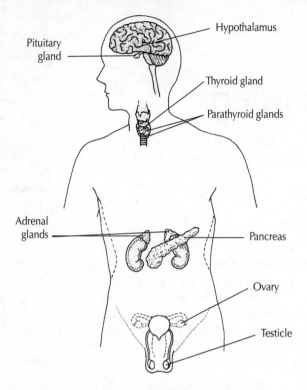

The endocrine system

The endocrine system is a group of glands and tissues that secrete hormones directly into the bloodstream to regulate many body processes. The major endocrine glands are the hypothalamus, the pituitary gland, the thyroid gland, the parathyroid glands, the adrenal glands, the pancreas, the ovaries (in women), and the testicles (in men).

● **Pancreas** The pancreas is a long, tapering gland near the back of the abdominal cavity, under the stomach. The pancreas secretes digestive enzymes, which help break down food, and produces insulin and glucagon, hormones that regulate the body's use of sugar (glucose), fats, and proteins.

● **Ovaries** The ovaries are two egg-shaped glands on either side of a female's uterus and directly below the fallopian tubes. The ovaries produce eggs and the female sex hormones estrogen and progesterone, which regulate the female reproductive system.

● **Testicles** The testicles are two egg-shaped glands suspended outside of a male's body inside a pouch of skin and muscle called the scrotum. The testicles produce sperm and the male sex hormone testosterone, which regulates the male reproductive system.

Hormone levels in the blood vary in response to factors such as stress, infections or other diseases or conditions, and changes in the chemical composition of the blood. The amount of each hormone released into the bloodstream depends on the body's changing needs and is regulated by feedback mechanisms. In some cases, the level of one hormone in the blood affects the level of another hormone. For example, the pituitary gland produces thyrotropin (also called thyroid-stimulating hormone, or TSH), which regulates the production of hormones by the thyroid gland. If the hypothalamus detects variations in the blood level of thyroid hormones, it signals the pituitary gland, which adjusts its production of thyrotropin. The change in thyrotropin levels causes the thyroid to modify its production of thyroid hormones.

Disorders of the Pituitary Gland

The pituitary gland is the most important endocrine gland. It is located at the base of the brain and secretes hormones that regulate the activity of the other endocrine glands and control many body processes. The pituitary is divided into three parts: the anterior (front) lobe, the intermediate (center) lobe, and the posterior (rear) lobe.

The anterior lobe of the pituitary produces the following six hormones:

● Growth hormone (GH), which regulates body growth and development.
● Prolactin, which stimulates female breast development and milk production.
● Thyrotropin (also called thyroid-stimulating hormone, or TSH), which stimulates the thyroid gland to secrete more thyroid hormones.
● Corticotropin (also called adrenocorticotropic hormone, or ACTH), which stimulates the outer

layer of the adrenal glands to secrete cortico-steroid hormones.

- Follicle-stimulating hormone (FSH), which regulates the maturation of eggs in the ovaries and sperm in the testicles.
- Luteinizing hormone (LH), which stimulates the ovaries and testicles to secrete sex hormones and is a factor in the maturation of eggs and sperm.

The intermediate lobe of the pituitary gland produces one hormone, called melanocyte-stimulating hormone (MSH), which stimulates disper-sion of cells called melanocytes in the skin and regulates their production of melanin (the pigment that gives skin, hair, and eyes their color).

The posterior lobe of the pituitary produces the following two hormones:

- Arginine vasopressin (AVP; also called anti-diuretic hormone, or ADH), which acts on the kidneys to increase the reabsorption of water and helps regulate blood pressure.
- Oxytocin, which stimulates contractions of the uterus during childbirth and stimulates the flow of milk for breastfeeding.

The release of hormones from the anterior lobe of the pituitary gland is controlled by the hypothalamus, the area of the brain directly above the pituitary. The hypothalamus forms a link between the nervous system and the endocrine system. Because of this link, psychological factors (such as emotions) and environmental events (such as the changing of the seasons) can influence the secretion of hormones and the balance of chemicals in the body. For example, severe stress causes the pituitary to secrete corticotropin, which, in turn, stimulates the adrenal glands to secrete corticosteroid hormones, which help the body cope with the stress.

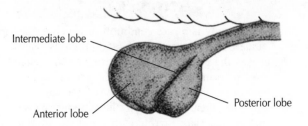

Intermediate lobe

Anterior lobe

Posterior lobe

The pituitary gland
The pituitary is a pea-sized gland that hangs from the base of the brain. It produces hormones that regulate the activity of the other endocrine glands and control many important body processes. The pituitary has three hormone-producing sections—the anterior lobe, the intermediate lobe, and the posterior lobe.

Pituitary Tumors

The pituitary gland is divided into three sections—the anterior (front) lobe, the intermediate (center) lobe, and the posterior (rear) lobe. Pituitary gland tumors usually develop in the anterior lobe. The exact cause of pituitary tumors is not known, but evidence suggests that they may result from mutations in specific genes involved in cell growth.

There are two main types of pituitary tumors—pituitary adenomas and craniopharyngiomas. Pituitary adenomas are overgrowths of cells in the pituitary gland that are usually noncancerous. Although most of these tumors are less than ½ inch in diameter, they grow in a confined space and can press on and damage surrounding nerves, blood vessels, and other tissues.

Symptoms
About half of all pituitary adenomas secrete abnormal amounts of the hormone prolactin. These tumors (called prolactinomas) may cause no symptoms, or they may cause erection problems (see page 486) in men or absence of menstrual periods or breast swelling and abnormal milk production in women. Pituitary adenomas may also secrete other hormones, leading to acromegaly (see next page), gigantism, or Cushing's disease (see page 898).

Craniopharyngiomas do not cause overproduction of any hormones but, as they enlarge, they can press on the anterior lobe, causing hypopituitarism (see page 887), or on the posterior lobe, causing diabetes insipidus (see page 887). A craniopharyngioma can also press on the optic nerves, causing headaches, double vision, and eventually blindness.

Diagnosis
Diagnosis of a pituitary tumor is based on the symptoms and a physical examination. Your doctor will recommend blood and urine tests to measure the levels of a number of hormones and to evaluate the functioning of the pituitary gland. High levels of some hormones can be a sign of a tumor. If

Hormone-Producing Tumors

Some cancerous tumors may secrete hormones or chemicals that imitate hormones, causing symptoms similar to those that result from overactive endocrine glands. For example, lung cancers may secrete hormones that are similar to corticotropin (the pituitary hormone that stimulates the adrenal glands), parathyroid hormone, or arginine vasopressin (antidiuretic hormone). Carcinoid tumors of the intestine (see page 761) also may secrete these hormones. Tumors of the islet cells in the pancreas (which produce insulin) also often secrete abnormal hormones. Because a wide range of tumors may secrete similar hormones, it can be difficult to identify the tumor that is causing the problem. However, a doctor will make a thorough evaluation of any suspected hormone-producing tumor. Surgery or radiation therapy to remove or destroy the tumor may help relieve the symptoms.

your vision has been affected, the doctor will recommend visual field testing. To confirm the diagnosis, your doctor will order a CT scan (see page 112) or MRI (see page 113) of the pituitary gland to locate the tumor and evaluate it.

Treatment

Prolactinomas often can be treated successfully with dopamine agonists (such as bromocriptine), which control the growth of the tumor. Taking a long-acting dopamine agonist such as cabergoline twice a week can shrink the tumor, often making surgery unnecessary or easier to perform. Dopamine agonists are drugs that imitate the actions of the chemical messenger dopamine and suppress the secretion of growth hormone by the pituitary gland. However, the most effective treatment for some prolactinomas and all other types of pituitary tumors is surgery or radiation therapy or, in some cases, a combination of both.

Surgery to remove a pituitary tumor is a delicate procedure that is performed as the surgeon looks through a powerful microscope (microsurgery). The tumor is reached either through a nostril or through a small hole that the surgeon creates in the bridge of the nose. If the tumor is large and is pressing on the optic nerves, open-brain surgery may be required. There is a risk that the pituitary gland will be damaged during surgery, which can lead to hypopituitarism or diabetes insipidus, or both. These disorders are treated with lifelong hormone replacement therapy.

In some cases, the surgeon may destroy the tumor with extreme cold (cryosurgery; see page 22) or by inserting tiny radioactive implants (called radioactive pellets or seeds) into the tumor. If the tumor is large or if it is difficult to pinpoint, the doctor may use radiation therapy on the entire gland. Like surgery, radiation therapy can damage the pituitary gland. Although the long-term outlook depends largely on the size of the tumor, in many cases a complete cure is possible.

Acromegaly

Acromegaly is a rare condition in which a non-cancerous pituitary tumor (see previous page) causes the pituitary gland to produce too much growth hormone. Excess growth hormone causes bone deformities and enlargement of internal structures and organs, including the heart, kidneys, liver, spleen, pancreas, thyroid gland, and parathyroid glands. The condition usually occurs in adults between ages 30 and 50.

Symptoms

Symptoms of acromegaly include enlargement of the hands and feet, lengthening of the face, broadening of the head and neck, and enlargement of the lower jaw, brow, nose, and ears. The skin may thicken and darken, and coarse hair may appear on the arms, legs, and body. The tongue may enlarge and, in some cases, the voice may deepen or become hoarse. These changes develop gradually and may go undetected for many years.

Other symptoms of acromegaly can include tingling in the hands, increased sweating, fatigue, severe headaches, joint stiffness, and dull, persistent pain throughout the body. Enlarging tissues may press on the optic nerves, causing vision problems, especially with peripheral (side) vision. Most women with acromegaly experience irregular menstrual periods, and some may produce breast milk even though they are not breastfeeding. Some men who have acromegaly develop erection problems (see page 486). In some people, acromegaly can cause diabetes (see page 889).

Diagnosis

A diagnosis of acromegaly is based on the symptoms and a physical examination. If your doctor suspects that you have acromegaly, he or she will probably refer you to an endocrinologist (a doctor who specializes in treating disorders of the endocrine system). The doctor may perform an X-ray of your skull to check for thickening or enlargement of the bones in the skull. He or she may also take X-rays of your hands to look for deformities in the finger bones.

The doctor will recommend a blood test to determine the level of growth hormone and insulinlike growth factor 1 (IGF-1) in the blood. High levels of these substances confirm the diagnosis. The doctor will then perform a CT scan (see page 112) or MRI (see page 113) of the pituitary gland to determine the location of the tumor and evaluate it.

Treatment

Treatment for acromegaly begins as soon as possible after the diagnosis is confirmed. Your doctor may prescribe a dopamine agonist such as bromocriptine or cabergoline to control the growth of the tumor. Dopamine agonists are drugs that imitate the actions of the chemical messenger dopamine and suppress the secretion of growth hormone by the pituitary gland. The doctor may prescribe the drug somatostatin, which also inhibits growth hormone and is often used to treat acromegaly. If these drugs are not effective, your doctor will probably recommend surgery or radiation therapy to remove or destroy the tumor.

Pituitary tumors can be selectively removed, leaving behind only healthy tissue. If most or all of your pituitary gland is removed or destroyed, you will need to take hormone replacement therapy for the rest of your life. Surgery or radiation treatments to remove or destroy the pituitary tumor may help improve vision problems by relieving pressure on the optic nerves. Although successful treatment stops progression of the disease, the changes in your bones and your appearance are permanent.

Hypopituitarism

In hypopituitarism, the anterior (front) lobe of the pituitary gland is underactive and does not produce adequate amounts of one or more pituitary hormones. Because the pituitary is the master gland that produces hormones that control other endocrine glands and many essential body processes, underactivity of the pituitary can result in a wide range of problems throughout the body.

Some common causes of hypopituitarism

include severe head injuries, a pituitary tumor (see page 885) or a brain tumor (see page 682), treatment for a pituitary tumor or a brain tumor (such as surgery or radiation therapy), or an autoimmune disorder (in which the body's immune system mistakenly attacks the pituitary gland). In some cases, the disorder develops for no obvious reason.

Symptoms

Because the pituitary gland stimulates several other endocrine glands, the symptoms of hypopituitarism are a combination of the symptoms of disorders related to the other affected glands. These disorders include hypothyroidism (see page 903), Addison's disease (see page 899), infertility (see page 493), absence of menstrual periods (see page 846), and short stature.

Diagnosis

A diagnosis of hypopituitarism is based on the symptoms and a physical examination. Your doctor will probably perform blood and urine tests to measure the levels of pituitary hormones and evaluate the functioning of the anterior lobe of the pituitary gland. If the test results indicate that you have hypopituitarism, your doctor may recommend a CT scan (see page 112) or MRI (see page 113) to look for a pituitary tumor.

Treatment

The treatment for hypopituitarism involves taking oral and intravenous medications that replace the hormones of the pituitary and other affected endocrine glands. Hormone replacement therapy may be needed to treat underproduction of hormones by the thyroid gland, the adrenal glands, the ovaries (in women), or the testicles (in men).

Diabetes Insipidus

Diabetes insipidus is a disorder in which a deficiency of arginine vasopressin (AVP; also called antidiuretic hormone, or ADH) causes the body to produce large quantities of diluted urine (urine that contains a high percentage of water). AVP, which is produced by the hypothalamus and released by the posterior (rear) lobe of the pituitary gland, regulates the process of water reabsorption in the body and prevents the body from producing too much urine. In normal urine production, the kidneys filter water and other substances from the blood, reabsorbing nearly all of the filtered water and leaving only urine to be eliminated from the body. The reabsorbed water is returned to the bloodstream to maintain normal concentrations of minerals, proteins, and other chemicals in the blood and other body fluids. However, in diabetes insipidus, the kidneys do not reabsorb the filtered water, and it is eliminated from the body in urine.

Diabetes insipidus usually results from damage to the hypothalamus or to the pituitary gland caused by a severe head injury. The condition may also result from scarring or damage caused by surgery on the hypothalamus or the pituitary gland, or as a side effect of radiation therapy on the pituitary or surrounding tissue. In rare cases, diabetes insipidus is caused by pressure on the posterior lobe of the pituitary gland from a pituitary tumor (see page 885). In a form of the disorder called nephrogenic diabetes insipidus, the condition results from an insensitivity of the kidney tubules to AVP; the levels of AVP in the bloodstream are normal, but the kidneys do not respond properly to reabsorb water.

Diabetes insipidus may develop gradually or occur suddenly. If not treated promptly, the disorder can quickly cause dehydration, which can result in very low blood pressure and shock (see page 162).

Symptoms
The main symptoms of diabetes insipidus are excessive thirst and passing large quantities of urine (as much as 20 quarts a day). The need to drink and urinate is strong and constant throughout the day and night.

Diagnosis
A diagnosis of diabetes insipidus is based on the symptoms and a physical examination. If your doctor suspects that you have diabetes insipidus, he or she will probably recommend that you have a water deprivation test, which can be performed in the doctor's office. During the test, which takes several hours to complete, you will not drink any fluids. The doctor will measure your weight and the volume and concentration of your urine at regular intervals. If the volume of water in your urine remains high and your urine is diluted, you have a deficiency of AVP. To confirm the diagnosis, after the water deprivation test is stopped, the doctor gives you an injection of synthetic AVP (vasopressin). If your symptoms are relieved, you have diabetes insipidus.

Treatment
The first step in therapy for diabetes insipidus is to treat the underlying cause. The most effective treatment is vasopressin, taken either in nose drops or by mouth. The length of time you must take the drops or pills is determined mainly by the cause of the disorder. If diabetes insipidus was caused by a head injury, surgery, or radiation therapy, taking vasopressin may help the defective gland return to normal within a year, and your symptoms will disappear. If your symptoms don't go away, you will probably have to take the medication for the rest of your life. If the disorder is caused by a pituitary tumor, your doctor may recommend surgery or radiation therapy to remove or destroy the tumor. If you have nephrogenic diabetes insipidus, your doctor may recommend restricting your salt intake and taking medications that stimulate production of AVP, such as chlorpropamide, carbamazepine, or thiazide diuretics, to help your kidneys reabsorb water.

Disorders of the Pancreas

The pancreas is a thin gland, about 6 to 8 inches long, that lies sideways just behind the stomach. The pancreas has two major functions—to produce enzymes that help digest food, and to produce the hormones insulin and glucagon. Insulin and glucagon have an essential role in regulating the level of the sugar glucose in the blood. Insulin also helps regulate fat and protein metabolism.

Glucose is found in many foods, including some that don't taste sweet. Glucose is the major source of energy for all the cells in the body. Insulin stimulates cells in the body to absorb glucose from the blood for the energy they need, and insulin stimulates the liver to absorb and store the glucose that isn't used. In this way, insulin maintains glucose at a healthy level in the blood. Glucagon does the opposite—it helps raise the glucose level in the blood by stimulating the liver to release glucose (hypoglycemia; see page 897). Too much glucose in the blood can cause diabetes (see next page) and can damage organs and tissues throughout the body.

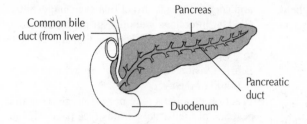

Common bile duct (from liver)

Pancreas

Pancreatic duct

Duodenum

The pancreas
The pancreas is a hormone-secreting gland about 6 to 8 inches long that lies close to the duodenum (the upper part of the small intestine that opens into the stomach) and is linked to the duodenum by the pancreatic duct. The pancreas secretes enzymes that aid digestion, and several hormones, including insulin (which helps the body use and store the sugar glucose).

Type 1 Diabetes

Type 1 diabetes, which used to be called juvenile or insulin-dependent diabetes, occurs when the pancreas stops producing the hormone insulin or does not produce the hormone in the amounts the body needs. The lack of insulin prevents cells from bringing in the sugar glucose for energy and prevents the liver from absorbing and storing glucose. If glucose cannot be used or stored, it builds up in the blood and spills over into the urine. An abnormally high level of glucose in the blood is the hallmark of diabetes.

In type 1 diabetes, insulin-producing cells in the pancreas (islet cells) produce very little or no insulin. Type 1 diabetes occurs mainly in young people, but can occur at any age. About 5 to 10 percent of the 17 million people in the United States with diabetes have type 1 diabetes. In most cases, type 1 diabetes results from an errant immune response in which the immune system mistakes the islet cells of the pancreas for invading organisms and attacks them, damaging or destroying them. Type 1 diabetes can also develop in people who have chronic diseases that can damage the insulin-secreting cells in the pancreas, such as cystic fibrosis (see page 958) or long-term alcohol abuse (see page 733).

Unable to use glucose for energy because of the lack of insulin, the body is forced to obtain energy from fat. As fat is burned, chemicals called ketones and keto acids are produced. A buildup of these substances is a life-threatening condition called ketoacidosis, characterized by dehydration and very high levels of glucose in the blood.

Over time, uncontrolled high blood levels of glucose can cause serious complications, including the eye disorder diabetic retinopathy (see page 1048), which can lead to blindness; peripheral neuropathy (see page 702) and other nerve diseases; and chronic kidney failure (see page 817). People with diabetes have a higher-than-average risk of developing atherosclerosis (see page 557), a major risk factor for stroke, heart attack, and high blood pressure. For people with diabetes, treatment of high blood pressure and elevated cholesterol is just as important as controlling glucose levels in avoiding heart disease and some of the other possible complications of diabetes. People with diabetes also have an increased risk of developing infections.

If you have diabetes, always tell your doctors or dentists before you have any treatments, so they can take any necessary precautions. Your doctor can give you a card to carry at all times that lists your name, address, the fact that you have diabetes, and instructions on how to help you if you become ill. Wear a medical identification bracelet or necklace indicating that you have diabetes, so that emergency medical personnel can treat you promptly and correctly if you are found unconscious, and to let people know that your symptoms are caused by low blood sugar

Children and Diabetes

Having a chronic illness such as diabetes can be especially difficult for children and can present challenges to their parents and caregivers. Young children may not understand why they must stick to a special diet and can't have candy and soft drinks like other kids. But parents and caregivers need to be firm and consistent in enforcing the child's diet. Many teenagers go through periods of rebellion, and teenagers with diabetes may react against the restrictions the disease imposes on them. In this case, it is essential to consult a psychiatrist or counselor who can work with the teen to help him or her cope with the emotional and social ramifications of having a chronic disease and to encourage him or her to regain control over it.

(hypoglycemia; see page 897). Such aids can help ensure that someone will be able to help in an emergency.

Symptoms

The symptoms of type 1 diabetes usually develop rapidly, within weeks or months. See your doctor right away if you have any of the following symptoms:

- Unusually frequent urination, sometimes as often as every hour or so, throughout the day and night.
- Unusual thirst from excessive loss of fluid; drinking sweetened beverages increases urination and makes the thirst worse.
- Fatigue, weakness, and apathy that can make it hard to get up in the morning.
- Significant weight loss, especially in children and young adults, because fat and muscle are burned for energy, and the glucose lost in urine is a major source of calories.
- Tingling in the hands and feet.
- Reduced resistance to infections, especially boils

and vaginal yeast infections (see page 880). Bladder infections and other urinary tract problems can develop from bacteria that are attracted to the glucose in the urine.
- Blurred vision resulting from excess glucose in the fluid of the eye.
- Erection problems (see page 486) in men and absence of menstrual periods (see page 846) in women.

Diagnosis

If you have symptoms of diabetes, your doctor will ask you for a urine sample to test for glucose and ketones; their presence in the urine indicates that you probably have diabetes. If only glucose is present in your urine, your doctor will ask for a blood sample to measure the amount of glucose in your bloodstream. A blood glucose test (see page 895) is necessary for a diagnosis because you can have some glucose in your urine without having diabetes. A diagnosis of diabetes is made if the blood glucose level is 126 milligrams per deciliter (mg/dL) or higher.

Long-Term Complications of Diabetes

When uncontrolled, both forms of diabetes can have long-term consequences, damaging blood vessels, kidneys, and nerves. The best ways to avoid the following serious complications are to keep your blood glucose level in a healthy range and to see your doctor regularly—even when you feel fine.

- **Heart disease** The changes in the body's chemistry brought on by an elevated glucose or insulin level can lead to the buildup of fatty deposits inside the arteries (atherosclerosis; see page 557). These changes can also make the blood clot more easily, leading to the formation of blood clots that can block blood flow and cause a heart attack or stroke. High blood pressure linked to diabetes can also lead to heart disease and stroke.

- **Nerve damage** An elevated level of glucose reduces the ability of nerves to carry messages to various parts of the body, including the feet and legs, bladder, digestive system, and reproductive system. Depending on the tissues affected, nerve damage (neuropathy) can cause symptoms that include loss of feeling; muscle weakness; tingling, burning, or jabbing sensations; vomiting; frequent bladder infections; and sexual problems.

- **Peripheral vascular disease** An elevated glucose level can cause narrowing of the blood vessels that

deliver blood to the feet and legs. Without a regular supply of nourishing oxygen-rich blood, the tissues that are farthest away from the heart can die. In severe cases, part or all of a foot or leg may need to be amputated.

- **Eye damage** Diabetes can damage the small blood vessels that supply the back of the eye, causing them to leak blood or other fluid into the eye. This condition, called diabetic retinopathy, is a major cause of blindness in people between ages 25 and 74. Having diabetes also increases a person's risk of other vision-robbing eye disorders, such as cataracts (clouding of the lens of the eye) and glaucoma (buildup of pressure from excess fluid inside the eye). For this reason, if you have diabetes, you should see an eye doctor (an ophthalmologist) every year for a complete eye examination.

- **Kidney disease** Diabetes can cause narrowing of the blood vessels that carry blood to the kidneys, reducing their ability to filter out and eliminate wastes from the body. Diabetes can also harm the kidneys by causing frequent infections of the urinary tract. Because kidney disease seldom causes noticeable symptoms until the kidneys are seriously damaged, see your doctor regularly for urine tests and blood tests to help evaluate the health of your kidneys.

Treatment

There is no cure for diabetes. Treatment involves a combination of a carefully controlled diet and daily injections of insulin (from two to four times a day) to replace the insulin your pancreas is not producing. Keeping your blood glucose level in a normal range can keep you healthy and help you avoid potentially serious complications, such as retinopathy and kidney failure. You will require treatment for diabetes all your life. To monitor the effectiveness of your treatment, you will learn how to measure your blood glucose level at home. Self-discipline, along with the support and help you get from your health care team, is extremely important if you are to control your diabetes successfully.

If you maintain good control over your blood sugar level, you can expect to lead a full and healthy life. Intensive therapy with multiple daily injections of insulin and the insulin pump allow you flexibility with your meals and exercise and work schedules. Hypoglycemia (low blood glucose; see page 897) can be avoided by testing your blood glucose regularly, eating appropriate snacks, and using small doses of short-acting insulin when necessary. Your risk of serious complications can be reduced by having regular medical checkups and following your doctor's recommendations. The following steps can help you stay healthy:

- Exercise regularly.
- Follow the diet your doctor or dietitian recommends.
- Maintain good control of your blood glucose level with frequent blood sugar tests at home and regular (usually every 3 months) hemoglobin A1C tests (see page 895).
- Keep your blood pressure at a healthy level—lower than 120/80 millimeters of mercury (mm Hg).
- Keep your LDL (harmful) cholesterol lower than 100.
- Take ACE inhibitors or any other heart disease or blood pressure medications your doctor prescribes.
- Don't smoke cigarettes or cigars.

Ask your doctor the best way to engage in strenuous activities such as fast-paced sports, because exercise burns up glucose and may bring on hypoglycemia. Before exercising, your doctor may recommend that you eat extra food or adjust your dose of insulin.

Any illness, from a minor cold to a heart attack, puts stress on the body and therefore increases the amount of insulin needed. You must follow the timetable of meals and snacks recommended by your doctor to keep the supply of glucose in your blood steady. This routine will also help ensure that your regular doses of insulin always act on approximately the same amount of glucose. If you are not able to eat according to your usual schedule, take glucose drinks and monitor your blood sugar, but do not reduce your dose of insulin. Talk to your doctor immediately if your blood sugar level increases, for any reason, beyond the goals or ranges you and your doctor have discussed.

If diabetes causes the blood vessels in the legs to narrow, you can have cramps, cold feet, pain when you walk or climb stairs, and skin sores that don't heal. Eventually, the lack of circulation can lead to death of tissue (gangrene; see page 601) in the feet and legs, which may require amputation. The feet are especially prone to injury, so it is important to take good care of them (see next page). If any cut fails to heal within 10 days, see your doctor immediately. Any sore or ulcer must be examined promptly by your doctor.

Insulin

Many different types of insulin are available for people with diabetes, and the type of insulin and the schedule that your doctor prescribes will depend on many factors, including your age and the severity of your diabetes. The insulin most frequently prescribed is identical to human insulin, produced in bacteria or yeast. Insulin can currently only be injected or infused, although studies are under way to determine the effectiveness and safety of insulin formulations that can be inhaled, eaten, or absorbed through the skin or mucous membranes. Several modified versions of human insulin are available that produce effects rapidly or over a longer time.

The best control is usually achieved by giving yourself injections once or twice a day of a long-acting insulin and injections of a rapidly acting insulin at mealtimes. Your doctor will show you how to inject the insulin just under the skin of your thigh, arm, or abdomen. Most people learn to do this expertly within a few days. (If you have a child with diabetes, you will need to administer the injections until the child is about 10.) Always make sure that you obtain the same type and strength of insulin each time you renew your prescription.

Taking Care of Your Feet

If you have diabetes, you are at risk of damage to the nerves and blood vessels in your feet, which can reduce their sense of feeling and limit the circulation of blood to them. If you don't have feeling in your feet, you can injure them and not realize it. In addition, the reduced flow of blood to the feet can make injuries heal slowly or not at all, which can cause the tissue to die (a condition called gangrene). In severe cases, amputation is necessary to save the rest of the foot and leg. The following steps can help you avoid these serious but common complications of diabetes:

● Inspect your feet every day for scratches, cuts, blisters, ingrown toenails, or warts on the soles (called plantar warts; see page 1060); using a mirror can help you see the bottoms of your feet better. If you notice anything unusual, see your doctor right away.

● Immediately report to your doctor any signs of infection, burning, tingling, or numbness in your feet.

● Do not cut or treat corns or calluses yourself. Have a doctor remove them.

● Make sure your doctor examines your feet at each visit.

● Wash your feet every day and dry them well, especially between the toes.

● Shake out your shoes before putting them on to make sure there aren't any pebbles or other objects that could cause a cut or blister.

● Wear comfortable, well-cushioned shoes that do not pinch at the toes or scrape at the heel. Try wearing shoes that are a half size larger than you normally wear. Never wear shoes with high heels.

● Break in new shoes slowly.

● Change your socks every day. Wear socks that wick away moisture. Smooth your socks or panty hose over your feet carefully, leaving no lumps that could cause chafing or blisters.

● Put a moisturizer on your feet nightly if your skin is dry.

● Never walk barefoot, even in your own home.

● Don't smoke. Smoking reduces blood flow to your feet.

● To prevent ingrown toenails and infections, be extra careful when you trim your toenails. Cut your nails straight across from side to side (ask your doctor to show you how). If you have numbness in your feet, you should not trim your own nails.

● To prevent scalding, do not test the water temperature in your bath with your feet.

● Have a podiatrist examine and care for your feet regularly.

In addition to the standard insulin syringe, a variety of disposable penlike devices are available. These devices allow you to inject insulin by turning a dial to select the dose. Each device can hold about 150 to 300 units of insulin. In some cases, the pen is prefilled with insulin; in others, a disposable cartridge is used, providing added convenience to people who take multiple injections a day. Always inspect your pens and cartridges to make sure that you have been given the correct kind of insulin (rapidly acting, long-acting, or mixed).

An alternative to multiple daily injections of insulin is a course of treatment called continuous insulin therapy, which uses an external, wearable device (called an insulin pump) to infuse specific amounts of insulin automatically and continuously through a thin plastic tube inserted under the skin, usually on the abdomen. Several small, highly reliable insulin pumps are currently available that are about the size of a pager and can hold up to a 3-day supply of insulin. The pumps are about as effective as daily injections, but many people find the pumps more convenient and comfortable. Because the pumps do not sense blood glucose levels, you still need to do frequent blood sugar tests for best results. (Implantable insulin pumps remain experimental.)

Checking blood glucose levels

Many people with diabetes find it helpful to check their blood glucose levels at home daily even if they are only taking oral glucose-lowering medications (hypoglycemics; see page 896). People who are taking insulin may need to check their blood sugar three to seven times a day or as often as their doctor recommends. You can test your blood sugar level with a machine that provides a digital readout. A pricking device that comes with the machine enables you to take your blood sample quickly and easily. Some newer devices allow you to take blood samples from skin areas other than the fingertips. The results obtained by the machine provide valuable information on how well your diabetes is being controlled and will enable you and your doctor to take steps to improve this control by adjusting your diet, insulin injections, or treatment with drugs when your sugar level fluctuates. Some newer machines allow you to download the information to a computer for analysis.

Having regular hemoglobin A1C tests (see page 895) can track your average blood sugar over the last 3 to 4 months, which can help you and your doctor evaluate how successfully your blood sugar level is being controlled. Your doctor will encourage you to know your hemoglobin A1C test numbers and strive to keep them as close to the normal range (less than 8 percent) as you can without triggering excessively low blood sugar reactions. These tests are available for home use.

Continuous blood glucose monitoring

Several useful devices are available that can continuously monitor glucose levels in the tissues beneath the skin instead of glucose in the blood. Fluid in tissues (called interstitial fluid) can provide extremely useful information about blood sugar. Some of these devices have an alarm that alerts you when your blood sugar level is very high or very low or if it is changing rapidly. Other devices track the blood glucose level to provide a retrospective analysis to help determine how well the blood sugar is being controlled between meals and during sleep; treatment can then be adjusted if necessary. Doctors are hopeful that in the future these devices will be attached to an automatic insulin delivery system that provides insulin on demand in response to glucose levels.

Pancreas transplants

Pancreas transplantation has become a widely used approach to treating type 1 diabetes, usually when a person also has advanced kidney disease. A kidney transplant (see page 820) is usually done at the same time. Although pancreas transplantation techniques continue to improve, a pancreas transplant is a technically complex surgical procedure with significant potential complications. However, many people who have type 1 diabetes and have a successful pancreas transplant are able to lead long, healthy lives after the transplant. They no longer need insulin injections or have repeated episodes of too-

high or too-low blood sugar, and their risk of long-term complications such as diabetic retinopathy (see page 1048) is reduced.

For a pancreas transplant, the diseased pancreas and the upper part of the small intestine (duodenum) to which it is connected are removed through an incision in the upper abdomen. The donor pancreas and duodenum are inserted in place and attached to the recipient's blood vessels and bladder. The procedure usually takes about 5 to 7 hours, and the person is hospitalized for about 2 to 3 weeks to enable doctors to monitor the transplant.

Experimental treatments

Because type 1 diabetes is an autoimmune disease that results when the immune system mistakenly attacks the insulin-producing cells in the pancreas, researchers are looking for ways to intervene to prevent the abnormal immune response from occurring in the first place or to control or reverse diabetes once it develops. Several promising studies are under way.

Because of the complexity of pancreas transplant surgery and successfully suppressing the immune system to prevent organ rejection, researchers are looking for ways to transplant just

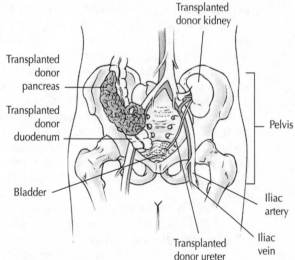

Pancreas transplant

In most cases, a pancreas transplant and a kidney transplant are performed at the same time. The donor pancreas and duodenum usually are implanted first, in the right lower abdomen, and connected to the recipient's blood vessels and bladder. The donor kidney and ureter are then implanted in the left lower abdomen and connected to the recipient's blood vessels and bladder.

the insulin-secreting cells into people with diabetes to enable them to go without insulin.

Type 2 Diabetes

Nine out of ten people with diabetes have type 2. In type 2 diabetes, the body does not respond appropriately to the hormone insulin, and there may be a corresponding lack of insulin secretion to compensate for the degree of resistance. Insulin enables cells to take in and use glucose, a simple sugar that is the body's main source of energy, or store it as fat.

The incidence of type 2 diabetes is reaching epidemic proportions throughout the world as more and more people adopt a lifestyle of exercising too little and eating too much—and getting fatter. More than a third of the 15 million Americans who have type 2 diabetes do not know they have it because the disease has no noticeable symptoms in the early stages. More and more American children are developing type 2 diabetes because they are increasingly less active than children of previous generations; eating more high-fat, high-calorie fast foods; and becoming obese. Just a few years ago it was rare to see children affected by this form of the disease, which used to be called adult-onset diabetes. However, today one out of five children who develop diabetes has type 2.

As people gain weight, the extra weight causes their cells to become resistant to the effects of insulin. The pancreas responds by producing more and more insulin, which eventually begins to build up in the blood. High levels of insulin in the blood, a condition called insulin resistance, can result in problems such as high blood pressure and harmful changes in the levels of the different kinds of fats in the blood. Insulin resistance, which doctors sometimes refer to as syndrome X or the metabolic syndrome (see page 53), is the first step toward type 2 diabetes.

The second step toward type 2 diabetes is a condition called impaired fasting glucose (also referred to as impaired glucose tolerance or prediabetes), which occurs when the pancreas can no longer produce enough insulin to get glucose out of the bloodstream into cells. Glucose begins to build up in the blood. If not diagnosed and treated, it is this gradual rise in glucose that will eventually lead to type 2 diabetes, high blood pressure, and heart disease—in any order and in any combination. It is estimated that as many as 16 million Americans over age 40

have prediabetes. Uncontrolled, diabetes can lead to stroke, blood circulation problems, kidney failure, and blindness. Complications from diabetes are the major cause of limb amputations.

Risk Factors

You are at increased risk of developing type 2 diabetes if you have any of the following risk factors:

- You have a family history of type 2 diabetes—for example, a parent or sibling with the disease.
- You are obese—you have a body mass index (BMI; see page 11) of 27 or higher. Having too much body fat, especially around the abdomen, can make your cells resistant to the effects of insulin, causing glucose to build up in the blood.
- You are Native American or of African, Asian, or Hispanic descent.
- You are 45 or older. The risk of type 2 diabetes tends to increase with age.
- You have been diagnosed with impaired fasting glucose, detected by a blood test showing a glucose level between 110 milligrams per deciliter (mg/dL) and 126 mg/dL.
- You have high blood pressure, defined as blood pressure readings consistently higher than 120/80 millimeters of mercury (mm Hg).
- Your level of HDL (good) cholesterol is 40 mg/dL or lower, or your triglyceride level is 250 mg/dL or higher (see page 146).
- You developed diabetes during a pregnancy (called gestational diabetes; see page 521), or you gave birth to an unusually large baby (weighing more than 9 pounds).
- You get little or no exercise most days.
- You carry more weight around your abdomen than on your hips and thighs and your waist is 40 inches or larger (if you're a man) or 35 inches or larger (if you're a woman). Waistline obesity reduces the ability of insulin to get glucose into cells.

If you have any of these risk factors, talk to your doctor about having a blood glucose test for type 2 diabetes.

Symptoms

Because the elevated level of glucose in the blood develops gradually, symptoms often do not occur for several years and frequently go unnoticed.

Type 2 Diabetes

Q. *Both of my parents are overweight and both have type 2 diabetes. Does that mean I will get it too?*

A. Because your parents have this form of diabetes, which tends to run in families, you are at increased risk of developing the disorder. But this does not mean that you are destined to get it. Your genes only make you more susceptible than a person who doesn't have the genes. You can avoid type 2 diabetes by not becoming overweight like your parents, and by exercising regularly and eating a healthy diet.

Q. *My 6-year-old son is extremely overweight and I'm getting worried about his health. What can I do?*

A. You are right to be concerned about your son's health. Obesity during childhood begins the processes that can lead to heart disease, high blood pressure, and type 2 diabetes. Alarmingly, increasing numbers of American children are developing type 2 diabetes as teenagers and even younger. This form of diabetes used to occur only in people over 40. To help your son avoid diabetes, work closely with his doctor to develop a plan to help your son lose weight. The plan will include a nutritious, low-fat, high-fiber diet and ways to encourage your son to be more active.

Q. *I'm currently taking a medication that lowers my blood glucose level. Is there any way to control my glucose level without medication?*

A. Yes, there is, but it requires a great deal of effort on your part. Many people with type 2 diabetes have been able to go off their medication by losing weight and increasing their level of activity. If you want to give it a try, work closely with your doctor to develop a weight-loss plan, including a diet and exercise program that will be effective for you.

When symptoms develop, they include frequent urination; unusual thirst; weight loss, sometimes even while eating excessively; and blurred vision.

Diagnosis

To diagnose type 2 diabetes, doctors use blood tests to measure the level of glucose in the blood. Because a number of factors (such as the medications a person is taking) can affect blood glucose levels, a doctor usually uses more than one blood test to help make a diagnosis. Your doctor may recommend one or more of the following tests if he or she suspects you have diabetes or if you are at risk of developing it.

Fasting plasma glucose test

A fasting plasma glucose test measures your blood glucose level after you have fasted (have not had anything to eat or drink except water for at least 8 hours, usually overnight).

- A glucose level of less than 110 milligrams per deciliter (mg/dL) is considered normal.
- A glucose level between 110 and 126 mg/dL indicates the possibility of impaired glucose tolerance, which means that you are at high risk of developing diabetes. In this case, your doctor will recommend having another blood test.
- A glucose level of 126 mg/dL or more on one fasting glucose test indicates that you have diabetes. Another blood test will be given to confirm the diagnosis.

Oral glucose tolerance test

An oral glucose tolerance test measures the body's ability to use glucose. To prepare for this test you will be asked to eat a diet rich in carbohydrates (foods such as whole grains, dried beans, and vegetables) for 2 or 3 days and then to fast overnight, or for at least 8 hours, before the test. After having a fasting glucose test, you will be asked to drink a sweet liquid containing glucose. Then you will be asked to lie or sit quietly while samples of your blood are taken every half hour for the next 2 hours to measure the level of glucose.

- A glucose level of 200 mg/dL or higher between the first and last blood tests and still higher than 200 mg/dL on the last test indicates diabetes.
- A glucose level of 200 mg/dL or higher on any of the blood tests but less than 200 mg/dL on the last test indicates impaired glucose tolerance, which means that you are at high risk of developing diabetes.

Hemoglobin A1C test

A test called a hemoglobin A1C test (or glycohemoglobin test) measures the percentage in your blood of a particular type of hemoglobin (the substance in red blood cells that carries oxygen). If you have too much glucose in your blood, the extra glucose links with the hemoglobin. This blood test can determine the average level of glucose in your blood over the past 3 to 4 months. For this reason, doctors use it to monitor the effectiveness of treatment in people who have diabetes.

Treatment

Managing type 2 diabetes means keeping your blood glucose level as close to normal as possible. Helpful strategies include keeping your weight down or losing weight if you need to, exercising regularly, and eating a nutritious diet rich in vegetables, whole grains, and legumes such as dried peas and beans. Eat fruit in moderation, and limit fruit juice (because it can raise blood sugar quickly). Many people with type 2 diabetes can keep their blood glucose level in a healthy range by following these measures.

Your doctor may recommend that you also take medication, depending on factors such as how long you have had diabetes, how high your blood glucose level is, and other medications you are taking. Although your doctor may prescribe insulin injections, taking insulin is usually not part of the initial treatment of type 2 diabetes. Your doctor may ask you to test your blood glucose level frequently or to have a hemoglobin A1C test (see previous page) periodically to evaluate the effectiveness of your treatment. You will have frequent blood tests to determine if your treatment is effective in keeping your glucose level in the healthy range.

Medication

Many types of medication are available for treating type 2 diabetes. If you take too much of some glucose-lowering medications (particularly sulfonylureas), your blood glucose level can drop too low. This condition—called hypoglycemia (see next page)—can be serious. Like all medications, these drugs can cause side effects in some people. Tell your doctor immediately if you feel unusual in any way after you start taking a medication.

Metformin

Metformin reduces glucose level by decreasing the liver's production of glucose. The drug also helps cells take in glucose and use it. Metformin is the only drug for diabetes that does not frequently cause weight gain. It can sometimes cause gastrointestinal problems such as diarrhea and therefore should be taken with meals. It is available in several forms and is sometimes taken in combination with an insulin-stimulating drug and a thiazolidinedione medication (see right) such as rosiglitazone or pioglitazone.

Acarbose

Acarbose is a drug you take with the first bite of a meal. This medication limits the rise in glucose that usually occurs after eating by decreasing the amount of glucose your body produces.

Insulin-stimulating drugs

A class of drugs called insulin-stimulating drugs (including sulfonylureas and nonsulfonylureas) stimulates the pancreas to make more insulin, which, in turn, lowers the glucose level. These drugs sometimes stop working after a few months or years or if you gain weight or if your body is under stress, such as when you have a bad infection or have had a heart attack or surgery.

Thiazolidinediones

Thiazolidinediones (TZDs) are a newer class of drugs that improve insulin sensitivity and may have other beneficial effects. Like metformin, they seldom cause too-low glucose levels. They can be used alone or in combination with other sugar-lowering drugs, such as metformin, or even with insulin.

Insulin

Some people with type 2 diabetes who have difficulty lowering their glucose level with glucose-lowering pills need to have insulin shots, or a combination of glucose-lowering pills and insulin. Your doctor may recommend trying different combinations to see which works best for you. If you need insulin, your doctor will give you precise instructions about how to give yourself shots and how often to give them. Eating about the same amount of food every day at approximately the same time can make adjusting the doses of medication easier to maintain the delicate balance between the level of insulin and the level of glucose in your blood. Your doctor or a diabetes educator can design a program tailored to your lifestyle and preferences.

Prevention

Exercising regularly and keeping your weight in a healthy range (see page 11) are the two most effective measures you can take to avoid type 2 diabetes. Exercise and being at a healthy weight enhance your body's ability to use glucose. If you need to lose weight, do so; even a weight loss of as few as 10 pounds can significantly reduce your risk of developing type 2 diabetes. Eating a well-balanced diet that is low in fat, rich in nutrients such as vitamins and minerals, and high in fiber is also helpful. Try to eat a wide variety of vegetables, fruits, whole grains, and legumes (such as dried beans and lentils).

Hypoglycemia

Hypoglycemia is a low level of the sugar glucose in the blood, which deprives your muscles, cells, and brain of the energy they need to function. Hypoglycemia occurs almost exclusively in people who have diabetes, especially if they are taking insulin injections or oral hypoglycemic (glucose-lowering) medication. The condition can be triggered by taking too much insulin, by not following the prescribed meal schedule, or by engaging in unusually strenuous or prolonged exercise. Drinking alcohol also can cause low blood glucose. Alcohol blocks the liver's ability to increase its output of glucose in response to the low blood glucose level; this glucose-blocking effect on the liver can last for 24 hours after having one beer or one mixed drink. Hypoglycemia can also develop when a person with diabetes has cancer, a reaction to a medication, abdominal surgery, liver disease, or a high fever, or is pregnant. When severe, hypoglycemia can cause unconsciousness.

Attacks of hypoglycemia are almost always treated and reversed before they become serious. The major danger is that you might have an attack while you are swimming, operating machinery, or driving a car. If you have frequent attacks, don't engage in these kinds of activities. If not detected, nighttime attacks, especially in older people, can cause severe, sometimes permanent, brain damage.

Symptoms

The symptoms of hypoglycemia vary considerably from person to person, but they often start with a feeling of being hot and uncomfortable, which is followed by profuse sweating and rapid heartbeat. You may also have a feeling of panic and feel hungry. Other possible symptoms include dizziness, weakness, trembling, unsteadiness, blurred vision, slurred speech, tingling in the lips or hands, or headache. You may become aggressive or uncooperative without being aware of it; you may appear intoxicated. Hypoglycemia can sometimes cause seizures (see page 686), especially in children or in people who drink alcohol without eating. If symptoms occur during the night, they usually wake you up. Severe cases can cause unconsciousness; this is referred to as a diabetic coma.

Treatment

If you have an attack of hypoglycemia, your doctor will use it to teach you to recognize an oncoming attack and discuss ways to prevent it. If you are having frequent attacks, your doctor may reduce your dose of insulin or oral hypoglycemic medication. You should always carry glucose gel tablets, sugar cubes, or candy with you. At the first sign of an attack, eat or drink something sweet until you feel the attack has passed, which should take only a few minutes.

Wear a medical identification bracelet or carry a card in your wallet indicating that you have diabetes, and make sure that members of your family and your friends know the symptoms of hypoglycemia so that if you become disoriented or uncooperative they can give you something sweet. Tell them that if they give you even a small drink of fruit juice you will probably recover enough to then be able to eat properly. But make sure they know that they should never try to feed you if you are unconscious (in a diabetic coma), because you could choke. If your hypoglycemia is caused by a medication you are taking for another disorder, talk to your doctor; he or she may recommend discontinuing the drug or may prescribe an alternative.

An alternative to glucose tablets for hypoglycemic attacks is an injection of glucagon, a hormone that helps raise blood glucose level. The injection is especially helpful if an attack makes a person unconscious, because someone else can give the injection. Many people who have hypoglycemic attacks teach their family and friends how to inject the hormone into an arm or leg muscle. Because the glucose-raising effects of glucagon are temporary, you also need to take additional sugar to raise your sugar level. Make sure that your family members and friends know that if these measures are not effective or available, they should call 911 or your local emergency number or take you to the nearest hospital emergency department immediately. You will be given an injection of glucose, which raises blood sugar so fast you may even regain consciousness as the injection is given.

Continuous glucose monitors now enable people with diabetes to check their blood glucose level minute by minute, enabling their doctor to detect patterns of fluctuation in the level and recommend measures to maintain better control. The devices, some of which are worn like a watch or implanted, can give a warning to alert the person if his or her blood glucose gets too high or too low.

Disorders of the Adrenal Glands

The adrenals are a pair of small, triangular glands; one adrenal gland is on top of each kidney. Each adrenal gland has a central core (adrenal medulla) and an outer layer (adrenal cortex). The adrenal medulla produces two hormones— epinephrine and norepinephrine—that have an important role in controlling heart rate and blood pressure and the body's response to stress. The hypothalamus in the brain stimulates the adrenal glands to produce these hormones.

The adrenal cortex produces three different groups of corticosteroid hormones. The hormones in the first group regulate the concentration and balance of various chemicals in the body. The most important hormone in this group is aldosterone, which helps control blood pressure and regulates sodium and potassium levels in the body. The hormones in the second group have a number of functions, including helping to convert carbohydrates into energy-rich glycogen in the liver. (Glycogen has an essential role in regulating blood sugar levels.) Cortisol is the main hormone in this group.

The third group of hormones consists of androgens (male sex hormones) and estrogen and progesterone (female sex hormones), which regulate sexual development and the functioning of the reproductive system. Sex hormones are produced mainly by the testicles and the ovaries. Although both sexes produce male and female sex hormones, androgens are more prevalent in men and estrogen and progesterone are more prevalent in women.

The pituitary gland controls the production of most corticosteroid hormones. The only exception is aldosterone, which is stimulated by the hormone renin, produced by the kidneys.

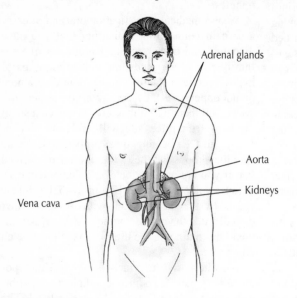

Adrenal glands

Aorta

Kidneys

Vena cava

The adrenal glands
The adrenal glands are on top of each kidney. The adrenal glands produce corticosteroid hormones, which help regulate metabolism (the chemical processes that take place in the body), and the hormones epinephrine and norepinephrine, which help control heart rate and blood pressure and the body's response to stress.

Cushing's Syndrome

Cushing's syndrome is a rare condition that results from an excess of corticosteroid hormones in the blood. The disorder usually results from taking large doses of corticosteroid drugs for long-term treatment of an inflammatory illness such as rheumatoid arthritis (see page 918) or asthma (see page 640). In rare cases, the condition develops when the outer layer of one or both adrenal glands (the adrenal cortex) produces excessive amounts of corticosteroid hormones. Overproduction of corticosteroid hormones can occur when a tumor in one of the adrenal glands or elsewhere in the body over-stimulates the adrenal glands. If the tumor that is causing the excess hormone production is in the pituitary gland in the brain, the condition is called Cushing's disease rather than Cushing's syndrome. Cushing's syndrome is most common in young to middle-aged women.

Symptoms
The symptoms of Cushing's syndrome usually appear gradually, over a period of several months. First, the face becomes large and round. Excess fat forms on the body, and a pad of fat develops between the shoulder blades. At the same time, muscles in the arms and legs lose mass and weaken. The skin may become thinner and may bruise easily. Over time, blood pressure increases and the

bones become thin and fracture easily (osteoporosis; see page 989).

Diagnosis

A diagnosis of Cushing's syndrome is based on the symptoms and a physical examination. The doctor will recommend blood and urine tests to measure the levels of cortisol, the major corticosteroid hormone. If cortisol levels are high, the doctor may recommend a 24-hour urine test to evaluate pituitary function and determine if there is a tumor in the pituitary gland. For a 24-hour urine test, you collect a sample of urine each time you urinate over a 24-hour period. Depending on the test results, the doctor may also recommend a CT scan (see page 112) or an MRI (see page 113) to look for a tumor in the pituitary or in the adrenal glands. If no tumor is detected, he or she may recommend an X-ray or CT scan of the lungs to check for lung cancer (some tumors in the lungs secrete corticosteroidlike hormones).

Treatment

If long-term corticosteroid treatment for another disorder is the cause of Cushing's syndrome, your doctor will either adjust the dosage of the medication you are taking or prescribe a different drug. If the disorder results from a pituitary tumor, the doctor may recommend surgery or radiation therapy to remove or destroy the tumor. If you have a tumor in one adrenal gland, the doctor will recommend surgery to remove the gland; your body should function normally with the remaining adrenal gland. In some cases, both adrenal glands are removed surgically. If both adrenal glands are removed, you will need to take corticosteroid drugs for the rest of your life to replace the hormones your body no longer produces. With successful treatment, most people with Cushing's syndrome are able to lead healthy, active lives.

Addison's Disease

Addison's disease is a potentially life-threatening condition in which the outer layer of the adrenal glands (the adrenal cortex) gradually slows production of corticosteroid hormones. The disease usually occurs when the adrenal cortex is damaged or destroyed as a result of an autoimmune disorder, in which the immune system mistakenly attacks the adrenal glands. In rare cases, tuberculosis (see page 663) can cause Addison's disease. Addison's disease can sometimes run in families and can be the first sign of a rare inherited disorder called adrenoleukodystrophy.

Symptoms

The symptoms of Addison's disease—including loss of appetite, weight loss, dizziness, fatigue, weakness, muscle aches, and anemia (see page 610)—usually develop gradually. Other symptoms can include mild indigestion, nausea and vomiting, diarrhea, or constipation. In some cases, the skin may darken noticeably and permanently. Some people become more sensitive to cool temperatures.

If Addison's disease is left untreated, symptoms of acute adrenal failure (such as severe abdominal pain or dizziness) may develop and the person may go into shock (see page 162). Undergoing surgery or having an injury or a severe infection or other illness can trigger this life-threatening condition. During a medical examination of a person with acute adrenal failure, a doctor will find that the person has low blood pressure and kidney failure.

WARNING!

Acute Adrenal Failure

Acute adrenal failure is a medical emergency that requires immediate medical treatment. If you are with someone who has Addison's disease or another disorder of the adrenal glands and he or she has symptoms of acute adrenal failure (such as severe abdominal pain or dizziness) or if he or she goes into shock, call 911 or your local emergency number, or take the person to the nearest hospital emergency department immediately.

Diagnosis

A diagnosis of Addison's disease is based on the symptoms and a physical examination. The doctor will recommend blood and urine tests to measure the levels of corticosteroid hormones and to evaluate kidney function. He or she also may recommend a blood test to look for antibodies (proteins the body may have mistakenly produced to attack the adrenal glands). The presence of antiadrenal antibodies indicates an autoimmune response.

Treatment

To treat Addison's disease, your doctor will prescribe oral corticosteroid medication to replace the corticosteroid hormones your body is not producing. (Doctors may prescribe intravenous corticosteroids for people who are extremely ill.) You will probably need to take these drugs for the rest of your life.

Your doctor will give you a medical identification card that indicates you have Addison's disease. Always carry this card with you so emergency medical personnel will know what treatment to provide in case of an emergency. Whenever you have an illness or infection, call your doctor as soon as possible. He or she may increase your dose of corticosteroids to prevent acute adrenal failure. If you are planning to have surgery, make sure the surgeon knows that you have Addison's disease. Most people who are treated for Addison's disease are able to lead healthy, active lives.

Aldosteronism

Aldosteronism is a rare disorder in which the cortex of the adrenal glands produces too much of the hormone aldosterone, which results in high blood pressure (see page 574). Aldosteronism can result from a tumor in one adrenal gland (called Conn's syndrome) or from an enlargement of both adrenal glands. The disorder also can be caused by an underlying disease or condition that reduces blood flow through the kidneys, such as congestive heart failure (see page 570).

Symptoms and Diagnosis
The symptoms of aldosteronism include elevated blood pressure, fatigue, tingling, muscle weakness, muscle spasms, and paralysis. Some people also may experience increased thirst and frequent urination.

A diagnosis of aldosteronism is based on the symptoms and a physical examination. The doctor will recommend blood and urine tests to measure aldosterone levels. If the results of the blood and urine tests show high levels of aldosterone, the doctor may recommend a CT scan (see page 112), an MRI (see page 113), or a radionuclide scan (see page 114) to look for a tumor that could be causing the disorder.

Treatment
If aldosteronism is caused by an adrenal tumor, the doctor may recommend surgery to remove the tumor, which often cures the disorder. If aldosteronism is not caused by a tumor, the doctor will prescribe medications to block the action of aldosterone and control high blood pressure. If drug treatment is not effective, the doctor may recommend surgery to remove part of the adrenal glands to reduce production of aldosterone. In rare cases, both adrenal glands are removed.

Pheochromocytoma

Pheochromocytoma is a very rare condition in which a noncancerous tumor in the core of an adrenal gland (the adrenal medulla) causes the gland to produce too much epinephrine and norepinephrine. These hormones, which are produced in the adrenal medulla, work with the nervous system to control heart rate and blood pressure.

Symptoms
The main symptoms of pheochromocytoma are significantly elevated blood pressure and a rapid, pounding heartbeat. Other symptoms may include light-headedness; pale, cold, and clammy skin; excessive sweating; rapid breathing; and chest pain. Some people may experience numbness and tingling in the hands, faintness, severe headaches, constipation, nausea and vomiting, or visual disturbances.

The elevated blood pressure may be persistent, or it may come and go along with other symptoms. The symptoms can be triggered by pressure on the tumor, medication, mild physical exertion, exposure to cold temperatures, or mild stress.

Diagnosis
A diagnosis of pheochromocytoma is based on the symptoms and the results of blood and urine tests that measure the levels of epinephrine and norepinephrine. If the blood and urine tests show an excess of these hormones, the doctor may recommend a CT scan (see page 112), an MRI (see page 113), or radionuclide scanning (see page 114) to locate the tumor.

Treatment
To treat pheochromocytoma, a doctor performs surgery to remove the tumor, which usually cures the disorder. Before surgery, the doctor may prescribe a combination of the blood pressure medications alpha blockers and beta blockers to lower the person's blood pressure.

Disorders of the Thyroid and Parathyroid Glands

The thyroid is a small, butterfly-shaped gland in the lower part of the neck, directly in front of the trachea (windpipe). The thyroid has two lobes that are joined by a thin strand of thyroid tissue called the isthmus. Under the control of thyrotropin (also called thyroid-stimulating hormone, or TSH), which is produced by the pituitary gland, the thyroid gland produces thyroid hormones that control the speed of metabolism (the chemical processes that take place in the body). In general, the higher the level of thyroid hormones in the blood, the faster the speed of metabolism. To produce thyroid hormones, the thyroid needs an adequate supply of iodine, which comes from food (especially fish and iron-fortified products) and water.

At each of the four corners of the thyroid gland, but unrelated to the thyroid gland itself, are four parathyroid glands, each about the size of a pea. The parathyroid glands produce parathyroid hormone, which works with a thyroid hormone called calcitonin and vitamin D to control the level of calcium in the blood. Calcium is essential for healthy bones and teeth and has a significant role in the functioning of nerves and muscles. Parathyroid hormone, calcitonin, and vitamin D raise the calcium level in the blood in several ways—by causing the intestines to absorb more calcium from food, by causing the body to excrete less calcium in urine, and by causing calcium to be released from bone tissue.

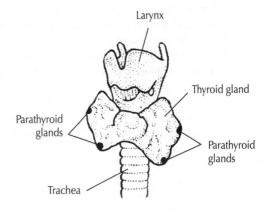

The thyroid and parathyroid glands
The thyroid gland is at the base of the neck, directly below the larynx (voice box) and in front of the trachea (windpipe). Thyroid hormones are essential for growth and metabolism (the chemical processes that take place in the body). The parathyroids are two pairs of pea-sized glands next to the thyroid gland. Parathyroid hormone helps control the levels of calcium in the blood.

Hyperthyroidism

Hyperthyroidism (also called Graves' disease) is a disorder in which the thyroid gland is overactive and produces excessive amounts of thyroid hormones. Activity of the thyroid gland is normally controlled by secretion of thyrotropin (also called thyroid-stimulating hormone, or TSH) by the pituitary gland. In hyperthyroidism, the control mechanism malfunctions—although the pituitary reduces its production of thyrotropin, the thyroid gland continues to produce large quantities of thyroid hormones. The resulting high levels of thyroid hormones in the blood generally speed up all of the chemical reactions in the body, causing both physical and psychological symptoms.

Hyperthyroidism can result from an autoimmune disorder in which the immune system mistakenly attacks the thyroid gland, causing it to become overactive. Thyroid nodules (see page 903) are another possible cause of hyperthyroidism. Thyroid nodules are noncancerous cysts in the thyroid gland that are filled with functioning thyroid tissue. The nodules produce thyroid hormones in addition to the hormones produced by the thyroid gland itself.

Older people and people who have high blood pressure (see page 574) or atherosclerosis (see page 557) have an increased risk of hyperthyroidism. Hyperthyroidism occurs more frequently in women than in men.

Symptoms
Although the symptoms of hyperthyroidism vary from person to person, most people experience a combination of several of the following symptoms:

- Nervousness and anxiety
- Irritability

- Difficulty sleeping
- Trembling of the body and hands
- Weakness
- Fatigue
- Confusion
- Decreased sensitivity to cold
- Increased sensitivity to heat
- Sweating
- Irregular heartbeat, rapid heartbeat, or palpitations
- High blood pressure
- Shortness of breath after mild exertion
- Frequent bowel movements (sometimes with diarrhea)
- Increased appetite combined with weight loss
- Light menstrual periods or absence of periods
- Prominent swelling in the front of the neck (called goiter)
- Puffiness around the eyes
- Bulging eyes
- Intense, constant stare
- Sensitivity to light
- Abnormally smooth skin
- Nail changes

In some people, high blood pressure or a rapid, irregular heartbeat may put additional strain on the heart and circulation, causing chest pain called angina (see page 559), arrhythmias (see page 580), or heart failure (see page 570).

Diagnosis

If you have symptoms of hyperthyroidism, your doctor will ask about your symptoms and examine you. He or she will probably arrange for you to have a blood test that measures the level of thyrotropin and indicates either high or low activity of the thyroid gland. The doctor may also recommend a blood test to measure the level of thyroid hormones in the blood. To confirm the diagnosis, blood tests may be done to check for antibodies (proteins the immune system mistakenly produces to attack the thyroid gland); the presence of antithyroid antibodies indicates an autoimmune response. Once hyperthyroidism is diagnosed, your doctor may arrange for a thyroid scan to determine whether part or all of your thyroid gland is affected. A thyroid scan is a type of radionuclide scan (see page 114), in which you swallow a small amount of radioactive iodine and lie under a special camera that detects the radiation in the thyroid gland.

Treatment

Before beginning treatment for hyperthyroidism, your doctor will probably prescribe blood pressure medications called beta blockers to slow your heart rate, to control trembling, and to reduce anxiety. Although these drugs will quickly relieve your symptoms, they will not affect the level of thyroid hormones in the blood.

To treat hyperthyroidism, along with the beta blockers, the doctor will probably prescribe antithyroid medications, which decrease the thyroid gland's production of thyroid hormones. In most cases, these drugs will control the disorder within about 8 weeks, but you will need to continue taking them—sometimes for a year or longer—until your doctor tells you to stop. Although the blood level of thyroid hormones may quickly return to normal, it may take several weeks for all of the symptoms to improve. The doctor also may prescribe corticosteroid medications to lower the blood level of thyroid hormones and reduce inflammation. Although some people are eventually cured with drug treatment, in most people, symptoms recur and additional treatment is required.

Following treatment with antithyroid drugs, the doctor may perform surgery to remove either a lump in the thyroid gland or, if it is overactive, most of the thyroid gland. In most cases, surgery cures the disorder. However, in rare cases, the disease recurs or the thyroid or parathyroid glands become underactive (hypothyroidism; see next page) as a result of the surgery. In such cases, doctors usually prescribe corticosteroids.

For some people, doctors may recommend treatment with radioactive iodine. In this procedure, the person swallows a small dose of radioactive iodine in the form of a clear, slightly salty liquid. Because iodine is an essential component of some thyroid hormones, the radioactive material concentrates in the thyroid gland, where it acts on the glandular tissue to slowly control the overactivity without exposing the rest of the body to radiation. In some cases, the thyroid gland may become underactive, and you may have to take medication to treat this condition.

Each treatment has advantages and disadvantages, and your doctor will work with you to determine the best course for you. With successful treatment, most people who have hyperthyroidism are able to lead a healthy, active life.

Hypothyroidism

Hypothyroidism is a common disorder in which the thyroid gland is underactive and does not produce enough thyroid hormones. As a result, all the chemical processes in the body slow down. The severe form of hypothyroidism is called myxedema. Hypothyroidism affects women more frequently than men.

The thyroid gland may become underactive for one of several reasons. Occasionally, treatment for hyperthyroidism (see page 901), which attempts to reduce production of thyroid hormones, causes an overactive thyroid gland to become underactive. A deficiency of thyrotropin, which regulates the activity of the thyroid gland, is another possible cause of hypothyroidism.

Because the hypothalamus controls the production of thyrotropin by the pituitary gland, a disorder in either gland can lead to a deficiency of this hormone. Without an adequate supply of thyrotropin, the thyroid gland cannot function properly. Hypothyroidism may also result from Hashimoto's disease (see page 928), an autoimmune disorder in which the immune system mistakenly attacks the thyroid gland, reducing or blocking the production of thyroid hormone. In some cases, the thyroid gland becomes underactive for no apparent reason.

Rarely, a child is born with a defective thyroid gland or without a thyroid gland, and has hypothyroidism (see page 404). If not detected and treated promptly, the condition can lead to short stature and irreversible mental retardation.

Symptoms

The symptoms of hypothyroidism develop slowly, over the course of many months or years. People who have hypothyroidism usually experience a combination of some of the following symptoms:

- Fatigue
- Slow heart rate
- Hoarseness
- Slowed speech
- Puffy face
- Constipation
- Confusion
- Depression
- Dementia
- Increased sensitivity to cold
- Decreased appetite combined with weight gain
- Drooping eyelids
- Dry hair
- Dry, scaly, thick skin
- Heavy, prolonged menstrual periods
- Loss of sexual desire
- Hearing loss
- Numbness and tingling in the hands and arms
- Drowsiness

Diagnosis

A diagnosis of hypothyroidism is based on the symptoms and a physical examination. The doctor will recommend blood tests to measure blood levels of thyrotropin and antithyroid antibodies (infection-fighting proteins that would indicate an autoimmune response). If a blood test shows a high level of thyrotropin, a diagnosis of hypothyroidism is confirmed. If the blood also contains antithyroid antibodies, the diagnosis is Hashimoto's disease.

Treatment

If you have hypothyroidism, your doctor will prescribe oral thyroid hormones, which you will need to take for the rest of your life. After a few days of treatment, your symptoms will improve; after a few months, you should recover completely. Myxedema is also treated with thyroid hormones.

Thyroid Nodules

A thyroid nodule is a small lump in the thyroid gland. Some thyroid nodules are cancerous, but most are harmless, noncancerous cysts filled with fluid or functioning thyroid tissue. The cause of thyroid nodules is not known, but doctors think they may result from mutations in genes that control tissue growth. Thyroid nodules usually develop as people get older, and they are much more common in women than in men. If you had radiation treatments to your head or neck as a child, you have an increased risk of developing a cancerous thyroid nodule.

Symptoms

A large thyroid nodule that contains functioning thyroid tissue may increase blood levels of thyroid hormones, causing symptoms of hyperthyroidism (see page 901) such as rapid heartbeat, trembling of the body and hands, increased sensitivity to heat, or sweating. A person may also have nail changes or bulging eyes and an intense, constant stare.

Diagnosis

Most thyroid nodules can be felt by a doctor during a physical examination. To evaluate the nodule, your doctor may perform a thyroid scan, which is a type of radionuclide scan (see page 114), in which you swallow a small amount of radioactive iodine and lie under a special camera that detects the radiation in the thyroid gland. Although a thyroid scan can detect nodules that contain functioning thyroid tissue, cancerous or fluid-filled nodules are not visible on the scan. Nodules that do not appear on a thyroid scan are usually evaluated by fine-needle aspiration, a diagnostic procedure in which a small amount of tissue and fluid are withdrawn from the nodule with a hollow needle and syringe and examined under a microscope for cancer cells.

Treatment

If a noncancerous nodule is small, your doctor may recommend monitoring it to see if it grows. If a fluid-filled nodule is large and unsightly, the doctor can reduce its size by removing some of the fluid with a needle and syringe. A nodule that contains functioning thyroid tissue can be destroyed by treatment with radioactive iodine. If a nodule is cancerous, the doctor will recommend surgery to remove the gland, and treatment with radioactive iodine to kill any remaining cancer cells. After the gland is removed, your doctor will monitor your condition regularly and you will need to take thyroid hormones for the rest of your life.

Hyperparathyroidism

Hyperparathyroidism is a disorder in which the parathyroid glands are overactive and produce too much parathyroid hormone. Along with vitamin D and a hormone called calcitonin produced by the thyroid gland, parathyroid hormone regulates the levels of calcium in the body. Overproduction of parathyroid hormone increases the amount of calcium circulating in the bloodstream by removing calcium from the bones. Loss of calcium from the bones can lead to osteoporosis (see page 989), a condition in which bones become weak and brittle and fracture easily. In an attempt to remove the excess calcium from the blood, the kidneys excrete greater-than-normal amounts of calcium in urine, which can lead to the formation of kidney stones (see page 814).

Hyperparathyroidism usually results from a small noncancerous tumor in one or more of the four parathyroid glands. In some cases, the disorder results from enlargement of the glands. The cause of this enlargement is not known. Hyperparathyroidism is more common in women than in men and, rarely, may run in families.

Symptoms

Symptoms of hyperparathyroidism can include muscle aches, muscle weakness, or frequent urination. Other possible symptoms are drowsiness, fatigue, depression, confusion, or seizures. Some people experience nausea and vomiting, abdominal pain, flatulence, or constipation.

Diagnosis

To diagnose hyperparathyroidism, a doctor will order blood tests to measure the levels of calcium, phosphorus (a mineral that has an essential role in bone formation), and parathyroid hormone in the blood. In some cases, the doctor may recommend an ultrasound scan (see page 111) or a radionuclide scan (see page 114) to determine which of the four parathyroid glands is causing the problem. Hyperparathyroidism can also be detected by genetic analysis to look for a rare genetic disorder called multiple endocrine neoplasia, which can lead to cancer.

Treatment

The usual treatment for hyperparathyroidism is surgical removal of a tumor if there is one, or of three of the four enlarged parathyroid glands. After surgery, the person may develop hypoparathyroidism (see next article), in which the parathyroid glands do not produce enough parathyroid hormone; he or she will then be treated for that condition.

If hyperparathyroidism causes kidney stones to form, a doctor may recommend treatment with extracorporeal lithotripsy (see page 816), a procedure in which shock waves pulverize the stones into a powder that can be passed out of the body in urine. Kidney stones also can be removed surgically.

Medications called bisphosphonates can help prevent bone loss resulting from hyperparathyroidism. Scientists are currently developing medications to prevent the parathyroid glands from secreting too much parathyroid hormone.

Hypoparathyroidism

Hypoparathyroidism is a rare disorder in which the parathyroid glands are underactive and do not produce enough parathyroid hormone. Along with vitamin D and a hormone called calcitonin produced by the thyroid gland, parathyroid hormone regulates the levels of calcium in the body. A deficiency of parathyroid hormone leads to low levels of calcium in the blood and in the tissues, which can affect the functioning of muscles and nerves. Hypoparathyroidism can occur alone or along with problems in other endocrine glands, such as the thyroid gland or the adrenal glands.

Hypoparathyroidism usually results when tissue is removed from the parathyroid glands in surgery performed to control hyperparathyroidism (overactivity of the parathyroid glands; see previous page). The disorder also can result from surgery performed on the thyroid gland to control overactivity of the thyroid gland (hyperthyroidism; see page 901) or to remove a cancerous tumor. In some cases, hypoparathyroidism has no obvious cause.

Symptoms

The main symptom of hypoparathyroidism is uncontrollable, painful, cramplike spasms in the face, hands, arms, and feet. Other symptoms include numbness and tingling in the face and hands, dry skin, and thinning hair. In rare cases, a person may have seizures. People who have hypoparathyroidism often develop a yeast infection in the mouth called oral thrush (see page 744). Women who have the disorder are susceptible to developing vaginal yeast infections (see page 880).

Diagnosis

Hypoparathyroidism is diagnosed by the symptoms and the results of a blood test to measure the level of parathyroid hormone in the blood. Low levels of parathyroid hormone indicate that the parathyroid glands are underactive.

Treatment

To quickly relieve the painful muscle spasms caused by hypoparathyroidism, your doctor will recommend intravenous injections of calcium. You will need to take calcium and vitamin D supplements for the rest of your life to help maintain normal levels of calcium in your body and to prevent symptoms of calcium deficiency. Your doctor will examine you and perform blood tests on a regular basis to evaluate the effectiveness of your treatment and to monitor the level of calcium in your blood.

11

Disorders of the Immune System

Your immune system is an elaborate system of proteins, cells, organs, and ducts that protects your body from infection by invading microorganisms such as bacteria, viruses, or fungi. When one of these microorganisms enters your body, white blood cells recognize it as foreign and move in to get rid of it. During this process, the white blood cells form a memory of a specific protein—called an antigen—that sits on the surface of the invading microorganism. This memory allows your immune system to recognize the microorganism in the future if you are exposed to it again. Doctors call this memory-forming ability immunity.

Protective immunity keeps you from developing some infections, such as measles, more than once. Your body recognizes the microorganism when it invades again and responds quickly to neutralize it. Immunity also explains how vaccines protect against infectious diseases. Exposure to a small amount of the inactivated microorganism contained in the vaccine creates an immune system memory that your body can use to defend itself if it encounters the microorganism again.

Your immune system fights infection in two important ways, using two types of white blood cells: B cells and T cells. B cells produce antibodies, which are proteins that circulate in the bloodstream. When an invading microbe enters the body, the antibodies target a specific antigen on the surface of the microbe. The antibodies bind to the antigen and either destroy it or change it to make it more attractive to the scavenger white blood cells that will eat it.

T cells play two roles in immune defense. Helper T cells, also called CD4-positive T cells, signal B cells to begin making antibodies. Helper T cells can also activate scavenger white blood cells to gobble up invading microorganisms. Killer T cells, also known as CD8-positive T cells, attack and destroy cells that have been infected by invading microbes.

A number of factors can contribute to the suppression of the immune system and make you susceptible to infection and disease. Stress and malnutrition, including excessive dieting, can adversely affect your body's ability to launch a defense against infection. Having major surgery or undergoing cancer treatment can also impair the immune system's ability to function. People who are infected with HIV experience a slow and devastating assault on their immune system that leaves them highly vulnerable to infections and diseases that healthy people can easily fend off.

The Lymphatic System

The organs of your immune system—strategically positioned throughout the body—are called lymphoid organs because they serve as stations for the growth and deployment of lymphocytes (white blood cells that mount the body's primary defense against infection). Lymphocytes recognize infectious agents and other potentially harmful substances and participate in the body's immune reaction against them. White blood cells form in the spongy tissue of the bone marrow. This nutrient-rich tissue is found in the center of the long, flat bones, such as those in the pelvis.

The white blood cells travel by way of the blood vessels to the lymphatic system—a circulatory system that is separate from the cardiovascular system. The lymphatic system circulates lymph, a clear liquid that carries white blood cells throughout the body. Round nodules called lymph nodes, or lymph glands, which lie along the lymphatic vessels, supply white blood cells to the bloodstream and remove bacteria and other potentially harmful particles from the lymph. When fighting an infection, the lymph nodes often become swollen. (You have probably noticed swelling of the lymph glands in your neck when you have an infection.)

A number of other key organs are also part of your immune system. The spleen, a fist-sized organ in the upper left part of the abdomen, produces infection-fighting antibodies and some types of white blood cells. Lying deep inside the upper chest behind the

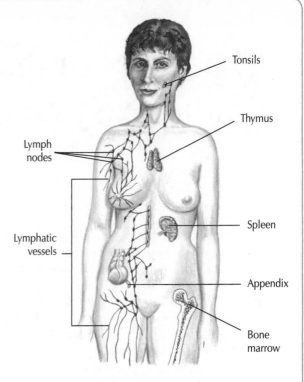

The organs of the immune system

breastbone, the thymus changes immature T cells into mature T cells. T cells are one of the two major types of lymphocytes. Your tonsils, adenoids, and appendix are clumps of lymphoid tissue that stand guard at key points in your body where infectious microorganisms are likely to try to enter.

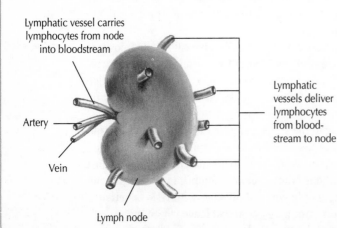

Lymph node

Lymph nodes play a major role in the body's immune response. Lymph nodes contain infection-fighting white blood cells called lymphocytes, which circulate throughout the body among the blood, lymph nodes, and lymphatic vessels and are always on guard against potentially harmful microorganisms. The lymphatic vessels carry lymphocytes from the lymph nodes into the bloodstream and deliver lymphocytes into the lymph nodes from the bloodstream.

HIV Infection and AIDS

The term AIDS—acquired immunodeficiency syndrome—refers to the most advanced stages of infection with HIV, the human immunodeficiency virus. By destroying cells that are part of the body's immune system, HIV progressively disables the body's ability to fight infection and some types of cancer. People infected with HIV often develop life-threatening infections that are called opportunistic because they seize the chance presented by the impaired immune system to take hold in the body. Such infections usually do not make healthy people sick.

HIV is a retrovirus, which means that, unlike other viruses that carry DNA as their hereditary material, HIV carries RNA. Retroviruses reproduce by turning their RNA into DNA using an enzyme called reverse transcriptase. When a retrovirus such as HIV infects a cell, it inserts its RNA into the cell along with reverse transcriptase. The resulting DNA contains the genetic instructions that allow the virus to replicate. HIV belongs to a subgroup of retroviruses called "slow" viruses. Infection by a slow virus is characterized by a long period—sometimes decades—between initial infection and the appearance of symptoms. Worldwide, roughly 40 million people are living with HIV; about 48 percent of adults infected with HIV are women.

HIV infection gradually impairs the functioning of the immune system by disabling and killing specialized immune system cells called CD4-positive T cells, or helper T cells, that signal other cells in the immune system to perform their special functions. Healthy people have 800 to 1,200 helper T cells per cubic millimeter (mm^3) of blood. After HIV infection, the number of helper T cells gradually decreases. When the number of helper T cells falls below 200 cells per mm^3, the affected person becomes especially vulnerable to opportunistic infections, such as some specific types of pneumonia and cancer.

How HIV Infects a Helper T Cell

When a particle of HIV encounters a CD4-positive T cell, it recognizes it by a molecule called a CD4 receptor on the cell's surface. The HIV particle binds with the CD4-positive T cell, which enables the HIV particle to enter the cell. Inside the cell, HIV converts its RNA into DNA. The newly made viral DNA enters the cell's nucleus, where it is spliced into the host cell's DNA. This processed HIV then moves out of the nucleus into the cytoplasm of the cell, where it uses the cell's protein-making machinery to make copies of itself. Once these new viral particles leave the cell, they become infectious and search for other CD4-positive T cells to invade.

People can become infected with HIV through contact with infected blood or other body fluids, usually by having unprotected sex with an infected partner or by sharing contaminated needles. Infected women can spread HIV to their babies during pregnancy or childbirth. Infected mothers can also transmit HIV to their babies in breast milk. Having a sexually transmitted disease (see page 477)—such as syphilis, genital herpes, or gonorrhea—makes a person more vulnerable to HIV infection during unprotected sex. HIV is not transmitted through casual contact, such as sharing towels or bedding, telephones, or toilet seats. It has not been shown that biting insects, such as mosquitoes or bedbugs, transmit HIV.

The only sure way of preventing HIV infection is to avoid behaviors that put you at risk, such as having unprotected sex and sharing needles. There is no reliable way to know if someone is infected with HIV because many infected people

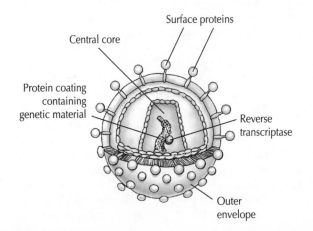

HIV

HIV is a microscopic spherical retrovirus. Its RNA, which contains its genetic information, resides inside a protective coating made up of proteins. HIV uses an enzyme called reverse transcriptase to convert its RNA into DNA inside the host cell it invades and uses the host DNA to make copies of itself.

have no symptoms for years. For this reason, you should use a latex condom each time you have sexual intercourse—vaginal, anal, or oral—unless you are in a monogamous relationship and you and your partner have both tested negative for HIV. Pregnant women who are infected with HIV can reduce the risk of spreading the infection to their babies by taking the drug zidovudine during pregnancy and labor. The infant must then be given zidovudine for the first 6 weeks of life.

Symptoms

Many people have no symptoms when they first become infected with HIV. Others experience a flulike illness that produces fever, headache, fatigue, and enlarged lymph glands about 4 to 8 weeks after becoming infected. The symptoms usually go away within a few weeks and the infected person often thinks that he or she has had the flu. During this time, affected people are extremely infectious because HIV is present in large amounts in blood and other body fluids.

In adults, additional symptoms may not appear for 10 years or more after exposure to the virus, although some people begin noticing symptoms within a few months or years. Children infected at birth usually show symptoms within 2 years. During this time, HIV is actively reproducing and destroying the helper T cells of the immune system.

As the immune system deteriorates, a wide range of symptoms begins to appear. The first sign may be swollen lymph glands that remain enlarged for more than 3 months. Other symptoms include lack of energy, weight loss, frequent fevers, profuse sweating, frequent yeast infections in the mouth or vagina, skin rashes, pelvic inflammatory disease (see page 871) that does not respond well to treatment, and short-term memory loss. Some people develop severe herpes infections (see page 482) or shingles (see page 936).

As the infection progresses, the level of helper T cells in the blood becomes very low, opportunistic infections begin to appear, and the diagnosis of full-blown AIDS is made. Signs of opportunistic infections that are common in people with AIDS include fever, shortness of breath, seizures, difficulty swallowing, confusion and forgetfulness, severe diarrhea, loss of vision, nausea, abdominal cramps, vomiting, extreme fatigue, severe headaches, and coma. Children with AIDS can develop the same opportunistic infections as adults or severe versions of common childhood bacterial infections such as tonsillitis or ear infections.

People with AIDS are especially susceptible to developing some cancers, usually those that are caused by viruses. For example, Kaposi's sarcoma (a cancer of the tissue under the skin or mucous membranes lining the mouth, nose, and anus) and cervical cancer (see page 875) are unusually common in people who have AIDS. Cancers of the immune system, such as lymphoma (see page 625), are also common in people with AIDS.

Diagnosis

Doctors diagnose HIV infection by testing the blood for the presence of antibodies (infection-fighting proteins the body has produced in response to exposure to HIV). The antibodies usually do not reach detectable levels for 1 to 3 months after infection.

In general, a person who is infected with HIV is thought to have developed AIDS when his or her level of CD4-positive T cells falls below 200 cells per cubic millimeter (mm^3) of blood. In addition, the person must have at least one opportunistic infection, such as Pneumocystis carinii pneumonia or Kaposi's sarcoma, for a diagnosis of AIDS.

Treatment

In the initial years of the AIDS epidemic, no drugs were available to fight the disease's destruction of the immune system, and few treatments were effective against the resulting opportunistic infections. AIDS was considered an untreatable, terminal condition, and many infected people died.

Over the past decade, however, researchers have developed several drugs that effectively treat HIV and the other infections and cancers it often produces. The drugs, called antiretroviral medications, slow the spread of HIV in the body and delay the onset of opportunistic infections by interfering with the virus's ability to reproduce. The two main types of antiretroviral drugs are reverse transcriptase inhibitors (which block the enzyme reverse transcriptase that the virus needs to convert its RNA into DNA inside the host cell) and protease inhibitors (which block the enzyme protease that the virus needs to reproduce itself). The two classes of drugs are frequently combined to produce a more potent and effective drug regimen.

No currently available drugs can cure HIV infection—the virus has become resistant to all the

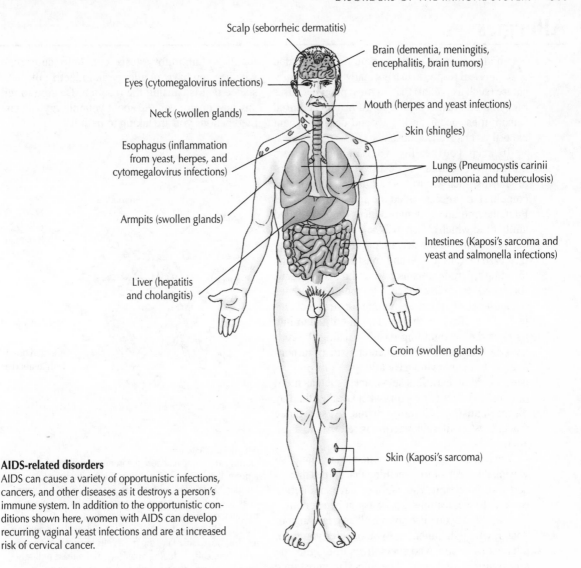

Scalp (seborrheic dermatitis)

Brain (dementia, meningitis, encephalitis, brain tumors)

Eyes (cytomegalovirus infections)

Mouth (herpes and yeast infections)

Neck (swollen glands)

Skin (shingles)

Esophagus (inflammation from yeast, herpes, and cytomegalovirus infections)

Lungs (Pneumocystis carinii pneumonia and tuberculosis)

Armpits (swollen glands)

Intestines (Kaposi's sarcoma and yeast and salmonella infections)

Liver (hepatitis and cholangitis)

Groin (swollen glands)

Skin (Kaposi's sarcoma)

AIDS-related disorders
AIDS can cause a variety of opportunistic infections, cancers, and other diseases as it destroys a person's immune system. In addition to the opportunistic conditions shown here, women with AIDS can develop recurring vaginal yeast infections and are at increased risk of cervical cancer.

drugs used so far. However, the medications can reduce the amount of virus circulating in the blood to nearly undetectable levels, and the drug combination has significantly lowered the number of deaths from AIDS. But as people with AIDS are living longer, they are developing other medical problems. Some people who have had AIDS for many years develop an abnormal fat distribution in their body, along with abnormalities in blood cholesterol and blood glucose levels. Also, all AIDS drugs have side effects, some of which can be serious. For example, some reverse transcriptase

inhibitors deplete the number of red and white blood cells, inflame the pancreas, or cause painful nerve damage. Protease inhibitors can produce nausea and diarrhea and can interact adversely with other drugs. Anti-HIV drugs can also cause muscle deterioration, weak bones, heart failure, and swelling of the liver.

A variety of new drugs to fight HIV infection and AIDS are under development, including medications that interfere with different stages of the life cycle of the virus. Vaccines against HIV are also under investigation.

Allergies

An allergy is an inappropriate or exaggerated physical response to a normally harmless substance (such as pollen) that, in most people, causes no symptoms. Allergies, also known as acquired sensitivities, occur on the second or subsequent exposures to specific substances.

To keep you healthy, your immune system normally recognizes and destroys invading microorganisms, such as viruses and bacteria, through a complicated process called the immune response. First, the immune system produces proteins called antibodies, which attach themselves to specialized cells called mast cells that are present in most body tissues. The antibodies and mast cells attack the invading microorganisms by bonding to antigens (proteins) on their surface. This bond stimulates the mast cells to release a number of strong chemicals. One of these chemicals, called histamine, irritates the surrounding tissue, causing the redness, swelling, and itching characteristic of inflammation. In people who have allergies, this process is triggered by harmless substances, such as mold or animal dander (tiny skin flakes), rather than by disease-causing microorganisms. A substance that causes an allergic reaction is referred to as an allergen.

You can have an allergic reaction to anything that you inhale or eat, or to something that comes in contact with your skin. You can also have an allergic reaction to medications or to wasp or bee venom.

If you think you may have an allergy, talk to your doctor, who will either treat you or refer you to an allergist (a doctor who specializes in diagnosing and treating allergies). The specific substance that is triggering your allergy may be difficult to identify. Laboratory tests can help determine whether you have an allergy and identify the substance that is causing the reaction. Be sure to tell any new doctor you see about your allergy and any medications you are taking to treat it.

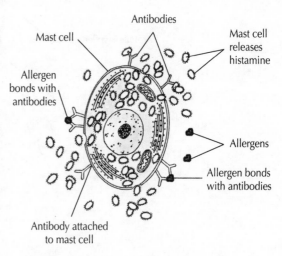

An allergic reaction

During an allergic reaction, the immune system responds to a normally harmless substance as if it were a harmful invader. During the first exposure to the substance (referred to as an allergen), the immune system produces antibodies that attach themselves to cells called mast cells. The next time the allergen enters the body, it bonds with the antibodies. This bond stimulates the mast cells to release many powerful chemicals, including histamine. The release of these chemicals from the mast cells causes the characteristic symptoms of an allergic reaction.

Diagnosing Allergies

Doctors and allergists use the following tests to help diagnose most types of allergies.

Skin Tests

Skin tests (also called patch tests or scratch tests) are most often used to test for allergies to airborne allergens or particular foods. In a scratch test, a small amount of the suspected allergen is pricked or scratched into the skin. A safer alternative (which reduces the risk of the allergen getting into the bloodstream) is a patch test, in which the suspected allergen is applied to a patch taped to the skin. Skin testing, especially scratch testing, is not usually performed on anyone who has had a life-threatening reaction to an allergen or who has a skin disorder (such as dermatitis) that could affect the results of the test. Any reaction (such as redness, swelling, or itching) usually indicates an allergic reaction to the substance being tested.

RAST Blood Test

The radioallergosorbent test (RAST) is the blood test most frequently used to detect all types of allergens. It can help identify the substance that is causing your allergic reaction by measuring the level of IgE antibodies in your blood after exposure to the substance. (IgE antibodies are proteins the body produces in most allergic reactions.) RAST can be done even if you are taking medications for the allergy or if you are having symptoms (such as dermatitis) that could alter the results of skin tests. A positive test result usually means that you are allergic to the substance being tested.

5-year period, the doctor administers a series of injections containing a small, carefully measured amount of the allergen to stimulate the immune system to produce protective antibodies. The allergen is given in increasing doses over the 3- to 5-year period until a sufficient number of antibodies has been produced to prevent the body from reacting to the allergen or to make it react less strongly, causing fewer symptoms. Desensitization is not used in all cases because it is not effective for everyone and because it can cause a life-threatening allergic reaction (anaphylactic shock; see page 916) in people who have a severe allergy.

Treating Allergies

The best treatment for any allergy is complete avoidance of the allergen. Sometimes it is possible to make an affected person less sensitive to an allergen in a process called desensitization. Desensitization is sometimes used to treat the symptoms of airborne allergies such as pollen or dust mites, and severe reactions to wasp or bee stings. Doctors usually recommend desensitization only if a person has mild to moderate symptoms more than once a year, and if the symptoms cannot be controlled with medication or by avoiding the allergen.

For desensitization, which is done over a 3- to

Allergies to Airborne Substances

Allergies to airborne substances are caused by contact with microscopic particles from pollen, mold, dust mites, smoke, or animal dander (tiny skin flakes) that are inhaled from the air. Airborne allergies include seasonal allergies such as hay fever (see next page). Some synthetic materials found in the home or workplace—such as paint, polyurethane, and artificial fibers—can also affect the respiratory system, causing allergic reactions in some people.

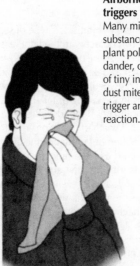

Airborne allergy triggers
Many microscopic substances—such as plant pollen, animal dander, or the feces of tiny insects called dust mites—can trigger an allergic reaction.

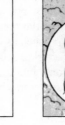

Dander on fur

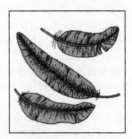

Dust mites

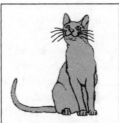

Pollen

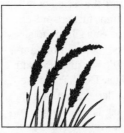

Dander on feathers

Extrinsic allergic alveolitis is the term used to describe a group of allergic lung diseases resulting from exposure to dusts of animal or vegetable origin. Some organic substances—such as barley and sugarcane—used on farms or in industry can cause severe allergic reactions, usually from exposure to molds or fungi. The allergic disorder known as farmer's lung (occupational lung diseases; see page 645) is caused by frequent exposure to a fungus that grows in moldy hay or grain. People who handle animals or who have frequent contact with birds may have severe reactions to their feathers, saliva, or droppings.

People who already have other types of allergies or who have family members who have allergies are more prone to having airborne allergies. Allergic reactions can occur when airborne allergens come in contact with a person's skin, eyes, or the mucous membranes of the nose. If the allergic reaction affects the airways of the lungs, causing wheezing and difficulty breathing, the disorder is a respiratory disorder known as asthma (see page 640).

Symptoms

Typical symptoms of airborne allergies include sneezing, a runny and itchy nose, a scratchy or sore throat, and itchy, red, swollen, watery eyes. You may have dark circles under your eyes because congestion in the nose interferes with the blood flow in the veins under the eyes. Some people (especially children) have a permanent crease in their nose or an upturned nose from constantly wiping an itchy or runny nose by pushing the nose upward. In rare cases, heavy exposure (such as to dusts generated during some manufacturing processes) can cause more severe symptoms including fever, muscle aches, fatigue, and symptoms of asthma such as difficulty breathing.

Diagnosis

If you have symptoms only during the spring or fall, you may have hay fever. Symptoms that are present all year are more likely to indicate an allergy to airborne substances found indoors, such as mold, animal dander, or dust mites. Your doctor may use skin tests (see page 912) or a blood test (RAST; see previous page) to determine what allergens are causing your symptoms. The doctor may take a sample of your nasal secretions for examination under a microscope to measure the number of eosinophils

in your nose. Eosinophils are a type of white blood cell that increases in number during an allergic reaction. Your doctor may also examine your nose for polyps (see page 634), which can cause symptoms similar to those of allergies.

Treatment

Because pollens and other airborne allergens are hard to avoid, your doctor may recommend over-the-counter antihistamines, which relieve symptoms by blocking the action of the histamine-releasing cells that produce the allergic symptoms. However, to be fully effective, antihistamines have to be taken regularly (usually daily for several years). Some people find the side effects of antihistamines, such as drowsiness and dryness in the nose and throat, more annoying than the allergy.

Other types of over-the-counter drugs may provide some relief. An over-the-counter nasal spray containing the medication cromolyn is about half as effective as prescribed corticosteroid nasal sprays but is much safer to use for long periods. Saline (salt solution) nose sprays can help clear the nose of airborne allergens. Doctors generally do not recommend decongestant nose drops or sprays because they can worsen symptoms, and they need to be taken more and more frequently to get the same effect. Take decongestants only if your doctor prescribes them and then only for short periods.

Hay Fever

Hay fever, or allergic rhinitis, is a type of seasonal allergy caused by contact with the light, easily blown pollen of grasses (such as Kentucky bluegrass), trees (such as oak, ash, and elm), and weeds (such as ragweed). Most people experience symptoms in the spring or fall, but exactly when a plant pollinates depends on its geographic location. Weather conditions don't affect the amount of pollen but influence the amount that gets distributed. For example, pollen counts are highest on warm, dry days and lowest on cold, wet days. If you have hay fever, stay indoors as much as possible with the windows closed when you are having symptoms or when pollen counts are high. Use air-conditioning and heating systems with built-in filters (smaller air-filtering machines may not be effective). Resist rubbing your eyes, which can make the irritation worse.

If over-the-counter medications don't relieve your symptoms, your doctor may prescribe an antihistamine that doesn't cause drowsiness. Eyedrops prescribed by your doctor can temporarily relieve eye irritation. Corticosteroid nasal sprays work well to relieve nasal congestion and the trickle of nasal secretions down the back of the throat (called postnasal drip). In rare cases, a doctor may also prescribe medications usually used to treat asthma—such as bronchodilators (see page 641) to open the airways, or corticosteroids taken by mouth or through an inhaler to reduce inflammation. If these medications don't control the symptoms or if they cause adverse reactions, desensitization (see page 913) therapy may be recommended.

Allergies to Food

A food allergy is an allergic reaction to particular foods or food additives. The reaction usually occurs immediately or within a few hours after eating. In celiac disease (see page 768), in which the small intestine is hypersensitive to the protein gluten, the reaction may not occur until days later. Food allergies can last a lifetime, but many food allergies diagnosed in childhood disappear as the child gets older. The most common foods that cause allergies are nuts (especially peanuts, walnuts, and Brazil nuts), legumes (such as soybeans), fish and shellfish (especially whitefish and shrimp), cow's milk, egg whites, and wheat. Food allergies tend to run in families.

Some people have abnormal reactions (such as indigestion; see page 749) to certain foods or beverages, but these reactions are not allergic because they don't involve the immune system. Lactose intolerance (see page 770) is an adverse reaction (but not an allergic reaction) to dairy products. Some substances, including sulfites in wine or monosodium glutamate (MSG) in food, can cause chemical disturbances in the body but are not true allergens.

Symptoms

Once the allergy-causing food is absorbed into the bloodstream, it can react with antibodies (infection-fighting proteins) in the blood vessels, causing headaches, rashes, itching and swelling in the throat and around the lips and mouth, a stuffy or runny nose, or shortness of breath or difficulty breathing. Other symptoms of food allergies include abdominal swelling and pain, gas, nausea, vomiting, and diarrhea. In some cases, a person may have a life-threatening allergic reaction called anaphylactic shock (see below and next page).

WARNING!

Anaphylactic Shock

If you experience any of the following symptoms (especially after eating an unfamiliar food, being bitten or stung by an insect, or having an injection of a medication), call 911 or your local emergency number, or go to the nearest hospital emergency department immediately:

- Severe itching or a rash over several areas of your body
- Swollen lips, tongue, or throat
- Excessive sweating or cold, clammy skin
- Difficulty swallowing
- Difficulty breathing
- Difficulty speaking
- Vomiting
- Confusion

Diagnosis

To diagnose a food allergy, your doctor may recommend that you keep a food diary so he or she can see what kinds of foods you have eaten when you experience symptoms. The doctor may also put you on an exclusion diet (also called an elimination diet) in which, one by one, you eliminate the foods from your diet that are suspected of causing your allergy, to see if you no longer have symptoms. Undertake an exclusion diet only under your doctor's supervision. Your doctor may also recommend a blood test (RAST; see page 913) or skin tests (see page 912) to identify the allergy-causing food.

Treatment

Avoiding the problem food is the usual treatment for a food allergy. Carefully read the labels on all foods you buy. Ask about the ingredients in dishes you are served when you eat away from home, such as peanut oil used in many Asian dishes. Always carry the drug epinephrine (adrenaline) with you in a self-injecting device. Epinephrine dilates the airways and makes breathing easier. At the first sign

Anaphylactic Shock

Anaphylactic shock (or anaphylaxis) is an extreme and sometimes fatal allergic reaction that requires immediate medical treatment. During an anaphylactic reaction, your body releases large amounts of histamine and other chemicals. These substances widen your blood vessels and cause a sudden drop in blood pressure. Your air passages narrow and may close completely, making it difficult or impossible to breathe. Anaphylactic shock may be triggered by any allergen, but most often occurs after an insect bite or sting, after eating a particular food, or after an injection of a medication.

If you are having a severe allergic reaction and you have never had one before, call 911 or your local emergency number. If you have had a severe allergic reaction before, always wear a medical identification tag around your neck or wrist that provides information about your condition. Also, your doctor will prescribe epinephrine (which improves breathing by widening the airways) in a self-injecting device. Carry the injection device with you at all times and give yourself an injection of epinephrine at the first sign of a severe allergic reaction.

If you are with a person who is having an anaphylactic reaction, call 911 immediately. If he or she becomes unconscious, lay him or her down with legs raised to improve circulation to the heart and brain.

of an adverse reaction to a food, immediately give yourself an injection and go directly to the nearest hospital emergency department.

Allergies to Medication

Some medications can trigger an allergic reaction. Drugs that are injected into a muscle or through a vein are most likely to cause allergic reactions because they enter the bloodstream directly. The medications that most often cause allergic reactions are penicillin and similar antibiotics. Oral medications are less likely to cause a reaction because some of the potential allergens are broken down during the digestion process. Many medications cause adverse reactions, or unwanted side effects, but because these reactions don't involve the immune system, they are not considered to be allergic reactions.

Symptoms and Diagnosis

The symptoms of an allergic reaction to medication include rash, wheezing, or shortness of breath. If the symptoms are severe, they can lead to a life-threatening condition called anaphylactic shock (see left).

To diagnose an allergy to a medication, a doctor evaluates the person's symptoms to make sure that they are not merely side effects of the medication. He or she will perform a blood test (RAST; see page 913) and skin tests (see page 912) to determine the cause and severity of the allergic reaction.

Treatment

Drug allergies can be treated in two ways. Avoiding the medication is the best treatment if the medication can be safely discontinued or if your doctor can substitute another drug. If you must have the drug that causes an allergic reaction and the reaction is relatively mild, your doctor may be able to treat the symptoms of the allergic reaction with another drug, such as an antihistamine or corticosteroid, to reduce inflammation. Be sure to tell any other doctors you see about your drug allergy so they won't prescribe it for you. Wear a medical identification necklace or bracelet that specifies the type of medication to which you are allergic.

Autoimmune Disorders

When bacteria or viruses attack your body, your immune system defends you from these invaders by detecting and killing them. But if your immune system is not working properly, it can mistake your body's own cells for foreign invaders and attack them. This process—the immune system attacking itself—is called autoimmunity. Doctors have not yet discovered exactly why the immune system treats some parts of the body as harmful invaders, but they think that certain people have a genetic predisposition to autoimmunity. Such susceptible people develop an autoimmune disorder when they are exposed to an environmental trigger such as an infection, certain drugs, or, in some women, pregnancy.

An autoimmune disorder can affect almost any

part of the body, and the specific symptoms depend on which organs are targeted. But when the immune system attacks, it almost always produces inflammation, and this inflammation can damage the body. Autoimmune disorders are unpredictable. In some people they last for a few months or years and then go away on their own. Other people experience periodic flare-ups—times when symptoms get worse—followed by intervals during which they feel better. Still others have a disorder that is active most of the time, lasts for years, and causes severe damage.

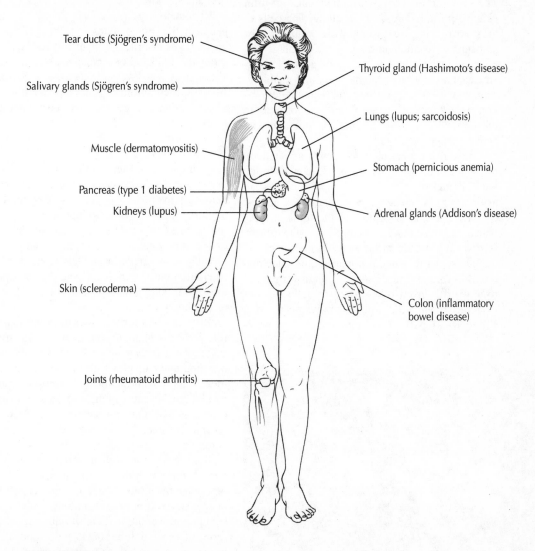

Tear ducts (Sjögren's syndrome)

Salivary glands (Sjögren's syndrome)

Muscle (dermatomyositis)

Pancreas (type 1 diabetes)

Kidneys (lupus)

Skin (scleroderma)

Joints (rheumatoid arthritis)

Thyroid gland (Hashimoto's disease)

Lungs (lupus; sarcoidosis)

Stomach (pernicious anemia)

Adrenal glands (Addison's disease)

Colon (inflammatory bowel disease)

**Autoimmune disorders affect
many parts of the body**

Autoimmune disorders cause the immune system to mistakenly attack cells and organs in the body as if they were invading microorganisms. Many different parts of the body can be affected. Some autoimmune disorders, such as rheumatoid arthritis, affect only specific parts of the body, such as the joints, while others are systemic, affecting the entire body. For example, some forms of lupus can cause serious damage to the lungs, heart, kidneys, and brain.

Rheumatoid Arthritis

Rheumatoid arthritis is a chronic autoimmune disorder that causes inflammation, pain, swelling, stiffness, and loss of function in the joints. In rheumatoid arthritis, the immune system attacks the membrane called the synovium, which lines joints. The synovium becomes inflamed, causing joint pain, warmth, redness, and swelling. The cells of the synovium begin to grow and divide abnormally, and start to invade and destroy the cartilage and bone inside the joint. The surrounding muscles, ligaments, and tendons become weak and unable to support the joint. Over time, untreated deterioration of joint and bone tissue produces deformities in the joint, making it difficult for a person to lead an active, independent life.

The joints that are most frequently affected are the small ones in the hands and feet, mainly the knuckles and toe joints, but rheumatoid arthritis can affect any joint, including the wrists, knees, ankles, or neck. It occurs less often in the spine or hips, which are much more susceptible to osteoarthritis (see page 996). Osteoarthritis results from stress on the joints over time and is not an autoimmune disorder. Certain characteristics distinguish rheumatoid arthritis from other types of arthritis. For example, rheumatoid arthritis always occurs in a symmetrical pattern—if one knee or wrist is affected, the knee or wrist on the other side of the body is also affected. Joint inflammation usually affects the wrist and finger joints closest to the hand. Unlike osteoarthritis, rheumatoid arthritis can affect parts of the body other than the joints, causing inflammation in the eyes, heart, lungs, and blood vessels, and changes in the tissues that lie just beneath the skin.

Rheumatoid arthritis affects more than 2 million people in the United States, two thirds of whom are women. The disorder occurs in all racial and ethnic groups and most often first appears in middle age, although it can develop in a person's 20s or 30s. Juvenile rheumatoid arthritis (see page 434) can affect children between the ages of 6 months and 16 years.

Symptoms

The symptoms of rheumatoid arthritis differ from person to person and can be more severe in some people than in others. The disorder sometimes begins with no obvious symptoms in the joints. Instead, the first symptoms may be listlessness, lack of appetite, weight loss, vague muscular pains, and possibly a low-grade fever. Only later do the characteristic joint symptoms appear. In other people, the joint inflammation flares up suddenly, with no prior symptoms.

Rheumatoid arthritis causes the joints to become red, warm, swollen, tender, painful, and stiff. The stiffness is usually most noticeable first thing in the morning and subsides with increased joint movement. People with rheumatoid arthritis sometimes feel fatigued because of the iron deficiency anemia (see page 610) that can accompany it. Occasional fever and a general sense of not feeling well are also common.

Some people with rheumatoid arthritis experience the effects of the disorder in parts of the body other than the joints. About one quarter of affected people develop bumps or nodules under the skin near pressure points, such as the elbows. Less common effects include neck pain and dryness of the eyes and mouth. In very rare cases, the blood vessels, the lining of the lungs, or the pericardium (the sac enclosing the heart) may become inflamed.

In severe cases, swollen, deformed joints can collapse and become partly or completely dislocated. This dislocation can cause great discomfort and problems with walking, especially if knee,

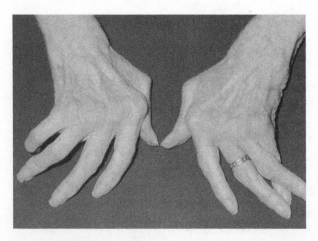

Rheumatoid arthritis in the hands
Rheumatoid arthritis can severely deform the joints of the hands, making routine daily activities difficult. The finger bones typically curve away from the thumb side of the hand.

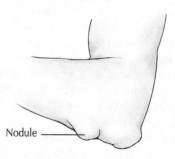

Rheumatoid nodule
Some people with rheumatoid arthritis develop small lumps of tissue called nodules under the skin near pressure points, such as the elbows.

ankle, or foot joints are affected. Tendons may become so weak that they snap, making it impossible to control certain movements.

Diagnosis

Early diagnosis of rheumatoid arthritis can help prevent joint deterioration, but the disorder can be difficult to diagnose in its early stages. No single test exists for diagnosing rheumatoid arthritis, and the symptoms can vary dramatically from person to person. The symptoms can mimic those of other joint problems, which the doctor will want to rule out. In addition, only a few symptoms may be present in the initial stages of rheumatoid arthritis, forcing the doctor to wait for the full range of symptoms to appear before confirming the diagnosis. For these reasons, doctors use a variety of tools to help make a diagnosis.

A thorough health history—your description of your symptoms and how they began—will help your doctor evaluate your condition and learn how it changes over time. Your doctor will also perform a physical examination of your joints, skin, reflexes, and muscle strength.

The doctor will probably order a blood test to detect rheumatoid factor, an antibody your immune system may have mistakenly produced. Rheumatoid factor is present in the blood of most—but not all—people with rheumatoid arthritis. Other diagnostic blood tests are often performed to detect inflammation, white blood cells, and anemia, which are often present with rheumatoid arthritis.

In later stages of the disease, doctors use X-rays of the joints to monitor the progression of joint damage.

Treatment

Doctors use many different types of treatment to relieve pain, reduce inflammation, and slow joint damage in people with rheumatoid arthritis. Some lifestyle activities—including a balanced program of rest when the disorder is active and exercise when symptoms subside—can help improve joint function. For example, swimming in a heated pool is good for stiff joints. Removable splints that you can strap onto your painful joints when they need rest, and self-help devices such as zipper pullers and bathroom safety bars, can help reduce the stress on painful joints. Using relaxation techniques (see page 59) to relieve emotional stress can help make living with rheumatoid arthritis a little easier. Your doctor may recommend that you apply heat to the affected joints and may refer you to a physical therapist, who can teach you some helpful exercises and provide splints for affected joints.

Nonsteroidal anti-inflammatory drugs were traditionally the mainstays of rheumatoid arthritis treatment in the early stages, and more powerful drugs were reserved for later, more severe stages. This approach has now been reversed, in the belief that stronger drugs taken early might prevent or limit additional joint damage. Drugs currently used to treat rheumatoid arthritis include hydroxychloroquine, sulfasalazine, and methotrexate. These drugs are powerful enough to interrupt the process that produces inflammation by blocking the interactions between immune system cells. A promising new class of genetically engineered drugs called tumor-necrosis factor (TNF) inhibitors are proving effective in both limiting inflammation and slowing the destruction of cartilage and bone, with few side effects.

Surgery can be helpful in the management of rheumatoid arthritis for relieving pain and improving joint function. Three types of surgery are available: joint replacement surgery (see page 999), reconstruction of affected tendons (most often in the hands), and synovectomy, in which the inflamed tissue of the synovium is completely removed.

Systemic Lupus Erythematosus

Systemic lupus erythematosus (usually referred to simply as lupus) is a chronic autoimmune disease that affects the skin, joints, muscles, and many other organs in the body. Lupus develops primarily in women during their childbearing years but can also affect men. In people with lupus, the immune system attacks multiple body systems, causing inflammation that damages organs and tissues.

There are three main types of lupus—systemic lupus, discoid lupus, and drug-induced systemic lupus. Systemic lupus, the most common type, produces inflammation in multiple body systems. Discoid lupus erythematosus (see page 1072) produces only a skin rash characterized by crusty skin patches on the face, neck, or chest that may scar. Drug-induced systemic lupus can be triggered by a wide variety of drugs, including beta blockers (see page 562) used for treating heart disease and high blood pressure. The drug-induced type of lupus disappears completely when the person stops taking the drug.

Systemic lupus affects women about 10 times as often as men and usually develops between ages 18 and 45. Blacks and Hispanics have an increased risk of developing the disorder. Lupus occurs more often in first-degree relatives (children, siblings, or parents) of affected people than in the general population, indicating that genes play a role. In other cases, the cause is unknown. Drug-induced lupus affects men more often than women because more men use the drugs that trigger the condition. Like all autoimmune disorders, lupus is not contagious.

Earlier diagnosis and better management of the disease have greatly improved the outlook for affected people in recent years. In the 1960s, only 40 percent of people diagnosed with systemic lupus were expected to live more than 3 years. Today, 80 to 90 percent of people with lupus live longer than 10 years after diagnosis, and many have a normal life expectancy.

Symptoms

The symptoms of systemic lupus vary greatly from person to person, and the course of the disease is unpredictable. The disorder's severity varies from mild cases (which require minimal treatment) to severe cases (in which potentially fatal damage occurs to organs such as the lungs, heart, kidneys, and brain). Lupus is characterized by periodic flare-ups of symptoms followed by improvement that can last for weeks, months, or years.

Early symptoms of lupus are usually vague and easily confused with other disorders. But the following symptoms usually appear over the lifetime of a person who has the disease:

- Fever over 100°F
- Painful, red, swollen joints
- A butterfly-shaped facial rash
- Coin-shaped skin rashes on areas exposed to the sun
- Anemia
- Pleurisy (inflammation of the pleura—the two membranes that line the lungs)
- Sensitivity to sunlight
- Hair loss
- Mouth or nose ulcers
- Seizures

Lupus and Pregnancy

Because lupus primarily affects women of childbearing age, pregnancy presents an especially difficult problem. In the past, doctors advised women with lupus not to have children because of the high risk of miscarriage caused by blood-clotting problems, but today only 25 percent of pregnancies in women with lupus end in miscarriage. Half of all pregnancies are completely normal and healthy, and another 25 percent result in premature births. Still, all pregnancies in women with lupus are considered high-risk and need to be managed by obstetricians who have experience with high-risk pregnancies.

The best time for a woman with lupus to get pregnant is when she is between flare-ups of the disease. About 20 percent of pregnant women with lupus experience a sudden increase in blood pressure, protein in the urine, or both. This condition is called preeclampsia (see page 526), a serious condition that can be fatal for both mother and baby if delivery is not done immediately.

The major risk to a baby of a woman with lupus is prematurity. About 3 percent of premature babies have a disorder called neonatal lupus, characterized by a rash, blood count abnormalities, and, in rare cases, a heartbeat abnormality. These symptoms clear up on their own in 3 to 6 months, except for the heartbeat problem, which is permanent but not dangerous.

About one third of all people with lupus have kidney damage, and some people experience a progressive loss of kidney function and kidney failure. Lupus affects the central nervous system in many ways. For example, many people experience headaches, confusion, difficulty concentrating, and strokes when antibodies attack nerve cells or blood vessels. Inflammation in the blood vessels (vasculitis; see page 927) occurs when infection-fighting white blood cells mistakenly enter the walls of the blood vessels, reducing blood flow and damaging the tissue. Vasculitis can produce numerous symptoms in multiple parts of the body, including any part of the heart—the pericardium (the sac enclosing the heart), the endocardium (the lining of the inside of the heart), and the heart muscle itself. People who have lupus are at increased risk of infections, and some people with lupus have blood-clotting problems.

Diagnosis

Lupus can mimic other conditions, so it can be very difficult to diagnose. To make a diagnosis of lupus, the doctor must see evidence of abnormalities in many different organs and body systems, including the skin, joints, kidneys, blood, lungs, nervous system, and the membranes lining the heart and other organs. The doctor obtains this evidence through a thorough physical examination and the person's description of his or her symptoms, including how and when they began. The doctor then looks for a relationship between the results of the physical examination and the person's symptoms.

If you have a number of the characteristic symptoms of lupus, the doctor will order blood and urine tests, as well as a series of specialized tests that evaluate how well your immune system is working. No one test can positively determine if a person has lupus but, taken together, the battery of laboratory tests can point to a diagnosis. In general, the tests are designed to detect the presence of autoantibodies (proteins that mistakenly identify cells in the body as invading harmful organisms and attack them). The most common tests used to diagnose lupus include:

- Complete blood cell count
- Liver and kidney screenings
- Blood tests for specific autoantibodies
- Urinalysis to detect kidney problems
- Erythrocyte sedimentation rate to measure levels of inflammation
- Chest X-rays to assess lung damage
- ECG (electrocardiogram) to detect heart problems

The results of these tests will determine what further tests might be helpful.

Treatment

Treatment for lupus depends on the severity of the disease, but most treatment plans use a combination of medications, exercise, rest, a nutritious diet,

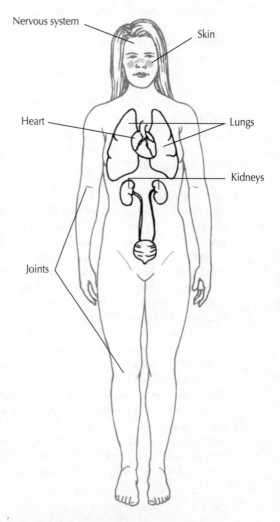

Organs and tissues affected by systemic lupus
Systemic lupus affects the skin as well as other organs and tissues throughout the body, causing inflammation in the lungs, heart, kidneys, joints, and nervous system.

and protection from the sun. The medications doctors prescribe for lupus are designed to relieve pain and inflammation and suppress the immune system to dampen its abnormal response. The disease remains mild in about one third of all affected people, requiring only nonsteroidal anti-inflammatory drugs such as aspirin, ibuprofen, or naproxen. More severely affected people need to take corticosteroid drugs such as prednisone, by mouth or by injection into a muscle. Corticosteroids taken at high doses for long periods can produce changes in appearance, such as acne, a rounded face, a swollen abdomen, and weight gain. If you are taking corticosteroids, do not stop taking them suddenly or you could go into shock. Your doctor will gradually reduce the dosage for you.

Antimalarial drugs were originally developed to treat malaria, but doctors soon found that they were also effective in relieving the joint pain and inflammation of lupus. Antimalarial drugs work especially well to relieve the skin rash that characterizes discoid lupus (which affects only the skin).

Up to 60 percent of people with lupus are sensitive to sunlight. Exposure to sunlight can stimulate flare-ups or worsen lupus-induced skin rashes. It is very important for people with lupus to protect themselves from the sun by wearing clothing that blocks the sun's rays such as long-sleeved shirts, long pants, and wide-brimmed hats. Applying sunscreen with a high sun protection factor (SPF 15 or above) half an hour before going outdoors will also help protect sensitive skin. Another way to minimize sun exposure is to avoid going out in the sun between 10:00 AM and 4:00 PM, when the sun's rays are strongest.

Several experimental treatments aimed at improving the function of the immune system have proven successful in treating lupus. Stem cell transplants (see page 624) are being tried in people with severe lupus, with promising results. People with end-stage kidney failure require treatment with kidney dialysis (see page 818) or a kidney transplant (see page 820); a person with lupus can have a transplant only when the disease is inactive.

Scleroderma

Scleroderma (which means hard skin) is a chronic autoimmune disorder in which the immune system mistakenly produces antibodies (infection-fighting proteins) that attack connective tissue throughout the body. The disorder is characterized by an overproduction of the protein collagen in the body's connective tissue, which results in thickening, hardening, and tightening of the skin, especially of the hands and face. There are two main types of scleroderma—localized (which affects only the skin and musculoskeletal system) and systemic (which causes a more widespread hardening of the skin and also affects internal organs, including the lungs, heart, kidneys, digestive tract, and blood vessels).

Scleroderma occurs much more frequently in women than in men, and its effects can range from mild to disabling to life-threatening. The cause of scleroderma is not known, and there is no known way to prevent it. Doctors think that genes play a role in the disorder, but it is not inherited. Environmental triggers or toxins, such as infection by a virus or exposure to organic solvents or adhesive materials, may also be factors. Some researchers theorize that, because the disorder affects women 7 to 12 times more often than men, female hormones such as estrogen may have an influence.

Symptoms

Symptoms of scleroderma usually appear between ages 20 and 40 and can vary, depending on the organs or tissues that are affected. In many people, the first symptoms of scleroderma occur when cold temperatures or stress trigger a condition called Raynaud's phenomenon (see page 924), in which spasms of the small blood vessels in the fingers and toes impair blood flow, causing the fingers and toes to become pale, cold, numb, and painful. Although Raynaud's phenomenon can be a symptom of scleroderma, not all people who have Raynaud's develop scleroderma.

Other hallmark symptoms of scleroderma include swelling in the fingers, hands, forearms, and face (and sometimes in the lower legs and feet), followed by a gradual thickening, hardening, and tightening of the skin. The muscles weaken and the joints stiffen, causing pain and limiting movement and flexibility.

Systemic scleroderma causes much more serious symptoms, including digestive symptoms such as difficulty swallowing, indigestion, and difficulty controlling bowel movements. Respiratory symptoms such as shortness of breath and a persistent dry cough can develop. If the disorder affects the heart, chest pain, abnormal heart rhythms (see page 580), or heart failure (see page 570) can occur. Damage to the kidneys can lead to high blood pressure, headaches, seizures (see page 686), infrequent urination, blood in the urine, or kidney failure (see page 816).

Diagnosis

To reach a diagnosis of scleroderma, the doctor will take a complete health history and perform a thorough physical examination, paying special attention to the appearance of the skin. The doctor will probably order a blood test to measure the level of a specific antibody produced only by people with scleroderma, which would indicate that the immune system is launching an abnormal attack against connective tissue throughout the body. To confirm the diagnosis, the doctor may recommend a biopsy, in which a sample of tissue is removed and examined under a microscope for excess collagen.

Treatment

There is no effective treatment for scleroderma, but self-help measures and medication can help relieve your symptoms and improve your quality of life. Relaxation techniques (see page 59) such as deep breathing or meditation can help you manage stress and reduce the frequency and severity of episodes. Stay warm and keep your hands and feet warm and dry to help prevent the painful constriction of the blood vessels in the fingers and toes. Your doctor may prescribe vasodilators (drugs that widen the blood vessels) and diuretics (drugs that help the body eliminate excess fluid) to improve circulation and reduce swelling in your hands and feet.

If you smoke or use other tobacco products, quit now. Chemicals in tobacco smoke can damage blood vessels and impair circulation. Smoking also lowers skin temperature, which can trigger an attack of scleroderma.

Exercise regularly to help maintain your flexibility and strength and improve your circulation. Ask your doctor to recommend some exercises that will work for you. To relieve inflammation, pain, and stiffness in your muscles and joints, your doctor may recommend over-the-counter nonsteroidal anti-inflammatory drugs (such as aspirin, ibuprofen, or naproxen) or may prescribe a corticosteroid medication. He or she will probably also recommend

physical therapy to help you retain your strength and mobility.

To relieve digestive symptoms, eat smaller, more frequent meals; avoid eating within 3 or 4 hours of bedtime; sleep with the head of your bed elevated; and take an over-the-counter antacid when you have symptoms. You should know, however, that while over-the-counter antacids can provide temporary relief of digestive symptoms such as heartburn, bloating, and indigestion, they also can mask symptoms of a more serious underlying disorder. If you use antacids, be sure to follow the instructions on the package. If you use antacids regularly, or if your symptoms persist or worsen, talk to your doctor.

For severe cases of scleroderma, doctors usually prescribe immune-suppressing drugs such as penicillamine or cyclophosphamide to relieve inflammation, reduce organ damage, and suppress the abnormal activity of the immune system.

Polymyositis and Dermatomyositis

Myositis means inflammation of the muscles. Polymyositis is a rare, chronic disorder that is characterized by inflammation of many muscles throughout the body. The disorder can occur at any age but is most common in children between ages 5 and 15 and in adults between ages 40 and 60.

Polymyositis occurs twice as often in women as in men. The cause of the disorder is unknown, but doctors think it is an autoimmune disorder in which the immune system mistakenly produces antibodies (infection-fighting proteins) that attack muscle tissues. In some cases, the disorder may be linked to some types of cancer (such as lung cancer). For reasons that are not fully understood, the normal, helpful antibodies the immune system has produced to attack the cancer cells also mistakenly attack the muscles. If polymyositis produces a skin rash, doctors call the disorder dermatomyositis.

Symptoms

The main symptom of polymyositis is muscle weakness, especially in the shoulders, upper arms, hips, and thighs. The muscle weakness may occur suddenly, without warning, or develop gradually over weeks or months. As the muscles weaken, you become less able to perform routine activities such as bathing, dressing, getting up from a chair, climbing stairs, or walking. Other symptoms of the disorder include muscle pain, joint pain and swelling, fever, fatigue, and weight loss. If polymyositis affects the lungs, it can cause shortness of breath and a persistent cough. If the disorder affects the muscles of the throat and esophagus, you can have difficulty swallowing and speaking. In addition to the characteristic symptoms of polymyositis, dermatomyositis produces a reddish rash on the face, shoulders, elbows, knuckles, knees, and ankles. In many cases, the symptoms of polymyositis and dermatomyositis come and go.

Diagnosis

To diagnose polymyositis or dermatomyositis, your doctor will ask about your symptoms, take a health history, and perform a physical examination. The doctor may recommend a muscle biopsy, in which a sample of muscle tissue is surgically removed and examined under a microscope. Blood tests that measure the levels of specific enzymes (proteins that promote or accelerate chemical reactions in the body) and antibodies produced by people with the disorder are also helpful in making a diagnosis. The doctor will probably order an electromyogram (an evaluation of the electrical activity of the muscles) and, in some cases, screening tests for cancer. He or she also may recommend an examination by a rheumatologist (a doctor who specializes in treating disorders of the joints, muscles, and connective tissues) or a neurologist (a doctor who specializes in treating disorders of the nervous system) to rule out other disorders.

Treatment

In some cases, polymyositis or dermatomyositis disappears on its own without treatment and does not return. However, in most cases, a doctor has to treat the disorder with high doses of a corticosteroid medication such as prednisone (taken by mouth) to relieve the inflammation, swelling, and pain. As the symptoms improve, the doctor will gradually reduce the dose, but most people will need to take low doses of corticosteroids for many years and, in some cases, for the rest of their lives to control the disorder. Corticosteroids usually are not an effective treatment for polymyositis or dermatomyositis that has been triggered by cancer.

If treatment with corticosteroids does not work, the doctor will probably prescribe immune-suppressing drugs (drugs that curb the abnormal activity of the immune system), such as methotrexate or azathioprine, in combination with or instead of the corticosteroids. If corticosteroids and immune-suppressing drugs are not effective in relieving the symptoms, the doctor may prescribe gamma globulin (the pooled antibodies of healthy donors) given intravenously (through a vein).

Your doctor will recommend that you get plenty of rest and limit activity when your symptoms flare up. He or she will work with you to develop a program of regular moderate exercise to help improve and maintain your flexibility, strength, and endurance.

Raynaud's Disease and Raynaud's Phenomenon

Raynaud's disease is a disorder in which the capillaries (the smallest blood vessels) in the skin constrict, reducing blood flow to the fingers and toes. In some cases, the nose, lips, and earlobes are also affected. The cause of Raynaud's disease is unknown, but doctors think it may be an autoimmune disorder, in which the immune system mistakenly produces antibodies (infection-fighting proteins) that attack the body's own tissues. Episodes of Raynaud's disease are usually triggered by exposure to cold air or cold water or by stress. Raynaud's disease occurs most often in women between ages 15 and 40.

Doctors call the disorder Raynaud's phenomenon when its underlying cause is known. Connective tissue diseases such as scleroderma (see page 922), systemic lupus erythematosus (see page 920), or rheumatoid arthritis (see page 918) often cause Raynaud's phenomenon. Atherosclerosis (see page 557), a condition in which arteries are narrowed by hardened fatty deposits called plaque, also may cause the disorder. In some cases, Raynaud's phenomenon occurs as a reaction to drugs that constrict the blood vessels, such as beta blockers (see page 562), some chemotherapy drugs used to treat cancer, and some over-the-counter cold medications and weight-control products. Regular use of vibrating equipment or machinery such as chain saws or pneumatic drills can damage the blood vessels in the hands, causing Raynaud's phenomenon. The disorder also occurs more frequently in smokers, probably because of circulation problems.

Symptoms

The main symptoms of Raynaud's disease are color changes in one or more of the affected fingers or toes. As the capillaries begin to constrict, the skin turns white. When blood flow is blocked, the skin turns blue. As the capillaries reopen and blood flow returns to normal, the skin turns red and then gradually returns to its normal color. The fingers or toes may throb and feel cold or numb. Some people may also experience a burning sensation. At first, episodes are infrequent and mild, but they eventually increase in frequency and severity. Prolonged episodes can result in nerve irritation, causing pain in the affected fingers or toes.

In later stages of the disorder, reduced blood flow causes the skin on the affected fingers or toes to tighten and become smooth and shiny. In some cases, small open sores form on the tips of the fingers or toes. The reduced blood supply usually damages muscles and nerves and eventually weakens the fingers and diminishes the sense of touch. When the disorder is persistent or severe, it can result in tissue death (gangrene; see page 601).

Diagnosis

A diagnosis of Raynaud's disease is based on the characteristic symptoms, a complete health history, and a physical examination. Although diagnostic tests are usually not necessary, the doctor may examine a sample of the nailfolds (the skin at the base of the fingernails) under a microscope to look for abnormalities in the capillaries. He or she may also order blood tests to check for antibodies and to measure the extent of inflammation in the body, both of which are signs of an immune response. The doctor may recommend tests to check for specific underlying diseases or conditions.

Treatment

Treatment for Raynaud's phenomenon depends on the underlying disease or condition. Treatment for Raynaud's disease focuses on reducing the frequency and severity of episodes and preventing damage to the tissues of the fingers and toes. Your

doctor will probably recommend the following measures to help reduce your symptoms:

- **Stay warm and dry.** Keep your home comfortably warm year-round. Wear a sweater to avoid becoming chilled indoors. Avoid going barefoot. Put cold beverages in insulated drinking glasses. Wear cotton gloves when handling refrigerated or frozen foods. Avoid going outdoors when the weather is cold. If you go outdoors on a cold day, put on several layers of loose clothing under your coat and wear a scarf, gloves, and warm, comfortable socks and shoes. Keep your hands and feet dry. Wear rubber gloves while washing dishes.
- **Manage stress.** Find positive ways to cope with or reduce stress in your life. Biofeedback or relaxation techniques (see page 59) such as deep breathing, meditation, or yoga may be helpful. It is also important to get enough sleep every day (see page 57). Try to avoid stressful situations that could trigger symptoms.
- **Eat a healthy diet.** Eat a balanced diet that is high in antioxidants (found in abundance in fruits and vegetables) and low in fat and cholesterol to improve your cholesterol profile (see page 146) and help prevent high blood pressure (see page 574) and atherosclerosis (hardening of the arteries).
- **Exercise regularly.** Exercise for 20 to 30 minutes at least three to four times per week to reduce stress, lower blood pressure, prevent atherosclerosis, and promote restful sleep. Moderate aerobic exercise, such as brisk walking, is very helpful.
- **Stop smoking.** Stop using all tobacco products. The nicotine in cigarettes, cigars, and chewing tobacco impairs circulation by narrowing blood vessels and raising the level of LDL (bad) cholesterol, which are factors in high blood pressure and atherosclerosis. Smoking also lowers skin temperature, which can trigger symptoms.
- **Avoid wearing tight-fitting jewelry, shoes, or socks.** Wearing tight-fitting watches, bracelets, rings, socks, or shoes can compress the vessels that supply blood to the fingers and toes.

See your doctor as often as recommended so he or she can monitor your condition, evaluate how well your treatment is working, and detect and treat other health problems early. If the self-help measures do not prevent episodes or relieve your symptoms, your doctor will probably prescribe calcium channel blockers (see page 563) to keep the blood vessels open. In most cases, this type of medication reduces the frequency and severity of episodes and promotes healing of sores on the fingers and toes. If calcium channel blockers are not effective, the doctor may prescribe alpha blockers (see page 563) to block the effects of norepinephrine, a hormone in the body that causes blood vessels to narrow. In some cases, doctors prescribe angiotensin-receptor blockers (see page 563) to widen the arteries and improve blood flow. To heal skin sores, the doctor will probably recommend nitroglycerin ointment, which you apply directly to your fingers or toes to increase the blood supply to the area and promote healing.

In rare cases, when the disorder is severe and continues to worsen, doctors recommend a surgical procedure called a sympathectomy, in which the sympathetic nerves (the nerves that stimulate constriction of the blood vessels) are cut to interrupt the nerve pathways and prevent the capillaries from constricting. However, relief of symptoms from the surgery may last for only a couple of years.

Sjögren's Syndrome

Sjögren's syndrome is an autoimmune disorder in which the body's immune system mistakenly attacks and damages the moisture-producing glands that manufacture tears and saliva. The disorder can affect glands in other parts of the body as well, causing dryness in the nose, throat, airways, skin, stomach, pancreas, intestines, or vagina. When the disorder extends beyond the moisture-producing glands it can affect the whole body, including the joints, lungs, kidneys, blood vessels, and nervous system.

There are two types of Sjögren's syndrome—primary and secondary. The primary form appears by itself, and the secondary form occurs along with another autoimmune disease, such as rheumatoid arthritis (see page 918) or systemic lupus erythematosus (see page 920). People with the secondary type are likely to have more health problems than people with primary Sjögren's syndrome.

People who develop Sjögren's syndrome probably have a genetic susceptibility to the disorder, but having a gene for the condition does not necessarily mean that you will develop the syndrome. Some sort of trigger must activate the immune system's faulty response; doctors think that this trigger may be a viral or bacterial infection. Once the infection stimulates the immune system to act, the suspected gene alters the immune system's response, sending fighter cells to the moisture-producing glands, where they cause inflammation that damages the glands. The fighter cells then continue their attack long after the infection has cleared up.

Sjögren's syndrome is one of the most prevalent of the autoimmune disorders, affecting people of all racial and ethnic groups. Roughly 2 million to 4 million people in the United States have the condition—about half with the primary type and half with the secondary type. Ninety percent of affected people are women, and the disorder most often first appears in a person's late 40s.

Symptoms

The symptoms of Sjögren's syndrome usually develop slowly. If you have the disorder, you may notice that your eyes are dry, red, and itchy, and feel gritty. You may have blurred vision and be sensitive to bright light, especially fluorescent light. Your mouth will feel dry, making it difficult to swallow, speak, and taste. You may develop a dry cough. The lack of saliva makes you more vulnerable to developing cavities in your teeth and yeast infections in your mouth (thrush; see page 744). You may also have frequent nosebleeds. Intercourse may be painful because of vaginal dryness.

Sjögren's syndrome can affect your entire body, causing skin rashes, thyroid problems, joint and muscle pain, and pneumonia (if bacteria from the mouth migrate to the lungs). Nerve problems can cause numbness and tingling in the fingers and toes, carpal tunnel syndrome (see page 699), and loss of feeling in the face. Many people with the disorder experience extreme fatigue. Sjögren's syndrome can also cause poor kidney function, digestive problems, and connective tissue disorders. About 5 percent of people with Sjögren's syndrome go on to develop the blood cancer lymphoma (see page 625).

Diagnosis

If you experience dry eyes and a dry mouth for more than 3 months, see your doctor for an evaluation. He or she will first take a detailed health history and ask you about your general health, your symptoms, and your family health history. After performing a complete physical examination, your doctor will order several tests of your eyes and mouth to check the severity of the dryness and determine if it has caused any damage.

The most effective test for detecting Sjögren's syndrome is called salivary gland biopsy of the lip. During this test, the doctor removes one of the tiny salivary glands from the inside of the lower lip and examines it under a microscope for a characteristic pattern of infection-fighting white blood cells, which indicates Sjögren's syndrome.

Your doctor may decide to do additional tests to determine if any other parts of your body are affected. These tests may include blood tests, such as a complete blood cell count, a blood glucose test, and tests that check for the presence of the abnormal antibodies (infection-fighting proteins) that are commonly found in people with Sjögren's syndrome. The doctor may also order a chest X-ray to check for inflammation in the lungs and a urinalysis to determine how well your kidneys are functioning.

Making an accurate diagnosis can take time because the symptoms of Sjögren's syndrome are similar to those of a number of other diseases. In fact, the time from the first appearance of symptoms to diagnosis usually ranges from 2 to 8 years.

Treatment

The treatment of Sjögren's syndrome depends on the extent of the problem and the particular symptoms a person has. Because no cure for Sjögren's syndrome exists, the main goal of treatment is to relieve symptoms, especially the dryness. To relieve eye dryness, doctors recommend eyedrops called artificial tears. At night, a thicker eye ointment can help protect the eyes for several hours. Another option is surgery that temporarily or permanently closes the tear ducts that drain tears from the eyes.

A saliva substitute can help relieve dry mouth temporarily, and medications are available that stimulate the salivary glands to produce saliva. It is very important to maintain good oral hygiene by flossing and brushing your teeth daily, because the absence of saliva makes your teeth more susceptible to cavities. See your dentist for check-ups and cleanings at least three times a year.

If Sjögren's syndrome has affected organs in other parts of your body, your doctor will treat those problems also. For example, nerve problems are treated with drugs to control pain and inflammation. Lung disorders, such as pneumonia or bronchitis, are treated with antibiotics or corticosteroids and nonsteroidal anti-inflammatory drugs.

Vasculitis

Vasculitis is inflammation of the blood vessels that can result from an underlying illness or can occur for unknown reasons. Vasculitis can affect any of the blood vessels in the body (capillaries, arterioles, venules, arteries, or veins) and can range from mild to life-threatening. Some forms of vasculitis are more prevalent in one sex than the other, or among people of a certain racial or ethnic background. Vasculitis can lead to arteritis (chronic inflammation of the arteries). In arteritis, inflammation causes the arteries to thicken, reducing the amount of blood they can carry to organs.

Following are brief descriptions of some of the diseases that cause vasculitis. Most of these diseases are rare and their causes are unknown, but many seem to be autoimmune disorders in which an abnormal immune response attacks cells in the body.

Polyarteritis nodosa

Polyarteritis nodosa is a rare autoimmune disease in which the immune system mistakenly attacks the small and medium arteries in the body, causing inflammation. The inflammation can affect any organ but commonly affects the skin, muscles, joints, peripheral nerves, intestines, or heart. Polyarteritis nodosa is most common in people of middle age, and affects three times as many men as women. Without treatment, the disease can be rapidly fatal.

Temporal arteritis

Temporal arteritis, also known as giant cell arteritis, is chronic inflammation of the temporal artery that runs over the temple, beside the eye. The temporal arteries are branches of the carotid arteries, which supply blood to the head and brain. Temporal arteritis usually occurs after age 50 and occurs twice as often in women as in men. Temporal arteritis can impair vision and cause permanent blindness if not treated.

Takayasu's arteritis

Takayasu's arteritis is inflammation of the aorta (the artery that carries blood away from the heart to the organs). Takayasu's arteritis is rare, affecting mostly Asian women under age 40.

Wegener's granulomatosis

Wegener's granulomatosis, sometimes called Wegener's arteritis or Wegener's disease, is a form of vasculitis that affects the sinuses, nose, ears, trachea, lungs, and kidneys. Wegener's granulomatosis can occur in people of all ages, but primarily occurs during middle age.

Symptoms

The symptoms of vasculitis vary, depending on the underlying illness, the part of the body in which the affected blood vessels are located, and the severity of the damage to involved tissues. In many cases, symptoms are general and resemble those of a viral infection.

Diagnosis

To diagnose vasculitis, a doctor will take a detailed health history and perform a physical examination. Because vasculitis can resemble other diseases and therefore may be difficult to diagnose, the doctor may recommend one or more of the following tests:

- Blood test (see page 145) to look for a low red blood cell count (which can indicate anemia), a high white blood cell count (which can indicate infection), or a low platelet count (which can indicate bleeding)
- Urine test (see page 150) to detect abnormal amounts of protein and red blood cells in the urine
- Angiogram (see page 110) to detect narrow or constricted arteries
- Biopsy to detect damage to tissues
- X-ray (see page 109) to detect damage to organs
- CT scan (see page 112) to detect damage to organs
- MRI (see page 113) to detect damage to the brain or other organs
- ECG (electrocardiogram; see page 559) to detect damage to the heart
- Echocardiogram (see page 561) to detect damage to the heart
- Ultrasound (see page 111) to detect damage to organs
- Lung function test (see page 647) to measure how well the lungs are working

Treatment

The treatment of vasculitis depends on the cause of the inflammation and the severity of any organ damage. For some forms of vasculitis, no treatment is necessary. For other forms, only the symptoms can be treated. Treatments for vasculitis can range from taking over-the-counter nonsteroidal anti-inflammatory drugs or corticosteroid drugs (for inflammation), to a procedure called plasmapheresis. Plasmapheresis removes potentially harmful inflammatory substances from the liquid part of the blood (plasma).

Hashimoto's Disease

Hashimoto's disease (also called Hashimoto's thyroiditis) is an autoimmune disorder in which the immune system mistakenly attacks the thyroid gland. Hashimoto's disease can lead to hypothyroidism (see page 903), a condition in which the thyroid gland becomes underactive and produces too little thyroxine, the thyroid hormone that regulates metabolism (all of the chemical processes that take place in the body). Although anyone can develop Hashimoto's disease, the disorder usually occurs in women between ages 30 and 50. The cause of Hashimoto's disease is unknown, but it tends to run in families.

Symptoms

Many people who have Hashimoto's disease have no symptoms. Others may develop symptoms of hypothyroidism, including an enlarged thyroid gland, increased sensitivity to cold, high cholesterol, loss of appetite accompanied by weight gain, a slow heart rate, and fatigue. Symptoms can also include dry skin, brittle fingernails, swollen ankles, or constipation. Some people may also experience muscle stiffness or weakness, muscle cramps, memory problems, or depression.

Diagnosis

To make a diagnosis of Hashimoto's disease, your doctor will take a health history, ask you to describe your symptoms, and perform a physical examination. The doctor will order blood tests to evaluate how well your thyroid gland is functioning and may recommend specialized blood tests to check for Hashimoto's disease.

Treatment

If Hashimoto's disease results in hypothyroidism, the doctor will prescribe synthetic thyroid hormone to relieve and control your symptoms. You will probably need to take the medication for the rest of your life. Your doctor will perform blood tests and physical examinations regularly to monitor your treatment and the functioning of your thyroid gland. He or she may need to adjust the dose of your medication from time to time, depending on your health and the results of the blood tests.

Polymyalgia Rheumatica

Polymyalgia rheumatica is a disorder that causes pain and stiffness in large muscle groups, primarily in the neck, shoulders, and hips. The disorder, which usually occurs after age 50, affects twice as many women as men, and the incidence increases with age. The cause of the disorder is not known, but it may have a hereditary component. It seems to be an autoimmune disorder brought on by a faulty immune response that attacks muscle cells. About 15 percent of people who have polymyalgia rheumatica develop a type of vasculitis called temporal arteritis (see page 927), also known as giant cell arteritis.

Symptoms

The main symptoms of polymyalgia rheumatica are moderate to severe pain and stiffness in the neck, shoulders, and hips, especially in the morning or after a period of inactivity. The pain and stiffness usually last longer than 30 minutes. Other symptoms may include slight fever, fatigue, depression, and weight loss. Symptoms of temporal arteritis include headaches, pain in the temples, jaw pain, and blurred or double vision. The disorder can lead to permanent blindness.

Diagnosis

To diagnose polymyalgia rheumatica, a doctor will take a detailed health history and order blood tests. One of these diagnostic blood tests, called the elevated erythrocyte sedimentation rate, measures how fast red blood cells fall to the bottom of a test tube. Rapidly falling red blood cells signal inflammation in the body. Because polymyalgia rheumatica can resemble other conditions, the doctor will want to rule out any other illnesses by ordering additional blood tests. If you also have symptoms of temporal arteritis, the doctor will recommend a biopsy of one of the temporal arteries at the side of your head to look for abnormal cells in the artery walls.

Treatment

Polymyalgia rheumatica frequently disappears by itself after a year or longer. With treatment, symptoms are usually relieved within 48 hours. Depending on the severity of symptoms, the doctor may recommend taking nonsteroidal anti-inflammatory drugs such as aspirin, ibuprofen, or naproxen, or he or she may prescribe low doses of corticosteroid drugs, which are very effective in relieving symptoms. To produce the best results, corticosteroids must be taken for 6 months to 2 years.

Sarcoidosis

Sarcoidosis is a chronic inflammatory condition in which small areas of inflamed tissue (called granulomas) form in organs or other tissues in the body. Although sarcoidosis usually affects the lungs and the lymph nodes (infection-fighting glands), it can also affect the heart, nervous system, muscles, joints, liver, kidneys, skin, or eyes. Most doctors think that sarcoidosis is an autoimmune disorder, in which the immune system mistakenly produces antibodies (infection-fighting proteins) that attack the body's own tissues. The disorder most often affects black adults between ages 20 and 40, which indicates a genetic component.

Symptoms

Many people who have sarcoidosis do not have symptoms. When symptoms occur, they can vary according to the organs or tissues that are affected. In many cases, a red, itchy rash develops on the face, arms, and legs. You may also have a fever, fatigue, loss of appetite, and weight loss. Arthritis-like swelling and pain sometimes occur, especially in the hands and feet. If your lungs are affected, you may have a persistent dry cough, shortness of breath, or mild chest pain. Damage to the heart can cause chest pain, an abnormal heartbeat (see page 580), or heart failure (see page 570). The lymph nodes or liver can become enlarged. You may experience weakness or pain in your muscles or joints. If your nervous system is affected, you may have trembling, loss of balance and coordination, paralysis, hearing loss, or seizures. The condition sometimes causes dry, watery eyes and impaired vision. If your kidneys are affected, you may develop kidney stones (see page 814).

Diagnosis

Doctors base a diagnosis of sarcoidosis on the symptoms, a health history, and a physical examination. Your doctor will probably order a chest X-ray to examine your lungs, and lung function tests (see page 647) to evaluate your lung capacity (the amount of air you can inhale in a single breath) and the ability of your lungs to transfer oxygen to the blood. He or she may recommend blood tests to measure the levels of calcium, angiotensin-converting enzyme (a substance in the blood that narrows blood vessels), and specific antibodies. People who have sarcoidosis usually have excess amounts of these substances in their blood.

You may also have a procedure called bronchoscopy (see page 661), in which the doctor uses a long, flexible viewing tube to look inside your lungs. During this procedure, he or she may perform a biopsy, in which a sample of the affected tissue is removed for examination under a microscope. Because tuberculosis causes similar symptoms, your doctor may perform a tuberculin skin test (see page 663) to rule out tuberculosis as a possible cause of your symptoms.

Treatment

In many cases, sarcoidosis does not require treatment and clears up on its own within a few years. For mild, arthritislike symptoms, your doctor may recommend taking over-the-counter nonsteroidal anti-inflammatory drugs such as aspirin, ibuprofen, or naproxen to relieve pain and inflammation in the joints. If you have mild respiratory symptoms, your doctor may monitor your lungs for several months with chest X-rays and lung function tests to determine whether the condition is improving or worsening.

If your symptoms are persistent or severe, or if the condition worsens, your doctor will probably prescribe corticosteroid medications such as prednisone to reduce inflammation, relieve shortness of breath or joint pain, and suppress the abnormal activity of your immune system. He or she may also recommend supplemental oxygen to help you breathe more easily. For some severe cases, doctors recommend a lung transplant (see page 658).

Antiphospholipid Antibody Syndrome

Antiphospholipid antibody syndrome is a condition in which blood clots spontaneously form in the veins and arteries. The cause of this condition is not known. The blood clots form when abnormal antibodies (infection-fighting proteins) in the blood interact with cells in the blood or in blood vessels, stimulating them to form a clot. The disorder can be present in some people with autoimmune disorders such as systemic lupus erythematosus (see page 920), rheumatoid arthritis (see page 918), or certain types of thyroid disease, but it can also occur in people who do not have an autoimmune disease.

Antiphospholipid antibody syndrome also may appear during a bacterial or viral infection such as syphilis (see page 483) or Lyme disease (see page 942), and disappear after the infection goes away. The abnormal antibodies can even be present in people without a medical condition. Certain drugs—such as the epilepsy drug phenytoin, antibiotics, cocaine, and antimalarial drugs—also can cause antiphospholipid antibodies to be produced in the blood. Discontinuing the drug will stop the abnormal blood clotting.

Antiphospholipid antibody syndrome carries special risks during pregnancy. Miscarriage early or late in pregnancy and stillbirth are common in women with the disorder. The placenta may be small and the fetus may have retarded growth. Affected women have an increased risk of a potentially dangerous condition called preeclampsia (see page 526)—a sudden increase in blood pressure, protein in the urine, or both during pregnancy. All pregnancies in women with antiphospholipid antibody syndrome are considered high-risk pregnancies.

Women with antiphospholipid antibody syndrome have an even higher risk of blood clots when taking birth-control pills, so they need to use other methods of birth control (see page 470). Smoking also dramatically raises the risk of blood clots in people who have the syndrome.

Symptoms

In a person with antiphospholipid antibody syndrome, blood clots appear in the leg or arm veins and can travel to the lungs, causing a life-threatening pulmonary embolism (see page 606). Other common symptoms include sudden vision loss, numbness or weakness in the face or limbs, purplish discoloration of the skin, seizures, stroke, or recurring pregnancy loss. Multiple strokes can lead to dementia (see page 689). All of these symptoms result from blood clots that develop in small or medium blood vessels. People with the disorder usually experience only a few of these symptoms.

Diagnosis

To diagnose antiphospholipid antibody syndrome, the doctor will take a complete health history, perform a physical examination, and order a series of blood tests to detect abnormal blood clotting and the antiphospholipid antibodies. The most important of these tests are the lupus anticoagulant test and the anticardiolipin antibodies test.

Treatment

The treatment of antiphospholipid antibody syndrome is tailored to each person. The presence of blood clots requires anticlotting medication such as heparin or warfarin, sometimes combined with aspirin. People with an autoimmune disorder may need to take corticosteroid drugs such as prednisone to suppress the abnormal immune system response.

Pregnant women with the disorder must also take medication to prevent blood clots in the veins that could travel to the brain or lungs. Baby aspirin, heparin, and immunoglobulin (human antibodies) are sometimes prescribed separately or in combination. Treatment during pregnancy significantly boosts the fetus's survival rate.

Chronic Fatigue Syndrome

Chronic fatigue syndrome (CFS) refers to a variety of symptoms that differ from person to person and can last for different lengths of time. People who have CFS generally have severe fatigue that is not improved by rest and that can worsen after physical or mental activity. Their level of activity is substantially lower than it was before the onset of the illness. The cause of CFS is not known, but doctors believe it may result from a combination of factors, including a viral infection, an abnormal immune response (possibly triggered by stress), or low blood pressure. In many cases, the symptoms of CFS last for months or even years.

Symptoms

Some symptoms of CFS resemble those of viral infections, such as a sore throat, tender lymph nodes, muscle pain, joint pain (without swelling or redness), and headaches that are different than usual. A person who has CFS can also experience significant impairment in short-term memory or ability to concentrate, feeling tired even after sleeping for several hours, and fatigue that can last 24 hours after physical exertion. Some people develop psychological problems such as anxiety (see page 718) or depression (see page 709).

Diagnosis

CFS is difficult to diagnose because the symptoms resemble those of many other disorders. Also, there are no laboratory tests or imaging procedures that can be used to help make a diagnosis. Your doctor will take a detailed health history and perform tests to rule out other possible causes of your symptoms. Before a diagnosis of CFS can be made, you must have experienced chronic fatigue for at least 6 months along with at least four of the symptoms described above.

Treatment

Although the cause of CFS is unknown, it is possible to treat many of the symptoms. For example, your doctor may prescribe aspirin, ibuprofen, naproxen, or another nonsteroidal anti-inflammatory medication to help relieve headache, muscle aches, and joint pain. Most people who have CFS recover; their symptoms go away and they eventually return to their usual level of activity.

12

Infections and Infestations

Infections are caused by organisms—including bacteria, viruses, fungi, and protozoa—that invade the body and multiply once they are inside. The course of an infection depends on several factors, including the nature of the infecting organism, its ability to cause disease, where it enters the body, how it spreads through the body, and the speed and effectiveness of the body's response to it. Disease-causing organisms require favorable conditions to cause infection—such as the right temperature, enough moisture, and a supply of nutrients. Viruses require suitable cells to invade and multiply in.

The immune system is a group of cells and proteins that can recognize foreign proteins (antigens) in the body, seek them out, and destroy them. The immune system attacks invading organisms either with white blood cells or proteins called antibodies. The immune system usually is able to mount an effective counterattack against invaders. The symptoms of an infection (such as fever, pain, and inflammation) are the results of this struggle.

Once infectious microbes enter your body, it takes time for them to multiply and cause symptoms. This period before symptoms develop is called the incubation period, which can vary from a few days to several months, depending on the particular disease-causing microbe. Doctors know the incubation periods for most common infectious diseases, making it possible to figure out when, where, and how a person acquired a particular infection.

After exposure to some kinds of organisms, the immune system is able to respond to future infections by those specific organisms and protect against them. Immunization is a way to induce this protective immune response without actually having the infection. Immunization can be active or passive. In active immunization, a person is given altered live or killed forms of a particular disease organism to trigger the same immune response that would occur from exposure to the actual organism. In passive immunization, a person is given injections of antibodies (infection-fighting proteins) produced by people who have recovered from an infection with a particular microbe. The antibodies are generally administered in a liquid derived from blood, called immunoglobulin.

Infections usually are limited to specific organs or tissues in which the infectious organisms are able to multiply. Some organisms are spread through the body in the

933

Viruses and Bacteria

Viruses and bacteria are the two microorganisms that cause most infections. Viruses cause infection by taking over the machinery of the cells they invade and making copies of themselves. In the process, the host cells are usually destroyed. The newly manufactured viruses invade other cells, continuing the cycle of multiplying inside the cells and destroying them. Viral infections may cause symptoms such as high fever, muscle pain, headache, and weakness. There are no effective treatments for most viruses, but some viral infections can be treated with antiviral drugs.

Bacteria live everywhere, including in and on the human body. Many types of bacteria are helpful in protecting the body from disease. They inhabit the skin and the mucous membranes that line the mouth, nose, intestines, and vagina, acting as barriers against potentially harmful invading microorganisms. Problems arise, however, when the beneficial bacteria in your body multiply in greater-than-normal numbers and cause infections or when harmful bacteria enter your body, such as through a cut in the skin or in food you eat. Some bacteria cause disease by producing toxins that damage cells.

Most of the harmful bacteria can be eliminated with antibiotics. However, antibiotics must be used appropriately, only for bacterial infections, and exactly as the doctor prescribes. If you stop taking a course of antibiotics before you finish the prescription, you risk having a recurrence of the infection. If you take antibiotics frequently or intermittently, you risk allowing bacteria to grow that will be resistant to the effects of the antibiotic and therefore harder to eliminate. Antibiotic resistance can also result when antibiotics are taken for viral infections such as a cold. Antibiotics are not effective against viral infections.

How viruses multiply

Viruses cause infection by invading cells in the body and taking over the cells' internal machinery to make copies of themselves. The viruses usually destroy the host cells in the process. The newly formed viruses leave the host cells, and go on to invade other cells, continuing to multiply.

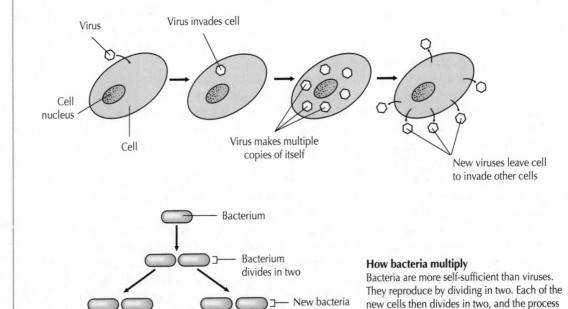

Virus

Virus invades cell

Cell nucleus

Cell

Virus makes multiple copies of itself

New viruses leave cell to invade other cells

Bacterium

Bacterium divides in two

New bacteria divide

How bacteria multiply

Bacteria are more self-sufficient than viruses. They reproduce by dividing in two. Each of the new cells then divides in two, and the process continues. Bacterial reproduction is so efficient that 1 million bacteria can develop from a single bacterium within 10 hours.

lymphatic system—a circulatory system that is an important part of the immune system (see page 908). If disease organisms gain access to the bloodstream, they can cause a life-threatening infection that affects the whole body.

Some infectious organisms are spread when they are coughed or sneezed into the air and breathed in; others are spread through physical contact such as a handshake. Still other organisms are spread in contaminated food or water.

Some microbes are transmitted to humans from animals or animal products (such as meat or eggs). If the spread of an organism that causes an infection can be stopped, the incidence of the disease may be reduced.

The parasites that cause infestations—such as worms, ticks, and lice—are larger than bacteria and viruses, and can be seen without a microscope. Infestations usually cause symptoms only at the site of infestation.

Generalized Infections

The infections in this section cannot be categorized easily, but one thing they have in common is that they produce symptoms throughout the body. Infectious mononucleosis and shingles are caused by viruses, while tetanus and toxic shock syndrome are caused by bacteria.

Infectious Mononucleosis

Infectious mononucleosis, often called mono for short, can be caused by either the Epstein-Barr virus or cytomegalovirus (see page 508). The infection can be transmitted from one person to another through oral contact such as kissing, and can spread to almost any organ. Mononucleosis is more common in teenagers and young adults (especially those who live in dormitories) and often occurs during stressful periods, such as during final examinations.

Symptoms

The early symptoms of infectious mononucleosis appear 4 to 6 weeks after exposure to the virus and resemble those of the flu (see page 649), including fever, headache, sore throat, swollen tonsils, and fatigue. Later symptoms may include painful, swollen glands in the neck, armpits, or groin (a condition called lymphadenopathy). Some people may also develop a rash over their entire body. In some cases, mono affects the liver and can cause jaundice (yellowing of the skin and the whites of the eyes; see page 785). If you have mono and you have a feeling of fullness in your upper left abdomen, you may have an enlarged spleen (an organ of the immune system that stores red blood cells and platelets). The symptoms of mono usually go away

within 2 to 3 weeks, but you may continue to feel weak for a couple of weeks to several months.

Diagnosis

If you have flulike symptoms that persist for more than a week, especially if you have swollen glands, a sore throat, and fatigue, your doctor will take a detailed health history and order blood tests to check for an increased number of white blood cells (which fight infection) and antibodies (specific proteins the body produces to fight the virus). You may have a test in the doctor's office (called a mono spot test) that gives immediate results. If the test result is negative but the doctor still thinks you may have mono, he or she will recommend an antibody test to make a definite diagnosis.

Treatment

Because infectious mononucleosis is caused by a virus, doctors do not prescribe antibiotics to treat it. Getting plenty of rest is essential. Your doctor may recommend taking an over-the-counter pain reliever such as ibuprofen or acetaminophen. (Do not give aspirin to a child or adolescent who has a fever from any cause, because aspirin has been linked to Reye's syndrome, a potentially fatal condition; see page 411.) The doctor also will probably recommend drinking plenty of water, especially while you have a fever. In severe cases, a doctor may prescribe corticosteroids to control swelling in the throat and tonsils. If your spleen is enlarged, your doctor will recommend avoiding any activities that could cause injury, such as contact sports. An injury to your upper left abdomen could cause your spleen to rupture, which can be life-threatening.

Tetanus

Tetanus, also called lockjaw, is a potentially life-threatening infection caused by clostridium bacteria that live in soil. The bacteria can enter the body through a cut in the skin that comes in contact with contaminated soil or through a wound caused by a contaminated object such as a nail or thorn. People who use drugs intravenously and share needles or who get tattoos or body piercings under unsanitary conditions are also at risk of infection. A toxin produced by the bacteria binds to the nerves in the spinal cord that control muscle activity and prevents them from functioning normally.

Symptoms

The symptoms of tetanus appear after an incubation period that can be as short as 3 days or longer than 3 weeks and can include headache, cramping and stiffness in the jaw (lockjaw), a stiff neck, and difficulty swallowing. Later symptoms include painful spasms and stiffness of the muscles in the neck, arms, legs, and stomach. Tetanus can affect the muscles involved in breathing, causing life-threatening breathing problems.

Diagnosis and Treatment

If you have not had a tetanus shot within the past 10 years and you get a puncture wound, call your doctor or your local emergency number, or go to the nearest hospital emergency department to have the wound cleaned and examined to determine the appropriate treatment.

If tetanus develops, you will be hospitalized immediately and given antibiotics and an injection of tetanus antitoxin. You may also be given sedatives (such as benzodiazepines) or muscle relaxants to prevent muscle spasms. You may need a mechanical ventilator to help you breathe. The goal of treatment is to keep your body functioning for several weeks while the disease runs its course. In some cases, tetanus can be fatal.

Prevention

To help prevent tetanus, always clean small cuts with soap and water and apply an antiseptic to the wound. It is especially important to clean cuts that occur outdoors (where contamination with clostridium bacteria is more common) or puncture wounds (because they are hard to clean and provide an environment favorable to the growth of bacteria).

Infants are immunized against tetanus during their first year of life. Booster shots are recommended at 10-year intervals throughout life (see page 145). Make sure that each family member is immunized against tetanus and has a booster shot every 10 years; keep a record of the dates when family members received their shots. Because immunization against tetanus is routine, tetanus is rare in the United States, with fewer than 100 cases each year.

Shingles

Shingles is a condition caused by the reactivation of the varicella zoster virus (the virus that causes chickenpox; see page 439) and occurs mostly in older adults. During a chickenpox infection, the virus can invade the nerve cells in the brain stem or spinal cord and be inactive for years. If the virus is later reactivated, it can multiply, causing a rash of blisters and intense pain on the skin over the affected nerve. You cannot acquire shingles from contact with an infected person. However, if you have never had chickenpox, you can get chickenpox from a person who has shingles, because both conditions are caused by the same virus.

Shingles can affect almost any part of the body, but often affects one side of the trunk. The disorder can be serious if it affects the face or eyes, because it can cause temporary facial paralysis and impaired vision. It can also spread to the auditory nerves, resulting in hearing problems. In some cases, the pain from shingles persists after the blisters heal. This condition, called postherpetic neuralgia, can last weeks, months, or years.

A weakened immune system seems to play a part in reactivation of the virus. For this reason, people who have an impaired immune system, such as those who have an HIV infection or AIDS or who are being treated for cancer, are at increased risk of developing shingles. These people are also at increased risk of having recurring episodes of shingles.

Shingles

Q. Can I get shingles from someone who has it?

A. You cannot get shingles from being around someone who has it. You can, however, get chickenpox, if you have never had it, from someone who has shingles because both are caused by the same virus.

Q. Both of my parents had shingles when they were in their 50s. Does this make me susceptible to getting shingles too?

A. No. Shingles does not have a genetic component. Anyone who has had chickenpox can develop shingles at any time, but the risk increases with age.

Q. Does stress cause shingles?

A. It's possible. Any condition or illness that weakens the immune system, even temporarily, can increase a person's risk of developing shingles. Stress can also weaken the immune system, making the dormant varicella zoster virus left in the body after a chickenpox infection more likely to be reactivated, causing shingles.

Symptoms

The symptoms of shingles include an itchy, tingling feeling or severe, burning pain in the affected area several days before a rash develops. A person may also have a headache, fever, or chills. The rash, which usually appears in a band or patch, can be itchy or painful and is contagious to people who have never had chickenpox. After a few days, the rash turns into small, fluid-filled blisters, which gradually become encrusted and less contagious. The blisters usually disappear after about 7 days and, in most cases, do not leave scars.

Diagnosis and Treatment

Your doctor can diagnose shingles from your symptoms. Laboratory tests can confirm the diagnosis.

To treat shingles and reduce your risk of developing postherpetic neuralgia, your doctor will prescribe an antiviral medication, such as acyclovir, within 72 hours of the appearance of the rash. If your face is affected, your doctor will recommend steps you can take to protect your eyes. To relieve pain caused by postherpetic neuralgia, the doctor may prescribe an antidepressant (see page 712) or a topical medication such as lidocaine. Some doctors may prescribe corticosteroids to help reduce the risk of postherpetic neuralgia.

Toxic Shock Syndrome

Toxic shock syndrome is a rare condition that can develop when staphylococcal or streptococcal bacteria release toxins into the bloodstream. Toxic shock syndrome caused by staphylococcal bacteria was linked in the early 1980s to the use of super-absorbent tampons, which were then taken off the market. In rare cases, toxic shock syndrome can result when streptococcal bacteria (which are ordinarily found on the skin) infect a skin wound or surgical incision. Toxic shock syndrome, when severe, can lead to a life-threatening drop in blood pressure that, if not treated promptly, can lead to shock (see page 162) and be fatal.

Symptoms

Symptoms of toxic shock syndrome caused by staphylococcal bacteria appear suddenly and include high fever, vomiting and diarrhea, and a sunburnlike rash over the entire body. Other symptoms include bright red eyes and throat, headaches and muscle aches, and confusion. The rash may peel as it heals.

Symptoms of toxic shock syndrome caused by streptococcal bacteria usually appear 2 to 3 days after exposure to the bacteria. Symptoms of a skin infection caused by streptococcal bacteria include oozing pus from the site of the infection, and pain, redness, and a feeling of heat around the infected area.

Blood Poisoning

If the blood becomes infected with bacteria that your immune system can destroy easily (such as from routine dental procedures, minor skin infections, or a small puncture wound), the condition is called bacteremia. Blood poisoning is a life-threatening infection that is caused by the rapid spread of bacteria (septicemia) and their toxins (toxemia) in the bloodstream. Symptoms of blood poisoning include fever, chills, loss of appetite, and fatigue. A blood test can help identify the type of bacteria that is causing the infection. Antibiotics are the usual treatment. Large numbers of bacteria or their toxins in the bloodstream may cause a potentially fatal condition called septic shock, in which low blood pressure and low blood flow can cause vital organs such as the liver, kidneys, heart, or brain to malfunction or fail.

If you have symptoms of toxic shock syndrome, call your doctor, 911 or your local emergency number, or go to the nearest hospital emergency department immediately.

Diagnosis

To diagnose toxic shock syndrome, a doctor takes a detailed health history and orders blood tests to check for abnormalities in the liver and kidneys and to rule out other possible illnesses. He or she may also test a sample of fluid from any pus-filled sores (boils) on the skin or infected cuts.

Treatment

Treatment for toxic shock syndrome requires a stay in a hospital. You will be given fluids intravenously (through a vein) and an antibiotic. Your blood pressure and the function of your liver, kidneys, and other vital organs will be closely monitored. If toxic shock syndrome is caused by a skin infection such as a boil or abscess, your doctor may drain the infected area. If toxic shock syndrome develops after surgery, a person will need to return to the hospital so the doctor can determine the cause and remove any dead tissue if necessary.

Infestations and Diseases Spread by Insect and Animal Bites

Infestations occur when parasites invade your body and live either on it (as lice do) or in it (as tapeworms do). Parasites that live on the skin usually cause no symptoms other than discomfort. Some parasites, such as ticks, can cause infections because they can carry disease-causing microorganisms. Parasites that live inside the body may go undetected because they sometimes cause vague symptoms that often go unnoticed. However, if parasites lodge in a vital organ or multiply rapidly, they can cause serious problems. Anyone, regardless of personal hygiene, can become infested with parasites.

Because the human body has only limited natural defenses against parasites, it is almost impossible to eliminate them without treatment. Most types of dangerous infestations are rare in the United States, and the parasite-destroying drugs that are available are highly effective.

Tapeworm

Tapeworms are parasites that sometimes infest pigs, cattle, and fish. A tapeworm can be transmitted to a person who eats infested pork, beef, or fish that has not been adequately cooked. Under poor sanitary conditions, tapeworm eggs can be transmitted in the stool of infested people or animals. Once inside the intestines, a tapeworm anchors itself by embedding its head in the intestinal wall. The tapeworm then absorbs food and may grow to more than 30 feet long. A pork tapeworm can cause brain damage (cysticercosis) and liver damage; a fish tapeworm can cause anemia (see page 610). Despite strict government regulations for meat-packing procedures, meat that contains tapeworms occasionally gets on the market. However, thorough cooking will kill any worms in the meat.

Symptoms

Segments of the tapeworm break off and are eliminated in stool. In the stool, the worm segments look like short pieces of narrow white ribbon. If the worm remains in the intestines, it often causes symptoms such as weight loss, occasional abdominal pain, loss of appetite, and irritation around the anus.

Diagnosis and Treatment

If your doctor thinks you may have a tapeworm, he or she will examine a stool sample and prescribe medication to kill the parasite. The treatment can take several days. You may need to have samples of your stool examined during this time until you pass the tapeworm's head (which indicates an end to the infestation) and follow-up stool tests after 1 month and again 3 months later to make sure the worm has been eliminated.

Scabies

Scabies (see page 126) is an infestation with tiny arachnids called mites that burrow under the skin and lay eggs. The mites can be spread through close physical contact such as sexual intercourse or from contact with infested clothes or bedding. Scabies most often affects the hands, wrists, armpits, buttocks, or genital area, rarely the head or face. The mites that cause scabies do not live long once they are removed from the skin.

Symptoms

The symptoms of a scabies infestation are caused by an allergic reaction to the insect's excrement and usually develop within 2 to 6 weeks in people who have never been exposed to scabies before, and within 1 to 4 days in people who have previously been exposed. Symptoms include intense itching (usually at night) and red, raised bumps on the skin. Constant scratching can cause sores and scabs to form.

Diagnosis

To diagnose scabies, a doctor may apply a blue or black felt-tipped pen to an affected area of the body (usually the area between the fingers). If you have scabies, the ink will seep into the burrows in the skin caused by the mites. The doctor will wash the ink off the surface of the skin to expose the burrows, apply a drop of mineral oil, and scrape the area to get a sample. The sample will be examined under a microscope to check for eggs, mites, and mite feces.

Treatment

To treat a scabies infestation, your doctor will prescribe a cream or lotion containing the insecticide permethrin or lindane for you to apply to your entire body below the neck. Follow the directions on the label or your doctor's instructions for application. Wash all infested areas of your body thoroughly before applying the cream or lotion. Do not apply lindane after a hot bath, which can increase the risk that it will be absorbed into the bloodstream, where it can be toxic. Immediately after beginning treatment, wash all contaminated clothing, bedding, and towels in very hot water and dry them in a hot dryer. Ironing everything can also help kill the mites. Spraying your furniture with gamma benzene hexachloride spray can help destroy mites, but be sure to follow the directions on the label carefully and avoid getting the spray in your eyes or on your skin, especially in open wounds or sores. Everyone you've had close contact with should also be treated for scabies.

Lice

Lice are tiny, wingless insects that can live on any part of the body and suck blood from the skin. The eggs of lice, known as nits, look like tiny white grains that cling to the hair. Infestations of body lice are rare and can be transmitted through close physical contact and by sharing infested clothing, towels, or bedding. Crab lice, or pubic lice (see page 485), live in pubic hair and are usually spread through sexual contact. Head lice infestations most often occur among schoolchildren. If your child has lice, report it to his or her school. Lice infestations are considered a public health problem, and it is necessary to trace them to their source to prevent them from spreading more.

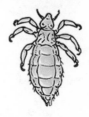

Louse (magnified)

Symptoms

The symptoms of a lice infestation include intense itching at the site of infestation, a feeling of something moving through the hair, and slight redness to severe inflammation of the skin caused by an allergic reaction to the bites. Lice bites pose a slight risk of infection.

Diagnosis and Treatment

If you have lice on your scalp or another part of your body, your doctor will recommend treating the affected area with a shampoo or lotion that contains permethrin. Carefully follow the instructions on the package. Then, using a fine-toothed comb or tweezers, remove as many nits as possible. Spray surfaces with a furniture spray that contains permethrin. Wash clothing, bedding, and towels in hot water, and dry them in a hot dryer. If possible, iron them. If any items cannot be cleaned, store them in a plastic bag for at least 2 weeks.

If lice are present on another part of your body, such as the genitals, inform your sex partner or anyone else with whom you have had close physical contact so he or she can also seek treatment.

Fleas

Fleas are tiny, wingless insects that live on and bite animals but that also can bite people. There are

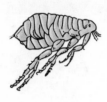

Flea (magnified)

many species of fleas, and each one is a parasite of a different animal. Flea eggs hatch in animal bedding about 7 days after they are laid. The fleas live in the bedding and feed off their hosts. Fleas do not stay long on the skin.

Flea infestations of humans are most common in developing countries and in places with crowded living conditions, close contact between people and domestic animals, or unclean conditions. Fleas can spread life-threatening diseases such as plague (see page 31).

Symptoms and Treatment

Isolated flea bites on the skin can cause a rash and intense inflammation (see page 126) for up to 2 days. If you suspect a flea infestation in your bedding, furniture, or rugs, spray the items with a flea pesticide or repellent. If the infestation is extensive and you are not able to eliminate the fleas, call a professional exterminator. To avoid flea infestations, use antiflea spray, powder, or shampoo on your pet, and spray pet bedding regularly. Flea collars for pets also can be helpful. Apply an insect repellent before going into a flea-infested area.

Chiggers

Chiggers (sometimes called red bugs or harvest mites) are a type of mite that lives in grasses, shrubs, and vines. Farmers, hikers, hunters, and others who spend time outdoors are most likely to get chigger bites. The larva (or immature mite) is barely visible ($\frac{1}{100}$ inch). It attaches to a hair follicle in an area of skin that is thin and moist (usually around the ankles, groin, or waistline), or wherever clothing is tight. The larva releases enzymes that dissolve the skin and then eats the liquefied cells. It feeds for 1 to 4 days in one spot and then drops off.

Symptoms

The most common symptom of chigger bites is intense itching in the affected area, especially at night. Some people may have an allergic skin reaction, such as hives (see page 1066) or an itchy, red, pimplelike lump. In some cases, blisters, swelling, or large red patches develop on the skin.

Treatment

To treat chigger bites, your doctor may prescribe medication such as antihistamines to relieve itching, corticosteroid creams to reduce irritation and allergic reactions, or antibacterials applied directly to the affected area to prevent bacterial infection.

Toxoplasmosis

Toxoplasmosis is a rare infection caused by the parasite Toxoplasma gondii. Found throughout the world, the parasite can infect virtually all warm-blooded animals, including livestock, birds, household pets, and humans, but cats are the major host and source of infection. Eating raw or undercooked meat is a less common source of infection. In the United States, about one of five people has been exposed to the parasite that causes toxoplasmosis, but most people have no symptoms because their immune system keeps the infection in check. The parasite remains in an inactive state inside muscle or brain tissue and usually causes no health problems.

Two groups of people—pregnant women and people who have a weakened immune system—have especially important reasons for avoiding infection with the parasite. A pregnant woman who contracts toxoplasmosis has a 40 percent chance of passing the infection to her fetus, a serious condition called congenital toxoplasmosis, which affects one or two babies of every 1,000 born in the United States each year. In people who have a weakened immune system (such as from an HIV infection or cancer or from taking immune-suppressing drugs), toxoplasmosis can cause life-threatening symptoms affecting the central nervous system and brain.

Cats, both domestic and wild, are the only hosts that produce the oocyst, the sexually mature and most infectious (to humans) stage of the parasite's life cycle. The parasite multiplies in the cat's intestine, and the oocyst is excreted in the cat's feces. Cats become infected when they eat contaminated rodents or birds, but infected cats have no symptoms.

Symptoms

Most healthy people who are infected with toxoplasmosis have no symptoms. Others experience swollen glands, muscle aches, and flulike symptoms that last for a few days to several weeks. Once you have been exposed to toxoplasmosis, you cannot get it again.

Women who develop toxoplasmosis more than 6 months before becoming pregnant are immune to the infection and cannot pass it on to their fetus. Women who contract toxoplasmosis during pregnancy have a higher-than-normal risk of having a miscarriage or stillbirth and can transmit the infection to the fetus. Infants born with congenital toxoplasmosis often appear normal at birth but develop symptoms such as blindness, deafness, seizures, and mental retardation months or even years later.

People who have a weakened immune system (such as those who are infected with HIV) cannot fight the infection and will experience headaches, confusion, fever, seizures, poor coordination, and nausea. Dormant toxoplasmosis infections can reactivate in people who have a weakened immune system, causing the same symptoms as those of a new infection.

Diagnosis

A blood test can detect the antibodies (infection-fighting proteins) that the body produces after infection by the toxoplasma parasite. If you plan to become pregnant, consider being tested for toxoplasmosis. If the test result is positive (meaning that you have been infected), there is no need to worry about passing the infection to a fetus during pregnancy. If the test result is negative, take precautions to avoid infection (see below). To find out whether a fetus is infected, doctors perform prenatal tests, including amniocentesis (see page 510) and an ultrasound scan (see page 509).

Treatment

Most people who are infected with toxoplasmosis need no treatment. Doctors treat infected people who have weakened immune systems with two antiparasitic drugs, pyrimethamine and sulfadiazine; pregnant women who have toxoplasmosis are treated with spiramycin. These drugs also lessen the severity of an infected infant's symptoms both at birth and later in life.

Prevention

If you are pregnant or have a weakened immune system because of a chronic illness such as AIDS, take the following precautions to avoid infection with the parasite that causes toxoplasmosis:

- If you have a cat, don't clean the litter box yourself. Have someone clean it for you every day to reduce the chances of being exposed to infectious toxoplasma oocysts (which take up to 2 days to become infectious). If you have to clean a litter box, put on rubber gloves before you do it and avoid inhaling the dust from the litter box. Dispose of the litter in a tightly wrapped and tied plastic bag. Wash the dust off the gloves with soap and water and rinse them before taking them off. Then wash and rinse your hands thoroughly.
- Don't eat raw or undercooked meat—especially lamb, pork, or venison—and don't feed it to your cat. Cook meat to an internal temperature of 160°F. Microwaving does not kill the toxoplasma parasite.
- Wash your hands thoroughly after handling raw meat.
- Don't taste meat while it is cooking.
- Keep your cat indoors so it doesn't come into contact with infected birds or rodents.
- Wear gardening gloves when working in the garden because outdoor cats defecate in soil. Avoid touching your mouth while gardening and always wash your hands after gardening.
- Stay away from children's sandboxes, or keep them tightly covered. Cats sometimes use them as litter boxes.
- Wash all fruits and vegetables well before eating them, even if they were grown in your own garden.

Rabies

Rabies is a life-threatening disease caused by a virus that is spread to humans through a bite or scratch from an infected animal. Once the rabies virus enters a human, it travels to the nerve nearest the bite and follows the nerve pathway to the brain. In the United States, rabies rarely occurs in dogs or outdoor cats because most are vaccinated annually. The wild animals that most often carry rabies are raccoons, skunks, bats, foxes, and coyotes.

Symptoms

The incubation period for rabies (the time it takes from being exposed to the virus until the appearance of symptoms) varies from 10 days to 2 years but is usually about 1 to 3 months. The earliest symptoms of rabies can resemble those of other viral infections and include fever and a general feeling of illness. After 2 or 3 days of feeling ill, a person becomes confused and agitated and has mouth and throat spasms; these symptoms usually last from 2 to 10 days. Trying to drink will worsen the spasms (this is why rabies is also called hydrophobia, which means fear of water). Death usually occurs within 3 weeks after the appearance of symptoms.

Diagnosis and Treatment

If you have been bitten or scratched by an animal that could have rabies, call your doctor, 911 or your local emergency medical number, or go to the nearest hospital emergency department immediately. A delay in treatment increases your risk of dying of rabies. If possible, the animal should be captured (but not destroyed) so tests can be performed to determine if it has rabies. You will probably be given an injection of immune globulin (proteins that fight the rabies virus) and a five-shot series of rabies vaccine to help prevent the disease from developing. The injections are usually given in the arm over a period of 28 days.

Avoiding Animal Bites

Take the following steps to avoid being bitten by an animal or infected with rabies:

- Don't keep wild animals as pets.
- Don't make any sudden moves or gestures toward an unfamiliar animal.
- Don't tease, provoke, or surprise an animal, especially when it is resting or eating.
- If confronted by an animal, back away slowly.
- If you have frequent contact with wild animals, talk to your doctor about having a rabies vaccination regularly.
- Have your pets immunized against rabies every year.

Lyme Disease

Lyme disease is an infection caused by bacteria that are transmitted to humans through the bites of infected ticks that live on animals such as deer, mice, rabbits, and raccoons. The ticks that carry Lyme disease can also carry ehrlichiosis (see page 945) and babesiosis (see page 944). Lyme disease can occur in anyone who is bitten by an infected tick.

Symptoms

A person who has been bitten by an infected tick usually develops a red spot on the skin that gradually increases in size (see page 126). The center of the spot returns to its normal color after a day or two, leaving a bull's-eye appearance on the skin that may be painless. In some cases, the skin clears up and the person has no other symptoms. However, in other cases, more red spots appear within a day or two and the person may have a headache, fever, swollen lymph glands, and pain in the joints and muscles. He or she may also feel generally ill and weak.

If Lyme disease is not treated, it progresses to a second stage of illness, in which the disease affects the nervous system and heart. Partial paralysis of the muscles served by the facial nerves and other affected nerves may occur. The person may also develop meningitis (see page 692), which is inflammation of the meninges (the coverings of the brain and spinal cord). Meningitis causes severe headache, sensitivity to light (photophobia), and generalized weakness. Rarely, an irregular heartbeat and inflammation of the heart and pericardium (the heart's covering) can occur.

If the second stage is not treated, a third stage will occur in which a person may develop chronic arthritis that affects the larger joints such as the knees.

Diagnosis and Treatment

A diagnosis of Lyme disease can be confirmed by blood tests.

Lyme disease is treated with doxycycline or another antibiotic (children are treated with amoxicillin). If Lyme disease is diagnosed and treated in its early stages, the outlook is good. Once chronic arthritis has developed, however, treatment is less successful. Additional treatment may be necessary if symptoms recur.

Rocky Mountain Spotted Fever

Rocky Mountain spotted fever is a potentially life-threatening infection caused by rickettsia bacteria that are transmitted through tick bites. Although ticks that carry the rickettsia bacteria are found all over the United States, the disease most frequently

Ticks

Ticks are parasites, usually found in wooded areas or tall grass, that feed on animals such as deer, mice, rabbits, and raccoons. A tick bite can be life-threatening because of the viruses and bacteria that ticks carry and transmit as they feed. There are several different types of ticks; each one can transmit a different disease. Some ticks can transmit more than one disease at a time. Diseases transmitted through tick bites include

Tick (magnified)

Rocky Mountain spotted fever, Lyme disease (see previous page), and encephalitis (see page 694). Some ticks also harbor a toxin that paralyzes the nerves in the legs and in the trunk. The paralysis is relieved by removing the tick.

A tick embeds its mouth into a person's skin, then swells as it feeds, sometimes to several times its original size. The skin around the bite hardens into a lump surrounded by a red halo. Usually, the lump subsides after the tick is removed but, in some cases, it can persist, especially if the tick's head remains in the skin after its body has been removed.

Take the following steps to avoid being bitten by ticks or to detect ticks as soon as possible:

- Use an insect repellent that contains DEET or permethrin. Carefully follow the instructions on the package.

- Wear light-colored clothing with a tight weave to see ticks more easily and avoid having them come in contact with your skin. Always wear shoes or boots, socks, long pants, and long-sleeved shirts. Tuck your pants into your socks, and tuck your shirt into your pants.

- Mow your lawn regularly. Clear out brush and leaf litter. Stack woodpiles neatly in a dry location,

preferably off the ground. Remove leaves and the remains of plants from your garden in the fall.

- After being outdoors, inspect your body thoroughly for ticks several times a day and at bedtime. Ticks often lodge in the hair, around the ankles, and in the genital area, so you may have to search for them.

- If you think that a tick has bitten you, see your doctor right away.

Removing a Tick

If you find a tick on your skin, remove it as soon as you can (before it becomes embedded in your skin), but resist the urge to hit it or to pull it out immediately with your fingers. Removal of the entire tick (including the head) is necessary because any part of a tick can continue to release infectious microbes.

To remove a tick from the skin:

- Do not touch the tick with your fingers. If possible, put on a pair of rubber gloves, or protect your fingers with a tissue. Do not use a lighted match or cigarette on the tick because doing so can cause the tick to embed itself farther into the skin or to release disease-causing microbes from its stomach.

- Using tweezers or small, curved forceps, grasp the tick's head (not just the body) as close to the surface of the skin as possible. (Try to remove the tick in one piece; if the tick's head breaks off, it could become embedded in the skin.) Pull on the tick gently; it may take a few minutes for the tick to loosen its grip.

- After you remove the tick, save it in a jar or small, sealable plastic bag to bring to your doctor. Remember not to touch the tick.

- Disinfect the bite with alcohol.

- Wash your hands thoroughly with soap and water.

- See your doctor right away. If the tick's head is still embedded in the skin, the doctor will remove it and recommend treatment.

occurs in the Southeast, from Maryland to Georgia. Rocky Mountain spotted fever usually occurs in the spring and summer in people who spend a lot of time outdoors.

A person who has been infected with the bacteria may not notice the tick bite that caused the disease. If you find a tick embedded in your skin, remove it as soon as possible (see above). The risk of becoming infected increases if the tick stays attached to your body for several hours or if you crush the tick while trying to remove it. Untreated, Rocky Mountain spotted fever can be fatal.

Symptoms

Symptoms of Rocky Mountain spotted fever develop from about 2 days to several weeks after exposure to the bacterium. Symptoms include severe headache, fever (up to 105°F), and severe muscle aches and weakness. Other symptoms can include chills, abdominal pain, nausea, spasms in the back, and mental confusion. Most people develop a characteristic rash (2 to 5 days after a bite) that usually begins as flat red spots on the palms of the hands and on the soles of the feet. The rash spreads to the wrists, ankles, legs, arms, and finally the trunk. Later stages of the disease include damage to the kidneys, liver, and lungs. Eventually, the person loses consciousness.

Diagnosis

Doctors diagnose Rocky Mountain spotted fever by taking two consecutive blood tests to check for antibodies (specific proteins the body produces to fight the bacteria). The second test is done 10 to 14 days after the illness begins to see if the level of antibodies has increased, which indicates an active infection.

Treatment

To treat Rocky Mountain spotted fever, your doctor will prescribe antibiotics as soon as the infection is diagnosed (because there is an increased risk of organ damage and death if treatment is delayed). If the disease is not treated right away, you may have to be hospitalized to treat any organ damage.

West Nile Virus Infection

West Nile virus is spread by the bites of infected mosquitoes and can infect people, birds, horses, and some other animals. The virus does not appear to spread from person to person or from animal to person but it may be transmitted through infected donor organs or in blood transfusions. In northern climates, most cases develop in late summer or early fall. In southern climates, the virus can be transmitted throughout the year. Most people who are infected have mild symptoms or no symptoms at all. However, in rare cases, the infection can cause severe symptoms and can be fatal. People over age 50 are more likely to have a severe infection. An estimated 1 in 150 people infected with the virus develops a severe form of the disease.

Symptoms

Symptoms of a West Nile virus infection usually develop from 3 to 14 days after the infecting mosquito bite. A mild case, called West Nile fever, is characterized by flulike symptoms such as fever, headache, body aches, and, sometimes, a rash on the trunk and swollen lymph nodes. The symptoms in mild cases usually last only a few days and don't cause any long-term health effects. Infection with West Nile virus may provide lifelong immunity to the virus.

The symptoms of more severe infections—West Nile encephalitis (inflammation of the brain), meningitis (inflammation of the membranes surrounding the brain and spinal cord), and meningoencephalitis (inflammation of the brain and the membrane surrounding it)—include headache, a high fever, a stiff neck, disorientation, muscle weakness, tremors, seizures, coma, and paralysis. These symptoms can last several weeks and their effects on the brain can be permanent or fatal.

Diagnosis

To diagnose a West Nile virus infection, a doctor will take a detailed health history to evaluate a person's risk of infection, such as being in an area where the virus has been detected. If your doctor thinks you may be infected or if you have symptoms, he or she will take a sample of blood and send it to a laboratory for microscopic examination to detect the virus.

Treatment

There is no specific treatment for a West Nile virus infection. Mild cases generally clear up on their own. For severe infections, people are usually hospitalized and given intravenous fluids and antibiotics (to prevent or treat secondary bacterial infections such as pneumonia). If breathing is affected, a person may need to use a ventilator to temporarily assist breathing.

Babesiosis

Babesiosis is a rare, potentially life-threatening disease caused by the Babesia microti parasite, which is spread to people through the bites of infected ticks that live on animals such as deer and mice. Babesiosis also can be transmitted through blood transfusions. The parasite that causes babesiosis attacks red blood cells.

Babesiosis can be mild or severe. Most people who are infected do not become sick. However, older people and people who have an impaired immune system or who have had their spleen removed (splenectomy) are at increased risk of developing a severe infection. If not treated, babesiosis can cause extremely low blood pressure, hemolytic anemia (see page 616), liver problems, and kidney failure in high-risk people.

Although babesiosis usually occurs in the coastal areas of the northeastern United States, cases have been reported on the West Coast and in the Midwest. The tick that carries Lyme disease (see page 942) and ehrlichiosis (see below) can also carry babesiosis, and a person can be infected with a combination of the diseases at the same time. If you find a tick embedded in your skin, remove it as soon as possible (see page 943).

Symptoms

Symptoms of infection with babesiosis may develop from 1 week to a month after a bite by an infected tick. Symptoms can include fatigue and a general sense of feeling ill. Later symptoms may include headache, fever, muscle and joint aches, and drenching sweats.

Diagnosis and Treatment

To diagnose babesiosis, your doctor will take a detailed health history and perform blood tests to check for antibodies (proteins the body produces to fight the parasite) or for the parasite itself. The disease can be difficult to diagnose in older people and in people who have other health problems.

Although most people do not need treatment for an infection with babesiosis, a doctor may prescribe a combination of antiparasitic medications for those at risk of severe illness or complications.

Ehrlichiosis

Ehrlichiosis is an infection caused by ehrlichia bacteria, which can be transmitted to people in tick bites. The infection has two forms—monocytic and granulocytic. Human monocytic ehrlichiosis is caused by a type of ehrlichia bacterium that attacks the infection-fighting white blood cells called monocytes. The bacterium that causes the granulocytic type, which also affects humans, attacks white blood cells called granulocytes. Human monocytic ehrlichiosis occurs mainly in the south central and southeastern parts of the United States. Human granulocytic ehrlichiosis occurs in the Northeast, the Midwest, and in northern California.

Some people who are bitten by a bacteria-carrying tick may not develop ehrlichiosis. However, older people, people who have an impaired immune system, and people who have had their spleen removed (splenectomy) are at increased risk of developing a severe infection. If you find a tick embedded in your skin, remove it as quickly as possible (see page 943).

Symptoms

The initial symptoms of ehrlichiosis may develop 5 to 10 days after a bite from an infected tick and include fatigue and a general feeling of illness. Other symptoms include fever, headache, and muscle and joint aches. People who develop a severe infection may also have nausea, vomiting, diarrhea, and a rash.

Diagnosis and Treatment

To diagnose ehrlichiosis, your doctor will take a detailed health history. He or she also may perform blood tests to check for antibodies (proteins the body produces to fight the bacterium) or for the bacterium itself. The doctor also may test your blood for a decrease in platelets (sticky cell fragments that enable blood to clot) and infection-fighting white blood cells. The blood test is performed when the symptoms begin and again 4 to 6 weeks later. A doctor will prescribe antibiotics to treat ehrlichiosis. Be sure to follow your doctor's instructions when taking the antibiotic to make sure you eliminate the infection.

Travelers' Infections

If you are planning a trip out of the country, make sure that you are adequately protected against any diseases that can occur in your country of destination. Many developing countries do not have adequate water or sewage systems. For this reason, diseases linked to contaminated water supplies— such as dysentery (see page 948), typhoid (see page 948), and polio (see page 695)—are common in many developing countries.

About 6 weeks before you leave on your trip, find out from your doctor which vaccinations are necessary for entry into the country and which are recommended. The US Centers for Disease Control and Prevention (CDC) is also a good source of information (www.cdc.gov). At least 1 month before you travel, see your doctor or go to a clinic that specializes in travelers' health and get any immunizations you may need; many vaccinations are not immediately available or must be taken well in advance of a trip. For example, if you plan to visit (even if only for a few hours) any of the countries in which malaria (see next page) is endemic (always present), you should begin antimalarial drug treatment before your trip and continue it after you leave the malaria-infested country. The length of the treatment time depends on the drug used. You can be immunized against typhoid and polio.

Depending on your destination, you may be advised to have one or more of the following vaccinations:

- Hepatitis A and B
- Yellow fever
- Meningococcal meningitis
- Rabies
- Polio booster
- Tetanus booster
- Measles booster

Tropical countries have insects, including mosquitoes and flies, that transmit diseases such as yellow fever (see page 949). If you swim or bathe in developing countries, or walk barefoot there, you risk becoming infested with parasitic worms such as schistosomes or hookworms. Schistosomes, or blood flukes, can be found in fresh water and can enter your body through the skin. In some cases, these parasites cause only a skin condition called dermatitis (see page 1062). In other cases, infestation with schistosomes results in a disease called schistosomiasis, or bilharziasis. In this disease, the parasites travel from the skin to the bladder and the intestines, from where they may spread to other parts of the body. The severity of the disease depends on the number of parasites that enter your body.

Hookworms are parasitic roundworms that are found in developing countries, particularly in areas with poor sanitation. Larvae of the parasite live in the soil, and your risk of infestation increases if your skin comes in contact with infested soil or if you eat or drink contaminated food or water. The hookworms enter the bloodstream and travel to the lungs. From the lungs they travel to the trachea, are swallowed, and end up in the small intestine. The worms then "hook" themselves to the lining of the intestine, where they feed on blood, causing blood loss. Severe infestations can result in anemia (see page 610).

While you are traveling in a developing country, the following precautions can help you stay healthy during your trip:

- Wash your hands before handling or eating food.
- Drink only bottled water or milk, or boil water to make it safe to drink. Alternatively, use both a water filter and iodine tablets to purify water and other liquids by the glassful. Avoid ice cubes. Carbonated beverages such as colas in sealed cans and bottles are usually safe.
- Do not use tap water for brushing your teeth.
- Avoid salads and reheated foods. Do not eat peeled fruit; always peel it yourself.
- If you plan to visit rural or remote areas, make sure that your clothing protects you adequately from insect bites, especially if you plan to sleep outside or travel at night (when insects can be most active). Wear long-sleeved shirts, long pants, and socks when traveling.
- Use an insect repellent containing DEET or permethrin (in a 35 percent solution for adults and a 6 to 10 percent solution for children).
- Stay in air-conditioned or well-screened areas.
- Don't use scented products such as lotions or perfumes, which can attract some insects.

Cholera

Cholera is a disease caused by bacteria that damage the intestinal lining. The bacteria are transmitted through polluted water, shellfish, or raw fruits and vegetables in places where sanitation is poor. Cholera seldom occurs in developed nations. When it does, it usually can be traced to visits to (or residence in) developing countries. However, every year the US Public Health Service reports a few cases of illness caused by contamination of American shellfish with bacteria related to the cholera bacillus.

Symptoms

The symptoms of cholera are abdominal pain and severe diarrhea. Cholera can cause such severe diarrhea that up to 4 gallons of fluid are lost in a day. A person who has cholera may have bowel movements resembling murky water that may be passed almost continuously. He or she may have muscle cramps, extreme thirst, and sudden vomiting, sometimes without the usual initial feeling of nausea. If dehydration is not treated immediately, cholera can be fatal quickly. If you are abroad or have just returned home and have extremely watery, continuous diarrhea that does not improve within a couple of hours, get medical help immediately.

Diagnosis and Treatment

If you have symptoms of cholera, see your doctor immediately. He or she will ask for stool samples to look for the bacteria in the stool. He or she may also order a blood test to look for antibodies (infection-fighting proteins) produced by the immune system to fight the cholera-causing bacteria.

The main treatment for cholera is to prevent or treat dehydration by replacing fluids. If the diarrhea is severe, you may need to be hospitalized. You will be given a rehydration fluid either orally or intravenously (through a vein) until your body chemistry is restored to normal. Your doctor also may prescribe an antibiotic.

Malaria

Malaria is a disease caused by any of four species of parasites called plasmodia that are transmitted from one person to another through the bite of an

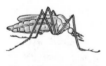

Mosquito (magnified)

Anopheles mosquito (the only carrier). Plasmodia enter the bloodstream only if the Anopheles mosquito that bites you has previously bitten a person who has malaria.

Once in the bloodstream, the plasmodia travel to the liver, where they multiply rapidly. After 9 to 16 days, thousands of plasmodia flow back into the bloodstream, where they destroy oxygen-carrying red blood cells, which can result in anemia (see page 610) and a high fever. Many plasmodia remain in the liver cells and continue the cycle of multiplying, entering the bloodstream, and destroying red blood cells. When the parasites inside the red blood cells mature, they rupture the cells and reenter the bloodstream. The destroyed red blood cells can form small clumps, which can block blood vessels, potentially leading to brain or kidney damage. One species of the plasmodia

causes an especially dangerous infection called falciparum malaria, which can cause massive, potentially fatal blood vessel blockages.

In most forms of malaria, a person usually has repeated attacks unless the disease is treated. Each attack signals the release of plasmodia into the bloodstream. If malaria is not treated, attacks can occur for years. However, as the immune system slowly builds up a defense against the disease, the attacks occur less and less frequently.

The Anopheles mosquito is found in the southeastern and western United States and in tropical and semitropical countries. Mosquito abatement programs have virtually eradicated malaria in the United States. With the exception of a few cases each year, nearly all cases of malaria in the United States are brought back by people who have traveled to other countries.

Symptoms

The symptoms of malaria depend on the type of plasmodium carried by the mosquito and usually appear about 8 to 30 days after a mosquito bite. A full day of headache, fatigue, and nausea is followed by 12 to 24 hours of chills alternating with fever. A sudden chill is followed by a stage of fever with no sweating, and rapid breathing. A drop in temperature accompanies a final sweating stage. Similar bouts occur whenever more plasmodia are released into the bloodstream, generally every 2 or 3 days.

Children with malaria are likely to have prolonged high fever without chills. The fever sometimes affects the brain, causing unconsciousness or seizures (see page 686).

In falciparum malaria, the most severe form, all the plasmodia are released from the liver into the bloodstream at the same time, resulting in a single extremely severe attack. The alternating chills and fever can last 2 or 3 days. If the person recovers, however, the attacks do not recur.

Diagnosis and Treatment

If you develop symptoms of malaria, see your doctor immediately. He or she will order blood tests. Because it is not always easy to detect the presence of plasmodia in the blood, you may need to have blood tests periodically. If blood tests show that you have malaria, the doctor will prescribe an antimalarial medication.

Prevention

To protect against malaria, when you are planning to visit an area in which the disease is prevalent, your doctor will prescribe antimalarial drugs. You need to start taking the drugs before your trip and continue to take them after you return. In many parts of the world, malaria parasites have become resistant to some of the more common drugs used against them such as chloroquine, but newer and more effective drugs are constantly being developed.

Amebic Dysentery

Amebic dysentery, also known as amebiasis, is an intestinal illness caused by infection with a microscopic parasite (ameba). Amebic dysentery is prevalent in developing countries that have poor sanitation. Contaminated water and lack of proper hygiene among food handlers can spread the organisms that cause amebic dysentery. In the United States, amebic dysentery is transmitted most frequently through oral-anal sex.

Symptoms

The main symptom of amebic dysentery is diarrhea, which can contain blood and may persist for weeks if not treated (resulting in weight loss). Other symptoms include abdominal cramps, excessive gas, and fatigue. After the diarrhea subsides, it may recur from time to time. In rare cases the organisms spread from the digestive tract into the bloodstream and settle in the liver, where they form abscesses (pus-filled sacs).

Diagnosis and Treatment

If you have symptoms of amebic dysentery, your doctor will ask for stool samples to look for the parasite in the stool. He or she also may order a blood test to look for antibodies (proteins the body produces to fight the parasite) or for the parasite itself. The doctor may also recommend a sigmoidoscopy (see page 144) to view the lower part of the colon directly. If you have amebic dysentery, the doctor will prescribe antiparasitic drugs to be taken for about 10 to 20 days. Make sure you wash your hands thoroughly after you use the toilet to avoid reinfecting yourself or spreading the infection to others. After the diarrhea has stopped, your doctor

will want to examine samples of your stool monthly until no infecting organisms are found.

Typhoid Fever

Typhoid fever is an infectious disease spread under unsanitary conditions from person to person or through contaminated food or water. Some people carry typhoid-causing bacteria in their body after they have the disease (even without having symptoms) and can infect others. Typhoid fever is rare in the United States, although the disease occurs occasionally in rural areas. Nearly all cases can be traced to recent travel or residence in a developing country. If you are planning to travel to a developing country, talk to your doctor. Depending on the country, he or she will probably recommend that you have a vaccination against typhoid.

Symptoms

The symptoms of typhoid fever begin suddenly with headache, loss of appetite, and vomiting followed by a persistent fever of about 104°F, chills, increasing weakness, diarrhea (usually bloody), and, often, delirium. Early in the disease, you may have a pink rash on your abdomen (called rose spots), which then fades. In severe cases, a person can have extensive gastrointestinal bleeding or rupture of the intestines, which can be life-threatening.

Diagnosis and Treatment

If you have recently returned from a developing country and have symptoms of typhoid fever, see a doctor immediately. If he or she suspects you could have typhoid fever, you will be admitted to a hospital isolation unit. You may have a blood test to look for antityphoid antibodies (proteins the body produces to fight the bacteria) or to detect the bacterium itself. A doctor may also take a stool sample to look for the bacteria. If you have typhoid fever, your doctor will prescribe antibiotics, which you will need to take for about 7 to 14 days. It may be several more weeks before your digestive tract is free of infectious bacteria; during this time, you can still transmit the infection to others. To make sure that you are free of typhoid bacteria, your doctor will examine a sample of your stool each month for at least 3 months (longer if you are a food handler).

Yellow Fever

Yellow fever is a disease caused by a virus that damages the liver and kidneys. The virus is transmitted through Aedes mosquito bites and occurs in South America and Africa. As with many viral infections, there is no effective treatment for yellow fever. A person who has recovered from yellow fever is immune to it for life. A vaccine is available to prevent yellow fever in people who are traveling to countries where the disease may be prevalent. However, the vaccination is not recommended for children younger than 6 months, pregnant women, or people who are allergic to eggs or who have a weakened immune system.

Symptoms

The symptoms of yellow fever, which develop 3 to 6 days after the infecting mosquito bite, can be mild to severe. A mild case produces symptoms that resemble those of the flu (see page 649). Symptoms of more severe cases include fever, headache, abdominal pain and vomiting, bleeding from the gums, frequent nosebleeds, easy bruising, blood in stool or vomit, and yellowing of the skin and whites of the eyes (jaundice; see page 785). Other possible symptoms include confusion, kidney failure, and coma.

Diagnosis and Treatment

To diagnose yellow fever, a doctor will perform blood tests to check for antibodies (proteins the body produces to fight the virus) or for the virus itself.

There is no treatment for yellow fever. You will be given a rehydration fluid either orally or intravenously (through a vein) to replace lost fluids. If you develop a bacterial infection, your doctor will prescribe an antibiotic.

Dengue

Dengue is an infection caused by a virus that is transmitted through the bites of Aedes mosquitoes. Dengue infections occur in Central and South America, the Caribbean, the South and Central Pacific islands, Southeast Asia, China, India, the Middle East, and Africa.

Symptoms

The symptoms of dengue, which develop 8 to 10 days after the infecting mosquito bite, occur suddenly and resemble those of other viral infections, such as high fever, headache, nausea and vomiting, and joint and muscle pain. The joint and muscle pain is so severe that dengue is often called breakbone fever. A rash may appear 3 to 4 days after a fever develops. Dengue can last up to 10 days, but complete recovery can take 2 weeks to a month. In severe cases, dengue progresses to a life-threatening complication called dengue hemorrhage, which is characterized by severe bleeding that can be fatal.

Diagnosis and Treatment

To diagnose dengue, a doctor takes a detailed health history and orders blood tests to check for antibodies (infection-fighting proteins the body produces to fight the virus) or for the virus itself. If you have recently traveled to any area where dengue is prevalent and have symptoms, tell your doctor.

To treat dengue, doctors usually recommend bed rest, plenty of fluids, and a pain reliever such as acetaminophen. People with dengue should not take aspirin because aspirin interferes with blood clotting and can increase the risk of bleeding.

Leishmaniasis

Leishmaniaisis is a potentially life-threatening disease caused by a parasite that is transmitted through the bites of infected sand flies. In very rare cases, leishmaniasis can be transmitted through blood transfusions, and from a pregnant woman to the fetus. The most common types of leishmaniasis are cutaneous leishmaniasis, mucosal leishmaniasis, and visceral leishmaniasis. The majority of cases occur in countries in South America, South Asia, and Africa. Leishmaniasis is also found in some parts of Central America, Mexico, and the Middle East. Although very rare in the United States, cutaneous leishmaniasis infections have occurred in rural areas of southern Texas.

Symptoms

The symptoms of cutaneous leishmaniasis—skin sores that begin as small red or purple bumps—can appear weeks or months after a person has been bitten by an infected sand fly. The sores increase in size and develop a raised edge and central crater. The sores can cause scabs that may leave disfiguring scars. In some cases, untreated cutaneous leishmaniasis can spread, causing sores in the nose or mouth (mucosal leishmaniasis).

Symptoms of visceral leishmaniasis can include fever, swollen glands, weight loss, darkening of the skin, and an enlarged spleen or liver. Visceral leishmaniasis can destroy red blood cells (which deliver oxygen to tissues) and white blood cells (which fight infection) in the spleen, liver, and bone marrow, potentially causing anemia (see page 610).

Diagnosis
To diagnose cutaneous leishmaniasis, a doctor takes a detailed health history and examines the skin for the characteristic sores. If you have sores that have not healed, the doctor will take samples from the sores for examination in the laboratory. For all forms of leishmaniasis, blood tests are used to evaluate the levels of red cells, white cells, and platelets (cell fragments that enable blood to clot). You may have a blood test to look for antibodies (specific infection-fighting proteins the body produces to fight the parasite) or a test to detect the parasite itself in a tissue sample from a sore or from the bone marrow or lymph nodes.

Treatment
The skin sores of cutaneous leishmaniasis usually heal without treatment. However, a doctor may prescribe an antiparasitic or antifungal medication to treat cutaneous leishmaniasis or to prevent it from spreading to the nose and mouth. These drugs also are used to treat visceral leishmaniasis.

13

Genetic Disorders

Like eye color and hair color, some disorders can be transmitted from one or both parents to a child. Sometimes, normal genes change (mutate) as cells divide, or genes in a parent's egg or sperm are altered by environmental factors such as radiation to produce a genetic disorder in a child whose parents are both healthy. The child, who carries the genetic mutation in each of his or her cells, can then pass the mutated gene to the next generation.

Genetic disorders fall into three general categories—chromosome abnormalities, single-gene disorders, and disorders that result from an interaction of numerous genes and the environment. Chromosome abnormalities result from defects in the number or structure of chromosomes (structures that contain numerous genes). Single-gene disorders result from a single defective gene or pair of genes, are usually inherited, and are likely to recur in a family.

The way in which single-gene disorders are inherited depends on whether the defective gene is a dominant gene or a recessive gene on an autosome (one of the 22 chromosomes that are the same in males and females) or a gene on the X sex chromosome. To be affected by an autosomal dominant disorder, a person needs to receive only one copy of a dominant disease gene from one parent. Autosomal recessive disorders usually affect a person only if he or she has received two copies of the recessive disease gene, one from each parent. A person who has only one copy of a defective recessive gene is called a carrier. X-linked, or sex-linked, disorders are usually transmitted from mothers (who are unaffected carriers of the defective gene on their X chromosome) to sons, who are affected (because they don't have another X chromosome, as females do, to override the effects of the defective gene).

The most common chronic disorders—including heart disease, cancer, asthma, osteoporosis, and type 2 diabetes—usually result from the interaction of several genes with environmental influences such as diet and smoking. People who inherit genes that can make them susceptible to developing a particular disorder are not destined to get the disease unless they expose their body to the stresses that trigger the susceptibility genes. For example, people who inherit genes that make them susceptible to developing heart disease will not necessarily develop heart disease unless they eat a high-fat diet, smoke cigarettes, fail to exercise, or are overweight. Conversely, not having these susceptibility genes does not guarantee that a person will not develop a disease if he or she smokes or engages in other unhealthy habits.

If you have relatives who have had illnesses such as cancer or heart disease at a young age or who have died from such an illness at a young age, their illnesses were likely to have a strong genetic component. In this case, you might benefit from seeing a genetic counselor, who can help you understand your personal health risks and the steps you might take to reduce these risks. A genetic counselor can also explain how your family health history (see page 131) might affect your children.

Genetic disorders can affect different organ systems. Hemophilia, sickle cell disease, and thalassemia affect the blood; muscular dystrophy affects the muscles; cystic fibrosis affects the lungs; and Huntington disease and Tay-Sachs disease affect the brain and nervous system. Inborn errors of metabolism, such as Gaucher disease and galactosemia, are imbalances in the body's chemistry caused by a defective gene or pair of genes that a child inherits from one or both parents.

The severity of genetic disorders can vary from disorder to disorder, and the same disorder can differ in severity from one person to another. For example, Duchenne muscular dystrophy is always fatal during adolescence or early adulthood, while hemophilia can be treated successfully enough to enable an affected person to lead a relatively full life. Sickle cell disease and Marfan syndrome can be mild in one person and severe in another.

Genetic Counseling

The rapid increase in knowledge about genes, how they function, and how they cause disease is providing powerful new information about preventing, diagnosing, and treating genetic disorders. This information is also helping people evaluate their risk of inheriting a genetic disorder or of transmitting a disease-causing gene to a child. Of every 100 children born, two or three have a serious mental or physical disability that is genetic in origin or results from damage to, or faulty development of, the fetus during pregnancy.

A child may be born with a genetically influenced disorder from a number of different causes. For example, he or she may have inherited a copy of a defective gene from each parent and have a recessive genetic disorder such as cystic fibrosis (see page 958) or sickle cell disease (see page 613). A child may have an abnormal gene produced by a mutation in the egg or sperm of one of the parents. The occurrence of these spontaneous genetic mutations explains how parents who are completely healthy and don't carry a disease gene can have children with a genetic disorder such as muscular dystrophy (see page 972), hemophilia (see page 618), or neurofibromatosis (see page 968). A mistake during cell division before or just after fertilization can result in a chromosome abnormality such as Down syndrome (see page 955) or Turner syndrome (see page 957).

It is now possible, with many genetic disorders, to have a test to determine whether you are a carrier of a defective disease gene. Most people who suspect they may carry a defective gene wait until they are planning to have children before they are tested for the gene. However, if one child in a family has, for example, a recessive disorder such as cystic fibrosis, his or her relatives can be tested to see if they carry the cystic fibrosis gene in their cells.

If one or both parents are found to be carriers of a disease gene, genetic counselors can calculate the risk for each of their children of inheriting it and having the disease, depending on whether the abnormal disease gene is dominant or recessive. For some genetic disorders, an accurate risk calculation can be made.

Even for some congenital (present at birth) disorders of unknown origin, such as heart defects, genetic counselors are often able to estimate the risk that a subsequent child will be born with the condition. As with genetic disorders, tests may be performed during pregnancy to determine whether the fetus has a developmental defect. Many of these defects, including most congenital heart defects, can be corrected early in life. For other genetic disorders, however, it is more difficult to calculate the inheritance risk precisely.

If you suspect that you may carry a gene for an

inherited disorder, perhaps because a particular illness appears to run in your family, talk to a genetic counselor, who can help you evaluate your risk of passing the disorder on to a child. Also, if you have a stillborn child, ask your doctor if your child might have had a genetic disorder. If a genetic disorder is a possibility, your doctor will refer you to a genetic counselor, who can help you understand your risks of having another affected child.

A genetic counselor will ask you for detailed information about the health of your and your partner's parents, brothers, sisters, cousins, and other close relatives. It will help if you gather this information beforehand and bring it with you in writing when you see the counselor. You will be asked to give the exact cause of death of relatives, and the age at which they died, especially those who died during infancy. The counselor will also consider your ethnic and racial background and your age, which can be risk factors for some disorders.

Many genetic disorders, including cystic fibrosis and sickle cell disease, can be diagnosed during pregnancy. Chorionic villus sampling, or CVS (see page 511), is a prenatal diagnostic test that can be performed early in pregnancy—between the 10th and 12th weeks. In this procedure, a sample of tissue is removed from the placenta and examined under a microscope. Another test, called amniocentesis (see page 510), may be performed later in pregnancy, at 14 to 18 weeks, to diagnose genetic disorders using cells suspended in the fluid in the amniotic sac.

These prenatal diagnostic tests pose a slight risk to the developing fetus, including infection of the uterus and miscarriage. A genetic counselor will help you evaluate the risks and benefits of having these tests and weigh them against your risk of transmitting a genetic disorder to a child. This information will enable you to make decisions about whether you are willing to undergo the possible risk to your fetus that the test might confer and whether you would choose to terminate the pregnancy if you learn that the fetus has a serious disorder.

A genetic counselor will discuss with you the potential severity of the particular genetic disorder you may be at risk of passing on to a child, treatments that may be available for the disorder, and the effectiveness of these treatments. Many people decide not to have prenatal diagnostic tests, and accept the possibility that their child may be born with a genetic disorder or defect. Other people who would not choose to terminate a pregnancy decide to have the test so they can be prepared to care for a child with a genetic disorder or birth defect.

Who Should Seek Genetic Counseling?

Genetic counseling can help people understand their chances of passing on a genetic disorder or birth defect to children or of developing a particular disorder themselves. Consider genetic counseling if you have any of the following risk factors:

- You (or your partner) have a family history of a genetic disorder or birth defect.
- You have a child who was diagnosed at birth with a genetic disorder or birth defect.
- Your doctor has told you that you may be at risk of having children with birth defects or genetic disorders.
- You are a woman over age 35 who is pregnant or planning to become pregnant. (Being over 35 increases a woman's risk of having a child with a chromosome abnormality such as Down syndrome.)
- You have had a baby who died in infancy or you have had two or more miscarriages.
- You have been exposed to toxic chemicals, high doses of radiation, or other environmental factors that might increase your risk of having a child with birth defects.
- You are planning to have children with a person who is a close blood relative, such as a first cousin.

Genetic Testing

As scientists identify more and more genes linked to diseases and disorders, people increasingly will be offered the option of having a test to determine if they carry a particular gene or genes for a specific disorder. The more you know about how diseases can be passed from one generation to the next, or how having specific genes may make you susceptible to developing a disease such as heart disease later in life, the better prepared you will be to make decisions about planning a family and to make good lifestyle choices. Following are brief descriptions of some of the genetic tests that are available.

Prenatal Testing

During pregnancy, women are given the option to have testing to determine if their fetus has a genetic abnormality or birth defect. One of these tests examines a pregnant woman's blood for the level of a protein called alpha-fetoprotein (AFP; see page 510). AFP is normally present in the blood, but a higher-than-average level of the protein indicates that the fetus may have a brain or spinal cord defect such as spina bifida. A lower-than-average level of AFP, when combined with altered levels of other proteins—human chorionic gonadotropin (hCG) and unconjugated estriol (uE3)—may indicate that the fetus has Down syndrome.

Chorionic villus sampling, or CVS (see page 511), removes a small sample of tissue from the placenta for analysis; amniocentesis (see page 510) takes a sample of amniotic fluid for analysis. Ultrasound (see page 509) uses high-frequency sound waves to produce an image of the fetus to detect any visible birth defects. Preimplantation testing analyzes the DNA of a fertilized egg or embryo in the laboratory to rule out any genetic abnormalities before implanting the embryo into a woman's uterus.

Screening of Newborns

Every state requires testing of all newborns for a variety of disorders 24 hours after birth and before they are released from the hospital. Some disorders have no immediate visible effects but can cause physical problems, mental retardation, or death unless they are detected and treated early. Newborn testing allows treatment for some disorders to be started early, when it is most effective. Required screenings vary by state, but most states require testing for phenylketonuria, or PKU (see page 962), hypothyroidism (see page 404), galactosemia (see page 964), and sickle cell disease (see page 613). Many states are expanding newborn screening to test for more than 40 disorders. Ask your doctor if this is an option in your state.

Carrier Detection

Some people carry genes for specific diseases that they can pass on to children. Genetic testing can identify people who are carriers of disease genes.

Once a person or couple find out that they are carriers of a genetic disorder, a genetic counselor can help them understand all of their reproductive options and provide them with information to help them make decisions about family planning based on the test results.

Routine screening is offered to people who are at increased risk of having the genes for specific recessive genetic disorders because of their race or ethnic origin. For example, screening for sickle cell disease is offered to people of African descent; screening for thalassemia (see page 616) is offered to people of Mediterranean descent such as Greeks and Italians; screening for Tay-Sachs disease (see page 960) and Canavan disease (see page 960) is recommended for Ashkenazi Jews; and screening for cystic fibrosis (see page 958) is recommended for people of European descent.

Presymptomatic Testing for Genetic Disorders

Sometimes a person inherits a gene or genes for a disorder that does not have an effect until later in life. For example, a person who inherits the gene for Huntington disease (see page 969) will usually be perfectly healthy until sometime after age 30, when his or her nervous system begins to degenerate, eventually leading to death. Because the Huntington gene is a dominant gene, if a person has the gene, he or she will develop the disease and has a 50 percent chance of passing the gene on to a child, who will also have Huntington disease.

Some people with a family history of Huntington disease choose not to have the genetic test for it because they don't want to know that they will develop a disease that is fatal and for which there is no treatment or cure. Other people decide to have the test because they do not want to live with uncertainty about their future or they want to make sure they are not at risk of passing the gene on to a child. If you have a family history of a genetic disorder that does not cause problems until later in life, talk to a genetic counselor about the benefits and risks of being tested for the gene.

A recessive genetic disorder called hereditary hemochromatosis (see page 961) is a common disease that affects many people and for which there is effective treatment. In hemochromatosis, the defective gene causes the body to store too much iron, which can lead to diabetes, cirrhosis of the liver, heart disease, and tissue damage. The disease can be managed by periodically removing or donating a specified amount of blood to reduce the level of iron in the blood. Because hemochromatosis is so common and the treatment is effective and relatively easy, some doctors believe that everyone should be tested for it.

Presymptomatic Testing for Common Disorders

Newer genetic tests are being developed to screen for genes that make a person susceptible to developing a particular disorder such as cancer later in life. These genes are called susceptibility genes because people who have them are not necessarily destined to develop the disease, but they are at higher risk of developing the disorder than are people who do not have the genes. One of the tests being offered is for women who are at risk of developing breast cancer or ovarian cancer because they have a family history of either disease. This test looks for two genes for breast cancer and ovarian cancer, called BRCA1 and BRCA2. Another test detects the susceptibility genes for hereditary nonpolyposis colon cancer, the most common form of colon cancer (see page 775), and for familial adenomatous polyposis (see page 774), which can lead to colon cancer. A test is available for some inherited forms of melanoma (see page 1069), the deadliest type of skin cancer.

As scientists link more and more genes to diseases, more screening tests will be made available to determine a person's risk of developing a specific disease. If a particular chronic illness runs in your family, your doctor is likely to offer you the option of a genetic test for the disorder and will discuss with you the benefits and risks of having the test. For a disease that can be prevented, such as type 2 diabetes (see page 894) or heart disease (see page 558), knowing that you are at risk of developing the disease may motivate you to take steps to reduce your risks.

Chromosome Abnormalities

Chromosome abnormalities result from defects in the number or structure of chromosomes, the structures that contain genes. These abnormalities can occur when an extra chromosome is present, if chromosomes unite in an abnormal way, or if a chromosome is missing or broken. The majority of chromosome abnormalities arise during the formation of the mother's egg or the father's sperm, during fertilization, or during cell division after fertilization; they are usually not inherited and, for this reason, they seldom occur twice in a family.

Chromosome abnormalities are some of the most common and severe types of genetic disorders. An irregularity in the number or structure of chromosomes can interfere in various ways with the development and functioning of a fetus. Only those fetuses with less serious chromosome abnormalities survive until birth; severely defective embryos result in miscarriage. Babies with chromosome abnormalities who do survive can have varying degrees of mental and physical impairment or may not have any noticeable effects.

Down Syndrome

Down syndrome is a common genetic disorder caused by a chromosome abnormality (see above) that usually originates during cell division when an egg or sperm is formed. Eggs and sperm normally have one chromosome from every pair. However, if a pair of chromosomes does not separate during cell division, an egg or sperm will have an extra chromosome. At fertilization, this extra chromosome is transferred to the fertilized egg, and the fetus will have the extra chromosome in every cell.

Down syndrome results from an extra copy of chromosome 21.

A person with Down syndrome has mental impairment and characteristic physical traits. The average life expectancy of people with Down syndrome is 15 to 20 years less than that of unaffected people; most do not live beyond age 55, although some people with Down syndrome live into their 70s and 80s. People with Down syndrome are at increased risk of developing Alzheimer's disease (see page 688) later in life.

Women who have children after age 35 are at

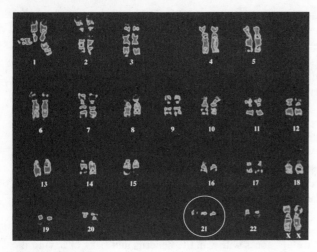

An extra chromosome
Normally, we all have 23 pairs of chromosomes—22 pairs of autosomes (which are the same in both males and females) and one pair of sex chromosomes (XX for females and XY for males). A child with Down syndrome is born with an extra copy of chromosome 21.

higher risk of having a baby with Down syndrome than are younger women. If you are planning to become pregnant and think you may be at risk of having a child with Down syndrome, genetic counseling (see page 952) can help you understand these risks.

Symptoms

The symptoms of Down syndrome can vary from mild to severe. Infants with Down syndrome have poor muscle tone, and their movements appear floppy. Their eyes slope upward at the outer corners, their ears and facial features tend to be small, and they have short necks, small hands, and short fingers. The back of their head and the bridge of their nose are flat. At birth, these physical features are often very subtle and can be recognized only by health professionals.

Many children with Down syndrome are small for their age and have delays in physical and mental development. They have some degree of mental retardation, with below-normal IQs ranging from 30 to 80. They tend to be friendly, good-natured, and affectionate, and get along well with others. Up to half of people with Down syndrome are born with congenital heart defects (see page 389). They may also have hearing loss and vision problems.

Intestinal obstruction can occur shortly after birth. Children with Down syndrome are more susceptible to developing leukemia (see page 621), pneumonia (see page 660), and ear infections (see page 417) than are other children.

Diagnosis

The physical characteristics of children with Down syndrome are usually recognized by health professionals at birth, although they are often not noticeable to parents. A doctor can confirm the diagnosis with a blood test to detect the extra copy of chromosome 21. Down syndrome can also be diagnosed in a fetus during pregnancy. If a blood test called AFP triple screen (see page 510), which is offered to all pregnant women, shows an increased risk of Down syndrome in the fetus, the doctor will recommend amniocentesis (see page 510) to confirm the diagnosis. Prenatal testing by amniocentesis or chorionic villus sampling, or CVS (see page 511), is generally also offered to pregnant women 35 and older, whose age puts them at increased risk of having a child with Down syndrome. Doctors may also recommend amniocentesis or CVS to women who have a family history of Down syndrome.

Treatment

In most respects, raising a child with Down syndrome is the same as raising any other child. Take advantage of all the special educational services offered in your community to help your child reach his or her full potential. For example, enrolling your infant in an early childhood development program can help him or her achieve his or her full developmental potential. Children with Down syndrome usually can learn most of the basic childhood skills, although more slowly than other children. Work with your doctor to learn about the special educational needs of your child and the services that are available in your community to meet these needs. Children with Down syndrome benefit from attending regular schools, where they can interact with and learn from other children and receive the same level of stimulation.

Your child's doctor will treat any physical complications of Down syndrome as they develop. Children with Down syndrome are at increased risk of instability in the neck region of their spine. For this reason, your child should have a neck X-ray at least once, especially before engaging in a new athletic activity, to make sure his or her spine is stable.

Turner Syndrome

Turner syndrome is a chromosome abnormality in which a female is born with a missing X chromosome (females normally have two X chromosomes). The missing chromosome affects the child's physical and sexual development. This abnormality occurs during fertilization, when one X chromosome (either from the mother's egg or the father's sperm) becomes lost.

Symptoms

A girl with Turner syndrome may have some minor physical variations at birth, including loose skin at the nape of the neck and a low hairline, drooping eyelids, swollen hands and feet, a broad chest, and a congenital heart defect called coarctation of the aorta (see page 393). As she gets older, she may be unusually short and will not mature sexually without treatment. She will not be able to have her own biological children because of the inability of her ovaries to make eggs. However, she may become pregnant by in vitro fertilization (see page 500) with an egg donated by another woman.

Diagnosis and Treatment

Turner syndrome can be diagnosed from chromosome analysis that detects the missing X chromosome. If your daughter has coarctation of the aorta or another type of congenital heart defect (see page 389), she may need surgery to correct it. When your child is about 3 to 5 years old, the doctor may recommend growth hormone treatment to increase her final adult height. When she is about 12 or 13, she will begin taking the female sex hormones estrogen and progesterone in pill form to stimulate her sexual development. She must continue taking these hormones until at least the age of menopause (usually at about 50).

Klinefelter Syndrome

Klinefelter syndrome is a chromosome abnormality that affects only males and makes them unable to produce sperm. Klinefelter syndrome results when a boy inherits an extra X chromosome, giving him two X chromosomes and a Y chromosome. The extra X chromosome interferes with the production of the male sex hormone testosterone.

If you have a son with Klinefelter syndrome and you are thinking about having more children, talk to a genetic counselor (see page 952) about your chances of having another child with the disorder. A genetic counselor can also help your son understand his genetic makeup and learn to cope with his infertility.

Symptoms

A boy with Klinefelter syndrome usually appears normal at birth but eventually grows tall and thin, may have a feminine build, and has a small penis and testicles. At puberty he may develop breast tissue that may continue to grow throughout adolescence. Adolescents with Klinefelter syndrome have normal erections and ejaculate normally, but their semen does not contain sperm. They usually have little facial hair. Some boys may have learning problems and a degree of mental retardation.

Diagnosis

Klinefelter syndrome can be diagnosed in a fetus using chromosome analysis. If the disorder has not been detected prenatally or during childhood, a doctor who recognizes the characteristic physical features in a child at puberty will recommend genetic testing. The diagnosis may be made in a younger child if a chromosome analysis is performed to find the cause of learning problems.

Treatment

Treatment for Klinefelter syndrome consists primarily of monitoring the boy's testosterone level each year, starting at age 12 or 13. If his testosterone level is low, he is given monthly injections of a synthetic form of testosterone to help promote normal physical and sexual development. (The testosterone supplements do not, however, give him the ability to make sperm.) As he gets older, he may need to have more frequent injections. If his breasts become enlarged enough to cause embarrassment, they can be reduced surgically.

Autosomal Recessive Disorders

M any genetic disorders are inherited as recessive disorders. A person with one copy of a recessive disease gene is called a carrier, and is usually unaffected by the gene because he or she has a healthy copy of the gene that overrides the effects of the defective gene. If two carriers of a defective recessive disease gene have children, each of their children has a 25 percent chance of inheriting both defective copies of the gene (one from each parent) and having the disease, a 50 percent chance of inheriting one defective copy and one healthy copy of the gene and being a carrier like his or her parents, and a 25 percent chance of inheriting two healthy copies of the gene and being neither affected nor a carrier. If only one of the parents has a defective copy of a recessive disease gene, all of their children will be healthy (although each has a 50 percent chance of inheriting a copy of the disease gene and being a carrier).

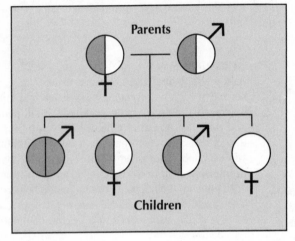

Parents

Children

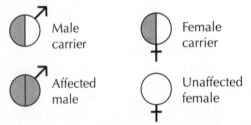

Male carrier

Female carrier

Affected male

Unaffected female

Recessive inheritance

In recessive inheritance, a person needs to inherit two copies of a defective gene to have a disorder—that is, he or she needs to inherit an abnormal recessive gene from each parent. A carrier has one healthy copy of the gene and one defective copy. Carriers are usually not affected because their healthy copy of the gene overrides the effects of the defective gene. If two carriers of a particular recessive disease gene have children, each child has a 50 percent chance of receiving a healthy copy of the gene from one parent and a defective copy from the other parent, and of being a carrier like his or her parents. Carriers can pass on a defective copy of a recessive gene through several generations without any of the children having the disorder. Each child of two carriers has a 25 percent chance of receiving two defective copies of the gene and having the disorder, and a 25 percent chance of receiving two healthy copies of the gene and being unaffected.

Cystic Fibrosis

Cystic fibrosis is an autosomal recessive genetic disorder that causes persistent lung and digestive problems. The genetic defect causes the lining of the airways leading to the lungs to produce excess mucus that clogs the lungs and makes the person vulnerable to chronic lung infections. The disorder also causes the pancreas (an organ that produces enzymes that help digest food) to fail to produce digestive enzymes.

Most people with cystic fibrosis live into their 20s or 30s; some people live into their 40s or longer. Survival can be significantly improved with early diagnosis; consistent, effective treatment to manage the fluid buildup in the lungs; and good nutrition. Researchers are experimenting with ways to replace the defective genes with healthy ones.

Symptoms

Some infants who have cystic fibrosis have symptoms right after birth, while others may not have symptoms for several months or years. In infants, an early sign may be foul-smelling stool that is pale and greasy. Because the child's body may not be absorbing sufficient nutrients from food, he or she may have inadequate weight gain or may lose weight. A child with cystic fibrosis may seem out of breath, have a constant cough that produces thick mucus, and have frequent lung problems, including pneumonia (see page 660), bronchitis (see page 655), and asthma (see page 640). He or she is more prone to dehydration, and his or her sweat may be excessively salty. Other complications include nasal polyps (see page 634) or rectal prolapse (see page 780). Damage to the pancreas can eventually lead to diabetes (see page 889).

Diagnosis

To diagnose cystic fibrosis, a doctor will order a sweat test, which can detect an abnormally large amount of chloride in the sweat, which is characteristic of cystic fibrosis. He or she may also order chest X-rays, a stool test, a mucus evaluation, and a blood test to detect the defective genes that produce cystic fibrosis. If prospective parents both carry the gene for cystic fibrosis, the disorder can be diagnosed during pregnancy with chorionic villus sampling, or CVS (see page 511), or amniocentesis (see page 510).

Treatment

To treat cystic fibrosis, a doctor prescribes pancreatic enzyme powders or pills to take with meals to aid digestion. Vitamin and nutritional supplements and a diet rich in calories and proteins help improve general health. A person may also need to take antibiotics for lung infections, decongestants to reduce congestion, and bronchodilator drugs to help open the airways. To help loosen and drain mucus from the lungs, the doctor will show you how to perform chest clapping (gentle pounding and pressing of the chest with a cupped hand) and postural drainage (see page 660).

Congenital Adrenal Hyperplasia

Congenital adrenal hyperplasia is a rare autosomal recessive genetic disorder that is present at birth. The disorder reduces the adrenal glands' production of the hormone cortisol, which has a role in many body functions. An affected person is missing or deficient in an enzyme that is necessary for the production of cortisol. Many enzymes are involved in cortisol production, and if any of them are absent or deficient, cortisol production decreases, usually triggering an overproduction of male sex hormones (androgens). The absent or deficient enzyme can also cause the adrenal glands to reduce their production of the hormone aldosterone, which is necessary for balancing the amount of salt in the blood.

Symptoms

The overproduction of male sex hormones can cause newborn girls to have ambiguous genitalia. The clitoris enlarges to the size of a small penis, and the external lips of the vagina may fuse to look like a scrotum. Newborn boys may look normal at birth but, without treatment, they display very early signs of puberty, sometimes as young as 2 or 3 years of age. Their penis enlarges, their voice deepens, pubic hair appears, and their body becomes muscular.

A deficiency in aldosterone can cause a severe loss of salt from an infant's body, resulting in dehydration, vomiting, and an abnormal heartbeat. This life-threatening condition occurs during the first few days or weeks after birth. If your child is vomiting and is severely dehydrated, take him or her to a hospital emergency department immediately for treatment. The signs of dehydration include pale, dry skin that looks loose; dry lips and tongue; a lack of tears; a decrease in urine output (fewer wet diapers in infants); and a sunken soft spot on the skull (if still present in a child). Other signs of dehydration include a rapid heartbeat, sunken eyes, lack of energy, and, in severe cases, behavior changes.

Diagnosis

Many states require a newborn screening test for the most common missing enzyme in congenital adrenal hyperplasia; for this reason, many affected children are diagnosed and treated early, before symptoms appear. In a child who has not been tested, a doctor can diagnose the disorder from the symptoms and the results of blood, urine, and hormone tests. He or she may also do an ultrasound scan of the child's adrenal glands.

Treatment

Children who have congenital adrenal hyperplasia are given drugs to replace the deficient hormones, returning their hormone levels to normal and decreasing their body's production of androgens. They continue taking the hormones for life. Baby girls with ambiguous genitalia need to have surgery to correct the appearance of their external reproductive organs. This reconstructive surgery is usually done between ages 1 and 3. With early treatment, a child will have normal sexual development and function, including normal fertility.

Tay-Sachs Disease

Tay-Sachs disease is a rare, devastating inborn error of metabolism caused by the lack of an enzyme called hexosaminidase A, which helps break down fats in brain and nerve cells. Without the enzyme, fats build up and destroy the central nervous system, causing paralysis and early death, usually by age 4 or 5. The disorder is most common among Ashkenazi Jews. Because the genetic defect is recessive, a child is affected only if both parents are carriers of the gene and the child inherits a copy of the gene from each parent.

All Ashkenazi Jewish couples are offered genetic testing to determine if they are carriers of the gene—nearly 1 in 29 Ashkenazi Jews is a carrier of the Tay-Sachs gene. If both parents are found to be carriers of the gene, they can have prenatal testing (see page 954) to determine if the fetus is affected. A genetic counselor can help them evaluate their risk of having a child with Tay-Sachs disease and can explain various family planning options they may want to consider.

Symptoms

Most newborns with Tay-Sachs disease appear normal at birth but begin losing muscle strength at about 3 to 6 months of age. They have difficulty turning over or sitting up, they stop smiling, they lose interest in their surroundings, and they have delayed mental and physical development. They may have seizures and severe constipation, and they gradually become blind, deaf, and paralyzed.

In a rare form of the disease, the symptoms don't appear until ages 2 to 5, and the disease progresses more slowly, but usually causes death by age 15.

Diagnosis

Tay-Sachs disease can be diagnosed before birth using chorionic villus sampling, or CVS (see page 511), or amniocentesis (see page 510). After birth, the disease can be diagnosed by a blood test that measures the level of the enzyme hexosaminidase A.

Treatment

Tay-Sachs disease has no treatment. Parents and caregivers focus on making the child as comfortable as possible. If you care for your child at home, your doctor and other trained health care specialists will help you learn how to meet your child's needs. If you cannot care for your child at home, an extended care center that has experience caring for children with Tay-Sachs disease is an option. You and your other children may benefit from talking with a mental health professional, who can help you cope with the emotional difficulties of having a child or sibling with a fatal disease.

Canavan Disease

Canavan disease is a rare, inherited brain disorder resulting from an enzyme deficiency that causes a normal substance called N-acetylaspartic acid to build up in the brain in much higher-than-normal amounts. The excess N-acetylaspartic acid destroys the protective covering (myelin sheath) around brain cells. As the myelin sheath degenerates, the white matter of the brain becomes spongy and develops spaces filled with fluid. N-acetylaspartic acid also builds up in the urine (where it does not pose any health risks).

The gene that transmits Canavan disease is recessive, which means that a child must inherit two copies of the defective gene (one from each parent) to have the disease. The disorder affects primarily people of Eastern European, Jewish (Ashkenazi) descent. For this reason, Ashkenazi Jewish couples are offered genetic testing before they start planning a family to determine if they are carriers of the gene. If you and your partner are carriers of the gene, a genetic counselor can help you evaluate your risk of having a child with the disorder and explain various family planning options you might want to consider.

Symptoms

Signs and symptoms of Canavan disease appear in early infancy and include a rapidly enlarging head circumference, loss of acquired motor skills, feeding problems, floppy or stiff muscle tone, and poor

Inborn Errors of Metabolism

Inborn errors of metabolism are genetic disorders that disturb the body's biochemical processes. Most inborn errors of metabolism are autosomal recessive disorders. The genetic defect can either produce a deficiency of a particular enzyme that controls a specific chemical reaction inside the body or prevent a particular enzyme from working properly. Many inborn errors of metabolism can be treated with a restricted diet, supplements of the deficient enzyme, or a medication that makes the enzyme work more effectively. The severity of these disorders can range from mild to severe. All states require testing of all newborns for some inborn errors of metabolism, including phenylketonuria, or PKU (see next page), shortly after birth. Additional newborn screening tests for more than 40 different inborn errors of metabolism, which are available through commercial laboratories, are gradually being added to state programs.

head control. Children with the disorder cannot crawl, walk, sit up, or speak. Over time, they may become mentally retarded, have seizures, and become blind. The symptoms vary from child to child and may progress in different ways, but most affected children do not live beyond age 10.

Diagnosis and Treatment

To diagnose Canavan disease in a child, doctors use a urine test that measures the amount of *N*-acetylaspartic acid in the child's urine. Before birth, prenatal diagnostic tests such as chorionic

---

WARNING!

In an Emergency: Inborn Errors of Metabolism

A person who has an inborn error of metabolism can become seriously ill very quickly. In extreme cases, he or she can lapse into a coma and die. If your child has an inborn error of metabolism and is in a crisis, act quickly by doing the following:

- Don't give your child anything to eat or drink.
- Call the doctor and take your child to a hospital emergency department immediately.
- Tell emergency department personnel what disease your child has and describe his or her symptoms.
- Tell emergency department personnel what your child ate or drank before becoming ill, what type of medication he or she takes regularly, and the medicine's dosage.

---

villus sampling, or CVS (see page 511), or amniocentesis (see page 510) can determine if the fetus has Canavan disease. At-risk people who are planning a family can have a blood test to detect the defective gene.

There is no cure or effective treatment for Canavan disease. Care focuses on treating the symptoms as they develop and making the child as fully functioning and comfortable as possible.

Hereditary Hemochromatosis

Hereditary hemochromatosis (also known as iron overload) is an inborn error of metabolism that causes the body to absorb and store too much iron. Because hemochromatosis is an autosomal recessive disorder, a person needs to inherit a copy of the defective gene from both parents to have the disease. Hemochromatosis is the most common genetic disorder in the United States, affecting mostly whites of northern European descent (especially Irish and German), although people in other ethnic groups can also be affected. One in eight people has one copy of the defective gene, and nearly 1 in 200 has two copies of the defective gene and has the disease, although many people with the disease never develop an overload of iron. Males are five times more likely than females to develop symptoms of hemochromatosis and tend to develop problems from the excess iron at a younger age, possibly because women naturally lose iron during menstruation, pregnancy, and breastfeeding.

Iron is an essential nutrient that the intestines absorb from food to make up part of hemoglobin, the pigment in red blood cells that transports oxygen from the lungs to the rest of the body. In people with hemochromatosis, the intestines absorb twice as much iron as normal. When the body cannot eliminate excess iron, it is stored in tissues, particularly in the liver, heart, and pancreas. Over time, a buildup of iron can cause organ damage and lead to serious problems such as arthritis, liver disease, heart abnormalities, erection problems, early menopause, abnormal pigmentation of the skin (making it look gray or bronze), diabetes, or thyroid deficiency. If the disease is treated early, before organ damage occurs, a person can lead a healthy life.

Because the genetic defect that causes hemochromatosis is so common and the disorder is easy to treat successfully when diagnosed at an early stage, many doctors recommend that all people be screened for the disorder. Testing is definitely recommended for people who have a sibling, parent, child, or other close relative with hemochromatosis.

Symptoms

Although a person has the genes for hemochromatosis from birth, he or she rarely has noticeable symptoms until adulthood, usually between ages 30 and 60. In men, symptoms of hemochromatosis tend to develop between ages 30 and 50; in women, symptoms usually appear after age 50. The disorder often goes undiagnosed because the symptoms can be vague and similar to those of many common disorders, such as osteoarthritis (see page 996). The most common initial symptoms are joint pain, fatigue, lack of energy, abdominal pain, loss of sex drive, and heart problems. Ask your doctor about being tested for hemochromatosis if you have any of these symptoms. Many people have no symptoms when the disease is diagnosed.

Diagnosis

Doctors diagnose hemochromatosis from a person's health history, a physical examination, and blood tests to measure the amount of iron stored in the body. If a blood test shows a higher-than-normal level of iron, the doctor will probably confirm the diagnosis with a genetic test to detect the disease-causing gene mutation. To evaluate the buildup of iron in the liver and to determine if the liver is damaged, he or she may recommend a liver function test and, if the results are abnormal, a liver biopsy (microscopic analysis of a sample of tissue taken from the liver).

Treatment

Hemochromatosis is usually treated by a doctor who specializes in liver disorders (a hepatologist), digestive disorders (a gastroenterologist), or blood disorders (a hematologist). You may need to see a number of specialists, depending on the organ systems that are affected.

Treatment, which is simple, safe, and inexpensive, involves removing blood to reduce the level of iron. Depending on the degree of your iron overload, you will probably have a pint of blood taken once or twice a week for several months to a year or more. After every four blood donations (called phlebotomies), you will have a blood test to measure the level of iron in your blood. Once your iron level is in the low-to-normal range, you must try to maintain the level by giving a pint of blood every 1 to 4 months throughout your life. An annual blood test can help determine how frequently you need to give blood.

Your doctor will recommend that you take daily vitamin supplements that do not contain iron and limit your consumption of vitamin C to 500 milligrams daily (because vitamin C increases the body's absorption of iron). You should also limit your intake of alcohol to avoid liver damage.

Phenylketonuria

Phenylketonuria (PKU) is an inborn error of metabolism, a genetic disorder in which the body cannot process the amino acid phenylalanine. Amino acids are the building blocks of proteins, which the body needs to develop and function. Normally, excess amounts of the amino acids in foods we eat are broken down or excreted. However, in people with PKU, phenylalanine is not processed normally and it builds up in the blood, causing brain damage. Phenylalanine is present in protein-containing foods such as milk products, eggs, meat, and fish.

Symptoms

Newborns with PKU may appear normal for the first several weeks or months of life. However, if the disease is not detected and treated, they gradually lose interest in their surroundings and eventually begin to show signs of mental impairment. By the time they are 1 year old, they may have delayed mental development. Untreated children may have jerky arm or leg movements, be restless and destructive, and may give off a musty odor from the accumulation of phenylalanine in their body. Some children with PKU have seizures (see page 686). Children with PKU generally have lighter hair, skin, and eye color than other members of their family.

Diagnosis

All states require testing of newborns for PKU shortly after birth (see page 954). A few drops of blood are taken from a needle prick in the baby's heel, and the blood is analyzed in a laboratory for phenylalanine. If the level of phenylalanine is higher than normal, the doctor will recommend more sensitive tests to confirm the diagnosis.

Treatment

If your child is found to have PKU, the doctor will prescribe a diet that severely restricts foods containing phenylalanine. (Some phenylalanine must be in the diet because a certain amount of the amino acid is essential.) Children with PKU can be breast-fed or given regular formula in limited amounts supplemented with a special phenylalanine-free formula. After a baby begins to eat specially selected solid foods, he or she must continue to consume the special formula as his or her major source of protein. People with PKU need to see their doctor regularly for tests to measure the level of phenylalanine in their blood and to make adjustments in their diet when necessary. They will need to follow the restricted diet throughout life, but will otherwise be able to lead a normal life.

If you are a woman who has PKU and you are thinking about becoming pregnant, talk to a genetic counselor (see page 952). You need to be especially conscientious about following the special diet before you become pregnant and during your pregnancy because a high level of phenylalanine in your blood could cause brain damage in the fetus.

Gaucher Disease

Gaucher disease is a rare, potentially fatal inborn error of metabolism characterized by reduced levels of a protein necessary for breaking down a particular fat in the body. This fat then accumulates in cells (called Gaucher cells), displacing healthy, normal cells in bone marrow and causing enlargement of the liver and spleen, organ dysfunction, and bone deterioration.

Gaucher disease has three different forms—type 1, type 2, and type 3—all of which follow an autosomal recessive pattern of inheritance (see page 958). The most common form, type 1, can develop at any age and does not involve the central nervous system. Type 1 can affect people of all ethnic groups, but it is the most common genetic disease among Ashkenazi Jews. Types 2 and 3 involve the central nervous system. Type 2, which occurs during infancy, is the most severe, usually causing death by age 2. Type 3 generally progresses slowly, with increasing damage to the nervous system that leads to a decline in mental and physical functioning. Usually, only one form of the disease will affect a particular family.

Symptoms

The symptoms of all three forms of Gaucher disease can vary widely from one person to another. Type 1 can cause bone problems including pain, reduced bone density and strength, fractures, and bone cell death. The disease can also affect the blood, causing anemia (see page 610), which can lead to general weakness and failure to thrive, and blood-clotting problems, which can cause easy bruising and bleeding. A person with this form of the disease also may have an enlarged liver, which can lead to liver dysfunction, and an enlarged spleen. Children with type 1 may have growth retardation, and adolescents may have delayed puberty. Fatigue and chronic pain can compromise the quality of life of people with Gaucher disease.

Type 2, which occurs in infants, causes a swollen abdomen from spleen and liver enlargement, mild anemia, inability to swallow, and a characteristic bending backward of the head. These children frequently have seizures, and most die by age 2.

Type 3 involves the central nervous system. People with type 3 may have poor coordination, decreased sensation and muscle function, abnormal eye movement, and behavior changes. Their mental function deteriorates gradually, usually over many years.

Diagnosis

Doctors can diagnose Gaucher disease before birth using amniocentesis (see page 510) or chorionic villus sampling, or CVS (see page 511). Prenatal testing is usually done only if a couple has previously had an affected child and therefore has a 25 percent chance of having another child with Gaucher disease. Before having children, some Jewish couples choose to be tested for the genetic mutation that most often causes Gaucher disease. If both partners are found to carry the gene, they may choose to have prenatal testing during a pregnancy to determine if the fetus has two copies of the Gaucher gene (one from each of them) and therefore will have the disease.

In a person who has symptoms of Gaucher disease, a doctor may take a sample of bone marrow (tissue inside bones that manufactures all the different types of blood cells). He or she withdraws the fluid with a needle and has it analyzed under a microscope for the presence of Gaucher cells, which are large cells filled with fat. The doctor may also perform a blood test to measure the deficient level of the protein.

Treatment

To treat Gaucher disease, doctors replace the missing protein with a synthetic one, which is given intravenously (through a vein). This treatment is very effective in reversing the enlargement of the liver and spleen, preventing bone disease, and improving the quality of life of people with type 1 disease. Treatment may not be as effective for people who have type 2 or type 3 Gaucher disease. For people with any form of Gaucher disease, doctors recommend regular examinations, blood tests, and imaging procedures to monitor the progression of the disease and the effectiveness of the treatment.

Galactosemia

Galactosemia is an inborn error of metabolism that results from the partial or complete lack of an enzyme (called galactose 1-phosphate uridyltransferase, or GALT) that converts the sugar galactose into glucose (which the body uses for energy). Normally, when a person eats a food containing the sugar lactose (such as dairy products), the body breaks down the lactose into galactose and glucose. If galactose cannot be converted into glucose, it accumulates in the blood and can damage organs. Untreated, galactosemia can cause an enlarged liver, kidney failure (see page 816), cataracts (see page 1041), and brain damage, and is fatal.

The most severe, classic form of galactosemia is a recessive genetic disorder, which results when a child inherits two copies of the defective gene, one from each parent. A less severe form of galactosemia, called Duarte galactosemia, results when a child inherits a copy of the gene for the classic form from one parent and a copy of the Duarte gene from the other parent. In Duarte galactosemia, the enzyme is partly active and able to convert some galactose into glucose.

If you have a child with galactosemia, seek genetic counseling (see page 952) to learn your chances of having another child with the disorder.

Symptoms

The symptoms of untreated galactosemia begin to appear shortly after birth when a newborn drinks breast milk or formula. Early symptoms include yellowing of the skin and the whites of the eyes (jaundice; see page 785) and vomiting. The baby may be irritable, have diarrhea, fail to gain weight, and develop severe infections. Without treatment, a child with galactosemia can develop cataracts or mental retardation.

Diagnosis

Both forms of galactosemia can be diagnosed during newborn screening tests (see page 954). Galactosemia can also be diagnosed during pregnancy with chorionic villus sampling, or CVS (see page 511), or amniocentesis (see page 510) if both parents are carriers of the gene. If your child has not been tested and he or she has symptoms of galactosemia, your doctor will order blood and urine tests to diagnose the disorder.

Treatment

The treatment of galactosemia involves excluding all foods from the diet that contain lactose or galactose—including breast milk, dairy products, and most legumes. Even when a child is started on a restrictive diet at birth, the disorder can cause long-term complications, including speech and language problems, delays in developing fine and gross motor skills, and learning disabilities. For unknown reasons, girls with galactosemia usually have premature ovarian failure that results in infertility.

Homocystinuria

Homocystinuria is an autosomal recessive genetic disorder, an inborn error of metabolism that usually results from a deficiency of an enzyme called cystathionine beta synthase. This enzyme enables the body to properly digest an amino acid in food called methionine. Amino acids are the building blocks of proteins and are essential for healthy growth and development. The inability to properly digest methionine leads to buildup of a protein called homocysteine in the blood, which can interfere with a baby's growth and development.

Many states now test all newborns for homocystinuria. If not diagnosed and treated early in life, more serious symptoms, such as eye abnormalities and mental retardation, can develop by age 3. If you or your partner has a family history of homocystinuria and you are thinking about having children, talk to a genetic counselor about your risk of passing the disorder on to children. Your children are at risk of inheriting the disorder only if both of you carry a copy of the gene for homocystinuria. The disorder can be diagnosed during pregnancy with chorionic villus sampling, or CVS (see page 511), or amniocentesis (see page 510).

Symptoms

Newborns with homocystinuria appear normal, but they may fail to grow or gain weight at the normal rate and they may not achieve the expected developmental milestones (see page 377). By about age 3, more noticeable symptoms develop, including partial dislocation of the lens of the eye and severe nearsightedness. Many children experience progressive mental retardation and some may have seizures. They tend to be thin and unusually tall, with long legs and arms and long, thin fingers and toes. They may have progressive curving of the spine (scoliosis; see page 433), chest abnormalities (such as a breastbone that protrudes or caves in), and loss of bone density (osteoporosis; see page 989) throughout the body. Their blood tends to clot easily, which can be life-threatening if a blood clot blocks a blood vessel.

Diagnosis

Homocystinuria can be diagnosed from a physical examination, a health history, and various imaging and laboratory tests. A doctor may notice during a physical examination that a child has dislocation of the lens of the eye and nearsightedness. In this case, he or she will refer the child to an ophthalmologist for a more thorough eye examination. A child with homocystinuria may also have a history of blood clots. To confirm the diagnosis, a doctor

may recommend X-rays of the bones to detect osteoporosis, a blood test to determine if the levels of methionine and homocysteine are high, a urine test to detect homocysteine, or a liver biopsy or skin biopsy to look for a deficiency of the enzyme cystathionine beta synthase.

Treatment

There is no cure for homocystinuria, but many people can control the disorder with a restricted diet. Infants are given a formula that is low in methionine. A low-protein diet must be followed throughout life. High doses of vitamin B6 along with a folic acid supplement (400 micrograms daily) can help lower the level of homocysteine in the blood in some people. For other people, supplements of a nutrient called betaine is used to reduce the level of homocysteine.

Alpha₁-Antitrypsin Deficiency

Alpha$_1$-antitrypsin deficiency is a recessive genetic disorder that causes the liver to make defective or inadequate amounts of the protein alpha$_1$-antitrypsin. Alpha$_1$-antitrypsin normally protects the lungs against an enzyme (neutrophil elastase) released by white blood cells when fighting infections. When the lungs do not have enough alpha$_1$-antitrypsin, they become damaged by the enzyme and lose their ability to properly expand and contract. Smoking worsens the lung damage by irritating lung tissue, prompting the release of more of the harmful enzyme.

If alpha$_1$-antitrypsin is defective, the liver cannot release it into the bloodstream and it stays in the liver, damaging it over time and eventually causing cirrhosis (see page 790). Not all people with alpha$_1$-antitrypsin deficiency have liver problems, but 12 to 15 percent of affected adults and a small percentage of young children with the disorder develop cirrhosis. Liver disease can occur at the same time as lung disease.

There are several different forms of alpha$_1$-antitrypsin deficiency that have varying degrees of severity, depending on the specific gene a person inherits. The condition is rare, affecting fewer than 100,000 people in the United States. However, an estimated 95 percent of affected people remain undiagnosed. To have alpha$_1$-antitrypsin deficiency, a person must inherit one abnormal copy of the gene for the disorder from each parent. Inheriting only one defective gene makes a person an unaffected carrier—that is, he or she does not have the disorder but can pass the gene on to a child.

Symptoms

The primary symptom of alpha$_1$-antitrypsin deficiency is shortness of breath during daily activities. Eventually, the person develops chronic emphysema (see page 656) by the third or fourth decade of life (earlier if he or she smokes). People who develop cirrhosis of the liver may have nausea, flatulence, weight loss, weakness, and abdominal pain.

Diagnosis

Alpha$_1$-antitrypsin deficiency can be difficult to diagnose because the symptoms can mimic those of asthma (see page 640) or chronic bronchitis (see page 655), but a diagnosis of emphysema at an early age raises a red flag. A simple blood test can measure levels of alpha$_1$-antitrypsin. If blood levels fall below 45 percent of normal, the doctor will order additional blood tests to identify the defective gene. The doctor will also order other tests of the lungs, including a pulmonary function test that measures how well the airways are working, a blood gas analysis that gauges the amount of oxygen in the blood, a chest X-ray, and exercise testing. An electrocardiogram (see page 559), which measures the electrical activity of the heart, may also be performed to confirm the diagnosis and determine the level of breathing incapacity.

Doctors use blood and urine tests to test liver function in people suspected of having alpha$_1$-antitrypsin deficiency. If a person has cirrhosis, the doctor may be able to feel abnormalities in the liver during a physical examination. A CT scan (see page 112), ultrasound scan (see page 111), and a radioisotope scan (see page 114) of the liver and spleen can also detect liver damage.

Treatment

Treatment of alpha$_1$-antitrypsin deficiency focuses first on protecting the lungs from damage. The single most important step to take to preserve lung function is to avoid smoking. People who have alpha$_1$-antitrypsin deficiency should get yearly immunizations for influenza (see page 649) and pneumonia (see page 660) and see their doctor at the first sign of a cold or other respiratory problem (when white blood cells travel to the lungs to fight infection). Drinking alcohol can accelerate the liver damage. To counteract the weight loss caused by the liver damage, affected people need to consume a sufficient amount of calories.

To reduce shortness of breath, doctors may prescribe medication such as bronchodilators (to expand the airways) and inhaled corticosteroids (to fight inflammation). Weekly intravenous infusions of alpha$_1$-antitrypsin (derived from pooled human blood) can be given intravenously (through a vein). Some people with the disorder may need supplemental oxygen.

Autosomal Dominant Disorders

A dominant gene, whether it's a gene for eye color or a disease, will determine the characteristic or disorder no matter what type of corresponding gene is on the matching chromosome. For example, the gene for brown eyes is dominant. If a child inherits a gene for brown eyes from one parent and a gene for blue eyes from the other parent, the child will have brown eyes. If both parents have brown eyes, each could also have a gene for blue eyes and, if each parent transmits the blue-eye gene to a child, the child will have blue eyes. In the same way, a person who receives a defective copy of a dominant disease gene, such as the gene for Huntington disease (see page 969), will have the disease. If one parent has a dominant gene for a disorder, each of his or her children has a 50 percent chance of inheriting the gene and also having the disease.

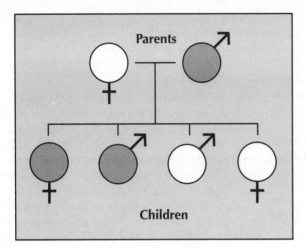

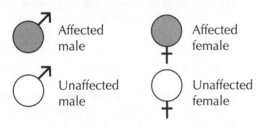

Dominant inheritance

In dominant genetic traits and disorders, a person needs only one copy of the dominant gene to have the trait or disorder. A person who has a dominant trait such as brown eyes or a dominant genetic disorder such as Marfan syndrome has a one-in-two (50 percent) chance of passing the gene to each child. He or she also has a 50 percent chance of passing the healthy copy of the gene to each child, who will be unaffected. Most dominant traits and disorders affect males and females with equal frequency. A child can be born with a dominant disorder either by inheriting the gene from a parent who is also affected or as a result of a new gene change (mutation) that occurred in a parent's egg or sperm cell before conception.

Marfan Syndrome

Marfan syndrome is a rare inherited genetic disorder that affects connective tissue throughout the body, including in the bones, lungs, eyes, heart, and blood vessels. People with Marfan syndrome do not produce normal amounts of an essential component of connective tissue called fibrillin, which binds cells together and strengthens tissues. The disorder affects people of both sexes and of all racial and ethnic groups. With appropriate treatment and regular monitoring by a doctor, most people with Marfan syndrome live into their 70s and longer.

If you or another member of your family has Marfan syndrome, genetic counseling (see page 952) can help you determine your risk of passing the disease on to a child.

Symptoms

The symptoms of Marfan syndrome can vary greatly from one person to another. In mild cases, the symptoms may not be noticeable until age 60 or later. In rare, severe cases, serious problems may be evident at birth. People with Marfan syndrome usually begin to develop characteristics of the disorder at about age 10. The lack of fibrillin in the body causes the tissues to stretch, making the person grow tall and thin and making the joints loose and able to move beyond their normal range and dislocate easily. The bones in the arms, legs, and fingers become longer than normal and look out of proportion to the rest of the body. The breastbone may stick out or look caved in, and the spine may be curved from scoliosis (see page 433). The face may look long and narrow, the teeth may be crowded together, and the roof of the mouth may be highly arched.

Most people with Marfan syndrome have abnormal heart valves that may produce a murmur (unusual heart sound) or irregular heartbeat. The aorta (the major blood vessel in the body), which contains an abundance of fibrillin, can weaken. Without treatment, this weakness can cause the aorta to stretch and balloon out to form an aneurysm (see page 599) or tear, causing bleeding into the chest or abdomen and sudden death. Most people with Marfan syndrome are nearsighted, and about half have a dislocation of the lens of the eye.

Detachment of the retina (the light-sensitive lining at the back of the eye) also can occur. The syndrome can make a person prone to sudden lung collapse.

Diagnosis

Marfan syndrome is difficult to diagnose because there are no specific laboratory tests for the condition and because the symptoms can vary greatly among people who have the disorder. A doctor usually diagnoses Marfan syndrome by a complete physical examination. If a doctor suspects that a person has Marfan syndrome, he or she may order an echocardiogram (see page 561) and an eye exam to look for the characteristic abnormalities of the disorder.

Treatment

A doctor may prescribe heart medications such as beta blockers (see page 562) to reduce the rate of stretching of the aorta and to decrease the risk of complications. Heart surgery may be necessary if an aneurysm develops or to repair or replace defective heart valves. Some spine deformities can be corrected with a brace or with surgery.

Neurofibromatosis

Neurofibromatosis is a genetic disorder that causes tumors (abnormal masses) to grow along the nerves, including the nerves in the brain. Tumors can also appear under the skin and in the bones. The disorder is the result of a single defective gene that has been inherited from a parent or that became abnormal through a spontaneous mutation (change) in a gene. Most of the tumors produced by the disease, which can grow throughout the body, are not cancerous. However, in rare cases, a tumor in the brain or spinal cord becomes cancerous.

Neurofibromatosis has two forms—type 1 and type 2. Neurofibromatosis type 1 (NF1) is one of the most common genetic disorders, affecting 1 in 4,000 people in the United States. Fifty to 70 percent of cases of NF1 are inherited from a parent; the remaining 30 to 50 percent result from a spontaneous genetic mutation in a parent's egg or sperm. Neurofibromatosis type 2 (NF2) is much rarer than NF1 and causes tumors to grow around the auditory (hearing) nerves on both sides of the brain and elsewhere in the brain. These tumors can cause brain damage and can be life-threatening.

If you have neurofibromatosis, see a genetic counselor (see page 952) to learn your risk of passing the disorder on to a child.

Symptoms

Most people with NF1 have only mild symptoms and live normal lives, but others have severe symptoms. The most common sign of NF1 is the appearance of flat, light-brown spots on the skin called café au lait (French for "coffee with milk") spots, which can appear at birth or in early infancy. Children with NF1 usually have six or more of these spots on their body, each spot measuring more than $1/5$ inch. By puberty, the spots begin to grow to about $1/2$ inch in diameter. Tumors begin to grow around nerves throughout the body during adolescence and appear as small lumps or bumps under the skin.

A person with NF1 may also have freckles in his or her armpits and groin area, abnormal tissue in the iris (the colored part of the eye), poor vision resulting from the growth of tumors on the nerves behind the eyes, and deformed bones in the spine or legs. Some people with NF1 also have learning disabilities (see page 415) or develop a seizure disorder (see page 686).

NF2 causes progressive hearing loss, beginning during adolescence, as tumors grow around the nerves involved with hearing. A person with NF2 also may have ringing in the ears (tinnitus; see page 1020), problems with balance, skin growths, and vision problems caused by thickening of the lens of the eye. Tumors in the head can cause headaches, numbness, and pain in the face. In rare, severe cases, brain tumors caused by NF2 can be fatal.

Diagnosis

If a doctor knows that one of a child's parents or another family member has neurofibromatosis, he or she can sometimes test for the disorder in the fetus before birth (prenatal testing; see page 954). To diagnose the disorder in a child who develops the symptoms of either type of neurofibromatosis after birth, a doctor may order X-rays, an eye examination, vision and hearing tests, or a CT scan (see page 112) or MRI (see page 113) of the brain. The results of these tests and a physical examination, along with the child's family health history, can confirm or rule out a diagnosis of neurofibromatosis.

Treatment

If your child has been diagnosed with neurofibromatosis, he or she should have regular checkups and examinations to monitor the progression of the disorder and treat any new symptoms. For disfiguring or painful tumors under the skin, a doctor may recommend removing them surgically, although the tumors may grow back. Tumors that affect hearing or vision may require treatment to preserve these senses.

Bone deformities such as scoliosis (see page 433) can be treated with surgery, a brace, or both. In the rare cases in which the brain or spinal cord tumors become cancerous, doctors recommend surgery along with radiation therapy (see page 23) and chemotherapy (see page 23).

Huntington Disease

Huntington disease is a devastating, degenerative brain disorder caused by a dominant genetic defect that destroys cells in a part of the brain called the basal ganglia, which slowly destroys a person's ability to think, walk, and talk. The onset of the degenerative process usually begins between ages 30 and 50, but it occasionally develops in young children and in the elderly.

Huntington disease affects people of both sexes and all races throughout the world. Because symptoms usually do not appear until middle age, many people are not aware they have the gene until after they have children (who have a 50 percent chance of also having the gene). A test is available that can identify people who have the Huntington gene. If the disease has occurred in a member of your family, including in cousins, aunts, or uncles, and you are considering having the test or are unsure what to do, a genetic counselor (see page 952) can help you evaluate your risk of having the gene and can explain the risks and benefits of testing.

Symptoms

The symptoms of Huntington disease vary widely from person to person, even in the same family. Early symptoms can include emotional problems such as depression, mood swings, irritability, and anxiety. Behavioral changes can include aggressive outbursts, impulsiveness, demanding behavior, and withdrawal from friends and family. Sexual desire may be absent or exaggerated. As the disease progresses, a person becomes increasingly less able

to concentrate and his or her short-term memory declines. Physical symptoms begin as nervous twitching, fidgeting, or restlessness. The person's handwriting may change, and he or she may be less able to perform skills that require coordination and concentration, such as driving. Over time, the person will develop more noticeable involuntary movements of his or her head, trunk, and limbs. The person slowly loses the ability to walk, speak, and swallow. Eventually, he or she can no longer function independently and dies from complications such as choking, infection, or heart failure.

Diagnosis

To diagnose Huntington disease, doctors take a detailed family health history and perform comprehensive physical, neurological, and psychological examinations. A doctor also may recommend an MRI (see page 113) or CT scan (see page 112) of the brain. A genetic test to detect the Huntington gene may be done to help confirm or rule out the disease.

Treatment

Huntington disease has no cure. Available treatments do not stop the progression of the disease, but medication can help treat symptoms such as depression and anxiety and help reduce involuntary movements. Doctors try to minimize the use of drugs because they can have side effects, and drugs that are effective at one stage of the disease may not be effective at another.

If you have Huntington disease, work with a neurologist who is familiar with the disease and a team of health care professionals such as occupational therapists and speech therapists, who can help you maintain your quality of life. Because people with Huntington disease burn more calories than normal and can have difficulty chewing and swallowing, they need to work with a nutritionist to avoid losing too much weight. Maintaining weight and muscle can help reduce involuntary movements and other symptoms. Support groups are valuable sources of emotional support and shared knowledge for people with Huntington disease and their families.

Ehlers-Danlos Syndrome

Ehlers-Danlos syndrome is a group of inherited disorders that result from genetic defects that affect connective tissue, the tissue that gives support and strength to other tissues. The six major types of Ehlers-Danlos syndrome are distinct disorders with distinctive symptoms, but most are characterized by problems with the skin and joints. Although a person is born with the Ehlers-Danlos gene, the disorder may not become apparent until later in life or after exposure to an environmental stress such as surgery or an injury. If you or a family member has the disorder, talk to a genetic counselor (see page 952) about the risk of passing the defective gene on to a child.

Symptoms

Because Ehlers-Danlos syndrome can result from mutations in several different genes, the symptoms vary widely from one form of the disorder to another. Generally, people with Ehlers-Danlos syndrome have some degree of joint looseness, abnormal scar formation, slow healing of wounds, and fragile, small blood vessels (which can cause easy bruising). The looseness in the joints may make them prone to dislocation and chronic pain. The skin can be soft and velvety and stretch more than usual (but return to normal after being pulled). Some forms of Ehlers-Danlos syndrome can cause problems with the spine, such as curving, or with the eyes, such as an abnormally shaped cornea (the clear, protective covering at the front of the eye). The uterus, intestines, and large blood vessels may be weak and susceptible to rupture.

Diagnosis

Doctors diagnose Ehlers-Danlos syndrome from a physical examination, a person's health history, and his or her family health history. Some forms of Ehlers-Danlos syndrome are diagnosed from laboratory analysis of a sample of skin (biopsy) to determine the chemical makeup of the connective tissue. For some forms of Ehlers-Danlos syndrome, genetic testing (see page 953) is available to confirm the diagnosis.

Treatment

The treatment of Ehlers-Danlos syndrome depends on the symptoms. If you have loose joints, your doctor may recommend avoiding activities that can make your joints lock or overextend or increase the wear and tear on them, increasing your risk of developing osteoarthritis (see page 996) at a younger age than usual. Activities you might be asked to avoid include gymnastics, ballet, figure skating, long-distance running, and competitive sports involving running. Your doctor may recommend a brace to stabilize your joints.

In some people, surgery is necessary to repair damaged joints. Your doctor may refer you to a physical or occupational therapist, who can help you strengthen your muscles and teach you how to use and protect your joints properly. To reduce bruising and improve wound healing, some doctors recommend vitamin C supplements for people with Ehlers-Danlos syndrome (however, don't take vitamin C without talking to your doctor first).

If your child has Ehlers-Danlos syndrome, he or she needs to avoid contact sports and other physically stressful activities that could result in injuries and increase the risk of chronic pain later in life. Also, make sure your child knows not to show off the unusual positions he or she can put his or her joints into, because doing so can damage the joints. Make sure that other family members and your child's friends and teachers have knowledge about Ehlers-Danlos syndrome that will enable them to help your child if necessary.

X-Linked Disorders

X-linked disorders, also called sex-linked disorders, are genetic disorders that are transmitted by a defective gene on an X chromosome. The X and Y chromosomes determine sex. Females have two X chromosomes; males have one X chromosome and one Y chromosome. All egg cells contain an X chromosome. If a sperm that fertilizes an egg carries an X chromosome, the resulting embryo will have two X chromosomes and will be female. If a sperm carries a Y chromosome, the embryo will have an X and a Y chromosome and will be male.

Most X-linked traits and disorders are recessive and are passed from mothers to sons. Women are rarely affected by X-linked disorders because their other X chromosome has a healthy copy of the gene, which overrides the effects of the disease gene. However, females can be carriers of an X-linked disorder, and they have a 50 percent chance of transmitting the X chromosome with the disease gene to a son, who will have the disease. Boys who receive an X-linked gene from their mother will be affected because they have only one X chromosome (and a Y chromosome from their father).

The daughters of female carriers of X-linked disease genes also have a 50 percent chance of

inheriting their mother's X-linked disease gene; they, however, will be unaffected carriers. An X-linked recessive disease gene can be transmitted through many generations of a family by healthy carrier mothers before it becomes apparent when, for the first time, a boy in the family is born with the disease.

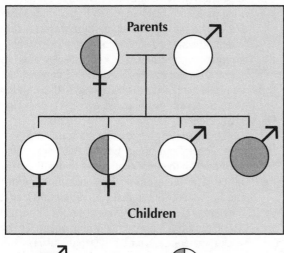

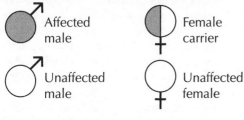

X-linked inheritance
Disorders that are caused by defective genes on the X sex chromosome generally are transmitted from mothers to sons, who receive one X chromosome (only from their mother). A woman who has the defective gene on the X chromosome is usually unaffected. She has a 50 percent chance of passing the gene on to a son, who will be affected, and a 50 percent chance of passing the gene on to a daughter, who will be an unaffected carrier like her mother.

Fragile X Syndrome

Fragile X syndrome is caused by a defective gene on the X sex chromosome that narrows the affected part of the chromosome and makes it look fragile. Fragile X syndrome is the most common inherited form of mental retardation. Males are more likely to have the disorder and to have more severe symptoms than females. Because females can have one defective X chromosome and one healthy X chromosome, they can be carriers of fragile X and either have no symptoms or have a mild form of the disease. They have a 50 percent chance of transmitting their defective X chromosome to a son, who will be affected. If you have a family history of

fragile X syndrome or if you have a child with fragile X syndrome, you can benefit from talking to a genetic counselor (see page 952), who can evaluate your risk of transmitting the disorder to a future child.

Symptoms

Physical features that are characteristic of fragile X syndrome may be evident at birth, but the first noticeable sign is usually developmental delay that is apparent by age 2 or 3. Most boys have some degree of mental impairment, ranging from below-average intelligence to severe mental retardation. The severity of the mental impairment may become more apparent with age. About 20 percent of boys have symptoms similar to those of autism (see page 731), including difficulty interacting socially, avoiding eye contact, hand-biting, and hand-flapping. About 30 percent of girls who carry the gene have some degree of mental retardation.

The physical features of fragile X—which are often unnoticeable and are not a health problem—can include large ears, a long face, crossed or wandering eyes, a prominent jaw and forehead, enlarged testicles, and loose joints. The features are usually more subtle in girls.

Diagnosis

If your child is not developing at the normal rate or if your doctor knows that you or your partner has a family history of fragile X syndrome, he or she will order a blood test to look for the defective gene. For prospective parents who have a family history of fragile X syndrome, a diagnosis of fragile X in the fetus can be made during pregnancy with chorionic villus sampling, or CVS (see page 511), or amniocentesis (see page 510).

Treatment

Fragile X syndrome has no specific treatment. Your doctor may prescribe medication for your child to treat behavior problems, which are common in boys with fragile X. Make sure that your child has access to special education services and interventions available in your community to help him or her reach his or her full potential.

Muscular Dystrophy

Muscular dystrophy is a group of inherited genetic disorders that cause muscle weakness that worsens over time. A person's muscles waste away as muscle cells die and are replaced by fat and connective tissue. Although there are nine different types of muscular dystrophy, the two most common are Duchenne muscular dystrophy and Becker muscular dystrophy. They are the same disease, except that Duchenne muscular dystrophy develops at an earlier age and progresses more rapidly. Some of the other forms of muscular dystrophy may not produce symptoms until adulthood. Because the disorder is carried on the X chromosome, boys are more likely to be affected than girls.

Symptoms

The symptoms of muscular dystrophy usually are not apparent until about age 3, although infants may have slow development and muscle weakness. The child begins to lose strength in his or her legs and hips from the gradual wasting away of muscle and may walk with feet wide apart to maintain balance. He or she may have trouble climbing stairs. Frequent falls and difficulty getting up or standing up straight are common. The calf muscles often look larger than normal because fat and connective tissue have replaced muscle. By age 10, a child may need braces for walking and, by age 12, may require a wheelchair.

The disease progresses to the muscles in the arms, neck, and upper half of the body, causing the bones in the chest and spine to develop abnormally. The bone deformities combined with the muscle weakness can make breathing difficult and can interfere with the functioning of the heart. Some children have mental impairment. Children with Duchenne muscular dystrophy usually die of pneumonia (see page 660) or other lung problems by late adolescence. Becker muscular dystrophy produces similar symptoms but they don't appear until about age 7 and progress slowly. However, Becker muscular dystrophy is usually fatal by age 40.

If you have a child with muscular dystrophy, you and other members of your family would benefit from genetic counseling (see page 952) to learn your risks of transmitting the gene to future children.

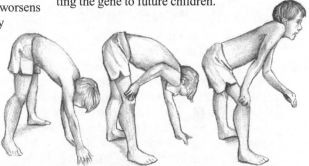

Leg muscle weakness in muscular dystrophy
Because muscular dystrophy causes muscle weakness in the legs, a child with muscular dystrophy uses his or her arms and hands to get up to a standing position from sitting on the floor.

Diagnosis

If a child has symptoms of muscular dystrophy, the doctor will order a blood test that can detect levels of specific proteins in the blood. He or she may also order a test called electromyography, which evaluates the electrical activity in muscles. To confirm the diagnosis, the doctor may recommend a biopsy (in which a sample of the child's muscle tissue is sent to a laboratory for examination) or genetic testing of a sample of the child's blood.

Treatment

Muscular dystrophy has no specific treatment. Doctors and caregivers usually focus on relieving the symptoms, helping the child perform activities of daily living, and making his or her life as comfortable as possible. The effects of muscular dystrophy can be reduced significantly by staying active and keeping the body as flexible, upright, and mobile as possible. A physical therapist will work with the child to teach him or her to perform range-of-motion exercises to prevent the tendons (bands of tissue that support the joints) from shortening and causing the joints to stiffen. Braces on the hands and lower legs can also help keep the limbs stretched and flexible. Most children with Duchenne muscular dystrophy need a wheelchair full-time by about age 12, which helps them remain active and independent. In some cases, doctors prescribe corticosteroids, which may help slow the loss of muscle function and increase strength. Ask your doctor or the local chapter of the Muscular Dystrophy Association about support groups, summer camps, and other services that might be available in your community for people with muscular dystrophy and their families.

14

Disorders of the Bones, Muscles, and Joints

Bones, muscles, and joints provide the body a supportive framework that allows flexibility of movement. All movement, including the movement of the organs inside the body, is carried out by muscles, which can do their job because they are composed of tissues that can contract.

Voluntary muscles, such as those in the arms and legs, are under conscious control. For example, if you want to bend your elbow, your brain instructs your biceps muscle to contract; if you want to straighten your arm, your brain signals your biceps muscle to relax and instructs your triceps muscle to contract. These brain signals are sent through the nervous system. Involuntary muscles, such as those in the heart and the digestive tract, function without your conscious control or awareness.

The 206 bones of the skeleton serve mainly as a support system for the body. Some bones also cover and protect organs. For example, the skull protects the brain, and the rib cage and bones of the spine (vertebrae) shield the heart, lungs, and, to some extent, upper abdominal organs such as the stomach, liver, and kidneys.

Bones are composed of living cells embedded in a dense framework of collagen (the protein that provides structure and strength to tissues) and saturated with the minerals calcium and phosphorus. This framework both stores these minerals and supplies them to the rest of the body when needed. Inside some bones is a soft core of bone marrow, which manufactures blood cells. Some bones, such as those of the skull, are joined closely together in childhood by virtually immovable connective fibers called sutures.

Joints are the movable connections between bones that enable the bones to move in relation to each other. There are many different types of joints in the body. The vertebrae (the bones in the spine) can move only slightly in relation to each other, but provide enough flexibility over the entire spine to allow the back to bend. Hinge joints, such as those in the fingers, permit movement primarily backward and forward. Ball-and-socket joints such as the shoulders and hips are more versatile than hinge joints and allow the limbs to bend, twist, turn, and move in almost any direction.

How the Skeleton and Muscles Work Together

Skeletal muscles are attached to two or more bones. When a muscle contracts, the bones to which it is attached move. Muscles usually work in coordinated groups; contraction of one muscle causes relaxation of another. Some muscles stabilize nearby joints.

Head and neck muscles
Contractions of the head and neck muscles produce facial expressions and head movements and are responsible for speech and swallowing.

Arm muscles
The bulk of arm muscles is at the shoulder and below the elbow. Long tendons connect the muscles in the forearm to the wrist and fingers.

Abdominal muscles
The large group of muscles in the abdomen assists in the regular movements of breathing, balances the muscles of the spine during lifting, and holds the abdominal organs in place.

Leg muscles
Leg muscles are among the most powerful in the body and are strongly attached to bone, especially at the hip.

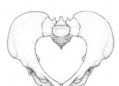

Male pelvis

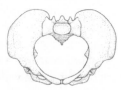

Female pelvis

Heart

Intestines

Male and female pelvis
Except for the pelvis, most of the bones in the female skeleton are the same shape as the bones in the male skeleton but are usually a little smaller. The female pelvis is usually broader than the male pelvis and has a larger space in the middle, to accommodate the head of a baby as it passes through the pelvis during childbirth.

Involuntary muscles
Involuntary muscles are not under conscious control—they do not contract or relax in response to your decision to move them. Instead, they work automatically under the influence of the autonomic nervous system. Involuntary muscles include muscles that push food through the digestive tract and muscles that control sweating and blood pressure.

Joint Movements

The finger joints are typical hinge joints and move primarily in one plane—backward and forward. Elbow joints move in the same way. A ball-and-socket joint such as the shoulder or hip allows movement in two planes—backward and forward and sideways. A ball-and-socket joint also allows the limb to rotate. Most actions of the arms and legs involve a combination of these movements.

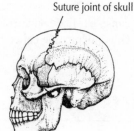

Little or no movement

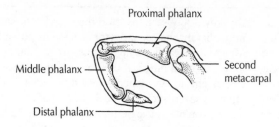

Proximal phalanx

Middle phalanx

Distal phalanx

Second metacarpal

Hinge joint (right index finger)

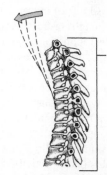

Flexible joints of vertebrae

Limited movement

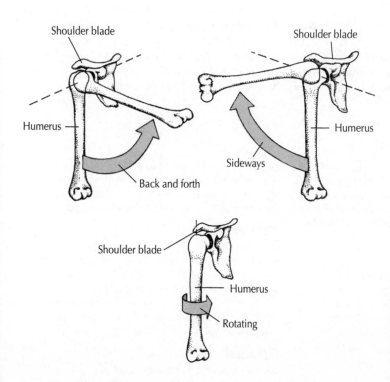

Shoulder blade

Shoulder blade

Humerus

Humerus

Sideways

Back and forth

Shoulder blade

Humerus

Rotating

Movement of a ball-and-socket joint (shoulder)

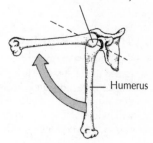

Ball-and-socket joint

Humerus

Maximum movement

Different types of joints

Some joints (such as the fibrous sutures that join the bones of the skull in adults) weld the bones into one rigid structure and allow no movement. Other joints provide limited movement. Each vertebra can move only slightly but, over the whole spine, the vertebrae allow considerable flexibility. Joints such as the shoulders and hips provide a wide range of movement.

Suture joint of skull

Each joint is a complicated structure held together on the outside by fibrous bands called ligaments. Under each ligament is a capsule made of fibrous tissue surrounding the joint. The capsule is lined on the inside by a slippery, fluid-filled membrane called the synovial membrane; the synovial fluid lubricates the joint. Where the bone ends meet, the surfaces are covered by a tough, rubbery tissue called cartilage. Cartilage acts as a shock absorber, or cushion, between the bones, allowing them to move against each other smoothly.

Sports Injuries

Exercise involves the risk of injury, but the health benefits of exercise far outweigh the risks. Anyone who exercises vigorously has an increased risk of injuring his or her muscles, ligaments (tough elastic bands of tissue that hold bones together), bones, and joints. Sports injuries frequently occur in athletes at the beginning of a sports season and in people who are new to a sport or who start an exercise or activity after a long period of inactivity. Exercising without warming up first can also contribute to injuries.

Taking precautions such as stretching before exercising can help you avoid injury. If you are injured, stop the activity right away to determine the extent of the injury. If you're not sure how serious your injury is, or if you are disoriented, even for only a few seconds, stop the exercise or sport immediately and see a doctor as soon as possible. Many injuries require no treatment other than rest. You may need physical therapy to treat damaged tissues and to strengthen affected muscles. If the injury is severe, you may need surgery. If an injury recurs, you may have permanently damaged a ligament or bone and may have to give up the sport or activity or risk developing a chronic condition such as osteoarthritis (see page 996). To help prevent an injury from worsening or becoming permanent, get an accurate evaluation of the damage from a doctor. He or she will probably order X-rays, a CT scan (see page 112), MRI (see page 113), ultrasound (see page 111), or arthroscopy (see page 1001) to determine the extent of the injury.

The RICE Routine

If you have a minor muscle or ligament injury such as a strain or sprain, RICE—which stands for rest, ice, compression, and elevation—is usually the best way to treat it. Performing the RICE routine will help relieve any pain or swelling and enable you to recover more quickly.

Rest

Rest the injured area and avoid moving it or putting any unnecessary weight or pressure on it. Use a sling to rest an injured shoulder or arm, and crutches to take weight off an injured leg. Rest reduces bleeding from damaged blood vessels, minimizes the risk of more damage, and enables tissues to heal.

Ice

Apply an ice pack to the injured area as soon as possible. Apply the ice every hour you're awake for 20 minutes for the first 24 to 48 hours after an injury. Cold helps relieve pain and minimize bruising and swelling by stopping internal bleeding and the accumulation of fluids in the injured area.

Compression

Wear a compression bandage around the injured muscle or joint for at least 2 days. Extend the bandage well above and below the injured area and try to apply the pressure evenly but not too tightly. The bandage is too tight if it causes numbness and tingling or increases the pain. Compressing the injured area helps reduce bleeding and swelling.

Elevation

Keep an injured leg above the level of your heart as much as possible. Elevate an arm or hand with a sling. Elevating the injured area helps drain fluid from the area and reduces bleeding and swelling.

Dislocated Shoulder and Separated Shoulder

A dislocated shoulder occurs when the top of the humerus (the bone of the upper arm) pops out of the joint. A separated shoulder occurs when ligaments that hold the collarbone to the shoulder blade are stretched or torn. Both injuries cause sudden, severe pain, swelling, and bruising, and the shoulder has an abnormal shape and limited movement. These injuries usually result from a fall or a direct blow to the shoulder.

To prevent a dislocated or separated shoulder:

- Ease into your workouts.
- Avoid situations that could cause shoulder injury.
- Wear layers of clothing or padding to help cushion a fall.
- Work with a trainer or physical therapist to strengthen the muscles, ligaments, and tendons of your shoulder.

Swimmer's Shoulder

Swimmer's shoulder is a strain or minor tear in a muscle between the neck and the top of the arm that causes pain in the top, front part of the shoulder. The injury results from a repetitive motion by the shoulder over time.

To prevent swimmer's shoulder:

- Work with a trainer or physical therapist to strengthen your shoulder muscle and the supporting ligaments and tendons.
- Ask a swimming instructor about proper technique.

Golfer's Elbow and Tennis Elbow

Golfer's elbow is inflammation of or a minor tear in the tendon that attaches the muscles that run down the inside of the forearm to the humerus (the bone of the upper arm) at the inner part of the elbow. The injury causes pain inside the elbow, limiting its movement. Golfer's elbow usually results from an incorrect repetitive use of the elbow, such as in an improper downward golf stroke or from hitting the ground during the swing.

Tennis elbow is inflammation of or a minor tear in the extensor tendons of the wrist. The wrist tendons attach the long muscles that run down the outside of the forearm to the humerus at the outer part of the elbow. The injury causes pain in the outside of the elbow and limits movement of the elbow. Tennis elbow usually results from snapping the wrist on a serve or using an improper backhand stroke or equipment, such as a grip that is too large or too small, a racket that is stiff or too heavy, or strings that are too loose.

To prevent golfer's elbow or tennis elbow:

- Work with a trainer or physical therapist to strengthen the muscles, ligaments, and tendons in your hand, wrist, and forearm.
- Get recommendations from a golf or tennis pro about proper equipment and technique.
- Wear an elbow brace, which helps constrict the muscles and reduce tension in the elbow.

Elbow Bursitis

Bursitis of the elbow caused by a sports injury is inflammation and swelling of the bursa (a fluid-filled sac) at the base of the elbow resulting from a fall or a direct blow to the elbow. The swelling is usually not very painful and seldom affects the elbow's range of motion.

To prevent elbow bursitis:

- Rest your elbow in a splint, or wrap it in an elastic bandage if the area is swollen.
- Use elbow pads to protect the bursa when you exercise.

Baseball Finger

Baseball finger is a partial to complete tear in a tendon (a fibrous band that joins muscle to bone) at the joint at the end of the finger caused by a sudden blow to the end of the finger. The injury causes immediate pain, swelling, and bruising at the tip of the finger, and the fingertip cannot be straightened.

To prevent baseball finger:

- Learn catching techniques that don't expose the tips of your fingers to injury.
- Work with a trainer or physical therapist to strengthen the tendons in your finger.
- Avoid playing 16-inch softball.

Skier's Thumb

Skier's thumb is a partial to complete tear in the ligament that attaches the thumb to one of the bones in the palm. The injury causes immediate pain and swelling at the base of the thumb. Skier's thumb occurs when the ski pole forces the thumb away from the fingers during a fall.

To prevent skier's thumb:

- Work with a trainer or physical therapist to strengthen the tendons and ligaments in your hand.
- Learn how to manipulate the ski pole in a fall to avoid injuring your thumb.

Hip Pointer

A hip pointer is severe bruising or a tear in the muscle that attaches to the top of the hipbone at the waist. The injury causes pain and bruising of the hip. A hip pointer usually results from a direct blow to or fall on the hip.

To prevent hip pointer:

- Wear proper padding around the hips when you engage in contact sports.

Runner's Knee

Runner's knee refers to damage to the cartilage that covers the undersurface of the kneecap. The resulting discomfort can range from a dull ache to sharp pain on or behind the kneecap when the knee is bent. The knee may also be swollen and may grind or pop. Runner's knee results from sudden stress on the knee, usually brought on by a change in the running routine or in the running surface.

Runner's knee sometimes refers to pain on the outside of one or both knees caused by a tear in connective tissue that runs from the hip to the top of the tibia (the inner, thicker bone in the lower leg). The pain is worse when the foot hits the ground at an angle. In this type of runner's knee, the knee may also be swollen or may grind or pop.

To prevent runner's knee:

- Use good judgment when increasing your running mileage and the intensity of your workout or when running on a different surface.
- Work with a trainer or physical therapist to strengthen and stretch the muscles, ligaments, and tendons in the legs.

- Wear shoes that fit properly and that are appropriate for the sport or activity; replace them when they wear out, especially when the heels wear down.
- Put shoe inserts in your running shoes to help your feet strike the ground at the correct angle.

Torn Knee Cartilage and Torn Knee Ligament

Torn cartilage in the knee is a partial to complete tear of one of the pads of cartilage inside the knee caused by a severe twist of or forceful blow to the knee. The injury causes pain in the knee, and the knee may be swollen or may grind, buckle, lock, or pop.

A torn ligament in the knee is a partial to complete tear in one of the two ligaments that crisscross inside the knee. The injury is caused by a sudden strain or twist of the knee, or a blow to the knee. Symptoms include swelling, pain, and limited movement in the knee.

To prevent torn knee cartilage or torn knee ligament:

- Work with a trainer or physical therapist to strengthen the muscles in the upper part of your leg, which will stabilize your knees.

Pulled Hamstring Muscle

A pulled hamstring is a partial to complete tear in the large muscle at the back of the thigh. The resulting pain ranges from a dull ache to severe pain that makes it difficult to walk, sit, or bend over. A pulled hamstring usually occurs in runners during a sprint and in people who have overdeveloped or naturally tight hamstring muscles.

To prevent a pulled hamstring muscle:

- Warm up before exercising or running.
- Work with a trainer or physical therapist to strengthen the muscles in the upper part of your leg.

Calf Muscle Tear

A calf muscle tear is a partial to complete tear in the calf muscle. Symptoms include sharp pain, swelling, and possibly a snapping sensation in the middle of the calf. The injury usually occurs when people who are not used to athletic activity jump and land on their toes.

To prevent calf muscle tear:

- Wear heel lifts in your athletic shoes to reduce tension in your calf muscles.
- Warm up your calf muscles by stretching for a few minutes before exercising.

Shin Splint

A shin splint can be one of several injuries that cause pain in the front, lower part of the leg—a small muscle tear, a stress fracture, a small tear in or inflammation of the membrane covering the bone, or overdevelopment of the leg muscles. All of these injuries result from overuse of the leg muscles.

To prevent shin splints:

- Ease into your workouts.
- Work with a trainer or physical therapist on exercises to strengthen the muscles surrounding your ankles.
- Wear arch supports to help relieve stress on the lower part of your leg.

Achilles Tendinitis

Achilles tendinitis is inflammation of the tendon that attaches the calf muscles to the heel. Symptoms can range from mild discomfort to severe pain and swelling in the lower, back part of the leg, about 2 inches above the ankle. Achilles tendinitis results from constant or sudden stress to the tendon.

To prevent Achilles tendinitis:

- Ease into your workouts.
- Wear heel lifts in your athletic shoes to relieve pressure on your heels.
- Wear shoes that fit properly (overly stiff heels can cause or worsen Achilles tendinitis) and that are appropriate for the sport or activity; replace them when they wear out.
- Work with a trainer or physical therapist on exercises to strengthen your calf muscles and stretch your Achilles tendon.
- Run on soft surfaces such as dirt or wood tracks—not on concrete.

Sprained Ankle

A sprained ankle is a partial to complete tear in the ligaments on the inside or outside of the ankle that occurs when the ankle is twisted. It is the most common musculoskeletal injury. Symptoms range from mild to intense pain. You may feel a popping or tearing sensation in your ankle, and the top of the foot may swell and bruise.

To prevent sprained ankle:

- Ease into your workouts.
- Tape your ankle or put an elastic bandage on it before you exercise to make it more stable.
- Wear shoes that fit properly and are appropriate for the sport or activity; replace them when they wear out. The heel counter of the shoe (the part of the shoe that wraps around the heel) should provide support for your ankle. Good shoes have a heel cup (a molded insert), which provides stability to the ankle. Shoes that lace up give the ankles more support than shoes that slip on or close with fasteners.
- Work with a trainer or physical therapist to strengthen the muscles around your ankle and lower calf.

Pain in the Front of the Foot

Pain in the front third of the foot can be caused by Morton's neuroma, which usually results from swelling of a nerve between the third and fourth metatarsals (two of the five long bones in the middle of the foot between the tarsals at the back of the foot and the phalanges, which form the toes). The pain usually is more noticeable on the top of the foot but may also develop in the ball of the foot or on the bottom of the toes. In severe cases, the toes may become numb. The injury usually results from wearing poorly fitting shoes or putting pressure on the feet (such as during long-distance running).

To prevent pain in the front of the foot:

- Ease into your workouts.
- Go without shoes or constricting socks as often as possible.
- Wear shoes that give your feet room to move.
- Wear foot pads (called metatarsal pads) specially made to cushion and protect the ball of the foot.

Heel Pain

Most heel pain occurs when the band of tissue that runs from the heel to the base of the toes becomes inflamed (a condition called plantar fasciitis). Heel pain usually results from overuse, wearing shoes with a stiff heel, or running on hard surfaces. Treating plantar fasciitis usually relieves the pain. The heels may be swollen and bruised and may hurt more when you stand on your toes. Plantar fasciitis can feel like walking on pebbles.

To prevent heel pain:

- Ease into your workouts.
- Work with a trainer or physical therapist to strengthen your calf muscles and stretch the connective tissue at the bottom of your foot by stretching your big toe toward you with your hand.
- Wear shoe inserts or heel pads to relieve pressure on your heels.
- Wear shoes that fit properly (overly stiff heels can cause or worsen heel pain) and that are appropriate for the sport or activity you are engaging in; replace your shoes as soon as they wear out.
- Run on soft surfaces such as dirt or wood tracks—not on concrete.

Stress Fracture in the Foot or Lower Leg

A stress fracture in the foot is a hairline crack in one of the bones of the foot that results from sudden or constant pressure on the foot or from a change in running routine or running surface. A stress fracture causes intense, burning pain at the site of the fracture, usually in the second metatarsal (one of the five long bones in the middle of the foot between the tarsals at the back of the foot and the phalanges, which form the toes).

To prevent stress fractures:

- Ease into your workouts.
- Wear shoes that fit properly and that are appropriate for the sport or activity, and replace them when they wear out.
- Run on soft surfaces such as dirt or wood tracks—not on concrete.

Disorders of the Muscles, Tendons, and Ligaments

Muscle is a type of body tissue that is composed of special elongated cells that contract to produce movement. Some muscles are connected to bones by bands of fibrous tissue called tendons. In some parts of the body, the tendons are very short or their fibers mesh with the muscle tissue. In other areas (especially in the hands and feet) tendons form long, tough cords. Ligaments are tough, slightly elastic bands of fibrous tissue that bind the ends of bones together. Muscles, tendons, and ligaments can be damaged by injury and sometimes by disease.

Cramp

A cramp is a painful spasm in a muscle. Some people are awakened at night regularly by sudden, severe cramps, usually in the legs or feet. Exercising more than usual or sitting, standing, or lying in an uncomfortable position for a prolonged period can cause muscle cramps. In most cases, cramps are not a cause for concern. However, if you think your cramps may be related to an underlying disease or disorder, see your doctor.

Symptoms

If you move a cramped muscle, it will contract violently (you will be able to see it), causing sudden pain. The cramped muscle will feel hard and tense to the touch. Unlike the pain from a sprain or broken bone, if you take a few steps on a cramped leg or foot, the pain is relieved temporarily. An ordinary cramp seldom lasts longer than a few minutes.

Treatment

Muscle cramps usually clear up quickly on their own. You can speed the process by massaging and gradually stretching the cramping muscle. Applying a heating pad can help relieve muscle tightness.

Preventing Cramps

If you have cramps often, warm up before you exercise by stretching. Drink lots of water before and during exercise. Eat foods that are high in potassium and calcium—such as bananas, fresh vegetables, milk, yogurt, and cheese—which helps improve muscle function. See your doctor if you have persistent or recurring muscle cramps.

Strained or Torn Muscle

If a muscle is overstretched, the muscle fibers are strained and some may tear. If a muscle is strained, it contracts and may swell from internal bleeding. Occasionally, a muscle may rupture or tear completely. Almost everyone has strained a muscle at some time. People who are active in sports are particularly susceptible to muscle strains.

In most cases, recovery from a strain is quick and complete with no loss of movement. Generally, the older you are, the more damage you can do to a muscle and the more slowly it will recover. A strain that tears muscle, however, may permanently impair the functioning of the muscle unless it is treated successfully.

Symptoms
The main symptom of a muscle strain is pain when the injury occurs. The strained muscle feels tender, may become swollen, and will not function efficiently until the pulled fibers heal. If the muscle is torn, it will not function at all. A muscle that gradually becomes stiff, painful, and tender (often overnight) has probably been strained, and a few of its fibers may have torn. If you are in a great deal of pain or if the affected area becomes badly swollen, see your doctor.

Diagnosis and Treatment
The doctor will evaluate the severity of your injury and may take X-rays to rule out a fracture. If the muscle is strained and does not seem to be severely damaged, he or she will probably recommend doing the RICE routine (see page 978) at home. For a more serious strain or a tear, the doctor may prescribe a pain reliever or recommend immobilizing the muscle to allow it to heal by, for example, using crutches for a leg injury or a sling for an arm injury. The doctor may also recommend physical therapy. As the pain and swelling subside, the therapist will show you how to gradually start exercising the injured muscle to help restore its movement and strength. If the muscle is torn, surgery may be necessary to repair it.

Sprained Ligament

If excessive demands are made on a joint, the ligaments that hold the neighboring bones together and keep the joint in position may be stretched or torn.

This type of injury is called a sprain. Any ligament can be sprained, but the ligaments at the knees, ankles, and fingers are the most susceptible because they generally receive the greatest force.

Minor sprains cause no damage, but a joint will weaken eventually if its ligaments are repeatedly stretched and torn. For example, if the ankle joint is sprained often, it may begin to give way occasionally for no apparent reason. If a sprain is so severe that all the supporting ligaments are torn, the joint may be misshapen.

Symptoms
The amount of pain and tenderness from a sprained ligament depends on the extent of damage to the soft tissues that support the joint. A sprained ligament can often continue to function but is painful to use. The injury may also cause swelling and skin discoloration. If the pain from a sprain is severe or if it lasts for more than 2 or 3 days, see your doctor.

Diagnosis and Treatment
The doctor will examine your joint and may take X-rays to rule out a fracture. If you have a mild sprain and the muscle does not seem to be severely damaged, he or she probably will recommend performing the RICE routine (see page 978) at home. After a day or so, start to exercise the joint as much as possible without forcing it to bear weight. When you are not exercising the strained muscle, keep it elevated to reduce the swelling.

If you have a severe sprain, your doctor may put a cast or splint on it. Occasionally, surgery is necessary to repair torn ligaments. After ligament surgery, your joint will be immobilized in a protective brace for a short time and you will be encouraged to use the joint to avoid stiffness. Ultrasound therapy, in which high-frequency sound waves are directed at the injured area, is used for some sprains to improve circulation and promote healing. Physical therapy can usually help strengthen the joint and enable it to heal more quickly.

Torn or Severed Tendon

Tendons are long, fibrous cords that connect muscles and bones, such as those that move the fingers and toes. The muscles that move the fingers are in the forearms and hand; those that move the toes are in the calves and feet. If you cut or severely injure your forearm or hand or your calf or foot, one or more tendons may be partly torn or completely severed. The Achilles tendon, which connects the calf muscles to the end of the heelbone, is the most frequently torn tendon.

Symptoms and Diagnosis

If you cut or severely injure a tendon, you will be in extreme pain and may be unable to move one or more of your fingers or toes. Go to the nearest hospital emergency department as soon as possible if you think you may have severed a tendon.

Treatment

Depending on the severity of the injury, a surgeon may immediately reconnect the severed ends of the tendon. Tendons are elastic and are under constant tension. When a tendon is severed, the two segments snap away from each other and may be difficult to retrieve. A large incision may be required to find them and reattach them. Tendon repairs are usually successful, although in some cases an affected finger or toe may be stiff and less movable than it was before the injury.

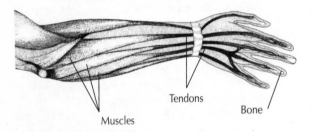

Muscles   Tendons   Bone

Tendons
Tendons are strong, flexible bands or cords of tissue that join muscles to bone. Tendons are made up mostly of bundles of collagen (a fibrous protein) and contain some blood vessels.

Tendinitis

Tendons are strong, elastic bands of tissue that connect muscles to bones. Tendinitis is inflammation of a tendon caused by injury or overuse. Tendons are usually slow to heal because they have a limited blood supply and because the muscles most often affected by tendinitis are constantly in use. Tendinitis can occur anywhere a tendon joins muscle to bone, but usually occurs at the shoulders or heels or on the outside or inside of the elbows (golfer's elbow or tennis elbow; see page 979).

Symptoms

In tendinitis, the affected area is swollen, tender, and painful. When the tendon heals, inflamed fibers may leave a painful scar. The pain usually goes away in a few weeks or months, but it can persist and become worse, especially in older people whose tissues heal more slowly and sometimes imperfectly.

Treatment

If you have tendinitis, your doctor will recommend resting the affected arm or leg by putting the arm in a sling or asking you to stay off the leg for a few days. Take aspirin, ibuprofen, naproxen, or ketoprofen to help relieve the pain and reduce inflammation and swelling (acetaminophen has no effect on inflammation). After a few days, exercise the joint gradually to prevent it from getting stiff. If the pain persists or gets worse, your doctor will recommend X-rays of the arm or leg to rule out a fracture. He or she may also inject a corticosteroid drug and a local anesthetic into the affected area to reduce inflammation and relieve pain. Treatment may consist of other measures, such as applying ice to the area or using ultrasound (high-frequency sound waves) to reduce inflammation and speed healing. Doing gentle, controlled exercises that stretch and strengthen the muscles will also help relieve the pain and inflammation.

Tenosynovitis

Tendons are strong, elastic bands of tissue that connect muscles to bones. Some tendons in the hands, wrists, feet, and ankles are enclosed in a fibrous tissue called a tendon sheath, which allows the tendon to slide over a joint. Tenosynovitis is inflammation of the inner lining of the tendon sheath. When the inner lining of the sheath becomes inflamed, it can form a knot or cause swelling.

The exact cause of tenosynovitis is not known, but it usually results from overuse of a wrist or finger, primarily from using the fingers repeatedly with the same motion, such as when using a computer keyboard. People who have rheumatoid arthritis (see page 918), gout (see page 1004), or diabetes (see page 889) seem to develop tenosynovitis more often than others. Tenosynovitis is sometimes caused by an infection from a puncture wound.

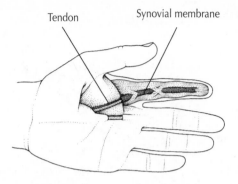

The synovial membrane
Some tendons, such as those in the hand, are covered by a membrane called the synovial membrane. The synovial membrane secretes a fluid (synovial fluid) that lubricates tendons and joints.

Symptoms and Diagnosis

You may hear a grating noise or feel a crackling sensation when you bend or straighten the tendon. The area over the tendon may become tender and swollen. In one form of tenosynovitis called trigger finger, a tight tendon sheath makes it hard to straighten the finger once it is bent. The tendon becomes jammed for a few moments before it suddenly pushes past the swelling and the finger straightens with a sudden jerk.

A doctor can usually diagnose tenosynovitis by examining the affected area and asking questions about the pain. Call your doctor immediately if the tenosynovitis may have been caused by an infection from a wound or if the affected area is warm, increasingly painful, and difficult to move.

Treatment

Mild cases of tenosynovitis can usually be treated by resting the affected area (such as by wearing a splint) and taking a nonsteroidal anti-inflammatory drug to reduce the swelling and relieve the pain. Your doctor may recommend ways to avoid overusing the tendon, such as changing your work habits. Noninfectious tenosynovitis can sometimes be treated with an injection of a corticosteroid drug to reduce the inflammation. Tenosynovitis caused by an infection requires prompt treatment with antibiotics to clear up the infection and possibly surgery to release pus from the affected area. If tenosynovitis persists, a simple surgical procedure to open the constricting tendon sheath will allow the tendon to move freely again.

Fibromyalgia

Fibromyalgia, also called fibrositis or myofascial pain, is chronic stiffness and pain in fibrous tissues, usually deep inside the muscles. The cause of fibromyalgia is unknown, but some doctors think it may result from an injury to the central nervous system or from a viral infection. The attacks of pain and stiffness seem to be associated with emotional stress. Although muscles knot up during an attack of fibromyalgia, the muscles themselves are not damaged in any way. Fibromyalgia is common, especially in people who are past middle age, and usually clears up on its own.

Symptoms

During attacks of fibromyalgia, you are likely to have localized pain and slight swelling in the affected muscles. The tenderness seems to occur in

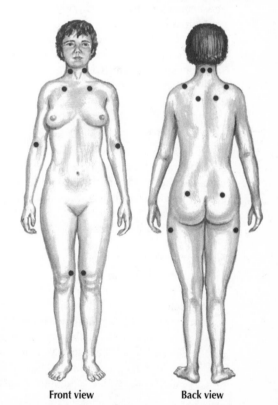

Front view   Back view

Sensitive areas of fibromyalgia
A person is diagnosed with fibromyalgia if he or she has chronic pain in at least 11 of 18 specific sensitive areas, called tender points, on the body (dots). Some people with fibromyalgia also have pain elsewhere in their body.

specific areas called tender points throughout the body. Backache is common. People who have fibromyalgia are often tired because the pain interrupts their sleep. They also may have other symptoms, including anxiety or digestive disturbances such as irritable bowel syndrome (see page 765).

Diagnosis and Treatment

Because symptoms of fibromyalgia are similar to those of other disorders, it is difficult to diagnose. Your doctor may make a diagnosis of fibromyalgia if you have had pain in at least 11 of the 18 sensitive areas in the body for longer than 3 months.

Soaking in a hot bath and massaging sore muscles can provide some relief. Exercise such as walking or swimming increases muscle strength and helps reduce pain and stiffness. Taking aspirin or another nonsteroidal anti-inflammatory drug can help relieve the pain. Your doctor may prescribe antidepressants, stronger pain relievers, or muscle-relaxant drugs to loosen muscles and help you sleep. A doctor may prescribe injections of a local anesthetic into the sensitive areas to relieve pain, sometimes with a corticosteroid drug to reduce inflammation.

Ganglion

A ganglion is a lump under the skin of the wrist or upper surface of the foot. A ganglion develops when a jellylike substance accumulates in a joint capsule or tendon sheath (the tissue surrounding a tendon) and causes it to balloon out.

Symptoms

The size of ganglia can vary. They may be soft or hard and are usually painless or only mildly painful. A ganglion on the wrist does not interfere with wrist movement, but a ganglion on the foot can make it difficult to wear some types of shoes. Although a ganglion is harmless, you should have your doctor look at it. A swelling of any kind could be a sign of a more serious condition.

Diagnosis and Treatment

A doctor can diagnose a ganglion by its appearance and feel. Your doctor may remove the jellylike substance from the ganglion with a syringe (aspiration) and inject the ganglion with a corticosteroid

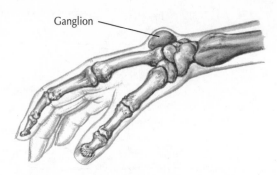

Ganglion
The wrist is one of the most common sites for ganglia. The cystlike swelling can vary from the size of a pea to, in rare cases, the size of a golf ball.

drug to reduce inflammation. Aspiration is effective only about half the time. In rare cases, ganglia that are especially painful are removed surgically. Do not try to eliminate a ganglion by smashing it with a book or other object; this folk remedy is ineffective and painful.

Dupuytren's Contracture

In Dupuytren's contracture, also called palmar fasciitis, a layer of tough, fibrous, connective tissue that lies directly under the skin on the palm of the hand thickens and shrinks over time. This shrinkage eventually causes fingers, most often the ring finger and little finger, to permanently fold in toward the palm at the knuckles. One or both hands and sometimes the bottom of the foot may be affected. The cause of Dupuytren's contracture is unknown.

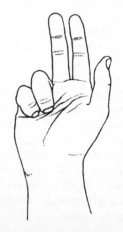

Dupuytren's contracture
In Dupuytren's contracture, the fingers of one or both hands are fixed in a bent position. The ring finger and little finger are the most frequently affected.

Symptoms and Diagnosis

Although Dupuytren's contracture is not usually painful, it stiffens the fingers in a flexed position and weakens the grasp. You may also have thickened skin pads over your other knuckles and on the balls of your feet. See your doctor right away if you have any of these symptoms. A doctor can diagnose Dupuytren's contracture by its appearance.

Treatment

If Dupuytren's contracture is treated early enough, the stiff fingers can be unbent surgically in a procedure that either removes or cuts through the thickened tissue. With physical therapy, you can regain the use of your hand. If untreated, the condition can become permanent. In some cases, the contracture recurs after treatment.

Muscle Tumors

Tumors in muscles are rare and are usually not cancerous. It is not known why muscle tissue seems to resist tumors. When cancerous tumors do develop in muscles, however, they are difficult to treat, and tend to grow and spread quickly.

Symptoms and Diagnosis

Usually the only sign of a growth in a muscle is pain or a detectable lump. In some cases, the tumor may grow moderately over a long period. If the growth is cancerous, it enlarges rapidly and may become more painful. A large muscle tumor can interfere with muscle contraction. See your doctor without delay if you develop an unexplained lump anywhere on your body.

The doctor will examine you and may recommend X-rays, a CT scan (see page 112), or an MRI (see page 113) of the affected area. He or she may also recommend a biopsy (in which tissue samples are taken from the lump and examined under a microscope).

Treatment

If you have a noncancerous tumor, your doctor will want to check it periodically for any changes. If you have a cancerous tumor, possible treatments include surgery, chemotherapy (see page 23), or radiation therapy (see page 23), or a combination of these, depending on the type of tumor and its location and size.

Bone Disorders

Bone is living, constantly changing, tissue that consists of several different types of cells embedded in a framework of collagen (a protein that provides structure and strength). The soft parts of bone that contain dense deposits of calcium salts make bone different from other connective tissue and give bone its strength.

Most bones develop from continuously growing pieces of cartilage that gradually harden. Some bones, such as the skull and the collarbone, form in membranes that develop in the skin of embryos. Inside some bones are spaces occupied by marrow, a tissue that contains the cells that form all the different types of blood cells in the body.

Fractures

A fractured, or broken, bone occurs when a bone is stressed by a force greater than it can withstand. Bones that are weakened by a bone disease such as osteoporosis (see page 989) or bone cancer (see page 995) are especially vulnerable to fracture. The bones most likely to break are those in the wrists, hands, and feet. Fractures of other bones (such as the arm bones, leg bones, spine, and hip)

are usually the result of a powerful force such as a vehicle collision.

The older you are, the more likely you are to break a bone. Children have resilient bones that tend to bend rather than snap. The bones of older people fracture more easily as they lose calcium and become weak and brittle. Also, problems with balance and coordination in older people can cause falls, making fractures more likely.

Fractures are classified as closed or open. A

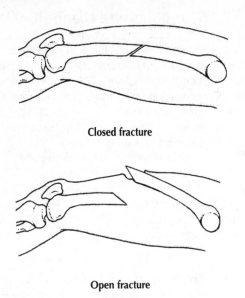

Closed fracture

Open fracture

Types of fracture
In a closed fracture, the skin is intact. In an open fracture, the broken bone protrudes through the skin.

closed fracture is one in which the bone is broken but does not protrude through the skin. In a closed fracture, surrounding muscles and other tissues usually are not damaged. In an open fracture, surrounding muscles and other tissues have significant damage, and the fractured bone breaks through the skin.

If a fracture is not treated, or if treatment is delayed, complications can occur. For example, the broken pieces of bone may begin to rejoin when they are still out of alignment and the bone may have to be separated or rebroken and realigned surgically. In an open fracture, the bone may become contaminated with bacteria, leading to infection and complicating the healing process. It is possible for a fragment of broken bone, cut off from its blood supply, to die, collapse, and gradually be absorbed by the body. Another complication associated with fractures is damage to neighboring tissues. Sharp fragments of bone may compress or sever nearby blood vessels or nerves. Fractures of the skull or spine can damage the brain or spinal cord. Occasionally, a fractured bone damages internal organs. For example, a broken rib can puncture a lung and cause pneumothorax (see page 644).

Symptoms and Diagnosis

A fracture makes the area around it look swollen, bruised, and sometimes misshapen. If you fracture a bone, you will probably be in severe pain, which is increased by any pressure to the area or attempt to move that part of the body. A minor fracture may cause only mild symptoms and can be mistaken for a sprain (see page 983).

If you or someone you know has a possible fracture, perform first aid (see page 167) and seek medical help immediately at the nearest hospital emergency department. Do not give an injured person anything to eat or drink. Having food or liquids in the stomach may delay treatment if a surgical procedure is necessary. Surgery may require general anesthesia, and it is safer to wait 6 to 8 hours after a person has had anything to eat or drink before having anesthesia. If you have signs of a fracture, the doctor will confirm the diagnosis with an X-ray of the injured area.

Treatment

To treat a fracture, a doctor realigns the broken pieces of bone (if they are in the wrong position) in a procedure called reduction, which may be performed using local or general anesthesia. The doctor may need to cut open the tissues around the fracture to reposition the bones correctly.

Plaster casts or lightweight plastic or resin casts and splints are usually used to hold the bone fragments together in correct alignment while they heal. Some bones are held together naturally and don't need a cast or splint. For a broken rib, nearby unbroken ribs and chest muscles may hold the broken rib in place. Your doctor can stabilize a fractured finger or toe until it heals by bandaging it to the adjacent finger or toe. In many cases, the broken ends of a fracture in an arm or leg are held in position internally by one or more metal screws, rods, or plates. Internal immobilization of an arm or leg allows the injured arm or leg to be used within a few days of the injury rather than weeks or months.

In children, fractures of the thighbone are often treated by putting the child in a body cast or by gradually applying tension to the bone to realign it using a system of weights and pulleys (called traction) and then putting the leg in a cast. Traction allows the broken ends of the bone to grow together correctly.

Because of the possibility of muscle atrophy (the wasting away of a muscle from disuse), it is important to use an injured arm or leg as soon as possible after immobilization. Follow your doctor's advice about when and how to move and exercise your injured arm or leg. Keep nearby joints as active as possible without disturbing the broken bones. Maintaining blood flow to the injured area helps prevent swelling and promote bone healing to heal.

The healing time for a fracture depends on many factors, including the bone that is fractured, the number of bone fragments, the person's age, and whether the fracture is open or closed. A child's broken finger may heal completely in 2 weeks, while an adult's tibia (the inner, thicker bone in the lower leg) may take 3 months or longer to heal.

Occasionally a fracture does not heal. In this case, a doctor may need to perform a bone graft to promote healing. In a bone graft, small pieces of bone are taken from a bone bank (a collection of bone donated for transplantation) or from the person's body (often the pelvis) and packed around the break. In some cases, doctors use an artificial bone substitute for the graft. Electrical stimulation of the fracture with a weak electric current is sometimes used to accelerate bone healing.

Bunion

A bunion (which doctors call hallux valgus) is an enlargement of the bone at the base of the big toe. Bunions are common and tend to run in families.

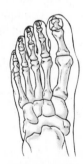 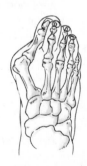

Normal left foot   **Right foot with bunion**

Bunion
In the bone deformity known as a bunion, the bone at the base of the big toe is enlarged, causing the big toe to turn toward the other toes.

The persistent pressure of a shoe on a bunion often leads to painful inflammation of the bursa (a fluid-filled sac that acts as a cushion at pressure points on the body) at the base of the joint (bursitis; see page 1002). Shoes that are tight or that fit poorly, especially shoes with high heels and pointed toes, can make bursitis worse.

Symptoms and Diagnosis
A bunion causes the big toe to point toward the other toes and the bones at the base of the big toe to enlarge and protrude out. If inflammation (bursitis) develops, the area becomes red, warm, swollen, and painful. Bunions are diagnosed by their appearance.

Treatment
If you have a bunion, wear soft, wide, low-heeled shoes or use soft, cushioned, cotton-flannel bandages (which can be cut to size) to take pressure off the affected area. Taking aspirin or another non-steroidal anti-inflammatory drug can help relieve pain and reduce swelling. If these treatments fail to relieve the pain or if walking is difficult, your doctor may refer you to an orthopedic surgeon. The surgeon may perform a procedure called a bunionectomy, in which the deformed bone is cut and straightened. After surgery, you may need to wear a cast or a special shoe for 3 to 6 weeks to protect the foot.

Osteoporosis

Bone is living tissue that undergoes constant change—breaking down and rebuilding. Its central core is a light, flexible, strong structure composed of vertical and horizontal links that resemble interlacing ladders. In osteoporosis, bone loses the horizontal rungs, making it thin, porous, weak, and prone to fracture. In healthy bone, the breakdown of bone tissue and the formation of new, replacement bone are balanced. In osteoporosis, the breakdown of bone tissue occurs faster than the formation of new replacement bone.

Risk Factors
Aging is the most common cause of osteoporosis in both men and women. Women are especially susceptible to osteoporosis after going through menopause (see page 851) because the female hormone estrogen, which declines substantially at

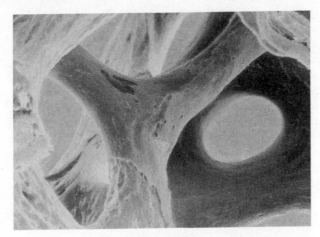

Healthy, dense bone

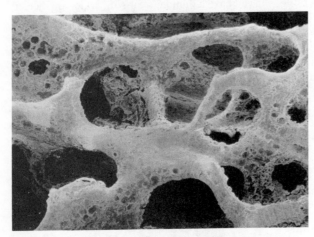

Bone weakened by osteoporosis

Osteoporosis
Healthy bone has dense, strong tissue. Bone weakened by osteoporosis gradually becomes thinner and weaker and susceptible to fractures. Bone thins from the loss of its structural protein, collagen, and its strengthening mineral, calcium.

menopause, plays a key role in helping bones absorb and retain calcium, which keeps them strong. Also, women tend to have smaller bones than men and, therefore, less bone to lose before problems develop. In addition to being older and being female, the following factors put you at increased risk of developing osteoporosis:

- Being thin, having a low body mass index (see page 11), or having small bones.
- Having a family history of osteoporosis.
- Being past menopause (either naturally or from

having had your ovaries removed surgically) and not taking a bone-strengthening medication (see page 993).
- Being a younger woman whose periods have stopped abnormally from excessive exercise or excessive weight loss from an eating disorder (see page 725) such as anorexia or bulimia. If you are not menstruating, your body is not producing estrogen and you could be losing bone tissue, which increases your risk of developing osteoporosis at a young age.
- Eating few calcium-rich foods and not taking calcium supplements.
- Having long-term therapy with medications (such as corticosteroids) that affect the bones (see page 992).
- Being a male with a low testosterone level.
- Getting little exercise.
- Smoking or a history of smoking.
- Drinking alcohol excessively.
- Being white or Asian.
- Having a gastrointestinal disorder such as a peptic ulcer (see page 755) or lactose intolerance (see page 770), which can interfere with the body's ability to absorb calcium.
- Having a history of fractures.

Symptoms
If you have osteoporosis, you may notice that you are shorter than you used to be, your posture is somewhat stooped, or your shoulders are rounded because the bones in your spine (vertebrae) have weakened. Other than these, osteoporosis seldom causes noticeable symptoms until a bone breaks. Osteoporosis can affect any bone, but the bones most likely to fracture are those in the hip, spine, and wrist. The hip and wrist usually break as the result of a fall, but the vertebrae can weaken gradually and fracture from a routine movement such as bending over. If one or more vertebrae break, you will have sudden, severe back pain.

Diagnosis
To diagnose osteoporosis, doctors perform a physical examination to check for a change in posture or loss of height. No test is available to accurately measure overall bone strength, but your doctor will recommend an imaging test that measures bone density (see next page) in different parts of the body. (Regular X-rays do not show bone loss unless the loss is severe.)

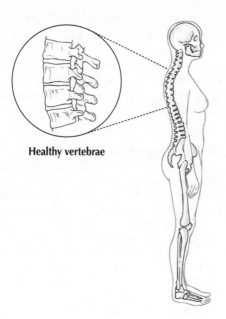

Healthy vertebrae

Healthy spine

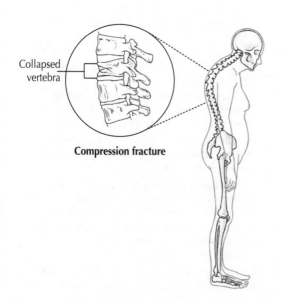

Collapsed vertebra

Compression fracture

Spine with osteoporosis

Compression fracture from osteoporosis

A bone in the spine (vertebra) weakened by osteoporosis may, over time, develop tiny cracks. Eventually, the weakened bone can collapse, causing a compression fracture. Compression fractures can make the upper part of the spine curve, affecting posture and reducing height.

Q & A

Osteoporosis

Q. *My 18-year-old daughter is an athlete and works out rigorously every day. She hasn't had a period in 6 months. Could this be a problem for her health?*

A. Your daughter should see a doctor right away. She is at risk of developing osteoporosis at a young age. Many young women who exercise strenuously and fail to consume enough calories stop menstruating, which means that their body is not producing the female hormone estrogen in normal amounts. Estrogen is essential for building bones, and bones reach their peak strength and density in adolescence. Your daughter may need to take birth-control pills to restart her estrogen production and periods. The doctor may also recommend that she decrease her workout regimen, consume more calories, and take in 1,300 to 1,500 milligrams of calcium every day.

Q. *My mother and my sister both have osteoporosis. I'm 40 years old and I'm starting to worry that I might develop it too. Is there anything I can do now?*

A. Because of your family history of osteoporosis, you are at increased risk of developing it. The first thing you should do is have a bone density test to evaluate the strength of your bones, which can help determine your risk of developing osteoporosis or breaking a bone. If your bone density is lower than normal for your age and build, your doctor will probably recommend a number of strategies to prevent you from losing more bone and, possibly, help you build more bone. For example, getting a sufficient amount of calcium (about 1,500 milligrams each day) and doing as much weight-bearing exercise (such as walking) as you can each day will help keep your bones strong. Also, your doctor may prescribe a medication that helps maintain bone density or promotes bone growth.

Bone Density Tests

The only way to determine if you have osteoporosis or are at risk of developing it is to have a test that evaluates the density of your bones, primarily in the spine, hip, or wrist (the most common sites of fracture). Some newer tests are able to measure bone density in the middle finger and heel or tibia (the inner, thicker bone in the lower leg). All bone density tests are painless, noninvasive, and safe; most use low-dose radiation or ultrasound. Your bone density is compared with two standard measurements—the bone density normally expected in someone your age, sex, and size; and the peak bone density of a healthy young adult of the same sex.

This information helps your doctor evaluate your risk of developing osteoporosis and fractures and determine if you need treatment. You may have to repeat the test periodically to assess the rate at which you are losing bone or to monitor the effectiveness of any bone-strengthening treatment you are undergoing. The following are the most common bone density tests:

Dual-energy X-ray absorptiometry
DEXA is an imaging technique that can measure bone density anywhere in the body. The spine and hip, and the wrist, heel, or finger are the sites most often tested. DEXA uses a very low dose of radiation and can detect bone loss of as little as 1 percent.

Single-energy X-ray absorptiometry
Single-energy X-ray absorptiometry measures bone density in the wrist or heel.

Quantitative ultrasound
Quantitative ultrasound uses sound waves to measure bone density at the heel, tibia, and kneecap.

Quantitative CT scan
A quantitative CT scan is usually used to measure bone density in the spine but can also be used at other sites, such as the wrist.

Radiographic absorptiometry
Radiographic absorptiometry uses an X-ray of the hand and a small metal wedge to calculate bone density.

Osteopenia
If the results of your bone density test fall below the normal range for a young adult, your doctor may tell you that you have osteopenia, a term that describes low bone mass. Osteopenia is not a disease, but it indicates that you may be at increased risk of developing osteoporosis. Your doctor will recommend steps you can take to prevent osteoporosis, such as taking calcium supplements and doing weight-bearing exercises.

Treatment
If you have osteoporosis, your doctor will discuss with you the various treatments available to stem further bone loss and to help build up bone. He or she will suggest that you get as much weight-bearing exercise as possible to help keep your bones strong. Your doctor may also recommend that you wear pads called hip protectors, which fit tightly around each hip. Each day, you should take in at least 1,500 milligrams of calcium (1,000 milligrams if you are a woman who is taking estrogen) and between 400 and 800 international units (IUs) of vitamin D (which helps your body absorb calcium). Many calcium supplements now contain vitamin D.

Medications and Bone Loss
A number of medications can contribute to bone loss in both women and men, primarily by reducing the body's ability to absorb calcium from the intestines. If you are taking one of the following medications regularly, ask your doctor if it could be affecting your bone density. You may be able to take the medication in a different way (such as through an inhaler or by injection) to bypass the intestines, which prevents the medication from having an effect on the bones.

- **Corticosteroids** Long-term therapy with glucocorticoids for inflammatory conditions such as rheumatoid arthritis, asthma, lupus, and inflammatory bowel disease can stimulate cells that destroy bone and inhibit cells that build bone.
- **Antiseizure medications** High doses of the antiseizure medications phenytoin and phenobarbital for treating epilepsy reduce the body's ability to use vitamin D, which helps the body absorb calcium.
- **Cholestyramine** The cholesterol-lowering medication cholestyramine reduces the body's ability to absorb vitamin D.
- **Thyroid hormone** High doses of thyroid hormone used for treating hypothyroidism increase the rate of bone loss.
- **Gonadotropin-releasing hormones** Long-term treatment with gonadotropin-releasing hormones for endometriosis by women who already have low bone density can decrease bone density more by reducing the woman's natural level of estrogen.
- **Antacids containing aluminum** Taking large quantities of antacids that contain aluminum can weaken bones because the aluminum replaces calcium in bones.
- **Cyclosporine** Therapy with cyclosporine to prevent organ rejection after a transplant interferes with the growth of new bone.
- **Heparin** The anticlotting medication heparin can weaken bones by reducing bone growth factors in the blood.

Medication

Some prescription drugs are available for preventing and treating osteoporosis by slowing or stopping bone loss, increasing bone density, and reducing the risk of fractures. Your doctor may prescribe one of the following medications:

Bisphosphonates

Bisphosphonates such as alendronate and risedronate slow bone loss and increase bone density in the spine and hips in women and men who have osteoporosis, including osteoporosis that develops from long-term use of corticosteroid medications such as prednisone or cortisone. To reduce digestive system side effects, take these medications on an empty stomach first thing in the morning with a glass of water. Remain upright, and don't eat or drink anything or take any other medications for at least half an hour after taking bisphosphonates.

Calcitonin

Calcitonin is a naturally occurring hormone (produced by the thyroid gland) that is involved in calcium absorption and bone metabolism. In women who are at least 5 years past menopause, a synthetic form of calcitonin taken in a nasal spray once a day or in an injection every day or every other day slows bone loss and increases bone density in the spine. Calcitonin also appears to relieve the pain associated with fractures.

Estrogen

When a woman's natural production of estrogen slows at menopause (or after surgical removal of the ovaries), taking low-dose estrogen and progestin in hormone therapy (see page 853) can slow bone loss, increase bone density, and reduce the risk of fractures in the hip and spine. Some estrogen compounds are even more effective when combined with bone-building drugs such as alendronate.

Selective estrogen receptor modulators

Selective estrogen receptor modulators (SERMs) such as raloxifene and tamoxifen, which are used for preventing and treating breast cancer (see page 857), also are used for preventing and treating osteoporosis. These medications, which are taken in pill form once a day, prevent bone loss and increase bone density in bones throughout the body. SERMs seem to have the beneficial effects of estrogen on bone without its potentially harmful effects on the uterus or breasts.

Parathyroid hormone

Parathyroid hormone is a naturally occurring hormone produced by the parathyroid glands (the two pairs of pea-sized glands next to the thyroid gland in the neck). Parathyroid hormone stimulates new bone formation by increasing the number and activity of bone-forming cells called osteoblasts. The medication, taken in daily injections, significantly increases bone density in the spine and hip and in bones throughout the body in postmenopausal women and in men and women who have osteoporosis from long-term treatment with glucocorticoids.

Vertebroplasty

Your doctor may recommend a nonsurgical procedure called vertebroplasty to treat a collapsing or fractured vertebra caused by osteoporosis. In this procedure, the doctor administers a local anesthetic and a contrast medium (dye) into the site of the fracture and, using X-rays to guide the needle, injects a liquid that contains bone cement. Antibiotics may be given at the injection site or intravenously (through a vein). The liquid cement hardens over 10 to 20 minutes and stabilizes and strengthens the fractured vertebra. The procedure can relieve back pain by preventing further collapse of the bone.

Preventing Osteoporosis

Because bone changes in response to environmental factors (such as what you eat and the amount of exercise you get), you can take steps to keep your bones strong. The following measures can help you avoid osteoporosis:

Calcium

Taking in a sufficient amount of calcium (see page 5) helps build and maintain bone strength throughout life. Good sources of calcium include low-fat or fat-free dairy products (such as skim milk), fish with edible bones (such as sardines), and green, leafy vegetables. Too many children get a substantial portion of their daily calories from fruit drinks, soft drinks, and high-fat, high-calorie snacks instead of from calcium-rich foods such as dairy products. Encourage your children to eat foods that are rich in calcium.

Vitamin D

Vitamin D helps the body absorb and use calcium. Oily fish such as salmon, vitamin D–fortified milk, and eggs are good sources of vitamin D. Although your body makes some vitamin D when you expose your skin to sunlight, you need to get most of your vitamin D from your diet or from supplements.

Weight-bearing exercise

Weight-bearing exercise such as walking, climbing stairs, and jogging stimulates new bone growth by putting stress on the bones. Lifting weights and doing exercises such as push-ups have the same effect. It's never too late to start exercising. If you have been diagnosed with osteoporosis, your doctor will probably recommend low-impact exercises such as walking and ask you to avoid activities such as tennis and golf that involve twisting.

Medication

Most of the medications used to treat osteoporosis (see previous page) are also used to prevent it when taken before significant bone loss has occurred.

Osteogenesis Imperfecta

Osteogenesis imperfecta, sometimes called brittle bone disease, is a genetic disorder that causes bones to break easily, often for no apparent reason. The disorder results from a genetic defect that affects the body's production of collagen, the major protein in connective tissue that provides structure and strength to the skeleton. A person with osteogenesis imperfecta has abnormal collagen or has less collagen than normal.

Osteogenesis imperfecta has four forms, which can vary greatly in severity from one person to another. Type I is the mildest, most common form; type II is usually fatal at or within a year of birth; type III is progressively deforming; and type IV is moderately severe. People with the same type of osteogenesis imperfecta, even members of the same family, can have different symptoms that differ in severity.

The genetic defect occurs in a dominant gene that is either inherited or is the result of a spontaneous mutation (change) in a parent's egg or sperm cell before conception. For this reason, a person who has the disorder has a 50 percent chance of passing the gene (and therefore the disorder) on to each of his or her children. If you or a relative has osteogenesis imperfecta, talk to a genetic counselor (see page 952) to learn your risk of transmitting the disorder to a child.

Symptoms

The most obvious symptom of osteogenesis imperfecta is bones that break easily. Other symptoms of the most common form (type I) include loose joints and poor muscle tone; a blue, purple, or gray tint to the whites of the eyes; a triangular face; curvature of the spine; bone deformities; a gray tint to the teeth; or hearing loss beginning in the person's 20s or 30s. The less common, more severe forms can cause bone deformities, short stature, a barrel-shaped rib cage, or respiratory problems. The most severe form (type II) can be fatal at or shortly after birth, often because the child is born with underdeveloped lungs.

Diagnosis and Treatment

Doctors can usually diagnose osteogenesis imperfecta from the symptoms. The diagnosis is sometimes confirmed by a chemical analysis of the person's collagen or by a genetic test (see page 953). There is no cure for osteogenesis imperfecta. The goal of treatment is to prevent or control the symptoms and help the person achieve optimal bone and muscle strength to reduce the risk of fractures and to be as independent as possible. Many people with severe forms of osteogenesis imperfecta must have surgery to strengthen their bones, dental and orthodontic procedures to correct and improve the appearance of their teeth, and physical therapy to enhance movement. In a surgical procedure called rodding, a metal rod is inserted through the length of the long bones to strengthen them and prevent or correct deformities. People with severe disability often must use wheelchairs, braces, or other mobility aids.

If you have osteogenesis imperfecta, exercise as much as possible (walking and swimming are good choices). Exercise strengthens your muscles and bones and helps you avoid fractures. Ask your doctor about other safe and appropriate exercises. Maintain a healthy weight, eat a nutritious diet, and don't smoke. An excessive intake of alcohol, caffeine, or corticosteroid medications can deplete bones and make them more fragile.

Osteomalacia

Osteomalacia, also called adult rickets, is softening and weakening of the bones. Osteomalacia results from the body's inability to absorb calcium or to deposit mineral salts on the protein structure of bone, usually because of a deficiency of vitamin

D. Without vitamin D, the body cannot absorb calcium and phosphorus from food. Both calcium and phosphorus are required for healthy bone growth, strength, and maintenance. Osteomalacia is rare in the United States.

The elderly, people in nursing homes, people who have darker skin (melanin blocks the action of ultraviolet light from the sun in the skin and interferes with the skin's ability to make vitamin D), people who have lactose intolerance (see page 770), or people who drink large amounts of alcohol are at risk of vitamin D deficiency. Vitamin D deficiency can sometimes result from chronic kidney failure (see page 817) or a condition such as celiac disease (see page 768) that interferes with the absorption of nutrients.

Symptoms

The symptoms of a vitamin D deficiency, such as bone pain and tenderness, can be mistaken for the symptoms of rheumatoid arthritis (see page 918). Other symptoms include muscle cramps, tingling, and weakness. You may feel tired and stiff and find it difficult to stand. In more severe cases, weakened bones may break easily.

Diagnosis

If you have symptoms of osteomalacia, your doctor may recommend blood and urine tests, X-rays, and possibly a biopsy (in which samples of cells are removed and examined under a microscope). Osteomalacia is much less common than osteoporosis but, because the two conditions look identical on X-rays, a biopsy is the only way to make an accurate diagnosis.

Treatment

If you have osteomalacia, your doctor will probably prescribe a vitamin D supplement and treat any underlying disease that is contributing to the problem. You can also get vitamin D from fortified milk, cereal, egg yolks, liver, and fatty fish (such as tuna, mackerel, or salmon) and by exposing your skin to moderate amounts of sunlight.

Paget's Disease of the Bone

In Paget's disease of the bone, also called osteitis deformans, the normal process of bone breakdown and formation is disturbed. Paget's disease causes an increase in the rate at which bone breaks down and causes abnormal bone to form in its place. This new bone, although thicker and larger than the healthy bone, is weaker and more fragile.

Paget's disease can occur in part or all of one or many bones; the hip and the tibia (the inner, thicker bone in the lower leg) are the most common sites. The thighbone, skull, spine, and collarbone are also frequently affected. Men seem to develop Paget's disease more often than women. For unknown reasons, Paget's disease is more common in some geographic areas than in others. Doctors think that a virus may be responsible because viruslike particles have been found in some bone cells of affected people.

Symptoms

Although Paget's disease of the bone does not always produce symptoms, the most common symptom is constant bone pain that is worse at night. Affected bones become large and misshapen and feel warm and tender. Depending on the bones involved, your head or feet may enlarge. You may appear shorter and your legs may be bowed. Headaches are common.

Bones weakened by Paget's disease are more likely to fracture. In rare cases, a cancerous bone tumor develops in the abnormal bone, or the skull presses on the auditory nerve (which carries signals from the ear to the brain) at the point where the nerve passes through the skull, causing deafness. Because the heart is strained from trying to maintain the greatly increased blood flow through the diseased bones, heart failure (see page 570) can occur.

Diagnosis and Treatment

If you have symptoms of Paget's disease, your doctor will examine you and may order X-rays, a CT scan (see page 112), and blood and urine tests to confirm the diagnosis. Nonsteroidal anti-inflammatory drugs such as aspirin, ibuprofen, or naproxen can help relieve the pain. If the pain is severe, your doctor may prescribe drugs such as mithramycin or etidronate, or give you injections of calcitonin to inhibit the breakdown of the bone.

Bone Tumors

Most bone tumors are cancers that have spread from elsewhere in the body, such as the breast or prostate gland. Tumors that result from cells that have spread from other parts of the body are called secondary tumors. Tumors that originate in bone are called primary bone tumors. Primary bone tumors are rare and usually are not cancerous. Noncancerous bone tumors include osteochondromas, osteomas, and cysts. Osteochondromas consist of bone and cartilage and tend to develop close to joints such as the knee or elbow. Osteomas are hard knobs of bone that can form on any bone but usually form on the skull. Cysts may develop in long bones, making the bones more susceptible to fracture.

Symptoms and Diagnosis

If you develop a lump on a bone (or anywhere else on your body), see your doctor right away. He or she will examine you and may order X-rays, blood tests, a CT scan (see page 112), or an MRI (see page 113) to evaluate the lump.

Treatment

Noncancerous bone tumors such as osteochondromas and osteomas do not require treatment unless they are causing symptoms. Those that cause symptoms are usually removed surgically. Bone cysts may be treated by removing the fluid from the cyst and injecting some of the person's own bone marrow and bone tissue to rebuild the bone.

Primary bone tumors can usually be treated successfully with chemotherapy (see page 23) and by replacing the part of the bone that contains the tumor with a bone graft from another part of the body or from a human graft obtained from a bone bank. If the bone of an arm or leg is affected by a primary bone tumor, and the tumor does not initially respond to chemotherapy and radiation therapy (see page 23), the arm or leg may need to be amputated, followed by chemotherapy.

Secondary bone cancer is usually treated with chemotherapy and analgesic drugs for pain relief. Radiation therapy may also provide relief from some symptoms. If a secondary tumor has become large enough to fracture the bone, a doctor may treat the break by inserting metal plates and rods and filling any empty, dead spaces in the bone with bone cement to provide stability. A bone graft from a bone bank or from another part of the body (such as the hip) may also be used to stabilize the bone and prevent fractures. If the tumor is in the spine, a rib graft may be used. Rib grafts have an advantage over regular bone grafts because the rib can be transferred to the spine while still connected to its blood supply, which enhances healing and reduces the risk of infection.

Joint Disorders

Joints provide a range of movement to parts of the body. Because you use one or more joints every time you move, you will quickly notice if any are not working properly. A highly movable joint, such as the hip, is bound together by fibrous bands called ligaments. Inside the ligaments is a fibrous joint capsule lined on the inside by the synovial membrane, a thin membrane that continuously produces tiny amounts of fluid to lubricate the joint. A tough, smooth tissue called cartilage covers the ends of the bones inside the joint, cushioning the bones and enabling them to glide easily against each other.

Osteoarthritis

Osteoarthritis, also called degenerative joint disease, occurs when cartilage (the tough, smooth tissue that covers the ends of bones in a joint) breaks down and gradually becomes rougher and thinner. Swelling can occur if the lining of the joint (called the synovial membrane) becomes irritated and produces excess fluid that collects inside the joint. As the cartilage wears away, growths of bone called bone spurs may form around the edges of the joint, making it look knobby and swollen. As the process continues, more cartilage wears away, causing the bones that meet at the joint to rub against each other. Because bone is very sensitive, this rubbing together can cause extreme pain and severely reduce movement in the joint. The joints that are most often affected by osteoarthritis include the knees, hips, back, neck, toes, and fingers.

Risk Factors

Osteoarthritis, which affects both women and men, is the most common joint disorder. Women usually develop it in their hands and knees, while

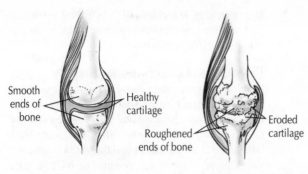

Smooth
ends of
bone

Healthy
cartilage

Roughened
ends of bone

Eroded
cartilage

Healthy joint   **Joint with osteoarthritis**

Joint damaged by osteoarthritis
In a healthy joint (left), cartilage on the end of each bone cushions the bones and allows them to glide easily against each other. In a joint that has been damaged by osteoarthritis (right), the cartilage is damaged and the bones rub against each other, making movement painful.

men tend to develop it in their hips, knees, and back. The following factors can increase your risk of osteoarthritis:

- **Age**   People age 45 and older are most often affected by osteoarthritis. Most people over age 60 have some degree of osteoarthritis. Although age is an important factor in osteoarthritis, the disease is not an inevitable result of aging.
- **Heredity**   Some people inherit genes that make them more susceptible than other people to developing osteoarthritis.
- **Being overweight**   People who are overweight are more likely to develop osteoarthritis because extra weight can strain the joints, especially the knee joints. If you already have osteoarthritis, being overweight can make your symptoms worse.
- **Injury or overuse**   Osteoarthritis usually results from injury to a joint. A serious injury to a joint such as a fracture or an infection can damage the tissue in the joint, which can cause osteoarthritis in that joint. Overusing a joint can also lead to osteoarthritis.
- **Lack of activity**   You are more likely to develop osteoarthritis if you rarely exercise. Inactivity can cause a joint to become stiff and painful and reduces flexibility.

Symptoms

In many people, osteoarthritis does not cause symptoms. (Osteoarthritis is often detected when X-rays are taken for some other reason.) When symptoms develop, they may be mild, with only one or two joints affected at first. Over time, symptoms may become severe and eventually make normal movement difficult. See your doctor if you have any of the following symptoms for longer than 2 weeks:

- **Pain or stiffness in or near a joint**   The pain of osteoarthritis can be deep and aching in or near the affected joint. It can come and go and increase or decrease in severity, depending on the time of day or the type of activity. The pain may be worse at the end of the day or after extreme use such as exercise. The joint is often stiff in the morning and after other long periods of inactivity.
- **Swelling in a joint**   Swelling occurs in the joint when the synovial membrane becomes irritated and produces fluid that collects inside the joint. As more cartilage wears away, growths may form on the ends of the bones and make the joint look knobby and swollen.
- **Crackling and grating when you move a joint**   You may hear crackling and feel a grating sensation (called crepitation) when you move a joint that is affected by osteoarthritis. In most cases, crepitation results from swollen synovial membranes rubbing inside the joint. In severe cases, it can result from bone rubbing against bone.
- **Mild inflammation in a joint**   Inflammation in a joint causes swelling, redness, warmth, and tenderness.

Diagnosis

A doctor can diagnose osteoarthritis by the symptoms and the person's health history. He or she will feel the affected joints for swellings such as bony growths, move or try to stretch the sore joints to see if their movement is limited, and listen and feel for crepitation. X-rays or an MRI can show if and how badly a bone is damaged and the extent of pressure on the nerves.

If the diagnosis of osteoarthritis is still uncertain, the doctor may test a sample of blood or of fluid withdrawn from inside the affected joints. Testing fluid from the joints or testing blood may help rule out other diseases and determine the type of arthritis that is causing the symptoms (osteoarthritis causes no blood abnormalities). Your doctor may refer you to a rheumatologist (a doctor who

Symptoms of Cervical Osteoarthritis

The symptoms of cervical osteoarthritis (which affects the joints in the neck) are the same as the symptoms of osteoarthritis in other parts of the body. In addition, pressure on nerves in the neck can cause headache, dizziness, and muscle weakness, tingling, and numbness in the shoulders, arms, hands, or legs. If the nerves that control the muscles of the bladder are pinched, a person with cervical osteoarthritis may have problems with bladder control.

specializes in treating disorders of the joints) to help determine the diagnosis. Some types of arthritis become obvious only as they develop over time.

Treatment

Osteoarthritis cannot be cured, but it can be treated. A rheumatologist can design a treatment program to help manage the condition. Beginning treatment as early as possible can help reduce long-term damage to the joints and bones. The goal of treatment is to reduce pain and stiffness, allow for greater movement, and slow the progression of the disease. A combination of several of the treatments described below usually works best. It can take time to find the most effective combination. Work with your doctor to develop the treatment plan that will be most helpful for you.

Weight loss

Weight loss and exercise are usually the first treatments recommended for osteoarthritis. Losing weight can help relieve the pressure and strain on your joints, thereby reducing the damage to tissues inside the joints. Weight loss can also help reduce pain and stiffness in the affected joints, especially the joints in the hips, knees, back, and feet. Avoiding weight gain as you get older or losing excess weight can help prevent osteoarthritis or reduce your symptoms.

Exercise

Regular exercise can be very effective for relieving the pain and stiffness of osteoarthritis and may help slow the progression of the disease. Exercise also helps you reach or maintain a healthy weight, which reduces stress on your joints. Pick an exercise program that works for you and fits your lifestyle and physical abilities. Doctors generally recommend a combination of stretching exercises, mild

strengthening exercises (such as lifting weights), and low-impact aerobic exercises (such as swimming, walking, or bicycling).

Physical and occupational therapy

Your doctor may recommend that you work with a physical therapist to prevent or reduce joint stiffness. A physical therapist will help you improve the range of motion in your affected joints and strengthen the muscles around the joints to give the joints support. He or she can also provide splints, canes, crutches, walkers, and other mobility aids if you need them.

An occupational therapist will help you learn new ways to perform everyday activities such as bathing, dressing, walking, and climbing stairs. You will learn to move in ways that reduce discomfort and put less strain on your joints. An occupational therapist can help you make changes in your home or office that will enable you to get around and perform routine tasks more easily and safely.

Hot and cold treatments

Applying heat or cold directly to the affected joints can temporarily relieve pain, stiffness, and occasional swelling. Finding the most effective treatment for you may require trial and error. Do not apply either heat or cold for longer than 20 minutes at a time, and allow your skin to return to normal temperature between applications. Do not use pain-relieving creams or rub your skin when using hot or cold treatments; you could injure your skin and not realize it because your sensation of pain is reduced.

Heat is usually used to relax muscles and warm them up before exercising. Heat up your sore joints with a heating pad or hot pack or by sitting in a hot tub or heated pool. Many people who have osteoarthritis find that a hot shower in the morning is all they need to loosen their stiff joints.

Applying cold can be helpful for short-term pain relief. Cooling a sore joint reduces pain by numbing the area. Never apply ice or cold packs directly to your skin—wrap them in a towel first. Use cold treatments carefully; the lack of feeling may cause you to overuse the sore joint.

Medication

Because of the potential side effects of many drugs that are used for treating osteoarthritis, medication is usually recommended only after other treatments such as weight loss and exercise have been tried and have not been effective. Arthritis medications generally are used to reduce pain and tenderness in the joints. No drugs are available that can stop the progression of the disease or cure it.

Many medications that are used to relieve osteoarthritis pain are available over the counter; some of the stronger ones are available only by prescription. All drugs used to treat osteoarthritis can cause side effects. If you are taking a medication for arthritis, tell your doctor immediately if you have any unusual symptoms. You may not have any problems until after you have been taking the medication regularly for a long time.

Topical medications

Creams, rubs, or sprays can be applied to the skin over a sore muscle or joint to temporarily relieve pain. Creams containing capsaicin (a substance found in hot peppers) reduce pain by blocking the ability of the nerve endings around the joint to send pain messages to the brain. Many of these medications are available over the counter. (Do not touch your eyes, nose, or genitals after applying capsaicin cream.)

Pain relievers

Drugs containing acetaminophen are usually prescribed for osteoarthritis because they don't cause stomach irritation like some other pain relievers such as aspirin. Acetaminophen is most effective when it is used regularly. However, acetaminophen does not relieve inflammation, and you should not take it regularly if you consume three or more alcoholic beverages a day because the combination can damage the liver.

Nonsteroidal anti-inflammatory drugs

Nonsteroidal anti-inflammatory drugs (NSAIDs) such as aspirin, ibuprofen, naproxen, and ketoprofen are often used to relieve the pain and inflammation of osteoarthritis. Many NSAIDs are available over the counter, but stronger ones require a doctor's prescription. NSAIDs such as celecoxib and rofecoxib may cause less stomach irritation than some of the older medications and are very effective for many people.

Corticosteroids

Corticosteroids are sometimes given in injections to reduce the inflammation and pain of severe osteoarthritis. A doctor injects the corticosteroid directly into the affected joint. Because corticosteroids can cause serious side effects, such as

damage to bones and cartilage, the injections are given no more than a few times a year.

Glucosamine and chondroitin

A combination of the over-the-counter supplements glucosamine and chondroitin may help relieve osteoarthritis pain and increase mobility. These supplements seem to work together to strengthen cartilage.

Viscosupplementation

Viscosupplementation is a nonsurgical procedure that is usually recommended for people with osteoarthritis who do not yet need surgery. In viscosupplementation, a doctor injects a sterile mixture of a synovial fluid substitute and saline solution into a joint (usually the knee joint) three times a day for 2 weeks. The synovial fluid substitute, which supplements the person's own synovial fluid, helps lubricate the joint and rejuvenate damaged cartilage. The procedure may have to be repeated.

Surgery

An orthopedic surgeon (a doctor who specializes in surgery on bones) can determine if surgery is necessary to relieve the pain from osteoarthritis and restore movement to a joint. Surgery is recommended only for severe, disabling osteoarthritis for which other treatments have been unsuccessful. (Most people who have osteoarthritis never need to have surgery.) If your doctor recommends surgery, get a second opinion from another doctor. Surgery may be done to prevent the joint from becoming deformed, to correct a deformity, to remove pieces of bone or cartilage from around the joint to allow greater movement, or to replace a damaged joint with an artificial one.

Arthroplasty

Artificial devices are available to replace almost any joint in the body. Arthroplasty, or joint replacement surgery, is most often done to repair hips (see next page) and knees but also is used to repair shoulders, elbows, fingers, ankles, and toes. A successful joint replacement relieves pain and restores most of the joint's movement.

During joint replacement surgery, the surgeon first removes all the damaged bone from the joint. Artificial joint components made of metal and plastic are then cemented to the healthy bone that remains. The joint components are usually attached to the bone tissue with acrylic cement. For younger people who are more active or for older people who have strong bones, doctors sometimes use artificial joints that do not require cement to stay in place. These artificial joints are designed with spaces into which the person's own bone can grow, holding the artificial joint in place more naturally. By avoiding the use of cement, which can weaken over time, these types of artificial joints usually stay in place longer than those that are held in place with cement.

Recovery from joint replacement surgery depends on several factors, including a person's general health and level of activity before the surgery. For this reason, it is not a good idea to put off the surgery for long. The more active you are before your surgery, the faster your recovery is likely to be. Hip replacement and knee replacement surgery require more time for recovery than replacement of smaller joints, such as those in the fingers, wrists, toes, or ankles.

Although complications from joint replacement are rare, the new joint can become infected or slip out of place. For this reason, your doctor will ask you to come in regularly for checkups so he or she can monitor your healing and recovery. To reduce the risk of blood clots, your doctor may prescribe anticlotting medication.

Joint replacement surgery is serious and will cause a short period of disability during recovery. Complete recovery can take from 3 to 6 months. Most people who have a hip or knee replaced will need physical therapy to help regain their mobility. A physical therapist will recommend special exercises to help you build up the muscles around your new artificial joint. Physical therapy starts in the hospital shortly after surgery and continues after you are home.

Hip Replacement

Hip replacement is a surgical procedure in which a damaged hip joint is removed and replaced with an artificial ball-and-socket joint made of metal and plastic. The procedure usually takes about 2 to 3 hours. You will be hospitalized for about a week after the surgery and will start physical therapy in the hospital. You will be encouraged to try to begin walking with support within a day or two after surgery. A physical therapist will teach you how to perform exercises to help strengthen the hip and teach you how to move the joint to avoid injuring your new hip.

At home, maintain a stretching and exercise program to help keep your new joint working properly. Full recovery can take up to 6 months, depending on your overall health, whether you have any complications (such as infection, blood clots, or joint dislocation), the success of your rehabilitation, and other factors. Hip replacements generally last from 15 to 20 years. Young or active people who have had hip replacements may eventually need to have surgery to repair or replace the artificial joint because of wear or loosening of the implant.

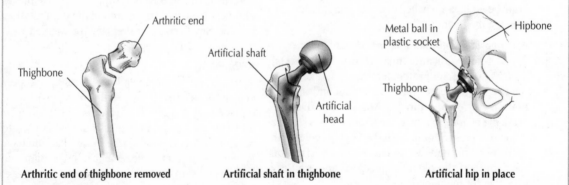

Arthritic end of thighbone removed

Artificial shaft in thighbone

Artificial hip in place

Hip replacement surgery
In a hip replacement, the surgeon removes the end of the thighbone affected by arthritis (left) and creates a hollow channel in the bone. A metal shaft (with a ball at the head) is inserted into the channel in the thighbone (center). The surgeon creates a cavity in the hipbone and implants a plastic socket in the cavity. The metal ball is fitted into the plastic socket (right), forming an artificial hip joint that works like a natural ball-and-socket hip joint.

Arthrodesis

A surgical procedure called arthrodesis, or joint fusion, sometimes is used to correct severe joint problems caused by osteoarthritis. In this procedure, the surgeon makes the affected joint permanently immobile by using a bone graft and inserting metal screws, plates, and rods to hold the joint in place. Arthrodesis is performed only when the pain from osteoarthritis is so severe that immobilizing the joint is an improvement. This procedure is usually performed on smaller joints such as those in the fingers, toes, ankles, or feet.

Osteotomy

Osteotomy is a surgical procedure most often performed on younger people who have a joint (usually a hip or knee) that has been unevenly damaged by osteoarthritis. The procedure is done to relieve stress on the cartilage and prevent further damage to the joint. During an osteotomy, the surgeon removes a small wedge of bone near the affected joint. Removing the piece of bone realigns the bone and improves the contact between the remaining, healthy areas of cartilage in the joint. In younger people, this procedure can delay joint replacement surgery for years.

Arthroscopy

Arthroscopy, or "scoping" a joint, is an outpatient procedure that is used to examine and sometimes repair joints. The procedure is performed most often on knees and shoulders but can be done on other joints, including the hip. For arthroscopy, the doctor inserts a viewing tube (arthroscope) through a small incision into the fluid-filled space in the affected joint. Through the arthroscope the doctor can see any tissue damage and make necessary repairs. Although the repair may provide temporary relief of symptoms, it does not stop the progression of arthritis.

Cartilage transplantation

Unlike bone, cartilage that is injured does not rejuvenate. Cartilage injuries commonly occur with ligament injuries. Damaged cartilage can increase friction in joints, sometimes leading to osteoarthritis. Cartilage transplantation uses live cells from donated cartilage. The donated cartilage must be transplanted within 72 hours. The graft is made of cartilage and bone (the person's bone heals into the donated bone supporting the cartilage).

Dislocated Joint

A joint is dislocated if the bones that normally connect in the joint are pulled apart, usually by a severe injury. Dislocations that are not caused by injury may be present from birth (such as congenital dislocation of the hip; see page 401) or may occur as a complication of rheumatoid arthritis (see page 918).

A dislocation can occur repeatedly in a joint that has been weakened by an earlier injury. The jaw and shoulder joints are especially susceptible to recurring dislocation. Dislocation of vertebrae can damage the entire spinal cord, sometimes causing paralysis of areas of the body below the level of the injury. Dislocation of a shoulder or hip can cause paralysis of an adjacent arm or leg by damaging the main nerves to the arm or leg. Some joints that have been dislocated can eventually become susceptible to osteoarthritis (see page 996).

Symptoms and Diagnosis

A dislocated joint is usually painful, swollen, and discolored, and cannot be moved. See your doctor or go to the nearest hospital emergency department immediately if you think you have dislocated a joint. During this time, protect the injured area and keep it immobile. Do not eat or drink anything, because you may need to have general anesthesia to have the joint repositioned. Don't let anyone try to manipulate the joint or attempt to reposition it. You could damage nerves or blood vessels or worsen an accompanying injury such as a fracture. A doctor will usually X-ray the joint and surrounding area to make a diagnosis and to evaluate the dislocation.

Treatment

A dislocated joint usually becomes so swollen and painful that repositioning may have to be done with the person under general anesthesia. Sometimes a dislocated joint needs to be repositioned surgically. Your doctor may recommend surgery to tighten the ligaments if one of your joints has become very weak from repeated dislocation.

After repositioning, if the blood vessels, nerves, and bones are in place and undamaged, the joint will probably be immobilized in a brace for 3 to 6 weeks to allow any damaged tissues to heal. Follow your doctor's instructions about when and how to use your joint again to avoid reinjuring it. After the swelling has subsided, your doctor may recommend exercises to help strengthen the joint.

Ankylosing Spondylitis

Ankylosing spondylitis is a disease that causes inflammation of and damage to the joints, usually the joints of the spine and the hips. After the inflammation subsides, growths of bone called bone spurs gradually develop on each side of the joint and fuse, preventing the joint from moving. The condition occurs most often in men between ages 20 and 40. The cause is unknown.

Symptoms

Ankylosing spondylitis often starts with pain in the lower back that spreads to the buttocks. The pain and stiffness are usually most severe in the morning. Other symptoms include chest pain, difficulty breathing, slight fever, fatigue, jaw pain, and weight loss. The eyes may become red and painful. In some people, a stiff spine makes the head tilt permanently toward the chest.

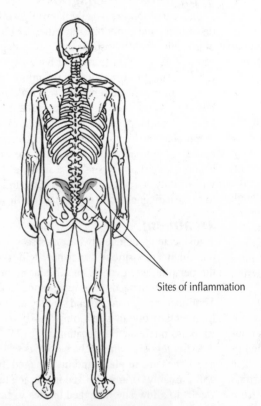

Sites of inflammation

Inflammation in ankylosing spondylitis
The sacroiliac joints (the joints between the spine and the pelvis) are commonly affected by ankylosing spondylitis, causing stiffness and pain that worsen after rest.

Diagnosis

If you have symptoms of ankylosing spondylitis, your doctor will perform a physical examination. During the examination, the doctor may press on the affected joints to check for pain, move your arms to evaluate the range of motion of your back, and ask you to take a deep breath to see if you have difficulty expanding your chest. He or she may order blood tests and X-rays of your back and hips to confirm a diagnosis of ankylosing spondylitis.

Treatment

Your doctor may prescribe nonsteroidal anti-inflammatory drugs to relieve pain and reduce inflammation. He or she may refer you to a physical therapist, who will teach you how to perform daily activities and exercises that will correct your posture, improve your mobility, and keep your back muscles strong. Exercise and deep breathing will help your chest expand normally. To help keep your spine straight at night, the doctor or physical therapist may also recommend sleeping on a firm mattress without a pillow.

If the inflammation and pain are severe, your doctor may inject a corticosteroid drug into the affected area to reduce inflammation. In severe cases, a doctor may perform a surgical procedure that straightens bent, fused bones by removing some of the damaged bone.

Bursitis

Bursitis is inflammation of a fluid-filled sac (bursa) around a joint. A bursa acts like a cushion to take pressure off the surface of a bone or reduce friction around a tendon or muscle. In bursitis, the bursa becomes inflamed and swollen with excess fluid because it has been damaged or irritated by prolonged pressure, an injury, or repetitive movement. The most common sites for bursitis are the elbows (from leaning or falling on the elbow) and knees (from kneeling for long periods), but the shoulders, hips, and heels also can be affected. Bursitis can also occur as a complication of a deformity of the joint at the base of the big toe called a bunion (see page 989).

Symptoms and Diagnosis

In bursitis, the area around the bursa is painful and swollen, and the pain is usually more severe when

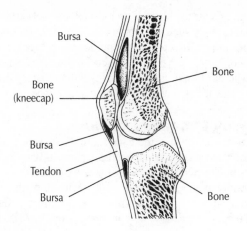

Bursae in the knee
Bursae (fluid-filled sacs for cushioning joints) in the knee are located between the tendon and the bone.

much of your working day kneeling, as carpet layers or roofers do, wear knee pads to reduce pressure on the bursae of your kneecaps. To prevent bursitis in your elbow, avoid resting your elbows on the table or desk while working or studying. Wear elbow and knee pads during athletic activities to cushion your elbows and knees from falls that could cause bursitis. Bursitis in the heel can result from wearing shoes that are too tight or that don't fit properly, or from running long distances. Wearing high heels or shoes that are too tight can irritate bunions and cause bursitis in the joint at the base of the big toe.

the joint is moved. The skin over the bursa may feel warm and look red. If the symptoms persist, see your doctor. He or she will examine the joint to confirm the diagnosis and may remove fluid from the swelling with a needle or order X-rays to rule out other possible causes.

Treatment
Bursitis usually subsides on its own after a few days. Rest the affected area and use an ice pack to ease the pain and help absorb the excess fluid into your bloodstream. Take a nonsteroidal anti-inflammatory drug such as aspirin to help relieve pain and reduce inflammation.

If your symptoms persist, your doctor may remove the excess fluid through a needle and apply a bandage tightly over the area to prevent fluid from reaccumulating in the area. If the fluid contains pus, the doctor will prescribe antibiotics to help fight a bacterial infection. He or she may also inject a local anesthetic to relieve pain and a corticosteroid drug to reduce inflammation. Surgery to remove a bursa, called a bursectomy, is performed only if bursitis recurs repeatedly or if the bursa is infected and the infection seems to be spreading.

Preventing Bursitis
Bursitis tends to develop in joints that are repeatedly placed under a lot of pressure. You can prevent bursitis by taking steps to protect your joints from prolonged pressure. For example, if you spend

Baker's Cysts

Baker's cysts are fluid-filled sacs that form behind the knee. The cyst usually develops from inflammation of the knee joint that causes the membrane around the joint to swell backward and, sometimes, down into the calf muscles. Inflammatory conditions such as rheumatoid arthritis (see page 918) and osteoarthritis (see page 996), or overuse of the knee can cause Baker's cysts to develop.

Symptoms
Baker's cysts usually produce no symptoms, but movement can cause pain behind the knee or upper calf. If the cysts become inflamed or rupture, however, they can cause persistent discomfort or pain.

Diagnosis
A doctor usually can diagnose Baker's cysts by their appearance and feel. Because the cysts can cause pain and swelling behind the knee and in the upper calf, a doctor may want to rule out a blood clot (deep vein thrombosis; see page 605), which has the same symptoms. He or she may recommend an ultrasound (see page 111) or MRI (see page 113) of the knee.

Treatment
If the cyst is not causing symptoms, a doctor may recommend monitoring it for a few months to see if it goes away on its own. If it is large or is causing pain or other symptoms, the doctor will probably recommend removing it surgically in an outpatient procedure. If an abnormality in the joint itself caused the cyst, the abnormality may need to be corrected surgically to prevent another cyst from forming.

Frozen Shoulder

Frozen shoulder is a condition in which the joint capsule (the tough, fibrous tissue that encloses a joint) becomes thick, inflamed, and forms scar tissue. Frozen shoulder usually begins with a minor injury or condition such as tendinitis (see page 984) or bursitis (see page 1002) that causes chronic pain and makes it difficult or impossible to move the shoulder. This lack of use leads to more stiffness, which progresses to further disuse, weakening of the tissues, and loss of function of the shoulder.

Symptoms and Diagnosis

At first, a frozen shoulder is difficult to move, and the slightest movement causes pain. The discomfort may be worse at night. The pain may eventually subside, but the shoulder will be permanently impaired unless it is treated. To diagnose frozen shoulder, the doctor moves your arm to evaluate the range of motion of your shoulder joint.

Treatment

If you have frozen shoulder, your doctor may prescribe a nonsteroidal anti-inflammatory drug such as aspirin to help relieve the pain and reduce inflammation. He or she may refer you to a physical therapist, who will teach you how to improve the mobility of your shoulder with exercises. (A frozen shoulder should be kept in motion as much as possible.) At each session, you will be given ultrasound therapy, in which high-frequency sound waves are directed at the injured areas, in combination with intense massage to help loosen the scar tissue that has caused the pain and immobility. Your doctor may inject a corticosteroid drug into your shoulder to reduce inflammation if the condition persists. In severe cases, the doctor may need to manipulate the shoulder while the person is under general anesthesia or perform a surgical procedure to loosen the scar tissue.

Septic Arthritis

Septic arthritis is a type of infectious arthritis that is usually caused by a bacterium but can also be caused by a fungus. The condition can result when bacteria enter the joint through a wound, when bacteria spread from a generalized infection such as tuberculosis (see page 663), or when bacteria travel through the bloodstream from an infection elsewhere in the body such as a boil on the skin. Usually only one joint is affected. The condition tends to occur in people who have a weakened immune system or who have joint damage from an inflammatory disorder such as rheumatoid arthritis (see page 918).

Symptoms and Diagnosis

In septic arthritis, the bacteria multiply inside the joint and cause redness, warmth, pain, and swelling. A person with septic arthritis usually has a fever (which can be as high as 104°F) with shaking and chills. If you have symptoms of septic arthritis, your doctor can diagnose it by analyzing samples of your blood and synovial fluid (taken from inside the joint) for the presence of bacteria.

Treatment

Septic arthritis is treated with antibiotics. Your doctor or a surgeon may open the joint to drain the infected synovial fluid to relieve the pressure and pain. Once the infection has cleared up, your doctor will recommend exercises you can do to prevent the joint from becoming permanently stiff.

Gout and Pseudogout

Gout is a common joint disease in which deposits of uric acid crystals in a joint (usually the joint at the base of the big toe, but also the joints of the knees, elbows, ankles, wrists, or fingers) cause painful inflammation. Uric acid is a waste product that normally passes through the kidneys and out of the body in urine. If your body is producing too much uric acid or if your kidneys are not working properly, uric acid crystals accumulate in the spaces in a joint (usually only one joint is affected). Although gout most often occurs in people over age 70, a hereditary form of the disease can affect males shortly after puberty. People who take diuretics (medications that eliminate excess fluid from the body) are at increased risk of developing gout.

Pseudogout (also called calcium pyrophosphate deposition disease, or CPDD) occurs when the attacks of arthritis are caused by calcium pyrophosphate dihydrate crystals rather than uric acid crystals. Like gout, pseudogout usually develops later in life, although it can develop in younger people, especially those who have thyroid disorders. The cause of pseudogout is unknown.

Symptoms

The symptoms of gout or pseudogout are severe pain, redness, warmth, and swelling in the affected joint. The person often has a fever, which can be as high as 101°F. Attacks occur suddenly, but people who have frequent attacks learn to recognize the early signs of an oncoming attack.

Diagnosis

See your doctor if you have symptoms of gout, even if the symptoms subside. Your doctor will examine the affected joint and may withdraw a sample of fluid from the joint to determine if the pain is caused by an accumulation of uric acid or of calcium pyrophosphate dihydrate crystals.

Treatment

If you have had only one attack of gout, your doctor will recommend taking a nonsteroidal anti-inflammatory drug other than aspirin, such as ibuprofen or naproxen. Aspirin is not used to treat gout because it can interfere with the excretion of uric acid crystals in urine. However, aspirin can be used to treat pseudogout. Your doctor may prescribe colchicine to reduce inflammation and relieve pain. He or she may also inject a corticosteroid drug into the affected joint to reduce inflammation. No other treatment is usually necessary.

If you have frequent attacks of gout, your doctor may prescribe drugs such as allopurinol, probenecid, or sulfinpyrazone to help prevent attacks. He or she will also recommend that you drink more water to dilute your urine and that you stop drinking alcohol, which can inhibit the body's ability to eliminate uric acid. Avoid eating protein-rich foods, especially organ meats such as liver or kidneys, because protein can increase the uric acid level in the blood. In rare cases, a doctor may recommend surgical removal of the uric acid crystals that have accumulated in a joint.

Temporomandibular Disorder

Temporomandibular disorder, or TMD (formerly called temporomandibular joint syndrome), is a disorder that affects the jaw muscles and the joints

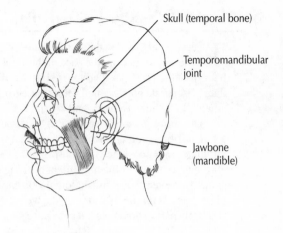

Temporomandibular joint
The temporomandibular joint is a hinged joint on each side of the head where the lower jawbone (mandible) connects with the temporal bone of the skull.

on either side of the jaw (the temporomandibular joints). TMD affects twice as many women as men.

Symptoms and Diagnosis

In TMD, the joints or, more often, the jaw muscles cause pain. In some cases, the pain can extend to the ear or even as far as the shoulder. It may be difficult to open the jaw fully, and your jaw may make clicking or snapping noises.

If you have symptoms of TMD, your doctor will examine your face and jaw. He or she may recommend X-rays and laboratory tests to rule out other disorders, but tests performed on people with TMD often reveal no physical abnormality.

Treatment

To treat TMD and relieve painful spasms, your doctor may recommend massage, heat therapy or ice packs, anesthetic injections or sprays, and pain relievers. He or she will tell you to eat soft foods and avoid extreme movements of your jaw, such as yawning widely or opening your mouth wide to eat, or clenching or grinding your teeth. Ask your doctor or dentist if you should use a nightguard (see page 1111) to reduce clenching or grinding of the teeth. Using a nightguard may also help ease muscle tension around the jaw and prevent damage to the teeth.

Back and Neck Problems

The spine, also called the spinal column or backbone, stretches from the base of the skull to the bottom of the buttocks. The spine consists of more than 30 separate bones called vertebrae. Strong ligaments link the vertebrae, and flexible, flattened disks lie between them. Each disk is constructed of a tough, fibrous outer covering wrapped around a jellylike inner substance, which provides enough elasticity to permit some movement over the entire spine. However, this construction also limits flexibility. For this reason, if you twist the wrong way or strain any part of your spine, it can cause pain in the vertebrae and the muscles and ligaments that connect the vertebrae.

The back is also especially susceptible to pain because the spinal cord, which is a major part of the central nervous system, is in a channel that runs the length of the spine. Peripheral nerves pass through narrow side channels of the spine on their way to and from the rest of the body. As a result, any problem with a vertebra, supportive ligament, or disk can affect nerves that supply the arms and legs and lead to pain and weakness in an arm or leg.

Common Sites of Back Pain

Back pain is usually centered in three common places: the lower back, the coccyx, and the area around the sciatic nerve. See your doctor whenever you have back pain that persists for more than 3 or 4 days.

Lower Back Pain

Pain in the lower part of the back is centered in the small of the back and spreads out from there. It is often caused by unusual exertion, such as moving furniture or digging in the garden. It may develop suddenly or gradually and can be mild or severe. Sometimes you may be completely unable to move. Doctors disagree about the exact cause of lower back pain, but it probably results from a combination of pulled or strained muscles (see page 983), muscle spasms, and sprained ligaments (see page 983).

Coccyx

Pain in the area of the coccyx, at the base of the spine, can be continuous and worsen when you sit. Pain in the coccyx may be caused by falling on or otherwise hitting the base of the spine. Women may temporarily experience pain in this area after giving birth. You may be able to relieve the pain by sitting on a soft cushion designed specifically for this purpose.

Sciatic Nerve

The sciatic nerve is the longest nerve in the body. It branches out to the lower part of the body through the buttocks and down each leg. Sciatica is pain caused by pressure on the sciatic nerve as it leaves the spinal cord. The pressure is usually caused by a prolapsed disk (see next page) or osteoarthritis (see page 996) in the spine. You may feel burning pain shooting into your buttocks and down the back of your thigh, along with numbness and tingling. The pain may get worse if you cough, sneeze, or move your back in any way.

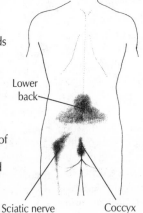

Lower back

Sciatic nerve

Coccyx

Common sites of back pain

Nonspecific Backache

Backaches are a common health problem. The pain occurs most frequently in the lower back, around the coccyx (a small, triangular bone at the base of the spine), and around the sciatic nerve (the longest nerve in the body, which extends from the lower end of the spine to the foot).

The vast majority of backaches have no specific cause—many different factors can be involved. Most nonspecific backaches are caused by muscle strain and injury to the surrounding ligaments (bands of tough, elastic tissue that hold bones together) or joints in the spine. The pain may begin after lifting a heavy object, falling, holding your body in an awkward or cramped position for some time, or performing an exercise or activity that you have never done before. Some people have back pain when they are under stress, just as other people get tension headaches.

Symptoms

A nonspecific backache is often very painful and can interfere with your daily routine. The pain, usually with stiffness, may develop slowly or suddenly, may be continuous or occur sporadically, or may occur only when you are in a particular position. Coughing, sneezing, or bending and twisting your back may worsen the pain. The pain may be localized in only one region of the back or travel from one area to another.

Diagnosis and Treatment

The cause of a backache can be difficult to determine. After examining your back, your doctor may order X-rays of your spine to rule out osteoarthritis (see page 996) or another disorder. The doctor probably will recommend the self-help measures at right to try for a few days to see if the pain goes away. Gentle massage performed by someone who is well trained and experienced may provide temporary relief of your symptoms. If the pain persists for more than 3 or 4 days, your doctor may prescribe pain relievers or a muscle-relaxing drug. Although nonspecific backaches may recur, they usually heal without treatment or complications. Exercising to stretch and strengthen the abdominal and back muscles can help prevent recurring backaches (see next page).

Prolapsed Disk

Between each vertebra is a disk made up of a fibrous outer layer surrounding a jellylike inner substance that provides cushioning. If a disk begins to degenerate and becomes less supple (usually because of overuse or pressure), the disk may move from its normal position (prolapse). This action squeezes some of the jellylike substance out through a weak point in the harder outer layer, resulting in loss of the cushioning and causing painful pressure on a nerve. This condition is called a prolapsed disk (sometimes referred to as a herniated, ruptured, or slipped disk). The disks in the lower back are especially susceptible to prolapse. A prolapsed disk between the vertebrae of the neck can put pressure

Protecting Your Back

It is impossible to protect yourself completely from back problems, but you can reduce the strain on your back by following these tips:

- Maintain correct posture. Don't slouch when standing or sitting. Keep your head up, your shoulders straight, and your chest forward. When you stand, try to balance your weight evenly on your feet.
- Avoid awkward movements such as bending over and twisting at the same time.
- Learn the techniques that can help you avoid injuring your back when lifting heavy objects. Keep your back straight, bend your knees, and grasp the object firmly (make sure it is close to you). Because your legs are stronger than your back, let your legs do the work, and straighten them to lift the object.
- Avoid wearing high heels; the higher they are, the more they force your posture into an unnatural position that strains your back. Wear low-heeled, comfortable shoes.
- Sit properly. Don't slump, and don't cross your legs. Select a firm, high-backed chair that supports your lower back, or use a cushion to support the small of your back. Adjust your workstation if necessary. Your feet should be flat on the floor or on a footrest, with your knees bent comfortably at right angles. In your car, your knees should be higher than your hips, and you should be able to reach the pedals without stretching.
- Sleep on a firm (but not hard) mattress, or put a stiff board under your mattress (between the mattress and box spring).
- If you are overweight, try to lose weight (see page 53); excess weight puts strain on your back.
- Relax. Tension leads to bad posture and causes muscle fatigue.

on a nerve root and cause pain and tingling down the arm. Episodes of pain from a prolapsed disk may recur, sometimes resulting in chronic back or neck pain. The most serious complication is damage to the nerve roots of the spinal cord.

Symptoms

The symptoms of a prolapsed disk may develop suddenly or gradually. If you have a prolapsed disk in your neck, you may wake up with a sore neck or

Back-Strengthening Exercises

Exercises that strengthen your abdominal muscles can help keep your back muscles flexible and prevent back injury. Try to do these exercises at least three times a week. If the exercises cause any pain while you are doing them, or if you have pain or feel stiff the next day, talk to your doctor—you could be overdoing it or not doing the exercises properly.

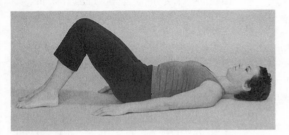

Pelvic tilt
Lie on your back with your knees bent, feet flat on the floor, and your arms at your sides. Tighten your abdominal muscles as you press your lower back into the floor. Hold for 5 seconds. Release. Do one to three sets of 10.

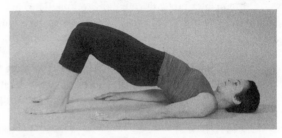

Bridging
Lie on your back with your knees bent, feet flat on the floor, and your arms at your sides. Tighten your abdominal and buttock muscles as you lift your buttocks off the floor. Hold for 5 seconds and slowly return to the starting position. Do three sets of 10.

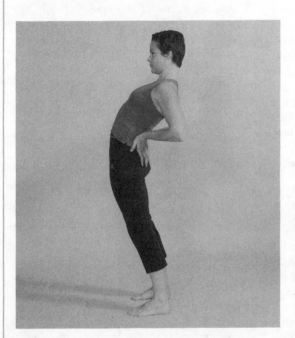

Extension
Stand with your feet comfortably apart, knees straight, and hands against the back of your pelvis. Arch your shoulders backward as far as you can comfortably while pushing your pelvis forward with your hands. Don't arch your neck back—continue looking straight ahead, keeping your head centered. Do one set of 10.

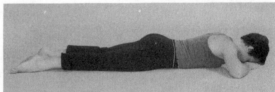

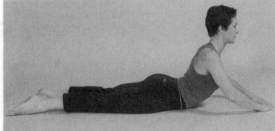

Prone press-ups
Lie on your stomach with your elbows bent and hands meeting in front of you. Rest your forehead on your hands (top). Slowly straighten your arms, raising your torso from the waist while keeping your pelvis on the floor (bottom). Relax, allowing your back to sag from your shoulders and pelvis. Hold this position for 5 seconds. Return to starting position. Do one set of 10.

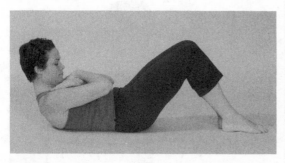

Curl-ups
Lie on your back with your knees bent, feet flat on the floor, and your arms crossed with hands on the opposite shoulder. Tighten your abdominal muscles and press your lower back into the floor as you lift your head and shoulders from the floor, keeping your chin tucked and looking at your abdomen. Hold for 5 seconds, then release. Do three sets of 10.

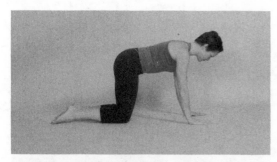

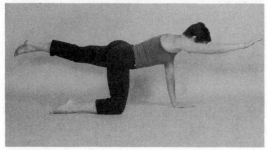

Extension
Get on your hands and knees on the floor, centering your shoulders over your wrists (top). Keeping your back straight and your abdomen lifted, lift one leg and the opposite arm at the same time, straightening the leg and lifting the arm forward and upward (bottom). Hold for 5 seconds. Return to the starting position and repeat with the other arm and leg. Do three sets of 10.

gradually become aware of numbness, tingling, or weakness in your arm. You may suddenly feel intense pain in your back, often along with burning pain down one or both legs, when you bend over or lift something. You may have back and leg pain that comes and goes and worsens over several weeks. If the prolapsed disk is in the lower part of your back, you may develop symptoms of sciatica (see page 1006).

Self-Help for Backaches

Whatever the cause of your backache, you can take steps to ease the pain and speed healing. But if your backache persists for more than 3 or 4 days, see your doctor.

- Use pain relievers such as aspirin, ibuprofen, naproxen, or ketoprofen.
- For the first 24 to 48 hours, apply cold packs for 10 to 20 minutes at a time to reduce swelling and relieve pain. After a day or two, apply heat to the painful area to relax the muscles and promote healing.
- Lie flat on your back on a firm mattress or on the floor. If you are lying on your back, don't use a pillow, or use only a single, flat pillow under your head. You might get relief by putting a pillow under your knees. If you are lying on your side, try putting a pillow between your knees and one under your head to keep your spine straight. Lying on your stomach is usually not recommended if you have a backache. While resting your back during the day, don't stay in bed for prolonged periods; get up and walk around for at least a few minutes every hour or two.
- For some types of back pain, doctors recommend wearing a special brace that supports the back.
- An osteopathic physician, a chiropractor, or a physical therapist may be able to manipulate the vertebrae of the spine enough to take pressure off the adjacent nerves and relieve pain temporarily.

Diagnosis and Treatment

If you have symptoms of a prolapsed disk, your doctor will carefully examine your back and legs and may order X-rays, a CT scan (see page 112), an MRI (see page 113), and tests of the nerves of your spine.

How a Prolapsed Disk Causes Pain

The flexible disks between your vertebrae act as shock absorbers. Each disk has a hard outer layer and a jellylike core. When your back is strained, pressure may push some of the jellylike core through a weak point in the hard outer layer. If the jellylike core presses against a nerve where it leaves the spinal cord, it can cause pain.

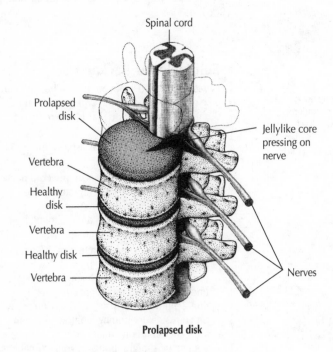

Spinal cord

Prolapsed disk

Jellylike core pressing on nerve

Vertebra

Healthy disk

Vertebra

Healthy disk

Vertebra

Nerves

Prolapsed disk

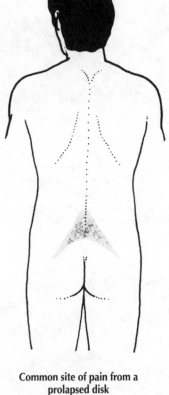

Common site of pain from a prolapsed disk

Treatment of a prolapsed disk varies, depending on the location of the prolapse along the spine. Resting flat on your back is usually the best treatment. Applying heat to the painful area may help relieve the pain. If the prolapsed disk is in your neck, you may need to wear a support collar for several weeks.

Your doctor may inject a corticosteroid drug into the area of the compressed nerve to reduce inflammation, or inject an anesthetic into the lower part of your spine to relieve pain. He or she may recommend traction, a technique to align the bones by gradually applying tension through a system of weights and pulleys. In some cases, doctors inject a substance called chymopapain into the disk. Chymopapain dissolves the disk's jellylike center, causing the disk to shrink and relieving pressure on the nerve. However, some people have a severe allergic reaction to chymopapain.

If your symptoms persist and the pain is severe, surgery may be an alternative. Your doctor may remove a small piece of bone from the adjacent vertebra to relieve pressure on the nerve. If several disks are involved, a procedure called spinal fusion may be recommended to permanently immobilize the adjacent vertebrae. It is always a good idea to get a second opinion before having back surgery.

Disorders of the Ear

The ear is the organ of hearing, and it also plays a role in maintaining balance. It has three parts—the outer ear, the middle ear, and the inner ear. The outer ear includes the part of the ear that we see—folds of skin and cartilage called the pinna—and the ear canal, a passage about ¾ inch long that leads from the pinna to the eardrum. The opening of the ear canal is surrounded by cartilage, which is covered with skin that contains wax-producing glands and hairs. The bone of the deeper part of the canal is lined with a very thin layer of skin. A thin membrane called the eardrum stretches across the inside end of the outer ear canal, separating the outer ear from the middle ear.

The middle ear is a small cavity between the eardrum and the inner ear that is bridged by three small, interconnected bones (the ossicles)—the hammer, the anvil, and the stirrup. The hammer is attached to the inner lining of the eardrum. A ligament (a band of fibrous tissue) attaches the stirrup to an opening (the oval window) that leads to the inner ear. The anvil lies between the hammer and the stirrup and is attached to both.

One of the openings in the middle ear leads into the mastoid portion of the temporal bone (the bone that contains all of the internal structures of the ear). Two openings lead into the inner ear. Another opening, the eustachian tube, leads to the back of the nose. The eustachian tube equalizes air pressure on the inside of the eardrum with the environmental air pressure. Sometimes the eustachian tube becomes blocked and then clears again; this sudden equalization of air pressure feels as if your ear has popped.

The inner ear consists of several fluid-filled chambers—the cochlea (which is involved in hearing) and the semicircular canals and vestibule (which are involved in balance and together form the vestibular labyrinth). The vestibular labyrinth and the cochlea relay hearing and balance information from the inner ear to the brain via the vestibulocochlear nerve.

How the Ear Works

How You Hear

Sound starts as a disturbance of the air, which produces sound waves. The outer ear collects the sound waves and funnels them into the middle ear, which consists of the eardrum, the hammer, the anvil, the stirrup, and the eustachian tube. The sound waves hit the eardrum and make it vibrate. The vibrations then pass into the inner ear, which consists of the semicircular canals, the vestibule, and the cochlea. Tiny hairs that line the cochlea convert the vibrations in the fluid into electrical nerve impulses, which are transmitted to the brain via the vestibulocochlear nerve. The cochlea also transmits information about balance to the brain via the cochlear nerve.

Most sounds reach you through this process, which is supplemented by vibrations that are conducted through the bones of the skull to the inner ear. You hear your own voice mainly through this supplemental type of hearing.

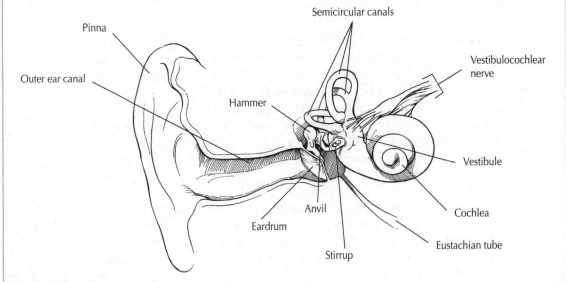

Semicircular canals

Pinna

Outer ear canal

Hammer

Vestibulocochlear nerve

Vestibule

Anvil

Eardrum

Cochlea

Stirrup

Eustachian tube

How You Keep Your Balance

Your brain constantly monitors the position and movement of your head and body to enable you to keep your balance. A structure called the vestibular labyrinth in the inner ear monitors the movement of the head by means of three semicircular canals that sit at right angles to each other. Whatever way you move your head—nod it, shake it, or tilt it—at least one of the semicircular canals will detect the movement and relay the information to your brain. Other areas of the vestibule provide information to the brain about the pull of gravity. The brain processes this input with sensory information from your eyes, and from the muscles and joints in your body, to assess your exact position and the movements you need to make to keep your balance.

Vertigo is a false sense that you or your surroundings are moving. A person with vertigo may also experience nausea, vomiting, and loss of balance. Vertigo is usually a symptom of disorders of the inner ear, the part of the ear that senses movement and maintains balance.

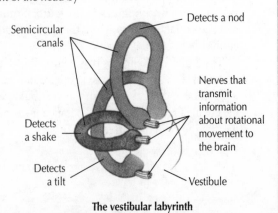

Detects a nod

Semicircular canals

Nerves that transmit information about rotational movement to the brain

Detects a shake

Detects a tilt

Vestibule

The vestibular labyrinth

Disorders of the Inner Ear

D isorders of the inner ear affect the extremely sensitive structures inside it—the cochlea and the vestibular labyrinth. The cochlea transforms sound vibrations into electrical signals that are transmitted to the brain along the auditory nerve. The vestibular labyrinth helps provide balance. If these structures are damaged, they cannot be repaired because they are too delicate for surgery. Damage to either structure can result in sensorineural hearing loss (see page 1016), which is usually permanent.

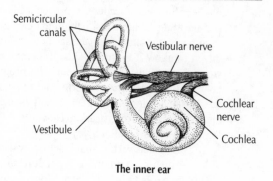

The inner ear

Ménière's Disease

Ménière's disease results from an increase in a fluid called endolymph inside the membranous labyrinth, the part of the ear that is involved with balance and hearing. The excess fluid causes the vestibular and cochlear portions of the membranous labyrinth to swell, which can affect balance and hearing. Ménière's disease usually affects one ear but can sometimes affect both ears.

Symptoms

The most common symptoms of Ménière's disease are hearing ringing or other noises in the ear (tinnitus; see page 1020) and muffled, distorted hearing, especially of low tones. Other symptoms can include a false sense that you or your surroundings are moving (vertigo; see previous page) and nausea and vomiting. The symptoms develop in episodes that may occur every few days, every few weeks, or every few years and can last from 20 minutes to several hours. A person may feel pressure in the affected ear before or during an episode.

Episodes of Ménière's disease usually become less severe over time, but some hearing loss and noises in the ear may persist between episodes. In some people, the disorder is mild and goes away on its own. The nausea and the vomiting tend to stop after the first few episodes. After several years, the dizzy spells usually stop; at this point, doctors consider the disease to have run its course. However, Ménière's disease usually leaves a person with severe hearing loss in the affected ear.

If you have symptoms of Ménière's disease, see your doctor or an otolaryngologist (a doctor who specializes in disorders of the ear, nose, and throat) immediately.

Diagnosis

To diagnose Ménière's disease, a doctor will take a detailed health history and examine your ears. A doctor is usually able to make a diagnosis from the health history, but he or she will probably recommend hearing (audiometry) tests (see page 1016) and may recommend balance tests. You may also have an MRI (see page 113) to rule out a brain tumor as a possible cause of your symptoms.

Treatment

To treat nausea and vomiting associated with Ménière's disease, a doctor will prescribe a medication such as meclizine. He or she may also prescribe a diuretic to reduce fluid accumulation in the membranous labyrinth, which may help prevent future episodes.

Your doctor may recommend measures you can take to help minimize your symptoms. For example, he or she may suggest lying still when you are having an episode. Because an increase in fluid in the ear causes Ménière's disease and too much salt can cause your body to retain fluid, the doctor may ask you to cut down on your salt intake.

If (even after treatment) fluid remains in the labyrinth and damages it or if you are incapacitated by your symptoms, your doctor may inject a drug called gentamicin into the middle ear to destroy the hair cells that play a role in vertigo.

Doctors sometimes recommend surgery on a part of the membranous labyrinth called the endolymphatic sac. In this procedure, a surgeon drills through the mastoid (the bone just behind the ear) either to decompress the endolymphatic sac or to insert a tube into it to allow it to drain. This procedure usually stops the episodes of vertigo and the progressive hearing loss at least temporarily and prevents further loss of hearing in the affected ear. In some cases, the procedure improves hearing. However, the symptoms usually return after a year or so.

If a person has vertigo that is seriously disabling, a doctor may recommend a procedure to cut the vestibular nerve (which is crucial for balance). For severe cases of hearing loss, a doctor may recommend a procedure called labyrinthectomy, in which the vestibular labyrinth (the part of the inner ear involved with balance and hearing) is destroyed.

Labyrinthitis

Labyrinthitis is inflammation of the fluid-filled chambers that control balance and hearing. The exact cause of labyrinthitis is not known, but it usually follows a viral or bacterial infection in the ear or upper respiratory tract.

Symptoms
The main symptom of labyrinthitis is a false sense that you or your surroundings are moving (vertigo; see page 1012). If you move your head even slightly, the vertigo gets worse. In most cases, the vertigo is accompanied by severe nausea and vomiting. Labyrinthitis may also cause ringing or other noises in the ear (tinnitus; see page 1020) or hearing loss (see page 1016). If you have severe vertigo, have someone take you to your doctor's office or the nearest hospital emergency department immediately.

Diagnosis and Treatment
To diagnose labyrinthitis, a doctor will take a detailed health history and examine your ears. You may also have hearing tests and a CT scan (see page 112) or an MRI (see page 113) to rule out other possible causes of vertigo.

If the vertigo is associated with labyrinthitis, your doctor may recommend that you try to stay still and avoid sudden changes of position during episodes. He or she may prescribe medications such as meclizine or diazepam to relieve the nausea and vomiting. To treat labyrinthitis caused by bacteria, a doctor prescribes antibiotics. For labyrinthitis caused by a virus, a doctor may prescribe medication to relieve the symptoms.

Otosclerosis

Otosclerosis is an abnormal growth of bone in the inner ear that prevents the stirrup (one of the tiny bones in the inner ear) from transmitting sound waves to the inner ear, resulting in conductive hearing loss (see page 1016) in the affected ear. In most cases, both ears are affected, either simultaneously or one after the other. As the disease progresses, some sensorineural hearing loss (see page 1016) may occur.

The cause of otosclerosis is not fully understood, but it tends to run in families. The disorder occurs more often in middle-aged women than in men, and in whites more frequently than in blacks. Hormonal changes during pregnancy can accelerate the hearing loss in some women. Without treatment, otosclerosis can result in significant conductive hearing loss, requiring a person to wear a hearing aid to hear normal conversation.

Symptoms
The main symptom of otosclerosis is gradual hearing loss. In rare cases, primarily in children, the hearing loss progresses quickly. Some people may also experience a false sense that they or their

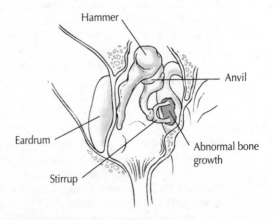

Otosclerosis
In otosclerosis, an abnormal growth of bone in the ear prevents the stirrup from properly transmitting sounds to the inner ear, causing hearing loss in that ear.

Noise and Hearing Loss

Sound is a series of air-pressure waves traveling through the atmosphere alternating between high pressure and low pressure. The loudness of sound is measured in units called decibels by an instrument called a decibel meter. Sounds that are softer than 10 decibels are very difficult for the human ear to hear, while sounds that are 120 decibels or more are usually painful to the ear. A sound loud enough to cause pain can damage your hearing, often permanently. "Noise" is a term usually used to describe a variety of loud sounds that a person finds unpleasant.

Prolonged exposure to noise (especially high-pitched noise) at or above 90 decibels can damage the sensitive hair cells lining the cochlea (the part of the ear that transmits sound information to the brain) and cause partial to severe hearing loss. Being constantly exposed to loud machinery (such as jackhammers or tractors) or listening to extremely loud music (whether on headphones or at a rock concert) can harm your hearing. A one-time or brief exposure to a loud noise (such as a gunshot or from fireworks) can cause temporary hearing loss.

The table below lists the decibel levels of some sounds and their effects on hearing.

How to Protect Your Hearing

Take the following precautions to prevent permanent damage to your hearing due to noise:

- Wear earplugs made of foam, plastic, wax, or rubber to mask noise.
- If you are exposed to a loud sound, eliminate the sound or cover your ears and get away from the source of the noise as quickly as possible.
- Keep the volume of music in your car and home at a comfortable level. If you wear headphones, set the volume at a level that is inaudible to others. If other people can hear the music coming from your headphones, it can damage your hearing.
- If you work in very noisy conditions, wear ear protectors that are designed to decrease sound volume by 40 to 50 decibels. If you need to communicate with coworkers while wearing ear protectors, a small microphone and earphones can be added to the ear protectors. Have your hearing tested frequently if your employer doesn't regularly test your hearing. If you think that the noise level where you work is too high, contact the person responsible for safety at your workplace, or your local health department or the office of the Occupational Safety and Health Administration (OSHA).
- If you hear ringing or other noises in your ear (tinnitus; see page 1020) after exposure to a loud noise, the noise was too loud. Take precautions to avoid exposure to the noise in the future.

Decibels	Type of Sound	Effect on Hearing
10	Barely audible	Safe
20	Ticking watch	Safe
30	Soft whisper at 16 feet	Safe
40	Suburban street (no traffic)	Safe
50	Interior of typical urban home	Safe
60	Normal conversation	Safe
70	Noisy restaurant	Safe
80	Loud music (including personal stereo)	Safe
90	Truck at 16 feet	Risk of injury
100	Typical rock concert	Risk of injury
110	Jet engine at 800 feet	Risk of injury
120	Jackhammer	Injury
130	Jet engine at 100 feet	Injury

surroundings are moving (vertigo; see page 1012) or hear ringing or other noises in their ears (tinnitus; see page 1020).

Diagnosis

If you have hearing loss, your doctor will take a detailed health history and examine your ears. He or she will refer you to an otologist (a doctor who specializes in disorders of the ear), who will examine your ears and perform simple hearing tests. You also may have specialized hearing tests (see next page) to confirm the diagnosis.

Treatment

If the hearing loss caused by otosclerosis is mild or occurs in just one ear, treatment may not be necessary, or you may only need a hearing aid (see page 1018).

If the hearing loss is severe, your doctor may recommend a procedure called stapedectomy. In stapedectomy, the stirrup is removed and replaced with an artificial bone made of plastic or metal to allow sound waves to reach the inner ear. If both ears are affected, one ear will be operated on first and given time to heal before the second one is operated on. Hearing after a stapedectomy usually does not improve immediately because a blood clot forms in the middle ear, and the eardrum swells. As the clot gradually disappears, hearing improves (usually about 2 to 4 weeks after the procedure).

People who have only a conductive hearing loss benefit more from stapedectomy than do people who have both conductive and sensorineural hearing loss.

Hearing Loss

Hearing loss is a worsening of hearing that can include muffled hearing or difficulty understanding or differentiating sounds or words. Hearing loss is a symptom of an underlying disorder. There are two kinds of hearing loss, conductive and sensorineural. Conductive hearing loss is caused by a mechanical failure that keeps sounds from reaching the inner ear, such as wax blockage (see page 1025) in the outer ear or fluid in the middle ear.

Sensorineural hearing loss refers to deafness that occurs when a damaged acoustic nerve fails to transmit sounds from the inner ear to the brain. Sensorineural hearing loss is usually caused by damage to the cochlea or to the auditory nerve (the cochlea and the auditory nerve convey sound information to the brain). Some sensorineural hearing loss is common as you get older. However, loud music, machinery noise, viral infections, heredity, or side effects from some medications can cause sensorineural hearing loss at any age. If you are under age 50 and have difficulty hearing, see your doctor.

Some people may have both conductive and sensorineural hearing loss. This combination hearing loss is the result of problems in the outer or middle ear and in the inner ear.

Diagnosis

To diagnose hearing loss, your doctor will take a detailed health history and examine your ears. He or she may refer you to an otolaryngologist (a doctor who specializes in disorders of the ear, nose, and throat) or an otologist (a doctor who specializes in disorders of the ear). You will have an examination of your ears, and you may have simple hearing tests. You may also be referred to an audiologist (a health care professional who specializes in hearing evaluation and treatment), who may perform more sophisticated tests such as those described below. These tests help diagnose the cause of hearing loss and evaluate the degree of hearing loss.

Audiometry tests

Audiometry tests evaluate a person's overall ability to hear, and determine whether hearing loss is conductive or sensorineural. These tests usually take place in a soundproof room. Pure tone tests measure a person's ability to hear tones and frequencies at different volumes. Speech tests measure a person's ability to distinguish and understand words spoken at different volumes. Impedance or compliance tests, also called tympanometry, measure the ability of the eardrum to reflect sound waves.

Pure tone test

The pure tone test consists of two parts. The first part of the test, called the air conduction test, measures how well you hear sounds conducted through the air. In this test, you listen through earphones, one ear at a time, to sound frequencies that range from low tones to high tones. For each frequency, the sound starts at an audible level and decreases in loudness until you can barely hear it. The softest level at which a tone can be recognized at least 50 percent of the time is your threshold for that frequency.

The second part of the test, called the bone-conduction test, measures how well sounds are conducted through the bones of your head. In this test, a special headphone is placed on the mastoid (the bone directly behind each ear) of one ear. To test one ear, the audiologist puts a competing, or masking, sound into the headphone of the ear that isn't being tested. As in the first part of the test, sound frequencies that range from low tones to high tones are sent through the headphone on the mastoid to find your threshold. The results of both tests are recorded on the same graph.

Speech reception test

The speech reception test measures how well a person can hear and understand words at different volumes. In this test, you listen through headphones to words spoken live or on a recording at different volumes, and you are asked to repeat them. The words start at an audible level and decrease in volume. Your speech reception threshold is the softest level at which you can recognize a two-syllable word at least 50 percent of the time.

Speech discrimination test

The speech discrimination test measures how well a person can distinguish words. In this test, you listen through headphones to a list of one-syllable words at a volume that is comfortable for you. You are asked to repeat the words. Your score is the percentage of words you have correct. A score of 90 percent or better indicates normal hearing.

Impedance test

In a healthy ear, the air pressure inside and outside the eardrum is the same. This equilibrium allows the eardrum to vibrate freely when sound waves hit it. The vibrations pass through the ear to enable us to hear, and reflect back into the air. Too much or too little air pressure on the inner side of the eardrum makes the eardrum too stiff to conduct sounds properly—more sound is reflected back, and less passes through to the inner ear.

The impedance test, or tympanometry, measures the ability of the eardrum to pass sound waves to the inner ear and detects abnormal air pressure in the middle ear, fluid in the middle ear, perforation of the eardrum, and disorders of the tiny sound-conducting bones of the middle ear. In this test, a probe covered with an airtight material (usually plastic) is inserted into the outer ear canal to seal the entrance to the ear. A transmitter in the probe pumps air through the probe to change the air pressure in the ear canal and then directs sounds to the eardrum. A receiver in the probe measures how well the eardrum absorbs the sounds. The probe has a tiny speaker (sound transmitter) and a tiny microphone (sound receiver). The difference between the sound transmitted and the sound received is the sound absorbed. Several measurements are made at different pressure levels.

Brain stem auditory evoked response test

The brain stem auditory evoked response test is a computerized hearing test that measures electrical responses in the brain stem (the part of the brain that controls basic functions) in reaction to sounds. In this test, electrodes are attached to the scalp and earlobes. You listen to clicking sounds through headphones, and a computer records the electrical activity of the brain in response to the sounds. The brain stem auditory evoked response test is used to evaluate the hearing of otherwise untestable people, such as infants, and is helpful in ruling out benign (noncancerous) tumors that can develop in the nerves involved in balance and hearing (called acoustic neuromas).

Treatment

Treatment of hearing loss depends on the cause. Conductive hearing loss can usually be corrected and hearing restored by treating the underlying

---

MY STORY | **Hearing Loss**

I noticed over the past few years that my father's hearing wasn't what it used to be. He would increase the volume on the TV and radio, and my mom would ask him to lower it because it was too loud. During conversations he often asked people to repeat themselves. I suggested that he have a hearing test, but he said his hearing was fine. He was once very active, but my mom said he started becoming more and more withdrawn and lost interest in social gatherings. He eventually stopped communicating with his friends and family because he was embarrassed about his hearing problem.

Now my father can hear again and has resumed his social life. He says his only regret was not having a hearing test sooner.

One day my mom called me and said my father had agreed to have a hearing test. After an ear examination and several tests, he was told he needed a hearing aid. The doctor told him that some hearing loss is common as a person gets older and referred him to an audiologist. The audiologist talked to my father about all the different kinds of hearing devices that are available and helped him choose the right kind of hearing aid. Now my father can hear again and has resumed his social life. He says his only regret was not having a hearing test sooner.

cause. For example, if earwax causes hearing loss, a doctor will remove the wax. Sensorineural hearing loss often cannot be corrected. However, in some people, devices such as a cochlear implant (see next page) can help restore some hearing. A number of other devices—such as hearing aids (see below), assistive devices (see next page), and alerting devices (see page 1020)—are available that can improve a person's hearing and his or her quality of life.

Hearing aids

Hearing aids are battery-powered devices that fit in the ear to electronically increase the volume of sound. Hearing aids contain a tiny microphone that transforms sounds into electrical signals, an amplifier that increases the strength of the signals, and a speaker that turns the signals into louder sounds. Some hearing aids are equipped with a device called a telecoil (also called a T-coil or T-switch), which converts electromagnetic fields into sound.

Hearing aids come in a variety of styles. Analog hearing aids are programmable or adjustable. Digital hearing aids are programmable and can be made to filter out some of the background noise and feedback that can occur with some analog hearing aids. Disposable hearing aids are available for people who have mild to moderate hearing loss.

It is important to choose both the right kind of hearing aid and one that fits properly. If you need a hearing aid, your doctor will refer you to an audiologist or a hearing aid dealer for an evaluation and fitting for a hearing aid. Tell your doctor or ear specialist immediately if you notice any deterioration in your hearing between regular checkups or after you get a hearing aid.

Behind-the-ear aid

A behind-the-ear aid contains a microphone, amplifier, and battery in a small, lightweight, plastic case worn behind the ear. The earphone, which is connected to the rest of the device by a short tube, fits into the outer ear and seals it to prevent amplified sound from being lost. People with varying degrees of hearing loss can benefit from behind-the-ear aids.

In-the-ear aid

An in-the-ear aid consists of a microphone, amplifier, and battery housed in a lightweight plastic case worn inside the ear. The aid is molded to seal the ear canal to prevent amplified sound from being lost.

These aids are less awkward to put in the ear than behind-the-ear aids, and the volume is easy to adjust. In-the-ear hearing aids are usually not recommended for children because the case has to be replaced as the child grows.

In-the-canal and completely-in-the-canal aids

In-the-canal aids, which remain only slightly visible when inside the ear, and completely-in-the-canal aids, which cannot be seen at all, are customized to fit inside the ear canal. People whose hearing loss ranges from mild to moderately severe can benefit from in-the-canal and completely-in-the-canal aids. These aids are not recommended for everyone, however, including children who are still growing. Some people may have difficulty inserting, removing, or adjusting in-the-canal aids, and excessive earwax or drainage from the ears can damage them.

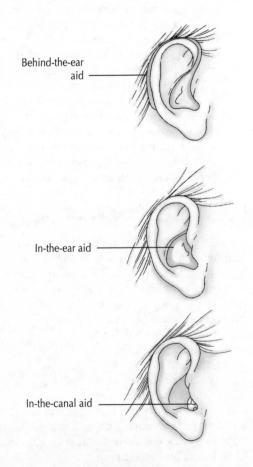

Behind-the-ear aid

In-the-ear aid

In-the-canal aid

Hearing aids

Implantable bone conduction hearing device

Some people—such as those whose ear canal has been narrowed by disease or surgery or who were born with a small ear canal that causes hearing problems—may not be able to wear a standard hearing aid. People who have chronic ear drainage or who are allergic to the plastic used in hearing aids may not be able to wear a standard hearing aid. For these people, an implantable bone conduction hearing device may be used to help improve hearing.

To implant a bone conduction hearing device, a surgeon makes an incision in the scalp behind the ear, drills a hole in the outer part of the skull, and screws a small device that contains a magnet in the hole. The person wears a microphone that converts sound waves into electrical impulses that stimulate the magnet, making it vibrate. The brain perceives the vibrations as sounds.

Cochlear implants

Some children are born with total sensorineural hearing loss, or nerve deafness, and some children and adults develop the disorder as a result of damage to the inner ear. To help a person with severe sensorineural hearing loss understand speech better, a tiny electronic device called a cochlear implant can be surgically implanted in the inner ear. Cochlear implants produce sound by stimulating undamaged nerves in the inner ear, not by amplifying sound as a hearing aid does. Cochlear implants do not restore normal hearing—they help a person distinguish speech sounds better. The benefits of cochlear implants have far exceeded expectations—most people who have cochlear implants even have some degree of hearing over the telephone (without lipreading cues). Previously used only for people with total hearing loss, the devices are being implanted in children younger than 1 year old and in adults who have some remaining hearing.

The devices are usually implanted in only one ear, but implanting them in both ears may be an option in the future. About 4 to 6 weeks after surgery to implant the receiver-stimulator (see illustration), the person is fitted with the externally worn parts of the device. Using a computer, technicians program the speech processor to make sure the frequency and pitch of the transmitted sounds are tailored to the person's needs.

Assistive devices

There are many different kinds of assistive devices. Assistive devices can improve a person's hearing, alert a person when a sound occurs, or help a person communicate.

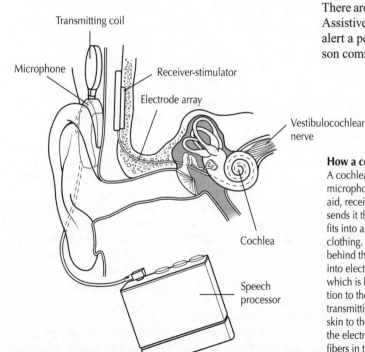

Transmitting coil

Microphone

Receiver-stimulator

Electrode array

Vestibulocochlear nerve

Cochlea

Speech processor

How a cochlear implant works

A cochlear implant has both internal and external parts. A microphone, which is worn like a behind-the-ear hearing aid, receives incoming sound from the environment and sends it through a thin cord to a speech processor, which fits into a pocket or can be worn on a belt or under or over clothing. (Newer, smaller speech processors can be worn behind the ear.) The speech processor converts the sounds into electrical signals that it sends to the transmitting coil, which is held in place against the skin by magnetic attraction to the receiver-stimulator implanted under the skin. The transmitting coil sends the electrical signals through the skin to the receiver-stimulator, which activates electrodes in the electrode array that stimulate specific groups of nerve fibers in the ear. The vestibulocochlear nerve transmits the signals to the brain, which interprets them as sound.

Assistive listening devices

Assistive listening devices are cordless devices that can be used with or without hearing aids to amplify sound, limit background noise, or overcome the effects of poor room acoustics. Headsets, earphones, or neckloops are used to send the sounds into the ears. Most assistive listening devices use one of three different technologies—FM, infrared, or inductive loop. An audiologist can help you decide what type of assistive device best suits your needs.

FM systems

FM systems transmit radio waves from a microphone used by a person who is speaking, to a receiver connected directly to a person's hearing aid or to a looped cord (worn around the person's neck). The looped cord picks up the signals and transmits them to the T-coil in the person's hearing aid. FM systems are portable and are used in classrooms, for meetings, and on tours. The microphone and transmitter are often built into the sound system at theaters, museums, or other public places. In such settings a person is given a receiver that connects to his or her hearing aid, or a special set of headphones to wear.

Infrared systems

Infrared systems use light waves to transmit sound from the transmitter to the receiver, which is worn by the user. Infrared systems are often used in homes (with TVs), theaters, and courtrooms. Bright sunlight can interfere with infrared systems.

Induction loop systems

Induction loop systems use electromagnetic fields to transmit sounds to a person's hearing aid. In induction loop systems, a loop of wire is installed around an area such as a classroom, theater, or home. Sound from a transmitting device (such as a microphone, sound system, or telephone) is turned into an electric current that is picked up by the loop of wire around the room. The loop transforms the electric current into electromagnetic energy, which stimulates a corresponding response in the T-coil of a person's hearing aid. The current then travels to the speaker in the hearing aid, where it is converted back into sound that can be heard.

Induction loop systems are used in places such as public buildings, conference halls, and theaters. Electromagnetic interference, such as from computer monitors and digital mobile phones, can interfere with induction loop systems.

Alerting devices

Alerting devices can make a person aware of sounds and help him or her communicate. Some alerting devices use light or vibrations to make a person aware of sounds. For example, the light on a lamp may flash to indicate that a doorbell is ringing, or a telephone may vibrate to indicate that it is ringing. Communication devices such as closed captioning on televisions allow a person to read what is being said, while devices such as text telephones allow conversations to be read rather than heard.

Tinnitus

Tinnitus is hearing ringing or other noises in the ear when there is no external source of sound. Tinnitus is a symptom, not a disease. It often results from an underlying condition such as an earwax blockage (see page 1025). The most common cause of tinnitus is hearing loss as a result of damage to the hair cells in the cochlea (which conveys sound information to the brain), usually caused by aging or exposure to loud noise (see page 1015). Taking some medications—such as aspirin or other nonsteroidal anti-inflammatory drugs, antidepressants, or some antibiotics—can also cause tinnitus. Some conditions—such as allergies, tumors that affect the auditory or facial nerves, or diabetes—can increase a person's risk of tinnitus.

Symptoms and Diagnosis

Tinnitus is characterized by hearing noises such as ringing, buzzing, or humming in one or both ears. The noise may vary in frequency and volume from high to low.

To evaluate tinnitus, your doctor will probably take a detailed health history, examine your ears, and ask you about any prescription or over-the-counter medications you are taking. He or she will probably refer you to an otolaryngologist (a doctor who specializes in disorders of the ear, nose, and throat) for an evaluation. You may have hearing tests (see page 1016), a CT scan (see page 112), X-rays (see page 109), or an MRI (see page 113) to rule out possible causes other than damage to your ear.

Treatment

The treatment of tinnitus depends on the cause. For example, if tinnitus is caused by a medication you are taking, your doctor will ask you to stop taking the medication or will recommend or prescribe a different one. Tinnitus caused by a medical condition can be corrected by treating the condition. Tinnitus that occurs as the result of aging or noise damage is difficult to treat. If a person has significant hearing loss, a hearing aid often can help. For people whose tinnitus causes insomnia, doctors may recommend supplements of melatonin (a hormone that regulates the body's sleep cycle) or sleep medication. Because tinnitus is usually worse when it's quiet, some people try devices called tinnitus maskers, which produce a variety of soft sounds—such as white noise—to help mask or cover up the noise heard in tinnitus.

Disorders of the Middle Ear

The most common disorders of the middle ear are infections and damage to the eardrum. Infections of the middle ear are often caused by bacteria or viruses, which enter the middle ear via the bloodstream, through a perforated eardrum, or along the eustachian tube from the back of the nasal cavity. A buildup of fluid in the middle ear is a frequent cause of hearing loss in middle ear disorders, especially in children.

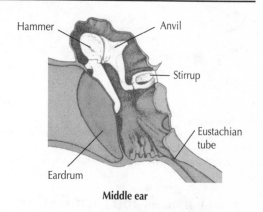

Middle ear

Barotrauma

Normally, because of air passing through the eustachian tube, the air pressure in the middle ear is the same as the air pressure in the outer ear. But if the eustachian tube becomes blocked—such as from a cold, sinus infection, or nasal allergies—an imbalance between the pressure in the middle ear and the pressure in the outer ear can result. This imbalance in pressure, called barotrauma, can stretch the eardrum, causing pain.

Barotrauma often occurs when a person who has a nose or throat infection travels in an airplane. The ascent of the plane lowers the air pressure in the cabin. If the eustachian tube does not open normally, air pressure in the middle ear becomes greater than the air pressure in the cabin. This trapped air is usually not a problem because it can be absorbed by the bloodstream or escape through the eustachian tube. However, when the airplane descends and the cabin pressure rises, the middle ear air pressure may not be equalized by the eustachian tube opening, and a vacuum develops in the middle ear. The vacuum causes the eardrum to stretch, which can be painful.

Symptoms

The symptoms of barotrauma can include moderate to severe pain in the ear, a plugged feeling in the ears, and hearing loss. You may also hear noises in the ear (tinnitus; see previous page) and feel dizzy. If the eardrum was stretched during an airplane trip, the pain usually stops when the plane lands, although the pain may persist even after the pressure inside and outside the ear is the same. Other symptoms, such as hearing loss, usually clear up within 3 to 5 hours.

Rarely, a severe imbalance in pressure can cause the eardrum to rupture (see next page), immediately relieving the pain and pressure. (You may notice a few drops of blood in your ear.) In most cases, the ruptured eardrum heals on its own. Barotrauma may also cause bleeding into the middle ear, which a doctor can see only with a lighted viewing instrument called an otoscope. The blood will reduce hearing for a few days until it is reabsorbed.

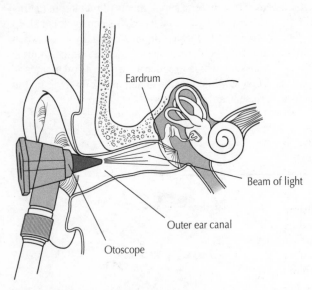

Ear examination
Doctors examine the ears with a lighted viewing instrument called an otoscope. Through the otoscope, a doctor can see many structures of the ear, including the ear canal and the eardrum.

Diagnosis and Treatment

To diagnose barotrauma, your doctor will take a detailed health history. He or she may examine the affected ear with an otoscope to look for blood in the middle ear. If you have a nose, sinus, or throat infection, your doctor may prescribe antibiotics. Your doctor will check the affected ear periodically.

Prevention

If you have a nose, sinus, or throat infection and you must fly, use a decongestant spray or oral medication before takeoff. Suck candy or chew gum, especially during the last 30 minutes of the flight, which will encourage frequent swallowing and help keep the eustachian tube open. You might also try forcing air up your eustachian tube by breathing in, holding your nose, and then trying to blow the air out while keeping your mouth closed.

Ruptured or Perforated Eardrum

The middle ear is separated from the ear canal by a thin membrane called the eardrum. The eardrum turns sound waves into vibrations that are passed along to the tiny bones of the middle ear. The eardrum can be perforated by a sharp object inserted into the ear (usually to relieve itching) or ruptured from a severe middle ear infection or a blow or other injury to the ear.

Symptoms

The symptoms of a ruptured eardrum can include pain in the ear, partial loss of hearing, or a slight discharge or bleeding from the ear. Other than the hearing loss, the symptoms usually last only a few hours.

Diagnosis and Treatment

If you have symptoms of a ruptured eardrum, cover the affected ear with a heating pad set on low, take an over-the-counter pain reliever, and see your doctor.

To diagnose a ruptured eardrum, a doctor will examine the affected ear with a lighted viewing instrument called an otoscope. If you have a ruptured eardrum, the doctor may place a temporary patch of paper over the eardrum to allow it to heal and to prevent bacteria from entering the middle ear. He or she may close a small perforation in a minor surgical procedure performed in the office. To treat or prevent an infection in the middle ear, the doctor may prescribe an antibiotic. He or she may periodically check the ear until it heals, which usually takes about 1 to 4 weeks.

After a ruptured eardrum has healed, hearing usually returns to normal. However, if the eardrum has not healed within 3 months, your doctor may recommend a procedure called tympanoplasty, in which a tiny piece of tissue is used to replace or repair the injured area of the eardrum. If any of the tiny bones of the ear are damaged, they can be repaired at the same time.

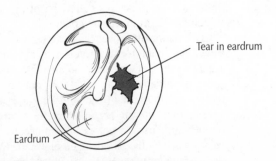

Ruptured or perforated eardrum
An object inserted into the ear, a middle ear infection, or an injury to the ear can cause a ruptured or perforated eardrum.

Acute Middle Ear Infections

An acute infection of the middle ear is a bacterial infection that usually follows a viral infection of the upper respiratory tract—such as a cold (see page 648), the flu (see page 649), or measles (see page 437)—that inflames the cells that line the middle ear cavity. Bacteria can enter the middle ear through a ruptured or perforated eardrum (see previous page). Persistent sinusitis (see page 651) often leads to a middle ear infection. Middle ear infections develop most often in children and frequently recur.

Symptoms

The symptoms of an acute middle ear infection can include a feeling of fullness or pain in the ear that may be mild or severe enough to interfere with sleep and daily activities. Other possible symptoms include chills, fever, sweating, and hearing loss in the affected ear.

If the infection is severe and is not treated, the pressure of pus collecting in the middle ear can rupture the eardrum (see previous page), producing a discharge of pus, sometimes with blood, that relieves the pain.

If you have symptoms of an acute middle ear infection, see your doctor. If treatment is delayed, the infection can spread to the mastoid bone (the bone behind the ear) and become a chronic infection (see right).

Diagnosis

To diagnose an acute infection of the middle ear, a doctor will examine your ear with a lighted viewing instrument called an otoscope. He or she also may take a sample of fluid from the ear for examination in a laboratory.

Treatment

To treat an acute infection of the middle ear, doctors usually prescribe antibiotics. In some cases, the eardrum ruptures and drains while a person is taking antibiotics. The pain usually subsides within a day or two, but fluid may be present for several weeks and cause hearing loss. If your child has an acute middle ear infection, the doctor will ask you to bring him or her in again for another evaluation within the next 6 weeks. If an acute infection of the middle ear is unusually prolonged and painful or if complications such as paralysis of a facial nerve (Bell's palsy; see page 696) develop, a doctor may recommend an outpatient procedure called myringotomy (see page 418) to remove the fluid, which helps clear up the infection.

Chronic Middle Ear Infections

Chronic middle ear infections are often the result of an ear infection that clears up but leaves a perforation or pocket that harbors bacteria and therefore is susceptible to infection. A ruptured or perforated eardrum (see previous page) that has not healed or an abnormal growth in the middle ear (cholesteatoma; see next page) can also cause a chronic infection of the middle ear.

In rare cases, the bones of the ear may become damaged, or scar tissue may fuse the bones together and prevent them from transmitting sound signals to the brain, causing permanent hearing loss.

Symptoms and Diagnosis

A chronic infection of the middle ear can produce grayish or yellowish pus that seeps from the ear periodically. The infection may cause some hearing loss, depending on how long the infection has been present.

If you have symptoms of a chronic middle ear infection, your doctor will refer you to an otolaryngologist (a doctor who specializes in disorders of the ear, nose, and throat). The otolaryngologist will examine your ear with a lighted viewing instrument called an otoscope and may perform a hearing test (see page 1016). He or she may also examine your ear with a microscope and may order a CT scan (see page 112) of your head to determine if the infection has spread.

Treatment

To treat a chronic middle ear infection, a doctor usually cleans out the ear and prescribes eardrops that contain an antibiotic (to kill the bacteria) and a corticosteroid (to reduce inflammation) or an oral antibacterial medication.

If the infection does not respond to medication, the doctor may recommend a surgical procedure called tympanoplasty to remove the remaining infected tissue and mend the tiny bones in the middle ear or replace them with plastic substitutes. He or she will then repair the eroded eardrum with a tissue graft. In many cases, the middle ear can be rebuilt to restore some hearing.

If a child has recurring middle ear infections, his or her adenoids (lymph tissue that lies on each side of the back wall of the nose and the upper part of the throat) may be acting as a reservoir for the infection-causing bacteria. In these cases, doctors sometimes recommend removing the adenoids or inserting tubes into the child's ears (myringotomy; see page 418).

Cholesteatoma

A cholesteatoma is an abnormal growth of the skin of the eardrum into the middle ear. The skin forms a cyst that fills with dead skin cells shed by the eardrum. Over time, the cyst becomes infected repeatedly and can erode the bone that lines the middle ear cavity and the delicate bones in the middle ear. A cholesteatoma can also erode the protective bone between the middle ear and the facial nerve, damage the areas of the middle ear responsible for balance and hearing, and damage the brain, including its covering and blood supply. A cholesteatoma may be congenital (present at birth), but it is usually caused by recurring middle ear infections.

Symptoms

The symptoms of a cholesteatoma can include headache, earache, weakness of the facial muscles, dizziness, and mild to moderately severe conductive hearing loss (see page 1016). In some cases, pus seeps from the ear. If a cholesteatoma erodes the roof of the middle ear cavity, you may have paralysis of the facial nerves, a false sense that you or your surroundings are moving (vertigo; see page 1012), or profound sensorineural hearing loss (see page 1016). A cholesteatoma that infects the brain can produce a pocket of pus between the membrane covering the brain and spinal cord and the bones of the skull or spine (epidural abscess; see page 695) or inflammation of the membranes that surround and protect the brain and spinal cord (meningitis; see page 692). An abscess also can form behind the ear.

Diagnosis

To diagnose a cholesteatoma, a doctor will take a detailed health history and examine the affected ear with a lighted viewing instrument called an otoscope. If the doctor suspects that you have a cholesteatoma, he or she will refer you to an otolaryngologist (a doctor who specializes in disorders of the ear, nose, and throat). The otolaryngologist will examine you and may perform hearing tests (see page 1016).

Treatment

To treat a cholesteatoma that is small or at an early stage, the otolaryngologist may remove it and thoroughly clean out the middle ear cavity in a relatively simple surgical procedure performed through the ear canal. If the cholesteatoma is large or at a later stage, damage to the middle ear may be extensive. In this case, removal of the cholesteatoma is more complicated, involving a procedure to rebuild the hearing structures, repair the broken eardrum, and clean out the mastoid bone (the bone behind the ear), often leaving it open to the ear canal. If your hearing is badly damaged by the cholesteatoma or its treatment, a hearing aid (see page 1018) may be helpful.

Cholesteatomas sometimes recur. For this reason, the otolaryngologist probably will want to examine your ears at least once a year.

Disorders of the Outer Ear

The lining of the outer ear canal is an extension of the skin of the visible ear. Most disorders of the outer ear are skin disorders. While the symptoms can be bothersome, disorders of the outer ear are generally not as serious as middle and inner ear disorders because they do not permanently affect the delicate mechanisms of hearing and balance.

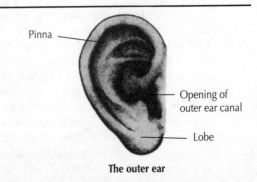

Pinna

Opening of outer ear canal

Lobe

The outer ear

Earwax Blockage

Glands in the outer ear canal produce wax to protect the canal from bacteria, dirt, and other debris. Usually, shedding of skin cells in the ear canal causes the wax and debris in the ear canal to fall out. However, in some people, excessive wax production, abnormal shedding of skin cells, use of hearing aids, or trying to clean the ear canals with cotton-tipped swabs can cause earwax to accumulate.

Symptoms and Diagnosis

The symptoms of an earwax blockage include a feeling that the ear is plugged, partial hearing loss, ringing in the ear, and sometimes earache. If you have symptoms of earwax blockage, do not try to remove the wax with a stick or swab—you could easily pack earwax against the eardrum and damage it.

See your doctor to rule out a more serious problem. He or she will examine your ears with a lighted viewing instrument called an otoscope.

Treatment

If you have an earwax blockage, the doctor may flush the ear with warm water and soften the wax with eardrops before removing it. If the wax is difficult to remove, he or she may dislodge it with a probe or electric suction device. If an earwax

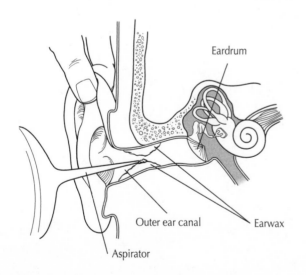

Eardrum

Outer ear canal

Earwax

Aspirator

Removing earwax
To remove earwax, a doctor injects warm water into the ear. The water flows through the ear canal, bounces off the eardrum, and flows back along the bottom of the canal, helping to clear out the wax.

blockage recurs, the doctor may recommend an over-the-counter liquid or prescribe eardrops to loosen and remove the earwax.

Infections of the Outer Ear Canal

Infections of the outer ear canal may be either local (such as a boil or abscess) or general (affecting the whole lining of the ear canal). General infections of the ear canal can result from persistent, excessive moisture in the canal, such as from swimming regularly or bathing.

Symptoms

The symptoms of an infection of the ear canal include pain when you touch the ear but not when you move your head. In some cases, yellowish green pus seeps from the ear and blocks the ear canal, which can result in temporary hearing loss.

Diagnosis and Treatment

If you have symptoms of an infection of the outer ear canal, keep your ear dry and do not try to wash it or clean it. Also, do not scratch or touch it. Place a clean cotton pad or heating pad over the ear and take an over-the-counter pain reliever. See your doctor.

To diagnose an infection of the outer ear canal, your doctor will examine your ear with a lighted viewing instrument called an otoscope. He or she may clean the ear with a suction device or a cotton-tipped probe, which usually relieves the irritation and pain. Because these infections are usually caused by bacteria, the doctor may prescribe eardrops that contain antibiotics (to clear up the infection) and corticosteroids (to reduce inflammation). If the canal is very swollen and narrow, he or she may insert a medicine-soaked wick to make sure the medicine reaches the ear canal.

Because you must keep the infected ear dry during treatment, the doctor will ask you not to swim and will recommend wearing a shower cap or using cotton covered with petroleum jelly as an earplug in the tub or shower.

If the infection does not clear up within a week, you may need to have the ear cleaned again. The doctor may then take a sample of pus to identify the bacterium that is causing the infection or to rule out a bacterial infection. He or she may also prescribe different eardrops or an oral antibiotic.

If the infection is caused by a fungus or if you develop an allergy to the medication, the infection may recur and require treatment for several weeks. In this case, your doctor may prescribe a corticosteroid cream, antifungal eardrops, or antibiotic eardrops. If the infection is caused by chronic itching or scaling, the doctor may prescribe corticosteroid eardrops and recommend precautions to take when you bathe or swim.

Tumors of the Outer Ear

Tumors of the outer ear may be either benign (noncancerous) or malignant (cancerous). On the visible portion of the ear, a noncancerous tumor may develop as a painless lump. In the ear canal, the tumor may be a hard growth of bony tissue called an osteoma.

Cancerous tumors on the visible part of the ear can resemble wartlike growths, benign tumors, or ulcers or sores that don't heal. Cancerous tumors of the outer ear are almost always skin cancers.

Symptoms
The symptoms of an osteoma can include pain, an accumulation of wax in the ear, and hearing loss. In most people, however, osteomas don't cause any symptoms.

In cancerous tumors of the outer ear, the ulcers or sores may bleed and eventually become painful. In advanced stages, cancerous tumors in the ear canal cause intense earaches and bloody drainage. If you have any of these symptoms, see your doctor immediately.

Diagnosis and Treatment
To diagnose tumors of the outer ear, a doctor will take a detailed health history and examine the affected ear. Treatment is usually not necessary for a noncancerous tumor that does not cause symptoms. However, if the tumor grows and causes pain or hearing loss, a doctor can usually remove it in a minor surgical procedure performed through the ear canal.

For a cancerous tumor on the visible part of the ear, a doctor will recommend surgery and radiation therapy (see page 23), alone or in combination. During surgery, the tumor and some of the visible portion of the ear are removed. Tumors in the ear canal may require a procedure called mastoidectomy, in which the mastoid bone (the bone behind the ear) is opened to remove any infected or cancerous tissue.

Eye Disorders

The eye is a complex and delicate structure. Each eyeball is a sphere about 1 inch in diameter, covered by three layers of tissue. The tough, white, outer layer, called the sclera, maintains the shape and size of the eyeball. Covering the sclera at the front of the eye is a transparent mucous membrane called the conjunctiva, which also lines the inside of the eyelids. At the front of the sclera is a transparent, dome-shaped, protective covering called the cornea.

The middle layer of tissue, which lies beneath the sclera, is called the choroid. The choroid contains blood vessels that supply the tissues of the eye with oxygen and nutrients. Toward the front of the eye, the choroid forms a circular ring with muscles called the ciliary body. Attached to the front of the ciliary body is the colored part of the eye, a circular curtain containing muscle fibers, called the iris. In the center of the iris is an opening called the pupil, through which light enters the eye. The dilating (widening) and constricting (narrowing) of the pupil, which are controlled by the muscle fibers of the iris, regulate the amount of light that enters the eye.

Directly behind the iris and pupil is a transparent, elastic structure called the lens, which is attached to the ciliary body. Contraction of the ciliary body muscles changes the shape of the lens and enables the eye to focus. The space between the cornea and the lens is filled with a clear, watery liquid called aqueous fluid. The

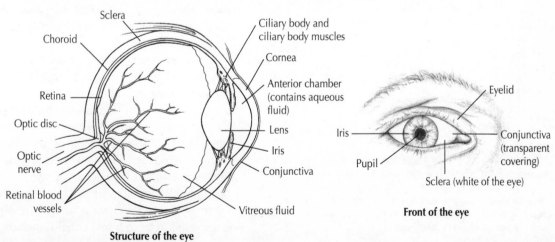

Structure of the eye

Front of the eye

Having Your Eyes Examined

If you are having vision problems, talk to your primary care doctor, or go directly to an eye care professional for diagnosis and treatment. The main types of eye care professionals are ophthalmologists (eye MDs), optometrists, and opticians.

Ophthalmologists are medical doctors with specialized training in the diagnosis and treatment of eye diseases and disorders. They perform eye examinations to evaluate vision and check for signs of eye diseases such as cataracts or glaucoma. Ophthalmologists are licensed to prescribe drugs, glasses, and contact lenses. They are also trained and licensed to perform eye surgery.

Optometrists are health professionals who are trained and licensed to diagnose and treat vision problems and to prescribe glasses and contact lenses. Optometrists are not MDs and are not licensed to perform eye surgery. In some states they are licensed to treat some eye diseases and prescribe certain drugs, such as eyedrops.

Opticians are eye care professionals who are trained to make and fit glasses and, sometimes, contact lenses, after they have been prescribed by an ophthalmologist or an optometrist. Opticians do not perform eye examinations.

How Often Should I Have My Eyes Examined?

To protect your vision, you should have regular eye examinations performed by an ophthalmologist every few years. If you are over age 40, your eyes should be examined every 2 years or as often as your doctor recommends. Some serious eye diseases, such as some types of glaucoma, produce no symptoms in the early stages and can be detected only by an eye examination.

For this reason, regular eye examinations are essential for maintaining good vision and eye health.

An Eye Examination

Before performing a thorough eye examination, an ophthalmologist asks you about your health history and your family's health history, and asks you to describe any vision problems you may be having. The examination itself usually consists of the following painless evaluations and tests:

● **Visual acuity test**   To test the acuity (sharpness) of your vision, the doctor asks you to read the rows of letters on an eye chart. The letters on the eye chart are of a standard, decreasing size, and the chart is set at a standard distance of 20 feet. To take the test, one eye is covered and you read as far down the chart as possible; then the other eye is covered and you read down the chart again. The results of a visual acuity test are given as two numbers (for example, 20/40). The first number refers to the distance at which you read the letters—20 feet. The second number refers to the distance at which a person with normal vision can read the smallest letters that you were able to read correctly at 20 feet. For example, the result 20/40 means that you were able to read letters at 20 feet that a person with normal vision would be able to read at 40 feet. Visual acuity may be different for each eye. Difficulty reading the chart may indicate a focusing disorder, usually nearsightedness (see page 1030) or farsightedness (see page 1032). It could also be a sign of a serious eye disease such as macular degeneration (see page 1046).

● **Outer eye examination**   The doctor examines the appearance of the outer eye, including the eyelids, eye-

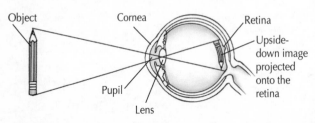

Vision
When you look at an object, light rays from the object pass through the cornea, pupil, and lens of the eye, which project an upside-down image of the object onto the retina. The retina converts the image into nerve impulses and transmits the impulses to your brain via the optic nerve. Your brain interprets the information it receives from the retina, and you see the object right side up.

space behind the lens is filled with a substance called vitreous fluid, which makes up the mass of the inside of the eyeball.

The inner layer of tissue, called the retina, lines the back of the inside of the eye. The retina includes a layer of light-sensitive nerve cells called rods and cones. The rods are very sensitive to light intensity and enable you to see in dim light. The cones detect color and detail. There are 125 million rods and 7 million cones in each eye. When you look at an object, light rays from the object pass through the cornea, pupil, and lens, and form an upside-down image of the object on the retina. The rods and cones transform the lashes, and orbits (the bony sockets in the skull that contain the eyeballs), and the surface of the eyeball, including the conjunctiva and sclera. He or she may direct a light toward and away from each eye to determine if the pupils open and close properly. To evaluate your eye muscles and the alignment of your eyes, the doctor asks you to focus on and follow a moving object, such as his or her finger. The ophthalmologist will also use a slit lamp (a powerful microscope that shines a bright light into your eye) to examine the front of the eye, including the cornea, anterior chamber, iris, lens, sclera, conjunctiva, and vitreous fluid under high magnification.

● **Visual field test**   To check your peripheral (side) vision, the ophthalmologist performs a visual field test, in which one eye is covered and you look straight ahead with the other while he or she moves an object (such as a pen) into and out of different areas of your field of vision. The doctor instructs you to respond as soon as you see the object, and he or she records your responses. In a computerized version of this test, you sit facing a screen (with your chin on a chinrest) looking straight ahead. The doctor instructs you to press a button each time you see a tiny flash of light. A computer records your responses and produces a printout for the doctor to evaluate.

● **Eye pressure test**   An ophthalmologist uses a test called applanation tonometry to measure the pressure inside your eyes. First, the doctor places a drop of a local anesthetic on each cornea to numb the eye, and then places a drop of an orange fluid called fluorescein in each eye. He or she then places the tip of an instrument called a tonometer against the cornea to measure the pressure inside the eyeball. You will not feel the tonometer against your eyeball. During the test, which is painless and takes only a few seconds, you will see a bright blue circle of light moving toward your eye. Sometimes a doctor performs a similar test called air tonometry, which uses a puff of air to measure the pressure inside the eyes, but this test is less accurate than applanation tonometry.

● **Inner eye examination**   The ophthalmologist dilates (widens) the pupils with eyedrops and looks through an ophthalmoscope (a viewing instrument that projects a bright light onto the back of the eye) to examine the structures of the inner eye, including the retina and the optic nerve.

If the doctor detects a focusing disorder, he or she may prescribe glasses or contact lenses. If you already wear glasses or contacts, he or she will probably change your prescription. If the doctor detects a more serious eye disease, he or she may order additional testing or may recommend treatment with medication or surgery.

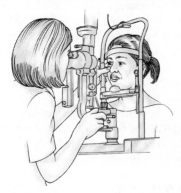

Slit lamp
A slit lamp is a powerful microscope with a light attached that enables a doctor to examine the structures at the front of the eye—the eyelid, cornea, sclera, conjunctiva, iris, and lens—under high magnification.

sensations of color, form, and light intensity that they receive into nerve impulses, which the retina then transmits along retinal nerve fibers to the optic nerve, a stalklike collection of nerves that connects the eye to the brain. The vision centers in the brain interpret nerve impulses received from each eye and integrate them into the single, right-side-up, three-dimensional image that you see. A wide variety of disorders can affect the eye and interfere with vision.

Focusing Disorders

In the eye, the cornea and lens work together to refract (bend) light rays from viewed objects and focus them on the retina, thereby producing an image. In normal vision, the light focuses directly on the retina, producing a sharp, clear image. However, if a person has a focusing disorder, the light focuses either behind or in front of the retina, producing a blurred image. The four most common focusing disorders are nearsightedness, farsightedness, astigmatism, and presbyopia.

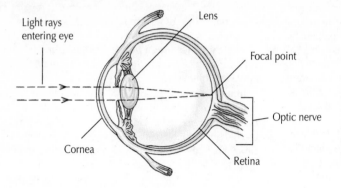

Light rays entering eye

Lens

Focal point

Optic nerve

Cornea

Retina

Normal vision
The cornea and lens of the eye act as convex (curved outward) lenses to refract (bend) light rays from a viewed object and focus them on the retina. The retina and the brain work together to transform these light rays into the image you see when you look at an object.

Nearsightedness

In nearsightedness (also called myopia), either the eyeball is too long from front to back, or the focusing power of the cornea and lens is too great. As a result, images of distant objects are focused in front of the retina and are blurred. Images of nearby objects are focused on the retina and are usually sharp and clear.

About one in every five Americans is nearsighted. The disorder usually begins to develop at about age 12 and may gradually worsen until about age 30. Nearsightedness tends to run in families.

Symptoms
The main symptom of nearsightedness is blurred vision when viewing distant objects. Constant straining to see faraway objects can produce headaches and eyestrain (aching in the eyes). If you have any problems with your vision, see an ophthalmologist (eye MD) for a thorough eye examination (see previous pages).

Diagnosis and Treatment
A diagnosis of nearsightedness is based on the symptoms, a family health history, an eye examination, and the results of vision tests.

To correct nearsightedness a doctor will prescribe glasses or contact lenses that move the focal point for distant objects backward onto the retina to bring them into clear focus. Although nearsightedness is not likely to worsen after age 30, you should continue seeing your ophthalmologist for regular eye examinations.

Doctors may recommend a surgical procedure called LASIK (see below) to correct nearsightedness in people who cannot or do not want to wear glasses or contact lenses.

LASIK
LASIK (which stands for laser-assisted in situ keratomileusis) is a surgical procedure that uses a laser (a highly concentrated beam of light) to reshape the cornea (the clear, protective covering at the front of the eye) to improve the focusing power of the eye. LASIK surgery is used to correct nearsightedness, farsightedness, and astigmatism.

LASIK can also be performed to produce monovision, in which one eye is corrected for far vision clarity and the other eye is left nearsighted or corrected for reading (near) vision clarity. The procedure is not recommended for children under age 18 because their eyes are still developing. It is also not recommended for people whose eyewear has a very weak correction or a very powerful correction or for people who have certain eye diseases, such as

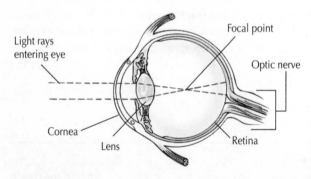

Light rays entering eye

Focal point

Optic nerve

Cornea

Lens

Retina

Nearsightedness
In nearsightedness, the cornea and lens focus the light rays from distant objects in front of the retina, producing a blurred image. Nearby objects are usually seen clearly.

Contact Lenses

Contact lenses are thin, transparent, plastic disks that fit closely over the cornea (the clear, protective covering at the front of the eye) to help correct focusing disorders, including nearsightedness (see previous page), farsightedness (see next page), or astigmatism (see page 1033).

The three main types of contact lenses are hard lenses, gas-permeable hard lenses, and soft lenses. Hard lenses are made of tough plastic and are inexpensive and durable, but many people find them uncomfortable and difficult to wear. Gas-permeable hard lenses are more comfortable than hard lenses but are less durable and more expensive. Soft lenses are the most comfortable and easy to wear but are the most fragile. Extended-wear soft lenses can be worn continuously for several weeks. However, continuous wear increases the risk of eye infections.

Before prescribing contact lenses, an ophthalmologist or optometrist will examine your eyes to determine if contact lenses are appropriate for you. For example, if you have dry eyes, you may not be able to wear contacts. If contacts are appropriate for you, the ophthalmologist will then decide which type of lens will work best for you. He or she will show you how to insert and remove your lenses and tell you how to care for them.

Proper Use and Care of Contact Lenses

Proper use and care of your contact lenses will help protect your eyes and vision and can prolong the life of the lenses themselves. Here are some helpful tips:

- Before touching your lenses, wash your hands with mild soap, rinse them thoroughly, and dry them with a clean, lint-free towel.
- Handle the same lens first every time to help prevent mixing up the right and left lenses.
- Clean and disinfect your lenses every time you remove them, using only sterile, commercial lens care products recommended by your ophthalmologist. Follow package directions.
- Keep the lens storage case clean and fill it with fresh disinfecting solution each time you remove your lenses.
- Inspect each lens for tears, cracks, or nicks before inserting it into your eye.
- Remove your lenses right away and call your ophthalmologist if you experience redness, irritation, discomfort, or pain in your eyes, or if you have vision problems.
- Remove your lenses before showering, swimming, or sleeping.
- Avoid getting cosmetics such as creams, lotions, or hair spray on your lenses.
- Talk to your doctor before using any over-the-counter or prescription eyedrops or ointments.
- See your ophthalmologist at least once a year (or as often as he or she recommends) to help prevent or detect possible problems, and ask him or her any questions you may have about using or caring for your contact lenses.

dry eye (see page 1037), or very large pupils. People with some disorders (such as autoimmune diseases) and people who take medications that might interfere with healing are not good candidates for LASIK. Not all people who have the surgery achieve 20/20 vision without glasses or contact lenses. If you use reading glasses, you may still need to use them after surgery.

An eye surgeon will examine your eyes and take a personal health history to determine whether you are a good candidate for the procedure. Because some types of contact lenses change the shape of the cornea, your doctor may ask you to stop wearing your lenses several weeks before this initial evaluation. He or she also may ask you to avoid wearing eye makeup, creams, lotions, or perfumes for several days before the surgery to minimize irritation to your eyes.

The procedure takes less than 30 minutes. Surgery can be done on both eyes at the same time (called bilateral simultaneous LASIK). Before surgery you will be given eyedrops to numb the eye, and you may be given an oral sedative to help you relax. The doctor will apply an eye clamp and suction device to the eye, which can cause some discomfort. He or she cuts a tiny flap in the cornea, uses a laser to reshape the targeted corneal tissue, and puts the flap back into position.

Immediately after the surgery, your eyes may burn, itch, and water, and your vision will probably be blurry. The burning and itching can last for a few hours. Your vision may be blurry until your eyes have healed. You may need to wear an eye shield to protect your eyes and to prevent the corneal flaps from dislodging. You may feel tired for a day or so after the surgery. If your eyes feel dry, your doctor will prescribe special eyedrops. Don't use anything in or around your eyes (especially right after surgery) that has not been approved by your ophthalmologist.

Complications from LASIK surgery include eye inflammation and infection. In people who undergo LASIK in both eyes at the same time, the same complication may occur in each eye. In this case, a doctor may prescribe medicated eyedrops. If any type of material gets beneath the corneal flap, the doctor may have to lift the flap, remove the material, and replace the flap.

Corneal refractive therapy

Corneal refractive therapy (also called orthokeratology or ortho-k) is a nonsurgical procedure that may temporarily lessen nearsightedness and astigmatism. In corneal refractive therapy, a series of rigid, gas-permeable contact lenses is used to gradually reshape (flatten) the cornea (the clear, protective covering at the front of the eye), improving vision. Each lens in the series is worn overnight every night for a period of 2 to 8 weeks, until optimal vision is attained. However, because corneal refractive therapy does not produce permanent results, retainer contact lenses must be worn for several hours every few days (or more often) to maintain the new shape of the cornea. If retainer lenses are not used, the cornea will gradually return to its original shape. Poorly fitting lenses can cause eye discomfort and distorted vision.

Farsightedness

In farsightedness (also called hyperopia), either the eyeball is too short from front to back or there is a weakness in the focusing ability of the cornea and lens. As a result, images of nearby objects can be focused behind the retina and are blurred. Images of distant objects are focused on the retina and are usually seen clearly. Farsightedness is usually congenital (present from birth) and tends to run in families.

Symptoms

The main symptom of farsightedness is blurred vision or eyestrain (aching in the eyes) when viewing nearby objects. However, in younger people, mild farsightedness often produces no noticeable symptoms. In older people, constant straining to

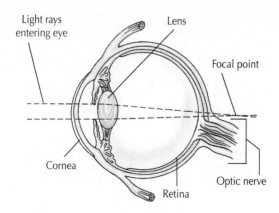

Farsightedness
In farsightedness, the cornea and lens focus the light rays from nearby objects behind the retina, producing a blurred image. Distant objects are usually seen clearly.

focus on nearby objects can produce headaches and eyestrain. If you have any problems with your vision, see an ophthalmologist (eye MD) for a thorough eye examination (see page 1028).

Diagnosis and Treatment

A diagnosis of farsightedness is based on the symptoms, a family health history, an eye examination, and the results of vision tests.

In younger people, mild farsightedness is often overcome by a natural process called accommodation, in which the ciliary body muscles (muscles surrounding the lens that help to control the shape of the lens) contract to thicken the lens and make it more convex. This brings the focal point for nearby objects forward onto the retina and produces a sharp, clear image. Farsighted people whose eyes can accommodate well usually do not need treatment.

To correct farsightedness, a doctor will prescribe glasses or contact lenses to boost the focusing power of the cornea and lens and move the focal point forward onto the retina to enable you to see more clearly. As you get older, usually beginning after age 40, the ciliary body muscles in the eye may gradually weaken. For this reason, you will probably need stronger glasses every few years. In some cases, ophthalmologists may recommend LASIK (see page 1030) to correct farsightedness.

Presbyopia

At rest, the lens in the normal eye is focused for distance vision. To focus on closer objects, the ciliary body muscles in the eye contract to thicken the lens and make it more convex (curved outward), a natural process called accommodation. With age, the lens of the eye hardens, gradually reducing its ability to accommodate (focus on nearby objects). This condition, called presbyopia, usually develops when a person is in his or her mid-40s, and gradually worsens as he or she gets older.

Symptoms

In presbyopia, a person can focus on nearby objects only by holding them at a distance. For example, to read, the person may need to hold a book or newspaper at arm's length from his or her eyes. If you find that close objects are slightly blurred unless you hold them away from you, see an ophthalmologist (eye MD) for a thorough eye examination (see page 1028).

Diagnosis and Treatment

A diagnosis of presbyopia is based on the symptoms, an eye examination, and the results of vision tests.

To correct presbyopia, your doctor will prescribe glasses to compensate for the inability of the lens to focus, which will enable you to see nearby objects clearly. You will need slightly stronger glasses every few years as you get older, until about age 65, to compensate for your decreasing focusing ability. After age 65, the lenses of the eyes stop changing.

If you are already wearing glasses to correct a focusing disorder, you can avoid the need for two pairs of glasses by getting bifocals. In bifocals, the upper part of each lens is for distance vision and the lower part is for close vision. Some types of bifocals gradually change strength from the middle of the lens to the bottom without a visible line between the lenses. Bifocal contact lenses are also available, or you may want to consider wearing a contact lens focused for distance vision in one eye and a contact lens focused for close vision in the other eye (called monovision).

Astigmatism

Astigmatism is distorted vision caused by an uneven curvature of the front surface of the cornea (the clear, protective covering at the front of the eye). This uneven shape prevents light from focusing properly on the retina.

Symptoms

Although mild astigmatism usually does not produce noticeable symptoms, more severe astigmatism may cause a person to see vertical, horizontal, or diagonal lines out of focus. Astigmatism commonly occurs along with farsightedness (see previous page) or nearsightedness (see page 1030), but in some people with astigmatism, vision may be blurred at all distances. If you have any problems with your vision, see an ophthalmologist (eye MD) for a thorough eye examination (see page 1028).

Diagnosis and Treatment

A diagnosis of astigmatism is based on the symptoms, an eye examination, and the results of vision tests.

Mild astigmatism usually does not need to be corrected. To correct more severe astigmatism and enable a person to see clearly, a doctor prescribes glasses or contact lenses that are shaped to the curvature of the cornea. The shape compensates for the unevenness of the surface of the cornea. In some cases, ophthalmologists recommend LASIK (see page 1030) to correct astigmatism.

Disorders of the Eyelids

The eyelids are movable folds of skin that cover and protect the visible surface of the eye. Muscles in the eyelids open and close them and work with fibrous and elastic tissue in the eyelids to keep them snug against the eyeball. A row of small glands, called meibomian glands, lubricates the edges of the eyelids. Rows of hairs (eyelashes), which also help protect the eye, grow from tiny pits called follicles at the edges of both the upper and lower eyelids.

Ptosis

Ptosis is a condition in which the upper eyelid droops and partially or completely covers the eye. Ptosis may be congenital (present from birth) and can run in families. However, it also can occur in anyone at any age if the nerve that controls the eyelid muscle or the muscle itself is damaged. The nerve can be damaged by an injury, an underlying disease such as diabetes (see page 889), or a brain tumor (see page 682). The muscle can be weakened as a result of muscular dystrophy (see page 972) or myasthenia gravis (see page 701) or as a natural result of aging. Ptosis may affect one or both eyes and may vary in severity over the course of each day.

Symptoms

Severe ptosis can prevent a person from seeing out of the affected eye. If ptosis is caused by a brain tumor, the person may have double vision.

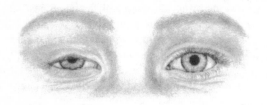

Ptosis
In ptosis, the upper eyelid droops and partially or completely covers the eye. In some cases, this condition may result from diabetes or a brain tumor, or it may be a symptom of a muscle or nerve disorder such as muscular dystrophy or myasthenia gravis.

Diagnosis and Treatment

A diagnosis of ptosis is based on the symptoms and an examination of the eye and eyelid. Ptosis usually improves after successful treatment of any underlying disease. In people whose vision is impaired as a result of ptosis, surgery can be performed to raise the drooping eyelid.

Stye

Like all hairs, eyelashes grow from tiny pits in the skin called follicles. When a follicle on the eyelid becomes infected, a swelling called a stye develops on the edge of the eyelid around the base of the eyelash (see page 128).

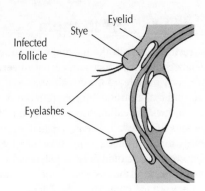

Stye
A red, painful swelling called a stye can develop on the edge of the eyelid when a hair follicle becomes infected. Styes often recur, and several may develop on the eyelid at the same time.

Symptoms

A stye is usually red and is often painful, especially when touched. Gradually, a white head of pus appears on the swelling. Several styes may develop at the same time if the bacteria that are causing the infection spread to other follicles. A stye usually bursts and drains within a few days after it forms, relieving the pain. The swelling usually subsides after about a week.

Treatment

To help a stye drain earlier, apply frequent warm, moist compresses as soon as it appears, to help draw the pus to a head. Do not squeeze the stye—allow it to open and release the pus on its own. Afterward, wash the eyelid carefully with mild soap or baby shampoo, using a clean, soft washcloth to remove all of the pus. Be careful not to spread the infection.

If a stye does not clear up in a week or so, if the swelling, redness, or tenderness spreads, or if a stye recurs, see your doctor. He or she will examine you, perform tests to determine what type of bacterium is causing the infection, and prescribe an antibiotic to treat the infection.

Chalazion

A chalazion is a painless swelling on the edge of the eyelid (see page 128) that results from inflammation of one of the meibomian glands, which lubricate the edge of the eyelid.

Symptoms and Treatment

Chalazions may be small or may grow large enough to cause blurred vision. Although small chalazions usually go away on their own within a month or two, you can speed the process by applying frequent warm, moist compresses to the affected area. For larger chalazions or chalazions that have become infected, a doctor may prescribe antibiotics, corticosteroid eyedrops, or surgery. To remove a chalazion, the doctor administers a local anesthetic, makes a small incision in the eyelid, and scrapes out the contents of the chalazion.

Papilloma

A papilloma is a slow-growing, benign (noncancerous) skin growth that can develop anywhere on the eyelid.

Symptoms and Treatment

The color of a papilloma can range from pink to skin-toned. Although a small, inconspicuous papilloma does not need treatment, a doctor may recommend surgery to remove a large, unsightly papilloma. Surgery is usually performed using local anesthesia in a doctor's office or in an outpatient facility.

Xanthelasma

In xanthelasma, yellow patches of fatty material (called xanthomas) accumulate beneath the skin of the eyelids (see page 128), especially near the nose. Xanthelasma usually occurs in older people and is often associated with elevated levels of cholesterol (a fatlike substance in the blood) and triglycerides (the main type of fat in the blood).

Treatment

Unsightly patches of xanthelasma can be removed surgically. However, they frequently recur, especially if a person's triglyceride and cholesterol levels remain high.

Entropion

In entropion, the edge of the eyelid—usually the lower lid—turns inward toward the eye (see page 128), causing the eyelid and eyelashes to rub against the surface of the eyeball. This continuous rubbing causes the eye to become inflamed and can damage the conjunctiva (the transparent membrane that covers the white of the eye and lines the eyelids) and cornea (the clear, protective covering at the front of the eye).

Entropion usually affects older people. As people age, the fibrous tissue on the lower eyelid loosens, allowing the muscle in the edge of the eyelid to contract abnormally and pull the edge of the eyelid in toward the eye. In some cases, an injury causes scarring on the inner surface of the eyelid, which can pull the edge of the eyelid in.

Symptoms

The symptoms of entropion include pain and redness in the eye, excessive tearing, and discharge and crusting of mucus. If not treated, entropion can lead to conjunctivitis (see page 1038), corneal ulcers (see page 1037), and vision problems.

Diagnosis and Treatment

A diagnosis of entropion is based on the symptoms and an examination of the affected eyelid. If the lower eyelid is turned inward, the doctor may recommend turning the eyelid outward to its normal position and holding it there for a few days by attaching one end of a piece of adhesive tape to the eyelid (below the eyelashes) and the other end to the cheek. In some cases, this corrects the condition. The doctor may prescribe eyedrops or ointments to help relieve the pain and inflammation. If entropion persists, an ophthalmologist may recommend surgery to turn the eyelid outward and prevent it from rubbing on the surface of the eyeball. The procedure is usually performed using local anesthesia in a doctor's office or in an outpatient facility.

Ectropion

In ectropion, the edge of the eyelid is turned outward and downward away from the eyeball (see page 128), causing the surface of the eye and the lining of the eyelid to become dry and inflamed. The abnormal position of the eyelid interferes with normal drainage of tears from the eye, causing them to run down the cheek. Losing tears this way can lead to inadequate lubrication of the eyeball, which can damage the cornea (the clear, protective covering at the front of the eye).

Ectropion usually occurs in older people, when aging stretches the tendons of the muscle in the lower eyelid that keep the eyelid snug against the eyeball. The condition can also occur at any age if a scar that has formed on the lower eyelid or cheek tightens or contracts, pulling the eyelid down. If ectropion is not treated, the cornea may be damaged and corneal ulcers (see next page) may form.

Symptoms, Diagnosis, and Treatment

The symptoms of ectropion include pain and redness in the eye, inflammation, discharge and crusting of mucus, infections, vision problems, and watering eye (see page 1038).

A diagnosis of ectropion is based on the symptoms and an examination of the affected eyelid. Because ectropion rarely goes away on its own, the doctor will probably recommend surgery to tighten the lower eyelid and move it back to its normal position beneath the eye. The procedure is usually performed using local anesthesia in a doctor's office or in an outpatient facility.

Blepharitis

Blepharitis is inflammation of the eyelids. The disorder occurs more often in people who have dandruff (see page 1075), oily skin, dry eye (see next page), rosacea (see page 1066), or seborrheic dermatitis (see page 1063). In some cases, a bacterial infection develops and makes the condition worse. Often, flakes from the eyelids enter the eye and cause an inflammatory condition called conjunctivitis (see page 1038).

In severe cases of blepharitis, small ulcers may develop on the edges of the eyelids and, in rare cases, the eyelashes may fall out. Persistent inflammation can lead to the development of corneal ulcers (see next page).

Symptoms, Diagnosis, and Treatment

The symptoms of blepharitis include redness, itching, and swelling of the eyelids; greasy, scaly, flaky upper and lower eyelids; and discharge and crusting of mucus around the eyes.

A diagnosis of blepharitis is based on the symptoms and an examination of the eye. To treat blepharitis, a doctor may recommend gently washing away the scaly flakes (morning and night) with a clean, soft washcloth moistened with a solution of warm water and mild, diluted baby shampoo. Rinse the affected area with warm water and pat it dry with a clean, soft towel. If the condition does not improve within 2 weeks, the doctor may prescribe an antibiotic ointment to rub into the edges of the eyelids after washing. He or she may also prescribe eyedrops containing a corticosteroid drug to relieve inflammation. Blepharitis often recurs after treatment.

Disorders of the Outer Eye

A sensitive, transparent mucous membrane called the conjunctiva lines most of the visible surface of the eye (except for the cornea) and the inner surface of each eyelid. A thin film of watery fluid (tears), which is produced by the lacrimal glands above each eyeball and by glands in the conjunctiva, lubricates and cleanses the eye and allows the lid to move over it smoothly as you blink. Tears drain away from each eye along two channels called the lacrimal canals. A tiny hole (lacrimal punctum) at the inner edge of each eyelid marks the opening of the channel, which leads to the lacrimal sac at the side of the nose. From there, the tears pass down the nasolacrimal duct into the nasal cavity.

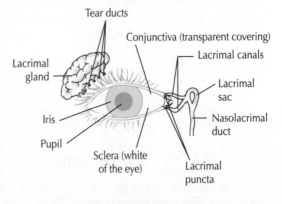

The outer eye

Dry Eye

Dry eye is a condition that results from inadequate tear production. Although dry eye often occurs in people who have rheumatoid arthritis (see page 918) or Sjögren's syndrome (see page 926), in many cases the condition occurs for no obvious reason. Dry eye usually develops in middle age and affects women more often than men. Usually both eyes are affected.

Symptoms

In dry eye, the conjunctiva (the transparent membrane that covers the white of the eye and lines the eyelids) may become red and swollen. The eye may feel irritated and gritty. Other possible symptoms include a dry mouth and joint pain.

Diagnosis and Treatment

A diagnosis of dry eye is based on the symptoms and an examination of the eye. To relieve discomfort, the doctor will probably prescribe eyedrops called artificial tears, which you may need to use for the rest of your life. In severe cases of dry eye, doctors may prescribe lubricating ointments or recommend a procedure to block the ducts that drain tears from the eye.

Corneal Ulcer

A corneal ulcer is an open sore or break in the surface of the cornea (the clear, protective covering at the front of the eye). In most cases, a corneal ulcer begins as a scratch or other injury to the cornea that becomes infected by a bacterium, virus, or fungus. An infection can also be spread from another part of the body, such as when a person with a cold sore (which is caused by the herpes simplex virus) touches his or her mouth and then touches his or her eyes. Conditions that interfere with normal lubrication of the eyes by tears—such as entropion (see page 1035), ectropion (see page 1035), or dry eye (see above)—or using extended-wear contact lenses can increase the risk of corneal ulcers. People whose eyes are exposed to a spray of particles, such as wood or metal shavings, are also at increased risk.

If a corneal ulcer is not treated promptly, a scar can form on the cornea and impair vision. An infected ulcer may perforate the cornea and allow the infection to enter the eyeball, causing blindness.

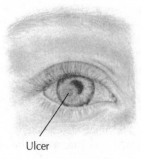
Ulcer

Corneal ulcer
A corneal ulcer is an open sore or break in the surface of the cornea caused by an infection. The ulcer may be visible as a whitish patch on the cornea.

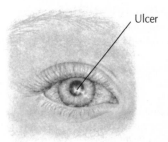
Ulcer

Dendritic ulcer of the cornea
A dendritic ulcer of the cornea is caused by a herpes simplex infection and is usually not visible to the naked eye. Staining the eye with special fluorescent eyedrops reveals the ulcer's branchlike structure.

Symptoms

The symptoms of a corneal ulcer usually include discomfort or pain in the eye, redness (see page 127), increased sensitivity to light, and impaired vision. The ulcer's effect on vision depends on its size and location. If a corneal ulcer is caused by a bacterial infection, the ulcer may be visible as a whitish patch on the cornea. An ulcer produced by a herpes simplex virus infection (dendritic ulcer) is usually not visible to the naked eye.

Diagnosis and Treatment

A corneal ulcer is diagnosed by the symptoms and an examination of the eye. If the doctor suspects that a dendritic ulcer may be present on the cornea, he or she may place special fluorescent eyedrops in the eye that stain and reveal the ulcer to confirm the diagnosis.

To treat a corneal ulcer caused by a bacterial infection, doctors prescribe antibiotics, given as drops, ointment, tablets, or injections. For a corneal ulcer caused by a herpes simplex virus infection, doctors prescribe antiviral medication in eyedrops or in an ointment. Corneal ulcers caused by fungi are treated with eyedrops that contain antifungal medication.

If scarring from corneal ulcers severely impairs a person's vision, a doctor may recommend a cornea transplant (see below), a surgical procedure in which the damaged cornea is removed and replaced with a healthy cornea from a donor. If an ulcer has perforated the cornea, immediate surgery is required to seal the hole and prevent the infection from entering the eyeball.

Cornea Transplants

A cornea transplant is a surgical procedure that is used to restore vision when the cornea has been permanently damaged as a result of injury, infection, disease, or degeneration. A surgeon performs a cornea transplant in a hospital operating room using either local or general anesthesia. The procedure lasts about 1 to 2 hours and does not usually require an overnight stay in the hospital.

To perform the transplant, a surgeon uses a special surgical instrument (called a trephine) that works like a cookie cutter to remove the central portion of the damaged cornea. He or she then places a clear cornea supplied by an organ donor into the opening in the damaged cornea and sews it into place with very fine thread. The stitches remain in the cornea for up to a year or longer, until the cornea has healed completely. You will need to wear a patch over the eye for a few days after surgery to keep it from moving and dislodging the stitches.

The ophthalmologist will examine your eye regularly to ensure that the cornea is healing properly. He or she will ask you to avoid rubbing or pressing on the eye and may recommend wearing a shield over the eye at night to protect it while you sleep. You will not be able to see clearly for several months after surgery, until the cornea heals. After the cornea has healed, the stitches are easily and painlessly removed at the ophthalmologist's office. You will need to wear glasses or contact lenses to see clearly.

Your immune system may try to reject the new cornea. For this reason, your doctor will ask you to watch carefully for any signs of rejection, such as redness or pain in the eye, increased sensitivity to light, or reduced vision. If you have any of these symptoms, call your ophthalmologist immediately so that he or she can begin treatment to combat the immune system's rejection of the transplanted cornea.

Watering Eye

A watering eye is an uncommon condition characterized by continuous tearing of the eye. Sometimes the condition occurs when a foreign object in the eye causes excessive tear formation. In other cases, a blocked nasolacrimal duct (the duct that drains tears from the eye into the nose), either as the result of an injury to the bone at the side of the nose or from long-term inflammation such as sinusitis (see page 651), prevents normal tear drainage. A blocked nasolacrimal duct can lead to an infection, as bacteria that would normally be washed from the eye build up inside the lacrimal sac. Watering eye usually occurs in people who are middle-aged or older.

Symptoms and Treatment

The symptoms of watering eye include excessive tearing and discharge from the eye. If an infection develops, redness and painful swelling occur on the affected side of the nose.

If the ophthalmologist finds a foreign object in the eye, he or she will remove the object, which should relieve the symptoms. If a nasolacrimal duct is blocked, the doctor may attempt to clear it by inserting a probe into the duct or by irrigating the duct with a sterile saline (saltwater) solution. If these measures are not effective, the doctor may recommend surgery to create an artificial nasolacrimal passageway that bypasses the blockage. If the blocked duct is infected, the doctor may prescribe antibiotics (in pills or in eyedrops) to clear up the infection before performing surgery.

Conjunctivitis

Conjunctivitis (also called pinkeye) is inflammation of the conjunctiva, the transparent membrane that covers the white of the eye and lines the eyelids (see page 127). Conjunctivitis is a common condition that can result from a bacterial or viral infection or from an allergy.

Both bacterial and viral conjunctivitis are extremely contagious and can be transmitted from eye to eye or to another person through contact with a contaminated finger, handkerchief, washcloth, or towel. Viral conjunctivitis is very common among young children and can occur with a viral infection of the upper respiratory tract such as a cold. Bacterial conjunctivitis occurs less often but can be more serious. Allergic conjunctivitis is caused by exposure to an allergen (such as pollen or cosmetics) that causes an allergic reaction in which the immune system produces antibodies (infection-fighting proteins) to attack the allergen.

If a pregnant woman is infected with the sexually transmitted disease genital herpes (see page 482), chlamydia (see page 477), or gonorrhea (see page 480), her newborn (up to about 3 days old) may develop a form of conjunctivitis called neonatal ophthalmia from coming into contact with the lining of the cervix during delivery. Neonatal ophthalmia is a potentially serious condition that can result in blindness if not treated.

Symptoms

In all forms of conjunctivitis, the normally clear conjunctiva turns pink or red and the eye feels gritty when you blink. The eye also has a discharge that forms a crust overnight. Bacterial conjunctivitis usually produces a thick, yellow discharge of pus; viral and allergic conjunctivitis usually produce a clear, watery discharge. Viral conjunctivitis also can cause a sore throat and swollen lymph nodes in front of the ears. Additional symptoms of allergic conjunctivitis include puffy, itchy eyes and a runny nose.

Diagnosis and Treatment

A diagnosis of conjunctivitis is based on the symptoms and an examination of the affected eye. If the doctor suspects bacterial conjunctivitis, he or she may take a sample of fluid or discharge from the eye for laboratory analysis.

To treat bacterial conjunctivitis, the doctor will recommend gently washing away any discharge with warm water and applying prescription antibiotic eyedrops or ointment to the eyes. The condition should clear up after 1 week. Viral conjunctivitis usually goes away on its own within 7 to 10 days. To treat allergic conjunctivitis, a doctor may recommend using nonprescription or prescription eyedrops to reduce the allergy symptoms. You will also need to identify and avoid exposure to the allergen to prevent future episodes of allergic conjunctivitis. To treat neonatal ophthalmia, a doctor may cleanse the baby's eyes and eyelids of any discharge, apply

antibiotic eyedrops to the eyes, and give antibiotics intravenously (through a vein).

To help prevent conjunctivitis from spreading, wash your hands frequently, and keep them away from your eyes. Use your own towels and washcloths and change them daily, and wash your towels, washcloths, sheets, and pillowcases in hot water.

Subconjunctival Hemorrhage

A subconjunctival hemorrhage is leaking of blood from a small blood vessel in the eye into the area between the conjunctiva and the sclera (the white of the eye). A subconjunctival hemorrhage may be caused by an eye injury or infection, or may develop as a result of coughing, sneezing, straining, or any other activity that increases the pressure in the blood vessels in the head and neck. A subconjunctival hemorrhage also may be associated with taking blood thinners. Sometimes a subconjunctival hemorrhage occurs suddenly, for no obvious reason.

Symptoms, Diagnosis, and Treatment

The main symptom of a subconjunctival hemorrhage is a bright red patch on the sclera. A diagnosis of subconjunctival hemorrhage is based on the symptoms and an examination of the eye.

In most cases, a subconjunctival hemorrhage is harmless and the red patch goes away on its own after about a week. However, if the patch results from an injury or is painful, call your doctor right away. You may have a serious eye injury or an underlying disorder that needs treatment. If you are taking anticoagulant drugs (blood thinners), talk to your doctor as soon as possible. He or she may need to reduce the dosage of the drug or prescribe another anticoagulant.

Scleritis

Scleritis is inflammation of the sclera (the white of the eye). The condition is rare and sometimes occurs along with rheumatoid arthritis (see page 918) or a digestive disorder such as Crohn's disease (see page 764). Scleritis usually affects people between ages 30 and 60. If the condition is not treated, the inflamed tissue could become perforated. Scleritis can affect one or both eyes.

Symptoms

The symptoms of scleritis include one or more dark red patches, widespread inflammation and redness in the white of the eye, and dull, aching pain in the eye. If the inflammation occurs at the back of the eye, vision may be impaired.

Diagnosis and Treatment

A diagnosis of scleritis is based on the symptoms and an examination of the eye. Mild or moderate cases of scleritis are usually treated with anti-inflammatory medications such as corticosteroids, taken in eyedrops or in tablets. In severe cases, doctors may prescribe immune-suppressing drugs, which dampen the abnormal immune response and relieve inflammation. If the sclera is perforated, surgery is necessary to repair the damage.

Uveitis

Uveitis is inflammation of the uvea, which consists of the iris (the colored part of the eye), the ciliary body (the ring of muscles that focus the lens), and the choroid (the layer of blood vessels beneath the retina). The condition is called iritis when the inflammation is confined to the iris, cyclitis when it is confined to the ciliary body, and choroiditis (see page 1052) when it is confined to the choroid.

Uveitis is rare, and the cause is usually unknown. However, in some cases, the disorder may result from an autoimmune disorder (in which the immune system mistakenly attacks body tissues) or from infection with a virus such as the herpes simplex virus or herpes zoster virus. Uveitis can occur at any age, but it occurs most frequently in young adults. The disorder can affect one or both eyes.

Because untreated uveitis can lead to serious complications—such as cataracts (see next page); glaucoma (see page 1042); the growth of new, abnormally fragile blood vessels on the retina; or blindness—early detection and treatment are crucial.

Symptoms and Diagnosis

The symptoms of uveitis include eye discomfort, pain, or redness; increased sensitivity to light; and blurred vision. The symptoms may be mild or severe. A diagnosis of uveitis is based on the symptoms and an eye examination.

Treatment

To treat uveitis, a doctor usually prescribes a corticosteroid drug in the form of eyedrops, an ointment, an injection, or a pill to relieve the pain and inflammation. Doctors may also prescribe eyedrops that dilate the pupil to prevent the back of the inflamed iris from sticking to the front of the lens, which could block the flow of fluid out of the eyeball, increasing pressure inside the eyeball. Even with effective treatment, the condition may recur.

Disorders of the Inner Eye

The lens is a transparent, elastic structure inside the eye that enables the eye to focus. It is directly behind the iris (the colored part of the eye) and is attached to a circular muscular ring called the ciliary body. When you look at an object, the ciliary body contracts, changing the shape of the lens and increasing the focusing power of the eye.

The membrane that lines the inside of the back of the eye is called the retina. The retina is covered with nerve cells—called rods and cones—that are specially adapted to detecting light. The cones, which detect fine detail and color, are located more densely in the macula, an area in the center of the retina at the very back of the inside of the eyeball. For this reason, you have to look straight at an object to see it clearly. The rods, which are sensitive to the intensity of the light entering the eye, are located throughout the retina.

When light passes through the cornea, pupil, and lens at the front of the eye, the light rays focus on the retina, which transforms them into nerve impulses. The impulses then pass along the optic nerve at the back of the eye to the areas of the brain that control vision, where they are perceived as images.

Cataracts

A cataract is clouding of the lens of the eye (see page 127). As protein fibers in the lens clump together, the clouding worsens and prevents some light rays from passing through the lens and reaching the retina, the light-sensitive membrane that lines the inside of the back of the eye. Because cataracts usually develop very slowly, early vision changes may not be noticeable. However, as the cataract grows denser, the person's vision gradually worsens. Cataracts usually do not cause pain.

There are several different types of cataracts. Congenital cataracts are present from birth, or cataracts may develop during childhood. In adults,

the most common type of cataract is an age-related cataract, which can begin to develop when a person is in his or her 40s or 50s. Most cataracts are age-related. Another type of cataract is a secondary cataract, which usually develops in people with a chronic disease, especially diabetes (see page 889). A traumatic cataract is a cataract that develops as a result of an eye injury.

Although the exact cause of cataracts is unknown, doctors think that factors such as smoking, excessive exposure to sunlight, uncontrolled diabetes, and long-term use of corticosteroid drugs (medications used to reduce inflammation from chronic diseases such as rheumatoid arthritis) may increase a person's risk of developing cataracts. If you are over age 60, you can help ensure early detection of cataracts by having your eyes examined by an ophthalmologist at least every 2 years (or as often as your doctor recommends).

Symptoms

The most common symptoms of cataracts include blurred, distorted, or multiple vision; sensitivity to glare from sunlight, lamps, or headlights; halos or rainbows around lights; poor night vision; and colors that look dull and faded. Gradual deterioration of vision makes everyday activities such as reading, watching TV, and driving more and more difficult. A person's eyeglass or contact lens prescription must be changed frequently to correct the progressive nearsightedness that may be associated with cataract formation.

Diagnosis

To diagnose cataracts, an ophthalmologist asks about your symptoms and your health history and performs a thorough eye examination. He or she will dilate (widen) your pupils with eyedrops and look inside your eyes with an ophthalmoscope (a viewing instrument that projects a bright light onto the back of the eye). The doctor uses a special microscope called a slit lamp to examine the lenses and look for any clouding. If the doctor detects a cataract, he or she will determine its type, size, and location.

Treatment

If you have a cataract, the doctor will work with you to determine the best course of treatment. In the early stages of a cataract, prescription glasses (bifocals), a magnifying glass for reading or other

---

Cataracts

Q. *My grandmother was an independent woman until she developed cataracts. After her vision became impaired, it seemed as though she needed help with just about everything. I am worried that the same thing might happen to me. Is there anything I can do to prevent cataracts?*

A. There's no surefire way to prevent cataracts, but you can do some simple things now to help reduce your risk of developing cataracts later in life. Because long-term exposure to sunlight may increase the risk of developing certain types of cataracts, always wear ultraviolet-blocking sunglasses and a hat with a brim when you're out in bright sunlight. Don't use sunlamps or tanning booths or beds. Eat lots of antioxidant-rich fruits and vegetables, which help protect the eyes. Other protective measures include not smoking, drinking alcohol only moderately, and keeping your blood pressure at a healthy level. In addition, if you have diabetes, controlling your blood sugar level is essential for protecting your eyes.

Q. *Recently my eye doctor told me that I have cataracts. Do I need to have them removed?*

A. Not necessarily. The decision is yours, and will probably depend on whether the cataracts are impairing your vision enough to prevent you from doing the things you like or need to do every day. Your eye doctor will work with you to determine the best course of treatment. If your cataracts are at an early stage, you may need only eyeglasses or a stronger correction for your glasses. You might also try improving the lighting in your home and at work and using a magnifying glass for close-up activities such as reading. If these measures are not helpful, your doctor will probably recommend cataract surgery.

Cataract Surgery

Surgery to remove a cataract and implant a replacement lens is performed frequently in the United States, with a very high success rate—good vision is restored in about 98 percent of people who have the procedure. Cataract surgery usually takes an hour or less, and most people are able to go home the same day. If you have cataracts in both eyes, you will have two separate procedures performed on different days.

The two major types of surgery to remove a cataract are phacoemulsification (also called phaco or small-incision cataract surgery) and extracapsular surgery. Your doctor will explain the advantages and disadvantages of each type of surgery so you can make an informed decision and choose the procedure that is best for you. Before surgery, your ophthalmologist will perform tests to measure the curve of the cornea and the size and shape of your eye to determine the strength of the replacement lens.

Preparing for Surgery

The doctor will ask you not to eat or drink after midnight on the day of surgery. To prepare your eye for surgery, you will be given eyedrops to dilate the pupil, and the area around your eye will be cleansed. If you choose to stay awake during surgery, you will be given a local anesthetic to numb your eye.

Surgery

In phacoemulsification, the surgeon looks at the eye through a special surgical microscope and makes a very small incision (about ⅛ inch long) on the side of the cornea. He or she then inserts a tiny probe through the incision and into the eye. The probe gives off ultrasound waves that break up the cataract, which is then sucked

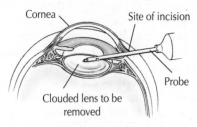

Breaking up a cataract

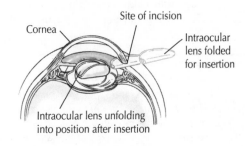

Inserting an intraocular lens

Phacoemulsification

In phacoemulsification, the surgeon makes a small incision in the cornea and inserts a tiny probe into the eye. The probe gives off ultrasound waves that break up the cataract, which is removed from the eye through a tiny suction tube. In most cases, the surgeon then inserts a replacement lens in the eye. The incision heals on its own and may not need stitches.

activities that require you to see things close up, or stronger lighting at home or at work may help you see better. However, when such measures are no longer helpful, your doctor probably will recommend surgery to remove the clouded lens and implant a substitute lens. If cataract surgery (see above) is an option, the doctor will explain the risks and benefits of the surgery.

Glaucoma

Glaucoma is a group of eye diseases in which damage to the optic nerve leads to loss of vision.

A leading cause of blindness in the United States, glaucoma is about three to four times more likely to occur in blacks than in whites, and the disease causes blindness in blacks about six times as often.

The most common type of glaucoma, called chronic open-angle glaucoma, usually develops gradually over a number of years. A clear, watery liquid called aqueous fluid flows in and out of a small space at the front of each eye (the anterior chamber) to bathe and nourish nearby tissues and remove wastes. In chronic open-angle glaucoma, the drainage angle (the channel through which aqueous fluid drains from the eyeball) malfunctions out of the eye through a tiny tube. After the replacement lens has been implanted, the incision may or may not be closed with stitches. Most cataracts are removed using phacoemulsification.

In extracapsular surgery, the surgeon looks at the eye through a special surgical microscope and makes an incision about $1/2$ inch long on the side of the cornea, removes the hard center of the lens through the incision, and removes the rest of the lens through a tiny suction tube. After a replacement lens has been implanted, the surgeon closes the incision with a few tiny stitches.

In both types of cataract surgery, the cloudy lens is usually replaced with a transparent, artificial intraocular lens. Phacoemulsification uses a folded lens that unfolds on its own after insertion. You cannot see or feel an intraocular lens, and it becomes a permanent part of the eye. In some cases, an intraocular lens cannot be used and a contact lens may be prescribed after surgery. In other cases, powerful eyeglasses may be prescribed.

Recovery

After surgery, a patch may be placed over your eye and your eye will be monitored carefully for signs of potential complications such as pain or bleeding. You will probably go home the same day. Your eye may be sensitive to light and touch and may itch and produce a sticky discharge. Your doctor will probably prescribe eyedrops or pills to promote healing and control pressure inside the eye and may recommend nonaspirin pain relievers (because aspirin may cause bleeding). You may need to wear protective glasses for a time and avoid sunlight and rubbing or pressing on your eye. Your doctor will ask you not to bend over or lift heavy objects, which can increase the pressure inside the eyes. Most people are able to return to their usual activities within a few days.

WARNING!

Do Not Take Aspirin After Cataract Surgery

Do not take aspirin (or any other nonsteroidal anti-inflammatory drugs) or drugs that contain aspirin to relieve pain after surgery because these drugs can cause bleeding. If you are experiencing discomfort or pain, talk to your doctor, who can recommend or prescribe a pain reliever that does not contain aspirin.

Your vision may be blurry for a few weeks after surgery, until the eye has healed. Most people with a lens implant still need to wear glasses for certain activities.

Possible Complications

Possible complications after cataract surgery include infection, bleeding, inflammation (which causes pain, redness, and swelling), increased pressure inside the eye, flashes of light, or loss of vision. These problems can usually be treated successfully when treated promptly. If you experience any of these symptoms, contact your doctor immediately. In some cases, the posterior capsule (part of the natural lens that is not removed in cataract surgery) may become cloudy months or years after cataract surgery, causing blurred vision. This condition, called an after-cataract, can be corrected with a surgical procedure that uses a laser to make a tiny hole in the cloudy membrane to allow light in, which improves vision. The procedure is brief and painless.

and the fluid does not drain properly, causing the normal pressure inside the eye to slowly rise. If not controlled, this abnormally high pressure can permanently damage the optic nerve and other parts of the eye, causing vision loss and, eventually, blindness.

In acute closed-angle glaucoma, the drainage angle unexpectedly becomes blocked by part of the iris, which causes a sudden, severe increase in pressure inside the eyes. If not treated promptly, the increased pressure can quickly lead to blindness in the affected eye. In low tension or normal tension glaucoma, the optic nerve is damaged for no obvious reason in people with normal pressure inside

the eyes, causing loss of peripheral (side) vision. Doctors do not fully understand this type of glaucoma.

Risk Factors

Although anyone can develop chronic open-angle glaucoma, your risk is increased if you have a family history of glaucoma or diabetes (see page 889) or if you are nearsighted (see page 1030), over age 60, or black and over age 40.

Early detection and treatment are the best ways to control glaucoma. If you are at increased risk of developing the disease, see an ophthalmologist (eye MD) for a thorough eye examination (see page

1028) at least every 1 to 2 years (or as often as your doctor recommends).

Symptoms

Chronic open-angle glaucoma usually does not produce symptoms in the early stages. However, as the disease progresses, the optic nerve is damaged, and blind spots begin to develop, especially in peripheral vision. Objects in the front of the visual field are seen clearly, but those to the side may not be seen. Gradually the visual field becomes more and more narrow until total blindness occurs. These symptoms also occur in low tension and normal tension glaucoma.

Acute closed-angle glaucoma occurs suddenly, without warning. The symptoms include redness of the eye, blurred vision, severe eye pain, severe headache, rainbows or halos around lights, and nausea and vomiting. This type of glaucoma is a medical emergency that requires immediate medical treatment to reduce pressure inside the eyeball.

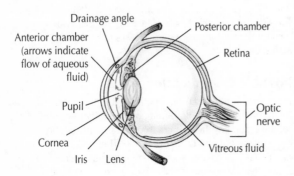

Healthy eye
In a healthy eye, a clear, watery liquid called aqueous fluid flows constantly through the pupil, between the iris and the cornea, and drains into veins. The fluid bathes and nourishes nearby tissues and removes wastes.

WARNING!

Acute Closed-Angle Glaucoma

If not treated promptly, acute closed-angle glaucoma can quickly lead to blindness. When glaucoma occurs suddenly, without warning, it is a medical emergency that requires immediate medical treatment. If you suddenly experience any of the following symptoms, call 911 or your local emergency number immediately, or go directly to the nearest hospital emergency department:

- Redness of the eye
- Blurred vision
- Severe eye pain
- Severe headache
- Rainbows or halos around lights
- Nausea and vomiting

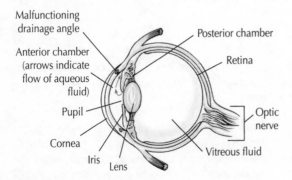

Chronic open-angle glaucoma
In chronic open-angle glaucoma, the drainage angle malfunctions and the aqueous fluid does not drain properly. As the fluid builds up, pressure inside the eyeball increases, potentially causing permanent damage to the optic nerve and other parts of the eye.

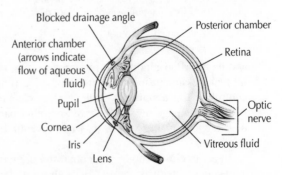

Acute closed-angle glaucoma
In acute closed-angle glaucoma, the entrance to the drainage angle becomes blocked, causing a sudden, severe increase in pressure inside the eyeball. Acute closed-angle glaucoma is a medical emergency that requires immediate medical treatment to clear the blockage and prevent blindness.

Diagnosis

In most cases, chronic open-angle glaucoma is detected by an ophthalmologist during a routine eye examination. If the doctor suspects that you may have glaucoma, he or she will examine your eyes to determine if the disease has affected your vision and will perform a visual field test and an eye pressure test (see page 1029). The doctor then dilates (widens) your pupils with eyedrops and looks inside your eyes through an ophthalmoscope (a viewing instrument that projects a bright light onto the back of the eye) to evaluate the retina and the optic nerve. He or she also looks through the cornea of each eye to examine the structure and condition of the drainage angle.

The doctor may perform a test called gonioscopy, in which he or she anesthetizes the eyes with eyedrops and places a special contact lens called a gonioscope on the cornea to closely examine the drainage angle of each eye for any changes or signs of blockage. In some cases, the doctor may take photographs (called disc photos) of the optic nerve in each eye at various intervals, to monitor the progression of the disease.

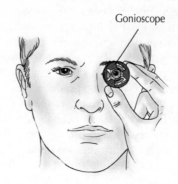

Gonioscope

Gonioscopy

In an examination called gonioscopy, an ophthalmologist anesthetizes the eye with eyedrops and places a special contact lens called a gonioscope on the cornea to examine the drainage angle for any changes or signs of blockage.

MY STORY   ## Glaucoma

I never had any trouble with my vision until I was about 45 and needed reading glasses. When I went in for an eye exam, one of the tests showed that I had signs of an eye disorder called glaucoma. The test found that there was an increase of pressure inside my eye, which, the doctor told me, can damage the nerves in the eye and eventually lead to blindness. I was shocked. I had heard of glaucoma before, and I seemed to recall that one of my grandparents had it, but I thought it happened just to older people.

Lucky for me, the doctor said that the glaucoma was at an early stage and that it could be treated by keeping the pressure inside the eye at a normal level. She prescribed some eyedrops for me to use every day, which, she explained, would lower the pressure in my eyes. She told me about the side effects of the medication—one of which is asthmalike symptoms. I put the eyedrops in my eyes religiously twice a day for about 2 months. Then I started having trouble breathing. I told the eye doctor about the breathing and she told me to stop taking the drops and to see my family doctor to be sure it was the medication and not a serious condition that was the cause of my breathing problems.

The eye doctor gave me different types of eyedrops to try that wouldn't affect my breathing, but they either did not control my glaucoma or they irritated my eyes. The eye doctor then suggested that I have laser surgery to control the pressure in my eyes. She explained that the procedure is painless and can be performed right in her office. I decided to go ahead with the laser surgery because I was having so much trouble with the medication.

My brother was not so lucky—he has glaucoma and didn't start his treatment early enough, and has lost some of his vision.

I'm glad I did. I no longer have to use eyedrops and my glaucoma is controlled. I see the eye doctor regularly to make sure everything is still OK. My brother was not so lucky—he has glaucoma and didn't start his treatment early enough, and has lost some of his vision. But he is using eyedrops now to prevent the glaucoma from getting worse.

Treatment

Although damage to the optic nerve caused by chronic open-angle glaucoma is permanent, treatment with medication and surgery can usually slow the disease or prevent it from progressing. An ophthalmologist will prescribe medication, usually given in eyedrops, that either reduces the pressure inside the eyeballs by slowing the flow of fluid into the eyes or improves fluid drainage from the eyes. Because pills may produce more serious side effects, they are prescribed only if the eyedrops are ineffective. You will need to take the medication for the rest of your life to control the pressure in your eyes. If the drugs lose their effectiveness over time or cause unpleasant side effects, a doctor may change the dosage or prescribe a different medication.

To treat chronic open-angle glaucoma that cannot be controlled with medication, the doctor can use a laser (a highly concentrated beam of light) to alter the shape of the drainage angle to make it easier for fluid to drain from the eye. This painless procedure usually is performed in the doctor's office or in an outpatient facility. In some cases, the effects of laser surgery may wear off over time and the procedure must be repeated. If glaucoma cannot be controlled with medication or laser surgery, an ophthalmologist may recommend a surgical procedure called trabeculectomy, in which an alternate outlet for aqueous fluid is created to lower the pressure inside the eyeball. This type of surgery is performed in a hospital.

Emergency treatment for acute closed-angle glaucoma involves a brief, painless surgical procedure called iridotomy. In this procedure, the doctor usually uses a laser to create a small drainage hole in the iris to change the shape of the structure of the eye and help fluid drain from the eye to relieve pressure inside the eyeball. Iridotomy usually is performed in the doctor's office or in an outpatient facility.

Macular Degeneration

Macular degeneration is a disease characterized by irreversible deterioration of the light-sensitive cells of the macula—the part of the retina (the light-sensitive membrane lining the back of the eye) that provides sharp focus in the center of the field of vision. The retina transforms light into electrical signals that travel along the optic nerve to the brain, which perceives them as visual images. Sharp central vision allows you to see fine details clearly, which is essential for such everyday activities as reading, driving, and recognizing colors and faces. As you age, the macula can deteriorate. This process can occur rapidly, or it can be slow and progressive. Macular degeneration often affects both eyes, one after the other. In the United States, age-related macular degeneration is the leading cause of blindness in people over 60.

There are two main forms of age-related macular degeneration—dry and wet. About 90 percent of people who have the disease have the dry form, in which the macula breaks down slowly, gradually resulting in blurred central vision. The other 10 percent have the wet form, which progresses more rapidly and carries a greater risk of vision loss. In the wet form, fragile, abnormal blood vessels grow under the retina and bleed and leak fluid, causing internal scarring and formation of a large blind spot in the center of the field of vision. Some hereditary forms of macular degeneration can affect children and adolescents. These forms of the disease are rare and can be referred to collectively as juvenile macular degeneration or dystrophy.

Risk Factors

Age is the greatest risk factor for macular degeneration, and the risk increases with age. In some people, the disease can occur as early as middle age but usually develops after age 60. People with a family history of macular degeneration are more likely to develop the disease. Risk factors include smoking, long-term exposure to sunlight, nearsightedness, coronary artery disease, high blood pressure, and a high cholesterol level. Women are at greater risk than men (loss of the female hormone estrogen at menopause may play a role). Whites are at greater risk than people of other races (people with light-colored eyes may be more susceptible to damage to the macula from prolonged exposure to sunlight or other forms of ultraviolet light).

Symptoms

The most common early symptom of dry macular degeneration is blurred vision. Distortion or a small blind spot may appear in the center of your field of vision, and you may be gradually less able to

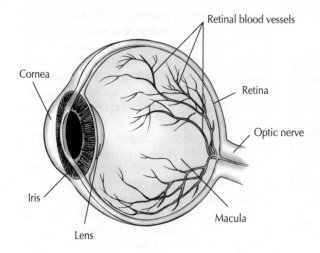

Retinal blood vessels

Cornea

Retina

Optic nerve

Iris

Macula

Lens

Location of the macula
The macula is the part of the retina that provides sharp focus at the center of the visual field. The macula enables you to see fine details, which are essential for activities such as reading and driving and for recognizing colors and faces.

distinguish fine details on, for example, faces or printed pages. Over time, the blind spot may become larger and darker. The disease may affect only one eye at first but, in most cases, the other eye is affected eventually.

In wet macular degeneration, fluid from the leaking blood vessels collects beneath the macula and lifts it, causing shapes to appear distorted and objects in straight lines (such as sentences on a page) to look crooked or wavy. Colors may appear faded. A blind spot in the center of the field of vision may develop quickly.

Neither dry nor wet age-related macular degeneration affects peripheral (side) vision or causes pain. A person may have difficulty seeing in bright light and may have problems adjusting from darkness to light. In people with dry macular degeneration, the disease progresses so slowly that they are not aware of any changes in their vision. In people with wet macular degeneration, the disease progresses rapidly and leads to the loss of sharp central vision in one or both eyes.

Diagnosis

To diagnose macular degeneration, an ophthalmologist (eye MD) will take a health history and ask you questions about your lifestyle—such as your diet and exercise habits and whether you smoke—

to help determine your risk of developing the disease. He or she will evaluate your central and peripheral vision, measure how well you can see at various distances, and may assess your ability to see color. The doctor will perform tests to determine how your eyes function, both separately and together. He or she will dilate (widen) your pupils with eyedrops and look inside your eyes with an ophthalmoscope (a viewing instrument that projects a bright light onto the back of the eye) to examine the retina. He or she also may take a series of photographs of the retina to establish a baseline that will allow him or her to track the progression of the disease.

A common early sign of dry macular degeneration is the appearance of tiny yellow deposits in the retina called drusen, which the ophthalmologist can easily see during an eye examination. The doctor may ask you to look at a pattern called an Amsler grid; if the lines of the grid look wavy or distorted, or if some sections of the grid appear blank, you may have macular degeneration. The ophthalmologist may perform tests called fluorescein angiography and indocyanine green angiography. In these procedures, a dye is injected into a vein in your arm, and a rapid series of photographs is taken as the dye moves through the blood vessels in the retina. This allows the doctor to evaluate the condition of the blood vessels in the choroid and in the retina.

Treatment

There is no cure for either form of age-related macular degeneration. Although there is currently no proven treatment for dry macular degeneration, this does not mean that you will lose your sight, because the disease progresses very slowly. The doctor may prescribe a supplement containing antioxidants and zinc and recommend changes in your diet that may help protect your eyes from additional damage and help slow the progression of the disease. Eat lots of fruits and vegetables, which are rich in antioxidants. Two antioxidants, lutein and zeaxanthin (which make up the pigment in the macula), are naturally protective of the macula.

Wearing sunglasses that block ultraviolet rays and sun visors may help prevent damage to the macula. Try vision aids such as magnifying glasses, bright lights, large-print reading materials, special lenses, and computer monitors with large print.

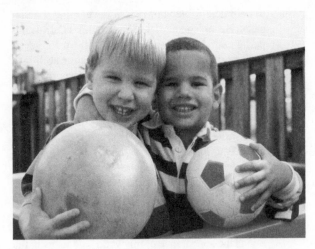

Normal vision

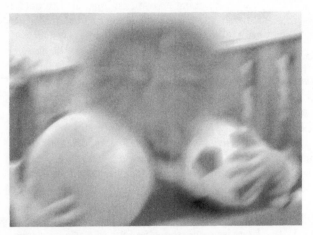

Blurred vision with large central blind spot

The effects of dry macular degeneration
Dry macular degeneration damages the macula, the part of the retina that provides sharp focus in the center of the visual field. An early symptom of dry macular degeneration is blurred vision, which makes it difficult to distinguish fine details on faces or printed pages.

Some people who have wet macular degeneration can be treated with laser photocoagulation, a type of surgery in which a highly concentrated beam of light is used to destroy abnormal blood vessels under the retina and stop vision loss. Laser photocoagulation is effective in about half of cases, but the results may last only for about a year. The procedure is usually performed using a local anesthetic in a doctor's office or in an outpatient facility; you return home the same day.

An outpatient procedure called photodynamic therapy sometimes is used for treating wet macular degeneration. In this procedure, the doctor injects a light-activated drug called verteporfin into the person's arm, and the drug collects in the abnormal blood vessels behind the macula. A special laser beam is aimed at the targeted area of the retina to activate the drug, which seals the leaking blood vessels and stops progression of the disease. If leaking recurs, the procedure needs to be repeated.

If you have dry macular degeneration, be sure to have your eyes examined by an ophthalmologist at least twice a year or as often as your doctor recommends. Ask your doctor about using an Amsler grid at home to monitor your vision daily to determine if your vision is getting worse. Your doctor will tell you how to use the Amsler grid.

If you have wet macular degeneration, frequent eye examinations will enable your doctor to detect any recurrence of leaking blood vessels. If you smoke, quit now. Smokers who have wet macular degeneration may have a greater risk of recurrence than nonsmokers because free radicals in cigarette smoke may damage the cells in the macula. If you notice any changes in your vision, see your doctor as soon as possible. Treatment of wet macular degeneration is most effective in the early stages.

Diabetic Retinopathy

Diabetic retinopathy is an eye disorder in which changes in the blood vessels of the retina (the light-sensitive membrane that lines the back of the eye) can lead to vision loss or blindness. The disorder occurs in people who have diabetes (see page 889), which can damage blood vessels, including those in the eye. Diabetic retinopathy is the leading cause of blindness in adults in the United States.

In some people who develop diabetic retinopathy, the blood vessels in the retina leak fluid. In others, abnormal new blood vessels grow on the surface of the retina and bleed and leak into the vitreous fluid (the substance that makes up the mass of the inside of the eyeball), preventing light from reaching the retina. The abnormal blood vessels also can produce scar tissue that pulls the retina away from the back of the eye, causing retinal detachment (see page 1050).

Anyone who has diabetes can develop diabetic retinopathy, and the longer you have diabetes, the more likely you are to develop this eye disorder. Nearly half of all people who have diabetes develop diabetic retinopathy. Good control of both blood sugar (glucose) levels and blood pressure and early detection and treatment of diabetic retinopathy can help slow progression of the disease and can help prevent vision loss and blindness.

Symptoms

Diabetic retinopathy often does not produce obvious symptoms in the early stages. As the disease progresses, symptoms may include blurred vision, seeing spots, vision that alternates between being

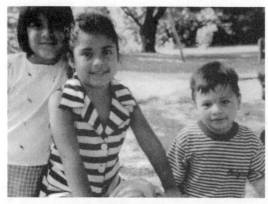

Normal vision

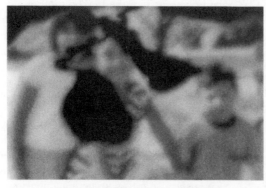

Vision impaired by diabetic retinopathy

The effects of diabetic retinopathy
Diabetic retinopathy damages the retina, the light-sensitive membrane that lines the inside of the back of the eye. As the disease progresses, vision becomes more and more blurred. If not treated promptly, diabetic retinopathy can eventually lead to permanent vision loss or total blindness.

normal and being diminished, pain in the eyes, or sudden loss of vision. If you experience any of these symptoms, contact your ophthalmologist immediately. Because visual symptoms may not develop until the disease is at an advanced stage, have eye examinations performed by an ophthalmologist every year (or as often as your doctor recommends).

Diagnosis

A diagnosis of diabetic retinopathy is based on the symptoms, a health history, and an eye examination. The ophthalmologist dilates your pupils with eyedrops and then examines your retinas while looking through an ophthalmoscope (a viewing instrument that projects a bright light onto the back of the eye). He or she looks for signs of diabetic retinopathy, such as changes in blood vessels, leaking blood vessels, abnormal new blood vessel growth on the retina, or damaged nerve tissue.

Treatment

To prevent diabetic retinopathy or to slow its progression, your doctor will recommend controlling the level of glucose in your blood with diet, exercise, and medication (insulin, in some cases). He or she will stress the importance of keeping your blood pressure within the normal range (see page 576).

In some cases, an ophthalmologist may recommend laser surgery, in which a surgeon directs a highly concentrated beam of light onto the retina either to seal leaking blood vessels or to shrink abnormal blood vessels. The procedure is done using a local anesthetic and can be performed in the doctor's office or in an outpatient facility; you return home the same day. Laser surgery can reduce the risk of severe vision loss from diabetic retinopathy, but it may not restore vision that has already been lost. After surgery you may lose some peripheral (side) vision, and your color and night vision may also be affected. In some cases, the surgery must be repeated.

For advanced cases of diabetic retinopathy in which leaking blood has filled the vitreous fluid, an ophthalmologist may recommend a type of microsurgery (delicate surgery performed under a microscope) called vitrectomy instead of laser surgery. In vitrectomy, the blood-filled vitreous fluid is removed and replaced with a clear saline (saltwater)

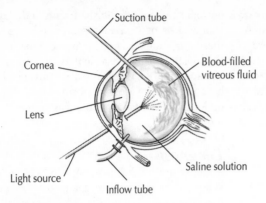

Vitrectomy
If leaking blood has filled the vitreous fluid, an ophthalmologist may recommend a surgical procedure called vitrectomy, in which the vitreous fluid is removed and replaced with a clear saline (saltwater) solution. A person cannot tell the difference between the saline solution and the vitreous fluid.

solution. Other than improved vision, you will not notice any difference between the saline solution and the vitreous fluid. Vitrectomy may take several hours to complete and is performed in a hospital using either local or general anesthesia. You may need to stay in the hospital overnight. Recovery time varies depending on the extent of the problem.

If the vitreous fluid has become clouded because of blood leaking from the abnormal blood vessels, an ophthalmologist may recommend a surgical procedure called cryosurgery that freezes the retina and shrinks the abnormal blood vessels. Cryosurgery is performed using a local anesthetic in a doctor's office or in an outpatient facility; you return home the same day.

If scar tissue causes the retina to become detached from the back of the eye (see below), surgery to reattach the retina may be combined with laser surgery or vitrectomy. The procedure is performed in a hospital using either local or general anesthesia and may take several hours.

Retinal Detachment

Retinal detachment occurs when the retina—the light-sensitive membrane that lines the inside of the back of the eye—lifts away from the choroid, the layer of blood vessels beneath the retina that supplies the eye with oxygen and nutrients. In most cases, detachment occurs after a hole or tear that has formed near the front edge of the retina allows

vitreous fluid (the substance that makes up the mass of the inside of the eyeball) to seep between the retina and the choroid, detaching the retina. The hole or tear forms either as a result of degeneration of the retina or because the vitreous fluid has shrunk away from the retina and torn it.

If not treated, this process continues until more and more of the retina lifts away from the choroid. Eventually, the retina is attached only at the front of the eye (to the ciliary body) and at the back of the eye (to the end of the optic nerve). Retinal detachment may affect both eyes, but rarely at the same time.

Retinal detachment is a rare condition, affecting middle-aged and older men and women in equal numbers. People who are nearsighted (see page 1030) have an increased risk of retinal detachment because the retina is stretched abnormally by the elongated shape of the eyeball. Other risk factors include eye injury and having a lens removed for treatment of a cataract (see page 1041). If the disorder is left untreated, a person can lose vision in the affected eye.

Symptoms
The early symptoms of retinal detachment include flashes of light and tiny spots and specks called floaters that drift across the visual field. As the condition progresses, you may lose part of your peripheral (side) vision in the affected eye, a symptom that often resembles a narrow purple or black curtain coming from the top, bottom, or side of the affected eye. If the detachment is not treated, more of the visual field is lost and the vision that remains becomes progressively blurred.

Diagnosis
A diagnosis of retinal detachment is based on the symptoms and an eye examination. The ophthalmologist dilates (widens) your pupils with eyedrops and then examines your retinas while looking through an ophthalmoscope (a viewing instrument that projects a bright light onto the back of the eye). He or she also tests your peripheral vision.

Treatment
If an ophthalmologist detects a hole or tear in the retina before detachment begins, he or she may repair the tissue using either cryosurgery (freezing) or laser photocoagulation (in which a highly concentrated beam of light is used to seal or destroy

the area around the tear). Both treatments are used to secure the retina to the eye and can be performed using either a sedative or a local anesthetic in a doctor's office or in an outpatient facility.

If detachment has already begun, an ophthalmologist may recommend a surgical procedure called scleral buckling, in which the fluid between the retina and choroid is drained to allow the retina to fall back into place against the choroid. The hole or tear in the retina is then sealed and a silicone band is sewn around the eye to securely attach the sclera (the white of the eye) to the retina.

In a procedure called pneumatic retinopexy, the doctor injects a small gas bubble into the vitreous fluid to push the retina back against the choroid. These procedures may be done either in a hospital or in an outpatient facility using either local or general anesthesia.

Your vision will probably return to normal if the procedure is performed before detachment has begun or if the detachment is limited to the front edge of the retina. If the detachment is more extensive and your central vision has been affected, your visual field and central vision may be permanently impaired to some extent.

After retinal detachment in one eye, there is a significant risk that the condition will develop in the other eye. For this reason, you should see your ophthalmologist as often as he or she recommends to watch for any weak areas in the retina.

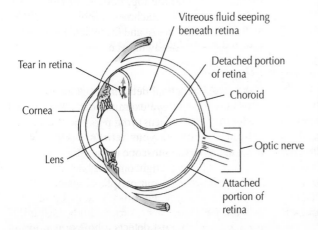

Retinal detachment
Retinal detachment occurs when a hole or tear in the retina allows vitreous fluid to seep between the choroid and the retina, causing the retina to lift away from the choroid, impairing vision.

Retinal Artery Occlusion

The retina (the light-sensitive membrane lining the back of the eye) receives its blood supply from the central retinal artery, a tiny blood vessel that enters the back of the eye through the optic nerve. Sometimes, usually in middle-aged or older people, the central retinal artery or one of its branches becomes blocked, cutting off the blood supply to the retina. The blockage may be caused by a thrombus (blood clot) or by an embolus (a tiny fragment of a blood clot or fatty deposit) that has traveled to the artery from the heart or from a blood vessel elsewhere in the body.

Symptoms
If the central retinal artery becomes blocked, the result is immediate blindness in the affected eye. If a branch of the artery is blocked, part of the visual field in the affected eye—usually the upper half or the lower half—is blacked out. If you suddenly lose all or part of your vision in one eye, see an ophthalmologist immediately or go directly to the nearest hospital emergency department.

Diagnosis and Treatment
A diagnosis of retinal artery occlusion is based on the symptoms and an examination of the affected eye. In rare cases, it may be possible to restore some of the lost vision by causing the clot or embolus to move farther along the blood vessel to a position where less of the retina is affected. This may be done by reducing pressure inside the eye, either with medication or by draining excess fluid, within a few hours of the appearance of symptoms.

Retinal Vein Occlusion

The central retinal vein carries oxygen-depleted blood away from the retina (the light-sensitive membrane lining the back of the eye). In rare cases, usually in middle-aged or older people, the central retinal vein or one of its branches becomes blocked by a thrombus (blood clot), which causes blood to leak from the blocked vessel, blurring vision.

Retinal vein occlusion may occur in chronic glaucoma (see page 1042) or with high blood pressure (see page 574). In rare cases, the disorder results from blood diseases in which the blood is thicker than normal and tends to clot more easily. Effective treatment of an underlying disease or condition, such as high blood pressure, can help prevent retinal vein occlusion.

Symptoms

If the central retinal vein becomes blocked, it usually causes sudden blurring of vision in the affected eye. When retinal artery occlusion (see previous page) occurs along with retinal vein occlusion, any blurring of vision is usually worse and more likely to be permanent. When retinal vein occlusion occurs alone, vision may improve as the clot is reabsorbed. However, permanent damage to the vein or retina frequently occurs.

Diagnosis and Treatment

A diagnosis of retinal vein occlusion is based on the symptoms and an examination of the affected eye. Sometimes retinal vein occlusion is detected by chance when an ophthalmologist examines the inside of the eyeball with an ophthalmoscope (a viewing instrument that projects a bright light onto the back of the eye) during a routine eye examination. In some cases, an ophthalmologist may recommend laser surgery (which uses a highly concentrated beam of light) to help close leaking blood vessels.

Choroiditis

Choroiditis is inflammation of the choroid, the layer of blood vessels beneath the retina (the light-sensitive membrane lining the back of the eye) that supplies the eye with oxygen and nutrients. In some cases, the retina and the vitreous fluid (the substance that makes up the mass of the inside of the eyeball) also become inflamed. Although the exact cause of the disorder usually cannot be identified, sometimes an infectious agent such as the bacterium that causes tuberculosis (see page 663) is the cause. In some cases, an abnormal immune response mistakenly produces antibodies (infection-fighting proteins) that attack the choroid and sometimes other parts of the eye.

Symptoms and Diagnosis

The symptoms of choroiditis include redness, discomfort, and blurred vision in the affected eye.

A diagnosis of choroiditis is based on the symptoms and an eye examination. An ophthalmologist will probably order blood tests to check for an infection, and possibly an ultrasound (see page 111) if he or she cannot see far enough into the eyeball with an ophthalmoscope (a viewing instrument that projects a bright light onto the back of the eye).

Treatment

To treat choroiditis, a doctor may prescribe corticosteroid drugs to relieve inflammation and pain and eliminate the blurred vision. If choroiditis is caused by an infection, the doctor may prescribe antibiotics.

Optic Neuritis

Optic neuritis is inflammation of the optic nerve, which disrupts the flow of signals from the retina to the brain and impairs vision. The condition usually develops between ages 20 and 40. In rare cases, optic neuritis results from an infection in the tissues that surround the optic nerve. Optic neuritis can occur in people who have multiple sclerosis (see page 696), which affects the nervous system.

Symptoms

The main symptom of optic neuritis is gradual or sudden blurring of vision in one eye. In severe cases, the blurring may progress to temporary blindness within a few days. Other symptoms include pain when moving or touching the affected eye, and seeing the color red as faded.

Diagnosis

A diagnosis of optic neuritis is based on the symptoms and an examination of the affected eye. The doctor may also order an MRI (see page 113) of the brain to examine the optic nerve and to rule out other neurological disorders.

Treatment

In most cases, optic neuritis clears up on its own. Sometimes a doctor prescribes high-dose intravenous corticosteroids to relieve inflammation and pain. Although some impairment of vision may persist, vision usually returns to normal within about 6 weeks. After treatment, optic neuritis may recur in the same eye or in the other eye.

Malignant Melanoma

Malignant melanoma (see page 1069) is a cancer that can affect the eyes as well as the skin, and is the most common type of cancer that occurs inside the eye. Malignant melanoma usually occurs in the choroid (the layer of blood vessels beneath the retina that supplies oxygen and nutrients to the eye) or the ciliary body (the muscles that focus the lens). However, it occasionally develops in the iris (the colored part of the eye).

Malignant melanoma affects only one eye and usually occurs in middle-aged or older people. Most tumors are detected during a routine eye examination by an ophthalmologist (eye MD). Others are brought to the doctor's attention because of a gradual loss of vision in the affected eye.

Symptoms

The symptoms of malignant melanoma of the eye can include a red, painful eye; a small flaw on the iris (the colored part of the eye) or conjunctiva (the transparent membrane that covers the white of the eye and lines the eyelids); a change in the color of the iris; poor vision in one eye; or bulging eyes.

Diagnosis

To diagnose malignant melanoma, an ophthalmologist will dilate (widen) your pupils with eyedrops and look inside your eyes with an ophthalmoscope (a viewing instrument that projects a bright light onto the back of the eye). He or she may order tests such as ultrasound (see page 111) or fluorescein angiography (see page 110) to determine the location and size of the tumor.

Treatment

Treatment for malignant melanoma may include radiation therapy (see page 23) to destroy the cancer cells or surgical removal of the affected eye (enucleation) to remove the tumor and help prevent the cancer from spreading. Because malignant melanoma can spread, your doctor will continue to monitor your condition after you have been treated.

Retinoblastoma

Retinoblastoma is a rare, malignant tumor of the retina that occurs in one or both eyes, usually in children between ages 2 and 3. Because retinoblastoma

is often inherited, you should seek genetic counseling (see page 952) before having children if you know that the disorder runs in your family. If you already have a child, have his or her eyes examined by an ophthalmologist soon after birth, and tell the doctor about your family history of retinoblastoma.

Symptoms

A child with retinoblastoma may have no symptoms or may have misaligned eyes (see page 1055). In some cases, the tumor may be visible through the pupil as a white area inside the eye.

Diagnosis and Treatment

Retinoblastoma can be diagnosed during an eye examination performed at birth or as part of a routine childhood health checkup. Early detection and treatment with medication, radiation therapy (see page 23), laser therapy (treatment using a highly concentrated beam of light), or cryotherapy (freezing) can be effective. If the cancer is advanced, the doctor may recommend surgical removal of the eye (enucleation) to remove the tumor and help prevent the cancer from spreading to other parts of the body. After the eye has been removed, the child may need to have radiation therapy and chemotherapy (see page 23).

Secondary Tumors

Cancer cells can spread through the bloodstream or the lymphatic system from a tumor in one area of the body to form a tumor in another part of the body, including in the eye.

Symptoms

If a so-called secondary tumor grows behind the eyeball, it can cause the eyes to bulge. The effects of a tumor on a person's vision can vary, depending on where in the eye the tumor is located, how fast the tumor is growing, and whether one or both eyes are affected. If a tumor grows inside the eye, it can cause blurred vision.

Treatment

A secondary tumor is treated separately from a primary tumor. A doctor may prescribe chemotherapy (see page 23) or radiation therapy (see page 23) to block the growth of or destroy a secondary tumor in the eye. Any loss of vision that occurs before treatment may be permanent.

Color Vision Deficiency

Color vision deficiency (also called color blindness) is a vision disorder in which a person sees colors differently than other people see them or has difficulty distinguishing shades of some colors. The disorder occurs when malfunctioning receptor cells for color in the retina (the light-sensitive membrane lining the back of the eye) transmit incorrect information about color to the brain.

Color vision deficiency is a common disorder that is usually inherited. Although women can carry the gene for the common form of color vision deficiency and pass it on to their children, men are more often affected by the disorder; about 8 percent of men in the United States have color vision deficiency. Difficulty distinguishing colors can develop when normal age-related changes in the lens of the eye cause it to darken, impairing a person's ability to see differences between some colors. The disorder can also result from a disease or injury that damages the eye or the optic nerve, or from degeneration of the retina or the optic nerve.

Symptoms
The symptoms of color vision deficiency can range from difficulty seeing the difference between shades of the same color to an inability to see all colors. Although the severity of color vision deficiency varies from one person to another, most people who have the disorder have a mild deficiency and have difficulty distinguishing shades of red and green.

Diagnosis and Treatment
A diagnosis of color vision deficiency is based on the symptoms, your family health history, and the results of color vision tests. Although there is no cure for color vision deficiency, your ophthalmologist can recommend steps you can take to deal with the problem, such as learning to recognize colors by brightness or location. For example, to read traffic signals, you remember that the red light is on the top and the green light is on the bottom. Some people who have difficulty distinguishing shades of red and green may benefit from using tinted prescription glasses.

Other Eye Disorders

The two bony sockets in the skull that contain the eyeballs are called the orbits. The eyeballs are supported in the orbits by soft tissue. Sometimes an underlying disease or condition, such as Graves' disease or a tumor behind the eyeball, causes one or both eyeballs to bulge forward in the orbits. In some cases, an infection that has spread to the soft tissue of the orbit from the sinuses or from a nearby boil causes inflammation that makes the eyeballs bulge forward. Muscles attached to the outside of each eyeball and to the inside back portion of each orbit give the eyes movement. If these muscles are not balanced, or if there is a defect in the nerves that control them, the eyes can become misaligned.

Exophthalmos

Exophthalmos is a condition in which one or both eyeballs bulge forward, exposing an abnormally large part of the front of the eye (see page 128). The most common cause of the condition is Graves' disease (see page 901), an autoimmune disorder that causes the thyroid gland to become overactive. Other possible causes of exophthalmos include a tumor behind the eyeball (see previous page) or inflammation of the tissue behind the eyeball (orbital cellulitis; see next page).

Symptoms
In exophthalmos, the eyes tend to feel dry. Eye movement may be restricted, which can cause double vision. In severe cases, the eye is pressed so far forward that the eyelids may not close completely and the front of the eye may become dry and feel gritty, causing pain and blurred vision.

Diagnosis
A diagnosis of exophthalmos is based on the symptoms, a health history, a physical examination, and an examination of the eye, especially the orbit (the

bony socket in which the eyeball sits). The doctor may order blood tests and recommend an ultrasound (see page 111), a CT scan (see page 112), or an MRI (see page 113) to help determine the cause.

Treatment

If exophthalmos is caused by Graves' disease, the doctor will treat Graves' disease. However, successful treatment of Graves' disease may not eliminate the bulging, and the ophthalmologist may prescribe corticosteroid drugs to relieve the inflammation and pain. If there is loss of vision, radiation therapy (see page 23) may be recommended.

An ophthalmologist may recommend surgery on the eyelids to help protect the exposed eyeball and prevent corneal ulcers (see page 1037) from developing. In severe cases, surgery may be necessary to increase the orbital space and relieve the pressure behind the eyeball. If a tumor is detected, the ophthalmologist will probably recommend a biopsy (in which samples of cells are taken from the tumor and examined under a microscope), or surgery to remove the tumor. Depending on the results of the biopsy, the doctor may recommend radiation therapy, chemotherapy (see page 23), or both.

Orbital Cellulitis

Orbital cellulitis is inflammation of the soft tissue of the orbit (the bony socket in the skull that contains the eyeball). The condition usually occurs when bacteria from a sinus infection (see page 651), from a penetrating injury to the orbit, or from a boil (see page 1060) spread and infect the orbit. There is a risk that the infection could spread to the brain and cause an abscess (a pus-filled cavity surrounded by inflamed tissue) or meningitis (see page 692), a potentially life-threatening infection of the meninges (the membranes that surround and protect the brain and spinal cord).

Symptoms

In orbital cellulitis, the swollen tissue pushes on the eyeball and causes it to bulge forward in the orbit (exophthalmos; see previous page). Other possible symptoms of orbital cellulitis include redness and severe pain in the eye, swollen eyelids, difficulty moving the eye, impaired vision in the eye, and fever. The eye may produce a discharge of pus.

Pressure on or inflammation of the blood vessels and nerves that supply the eye may lead to blurred vision or blindness.

Diagnosis and Treatment

A diagnosis of orbital cellulitis is based on the symptoms and an examination of the affected eye. The ophthalmologist (eye MD) will order blood tests to determine the cause of the infection and a CT scan (see page 112) of the affected orbit to determine the extent of the infection.

Treatment of orbital cellulitis consists of high doses of antibiotics given intravenously (through a vein). If infected sinuses are causing the problem, the doctor may recommend surgery to drain the sinuses. If the infection causes abscesses (pockets of pus) to form in the orbit, the ophthalmologist may recommend surgery to drain the pus from the abscesses.

Misaligned Eyes

Normally aligned eyes move together and look in the same direction at the same time, which is essential for normal vision. When eyes are misaligned, uncoordinated movements of the eye muscles cause each eye to look in a different direction. For example, when one eye looks forward, the other eye looks to the left or right (or up or down). The medical term for misaligned eyes is strabismus.

A child can be born with misaligned eyes, but this condition usually goes away on its own by the time a child is about 6 months old. The condition can also develop during childhood, usually between ages 2 and 7, when vision is still developing and the eye muscles are unbalanced and uncoordinated. Most children who have misaligned eyes do not see double because their brain ignores what one of the eyes sees. Because one of the eyes is not being used, it will gradually weaken. If the disorder is not treated, vision in that eye will be impaired (called amblyopia).

When the eyes become misaligned after childhood, the cause is usually an underlying disease or condition that affects either the nerves that transmit information between the brain and the eye muscles or, less frequently, that affects just the eye muscles. Possible underlying causes of misaligned eyes include diabetes (see page 889), high blood pressure (see page 574), temporal arteritis (see page

927), brain injury (see page 680), multiple sclerosis (see page 696), and myasthenia gravis (see page 701).

Many children are born with a fold of skin over the inner corner of each eye that covers part of the eyeball and may make the eyes appear misaligned. Their eyes are not misaligned, however; this is simply a normal variation.

Symptoms

In children, eye misalignment can be constant, or it can come and go. In addition to uncoordinated movement of the eyes, most adults who develop misaligned eyes experience double vision and sometimes problems with depth perception. They also may have symptoms of an underlying disorder that is causing the misalignment. Any child or adult who has misaligned eyes should be evaluated by an ophthalmologist.

Diagnosis

To diagnose misaligned eyes in a child, an ophthalmologist will perform an eye examination and may order tests to determine the cause. He or she will check for abnormalities in the eyes, in the movement of the eyes, and in the muscles that control eye movement.

To determine the underlying cause of misaligned eyes in an adult, an ophthalmologist asks about the person's symptoms and performs an eye examination. He or she may also order blood tests and a CT scan (see page 112) or MRI (see page 113). The ophthalmologist may recommend that you see your primary care doctor or a neurologist (a doctor who specializes in treating disorders of the nervous system) for further evaluation and treatment.

Treatment

Early treatment of eye misalignment improves a child's chances for normal vision. Children whose eyes are misaligned may need to wear an eye patch over the good eye and eyeglasses to ensure use of the misaligned eye and to strengthen vision in it. Surgery to tighten or loosen some of the muscles that control eye movement is frequently performed, especially in children under age 2. The procedure is usually performed on an outpatient basis, and the child stays in the hospital for a few hours after surgery. The child may need to wear an eye patch and glasses after surgery.

If a child's eyes become misaligned after age 2, an ophthalmologist usually prescribes glasses to correct the condition. The child may also need to wear a patch over his or her good eye for several hours each day to ensure use of the misaligned eye. In most of these children, the combination of a patch and glasses corrects the misalignment within a few years. In some children, surgery on the eye muscles may be needed to align the eyes.

In adults, successful treatment of an underlying disease or condition may eliminate the misalignment. Double vision may go away on its own within a few months. In some cases, an ophthalmologist may prescribe special glasses to correct the problem. In other cases, doctors may recommend surgery to tighten or loosen some of the eye muscles to coordinate eye movements.

Disorders of the Skin, Hair, and Nails

The skin is the largest organ of the body. It contains millions of tiny nerve endings (called receptors) that respond to pressure and changes in temperature to provide you with information about your surroundings. Your skin also contains many tiny glands. Sebaceous glands produce an oily substance called sebum that helps keep the skin's surface supple and prevent it from drying and cracking. When you are hot or have a fever, sweat glands produce a watery liquid that evaporates on the skin to cool your body, and small blood vessels in your skin dilate (widen) to allow heat to escape. When you are cold, your skin conserves heat by constricting (narrowing) the blood vessels.

Hair and nails are extensions of the skin and are composed mostly of keratin (the main constituent of the outermost layer of the skin). There are thousands of hair follicles in the skin. Follicles are pits of actively dividing cells that continuously make hairs. Relatively larger, thicker hairs grow on the scalp and pubic area; smaller, finer hairs (some that can barely be seen) grow elsewhere on the body. Fingernails and toenails, like hair, are continuously produced by actively dividing cells under the fold of skin at the base and sides of each nail.

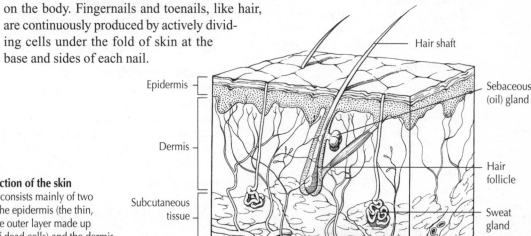

Cross section of the skin
The skin consists mainly of two layers—the epidermis (the thin, protective outer layer made up mostly of dead cells) and the dermis (the thicker layer containing blood vessels, nerves, oil glands, and hair follicles). The subcutaneous tissue is a layer of fat under the skin.

1057

Skin Disorders

Skin is composed of two layers. The surface layer that you see is a thin covering called the epidermis. Below the epidermis is a thicker layer called the dermis. The dermis contains most of the living elements of the skin, such as hair follicles and sweat glands. Below the dermis is a layer of fat called subcutaneous tissue.

The epidermis is a very active layer of cells. Cells at its base are continuously dividing to produce new cells. These cells gradually die as they fill up with a hard substance called keratin. As the cells die, they move up to the skin surface, where they are shed or rubbed away by movement (such as friction from your clothes or washing). In this turnover of cells, it takes an average of 1 month for a single epidermal cell to move from the base of the epidermis to its surface.

On parts of the body where pressure and friction are greatest, the epidermis is thicker, and it takes longer for cells to travel from the base to the surface. The normal turnover of cells can be disrupted by some skin disorders. For example, in psoriasis (see page 1064), new cells are produced at a faster rate than old cells are shed.

Birthmarks

Birthmarks are persistent (but not always permanent) areas of discolored skin that are present from birth. They may be pink, red, or purple marks caused by concentrations of blood vessels in the skin or tan or brownish black areas of intense pigmentation. Some birthmarks fade with time or disappear altogether. Birthmarks that bleed or that do not fade as a child gets older can be removed with laser surgery (see page 1088). Birthmarks can also be removed when a child is only a few weeks old.

Capillary mark
A capillary mark is a pink or pinkish brown spot that is present at birth but gradually fades and usually disappears before a baby is 18 months old.

Strawberry mark
A strawberry mark or hemangioma (see page 117) is a bright red, raised area up to 4 inches across that can occur anywhere on the body. It may be barely noticeable at birth, but it will grow rapidly for a few weeks and then increase in size proportionately with the child. Large strawberry marks may bleed easily if they are bumped or scratched. When the child is about 6 to 10 months old, small gray-white areas in the mark will spread and gradually replace the red tissue, and the area will flatten. Strawberry marks usually disappear by the time a child is 5 years old, leaving a pale spot.

Port wine stain
A port wine stain is a usually large, purplish red, sometimes raised area that occurs on the face (see page 117) or on an arm or leg. It generally persists throughout adulthood, although it may fade.

Café au lait spots
Café au lait spots are flat, irregularly shaped, small or large, tan or brown areas (see page 117) that are present on the skin at birth. They can occur in one or two spots or all over the body. In rare cases, the spots may become cancerous later in life.

Mongolian spots
Mongolian spots (see page 117) are bluish gray or bluish green flat marks of various sizes that are present at birth and resemble bruises on the buttocks or lower back. The spots occur most frequently in children of black, Asian, Native American, Hispanic, or Mediterranean descent, and usually disappear by the time a child is 1 year old.

WARNING!

Enlarging Strawberry Mark
Take your child to the pediatrician immediately if a strawberry mark that is near your child's eye, mouth, or nose seems to be growing. A hemangioma can interfere with vision, feeding, or breathing.

Abnormal Skin Pigmentation

Cells called melanocytes produce the pigment melanin, which gives color to the skin. The more melanin, the darker the skin. The amount of melanin your body normally produces is determined by your genes. Exposure to sunlight increases the production of melanin to protect the skin from harmful ultraviolet rays, making the skin look tan.

Moles

Moles are small, dark, raised areas of skin (see page 118) that are benign pigmented tumors. They are composed of dense collections of the pigment-producing cells in the skin called melanocytes. Moles are very common, especially in some ethnic groups. In rare cases, they can become cancerous (malignant melanoma; see page 1069). Benign moles can be surgically removed for cosmetic reasons.

Freckles

Freckles are tiny flat patches of pigmented skin that appear on sun-exposed areas and multiply with repeated sun exposure. They most often develop in people who are fair and have red hair. People who have freckles need to be especially careful about exposing their skin to the sun because they are at increased risk of developing skin cancer from sun exposure. If you have freckles, try to avoid the sun and always wear a sunscreen with an SPF of at least 15.

Age spots

Age spots (see page 118), medically referred to as solar lentigos, are darkened areas of skin that result from long-term exposure to the sun. They usually develop in middle age or later on the skin areas most frequently exposed to the sun, such as the hands, face, and chest. They may be up to an inch in diameter. For people who consider age spots unattractive, doctors can remove them with laser surgery, cryosurgery (freezing with liquid nitrogen), or chemical peels, or by cutting them out. Surgery is performed as an outpatient procedure and usually requires only one session. Age spots usually return because they are related to previous sun exposure. To help prevent the spot from returning after treatment, wear a sunscreen with an SPF of at least 15.

Dermatosis papulosa nigra

Dermatosis papulosa nigra is a noncancerous condition resembling seborrheic keratoses (see page 1063). It is characterized by brown or black mole-like or wartlike spots on the face and neck and occurs almost exclusively in people with dark skin.

Acanthosis nigricans and pseudoacanthosis nigricans

A thickening and darkening of skin folds around the neck or in the armpits or groin (called acanthosis nigricans) can be a symptom of cancer or a genetic disorder in people with dark skin. However, it usually is a noncancerous condition (called pseudoacanthosis nigricans) that is associated with obesity. Excessive sweating may occur in these areas, and the skin may itch.

Purpura and acquired angiomas

Purpura are purplish or reddish brown spots on the skin caused by leaks in the small blood vessels in underlying tissues. The spots can range from the size of a pinpoint (called petechiae) to 2 inches across, and can be flat or slightly raised. Purpura are linked to a number of disorders, from allergies (see page 423) to thrombocytopenia (see page 620), but their cause is unknown. They may result from an inherited weakness in the walls of blood vessels.

Harmless petechiae called cherry angiomas can appear on the trunk, upper arms, and thighs after age 30. They may bleed if injured. Cherry angiomas may result from loss of skin elasticity with age.

Dilated blood vessels known as spider angiomas, or spider veins, are most common on the face (especially around the nose), breasts, arms, and legs. Spider angiomas often occur in girls during puberty, in pregnant women, and in women who are taking oral contraceptives or hormone therapy, possibly because hormones such as estrogen weaken vein walls. Spider veins can also occur in people with liver disease and after sun exposure or injury to the skin.

Other pigmentation changes

Some diseases (such as Addison's disease; see page 899) and some medications (such as the acne medication isotretinoin or the antibiotic tetracycline) can cause the skin to darken. Other medications (such as birth-control pills) and some chemicals (such as perfumes) can intensify the effect of the sun on the skin and cause dark patches. Sometimes hormonal fluctuations during pregnancy or at menopause can cause changes in the skin, making patches of skin darker with sun exposure (a condition called chloasma). Cuts, abrasions, or acne sites that have healed can leave scars that stay discolored for a long time.

An excess amount of the bile pigment bilirubin can turn the skin yellow (jaundice; see pages 118 and 785), as can eating an excessive amount of foods that contain the orange pigment carotene (found in carrots, tomatoes, and some green vegetables).

Too much iron can turn the skin bronze (hemochromatosis; see page 961).

Boils

A boil (see page 122) is an infection of a hair follicle (a tiny pit in the skin from which a hair grows) by bacteria, usually staphylococcus. Boils are common and can result from poor hygiene or low resistance to infection. A carbuncle is the name for an unusually large boil or a group of boils that are joined together by small tunnels in the skin.

Bacteria from a boil may remain on the skin, possibly producing more boils. Bacteria from a boil can also contaminate food if a person does not wash his or her hands adequately before handling food (food poisoning; see page 783). In rare cases, the bacteria can travel through the bloodstream to other parts of the body, possibly causing a severe infection (blood poisoning; see page 937).

Symptoms

A boil starts as a red, warm, tender lump under the skin. Over a few days the lump becomes larger and more painful. As white blood cells (which fight infection), bacteria, and dead skin cells collect, the lump can develop a white or yellow head of pus. See your doctor if you have a large boil that doesn't open within 2 weeks or if you have recurring boils.

Diagnosis

A doctor can diagnose a boil by its appearance and by a skin culture. If you have recurring boils, your doctor may take blood and urine samples to rule out the possibility that your boils are a symptom of diabetes (see page 889) or of a weakened immune system.

Treatment

To eliminate a boil as quickly as possible, apply a cloth soaked in hot water to the boil every few hours, or soak the boil in a solution of warm water and white vinegar. Wash the area with an antiseptic cleanser and apply an over-the-counter antibiotic.

Your doctor may open the head of a boil with a sterile needle or make a small cut in the center to allow pus to drain. He or she may prescribe an antibiotic. Your doctor may recommend treating recurring boils for several weeks with a combination of topical cleansers and antibiotics and oral antibiotics.

A boil usually bursts under pressure from the accumulated pus, relieving the pain. The boil heals after the pus drains. Boils may go away on their own, or burst and dissolve under the skin.

Warts

A wart (see page 121) is a lump caused by the human papillomavirus in the top layer of skin. The virus invades skin cells and makes them multiply rapidly. Warts are spread through contact with a wart or with skin cells shed from a wart. Warts are common in teenagers and less common in children and adults. Facial warts occur most often in children and young adults. There are several different types of warts, each produced by a different strain of the virus. Most warts go away without treatment after a few years.

Symptoms and Diagnosis

The common wart is a rough, hard, usually painless lump that contains small black dots (which are clotted blood vessels). It usually grows on the hands but can grow anywhere on the body. A common wart on the bottom of the foot is called a plantar wart and can cause pain when it is pushed into the sole of the foot by the weight of the body. Flat warts are small, smooth warts that often appear in large numbers on the face but can occur anywhere on the body. Genital warts (see page 480) are spread through genital, anal, or oral sex and can occur in the genital area, around the anus, and in and around the mouth.

See your doctor if you are older than 45 and develop a wart (and have never had warts before) or if you have warts that are painful or that bleed or itch; you may have another skin disorder, such as skin cancer (see pages 1068 to 1070). You should also see your doctor if you have facial or genital warts or if a wart doesn't respond to treatment.

Treatment

Most warts eventually disappear on their own. The most common way to treat warts is to apply an over-the-counter wart remover. These medications either burn (using salicylic acid) or freeze (using a mixture of dimethyl ether and propane) the wart, destroying the cells containing the virus. But don't use over-the-counter wart removers to treat facial or genital warts; these types of medications are too harsh for the face and genitals.

A painless but time-intensive way to treat a common wart is to cover it with duct tape for 6 days, plane the wart down with an emery board or pumice stone, and reapply duct tape. Repeat the procedure every 6 days for up to 2 months or until the wart has completely disappeared. Doctors think that the technique works by softening the wart and possibly stimulating the immune system to fight the virus. Because this method is painless, it is especially recommended for children.

If these self-help methods are not effective, your doctor may try removing the wart by cutting it off, freezing it with liquid nitrogen (cryosurgery), or burning it off with lasers (see page 1088) or a high-frequency electric current (electrocautery). Treatment may have to be repeated. Alternatively, the doctor may prescribe a drug called imiquimod (which is usually used to treat genital warts) to treat common and flat warts. This medication is applied to the wart every day to every 3 days. Bleomycin (an anticancer drug injected in small amounts directly into the wart), cimetidine (an antihistamine), and tretinoin (a vitamin A derivative used in some acne preparations) sometimes are used to treat warts that are difficult to remove.

Molluscum Contagiosum

Molluscum contagiosum (see page 125) is a skin rash caused by a virus that is spread by close or intimate body contact, including sexual contact, with an infected person. The virus produces small, waxy-looking growths on the skin. The infection is relatively common in children; in adults, it is usually transmitted sexually. Scratching can spread the virus from one area of the body to another.

Symptoms
At first, the growths are firm, solid, and flesh colored. Eventually, they become softer and pearly, usually with a depression in the center. In some cases, a white, cheesy or waxy substance drains from them. The growths can appear on the face, trunk, arms, or abdomen. When transmitted sexually, the growths usually appear on the genitals and upper thighs.

Diagnosis and Treatment
A doctor can usually diagnose molluscum contagiosum by its appearance. A sample can be taken

from one of the growths for examination under a microscope (biopsy) to detect the virus and confirm the diagnosis. If not treated, the rash can spread or lead to bacterial infections, especially in people who have a weakened immune system. Doctors usually destroy the growths with heat (electrocautery) using a high-frequency electric current or cold (cryosurgery) using chemicals such as liquid nitrogen to kill the virus inside the growth. The treatment can cause temporary irritation or blistering but does not leave a scar. Some growths may reappear 2 to 3 weeks after treatment and need to be treated again. For a person with a weakened immune system, a doctor may prescribe an antiviral medication to help fight the infection.

Corns and Calluses

Corns and calluses are areas of skin that have thickened because of constant pressure and friction. Corns develop on the top or sides of the toes or between the toes. Calluses are larger areas of thickened skin that usually appear on the ball of the foot, on the heel, or over a bunion (see page 989), although they also can develop on the palms of the hands or on the tips of the fingers. Corns and calluses usually develop after wearing new or poorly fitting shoes. Wearing high heels can cause calluses from increased pressure on the ball of the foot. Calluses can develop on the hands in people who do heavy or infrequent manual work. Some people are susceptible to calluses and corns because they have less cushioning tissue between the bones and skin of their feet.

Symptoms and Diagnosis
The tissue under the thickened skin of a corn or callus can be tender. You probably don't need to see a doctor unless it becomes very painful. However, if you have a corn or callus and have a disorder such as diabetes (see page 889), which decreases sensitivity in the feet, see a doctor right away; poor circulation to the area can cause a deep ulcer to develop in the callus.

Treatment
You can relieve pressure on a corn or callus on your foot by going barefoot every chance you get and by using over-the-counter protective pads. Pads that contain salicylic acid can help dissolve thickened

skin. You can soften a callus on your feet or hands with a moisturizer. Gently rub away dead skin from the callus with a pumice stone or file, being careful not to press hard enough to inflame the sensitive tissue underneath. Wear comfortable shoes or protective gloves. The corn or callus should disappear within several weeks. If these measures don't work, your doctor may trim the corn or callus or use a strong chemical to dissolve it.

Dermatitis

Dermatitis is inflammation of the skin that can result from an allergy but in many cases occurs for unknown reasons. Many types of dermatitis are also known as eczema (see page 120). There are several types of dermatitis or eczema.

Atopic dermatitis

Atopic dermatitis (also called atopic eczema) is a skin reaction associated with allergies. In atopic dermatitis, the skin is much more sensitive than usual to many substances. Environmental factors seem to trigger atopic dermatitis in people who are genetically susceptible. Children are at increased risk of developing atopic dermatitis if they have a family history of other atopic diseases, such as hay fever (see page 914) or asthma (see page 640). Adults with atopic dermatitis have a susceptibility to developing contact dermatitis (see below) or irritant dermatitis (see above right).

Contact dermatitis

Contact dermatitis is a type of atopic dermatitis caused by a reaction to particular substances that have touched the skin. Some skin reactions related to contact dermatitis are relatively mild and do not occur in most people. For example, an allergic reaction to contact with a metal such as nickel may cause a red, flaky, itchy patch of skin where the metal (usually on jewelry such as a watch or earrings) touches the body (see page 120). The reaction may take weeks or months to develop.

Some people have more severe allergic reactions to contact with poison ivy and other plants. A delayed hypersensitivity reaction usually occurs 2 days after contact with the plant. The skin can become red and itchy (even in areas away from the point of contact) because small amounts of chemicals from the plant can be transferred from one part of the body to another. Tiny blisters eventually develop. The tiny blisters may join to form large blisters, which break and crust over.

Irritant dermatitis

Some people are especially sensitive to particular substances. Irritant dermatitis worsens during the winter (when the air contains less moisture) or with the use of soap and water because of excessive dryness of the skin. The skin of an older person tends to be dry, particularly on the legs, leading to mild redness, flaking, and irritation. People who take frequent hot showers or baths can develop irritant dermatitis. Dishwashing liquids, detergents, fabric softeners, household cleaners, and shampoos often irritate the skin on the hands (see page 120) and especially the skin over the knuckles.

Infantile eczema

Infantile eczema is a type of atopic dermatitis (see left) or seborrheic dermatitis (see next page) that is common in babies and young children and may indicate that the child will develop other allergies later in life. The skin reaction may range from a slight rash to small red pimples that ooze and crust over when scratched. Small areas of the body such as the cheeks and chin (see page 120) may be affected, especially in infants. In children, the rash often develops behind the knees or inside the elbows, but it can affect the entire body. The pimples may become infected, especially in the warm, moist diaper area (see page 120), where bacteria can live and grow rapidly.

Many infections that affect the skin (such as chickenpox; see page 439) can become severe in children with eczema. Infantile eczema can come and go for several years or go away completely without treatment after a few months. Most children outgrow it by puberty. However, in some children and adolescents, hormones, stress, and use of irritating skin-care products such as cosmetics or hair gels can cause the disorder to flare up.

> **WARNING!**
>
> ## Eczema and Allergy to Eggs
>
> If your child has eczema caused by an allergy to eggs, tell his or her pediatrician. The measles, mumps, and rubella vaccination (MMR; see page 376) is produced using eggs, so, to have the vaccination, your child may have to be slowly and gradually made less sensitive to the vaccine. Your doctor will recommend giving your child either increasing doses of the vaccine (which all children must receive) or diluting the vaccine and giving it in frequent small amounts.

Seborrheic dermatitis

Seborrheic dermatitis (see page 120) affects different people in different ways. In adults, the creases from the sides of the nose to the corners of the mouth may become red, flaky, and itchy. In men, this inflammation can extend to the beard area and the hair-covered areas of the chest and back. The condition also may affect skin creases in other parts of the body, such as those in the groin or armpits or under the breasts. Dandruff (see page 1075) is flaking of the skin of the scalp caused by a mild form of seborrheic dermatitis. The cause of seborrheic dermatitis is unknown, but it tends to run in families and comes and goes over several years. In infants, seborrheic dermatitis takes the form of infantile eczema (see previous page). On a baby's scalp, it is known as cradle cap (see page 387).

Symptoms

In dermatitis, the skin is usually dry, itchy, and red, possibly with flaking, scaling, or blistering. Sometimes dermatitis causes small bumps (papules) or small, rough bumps on the face, upper arms, and thighs (a condition called keratosis pilaris). In severe cases, dermatitis can result in blisters, darkening of the skin (hyperpigmentation), thickened skin from constant scratching and rubbing (lichenification), and bacterial infection from constant scratching.

Seborrheic Keratoses

Seborrheic keratoses are rough, round, or oval patches of dark skin (see page 121) up to about 1 inch across that have a crusty, greasy appearance. They can be flat or slightly raised. Seborrheic keratoses are common after middle age and are often mistaken for warts, moles, or cancerous tumors. The cause is unknown, but exposure to the sun is not a factor. Although seborrheic keratoses are not precancerous, they should be evaluated by a doctor because they can resemble cancerous tumors.

Diagnosis

If you have a mild form of dermatitis and know the cause, use the self-help measures at right. If you have a severe case of dermatitis or the self-help measures do not relieve your symptoms, see your doctor. He or she may refer you to an allergist or a dermatologist (a doctor who specializes in disorders of the skin), who may recommend skin and blood tests (see pages 912 and 913) to help determine the cause.

Self-Help for Dry Skin and Dermatitis

Skin can become dry for a number of reasons, such as overwashing or exposure to chemicals. Skin drying and irritation can usually be prevented and treated with the following measures:

- If possible, avoid contact with the substance that is causing your dermatitis.
- Don't rub or scratch the affected areas. Fill plastic bags with water and freeze them, then apply the frozen bags to the affected areas to relieve the itching.
- Ask your doctor to recommend an over-the-counter corticosteroid cream or ointment (to reduce inflammation and promote healing), a pain reliever, or an antihistamine (to reduce itching, swelling, and redness).
- Don't wash too often. Use a mild, superfatted soap and apply it with your hands or a clean sponge (not a washcloth or loofah, which are rough on the skin). Don't use bubble baths or bath oils. Try to keep showers and tub baths short (no longer than 5 minutes), and use cool or lukewarm (not hot) water. Pat (don't rub) your skin dry.
- Avoid saunas and steam baths.
- Protect your skin by using a moisturizer, especially right after bathing or showering.
- If dermatitis is on your hands, apply an unscented barrier hand cream frequently. Wear white cotton gloves under rubber gloves when working with a possible irritant.
- Don't use perfumes, scented sprays, or talcum powder on your skin; these products can irritate the skin and worsen dermatitis.
- Don't wear tight or poorly fitting clothes. Avoid rough, scratchy, or wool clothing, linens, blankets, rugs, or upholstery.
- Use mild laundry detergents, and rinse clothes in clear water twice. Don't use fabric softeners.
- Avoid excessive sweating. Dress lightly in cotton clothing.
- Keep the temperature of your home cool and stable. Use a humidifier to keep the humidity level constant.
- Avoid caffeine and alcohol; they can make itching feel worse.

Treatment

In addition to the self-help measures described on the previous page, your doctor may recommend a liquid cleanser (a substitute for both soap and water) that cleans and lubricates the skin. He or she may prescribe a more concentrated topical corticosteroid medication to speed up the healing process and an antihistamine to take before bedtime to reduce itching at night to help you sleep. Tacrolimus is a topical prescription ointment used to treat mild to moderate dermatitis that doesn't have the possible adverse side effects of topical corticosteroid preparations. Use only the creams or ointments that your doctor prescribes; using anything else may reduce the amount of natural oil produced by your skin. If you have a bacterial skin infection, your doctor will prescribe an antibiotic.

For mild cases of infantile eczema, try to prevent your baby from becoming too hot. Don't overdress him or her. Dress your child in cotton clothes that are washed and rinsed well. Do not use moisturizers on your child's skin that haven't been prescribed or recommended by his or her pediatrician. Your child's doctor may prescribe an antihistamine to prevent the release of substances called histamines that produce allergic symptoms such as itching. Severe infantile eczema is often treated with topical corticosteroid medications to relieve the inflammation. Your child's doctor may recommend eliminating foods from your child's diet that could be causing the eczema, such as cow's milk, wheat, orange juice, eggs, nuts, and chocolate.

Psoriasis

Psoriasis is a skin disorder in which new cells in the epidermis (the outermost layer of cells) are produced faster than old cells are shed, causing dead skin cells to accumulate in the affected areas. The cause of psoriasis is unknown, but it is probably a disorder of the immune system. An outbreak of psoriasis is often triggered by emotional stress, skin damage (such as that caused by severe sunburn), excessive consumption of alcohol, or taking some medications. A weakened immune system can trigger outbreaks. Psoriasis usually appears between ages 10 and 30, but it can occur at any age. The condition tends to run in families. Psoriasis can be disabling in the very young or very old if it is not treated. Occasionally a person who has psoriasis will have a form of arthritis (called psoriatic arthritis) that resembles rheumatoid arthritis (see page 918).

Symptoms and Diagnosis

The symptoms of psoriasis include pink or red raised patches of thickened skin covered by white or silvery scales (see page 123). Psoriasis may cause slight itching or soreness but usually causes

Side Effects of Topical Corticosteroids

Inflammation is a major feature of many skin conditions. Topical corticosteroids are medications that are applied to the surface of the skin to prevent or reduce inflammation and are useful for treating a number of skin conditions. If your doctor prescribes a corticosteroid preparation or if you use an over-the-counter topical corticosteroid, use it exactly as directed. Corticosteroids may cause the following adverse reactions:

- **Skin reactions (called steroid rashes)** These can be flushed skin, pus-filled spots, or a pink, flaky rash. The reactions should disappear when you stop using the corticosteroid.

- **Worsening of boils or other skin infections** Corticosteroids can make infections worse because they inhibit the immune system.

- **A rebound effect** The original skin disorder returns (sometimes in a more severe form) when you stop using the medication.

- **Permanent changes in your skin** If you use a corticosteroid preparation for several months (especially on the face, under the arms, or around the anus or groin), the skin in the affected area thins out, fine blood vessels under the skin can become conspicuous, and marks (similar to the stretch marks of pregnancy) may appear.

- **Diminished adrenal gland function** Corticosteroids interfere with the function of the adrenal glands by replacing (and preventing the release of) the naturally occurring hormones produced by the adrenal glands, which can be life-threatening.

- **Glaucoma and cataracts** Using corticosteroid creams around the eyes can cause increased fluid pressure in the eye that can cause eye damage (glaucoma; see page 1042) or clouding of the lens of the eye (cataracts; see page 1041).

no discomfort. You may have only one patch of scaly skin or many large ones. The most frequently affected areas are the knees, elbows, and scalp. Less often, patches may appear under the armpits and breasts, on the genitals, and around the anus. When psoriasis occurs on the hands and feet, it is usually in the form of painful cracks or small blisters. In some cases, the nails become thick and pitted and separate from the skin. A person with psoriatic arthritis also has stiff, swollen, and painful joints. Doctors can diagnose psoriasis by its appearance.

Treatment

Psoriasis is a chronic condition with no cure, but treatment usually is successful in clearing up outbreaks. If you have psoriasis, identify and avoid the factors that seem to trigger outbreaks. A number of treatments are available, depending on the severity of the disease. Exposing the skin to sunlight or light from an ultraviolet lamp can help clear up psoriasis. Narrow-band ultraviolet B lightbulbs are more effective than standard ultraviolet lightbulbs. Because a sunburn can make psoriasis worse (and cause skin cancer), your doctor will recommend safe techniques for sunbathing and for getting an adequate amount of ultraviolet light or sunlight to treat the psoriasis.

Topical treatments for psoriasis include over-the-counter or prescription coal tar or salicylic acid preparations, corticosteroid medications, a synthetic form of vitamin D called calcipotriene, a potent vitamin A derivative called tazarotene, and a medication called anthralin. The immune-suppressing medications cyclosporine and methotrexate (which slow cell division) and retinoid medications (vitamin A–like drugs) may be taken orally or injected to treat severe forms of psoriasis.

Medications that dampen the errant immune response that may cause psoriasis are given in injections to people whose psoriasis has not responded to treatment with other medications.

Acne

Acne is a common skin condition that results from inflammation of the hair follicles and sebaceous glands. Sebaceous glands produce an oily substance called sebum that lubricates the skin. If your body produces too much sebum and it becomes trapped in follicles, blemishes called blackheads

and whiteheads form. Bacteria that are normally present on the skin can invade the blocked follicle and multiply quickly, causing red, pus-filled lumps called pimples (see page 121). Acne is most common during puberty and adolescence because the level of male hormones rises in both boys and girls at this time, stimulating the sebaceous glands to increase sebum production. Acne usually clears up in the late teens or early 20s, although many people develop acne later in life.

Symptoms

Acne blemishes are usually concentrated on the face, but may appear on the neck, back, chest, buttocks, and sometimes the upper arms and thighs. As some blemishes heal, others appear. Pimples may leave dark, purplish marks on the skin, which usually fade. Severely inflamed pimples may take weeks to clear and can leave scars.

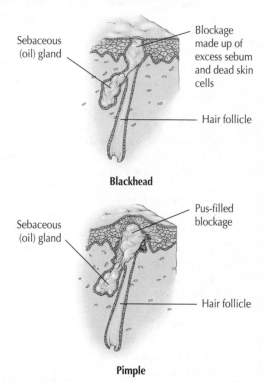

Blackhead

Pimple

Acne blemishes
An acne blemish can form when sebum and dead skin cells block the opening of a hair follicle. Blackheads (top) are blockages in which the collection of sebum turns dark because of oxidation and the presence of the skin pigment melanin. A blackhead can turn into a pimple (bottom) if the sebum that is unable to escape builds up along with bacteria and dead skin cells in the hair follicle, producing pus.

Treatment

If you have mild acne, keep your skin clean but don't scrub or pick it. Wash your skin with a mild, antibacterial soap twice a day. Try not to wash it more often unless it is very dirty or oily. Don't use moisturizers unless absolutely necessary, and then use only those recommended by your doctor—and only use them sparingly. Avoid wearing foundation makeup—if you feel you must, use a water-based makeup and always remove it completely. If you have oily skin, wash your hair with a dandruff or detergent shampoo, and don't use oily hair-care products.

Acne treatments work in one or more of the following ways—by reducing the production of sebum, by killing the harmful bacteria on the skin, or by speeding up the rate at which skin cells are shed (by removing keratin, the main component of the outer layer of skin). These treatments have made severe acne and scarring less common. Ask your doctor to recommend an over-the-counter acne preparation that contains salicylic acid (which loosens and helps remove the keratin blocking the pores) or benzoyl peroxide (an antibacterial medication that induces skin peeling).

Your doctor may refer you to a dermatologist (a doctor who specializes in disorders of the skin). The dermatologist may prescribe topical treatments such as a light chemical peel to loosen blackheads and prevent new blemishes, antibiotics (such as erythromycin, clindamycin, tetracycline, or sulfonamide) to kill the bacteria, medications that decrease bacteria (such as azelaic acid), or nicotinamide (a B vitamin that makes antibiotics more effective). He or she may prescribe stronger acne medications called retinoids (such as tretinoin, isotretinoin, adapalene, and tazarotene), which are derived from vitamin A. Retinoids have an antibacterial effect and loosen and remove keratin. Oral medications for acne include antibiotics (such as tetracycline, erythromycin, minocycline, and doxycycline), hormonal treatments (such as estrogen-containing birth-control pills or spironolactone), and the B vitamin nicotinamide.

Rosacea

Rosacea is a skin disorder in which the tiny blood vessels in the face (usually in the cheeks, nose, and forehead; see page 123) enlarge over weeks or months. The cause is unknown, but the following factors may play a role—genetic predisposition, environmental factors, a disorder of the immune system or blood vessels, tiny mites that live in hair follicles, or Helicobacter pylori (a bacterium that causes infection in the gastrointestinal system). The condition can be triggered by hot or caffeine-containing foods or beverages, alcohol, sun exposure, stress, exercise, cold wind, or hot baths or showers. Women are more often affected, but the disorder is often more severe in men.

Symptoms and Diagnosis

In rosacea, the entire face may be red, or it may be red only in streaks or patches. The skin affected by rosacea can have pus-filled bumps or pimples. In some cases, the nose is enlarged and bulbous, and thick, knobby bumps may develop on the nose (a condition called rhinophyma). Half of people who have rosacea also develop a form of the eye infection conjunctivitis (see page 1038). A doctor can diagnose rosacea by its appearance.

Treatment

Because rosacea cannot be cured, your doctor may refer you to a dermatologist (a doctor who specializes in disorders of the skin) to treat your symptoms and improve your appearance. He or she will prescribe topical or oral antibiotics such as clindamycin, tetracycline, doxycycline, erythromycin, or metronidazole. Sulfacetamide may be prescribed to treat conjunctivitis. Redness, enlarged blood vessels, and rhinophyma can be treated with laser surgery (see page 1088) or pulsed light therapy (which uses high-intensity pulses of light) to penetrate the skin and correct skin imperfections.

Hives

Hives are red, itchy lumps that develop on the skin, usually as a result of a mild allergic reaction (see page 912). They sometimes have a pale center and may join together to form large, irregular patches (see page 122). Hives are common and can appear anywhere on the body, brought on by factors such as an allergic reaction to foods or food additives, medications, plants, heat, cold, or sunlight.

In many cases, it is impossible to pinpoint the cause of hives. In rare cases, hives may be a symptom of a life-threatening disorder such as a severe allergic reaction or lupus (see page 920). In some people, stress, taking aspirin, or consuming caffeine can worsen hives.

In most cases, hives clear up on their own within a few hours. You will probably be able to identify and avoid the source of the problem if it is a particular food, plant, or medication. A food dye that is added to a wide variety of foods may be more difficult to identify and avoid. See your doctor or an allergist for skin tests (see page 912) to help identify the cause. He or she may prescribe an antihistamine to control your symptoms. Occasionally, hives persist or recur after treatment.

WARNING!

Hives May Be a Life-Threatening Allergic Reaction

If, soon after you develop hives, the tissues under the hives start to swell, especially on your face and around your lips or eyes, call 911 or your local emergency number or go to the nearest hospital emergency department immediately. You may be having a severe allergic reaction (anaphylactic shock; see page 915).

Impetigo

Impetigo is a highly contagious bacterial skin infection that is especially common in children. In infants, it can spread and infect the entire body. The bacteria (usually staphylococcus or streptococcus) enter through breaks in the skin such as cuts or scratches. In rare cases, if impetigo is caused by streptococcal bacteria and is not treated, a life-threatening condition called glomerulonephritis (see page 807) may develop.

Symptoms and Diagnosis

In impetigo, a small patch of tiny blisters appears on the body, frequently around the nose and mouth (see page 124). The blisters usually are not noticeable until they break, exposing red, moist, oozing skin, which gradually becomes covered by a tan crust. The infection spreads, and newly infected areas develop. Other symptoms of impetigo can include fever and swollen lymph glands. Doctors can diagnose impetigo from the symptoms.

Treatment

If you have impetigo, your doctor will prescribe a topical antibacterial medication or an oral antibiotic.

Wash away the crusts with antibacterial soap and water and a clean washcloth. To avoid spreading the infection, don't share washcloths, towels, or pillowcases. Children should stay home from school for at least 2 days after starting antibiotics. If not treated, impetigo can persist and spread.

Cellulitis

Cellulitis is a skin infection caused by bacteria such as streptococcus or staphylococcus. The bacteria enter through a break in the skin, such as a small cut or sore, and produce enzymes that break down the skin cells. Cellulitis can result from tinea (a fungus) skin infections such as athlete's foot (see page 1073).

Symptoms and Diagnosis

In cellulitis, a red, tender swelling develops on the body, usually on the legs (see page 125), and spreads gradually for a few days. Red lines may appear on the skin, running from infected areas along lymph vessels to nearby lymph glands. The lymph glands may swell, and a fever may develop. A doctor can diagnose cellulitis by the symptoms.

Treatment

To treat cellulitis, doctors prescribe oral antibiotics. In rare cases, treatment requires intravenous antibiotics. If cellulitis is not treated, bacteria can enter the bloodstream and cause blood poisoning (see page 937), which can be life-threatening.

Sunburn

Sunburn is inflammation of the skin from overexposure to the ultraviolet rays of the sun. The burned skin is red, hot, tender, and swollen. In severe cases, blisters may form and the skin may peel. You can get a sunburn more easily if you have light skin (although anyone can get sunburned). Having a disorder such as systemic lupus erythematosus (see page 920) or taking a medication such as tetracycline, doxycycline, or minocycline or a herbal supplement such as St John's wort can make the skin more sensitive to the sun's rays.

You can get sunburned at any time, even on an overcast or cold winter day. The sun's rays can reflect off surfaces such as snow, water, sand, or concrete. Sunburn is more likely to occur in places with intense sunlight, such as the southeastern and southwestern United States and places near the equator. People from northern latitudes who vacation in these areas are most susceptible to sunburn because they may not be aware of the sun's intensity at hours that are not usually dangerous at home.

Repeatedly or regularly exposing your skin to the sun breaks down the elastic tissues in the skin, making it age prematurely and become wrinkled. In addition, excessive sun exposure can produce red, roughened patches of skin called actinic (or solar) keratoses (see next page), which are especially common in people with fair skin. Actinic keratoses can become cancerous if not treated.

Preventing Sunburn

The ultraviolet rays in sunlight destroy cells in the outer layer of skin and damage tiny blood vessels beneath, possibly leading to skin cancer, premature wrinkling, and spider veins (dilated blood vessels). To avoid skin damage from the sun:

- Routinely apply a sunscreen with an SPF (sun protection factor) of 15 or higher to all uncovered areas of your body every time you go out during the day, especially before prolonged exposure to the sun. Reapply the sunscreen often throughout the day.
- Wear clothing with a high SPF to block light. High-SPF clothing has a tight weave. For example, plain cotton has an SPF of 7, cotton and polyester have an SPF of 15, polyester and lycra have 35, and cotton denim has 1,700.
- Wear a wide-brimmed hat that shades most of your face, neck, and shoulders. Baseball caps do not provide enough shade.
- Walk or sit in the shade when you're outside.
- Try to avoid the sun between 9 AM and 3 PM, when the ultraviolet rays are the strongest.
- Don't try to get a tan, and don't go to tanning salons. If you like the look of suntanned skin, apply an over-the-counter self-tanning product. Many of these products include a sunscreen.

Treatment

If you get a sunburn, take aspirin right away to help reduce the inflammation and relieve discomfort. Running cool water on the burned area or applying a cool cloth to the burn can help lower the temperature of the skin and reduce pain.

Basal Cell Carcinoma

Basal cell carcinoma is the most common skin cancer. In basal cell carcinoma, cells just beneath the surface of the skin are damaged and become cancerous, usually from long-term exposure to strong sunlight. Basal cell carcinoma is common on skin areas that are regularly exposed to the sun, such as the nose or the back or, in men, the chest. Unlike many malignant growths, basal cell carcinoma usually does not spread to other parts of the body. If it spreads, it does so over a number of years. A large, untreated basal cell carcinoma can eventually destroy surrounding tissue and cause disfigurement, but death from this cancer is rare.

Symptoms

In basal cell carcinoma, a small, flesh-colored, sometimes pearly lump with enlarged blood vessels appears on the skin (see page 119). The tumor grows slowly and develops a sore (ulcer) with a hard border and a raw, moist center that may bleed. Scabs may keep forming over the ulcer and the area may seem to heal, but the ulcer keeps returning.

Diagnosis and Treatment

If you have a basal cell carcinoma, your doctor will take a small sample from the tumor for examination under a microscope (biopsy). A basal cell cancer can be removed by cutting it out or destroying it with laser surgery (see page 1088), freezing (cryosurgery), burning with a high-frequency electric current (electrocautery), or radiation therapy (see page 23).

In a technique called Mohs surgery (see page 22), progressive layers of skin and surrounding tissue are sliced off parallel to the tumor and examined microscopically for the presence of cancer. The surgeon stops cutting off layers when he or she reaches a layer whose outer margins are free of cancer cells. Mohs surgery diminishes the amount of skin that has to be excised around a skin cancer and cuts down on the degree of disfigurement.

Doctors sometimes recommend a topical cream (fluorouracil or imiquimod) to treat superficial skin cancers in people who may not tolerate surgical procedures well, such as older people or people with a weakened immune system. However, treatment with topical creams is less effective and the cure rate is lower than that for surgery.

In some cases, basal cell carcinoma returns after treatment, usually within about 2 years, and treatment has to be repeated.

Squamous Cell Carcinoma

In squamous cell carcinoma, underlying skin cells are damaged, usually from many years of exposure to strong sunlight. Squamous cell cancers are common on body parts that are constantly exposed to the sun, such as the ears, hands, and mouth. Unlike basal cell carcinoma (see previous page), squamous cell carcinoma can spread to other parts of the body (metastasize) if untreated. You are most at risk of skin cancer if you have lived in a southern latitude or tropical area, worked outdoors for many years, have fair skin, or are middle-aged or older.

Symptoms

In squamous cell carcinoma, a firm, fleshy, hard-surfaced, sometimes scaly lump (see page 119) develops and grows steadily. In some cases, it looks like a wart or an ulcer. A squamous cell carcinoma can double in size in a few weeks.

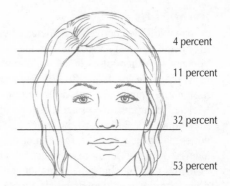

Squamous cell carcinomas on the face
Squamous cell carcinomas that appear on the face usually develop on the lower part of the face, particularly between the bottom of the nose and the chin.

another part of the body) to fill in the area that was cut away. When treated early, most squamous cell cancers are completely cured. However, because the cancer can recur, you should see your doctor regularly for follow-up examinations for at least 5 years.

Malignant Melanoma

Malignant melanoma (see page 119) is the most serious type of skin cancer because it can spread throughout the body quickly. Changes in the skin cells that make melanin (a skin-coloring pigment) can produce a life-threatening cancerous tumor. Melanoma usually develops in a mole or freckle that has formed after birth or in seemingly normal, unpigmented skin. In rare cases, melanoma occurs before adolescence, usually in a mole that has been present from birth. A melanoma can develop anywhere on the body (even on skin that is seldom exposed to the sun) and on any skin surface (including under a nail). However, having one bad sunburn in childhood, repeated sunburns over the years, or a family history of melanoma increases your risk of developing the cancer.

The incidence of melanoma is increasing faster than any other cancer, doubling in the United States since the 1970s. Doctors think this increase is related to the popularity of suntanning, tanning salons, and more leisure time in the sun. It also may be related to use of sunscreens (because people mistakenly think they can safely spend more time in the sun with sunscreen).

> ### Actinic Keratoses
>
> Actinic (or solar) keratoses are benign (non-cancerous) rough or thick patches of skin (see page 121) caused by overexposure to the sun. In rare cases, actinic keratoses develop into skin cancer, usually squamous cell carcinoma. For this reason, actinic keratoses are removed, usually by laser surgery (see page 1088), freezing (cryosurgery), or a topical medication such as fluorouracil, isotretinoin, or imiquimod.

Diagnosis and Treatment

If you have a lump on your skin that does not heal within 3 weeks, your doctor may take a small sample from the lump for examination under a microscope (biopsy). Most squamous cell cancers are removed by cutting them away. Other treatments include freezing (cryosurgery), burning with a high-frequency electric current (electrocautery), radiation therapy (see page 23), or Mohs surgery (in which progressive layers of the tumor and surrounding tissue are sliced off and examined for cancer cells until the layers are free of cancer; see page 22). You may need a skin graft (replacement skin taken from

Symptoms

A malignant melanoma can be black or brown and may begin as a flat spot or look like a mole. Often you can see other colors in the melanoma, such as gray, red, blue, or white. Sometimes a malignant melanoma may have no dark pigment at all. Melanomas appear asymmetrical (one half of the melanoma doesn't match the other half) and the edges may be jagged or blurred (a normal mole has a defined edge). Melanomas are usually larger than 1/4 inch in diameter but can be smaller and can grow almost imperceptibly in an existing mole.

WARNING!

ABCDs of Skin Cancer

See your doctor immediately if you notice any of these signs of skin cancer in a mole, or if a mole seems to be growing:

- **Asymmetry** If you draw an imaginary line down the middle of the mole, each side is a different size or shape.
- **Border** The mole has an irregular or blurred border.
- **Color** The mole has more than one shade or color (such as black, brown, blue, red, and white).
- **Diameter** The mole is larger than 1/4 inch (about the size of the tip of a pencil eraser).

Diagnosis and Treatment

If you have signs of melanoma, your doctor will remove part or all of the tumor for examination under a microscope (biopsy). If a diagnosis of melanoma is confirmed, the mole or tumor and some of the surrounding tissue is removed surgically. Usually a skin graft (replacement skin taken from another part of the body) is done at the same time to cover the area that was removed, especially if the melanoma is large. In addition, the doctor will test nearby lymph nodes (called sentinel nodes) to see if they contain cancer cells. If it is possible that the cancer has spread to other parts of the body, a doctor may recommend chemotherapy (see page 23) or immunotherapy (which strengthens the immune system to increase its ability to fight cancer cells; see page 22).

Varicose Ulcers

If you have stretched or twisted veins directly under the skin, especially in the legs (varicose veins; see

pages 125 and 602), you have poor circulation. Blood flow through the lower parts of your body (especially the calves, ankles, and feet) becomes sluggish, making small injuries or cracks in the skin less likely to heal, often causing them to enlarge and gradually become ulcers (sores). Varicose ulcers are more common in older people, pregnant women, and people who are obese or confined to bed.

Symptoms

Varicose ulcers are shallow sores that can become infected. They may heal and continuously recur or not heal at all. Varicose ulcers usually occur on the inside of the leg just above the ankle. The skin around the ulcer turns red and then brownish purple and is itchy and flaky. The ankles often swell.

Diagnosis and Treatment

A doctor can usually diagnose a varicose ulcer by its appearance. He or she may order an ultrasound (see page 111) of the legs to rule out another disorder.

If you have a varicose ulcer, your doctor will recommend that you avoid standing for long periods (but walk regularly), keep the affected area raised (preferably above the level of your heart) as often as possible (even while lying down), and wear an elastic support stocking during the day. He or she may show you how to clean the ulcer. Clean the ulcer often and keep it covered with a bandage.

If the ulcer is severe, the doctor may coat it with a medication specially formulated to soothe and heal wounds, and bandage it. You may need to have a skin graft (replacement skin taken from another part of the body) to cover the affected area and promote healing. If more serious complications develop, your doctor may prescribe a medication called becaplermin, which contains a natural blood factor that improves healing. If the ulcer gets worse, you may have to be hospitalized.

Epidermal Cysts

Epidermal cysts (also called sebaceous cysts) are benign (noncancerous) cysts that originate in the epidermis (the thin, protective outer skin layer made up mostly of dead cells). An epidermal cyst is formed when keratin (the hard substance that is the main component of the epidermis) blocks a sebaceous gland, producing a cyst that grows slowly over many years. Epidermal cysts are common and sometimes are associated with acne (see page 1065).

Symptoms

An epidermal cyst looks like a pale lump beneath the skin (see page 122), and may have a narrow pore that is visible on the surface of the skin. If the cyst becomes infected, it fills with pus and becomes red, inflamed, and tender and may eventually burst.

Diagnosis and Treatment

Doctors can diagnose an epidermal cyst by its appearance. If a cyst is not infected, no treatment is necessary, and the cyst may eventually go away on its own. If the cyst is infected, your doctor may prescribe antibiotics and ask you to apply warm, moist compresses to the area to release the buildup of pus. Alternatively, your doctor may inject the cyst with a corticosteroid medication, which will temporarily relieve the inflammation and pain. Sometimes a cyst breaks under the skin, causing redness and pain; eventually, scar tissue may form that can make the cyst difficult to remove surgically. Even if pus is released and the inflammation subsides, a cyst that has been infected should be removed surgically because it is likely to become infected again. Your doctor can remove the cyst in an outpatient procedure. However, if even a small part of an epidermal cyst is left behind, it can recur.

Pityriasis Rosea

Pityriasis rosea (see page 123) is a common skin disorder that affects primarily children and young adults. The cause is unknown, but some doctors think that a virus may be responsible.

Symptoms

Pityriasis rosea starts as one or more large, red, scaly spots, usually on the trunk. Over a few days, the spots grow and new ones appear on the trunk and upper part of the arms (in a T-shirt–like distribution). The spots become oval patches of copper-colored skin with scaly surfaces, and the rash may itch. You may have a mild sore throat as the rash develops.

Diagnosis and Treatment

Because the symptoms of pityriasis rosea can resemble the symptoms of other disorders, such as ringworm, your doctor will perform a physical examination to confirm the diagnosis. If you have pityriasis rosea, your doctor may recommend monitoring the rash for about a month to see if the spots go away on their own. In the meantime, he or she may recommend that you avoid taking hot showers or baths because the heat can dry the skin and make itching worse. You also can apply an over-the-counter cold cream to the rash. Your doctor may prescribe a corticosteroid medication to relieve the inflammation and an antihistamine to relieve the itching.

Keloids

A keloid is scar tissue that has grown excessively. Keloids can occur at the site of a surgical incision, burn, vaccination, piercing, severe acne, or even a small scratch, or they may occur spontaneously. Keloids are more common in people with dark skin.

Symptoms and Treatment

A keloid starts out like normal scar tissue but, after several months, grows and becomes larger and thicker (see page 122). Keloids can itch and cause discomfort.

Keloids sometimes stop growing or disappear without treatment. They cannot be removed surgically because scar tissue from the surgery can develop into another keloid. If you have a thin keloid, you can apply over-the-counter sheets of silicone gel to make it smaller. Your doctor may inject the keloid with a corticosteroid medication or prescribe a topical corticosteroid cream or ointment to stop the growth of scar tissue. Laser surgery (see page 1088) and, in rare cases, radiation therapy (see page 23) can be used to reduce the size of keloids.

Lichen Planus

Lichen planus is an inflammatory disease that is most common in middle-aged people. It can affect the mouth (oral lichen planus; see page 745) as well as the skin. Although the cause is not known, some doctors think that lichen planus is more common in people who have a weakened immune system or who are under stress. In some cases, lichen planus occurs as an allergic reaction to some medications.

Symptoms

The rash consists of small, shiny, reddish spots that appear suddenly (often on the wrists; see page 124); patches of thickened, discolored skin that gradually fade and leave a brown mark; or a lacy pattern of slightly raised tissue in moist areas such as the vulva or mouth. The rash may itch. Fingernails and toenails that are affected by lichen planus may be ridged.

Diagnosis and Treatment

If you have lichen planus, your doctor may refer you to a dermatologist, who can diagnose lichen planus by its appearance. However, because the symptoms of lichen planus resemble the symptoms of other, sometimes serious, skin disorders, the doctor may take a sample of skin cells for examination under a microscope (biopsy) to rule out cancer or other disorders. If a diagnosis of lichen planus is confirmed, the doctor will recommend a corticosteroid ointment to apply to the rash to reduce the inflammation; this medication usually clears up the rash. Treatment is repeated if the rash recurs.

Discoid Lupus Erythematosus

Discoid lupus erythematosus is a chronic skin disorder of unknown cause. The skin rash of discoid lupus resembles that of systemic lupus erythematosus (see page 920), but discoid lupus has none of the other symptoms of systemic lupus. Discoid lupus is more common in women than in men and usually develops between ages 30 and 40.

Symptoms

Discoid lupus usually takes the form of a red, itchy, scaly rash on the bridge of the nose and cheeks (often shaped like a butterfly; see page 124). However, circular patches of the rash may appear in other skin areas (particularly those exposed to the sun) with or without the butterfly rash on the face. When the patches of skin heal, they may be thin, pale, and scarred.

Diagnosis and Treatment

If you have symptoms of discoid lupus, your doctor will perform a physical examination and tests to rule out systemic lupus. If you have discoid lupus, the doctor will recommend protecting the affected areas of your skin with a sunblock or clothing. This is often the only treatment necessary.

If more treatment is needed, your doctor will prescribe an anti-inflammatory medication such as chloroquine or dapsone. A topical corticosteroid cream can help reduce inflammation and improve the appearance of the rash; however, long-term use of corticosteroids is not recommended because they can thin the skin and the symptoms recur when the medication is stopped.

Vitiligo

Vitiligo is a common disorder in which patches of skin lose their color (pigment), usually on the face and hands (see page 118) and in the armpits and groin. The condition seems to be an autoimmune disorder in which the immune system mistakenly attacks the pigment-producing cells in the skin. The loss of pigmentation is especially obvious in people who have dark skin. The condition may occur in cycles and then stop altogether.

Symptoms

In vitiligo, the irregular, unpigmented patches of skin often appear symmetrically on both sides of the body. The patches may grow, shrink, or stay the same size and, because they lack protective pigment, are especially sensitive to sunlight. In severe cases, the condition affects the whole body.

Diagnosis and Treatment

A doctor can usually diagnose vitiligo by its appearance. He or she may order a skin biopsy to rule out other disorders.

There is no cure for vitiligo. In rare cases, pigment returns to the skin. Makeup, self-tanners, dyes that color the skin, or tattooing small areas of skin with a skin-colored pigment can darken the lighter areas. It is important to protect these nonpigmented areas from sunburn (see page 1067) with a sunblock that has an SPF of at least 15. Topical corticosteroid medications or phototherapy (light therapy) can help temporarily return pigment to small areas. To even out their skin tone, some people choose to have the remaining pigment permanently removed from their skin with a chemical. In rare cases, skin grafts (transferring skin from one part of the body to another) are done, but they seldom result in a total return of pigment.

Tinea Infections

Tinea is a fungus that can infect the skin, hair, or nails. As the fungus grows, it spreads out in a circle, leaving normal-looking skin in the middle that makes the growth look like a ring. The skin at the edge of the ring is lifted up slightly and looks red and scaly. Because the infection can look like a worm under the skin, it is sometimes referred to as ringworm. On the feet, a tinea infection is called athlete's foot; in the genital area or groin, it is called jock itch. The fungus can spread easily from person to person by direct contact or in showers, bathrooms, or locker rooms, and can be transmitted to people from cats, dogs, or farm animals.

Athlete's foot

You can get athlete's foot (tinea pedis; see page 123) from direct contact with the fungus or contact with contaminated skin cells shed from an infected person. If the fungus spreads to the toenails, it makes them thick and crumbly. The fungus also can spread from the feet to the hands and fingernails.

Jock itch

When the tinea fungus grows in the genital area, usually in men, it is called jock itch (tinea cruris). The infection is especially common in athletes who wear elastic shorts or athletic supporters, which can make the groin area moist and warm (conditions favorable for fungus to grow).

Ringworm

Ringworm (tinea capitis) usually develops on the head and is most common in children. The fungus destroys the hair, leaving bald patches (see pages 123 and 1075).

Symptoms

In athlete's foot, the skin becomes red, flaky, and itchy. If the skin is moist (from water or perspiration), the top layer of skin becomes soggy and whitish. In jock itch, scaly, itchy patches of skin appear on the upper and inner thigh. Ringworm produces itchy, red areas on the scalp.

Diagnosis

Tinea infections can usually be diagnosed by their appearance. To confirm the diagnosis, a doctor may take a sample from the affected area and examine it under a microscope (biopsy) to look for the fungus.

In some cases, a sample of skin, hair, or nail is sent to a laboratory for analysis to confirm the diagnosis.

Treatment

Tinea infections, especially athlete's foot and jock itch, can usually be treated with an over-the-counter antifungal cream. Applying the cream twice a day for 2 to 4 weeks usually clears up the infection.

Your doctor will recommend self-help measures to help clear up the infection and to prevent recurring infections. For example, he or she will recommend drying your skin thoroughly (especially in the groin area and between your toes) after taking a bath or shower. Throw out worn-out shoes that might have fungal spores in them, especially if you have worn them without socks. Wear absorbent socks made of natural fibers (such as cotton) and change them daily. If the over-the-counter preparation you are using is not effective, your doctor may recommend another one.

In severe cases or for tinea infections on parts of the body other than the feet or groin (which can be harder to treat), a doctor may prescribe an oral antifungal medication.

Prevention

Keeping your skin clean and dry is the best protection against the tinea fungus. The following steps also can help you avoid a tinea infection:

- Change your socks and underwear every day, especially in warm weather.
- Try not to wear thick clothing for long periods in warm weather.
- In hot weather, wear sandals, open shoes, or shoes made of a breathable material that expose your feet to the air and allow perspiration to evaporate; go without shoes at home.
- Air out your shoes well between wearings.
- Avoid walking barefoot over surfaces (such as locker-room floors) on which the fungus often grows; use rubber sandals or shower shoes.
- Don't share towels, bathmats, or nail clippers with someone who might have athlete's foot.
- Throw out worn-out athletic or walking shoes, and never wear anyone else's shoes.
- Check your pets for areas of fur loss, and have your veterinarian check them regularly.
- Use a topical athlete's foot cream for about a week if you live with or have been in close contact with someone who has athlete's foot.

Cutaneous Anthrax

Cutaneous, or skin, anthrax is an uncommon infection of the skin by a spore-forming bacterium called Bacillus anthracis. The infection is most common in wild and domestic livestock (including cattle, sheep, and goats), but infections also can occur in humans. Cutaneous anthrax infections develop most frequently in people whose occupations expose them to infected animals or animal products (such as wool, hides, or hair)—including farm workers, veterinarians, and tannery and wool workers. However, outbreaks of skin anthrax also have occurred as a result of acts of bioterrorism (see page 30) in which letters intentionally contaminated with anthrax spores were sent through the mail. Treatment clears up nearly all cases of skin anthrax. If not treated, however, in one in five cases the infection can spread through the bloodstream and be fatal.

Symptoms and Diagnosis

Within about 2 weeks of contact with the anthrax bacterium, an itchy skin sore develops that looks like a mosquito bite. The area around the sore usually is swollen. The sore forms a blister and then an ulcer (open sore), which develops a black scab (see page 125) that dries and falls off within a couple of weeks. In some cases, a fever and headache develop, and lymph nodes in the area of the infection become swollen and painful.

To diagnose skin anthrax, a doctor performs a biopsy, in which a sample from a sore is examined under a microscope to look for the anthrax bacterium.

Treatment

If you have cutaneous anthrax, your doctor will prescribe one of several oral antibiotics that are effective against the bacterium, such as penicillin, doxycycline, or ciprofloxacin. (During a suspected outbreak, ciprofloxacin is the antibiotic that is likely to be prescribed.) You probably will have to take the medication for about 60 days, because it can take up to 60 days for anthrax spores to germinate (and potentially cause further infection). There is no known transmission of cutaneous anthrax from person to person.

Disorders of the Hair and Nails

Hair and nails are dead, hardened structures that are similar chemically to the surface layer of your skin. The substance that gives both hair and nails their hardness is a protein called keratin, which is found in smaller amounts in the top layer of the skin. Hair grows from follicles, which are pits of actively dividing cells that occur in varying numbers in the skin. Nails grow from special folds in the skin. Disorders that affect the hair and nails are usually cosmetic and generally not harmful to health.

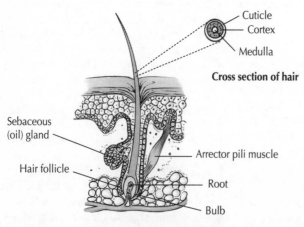

Cuticle
Cortex
Medulla

Cross section of hair

Sebaceous
(oil) gland

Hair follicle

Arrector pili muscle

Root

Bulb

Cross section of skin with hair follicle

Hair
Hair is a threadlike structure composed of dead cells filled with keratin (a type of protein). Shafts of hair grow from tiny pits in the skin called hair follicles. The root of the hair is embedded in the skin and, in its growing phase, is firmly enclosed by live tissue called a bulb. Hair is surrounded by sebaceous (oil) glands and arrector pili muscles, which pull hairs erect.

Each hair consists of a central, spongy, semi-hollow core called the medulla. The medulla is surrounded by a layer of long, thin fibers called the cortex. On the outside of each hair are several layers of overlapping cells called the cuticle.

Dandruff

Dandruff is a condition in which small, dead flakes of skin develop on the scalp when skin cells grow unusually fast. The two main causes of dandruff are a mild form of seborrheic dermatitis (see page 1063) and, less frequently, psoriasis (see page 1064) of the scalp. The hair itself is not affected.

Treatment

To treat dandruff, use an over-the-counter anti-dandruff shampoo as often as recommended on the label (usually every day or every other day). Make sure the shampoo contains one or more of the following ingredients: tar, selenium, sulfur, salicylic acid, zinc, or ketoconazole. For best results, lather twice each time you shampoo (the first time for 1 minute, then rinse, and the second time for 5 minutes). If regular use of the shampoo does not clear up your dandruff, your doctor may prescribe a corticosteroid lotion, or a lotion that contains a higher concentration of one of the ingredients in the anti-dandruff shampoo to apply to your scalp.

Ingrown Hairs

Ingrown hairs (also known as shaving bumps, razor bumps, or pseudofolliculitis barbae; see page 121) are hairs that become trapped in hair follicles. They usually result from close shaving but can occur for unknown reasons. Ingrown hairs are common, especially on the face in men and in people who have curly hair.

Symptoms and Treatment

Ingrown hairs cause small, hard bumps or swellings around hair follicles. The bumps can become inflamed and painful if they become infected.

To treat inflamed ingrown hairs, your doctor may recommend applying an over-the-counter acne medication that contains benzoyl peroxide (which loosens the hair by causing the skin to peel) or an over-the-counter antibiotic cream. Your doctor may prescribe a stronger acne medication such as tretinoin, or topical or oral antibiotics. If the problem is severe, your doctor may recommend that you stop shaving or have the hair in the areas that you normally shave permanently removed by electrolysis.

Preventing Ingrown Hairs

You can prevent ingrown hairs from shaving by following these tips:

- Before shaving, wash the area gently with mild soap and a soft, clean washcloth and rinse thoroughly. Apply a very warm washcloth to the skin but do not dry the skin.
- Apply a nonirritating shaving cream or gel, or one that contains benzoyl peroxide.
- Use a safety razor (not an electric razor) with sharp blades. Replace the blades often, preferably after every two shaves.
- Experiment to find the shaving technique that works best for you. Always shave in the direction in which the hair grows.
- Don't shave too closely; hold the razor lightly, and don't press too hard.
- Don't pull or stretch your skin while shaving, and don't shave twice over the same spot.
- After shaving, rinse the area thoroughly and pat it dry.

Pilonidal Cyst

A pilonidal cyst or abscess is inflammation of the sinus or space just above the cleft of the buttocks. The sinus becomes inflamed and fills with pus when one or more hairs become trapped beneath the skin. The condition is common in young men, especially in men who have a lot of body hair. It is thought to result from repeated friction, which pushes the hairs back into the skin.

Diagnosis and Treatment

A doctor can usually diagnose a pilonidal cyst by its appearance and the symptoms.

Your doctor may drain the sinus by removing the pus and trapped hairs. You must keep the area around the sinus clean and dry to prevent a recurrence. A pilonidal cyst that recurs (which is common) must be removed surgically.

Baldness

Baldness in older men is a natural process. Hereditary baldness tends to run in families on either the mother's or the father's side of the family. It is normal for women to have some hair loss throughout life. For men and women, hair loss may follow major psychological or physical stresses such as surgery or a debilitating illness or accident. But the hair usually grows back eventually.

In some people, hair loss can result from an overactive or underactive thyroid gland (see page 901), consuming an inadequate amount of protein, an iron deficiency (see page 610), or taking large doses of vitamin A. Having radiation therapy (see page 23) or chemotherapy (see page 23) or taking some medications (such as for arthritis, depression, heart disease, or high blood pressure) can also cause hair loss in some people. Hair follicles can be affected by any disorder that affects the skin, such as systemic lupus erythematosus (see page 920), lichen planus (see page 1071), or ringworm (see page 1073). Some people injure the roots of their hair by pulling on their hair to create a particular hairstyle. Some people constantly pull out their hair (including the eyebrows and eyelashes) as a nervous habit, sometimes stripping these areas completely of hair.

Alopecia areata

Alopecia areata is a disorder that usually causes patchy hair loss (although it can cause complete baldness). In alopecia areata, round, bald patches (see page 127) appear suddenly. The exposed scalp has normal skin and sometimes a few, fine, white hairs that may be abnormally narrow at the base. The cause of alopecia areata is unknown, but stress may be a factor in triggering it. A person with alopecia areata may also have pitted fingernails. In rare cases, a person has permanent hair loss all over the body, including in the armpits, pubic area, eyebrows, and eyelashes.

Baldness caused by alopecia areata often stops on its own within a few months, and the hair usually regrows eventually. To stimulate hair growth, a doctor may recommend applying minoxidil or a corticosteroid cream, or he or she may inject corticosteroids directly into the scalp or prescribe medication to help dampen the abnormal immune response. However, treatments for alopecia areata are not always effective.

Treatment

The treatment of baldness depends on the cause, the location of the hair loss, and on how extensive it is. Many people use hairpieces to cover a balding scalp. Hair-replacement surgery (see page 1096) is one of the most common cosmetic procedures performed on men.

Treatment with the topical over-the-counter medication minoxidil (available in a 2 percent solution for women and a 5 percent solution for men) produces a fine growth of downy hair in some men and women in 4 to 6 months. In 6 to 12 months, the new hair may eventually be about the same thickness as the rest of the hair. However, hair growth stops if the treatment is stopped. An oral medication called finasteride has been shown to be effective in about half of cases of male pattern baldness. It may take more than 6 months for the drug to produce noticeable results. To treat baldness in women, the blood pressure medication spironolactone is prescribed to lower the levels of the male hormones that are often linked to hair loss in women.

Unwanted Hair

Excessive hairiness (hirsutism) is usually not a sign of a health problem. However, you should see your doctor about excessive hair growth because hirsutism and hypertrichosis (hair growth in moles or in places not normally covered by hair) can result from a disorder or may be side effects of medication. In these cases, treating the underlying condition may correct the problem.

Temporary hair-removal methods include shaving, tweezing, waxing, and depilatory creams, lotions, or sprays. Hair can also be bleached to be less noticeable. Eflornithine, a topical enzyme inhibitor available by prescription, does not remove hair but slows the growth of unwanted facial hair in women. The only permanent methods of hair removal are electrolysis and laser hair removal.

Folliculitis

Folliculitis is infection of the hair follicles, which can occur anywhere on the skin or scalp. Most cases are caused by staphylococcal bacteria and usually result from hair-removal methods such as shaving, tweezing, or waxing. A type of folliculitis can develop from exposure to a bacterium called Pseudomonas aeruginosa, which can survive in hot tubs.

Symptoms

Folliculitis is characterized by an itchy, bumpy, red rash (see page 125) that appears within 2 days of exposure to the bacterium. The bumps may develop into dark red tender lumps (nodules) or may develop small, pus-filled blisters.

Diagnosis and Treatment

Your doctor will suspect folliculitis by the appearance of the rash or if you have used a hot tub within the past 3 days. For mild cases, treatment is usually unnecessary because the infection tends to clear up on its own. Your doctor may recommend a topical antibiotic cream or lotion to apply to the rash to eliminate the bacteria, and an oral or topical medication to reduce the itching.

For severe cases, a doctor may prescribe an oral antibiotic such as tetracycline, minocycline, ciprofloxacin, penicillin, or cephalosporin to take for 4 to 6 weeks. If you have chronic or recurring infections, your doctor will recommend letting your hair grow in the affected area for at least 3 months to help clear up the infection. If the folliculitis resulted from exposure to bacteria in a hot tub, your doctor will tell you how to control the pH (acid) and chlorine content of the water in the hot tub to eliminate bacteria and prevent more from growing.

Paronychia

Paronychia is infection of the cuticle or skin fold at the base or sides of a nail. The infection is usually caused by a bacterium (such as staphylococcus or pseudomonas) or a fungus (such as Candida) and is common in people who spend a lot of time with their hands in water. The infection comes on suddenly when it is caused by bacteria. A fungal infection, which is usually less painful, develops slowly and frequently becomes chronic.

Symptoms

The symptoms of paronychia include a swollen, red, and painful cuticle or nail fold (see page 127). The cuticle may lift away from the base of the nail; if you press on the nail, pus may come out. When the fold of the nail is affected, a blister of pus (called a whitlow) develops on the side of the nail. The skin around the nail may also be affected. The cuticle no longer protects the root of the nail, allowing the root to be damaged and deforming or discoloring the nail. In a fungal infection, the nail can become thick, white, and powdery.

Diagnosis and Treatment

A doctor can usually diagnose paronychia by its appearance. He or she may take a scraping from the nail to grow in a laboratory for examination under a microscope to identify the bacterium or fungus.

Your doctor will treat a bacterial nail infection (in its early stages) with antibiotics, and a chronic fungal nail infection with an antifungal cream. If you have a pus-filled blister, he or she may pierce the blister, which will relieve the pain and speed healing.

How to Keep Your Nails Healthy

The following guidelines can help you keep your nails healthy:

- Protect your nails and the skin surrounding them, especially when they are immersed in water, by wearing rubber or synthetic gloves over white cotton gloves (or rubber gloves into which you have sprinkled talcum powder).

- Don't use strong soaps on your hands or feet. Strong soaps can dry out the nails as well as the skin. Use a moisturizer after washing. Over-the-counter creams are available that are formulated to moisturize the nails and make them resistant to damage.

- Don't push back or cut your cuticles; they prevent germs from getting under your nail and causing infections.

- Nail polish remover makes nails brittle and weak. Don't use it more often than once a week.

- Keep nails short to prevent them from splitting.

- Trim your nails regularly. If you can't trim them yourself, have someone else, such as a family member or podiatrist, trim them.

- Cut your toenails straight across to avoid damaging the skin at the corners of the nail.

- Wear loose-fitting shoes and socks to avoid putting pressure on your toenails.

- If you have pain, redness, or swelling around a nail (especially if you have poor circulation or diabetes), see your doctor. Nail infections, particularly toenail infections, must be treated early to avoid complications.

Other Nail Problems

Nails can become abnormally shaped, discolored, or ingrown from a number of factors. Because some nail abnormalities can result from underlying disorders, always have any unusual nail condition evaluated by a doctor.

Deformed nails

Injury to the nail-forming area beneath the cuticle can lead to thickening of the whole nail. This thickening is most obvious in the toenails, where it results from poorly fitting shoes or decreased circulation from atherosclerosis (see page 557) or diabetes (see page 889). Many disorders such as psoriasis (see page 1064), lichen planus (see page 1071), and paronychia (see previous page) can cause the trimmed end of a nail to separate from the underlying skin. Iron deficiency anemia (see page 610) can make nails spoon-shaped. Congenital heart disease (see page 558), a chronic lung infection, or lung cancer (see page 646) can cause clubbing or knobby enlarged ends of the fingers and toes that also affect the shape of the nail (see page 127). Alopecia areata (see page 1076) may cause pitted fingernails. Poor nail growth can produce a temporary side-to-side groove in the nails.

Discolored Nails

Nails can be stained yellow or brown by tobacco or nail polish. Bruises can cause black and blue spots. The nail bed appears pale in anemia and bluish gray in some heart and lung disorders. If bacteria enter the space between the nail and the skin, the nail may turn blackish green. Small, black, splinterlike areas under the nails may indicate an infection of a heart valve. A vitamin or mineral deficiency or an injury to a nail can produce one or more small white patches in the nail (which will grow out with the nail).

Ingrown toenails

The nail of the big toe can curve under at the sides and catch in the skin, causing pain as the nail grows. If the nail continues to cut into the skin, infection can result because the area never has time to heal. Ingrown nails often result from pressure from poorly fitting shoes, from an injury, or from improper trimming.

Diagnosis and Treatment

See your doctor about a nail deformity or discoloration that doesn't grow out with the nail. Nails badly damaged by injury usually grow in again naturally in about 9 months.

See your doctor if you have an ingrown toenail. If the nail is not infected, he or she may place a piece of cotton between the nail and the toe, which usually relieves the pain. The cotton may be treated with a liquid (called collodion) that holds the cotton in place, protects the skin, and makes the cotton waterproof. If the nail is infected, your doctor may remove the ingrown edge of the nail and the toenail's fold next to it. To prevent ingrown toenails, follow the steps on the previous page to protect your nails.

18

Cosmetic Surgery

Plastic surgery includes both cosmetic surgery and reconstructive surgery. Doctors perform reconstructive surgery to correct abnormalities caused by birth defects, injury, or infection, or deformities from diseases such as cancer. For example, many women who have had a cancerous breast removed undergo reconstructive breast surgery (see page 860). Reconstructive surgery usually is covered by health insurance, although the extent of the coverage varies by policy.

This chapter focuses on cosmetic surgery—surgical procedures performed to enhance a person's physical appearance. Cosmetic surgery originally developed from reconstructive surgery and uses many of the same techniques. Health insurance usually does not cover the cost of cosmetic surgery because it is considered elective surgery. Read your health insurance policy carefully to find out what is and is not covered.

Set realistic goals when you are contemplating cosmetic surgery. Changing the way you look can enhance your appearance and might increase your self-esteem, but the final result may not completely match your preconceived image. The first time

How to Choose a Plastic Surgeon

All surgery involves risk. The most important step you can take to ensure a good result is to choose a skilled and experienced plastic surgeon. Make a list of potential surgeons recommended by your family doctor and friends and relatives who have had cosmetic surgery. Check to make sure that the surgeons have been adequately trained and are certified by the American Board of Plastic Surgery, which sets high standards of training and care in the specialty of plastic surgery. To be certified by the board, a surgeon must have completed at least 5 years of residency training after medical school (including 2 years in plastic surgery), passed comprehensive examinations, and been qualified to perform both cosmetic and reconstructive procedures.

Experience is another key qualification to look for in a plastic surgeon. Select a doctor who has performed the procedure you are interested in many times. Ask the surgeon how many times he or she has performed the procedure, and ask to see before-and-after photographs of previous patients.

Make sure that the facility where your surgery will be done meets strict safety standards. It should be certified by a national or state accrediting agency. All members of the American Society of Plastic Surgeons agree to operate only in certified facilities. Procedures performed in a licensed or accredited facility by a board-certified surgeon have the highest safety record.

you meet with your surgeon, he or she will evaluate your general health and carefully examine the part of your body you want to change. Be honest when talking about what you expect from your surgery. Your surgeon will explain your options and the risks and benefits of each. He or she will recommend the alternative that will most closely produce the results you are looking for.

Facial Surgery

Plastic surgeons perform plastic surgery on various areas of the face to give a more aesthetically pleasing appearance or to reverse signs of aging such as wrinkles or sagging skin. Cosmetic facial surgery encompasses a wide variety of procedures, including upper and lower eyelid surgery, forehead lifts, nose surgery, facelifts, facial implants, and collagen injections. Injections of botulinum toxin or collagen can improve the appearance of frown lines.

Nose Reshaping

Plastic surgeons perform surgery on the nose (known medically as rhinoplasty) to reshape the nose and correct breathing problems. Nose reshaping is the most commonly performed type of cosmetic surgery in the United States—more than 500,000 people have the procedure each year. Doctors recommend waiting to do nose-reshaping surgery until the nose has reached its full size, usually around age 14, unless a child's breathing is severely impeded. There is no upper age limit for nose reshaping. Many people request surgery on the nose at the same time as a facelift or other cosmetic surgery to correct age-related changes.

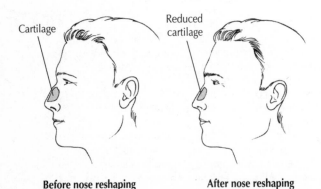

Before nose reshaping   **After nose reshaping**

Reshaping a nose
Excess cartilage in the bridge of the nose can produce an oversized or humped appearance (left). Cosmetic surgeons can reshape the nose by removing some of the cartilage (right).

The Procedure
Depending on the desired outcome, surgery can reduce or increase the bridge of your nose, decrease its size or width, make the nostrils narrower, or reshape the tip. Rhinoplasty can be either open or closed. In open rhinoplasty, the surgeon cuts the skin across the bottom of the center of the nose, separates the skin from the underlying bone and cartilage, reshapes the nose (by removing, adding to, or rearranging the underlying bone and cartilage), and then redrapes the skin. In closed rhinoplasty, the surgeon makes most of the incisions inside the nose, where they cannot be seen. In some cases, such as to narrow the nostrils, the surgeon may remove small wedges of skin from the area just under the nostrils. He or she closes the incisions with absorbable stitches (which don't need to be removed).

After completing the surgery, the surgeon often protects and stabilizes the nose with a splint and may place packs or soft nasal splints inside the nose to secure the positioning of the cartilage between the nostrils. The packing inside the nose is removed the next day, but the splint must stay in place for 5 to 8 days.

Most surgery on the nose is performed on an outpatient basis and takes 1 to 2 hours, although complicated procedures can take longer. Some procedures require general anesthesia, while others need only a local anesthetic combined with light sedation.

After Surgery
Your nose will feel sore after the surgery, and you will have temporary nasal stuffiness, along with swelling and bruising around your nose and eyes.

Incisions for rhinoplasty
To perform closed rhinoplasty, the surgeon makes most of the incisions inside the nose. Sometimes the surgeon removes small wedges of skin from the area just under the nostrils. The incisions are closed with absorbable stitches that do not need to be removed.

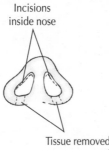

Incisions inside nose

Tissue removed to narrow nostrils

You may also have nosebleeds and headaches during the first week after surgery. To minimize swelling and bleeding, keep your head elevated, even while sleeping, and don't blow your nose for about a week after surgery. Avoid sun exposure for at least 8 weeks.

The main postsurgery risks are infection, bleeding, and broken blood vessels that leave permanent red spots on the skin of the nose. Nose reshaping alters the facial appearance so much that you may not look the way you expected, but more than 95 percent of people who have this type of surgery are satisfied with the outcome.

Most people who have had nose-reshaping surgery can resume their normal activities in 1 or 2 weeks. The final appearance of the nose may not be apparent until about a year after surgery.

Eyelid Surgery

Eyelid surgery, known medically as blepharoplasty, is one of the most common cosmetic surgery procedures, with about 100,000 men and women undergoing the procedure in the United States every year. Surgeons perform eyelid surgery to correct droopy, hooded upper eyelids and puffy lower lids that make the face look tired and older. In some people, the upper eyelids sag so much that they impair vision. (In this case, eyelid surgery may be covered by health insurance because it is not performed only to improve appearance.)

In blepharoplasty, the surgeon removes excess fat, skin, and muscle from the upper or lower lids, or both. Eyelid surgery does not remove dark circles from under the eyes, erase fine lines such as crow's feet, or lift sagging eyebrows. Sometimes doctors combine eyelid surgery with a forehead lift (see next page) or a facelift (see page 1083) to achieve better results.

People who should have a thorough medical evaluation before having eyelid surgery include those who have glaucoma (see page 1042), a detached retina (see page 1050), a thyroid problem such as hyperthyroidism (see page 901), high blood pressure (see page 574), diabetes (see page 889), or heart disease (see page 558).

The Procedure

Eyelid surgery is usually done on an outpatient basis using either a local anesthetic with sedation or general anesthesia. The surgery can take from 1 to 3 hours, depending on whether both the upper and lower lids are modified.

During surgery on the upper eyelids, the surgeon marks the natural creases and folds of the eyelids so he or she can make the incisions along those lines, hiding the scars in the folds. He or she makes the incisions and removes or repositions the surplus fat, muscle, and skin. When working on the lower eyelids the surgeon makes an incision either along the eyelash line or inside the lower lid, which leaves no visible scar, and trims away the excess fat, muscle, and skin. He or she then uses fine absorbable stitches (which do not have to be removed) to sew the incisions closed. Scarring from the incision will be hidden in the natural folds of the lids.

After Surgery

If you have had eyelid surgery, you can expect to have bruising and swelling, especially at the corners of your eyes, for about 2 or 3 weeks. A feeling of tightness in the eyelids is normal, and some people feel as if their eyelids are so tight they cannot close their eyes, but this feeling usually goes away in a few weeks. You will probably have some pain or discomfort. Your eyes may feel dry and may burn and itch for a few weeks, and you may have double vision or blurred vision during the recovery period. You may also have increased tearing and sensitivity to light and wind. In very rare cases, the lower eyelid can pull down and turn outward, requiring further surgery or longer recovery time to correct. The main risk after eyelid surgery is infection. Your doctor may prescribe an eye ointment to relieve drying, and pain medication to minimize your discomfort.

To immediately relieve some of the swelling, gently apply cold, wet cloths to your eyes. Keep your head elevated at all times—even while

Eyelid Surgery

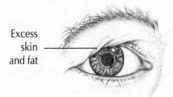

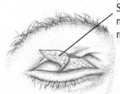

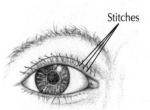

Upper eyelid surgery

Upper eyelid surgery can improve the appearance of drooping eyelids (left). The surgeon makes the incisions along the natural folds of the lids to hide the scars as much as possible and then removes excess skin, fat, and muscle (center). He or she then closes the incisions with fine absorbable stitches (right).

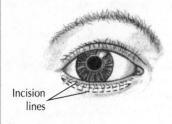

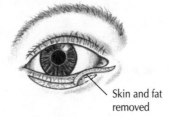

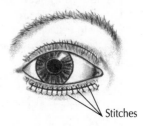

Lower eyelid surgery

During lower eyelid surgery, the surgeon makes an incision along the lash line or in a crease under the lower lid (left). (Some surgeons make the incision inside the lower lid, leaving no visible scar.) He or she then trims away the excess skin and fat (center) and closes the incision with absorbable stitches (right).

sleeping. Carefully clean your eyes every day as your doctor recommends to get rid of any sticky residue and to prevent infection. Don't wear contact lenses for at least 2 weeks after surgery or until your doctor says it is OK to do so. You probably can begin to read or watch TV 2 or 3 days after your surgery and you will probably be able to return to work within a week. But avoid strenuous activity, such as jogging, until 1 or 2 weeks after the procedure.

The improved appearance of the eyelids usually lasts for several years; for some people, the effects are permanent.

Forehead Lift

Forehead lift surgery, also known as a brow lift, is performed to alter the deep creases in the forehead, sagging of the brow over the eyes, and frown lines above the nose that often accompany aging. In a forehead lift, surgeons remove excess tissue from the forehead and redrape the skin to smooth out the forehead and decrease the presence of frown lines.

Most people who have forehead lifts are in their 40s, 50s, or 60s, although younger people may be good candidates if their brow droops excessively.

The Procedure

Surgeons can perform a forehead lift in two ways—endoscopic surgery or open surgery. Endoscopic surgery is the technique used most often. During the procedure, the surgeon makes several small incisions just behind the hairline and inserts a flexible viewing instrument called an endoscope into each incision. He or she then passes tiny surgical instruments through the endoscope to remove excess tissue. There is no need to redrape the forehead skin, and scarring is minimal.

In open surgery, a surgeon makes an incision either behind or directly at the person's hairline and removes excess tissue from the forehead. The incision can also be made inside one of the natural creases in the forehead; this option is usually used in men who already have deep lines in their forehead. After removing the excess tissue, the surgeon replaces the forehead skin over the brow and stitches it in place.

Open forehead lift surgery takes 1 or 2 hours; endoscopic forehead lift surgery may take a bit longer. Done on an outpatient basis, either procedure may be performed using a local anesthetic (with sedation) or general anesthesia.

After Surgery

You will probably experience headaches, swelling, and bruising during the first 3 weeks after surgery. You may also feel numbness and itching in your forehead and scalp for a few months. Some people lose some hair near the incision site, but the hair loss is usually temporary. Rare complications include infection, bleeding, and noticeable scarring.

The doctor will remove any stitches that are not dissolvable about 7 to 10 days after your surgery, at which time you will also be able to return to work and other routine activities. You can resume more vigorous activities after a few more weeks. You will need to limit sun exposure on your forehead for several months, even if you wear sunscreen. Prolonged bruising can be masked with makeup.

Reducing Frown Lines With Botulinum Toxin

Many people avoid surgery altogether by reducing their frown lines with injections of botulinum toxin type A, a protein made by the bacterium Clostridium botulinum. When a doctor injects the toxin into a facial muscle, it causes temporary paralysis of the muscle that lasts for several months. The paralyzed muscle is no longer able to pull the skin of the face into furrows, which relaxes wrinkling and smoothes out the skin. The procedure works best on forehead lines, crow's feet around the eyes, and lines between the eyebrows. The procedure takes about 10 minutes, and the wrinkle-relaxing results take effect in about 1 to 5 days.

Botulinum toxin should be injected using the lowest effective dose. Common side effects include mild swelling and numbness at the injection site, headache, bruising, a rash, nausea, and drooping eyelids, but these effects are temporary. Some people who have had botulinum toxin injections report temporary relief from migraine headaches.

Facelift

Plastic surgeons perform facelifts to restore a more youthful appearance to the face and neck by elevating the facial skin and removing excess tissue. A facelift can eliminate deep lines that run from the corner of the nose to the corner of the mouth, get rid of jowls at the jawline, and remove loose skin and fat from the neck. Features such as sagging eyebrows and eyelids or wrinkles around the mouth cannot be corrected by a facelift, but additional surgery to resolve these problems can be performed at the same time as or after a facelift. Most people who have a facelift are between ages 40 and 70, but older people can also be good candidates.

The Procedure

A facelift is usually an outpatient procedure that takes several hours. During the surgery, the surgeon makes incisions above the hairline (where they can be concealed) starting at the temples and extending down in front of and behind the ear to the lower scalp. The surgeon may also make a tiny incision under the chin to access the tissue in the neck. The surgeon first separates the skin from the underlying fat and muscle. If necessary, he or she may trim or suction fat from the neck and chin. Then the surgeon tightens the muscles and deeper connective tissues, draws the skin back tight, and trims off the excess skin. The incisions are closed with stitches. Tubes may be placed under the skin behind the ears to drain collected blood and fluid. The surgeon may also cover the person's head in loose bandages to minimize swelling; the bandages are removed in 1 to 5 days.

After Surgery

A facelift produces little pain or discomfort. After you go home, keep your head elevated to minimize swelling. You can be up and about in a couple of days, but you should not return to work for 10 days to 2 weeks. It may be 2 to 6 weeks before you can engage in strenuous activity. Bruising, stiffness, and puffiness are normal during the first few weeks, and your face may feel tight. The stitches are taken out after about 5 days.

The most common risks of facelift surgery are bleeding, infection, and facial scarring. Some people also experience unwanted hairline changes or feel that the new appearance of their face lacks symmetry. Occasionally, some of the nerves that

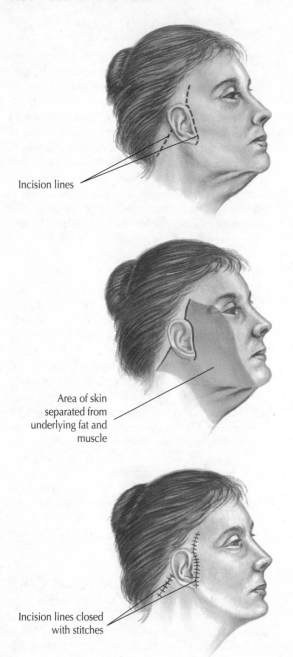

Incision lines

Area of skin separated from underlying fat and muscle

Incision lines closed with stitches

Facelift
During a facelift, the surgeon makes incisions above the hairline (where they can be concealed) starting at the temples and extending down in front of and behind the ear to the lower scalp (top). The surgeon first separates the skin from the underlying fat and muscle (center). Then the surgeon tightens the muscles and deeper connective tissues, draws the skin back tight, and trims off the excess skin. The incisions are closed with stitches (bottom).

serve muscles in the face are injured during surgery, resulting in numbness or weakness, which is usually temporary.

The firming effects of a facelift usually last from 5 to 10 years. Men may notice that they have to shave in new places, such as behind the ears, where beard-growing skin has been repositioned.

Facial Implants

Facial implants are used to reshape the face. Implants are commonly used in the chin, cheeks, lips, or jaw to remedy such features as a receding chin or sunken cheekbones, or to balance the proportions of the lower face. Facial implants come in a variety of sizes and shapes, and most are made of silicone. Once inserted, facial implants are usually permanent. Frequently, facial implantation is combined with other cosmetic surgery procedures to achieve better results.

The Procedure
Facial implantation is an outpatient procedure using either a local anesthetic or general anesthesia, depending on the implant. In any type of implant surgery, the surgeon makes a small incision near the desired location, forms a pocket between the skin and fat or muscle, inserts the implant, and then stitches the incision closed.

Chin implantation takes about 30 to 60 minutes. The incision is made either under the chin or inside the mouth at the base of the lower lip. To perform cheek implant surgery, the surgeon makes an incision either inside the lower eyelid or inside the upper lip. The surgery takes 1 to 1½ hours for both cheeks. In jaw implant surgery, which lasts 1 to 2 hours, the implant is inserted through an incision inside the lower lip. Lip implants, made of donor connective tissue or a synthetic gel, are injected or implanted directly into the lips.

After Surgery
Facial implant surgery produces temporary bruising and swelling. Activities such as eating and talking may be hampered for a brief period, depending on the site of the implant. The person may have to eat a liquid or soft food diet for several days. It may take months before the swelling goes down completely and the final facial configuration takes shape. While recovering, people who have implants

need to take special care when brushing and flossing their teeth.

Risks accompanying implant surgery include bleeding, infection, an asymmetrical appearance, numbness, and implants that shift out of place. If complications develop, the implant may have to be removed.

Collagen Injections

Collagen injection is a popular nonsurgical technique for giving the face a fuller, more youthful appearance by replacing the collagen that the skin naturally loses with age. Most collagen used for cosmetic purposes is a natural substance derived from the purified structural protein of cows. A few weeks before the procedure, the doctor tests the person for a possible allergic reaction to the collagen. Plastic surgeons most often inject collagen to treat frown lines, crow's feet, and the so-called laugh or smile lines that run from the nose to the mouth.

For the procedure, the doctor uses a tiny needle to inject the collagen (which is mixed with a local anesthetic) into the facial area being treated. More than one injection may be needed if the wrinkle is especially deep or long. The procedure can be completed in minutes, and you can go back to your daily activities immediately. The effects of collagen treatments last only a few months. Repeat treatments are needed to maintain the desired look.

Ear Surgery

Plastic surgery of the ear (medically known as otoplasty) is performed to position protruding ears closer to the head, decrease the size of overly large ears, repair earlobes that have been torn by injury, or replace an ear lost in an injury or missing at birth. Corrective surgery to fix protruding ears is usually done on children between ages 4 and 14. However, the surgery can be performed on older children and adults.

If your child has protruding ears and is not bothered by their appearance, wait until he or she expresses a desire for corrective surgery. Your child will be more cooperative during the process and happier with the results.

The Procedure

Ear surgery is usually an outpatient procedure. Younger children are usually given general anesthesia so they can sleep through the surgery. Older children and adults are usually given a local anesthetic combined with light sedation. The surgery takes about 2 to 3 hours.

The surgeon makes an incision behind each ear, in the crease where the ear meets the head. The surgeon may remove or remold the cartilage in the ear to reduce or reshape the ear, or simply bend the cartilage back toward the head. Then the surgeon sews the cartilage into its new position with absorbable stitches, which do not need to be removed.

The surgeon places protective dressings over the ears that must stay in place for a week. Sometimes a person has to wear a headband over the ears for the first month after surgery to hold them in place as they heal.

After Surgery

The doctor will recommend that the person get up and walk around a few hours after surgery. The incisions may hurt for a few days, but the doctor can prescribe medication to relieve the pain. The stitches usually dissolve in about a week, and the person will be able to return to school or work. However, he or she should be careful not to injure his or her ears. The scar is inconspicuous and will fade over time.

Rare complications of ear surgery include scarring caused by infection in the cartilage and a blood clot in the ear (which may go away on its own or can be drained with a needle).

Skin Rejuvenation

Skin rejuvenation or resurfacing refers to a number of techniques that can improve the appearance of your face by removing the top layers of skin. Your doctor will examine your skin to determine which rejuvenating technique will give you the best outcome. Before recommending a specific treatment, he or she will consider your skin type, how much sun damage or wrinkling you have, and the evenness of your skin color. The most common skin rejuvenation techniques include chemical skin peels, retinol treatments, dermabrasion, and laser skin resurfacing.

Chemical Skin Peel

A chemical skin peel is the application of a chemical solution to the skin to diminish fine wrinkles and sun damage and to even out irregular skin color by peeling away the top layers of the skin. It is the No. 1 nonsurgical facial cosmetic procedure performed in the United States. Chemical peels are safest when performed by plastic surgeons.

Chemical peels differ in their ingredients and strength. Light peels are short but effective procedures that require minimal recovery time. Light-to-medium skin peels usually use acidic chemicals such as alpha-hydroxy acids (AHAs) or trichloroacetic acid (TCA). Most deep peels use a very caustic chemical called phenol and are riskier than milder peels. Deep peels are usually performed on people who have severe or coarse wrinkles or precancerous growths. Phenol can be dangerous for people who have a history of heart disease. If you have a heart-related health problem, make sure you tell your doctor about it before you have a deep chemical peel.

The Procedure

Chemical peels using AHAs require no anesthesia or sedation. Your doctor will apply the AHA solution to your clean face with a sponge, pad, or brush, carefully avoiding the eyes, eyebrows, and lips. The procedure takes about 10 minutes.

For a chemical peel with TCA or phenol, you will probably be sedated, but you won't need anesthesia (the chemical solution itself contains an anesthetic). Before you have a TCA or phenol peel, your face will be thoroughly washed. A TCA peel takes about 30 minutes to complete. (You may need more than one application to achieve the results you want.) A phenol peel takes about 1 to 2 hours. During a phenol peel, your doctor will probably monitor your heart with an electrocardiogram (ECG; see page 559) to make sure the phenol is not affecting your heart.

After applying the solution to your face, the surgeon will wait about an hour for a protective crust to form naturally over your face. He or she will then coat your face with a layer of petroleum jelly or cover your face with strips of waterproof adhesive tape. The petroleum jelly or tape must stay in place for 1 to 2 days. If tape is used, a crust or scab will form after the tape is removed.

After the Procedure

AHA peels sometimes cause stinging, redness, flaking skin, dryness, irritation, and occasionally crusting of the skin, but these side effects are temporary. You won't need to use a facial cream or covering. Your doctor may recommend an AHA-based face wash or cream to apply at home once or twice a day for a few weeks. Most people see an immediate improvement in previously rough, dry, or sun-damaged skin. You will need to use a sunblock for several weeks after your peel.

A TCA peel can cause some tingling or even throbbing pain, for which your doctor can prescribe a pain medication. Depending on how deep the peel penetrated, you may also experience significant facial swelling, which will subside in about a week. You will see your new skin appear in a week to 10 days, when your skin should be healed enough to allow you to return to work. Be sure to avoid sun exposure and use a sunblock for the next several months.

Phenol peels cause significant swelling, and your eyes may be swollen shut for a few days. You will have to consume a liquid diet that you can sip through a straw for the first few days. Complete healing from a phenol peel can take many months, although you should be able to return to work in a couple of weeks. Your face will be healed enough by then to hide the facial redness with makeup.

After a phenol peel, the skin on your face will no longer be able to make pigment, which means that your face will never tan again and is more vulnerable to damage from the sun. You will have to protect your skin from the sun for the rest of your life. Phenol peels sometimes cause unwanted results, such as uneven skin color or scarring. However, most people who have phenol peels are satisfied with the dramatic improvement in their appearance. The effects of phenol peels can last up to 20 years.

Retinol Treatments

Retinol treatments are skin-rejuvenating techniques that you perform at home. Retinol is a prescription gel or cream containing tretinoin, a substance that is chemically related to vitamin A. Skin preparations containing retinol reverse some of the skin damage caused by sun exposure, including fine lines, wrinkles, and age spots. The gel form is generally stronger than the cream. Doctors often prescribe retinol to people who are planning to have a chemical peel (see previous page) to pretreat their skin—retinol thins out the top layer of skin, which allows the chemical peel solution to penetrate more deeply. Retinol also is prescribed to treat severe acne.

Applying Retinol

It is best to apply retinol right before going to bed. Wash your face with a mild soap or cleanser, pat your face dry with a towel, and then let your face completely dry for about 15 minutes. Gently apply a pea-sized drop of retinol to your entire face, avoiding your eyes. In the morning, apply a moisturizer containing a sunscreen with a sun protection factor (SPF) of at least 15. Avoid sun exposure between 10 AM and 3 PM, when the sun is strongest. Continue this routine for 8 months to a year. After that, your doctor will probably put you on a less frequent application regimen. The rejuvenating effects of retinol will last only for as long as you apply it.

After the Application

After a retinol application, your skin may become red, dry, and irritated, especially during the first few weeks after you start using it. If the irritation becomes excessive, your doctor may recommend decreasing the application to every other night or every third night. Because retinol thins out the skin and makes the skin more sensitive to the sun, you need to be vigilant about wearing sunscreen and minimizing sun exposure. During the first few months of application, your skin will have a rosy glow. Within about 6 months, the fine wrinkles and age spots will disappear.

Dermabrasion

Dermabrasion, also known as dermaplaning, is the removal of the top layers of facial skin for cosmetic purposes using a handheld instrument with a small, high-speed, rotating wheel that has a rough surface similar to fine-grade sandpaper. The procedure is especially effective for removing fine wrinkles, particularly the vertical lines around the mouth. It also works well for facial scars, including those resulting from acne. The technique is less effective for burn scars. Doctors can perform dermabrasion on selected areas of the face as well as on the entire

face. The final color of the treated area usually blends well with surrounding areas of skin.

The Procedure

Dermabrasion can take from a few minutes to more than an hour to complete, depending on the size of the area to be treated. If the treated area is small, a person may need only an anesthetic spray applied to numb the skin. Otherwise, either a local anesthetic with sedation or general anesthesia is used. Dermabrasion is almost always done on an outpatient basis. To perform the procedure, the doctor uses the rotating wheel to mechanically sand the parts of the face needing treatment.

After the Procedure

Dermabrasion usually causes temporary swelling, tingling, burning, itching, and redness of the skin. Your doctor can give you medication to relieve the pain. A crust forms over the treated area and then falls off within 3 to 5 days, revealing new skin growth underneath. For the first 6 to 12 months after treatment, the new skin will be lighter than surrounding skin, sensitive to the sun (and more vulnerable to damage from the sun), and incapable of tanning because of loss of pigment. You will need to protect your new skin from sun exposure. Avoid direct and indirect sunlight and wear a wide-brimmed hat and sunblock outdoors.

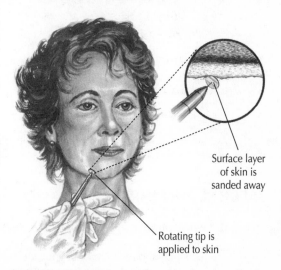

Surface layer of skin is sanded away

Rotating tip is applied to skin

Dermabrasion
Dermabrasion reduces fine lines, wrinkles, and acne scars by sanding away the top layer of skin using an instrument with a high-speed, rotating wheel. The wheel has a rough surface similar to fine-grade sandpaper.

The main risks of dermabrasion are infection, permanent scarring, and permanent skin-color abnormalities. Some people who have dermabrasion experience a recurrence of skin allergies or cold sores, brought on by the stress on the skin.

You will be able to hide the facial redness with makeup after about 2 weeks. The effects of dermabrasion are permanent, but the procedure does not prevent new age-related wrinkling.

Laser Resurfacing

Laser skin resurfacing is a newer technique developed to reduce or remove the upper layers of facial skin to improve its appearance. During the procedure, a surgeon uses a powerful beam of pulsing light to vaporize unwanted skin tissue. Laser resurfacing can improve facial wrinkles, lines around the lips, crow's feet, lower eyelid wrinkles, acne or surgical scarring, and uneven skin color. Laser

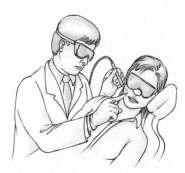

Laser resurfacing
During laser resurfacing, a surgeon uses a powerful beam of pulsing light to remove unwanted skin tissue. Both the surgeon and the patient wear protective goggles to shield their eyes from the light. Lasers can vaporize the sun-damaged top layer of skin, removing fine lines, wrinkles, and acne scars.

resurfacing carries fewer risks—such as scarring, infection, skin color loss, or bleeding—than chemical peels or dermabrasion.

Surgeons also use pulsed laser beams to remove broken veins in the face, spider veins on the legs, and unwanted body hair. When the laser beam is not pulsed but allowed to flow continuously, it can be used to cut the skin to remove skin cancers and warts and to perform cosmetic eyelid surgery (see page 1081).

The Procedure

Most laser skin resurfacing is performed in an outpatient setting using only a local anesthetic similar to that used in a dentist's office, although some surgeons prefer using general anesthesia for a full-face resurfacing. Using a wandlike handheld laser instrument, the surgeon burns off the upper layers of damaged skin. The concentration of the laser beam gives the surgeon precise control over the depth of penetration. Laser resurfacing takes about 1 hour.

After the Procedure

When the surgeon is finished, he or she may place a clear dressing over your face or give you an ointment to apply at home to help promote healing. Your doctor will tell you to change your dressings for 3 to 5 days, until your skin regenerates. Your skin may form a crust that will drop off in a few days. You probably won't have any pain or discomfort, but you may feel self-conscious about the way you look, so you may want to wait about a week before returning to work. Your facial skin will be red and then pink for several weeks to several months. Avoid unnecessary sun exposure and wear sunblock and a wide-brimmed hat when you go outside. The risks of laser resurfacing are low but can include skin color loss and, rarely, scarring.

Breast Surgery

Some women are unhappy about the way their breasts look. Some women feel that their breasts are too small and seek breast augmentation. Other women have breasts that are asymmetrical and want to correct the difference in size or shape. Breasts may lose their shape and firmness and begin to sag with age and after pregnancy and breastfeeding. A breast lift can elevate and reshape sagging breasts.

Women whose breasts are overly large can develop back and neck pain and indentations in their shoulders from bra straps. They may also be extremely self-conscious about the size of their breasts. Breast reduction surgery can relieve the physical and emotional discomfort produced by having large breasts.

Be aware that any surgery performed on your breasts will leave scars. However, your surgeon will conceal the incisions as much as possible by making them in the natural creases below the breasts or in other inconspicuous areas. Ask your surgeon to show you photographs of breast procedures he or she has performed so you can see the results. Some types of breast surgery, especially breast reduction, will make it impossible for you to breastfeed. Talk with your surgeon about these and any other questions or concerns you may have before deciding whether to proceed with surgery.

Breast Enlargement

Breast enlargement, medically known as augmentation mammoplasty, increases the size of a woman's breasts by surgically inserting breast implants for cosmetic purposes. Breast implants are made of a soft, pliable plastic (such as silicone) sac that contains a saline (saltwater) solution. The Food and Drug Administration (FDA) has restricted the use of implants filled with silicone gel to women who are in approved research studies.

Your surgeon will decide the best way to insert the implant after performing a physical examination. Implants can be inserted through an incision in the natural fold under the breast, or through an incision around the areola (the dark skin around the nipple) or in the armpit. The incision site depends both on your anatomy and on the experience of the surgeon. Implants can be located either on top of or underneath the muscles of the chest wall. Your surgeon will discuss which location is best for you.

Breast Augmentation

Breast augmentation uses saline-filled sacs made of silicone or another soft, pliable plastic to enlarge the breasts. After evaluating a woman's breasts, the surgeon will determine the best site for inserting the implants and for positioning them (under or over the chest wall muscle).

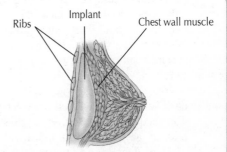

Implant inserted under chest wall muscle

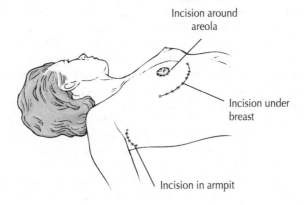

Incision around areola

Incision under breast

Incision in armpit

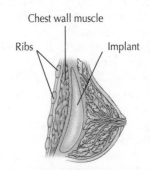

Implant inserted over chest wall muscle

Possible incision sites for breast enlargement
Many breast implants are inserted through an incision in the natural fold under the breast, but they can also be inserted through an incision around the areola (the dark skin around the nipple) or in the armpit.

Breast implant locations
Breast implants can be placed either under (top) or over (bottom) the chest wall muscle. Where to place the implant is a decision that you and your surgeon must make together.

The Procedure

Breast enlargement surgery can be done using general anesthesia, or local anesthesia combined with sedation. Most breast augmentation is done on an outpatient basis.

After making an incision, the surgeon will lift your skin and breast tissue to make a pocket either right behind the breast tissue or under your chest wall muscle. He or she will then insert the implant and center it under your nipples. The incision is closed with stitches. The surgeon repeats the process on the other breast. Gauze bandages may be placed over your breasts to help speed healing.

After Surgery

You will probably feel tired and very sore for the first few days after surgery, but your surgeon will encourage you to get up and walk around immediately after surgery. He or she will prescribe pain medication to relieve the discomfort. Your breasts will look bruised and swollen and your nipples may burn for the first 2 weeks after surgery. The stitches are removed a week to 10 days after surgery. The soreness and swelling usually last about 3 to 5 weeks.

You may be able to go back to work in a few days. Your surgeon will tell you when you can begin exercising or lifting. Your scars will stay noticeably pink for several months and then begin to fade, although they will never disappear completely.

The most common complication of breast enlargement surgery is capsular contracture, in which scar tissue around the implant contracts and becomes tight. The tightening scar squeezes the implant, making the breast feel hard. Surgeons can treat this condition by surgically removing the scar tissue or making parallel cuts in it to widen it and make it more elastic. Another option is to remove or replace the implant.

Other possible complications of breast enlargement surgery include excessive bleeding, infection, and numbness of the nipples or incisions. Sensation usually returns over time but loss of sensation can sometimes be permanent. Breast implants can break or leak after an injury or, occasionally, during routine activity. If an implant leaks, your body will absorb the saline solution contained in the implant, but the implant itself must be removed and replaced. Before having the surgery, make sure you talk with your surgeon about the risks and possible complications.

Breast Reduction

Breast reduction surgery is performed to remove breast fat and skin from very large, pendulous breasts that cause discomfort and restrict a woman's activities. The surgery makes the breasts smaller, less heavy, and in better proportion to the rest of the body. The best candidates for this surgery are women whose breasts are fully developed and who are seeking physical relief from symptoms caused by large breasts, in addition to an improvement in their appearance. Women who plan to breastfeed should not have breast reduction surgery because the surgery removes many of the milk ducts and can make breastfeeding impossible.

Before surgery, your surgeon may ask you to have a mammogram (see page 141). If the surgeon anticipates having to remove a large amount of breast tissue, he or she may recommend that you donate a unit of your own blood ahead of time in case you need a blood transfusion (see page 615) during surgery.

The Procedure

Breast reduction surgery may be done in a hospital or in an outpatient facility. It is always performed while the woman is under general anesthesia. The procedure takes from 2 to 4 hours.

Breast reduction techniques vary, depending on the amount of tissue to be removed. Using the most common technique, the surgeon makes an anchor-shaped incision around the areola (the dark area surrounding the nipple), down the middle of the bottom of each breast, and along the natural crease under the breast. The surgeon then cuts away excess fat, glandular tissue, and skin and moves the still-attached nipple to a higher position. Finally, he or she pulls the skin from both sides of the breast down and around the nipple and stitches the skin together along the original incision lines. If the breasts are extremely large, the surgeon may have to cut the nipples away and graft them into a new position on the breast. This technique causes the most loss of sensation in the nipple.

Liposuction (see page 1093) breast reduction, also called scarless breast reduction, is under study as a less invasive way to remove fatty breast tissue in women.

After Surgery

After surgery, gauze dressings will be applied to each breast, and your breasts will be wrapped in an elastic bandage or covered with a surgical bra. Small tubes may be inserted into your breasts to help drain

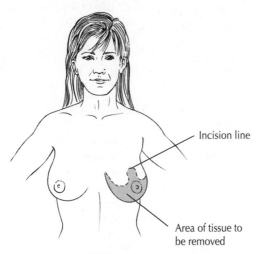

Incision line

Area of tissue to be removed

Before breast reduction

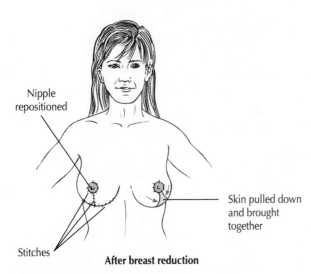

Nipple repositioned

Skin pulled down and brought together

Stitches

After breast reduction

Breast reduction
Breast reduction surgery makes large breasts smaller, less heavy, and in better proportion to the rest of the body. During the procedure, the surgeon makes an anchor-shaped incision in each breast, removes excess fat and skin, draws the skin together, and stitches it into place. The nipples are repositioned higher on the breasts. The surgery leaves permanent scars.

accumulated blood and fluids during the first 1 or 2 days. The doctor will ask you to get up and move around after a day or two. Your bandages can be removed 2 days after surgery, although you will have to wear the surgical bra day and night for several weeks until the swelling and bruising subside. The surgeon will remove your stitches in 1 to 3 weeks.

You will have pain for the first few days, especially when you move around or cough. Milder pain may last up to a week, and periodic shooting pains could persist for a few months. Your surgeon will prescribe pain medication to help relieve your discomfort. Loss of feeling in the nipples and breast skin is common but feeling usually returns in about 6 weeks, although some women report loss of feeling for up to a year. In some cases, the loss of feeling is permanent. Breast reduction surgery leaves permanent scars.

Follow your doctor's instructions about resuming your usual activities. Your breasts may take 6 months to 1 year to reach their final shape. It may take a while before you are comfortable with how your breasts look but, in general, most women are extremely satisfied with breast reduction surgery. The most common complications of breast reduction surgery include bleeding, infection, breasts that are not the same size, and permanent loss of feeling in the nipples and breasts. In rare cases, the nipple and areola can lose their blood supply, resulting in tissue death. Skin graft surgery can correct this problem.

Male Breast Reduction

Some men who have enlarged breasts (gynecomastia; see next page) may want to have the excess glandular tissue removed. The type of procedure used depends on the degree of breast enlargement. For male breast reduction, most doctors use liposuction (see page 1093) to suction out the excess fat and tissue in the breasts. Liposuction is often combined with surgery to remove the tissue in a procedure similar to female breast reduction (see previous page).

The Procedure

Male breast reduction is done as an outpatient procedure using either general anesthesia or a local anesthetic with sedation. For both liposuction and

Gynecomastia

Gynecomastia is excessive growth of the male breasts. In some cases, the breasts may even produce milk. Forty to 60 percent of all adult men have some form of gynecomastia. In adolescents, a mild degree of gynecomastia is normal. Most cases of gynecomastia in adults are caused by an excess amount of the female hormone estrogen in the blood. Men normally produce small amounts of estrogen, but some men produce an increased amount because of disorders such as obesity, a liver disease such as cirrhosis (see page 790), or hormone abnormalities. Gynecomastia also can be a side effect of taking some prescription medications, drinking excessive amounts of alcohol, or using marijuana. Rarely, gynecomastia is a symptom of breast cancer. In many cases, the cause is unknown. If the condition is caused by an underlying disorder, it usually subsides once the underlying disorder is treated. Most cases are not severe enough to require surgery.

surgery procedures, an incision is made in the lower half of the areola (the dark area surrounding the nipple). If the tissue is mostly fat, a small liposuction rod is inserted into the incision to remove excess fat and other tissue. If the tissue in the breast is more glandular, all the tissue directly under the nipple is removed surgically. The procedure usually takes 1 to 2 hours.

After Surgery

After breast reduction surgery, you may experience temporary swelling, bruising, numbness, soreness, or a burning sensation that can last from several days to 2 weeks. You can resume your usual activities within 3 to 7 days and engage in strenuous activities in 2 to 3 weeks. The swelling and bruising usually subside within 3 to 6 months. The doctor may recommend wearing a compression garment for several weeks after surgery to help relieve some of the symptoms. Besides the usual risks from surgery (such as infection), possible complications of breast reduction surgery include asymmetrical breasts, saggy skin, abnormal skin pigmentation, and excessive scarring.

Most men are very happy with the results of breast reduction surgery, which are permanent. However, the procedure may have to be repeated if too little tissue was removed from inside the breast or if excess skin remains after the surgery.

Breast Lift

A breast lift is cosmetic surgery that lifts and reshapes breasts that have sagged and stretched from pregnancy, breastfeeding, or aging. To perform a lift, excess skin is removed from the lower part of the breasts. Surgeons achieve the best results in women with small breasts because large, heavy breasts will begin to sag again after surgery. Breast lift surgery is not permanent, because no procedure can permanently halt the effects of gravity. If you plan to have children, consider delaying your breast lift until afterward because your breasts will probably stretch from pregnancy and breastfeeding.

The Procedure

A breast lift is usually performed on an outpatient basis while the woman is under general anesthesia. The procedure takes about $1\frac{1}{2}$ to $3\frac{1}{2}$ hours. During

Breast lift

A breast lift raises and reshapes breasts that have sagged and stretched from pregnancy, breastfeeding, or aging. To perform a breast lift, the surgeon makes an anchor-shaped incision on each breast and removes excess skin from the lower part of the breast. The nipple and areola are moved into a new position. The surgeon then pulls the remaining skin down and together to lift and reshape each breast.

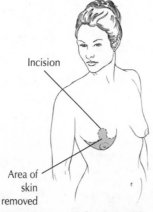

Incision

Area of skin removed

Before breast lift

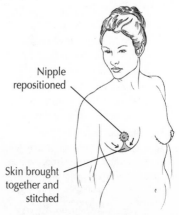

Nipple repositioned

Skin brought together and stitched

After breast lift

the procedure, the surgeon makes an incision that determines the boundaries of the area from which skin will be removed and locates a new position for the nipple. After removing the excess skin, the surgeon moves the nipple and areola into their new position and pulls the remaining skin down and together to lift and reshape each breast. Some women with small breasts choose to have breast implants inserted during breast lift surgery. If so, the surgeon inserts the implant in a pocket under the breast tissue or behind the chest wall muscle. The surgeon then stitches the incisions closed.

After Surgery

Gauze dressings and an elastic bandage or surgical bra will be placed over your breasts immediately after surgery. After a few days, you will wear a soft support bra over the gauze bandages day and night for 3 or 4 weeks. Your surgeon will examine your breasts and remove your stitches 1 to 2 weeks after the surgery.

Numbness and swelling will cause some loss of sensation in your breast skin and nipples. The numbness usually goes away in 6 weeks but may take a year or more to completely subside. Your scars will be lumpy and red for a few months and then will fade, but they will never disappear. Resume your activities gradually, according to your surgeon's instructions. You can probably return to work a week or two after your surgery.

Complications are unusual after a breast lift but can include bleeding, infection, unevenly placed nipples or asymmetrical breasts, or loss of a portion or all of a nipple. You can minimize these complications by carefully following your doctor's instructions after your surgery.

Body Contouring

C osmetic surgeons can reshape your body to change its appearance. Body-contouring techniques accomplish this goal by removing unwanted fat from problem areas. The top two body-contouring procedures are liposuction and abdominoplasty. The two techniques can be combined in one surgical procedure to produce even more dramatic results.

Liposuction

Liposuction, also called lipoplasty or suction lipectomy, reshapes the body by vacuuming out excess fat deposits. It is the most frequently performed cosmetic surgery procedure in the United States. Liposuction is not a substitute for weight loss but is designed to remove deposits of fat that persist despite diet and exercise. Using liposuction, a surgeon can remove unwanted fat from many parts of the body, including the abdomen, hips, buttocks, thighs, knees, calves, upper arms, chin, cheeks, and neck. The procedure works best on healthy people of normal weight who have firm, elastic skin.

Before surgery, your surgeon will evaluate your health, examine the fat deposits to be removed, and check the elasticity of your skin. Age is no barrier to liposuction, but older people tend to have looser skin and may not achieve the same effects as younger people. If liposuction is not appropriate for you, your surgeon may recommend an alternative method. For example, if you seek liposuction to reduce fat deposits in your abdomen, an abdominoplasty (see next page) might be more effective.

Liposuction techniques are available that give surgeons more precise control and make recovery time faster. One such technique, called ultrasound-assisted lipoplasty, uses an instrument that produces ultrasonic (sound wave) energy. The sound waves explode the walls of fat cells and liquefy the fat so it can be removed more easily. This technique works best on the hips, abdomen, thighs, and neck.

In a procedure called fluid injection, the surgeon injects a solution containing medication and an anesthetic into the fat deposits to help ease their removal. Depending on the technique the surgeon uses, the amount of injected fluid may equal or be up to three times the amount of fat to be removed.

The Procedure

Liposuction is almost always performed as an outpatient procedure. Liposuction performed to remove small amounts of fat from only a few sites can be done using a local anesthetic, with or without light sedation. More extensive areas of the body are treated using regional anesthesia such as an epidural block (see page 532), the same type of anesthesia used for pain management during delivery of a baby. Removal of a large amount of fat requires general anesthesia and intravenous fluids and, in some cases, a blood transfusion.

During a liposuction procedure, the surgeon makes a small incision in the skin over the area to be treated and inserts a narrow tube called a cannula under the skin. He or she pushes and pulls the tube through the underlying layer of fat and suctions the fat away with a vacuum pump or syringe. When one site is finished, the surgeon moves to the next area until all the designated areas are treated. The small incisions are closed with stitches. During and after surgery, you will be given intravenous fluids to replace the fluids that were suctioned out with the fat.

The amount of time needed to perform liposuction can vary substantially, depending on the volume of fat being removed, the number of body sites being treated, and the technique used. In general, liposuction takes from 1 to 4 hours.

After Surgery

To prevent fluid buildup, the surgical team will probably insert small drainage tubes under your skin. You may have to wear a tight-fitting elastic

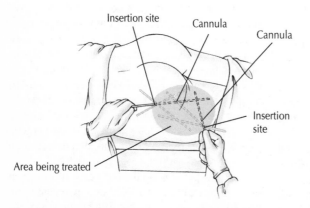

Insertion site
Cannula
Cannula
Insertion site
Area being treated

How liposuction is performed
During a liposuction procedure, the surgeon makes a small incision and inserts a narrow tube called a cannula under the skin. He or she pushes and pulls the cannula back and forth through the underlying layer of fat and suctions the fat away with a vacuum pump or syringe. When one area is finished, the surgeon moves on to the next until all the specified areas are treated.

garment over the treated area for a few weeks to help minimize swelling. Pain, burning, bleeding, bruising, and temporary numbness are common. Your doctor will probably prescribe medication to help relieve any discomfort, along with antibiotics to prevent infection. Most people who have liposuction can go back to work a few days after the procedure. The stitches are removed or will dissolve on their own in 7 to 10 days.

The risks of liposuction increase with the size and number of areas to be treated. Although complications are rare, they can include infection or the formation of clots of fat or blood that can travel to the lungs and cause sudden death. Other risks include excessive fluid loss that can lead to shock (see page 579), fluid accumulation in the lungs, burns or other damage to the skin or nerves, and injury to a vital organ. As with all cosmetic surgery, there may be imperfections in your final appearance, including baggy skin or an asymmetrical body contour. After the swelling goes down, you will begin to see the improvement in your body shape in 4 to 6 weeks.

Abdominoplasty

Abdominoplasty (also known as a tummy tuck) is a cosmetic procedure that removes excess skin and fat from the abdominal area and tightens the muscles in the abdominal wall to flatten a protruding abdomen. The procedure can also remove existing scars and stretch marks. Abdominoplasty is considered major surgery and leaves a permanent scar that can extend from hip to hip.

Cosmetic surgeons perform more than 50,000 abdominoplasties in the United States each year. The best candidates for the procedure are people who are generally healthy but who have a large amount of abdominal fat or loose abdominal skin that they cannot eliminate with dieting or exercise. The surgery may be especially beneficial to women whose abdominal muscles and skin have become stretched from multiple pregnancies. Older people whose skin has lost some elasticity may choose to have abdominoplasty to improve the contour of their abdomen.

People who have only a small amount of excess fat mainly below the navel may qualify for a partial abdominoplasty, in which a wedge of skin and fat is removed from the lower abdomen, leaving a smaller horizontal scar above the pubic hair. The abdominal muscles still can be tightened and liposuction (see page 1093) can be performed above the navel or around the waist to treat problem areas.

If you intend to lose a substantial amount of weight or if you plan to become pregnant, you should delay having abdominoplasty. Your abdominal muscles will stretch during pregnancy and undo the muscle tightening that is part of the procedure.

The Procedure

Many surgeons perform both types of abdominoplasty in outpatient facilities, but some prefer to do them in a hospital. Some surgeons prefer to use general anesthesia; others choose a local anesthetic combined with sedation. A full abdominoplasty takes 2 to 5 hours; a partial procedure can be done in 1 to 2 hours.

To begin the procedure, the surgeon makes a long, semicircular incision across the pubic area

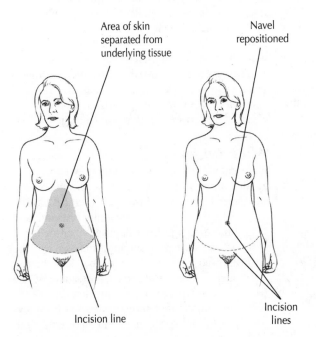

Area of skin separated from underlying tissue

Navel repositioned

Incision line

Incision lines

Abdominoplasty
To remove excess abdominal skin and fat, the surgeon makes a continuous incision that extends from one hip to the other. He or she then separates the skin from the underlying tissue up to the ribs and folds it out of the way (left). After removing excess fat, the surgeon pulls the abdominal skin back down and trims off the excess. A new opening is cut for the navel, and the skin is stitched into place along the incision lines (right).

from one hip to the other. In a full abdominoplasty, he or she makes a second incision around the navel to free it from the adjoining tissue. (The incision around the navel is not done in a partial abdominoplasty.) The surgeon then separates the skin from the underlying tissue up to the ribs and folds it out of the way. (In a partial abdominoplasty, the skin is separated only up to the navel.) The surgeon tightens the abdominal muscles by drawing them together and sewing them into place. He or she brings the skin flap back down, cuts away the excess skin, cuts a new hole for the navel, and stitches the navel in place. The large incision is then stitched closed and dressings are applied. The surgical team may insert a drainage tube into the abdomen to remove fluid from the site.

After Surgery

In the first few days after surgery, your abdomen will be swollen and painful. Your surface stitches can be removed in 5 to 7 days, but the deep sutures (the ends of which stick out through the skin) on your abdominal muscles will not come out for 2 or 3 weeks. Once your dressings are removed, you may have to wear an elastic support garment.

It will take several weeks or months before you feel completely back to normal. In general, the stronger your abdominal muscles were before the surgery, the faster you will recover. You can go back to work in 2 to 4 weeks, depending on the extent of the surgery. Light exercise, such as walking, during the first month or two will help you heal faster and help prevent blood clots from forming in your legs. Avoid vigorous exercise until your surgeon tells you it's OK.

Your scars will remain red and may even seem to get more noticeable for the first 6 months. It will take 9 months to a year before they fade into inconspicuous lines, but they will never disappear completely. You may have numbness for up to 2 years.

Complications from abdominoplasty are rare but can include bleeding, infection at the surgical site or in the lungs (pneumonia; see page 660), excessive scarring, irregularities in the shape of the abdomen, and blood clots that can travel to the lungs and cause sudden death.

The results of an abdominoplasty are long-lasting if you maintain your weight by eating sensibly and exercising regularly.

Hair Replacement Procedures

Hair loss (see page 1075) usually occurs in people who have a family history of baldness. More than 30,000 surgical hair replacement procedures are performed every year nationwide to fight hair loss. Most of these procedures are performed on men. Women can sometimes take advantage of hair replacement surgery but, because they lose hair from the entire scalp rather than just from the front and crown, hair replacement in women is more difficult and the outcome is often less successful. The most common surgical procedures used for hair loss are hair transplantation and scalp surgery, including tissue expansion, flap surgery, and scalp reduction surgery.

Hair Transplantation

Hair transplantation is the surgical transfer of grafts of skin from a hair-growing part of the scalp to a bald part. The process requires multiple sessions interspersed with months of healing. The entire process can take up to 2 years to complete. Common transplant methods include circular punch grafts that each contain 10 to 15 hairs, minigrafts of 2 to 4 hairs, micrografts of 1 or 2 hairs, slit grafts inserted into slit incisions in the scalp, and strip grafts, which are longer slit-type grafts. Surgeons may combine one or more of these techniques to achieve the best results.

Successful hair transplantation requires full, healthy hair growth at the back and sides of the head from which the surgeon can take the grafts. Because women generally experience uniform hair loss from all parts of their scalp, men (who tend to lose hair from only the front and crown) are usually better candidates for hair transplantation. Hair color and thickness can influence the results.

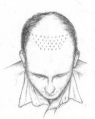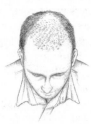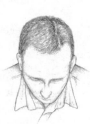

Hair transplantation
To transplant hair, doctors surgically transfer grafts of skin from a hair-growing part of the scalp to a bald area. The process involves multiple grafting sessions. Grafts of hair are inserted into tiny openings in the scalp (left). During subsequent sessions the surgeon fills in gaps between the original grafts with new grafts (center). After several grafting sessions over a period of up to 2 years, hair has filled in to form a natural hairline (right).

The Procedure

Before surgery, the surgeon will treat the areas from which hair will be taken (donor areas) and the areas to which hair will be grafted (recipient areas) with an anesthetic similar to the kind used by dentists. To perform a punch graft, the surgeon will use a tube-shaped instrument to punch out round skin grafts from the donor area. For the other techniques, surgeons use a scalpel to carefully remove small sections of scalp, which are then separated into tinier segments and transplanted to the recipient sites. The grafts are placed about $\frac{1}{8}$ inch apart. Later grafts will fill in the spaces in between.

The surgeon will usually close the scalp incisions with a single stitch but may use more if needed. The entire scalp will then be gently cleansed and covered with gauze bandages.

After Surgery

After each grafting session, you may experience aching, throbbing, and tightness in your scalp, which can be controlled with pain medication. You may also have some swelling, bruising, and fluid drainage. Your bandages will be taken off the day after surgery, and you will be allowed to carefully wash your hair the day after that. A week to 10 days after surgery, the surgeon will remove the stitches. During the first month after surgery, you will have several follow-up appointments so he or she can monitor your progress.

Avoid strenuous exercise for 3 weeks and abstain from sexual intercourse for about 10 days after the surgery because these activities can increase blood flow to the scalp and cause bleeding. The newly transplanted hair falls out about 6 weeks after surgery, which is normal. However, 5 or 6 weeks later, the hair will begin to grow back at a rate of about ½ inch per month. Many people who have had hair transplants need additional touch-up grafts to make the results look more natural.

Scalp Surgery

Scalp surgery can replace balding areas of the head with skin that grows hair using a number of specially developed techniques. The three most commonly used methods are tissue expansion, flap surgery, and scalp reduction surgery. Tissue expansion stretches the hair-bearing skin of the scalp so it can be used to cover bald areas. In flap surgery, the surgeon uses a flap of hair-growing skin from the side of the head to replace a section of scalp that was removed from the front hairline. Scalp reduction surgery is used to reduce bald areas at the top and back of the head by pulling areas of hair-bearing skin closer together. Sometimes surgeons combine two of these hair replacement procedures to produce better results.

The Procedure

In general, all three types of scalp surgery are done on an outpatient basis. Before scalp surgery, you will be given a sedative to make you feel relaxed. The surgeon will then inject a local anesthetic into your scalp.

Tissue expansion

In tissue expansion scalp surgery, the surgeon inserts a silicone balloon under a hair-bearing part of the scalp next to a bald area. He or she gradually inflates the balloon with a saline (saltwater) solution at intervals of 1 to 2 weeks to stretch the scalp. When the skin of the scalp is stretched sufficiently—usually after about 2 months—the surgeon removes the balloon and performs a second procedure to cover the adjacent bald area with the expanded hair-growing skin.

Flap surgery

Flap surgery is usually performed while the person is under general anesthesia, in either a hospital or in an outpatient facility. The surgeon cuts out and removes a segment of bald scalp from above the forehead. He or she then cuts a flap of hair-bearing skin from the scalp on the side of the head (leaving one end attached), repositions it over the first surgical site, and stitches it into place.

Scalp reduction surgery

During scalp reduction surgery, the surgeon cuts out a section of scalp in the shape of a Y, a U, or an oval. He or she then loosens the adjacent skin, gently pulls it together, and stitches it into its new position. Scalp reduction brings existing areas of hair growth closer together. The procedure often accompanies hair transplantation (see previous page). Scalp reduction sometimes must be repeated to achieve the best results.

After Surgery

After scalp surgery, a large gauze dressing will be applied to your head; you should leave it in place for 24 hours. When you go back to see the surgeon the next day, your scalp will be cleansed and your dressing will be changed. You cannot wash your hair for 1 week.

You can expect to have some tightness and swelling for up to 10 days, and bruises may appear around your eyes. Bleeding is a common problem after scalp surgery because the scalp is rich with blood vessels. Call your surgeon if the bleeding becomes excessive. Watch for signs of infection including redness and a discharge of pus.

Your newly transplanted hairs may fall out in a few weeks, which is normal, and will be replaced by new hair growth in 3 or 4 months. You are not likely to see the true results of your scalp surgery for 6 to 8 months.

19

Teeth and Gums

Teeth are living tissue. The pulp that forms the core of each tooth contains blood vessels that help nourish the tooth and nerves that sense heat, cold, pressure, and pain. Dentin, a substance that is harder than bone, surrounds the pulp. On the crown (the part of the tooth that you can see above the gum), a hard substance called enamel covers the dentin. Each tooth has one to three roots, covered by a sensitive, bonelike material called cementum. In healthy gums, the gum tissue fits tightly around the teeth, and the roots are embedded in sockets in the jawbone. A shock-absorbent material called periodontal ligament (a tough, elastic tissue that holds bones together) lines each tooth socket to support the root and prevent the skull and jawbone from vibrating when food is being chewed.

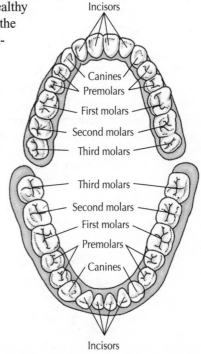

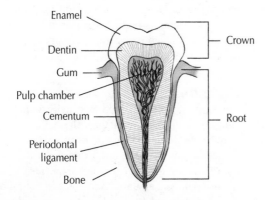

Structure of a tooth
The teeth are used for biting and chewing, and they also help give shape to the face and play a role in speech. This cross section of a premolar shows the many parts that make up a tooth.

Teeth start the digestive process
Adults have 32 permanent teeth that break food into pieces that can be easily swallowed and digested. The incisors cut, the canines tear, and the premolars and molars crush and grind. The four third molars (often called wisdom teeth) sometimes never emerge.

Although tooth enamel is the hardest substance in the body, acids produced in the breakdown of sugar and other simple carbohydrates you eat can erode the enamel and cause tooth decay. If not treated, decay can work its way through the dentin and into the pulp, which may cause a pocket of pus to form in the tissue around the tip of the root of a tooth (tooth abscess; see page 1104) and can eventually lead to loss of the tooth.

Tooth Decay

If you move the tip of your tongue over your teeth several hours after brushing them, you can feel patches of a slightly rough, sticky substance. This substance, called dental plaque, consists of mucus, food particles, and bacteria, and forms mainly between the teeth and where the teeth meet the gums. Bacteria in plaque break down the sugar in food and produce acid. Over time, the acid dissolves the calcium and phosphate in the tooth's enamel and can form tiny holes called cavities, which are tooth decay.

If the decay is not treated, the acid destroys the enamel and damages the dentin beneath it. Dentin contains tiny canals that lead to the pulp; the bacteria eventually reach the pulp, causing inflammation. Your body's immune system responds by sending white blood cells to the pulp to fight the bacteria. The blood vessels around the tooth dilate (widen) to accommodate the extra blood and white cells. The widened vessels press on the nerves entering the tooth, causing a toothache. The acid may also reach the nerves, causing more pain, especially if the decay reaches nerve endings in the dentin. If a large number of bacteria invade the pulp chambers, the nerve of the tooth usually dies, because the white blood cells cannot overcome the infection. Once the nerve dies, the pain stops, but a pocket of pus may begin to form in the tissue around the tip of the root of a tooth (tooth abscess; see page 1104).

For most people, tooth decay has no serious health risks if it is detected and treated early. However, some people, such as those who have heart disease, are at serious risk if bacteria from an infected tooth enter the bloodstream and travel to the heart. Because an infection can damage the heart valves and can lead to congestive heart failure (see page 570), people who are at risk need to take prescription antibiotics to eliminate the infection before having a tooth removed. People who have a blood clotting disorder such as hemophilia (see page 618) or who are taking anticlotting medication should consult their doctor before having a tooth removed because it might be difficult to stop the bleeding after the procedure. To prevent bleeding, the doctor may take precautions such as temporarily lowering the dosage of a person's anticlotting medication or prescribing a clotting factor (a protein in blood that is essential for blood clotting) to a person who has a clotting disorder. If bleeding occurs, a dentist can stop it by stitching the socket closed or by applying pressure to the socket with sterile gauze pads.

Symptoms

The early stages of tooth decay usually do not cause symptoms. In the later stages, the main symptom may be a mild toothache that occurs when you eat something sweet, sour, hot, or cold. As the cavity continues to grow, you may experience more intense pain and an unpleasant taste in your mouth that is produced by food and bacteria that are packed into the cavity.

In the final stage of decay, the pulp of the tooth becomes inflamed. If this occurs, you may have persistent pain after eating sweet, sour, hot, or cold food. You may also experience sharp, stabbing pains, sometimes in the jaw above or below the

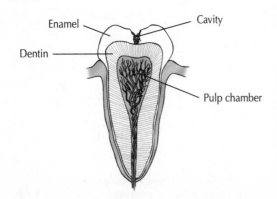

Cavities
If the enamel of a tooth has been eroded, bacteria in the mouth can destroy the dentin. If the decay is not treated, the bacteria can reach the pulp chamber, causing pain and inflammation.

decayed tooth. It may be hard to tell which tooth is causing the pain.

If you have a persistent unpleasant taste in your mouth, if you have a toothache, or if your teeth seem unusually sensitive to the foods you eat, see your dentist. Early detection and treatment of tooth decay can help you avoid more extensive treatment and can help prevent more serious problems such as an infected root canal or tooth loss.

Diagnosis

During a dental checkup (see page 1103) your dentist will examine your teeth for early signs of tooth decay; evaluate the condition of existing restorations, such as fillings, crowns, or bridges; and inspect your gums and mouth for signs of infection or other problems. He or she may also take X-rays to check for hidden signs of decay, such as cavities between the teeth or bone loss below the gum line.

Treatment

If a cavity is detected early, your dentist will clean and fill it to prevent further decay. If the decay is advanced, your dentist may recommend that you see an endodontist (a dentist who specializes in root canal treatment) for a root canal (see page 1104). In rare cases, a dentist will remove a tooth that is very badly decayed. Prevention is the best course for tooth decay.

Preventing Tooth Decay

You can keep tooth decay to a minimum by keeping your teeth and gums healthy (see next page). In addition to daily brushing and flossing and regular

dental checkups and cleanings, reduce your intake of sugary and starchy foods, avoid snacking between meals, use a fluoride toothpaste and mouthwash, and drink fluoridated water.

If you have young children, do not put them to bed with a bottle of milk, juice, or any other liquid that contains sugar. These liquids coat the teeth, promoting tooth decay. Your dentist will probably recommend that your children have topical fluoride treatments to prevent tooth decay every year starting at about age 3 to 4, even if your community's water supply is fluoridated.

Your dentist may recommend applying a clear plastic sealant to the biting surfaces of your teeth or your child's teeth to help prevent decay. The sealant provides a physical barrier that helps keep the teeth, particularly the molars, free of bacteria. To apply sealant to a tooth, the dentist cleans and polishes the biting surface of the tooth with a brush and then applies etching gel to the biting surface of the tooth to enable the sealant to bond to the tooth. He or she dries the tooth, brushes sealant into the grooves of the tooth, and aims a light wand at the sealant that causes it to harden immediately. The dentist examines the bite to make sure the sealant is not too thick. If it is, he or she will carefully buff the sealant down with a dental drill.

Once the sealant is set, a person can eat and drink as usual. The sealant will protect the treated areas of the teeth from cavities for about 5 years, but it will not protect untreated areas, such as the area between the teeth. Daily brushing and flossing and regular dental checkups and cleanings will still be necessary and will allow the dentist to examine the sealant and repair any chips or cracks.

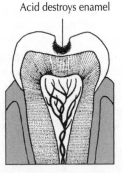
Acid destroys enamel

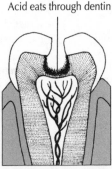
Acid eats through dentin

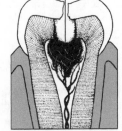
Decay reaches pulp

Untreated tooth decay

Keeping Your Teeth and Gums Healthy

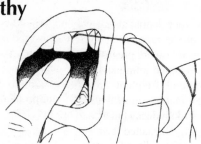

Even if you avoid foods and drinks that contain sugar and other simple carbohydrates, it is hard to avoid at least some tooth decay. However, you can keep tooth decay to a minimum and keep your teeth healthy by taking the following simple steps:

● **Brush your teeth thoroughly with a fluoride toothpaste for at least 2 to 3 minutes at least twice a day, every day.** Use dental floss every day to remove food particles and plaque from places you cannot reach with your toothbrush, such as between teeth and near the gum line. Your dentist or hygienist will show you how to brush and floss your teeth.

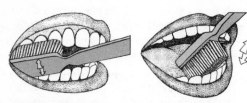

Brushing your teeth
Squeeze a pea-sized portion of toothpaste onto your toothbrush. As you brush, place your toothbrush at an angle, start at the gums, and gently move the brush back and forth, away from the gum line. Carefully brush the front, back, and chewing surfaces of each tooth. Use a soft-bristled brush to prevent damage to your gums. Do not push down too hard on the brush; let the bristles do the work. Gently massaging the gums with your toothbrush stimulates circulation and helps keep them healthy. Softly brushing your tongue will remove bacteria and help freshen your breath. An electric toothbrush helps you clean your teeth thoroughly while stimulating the gums. Replace your toothbrush or the brush head from your electric toothbrush every few weeks.

● **Cut back on sweets, avoid eating between meals, and eat a balanced diet.** Snacking on candy and other sugary foods and refined carbohydrates between meals is especially harmful because the bacteria in your mouth that break down these types of foods produce an acid that can dissolve tooth enamel. Try to avoid eating sugary foods completely. Avoid fruit roll-ups and other gummy snacks and candies that stick to the teeth. Have nuts or low-fat cheese for dessert instead of ice cream or cake. Cheese is especially good at neutralizing the acid that attacks teeth.

● **Strengthen your tooth enamel with fluoride.** Tap water in many communities contains added fluoride as a public health measure to help prevent cavities.

Flossing your teeth
Dental floss is a special thread that you slide between your teeth to remove plaque and food particles. To floss your teeth properly, take about 18 inches of floss and wind some of it around the middle fingers of each hand. Hold about 1 inch of floss between both index fingers, or between the thumb of one hand and the index finger of the other hand, or whatever way works best for you. Slide the floss between the teeth and, with a gentle up-and-down motion, rub the sides of each tooth. Use a clean section of floss for each tooth.

Bottled water with added fluoride also is available. Try to drink eight glasses of water every day. Because the enamel on their teeth is still forming, children under 13 should have fluoride applied to their teeth every year. Your dentist may recommend using a fluoride mouthwash or tablets and may apply a fluoride gel to your teeth. In addition, be sure your entire family uses a fluoride toothpaste.

● **Use disclosing tablets from time to time to monitor the effectiveness of your brushing and flossing techniques.** Disclosing tablets contain a nontoxic red vegetable dye that temporarily stains plaque so you can see how well you are brushing and flossing your teeth. After brushing and flossing, chew a tablet and swish it around in your mouth for about a minute, spit it out, and inspect your teeth. Areas with plaque will be stained reddish pink. To remove the plaque, brush and floss these areas again until the stains are gone. Because the dye also stains the mouth and tongue, you should use disclosing tablets right before going to bed.

● **See your dentist twice a year (or as often as he or she recommends) for an examination and cleaning.** Regular examinations will help ensure that your dentist can detect and fill any new cavity before the decay spreads and treat any gum disease before it becomes serious. Your dentist will take X-rays of your teeth every year or two to look for potential problems that can't be detected in an oral examination.

Going to the Dentist

See your dentist at least twice a year or as often as he or she recommends. (If you use tobacco products, if you are pregnant, or if you have diabetes or a weakened immune system, your dentist will recommend frequent oral examinations.) Regular examinations are necessary not only to detect and treat tooth decay but also to check your general oral health. Neglected teeth and gums are vulnerable to the various disorders described in this chapter and can increase your risk of developing infections that can enter the bloodstream and threaten your health. Dentures, like natural teeth, need to be checked regularly, and all dentures eventually wear down and need to be replaced. If you have a full set of dentures and have no problems with them, you still need to see your dentist regularly for oral examinations.

Dental Checkup

At your regular dental checkups, the dentist or hygienist will usually ask you questions about your general health before the dentist examines your teeth. This information is vital and may affect your treatment. For example, people who have some heart conditions and have a tooth removed, or any

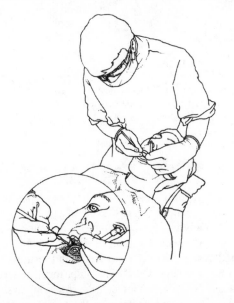

Dental examination
During a checkup, your dentist will examine your teeth for early signs of decay. He or she also will examine your gums and mouth for signs of disease or other problems. The dentist also may take X-rays to look for signs of decay that are not detectable from a visual examination.

other treatment that causes the gums to bleed, have an increased risk of bacterial endocarditis (see page 593). To prevent this complication in people who are at increased risk, a doctor may prescribe a course of antibiotics to eliminate any infection before the tooth is removed. Because stress can increase the level of glucose in the blood, people who have uncontrolled diabetes (see page 889) may become ill if they experience stress during treatment. The dentist will ask if you have any allergies, because people who have allergies may have a dangerous reaction to some drugs, such as penicillin. The dentist also needs to know about over-the-counter and prescription medications you are taking to help avoid possible harmful drug interactions. All dentists use universal precautions—such as wearing safety glasses, latex gloves, and a protective mask—to help prevent the possible spread of infection.

During an oral examination, the dentist first carefully inspects your mouth—including the tongue, the roof of the mouth, the insides of the cheeks, and the salivary glands—for signs of any diseases that are not confined to the teeth. For example, gums that are red, puffy, tender, or receding (pulling away from the teeth) indicate periodontal disease (see page 1114). A white discoloration of the inside of the mouth may indicate that you have oral thrush (see page 744), leukoplakia (see page 744), or oral lichen planus (see page 745). The dentist then examines your teeth with a mirror and a needle-shaped probe, looking for color changes that may indicate decay or cracks that may indicate the beginning of a cavity. He or she also examines your fillings to see if any parts have chipped off or if any new cavities are developing around the edges of a filling. If you have bridges or dentures, the dentist will check them for fit and examine their effects on your gums and any remaining teeth.

Why Your Dentist Takes X-Rays

Every year or two, your dentist takes bitewing X-rays (one or two X-rays of each side of your mouth are taken while you bite down on a piece of wing-shaped plastic to hold the X-ray film in place) to check for problems that he or she cannot detect during a visual examination. Every 3 to 5 years, your dentist should take a full set of mouth X-rays or a panoramic X-ray. He or she should also take X-rays of any teeth that have been treated with a

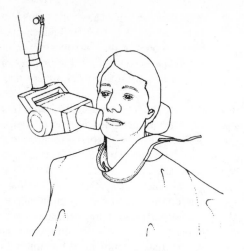

For root canal treatment the endodontist usually numbs the area around the affected tooth with a local anesthetic and places a rubber sheet called a dental dam around the tooth to isolate it from adjacent teeth. He or she then drills through the top of the crown of the tooth and into the pulp chamber. Next, the endodontist cleans out the root canal; disinfects it to kill the bacteria; fills the empty pulp chamber with a soft, rubberlike material to prevent recontamination; and seals the root canal. In some cases the endodontist inserts a metal post above the canal filling to reinforce the tooth. Your regular dentist will then place a crown over the tooth to restore its structure, function, and appearance.

Bitewing X-rays
One method of taking X-rays of the teeth uses a small piece of X-ray film that is covered by a protective wing-shaped plastic casing that is gripped firmly between the teeth.

root canal (see below) to look for a possible tooth abscess (see right). The dentist may also use X-rays to check the growth of your wisdom teeth or to determine how much bone is supporting your teeth if you have periodontal disease (see page 1114).

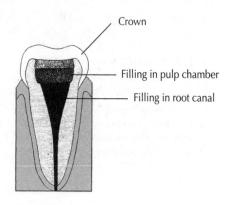

Crown

Filling in pulp chamber

Filling in root canal

Root Canal

At the core of every healthy tooth is the pulp, tissue that nourishes the tooth and makes it sensitive to heat, cold, pressure, and pain. However, the pulp may become infected or die after tooth decay penetrates it. The pulp may die after a blow to the tooth or, in some cases, for no obvious reason. If the pulp is infected or dead, root canal treatment is performed to save the tooth. Root canal treatment is usually performed by an endodontist (a dentist who specializes in root canal treatment).

A tooth with infected or dead pulp should be treated as soon as possible after it is detected because bacteria from the pulp can seep through the end of the root and cause a tooth abscess (see right). Although infected pulp may cause pain and swelling, it often produces no symptoms. Because a tooth with dead pulp can continue to function efficiently, it will not be removed unless it is badly decayed.

Root canal
When the pulp in a tooth becomes infected, a tooth abscess can form. The tooth must be treated by cleaning out the root canal, destroying any bacteria, filling and sealing the canal, and restoring the crown.

Tooth Abscess

A tooth abscess is a pocket of pus in the tissue around the tip of the root of a tooth. An abscess usually forms when a tooth is decaying, when its pulp is infected or dead, or when the gums have receded significantly from the teeth (periodontal disease; see page 1114). The pulp, together with invading bacteria, can infect the surrounding tissue. Until the pulp and bacteria in the tooth are removed, the infection will continue to spread.

If an abscess is not treated, it can eat away at the jawbone until it has worn a small canal, or sinus, through the bone and its overlying gum. Just before the canal reaches the surface of the gum, a painful swelling can form. The swelling may remain for weeks. However, in some cases, the abscess bursts, creating a drainage channel called a fistula. When this occurs, foul-tasting pus drains into the mouth, and the pain stops suddenly. The bacteria can invade adjacent bone and spread throughout the body, causing blood poisoning (see page 937).

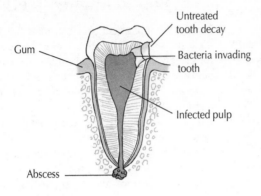

How an abscess forms
If tooth decay is not treated, the pulp can become infected, and pus may begin to form. Pus at the base of the tooth may form an abscess and seep out through the root of the tooth. Untreated, the infection can damage the jawbone.

Symptoms and Treatment

An abscessed tooth aches or throbs persistently, making biting or chewing extremely painful. The glands in the neck may swell and become tender and, if the abscess spreads, the affected side of the face may also swell. An abscess usually causes a fever and makes a person feel generally ill. If you have swelling around the tooth that spreads to your face or neck, see your dentist immediately. If your dentist is not available, call your doctor, who may prescribe an antibiotic. Then see your dentist as soon as possible.

In the meantime, take acetaminophen or ibuprofen to help relieve the pain. Rinse your mouth every hour with warm salted water, to speed the bursting of the abscess and help relieve the pain. When the abscess bursts, rinse your mouth again to wash away the pus. After the abscess has burst, see your dentist for treatment as soon as possible.

A dentist may remove an abscessed back tooth or primary tooth if it is thoroughly infected. In most other cases, the dentist will try to save the tooth. He or she will drill a small hole through the crown of the tooth into the pulp chamber. If the abscess has not yet burst, drilling the hole will release the pus and relieve the pain. The dentist then cleans out and disinfects the pulp chamber and root canals. During a later visit, after the infection has cleared up, the dentist will place a permanent filling in the pulp chamber, root canals, and drilled hole. About 6 months later the dentist will take X-rays of the area to make sure that new bone and tissue are growing into the cavity left by the abscess. If new tissue is growing in the cavity, further treatment is usually not necessary.

Sometimes, even after root canal treatment, bacteria remain in the tissue around the base of the root of the tooth and cause an abscess to form. If antibiotics cannot clear up the infection, your dentist may recommend that you see an oral surgeon or an endodontist (a dentist who specializes in root canal treatment). If you have already had root canal treatment but still have problems with a tooth, an oral surgeon may perform a procedure called apicoectomy. For apicoectomy, you are given a local anesthetic and the surgeon makes a small cut through the gum, drills away the bone that covers the tip of the root, and removes the infected tissue at the base of the tooth. In rare cases, apicoectomy may not be effective, and the tooth must be removed and replaced with a bridge (see page 1110) or an implant (see page 1111).

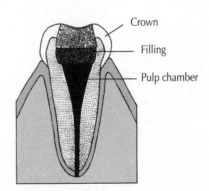

Treating an abscess
Your dentist may try to save an abscessed tooth by drilling a small hole through the crown to release the pus. He or she can then clean out and disinfect the pulp chamber and root canals and put in a temporary filling. During a later visit your dentist will remove the temporary filling and replace it with a permanent filling.

Discolored Teeth

A slight yellowing of the teeth occurs naturally with age. However, for a variety of other reasons, teeth sometimes become discolored. Smoking and chewing tobacco can stain tooth surfaces, and some foods and beverages (including blueberries, coffee, and red wine) also can cause stains. The death of the pulp of a tooth can turn the tooth gray. Some drugs, taken either in large doses or at specific times during childhood, can cause defective, discolored tooth enamel to form. Severe cases of some childhood infections, such as whooping cough and measles, can produce patches of discoloration on the teeth. Abnormally high levels of natural fluoride in drinking water, which occur in some areas, can lead to fluorosis, which causes white or brown marks on the teeth. Fluorosis does not occur, however, in areas where a controlled amount of fluoride is added to the water supply as a public health measure to reduce the incidence of tooth decay.

Treatment

To treat discoloration on the surface of a tooth, your dentist or dental hygienist will clean the tooth with a rotary polisher and polishing paste. Deeper discoloration can be treated by applying a bleaching gel directly to the teeth. Bleaching is safe and effective for healthy teeth and can be done at home or at the dentist's office. Healthy teeth with minor discoloration can be treated by bonding tooth-colored plastic material to the discolored area of the tooth. If a tooth is not in good condition overall but does not need a crown, a veneer made of porcelain laminate or acrylic resin can be bonded to the entire front surface of the tooth.

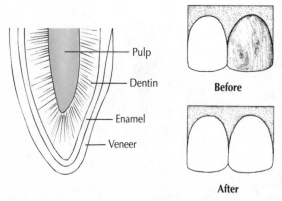

Before

After

Veneers
One possible treatment for a discolored tooth is to cover it with a veneer, a material such as porcelain laminate or acrylic resin that closely resembles the color of the teeth. The porcelain laminate is made in a lab and then glued onto the front surface of the tooth. The acrylic resin is applied to the tooth in thin layers.

Poorly Aligned Teeth

Ideally, the alignment (occlusion) of the teeth is a horseshoe-shaped arch that is exactly the right size for the jaws. In normal occlusion—the relationship between the upper and lower teeth when the mouth is closed—the upper teeth slightly overlap the lower teeth, and the cusps (points) of the molars mesh with the spaces between the opposing upper or lower teeth.

However, few people have perfectly aligned teeth. Because a person inherits genetic characteristics from each of his or her parents, sometimes the two sets of characteristics do not match, resulting in misalignment of the teeth (malocclusion). For example, if your teeth are too big for your jaws, your teeth can develop only by sloping backward or forward, by turning, by rotating, or by overlapping adjacent teeth. If your teeth are too small for your jaws, there will be some spaces between your teeth. If your lower jaw is smaller than your upper jaw, the teeth in your upper jaw may protrude, causing a type of malocclusion called an overbite. If your lower jaw protrudes slightly, your permanent upper front teeth may bite just behind the lower teeth, causing a type of malocclusion called an underbite. In some people, the position of the back teeth may prevent the front teeth from meeting properly, causing a type of malocclusion called an open bite.

Heredity is not the only cause of malocclusion. Crowding is sometimes the result of loss of primary teeth (baby teeth) through decay. For example, when primary molars are lost prematurely, the permanent molars move forward in the jaw to fill the gaps. Then, when the permanent premolars and canines appear, usually between ages 10 and 12, they are crowded or blocked out of the natural arch of the teeth. In some people, some permanent teeth may not appear at all.

In mild cases of crowding, a person has an increased risk of tooth decay and gum disease because it is more difficult to keep crowded teeth clean. In some people, severe crowding can lead to dental disease or difficulty chewing. Malocclusion can make some people self-conscious about their appearance. For them, orthodontic treatment not only can improve a faulty bite, but it can also improve their appearance and sense of well-being.

Treatment

If you are an adult with minor occlusion problems, such as a few crowded or twisted teeth, your dentist may recommend orthodontic treatment for cosmetic reasons or to prevent more serious problems. However, if your teeth are severely maloccluded, your dentist will probably recommend that you see an orthodontist for immediate treatment to prevent damage to or loss of your permanent teeth. An orthodontist is a dentist who specializes in treating malocclusion. Orthodontists undergo 2 to 3 years of additional training after graduating from dental school to obtain a certificate in orthodontics.

If you have a minor alignment problem, the orthodontist may remove some teeth or fit you with braces to correct the crowding or malocclusion. Many adults are choosing to wear braces and do not feel self-conscious about them. For some people, crowns (see page 1109) and bridges (see page 1110) can help correct the problem.

In some cases, severe malocclusion or jaws that protrude or recede may result from the size and shape of the jaw. In such cases, a person may need orthodontia or oral surgery to align the teeth and stabilize the bite. An oral surgeon can reposition or remove pieces of the jawbone and some teeth to correct the problem and create a normal occlusion.

If your child's teeth appear to be growing in crowded or misaligned, take him or her to a dentist for an examination. Depending on your child's age, the dentist may recommend that you take him or her to an orthodontist for evaluation and possible treatment. Orthodontia is usually most effective during childhood and early adolescence, when the teeth and jaws are growing and developing. Also, it is easier to move the teeth at this time because the bone that surrounds the teeth is soft and is still developing.

Before beginning treatment, the orthodontist takes X-rays of the teeth and jaw to determine if all of the child's permanent teeth have formed and are likely to emerge and to evaluate the development of the bones in the jaw, face, and head. The orthodontist also makes plaster casts of the teeth and jaw. If crowding is the problem, one possible treatment is to create a space by removing an adjacent tooth

Types of Malocclusion

Occlusion is the relationship between the upper and lower teeth when the mouth is closed. Malocclusion occurs when the upper and lower teeth are misaligned. Normal occlusion and four types of malocclusion are shown here.

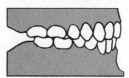

Normal bite

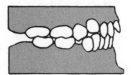

Crowded teeth

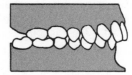

Overbite

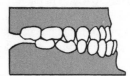

Underbite

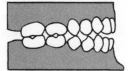

Open bite

that has already appeared. But the usual treatment for irregularly positioned teeth is to wear braces over a period of months or years.

Braces are either bands that are fitted around the teeth or brackets that are bonded directly onto the teeth. A wire is threaded from tooth to tooth. The wire applies gentle pressure that moves the teeth into the correct position. The bands, brackets, and wires are made of metal. To make braces less visible, brackets may also be made of ceramic or plastic material and may be clear or tooth-colored.

Fixed braces are often used when a child's upper incisors protrude and the canines are prominent and crowded. For severely crowded teeth, some premolars may be removed first so that the canines can be moved into the correct position. Once the canines are aligned, the incisors can be retracted to make them less prominent and to prevent spaces from forming between the front teeth. This type of treatment usually begins at about age 12 and takes about 18 to 30 months. The person (whether a child or an adult) returns to the orthodontist every 5 to 6 weeks to have the braces adjusted.

After the malocclusion has been corrected, the braces are removed and a removable device called a retainer is custom-made to hold the teeth in their new position. The retainer is used, usually at night, for several years to make sure that the surrounding tissue has enough time to stabilize. Often a permanent retainer is bonded into place on the back of the lower front teeth. Once the person's third molars (wisdom teeth) erupt or are extracted, the fixed retainer may be removed.

Braces and retainers can trap plaque, the sticky substance that forms on teeth from food particles, mucus, and bacteria in the mouth. Because plaque can cause tooth decay and gum disease, be sure to clean your teeth and braces thoroughly after every meal, and avoid candy and other sugary foods and snacking between meals.

Aligners—clear, removable pieces of plastic that are molded to fit over the teeth and that straighten the teeth without using brackets and wires—are an alternative to traditional braces. An aligner moves the teeth a very small amount and is worn day and night for about 2 weeks. You then replace it with the next aligner in the series, and continue this process until all of your teeth have been straightened. Aligners can be removed for eating, brushing, and flossing. The last aligner in the series is usually made of a thicker material, and you can wear it as a retainer to hold your teeth in their new position while the surrounding tissues stabilize. You may need to wear the retainer indefinitely to help ensure that your teeth don't move.

Dental Treatments

A variety of dental procedures can help keep your teeth and gums strong and healthy. Keeping your teeth and gums in good condition is an essential component of good health.

Cleaning and Polishing

If your teeth are coated with calculus (also called tartar), a chalky mineralized deposit of hardened plaque, the dentist or hygienist will remove the calculus with handheld instruments called scalers. Because they must be used both above and below the gum line, scalers can cause the gums to bleed

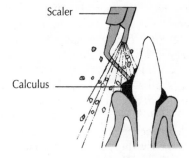

Cleaning teeth

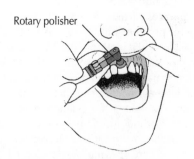

Polishing teeth

Cleaning and polishing the teeth
Along with daily brushing and flossing, regular professional cleaning and polishing can help prevent tooth decay and periodontal disease. A dentist or hygienist uses a number of different instruments to remove calculus both above and below the gum line.

Filling a Tooth

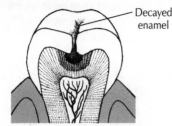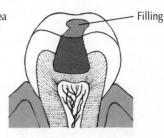

The dentist fills a tooth if the enamel has been damaged (left). If the tooth is not filled, bacteria can reach the dentin inside the tooth and destroy it, and then attack the pulp. To prepare a tooth for filling, the dentist drills through the enamel and removes all traces of decay (center). He or she then shapes the hole to prevent the filling from falling out. The hole is then filled with a mixture of silver, tin, and mercury (right). If a filling will be visible, the dentist may use a white filling material made of quartz in a plastic resin.

slightly. After scaling, the dentist or hygienist polishes the teeth, because a smooth surface slows the formation of calculus.

Fillings

When a tooth is partly decayed or chipped, the dentist replaces the damaged area with a filling (see above). White fillings often are used on front teeth. Silver amalgam—a mixture of silver, tin, and mercury—is generally used on back teeth. If the treatment is likely to cause discomfort, the dentist will inject the gum with a local anesthetic. The dentist removes any decayed area and shapes the hole to retain the filling securely. If a front tooth is chipped, the dentist roughens the surface and bonds the filling to it. If a tooth is badly damaged or discolored, the dentist may use laminate veneers or acrylic resins to restore the appearance of the entire visible surface of the tooth. If the dentist uses a local anesthetic, be careful to avoid biting your lip or tongue while it is still numb.

Crowns

When a tooth is severely decayed, broken, fractured, brittle, or discolored, the dentist usually recommends an artificial crown for it if the base of the tooth and the roots are in good condition. The dentist prepares the damaged tooth by reducing the size of the natural crown so an artificial crown can fit over it. He or she then takes an impression of the prepared tooth and sends the impression to a dental laboratory, where an artificial crown is fabricated.

Generally, a white porcelain crown is fitted on a tooth that can be seen. On back teeth, gold or a less expensive material is used. Porcelain that is fused to metal can also be used for crowns on back teeth. The treatment usually requires two visits—the first to prepare the tooth, and the second to fit and adjust the crown. Between visits the person usually wears a temporary crown fitted by the dentist. The life of a permanent crown is usually about 5 to 8 years, but may be extended in people who do not grind

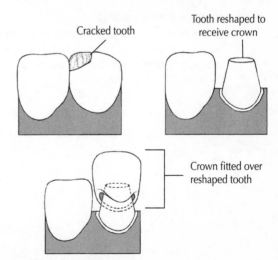

Fitting a tooth with a crown
A broken, cracked, or heavily filled tooth can be repaired with a crown. The remaining part of the tooth is reshaped to receive the crown. The crown, a hollow shell, is fitted over the old tooth and cemented on.

their teeth or bite their fingernails and who avoid chewing on hard foods or ice.

Bridges

If you have a gap of up to about four teeth, with healthy natural teeth on both sides of the gap, your dentist may recommend using an artificial tooth or teeth called a bridge to fill the gap (see below). A bridge helps prevent the remaining teeth from shifting or tilting out of place. The dentist will prepare the two natural teeth on either side of the gap for crowning. He or she then cements the two crowns to the prepared teeth. Enough of a gap should remain between the base of the bridge and the gum ridge to allow you to clean the area properly. Bridges at the front of the mouth are made of an alloy faced with porcelain; bridges at the back of the mouth are usually made of gold or less expensive alloys. Resin-bonded bridges are used when the two teeth on either side of the gap are healthy. Instead of filing these healthy teeth down, a bridge is made to fit around them and is cemented into place with a special glue. Putting in a bridge normally requires three or four visits to the dentist. If you have a bridge, see your dentist regularly to make sure it fits properly. If you have pain, sores, or bleeding in your mouth, see your dentist immediately.

Removing a Tooth

Although dentists try to save teeth whenever possible, they sometimes have to remove them. For example, a tooth may be too decayed or badly broken to be saved with a root canal or a crown, or it may be causing crowding or misalignment (see page 1106). A tooth may be loose because of advanced gum disease, or it may be preventing

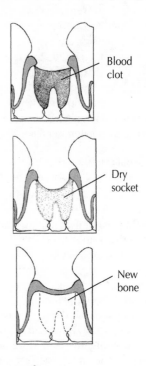

Blood clot

Dry socket

New bone

After removing a tooth
After a tooth has been removed, a blood clot usually forms in the empty tooth socket in the gum (top). In some cases, the blood clot breaks down, resulting in what is called a dry socket (center). Eventually, new bone grows into the empty socket and is covered by gum tissue (bottom).

Bridges

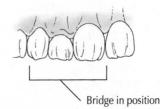

Missing tooth

Reshaped teeth

Bridge

Crowns

Bridge in position

If a tooth is missing (left), the gap can be filled with an artificial tooth called a bridge. The two teeth on either side of the gap are reshaped to enable them to accept crowns and anchor the bridge (center). The crowns are cemented to the reshaped teeth, holding the bridge in place (right).

another tooth from emerging from the gum.

Before removing a tooth, the dentist usually uses a local anesthetic to numb the tooth and gum. A general anesthetic or a sedative may be used for young children, to remove badly impacted third molars (wisdom teeth), to remove several teeth at once, or for people who are extremely anxious. After a tooth has been removed, be careful not to dislodge the clot that forms in the wound. If the socket bleeds persistently, bite on a clean, tightly folded handkerchief or gauze pad to stop the bleeding. Keep the pad in place for half an hour by clenching your teeth. If the bleeding does not stop, see your dentist immediately.

Dentures

If several teeth are missing, a partial denture is required to replace them. A full denture replaces all of the natural teeth. Dentures are made of tough plastic or of metal and plastic combined.

On a partial denture, the baseplate (artificial gums) often has clasps that fit around the natural teeth to help keep the denture in place. Full lower dentures stay in place by resting on the gum ridge and full upper dentures by suction to the roof of the mouth.

Fitting a denture usually requires several visits to the dentist. During the first visit, the dentist takes impressions of the gums and evaluates the relationship between the upper and lower jaws. He or she will also discuss the size and color of the dentures. In most cases, the dentist makes a preliminary denture and uses it to make any necessary adjustments. After the final denture is made, the dentist fits and adjusts it to enable the person to bite

evenly and comfortably. At first, talking and eating while wearing dentures may seem difficult, but most people adapt to them fairly quickly.

People who wear dentures should remove and clean them every day to promote good oral health and allow the gum tissues to rest. Dentures can be cleaned with a denture cleanser or with ordinary toothpaste and a toothbrush designed for cleaning dentures. People who wear dentures also should continue to see a dentist regularly so that he or she can monitor the condition of the mouth and gums, evaluate the dentures for continued good fit, and reduce the risk of denture problems (see page 1113). Poorly fitting dentures can cause chronic irritation and inflammation, which can lead to oral cancer (see page 747).

Nightguards

Nightguards are hard, transparent pieces of plastic that fit over the upper or lower biting surfaces of the teeth. Nightguards help prevent damage to the teeth caused by bruxism (clenching and grinding of the teeth, usually during sleep) or help relieve earaches, jaw aches, and headaches that can result from poorly aligned teeth (see page 1106) or temporomandibular disorder (see page 1005). To make a nightguard, a dentist takes impressions of the upper and lower teeth to make models of the teeth, from which a nightguard is made. The dentist makes the final adjustments to the nightguard in the person's mouth to make sure that it fits properly. For a nightguard to be effective, a person must wear it every night while sleeping. To clean a nightguard, soak it in a solution of denture cleanser according to package directions.

Implants

Implants can be used to replace one or more teeth without using neighboring teeth for support. To insert an implant, an oral surgeon cuts through the gum tissue where the tooth is missing to expose the bone beneath the gum. He or she then drills a hole into the bone and places a tiny titanium post into the hole and covers it with gum tissue. In about 6 months, after the tissue has healed, the oral surgeon cuts the gum and exposes the top of the post. Implants act as roots to which a dentist can securely attach crowns or bridges without using adjacent teeth. Because dentures that are attached to implants are more stable than traditional dentures, they make talking and eating much easier.

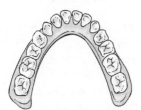

Full denture
Full dentures are used when all of the teeth are missing. A full upper denture is held in place by suction to the roof of the mouth; a lower denture rests on the gum ridge.

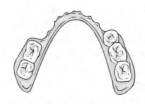

Partial denture
Partial dentures are used to fill gaps when some of the teeth are missing. Partial dentures are usually held in place by attaching them to healthy teeth that are adjacent to the gap.

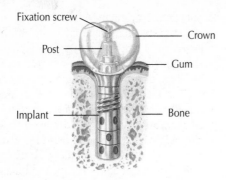

Dental implant
A dental implant is a tiny metal post that is implanted surgically into the jawbone to act as a root for a crown or bridge.

Missing Teeth

Teeth may be missing for a number of reasons. Sometimes permanent teeth do not come in after a child's primary teeth (baby teeth) come out. In adults, teeth are lost usually from decay or injury. A tooth also may be missing in an adult if the tooth has failed to develop, which occurs most often with the upper teeth, the incisors, the premolars, and the third molars (wisdom teeth). Also, the teeth may be impacted (blocked under the gum, usually because of overcrowding), which prevents them from emerging through the gum. The teeth that are most often impacted are the upper canines, premolars, and wisdom teeth.

Even one missing molar can cause problems. For example, when you chew, your jaw moves from side to side and up and down. If a molar fits into an empty space in the row of teeth above or below it, your jaw will not move easily from side to side. Because this condition can prevent you from chewing properly, your dentist will probably remove the molar or grind down high points (called cusps).

The remaining teeth naturally tend to tip toward the spaces left by missing teeth. To do so, they may emerge too much from the gum or grow at an angle, causing the teeth to be poorly aligned (see page 1106), which prevents the teeth from coming together properly when you bite or chew. A faulty bite places extra stress on your teeth and jaw; this stress can lead to temporomandibular disorder (see page 1005), a condition that causes discomfort and pain in the joints of the jaw. Misalignment can also wear down some teeth.

If teeth grow into gaps at an angle, the surfaces of the teeth may be difficult to clean. Plaque can build up in hard-to-reach places and lead to tooth decay and periodontal disease (see page 1114).

Treatment
If you think that your child is missing a primary tooth or a permanent tooth, take him or her to the dentist for an examination. You should also see your dentist if you have any missing teeth since childhood or are experiencing any problems caused by missing teeth.

A dentist may recommend treating a missing tooth with a bridge (see page 1110), a removable partial denture (see previous page), or a dental implant (see previous page). Your dentist may also refer you to an orthodontist, a dentist who specializes in treating irregularly positioned teeth. To treat any pain in the jaw caused by poorly aligned teeth, your dentist may fit a nightguard (see previous page) over your upper or lower teeth and gums or may grind down the high spots in your teeth to correct your bite.

Problems Caused by Wisdom Teeth

The last teeth at the back of your mouth are the third molars, or wisdom teeth. The four wisdom teeth usually appear between ages 17 and 21, but some people don't develop all four wisdom teeth. If one of your wisdom teeth fails to emerge, you probably will not have any symptoms. Missing wisdom teeth are not a cause for concern unless they have failed to emerge because they are impacted (blocked under the gum, usually because of overcrowding).

Wisdom teeth are difficult to clean and, therefore, decay more easily than other teeth. For example, if a wisdom tooth emerges at an angle, the space between the wisdom tooth and the next tooth can trap plaque and food particles, causing tooth decay or periodontal disease (see page 1114). Often a wisdom tooth fails to emerge properly because it becomes impacted, sometimes by the adjacent tooth. In this case, a pocket can form around the impacted tooth and collect plaque and food particles. Bacteria in the pocket may cause bad breath and an unpleasant taste in your mouth and can eventually cause an infection (called pericoronitis) around the impacted tooth.

Symptoms of pericoronitis include pain when you bite down on the tooth or the gum partially covering the tooth, and redness and swelling of the gum around the tooth. If you have any of these symptoms, see your dentist or doctor as soon as possible.

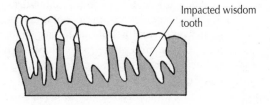

Impacted wisdom tooth

Impacted wisdom tooth
This impacted wisdom tooth is blocked as it grows at an angle against the adjacent tooth. Wisdom teeth are usually removed to prevent tooth decay or periodontal disease.

Treatment

The long-term solution for an impacted wisdom tooth is to remove it, which is the only way to treat a recurring infection or prevent future infection. If you have an infected impacted tooth, using a topical over-the-counter anesthetic, taking aspirin, and rinsing the area around the tooth with warm salted water can relieve pain until you can see your dentist.

Your dentist will take X-rays to determine the position of the tooth. If there is no sign of infection and the tooth can be easily removed, your dentist will extract it after injecting a local anesthetic. If the area around the tooth is infected, he or she will prescribe an antibiotic to eliminate the infection before removing the tooth

If the tooth lies at an angle that would make it difficult to extract (or if you have other impacted wisdom teeth that need to be removed), your dentist may refer you to an oral surgeon who can more easily remove the tooth (or teeth). You will probably be given a local anesthetic and possibly a sedative. However, general anesthesia is sometimes required.

Denture Problems

Most dentures, or false teeth, look natural and fit well, but no denture is as efficient and comfortable as your own teeth. With natural teeth, the stresses of biting and chewing are absorbed by the teeth, the roots of the teeth, and the periodontal ligament (a tough, elastic, shock-absorbent tissue that holds bones together and lines the tooth sockets in the jawbone). With dentures, the stresses are absorbed in unnatural ways. The most critical of these stresses is the pressure that the baseplate (the false gums of the dentures) places on the ridges of the natural gums, especially if the dentures are worn both day and night. This pressure can cause inflammation of the gums and eventually can lead to mouth ulcers and to degeneration of the jawbone under the gum tissue.

The base of a partial denture also places abnormal pressure on the natural teeth that are used to anchor the denture base. Partial dentures, especially poorly fitting ones, can trap plaque and food particles, causing tooth decay in the remaining teeth and possibly leading to periodontal disease (see next page). If you wear dentures and have been taking antibiotics, your risk of developing a yeast infection in the mouth called oral thrush (see page 744) is increased.

Symptoms

The early symptoms of excessive pressure on the ridges of the gums are pain when the dentures are in place, especially when you are eating, and white and patchy or red and inflamed gums. If the inflammation persists, your gums may become deep red and soft and may bleed easily—for example, after rubbing them with your toothbrush. An open sore may form on any spot where your dentures rub your gums. After a denture has been worn for many years, hard, pale pads called dental granulomas may form at the main pressure points on the gums, especially near the edges of the denture.

Other symptoms develop when the gums and jawbone shrink, which usually occurs after a few years of continuous pressure, even if the denture has caused no other problems. When the gums and jawbone shrink, you must close your mouth more to bite properly, and even more if your dentures are worn down. Common symptoms of gum and jawbone shrinkage are loose dentures, sunken cheeks, and a protruding lower jaw. You may have pain in the joints of the jawbone from the extra movement needed to bite down. The appearance of your mouth may change a great deal. Also, persistent irritation from friction, inflammation, and pressure can lead to infection or sometimes to cancerous changes in the tissue of the gums.

Treatment

If you have full dentures, have your dentist check their fit and any effect they have on your gums. You should have an oral examination at least once a year. If you have a partial denture, see your dentist regularly to make sure it fits properly and to safeguard your natural teeth and the general health of your mouth. If you have pain, sores, or bleeding in your mouth, see your dentist immediately.

Always remove your dentures at night, to rest your gum tissues and to allow you to adequately clean your mouth and dentures. Many dentures must be kept in a glass of water; they can warp if they dry out. It is normal for partial dentures to feel a little tight when you insert them in the morning, but the feeling passes quickly. Thoroughly clean your dentures daily, according to your dentist's or hygienist's instructions, and clean your natural teeth and gums thoroughly, especially around the base of the teeth. If you wear dentures and have a sore mouth, keep your dentures clean and soak them overnight in a cleaning solution designed for this purpose. You should also clean and massage your gums with your finger, a damp cloth, or a soft brush.

How long dentures last can vary, depending on the condition of the gums and jawbone, the denture material, and how well the dentures fit. When your dentures become worn or your gums and jawbone shrink, your dentist will make new dentures. However, if your dentures are not too worn, the dentist may be able to adjust the existing denture baseplate to the new shape of your gums. This process is called relining.

To clear up gum inflammation caused by a fungus, your dentist may prescribe an antifungal medication and teach you how to take better care of your gums and dentures to avoid future problems. Some people have problems coping with dentures and never fully adjust to them. And as some people who wear dentures get older, they find it difficult to adjust to a new set of dentures when their old dentures are replaced.

Periodontal Disease

Gingivitis is an early stage of periodontal (gum) disease. It is caused by plaque, a sticky deposit of bacteria, mucus, and food particles that forms at the base of the teeth. Plaque irritates the gums, causing inflammation and swelling. Gingivitis also may result from a vitamin deficiency, some medications, and some glandular disorders and blood diseases. Gingivitis can be treated easily and reversed. However, if it is not treated, gingivitis can progress to a more severe form of periodontal disease called periodontitis, which is the leading cause of tooth loss in adults in the United States.

About 75 percent of American adults over age 35 have some form of periodontal disease. Pregnant women and people who have diabetes are particularly susceptible to developing gingivitis because changing hormone levels can affect the condition of the gums. Smoking and chewing tobacco are major causes of periodontal disease and tooth loss.

However, periodontal disease may not affect only the teeth and gums—it may also be a risk factor for heart disease. The bacteria that cause periodontitis have been found in the bloodstream of some people with periodontal disease. These bacteria can cause blood platelets to accumulate and stick together in arteries, setting the stage for heart attack and stroke.

Preventing gingivitis
When plaque builds up, bacteria in its deeper layers die and mineralize and harden to form a material called calculus, which can lead to gum inflammation and swelling, or gingivitis. Proper brushing and flossing and regular dental checkups and cleanings help prevent the formation of calculus.

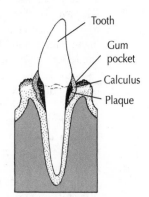

Tooth

Gum pocket

Calculus

Plaque

Symptoms

Healthy gums are firm, pink, and have natural variations in shade. When a person has gingivitis, his or her gums become red, soft, shiny, and swollen. The gums bleed easily, even from gentle brushing or flossing. If you have any of these symptoms, see your dentist as soon as possible.

Periodontitis develops if gingivitis is not treated. In periodontitis, the gums begin to pull away from the teeth, and pockets form between the teeth and gums. The pockets trap more plaque, the gums become more swollen, and the pockets deepen. The pockets between the teeth and gums gradually deepen, and the bacteria in the plaque inside the pockets cause a persistent, unpleasant taste in the mouth and bad breath. As the disease progresses, the teeth begin to loosen in their sockets. Eventually, more and more cementum (the sensitive, bonelike material that covers the roots of a tooth) is exposed, and the tooth aches when you eat very hot, very cold, or sweet or sour food. Sometimes a tooth abscess (see page 1104) forms deep inside a pocket and damages the jawbone.

Diagnosis

To diagnose periodontal disease, your dentist will check the gums for bleeding, measure the depth of any gum pockets, assess the looseness of the affected teeth, and take X-rays to determine the condition of the underlying bone. These factors are important for determining treatment.

Treatment

You can help prevent periodontal disease by keeping your teeth and gums healthy (see page 1102). If you already have gingivitis, try to brush and floss your teeth more carefully and thoroughly.

For more severe cases of gingivitis, the dentist removes any plaque and calculus from the base of the teeth. During a procedure called scaling, the dentist uses a handheld instrument called a scaler to remove plaque and calculus above and beneath the gum line. Ultrasonic scaling uses a high-frequency current to remove plaque and calculus. In a process called root planing, the dentist removes bacteria and other microorganisms by smoothing the surface of the root. In another technique, called subgingival debridement, the dentist removes tooth surface irritants from beneath the gum line to prevent infection in the treated area.

Some people need to have their teeth cleaned professionally every few months despite careful tooth care. For these people, dentists often recommend an antibacterial mouthwash. Most cases of gingivitis respond well to treatment, and the gums gradually return to their usual healthy condition. It is up to you to take the steps necessary to prevent another case of gingivitis.

Periodontitis can often be treated and reversed before it reaches an advanced stage. See your dentist as soon as possible if you have any symptoms such as red, swollen gums. If the disease is at an early stage, your dentist can help keep it under control by treating any pockets, which encourage plaque to form. He or she may place inserts that contain antibiotics or anti-inflammatory drugs directly into the pockets to fight the infection. If treatment with antibiotics begins early, no other treatment may be necessary. Ask your dentist if you should use toothpastes and mouth rinses that contain medication or antimicrobial agents. If you smoke or chew tobacco, stop; using tobacco products causes inflammation of the gums and promotes periodontitis.

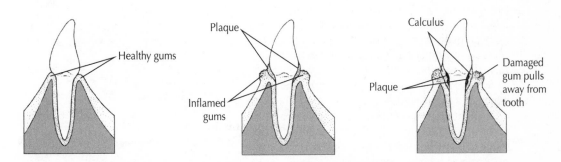

Gum disease caused by neglect
Inadequate brushing and flossing allows plaque to build up, which promotes gum disease. Without treatment, the disease progresses and can eventually lead to tooth loss. Healthy gums (left) fit firmly around the necks of the teeth and do not bleed easily. Plaque that builds up between the teeth and gums can cause painful inflammation (center). Untreated plaque can harden to form a substance called calculus, which can cause the gums to recede (right). The bacteria in calculus can cause severe damage to the teeth, gums, and jawbone.

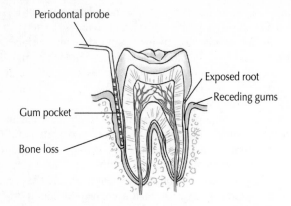

The bacteria that cause periodontitis can be transmitted among family members, so, if one member of your family has periodontal disease, all other family members should also see a dentist for a checkup and evaluation.

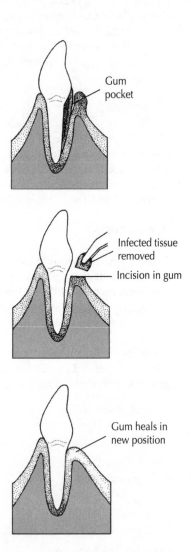

Evaluating periodontal disease
The bacteria in plaque can destroy the bone and gum tissue that surround and anchor the teeth. If not removed, plaque forms a hardened material called calculus, which can pry the gum away from the tooth, loosening it. Eventually the tooth may have to be removed. To evaluate the severity of periodontal disease, a dentist inserts an instrument called a periodontal probe between the tooth and gum (beneath the gum line) to measure and record the depth of the gum pockets. In general, the deeper the pocket, the more severe the disease.

If the pockets between the teeth and gums are very deep, you may need periodontal surgery. A gingivectomy is a minor surgical procedure performed in the office by a periodontist (gum specialist) in which the soft tissue wall of the pocket is removed. If the bone has been damaged, you may need to undergo a procedure called osseous surgery, in which the periodontist removes infected tissue and reshapes the gum and bone. After the surgery, the gum line is covered with a protective coating called a periodontal pack, which is left in place for 1 to 2 weeks until the gum heals. You can eat and drink normally with a periodontal pack in place. In some cases, the periodontist or an oral surgeon performs a procedure called regenerative surgery, which uses special inserts to try to regrow the jawbone and supporting tissue.

Cementum that has been worn away can be replaced by bonding a synthetic material to the tooth. Cementum that is especially sensitive can be protected with a layer of sodium fluoride or a prescription toothpaste that protects against sensitivity. Very loose teeth can be anchored.

Gingivectomy
The buildup of plaque and calculus between the teeth and gums forms a deep pocket (top) between them. During treatment, the pocket is cleaned and the soft-tissue wall of the pocket is removed (center). The gum heals close to the tooth after the procedure (bottom).

Glossary

This glossary defines some common medical terms you'll find in this book. Italicized words within definitions refer you to other terms in the glossary for additional information.

A

abscess   A *pus*-filled cavity surrounded by inflamed tissue that usually forms as a result of a bacterial infection.

acquired immunodeficiency syndrome   See *AIDS.*

acupuncture   A Chinese medical technique in which a practitioner inserts very fine needles into specific sites in the skin to achieve a particular result, such as pain relief. Sometimes the needles are twirled, warmed, or stimulated electronically. In the United States, acupuncture is used mainly to treat back pain, *migraines,* and other pain disorders.

acute   Describes diseases or conditions that occur suddenly, last for only a short time, and often produce severe symptoms.

adenoma   A *benign* tumor that arises from glandular tissue.

adhesion   A band of scar tissue that joins adjacent organs and tissues that are normally separated. Adhesions are often painful and usually develop in the abdomen.

adrenal glands   A pair of small triangular glands located directly above the kidneys. The adrenal glands produce *hormones* that affect nearly every system in the body.

adrenaline   See *epinephrine.*

advance directive   A legal document to help ensure that health care decisions made on a person's behalf are consistent with his or her preferences. Examples of advance directives include *do-not-resuscitate orders, durable powers of attorney for health care,* and *living wills.*

aerobic exercise   A physical exercise that requires the heart and lungs to work harder to meet the muscles' continuous demand for oxygen. Examples of aerobic exercise include brisk walking, jogging, biking, swimming, skating, and dancing.

afterbirth   See *placenta.*

AIDS   Acquired immunodeficiency syndrome. A disorder of the *immune system* caused by infection with *HIV.* AIDS impairs the immune system, making people with the infection vulnerable to a wide variety of *opportunistic infections* and cancers.

allergen   Any substance—such as animal dander, pollen, or a specific food—that is harmless to most people but causes an *allergic reaction* in some people.

allergic reaction   An inappropriate *immune system* response that occurs when an *allergen* enters the body.

allergic rhinitis   Also called hay fever. Inflammation of the *mucous membrane* that lines the nose, caused by an *allergic reaction.* Symptoms include coughing, sneezing, stuffy nose, and itchy, watery eyes.

allogeneic bone marrow transplant See *bone marrow transplant.*

allogeneic stem cell transplant See *stem cell transplant.*

Alzheimer's disease A progressive, incurable condition that destroys brain cells, causing gradual loss of intellectual abilities and extreme changes in personality and behavior.

amino acids The basic components of *proteins.* Twenty different amino acids make all of the proteins needed by the human body. The eight essential amino acids are found in food; the body makes the 12 nonessential amino acids as needed.

androgens Male sex *hormones* produced mainly in the testicles. Androgens stimulate the development of the male sex organs and secondary sexual characteristics such as growth of facial hair and deepening of the voice.

anemia A blood disorder caused by a deficiency of *red blood cells* or *hemoglobin.* Anemia reduces the ability of the blood to supply oxygen to tissues and remove carbon dioxide from the body.

aneurysm An abnormal ballooning of a weakened area in the wall of an *artery.* An aneurysm can rupture and cause a *hemorrhage.*

anorexia nervosa Also called simply anorexia. A potentially life-threatening eating disorder characterized by an abnormal fear of being fat, prolonged avoidance of food, excessive weight loss, and obsession with exercise. Anorexia occurs most frequently among young women.

antibodies Also called immunoglobulins. *Proteins* in blood and tissue fluids that protect the body from *antigens.*

antigens *Proteins* such as *microorganisms* or *toxins* that trigger the *immune system* to produce *antibodies* to fight them.

antioxidants *Molecules* that protect against cell damage caused by *free radicals.*

apheresis Also called pheresis. A procedure in which blood is removed, run through a machine that removes selected components such as *platelets, white blood cells,* or *stem cells,* and then reinfused

into the person. The removed blood components are stored and later used in blood *transfusions* or *stem cell transplants.*

apnea Involuntary cessation of breathing that may be intermittent and temporary, or prolonged.

apnea, sleep Intermittent, temporary cessation of breathing during sleep. The condition often occurs in people who are overweight.

arrhythmia An abnormally fast or slow *heartbeat* or an irregular heartbeat. The two main types of arrhythmias are *bradycardia* and *tachycardia.*

artery A blood vessel that carries oxygen-filled blood away from the heart to the organs and tissues.

arthritis See *osteoarthritis.*

arthroplasty Also called joint replacement. A surgical procedure in which a damaged *joint* is replaced with an artificial joint made of metal and plastic. Arthroplasty is performed most often on the knee and hip, but is also used on the ankles, hands, wrists, and toes.

artificial respiration See *artificial ventilation.*

artificial ventilation Also called artificial respiration or assisted breathing. Introduction of air—either with mouth-to-mouth resuscitation or with a machine called a *ventilator*—into the lungs of a person who has stopped breathing.

aspiration A procedure in which fluid or tissue is removed from a body cavity with an instrument such as a needle and syringe. Aspiration also refers to accidentally inhaling an object or substance, such as food.

asymptomatic Without signs or symptoms of disease. Two conditions that are often asymptomatic, especially in the early stages, are *high blood pressure* and type 2 *diabetes.*

atheroma See *plaque, arterial.*

atherosclerosis The buildup of hardened fatty deposits called arterial *plaque* inside *artery* walls. Atherosclerosis can narrow the blood vessels, reducing or blocking blood flow to organs and tissues and increasing the risk of *heart attack* or *stroke.*

atrophy Shrinking or wasting of an organ or tissue as a result of disease or lack of use.

autoimmune disease A disease in which the *immune system* mistakenly produces *antibodies* that attack the body's own cells and tissues. Rheumatoid arthritis is one type of autoimmune disease.

autologous blood donation   Donation of a person's own blood before scheduled elective surgery to ensure that the blood is available if a *transfusion* is necessary during or after surgery.

autologous bone marrow transplant   See *bone marrow transplant.*

autologous stem cell transplant   See *stem cell transplant.*

autopsy   Also called a postmortem. The examination of a body after death to determine the cause of death. An autopsy is performed if death seems to have occurred under suspicious circumstances or if the family of the deceased requests it, or to provide information for research or medical education.

B

bacteremia   A life-threatening condition in which *bacteria* are present in the bloodstream.

bacteria   Single-celled *microorganisms* that multiply by division. Bacteria are classified according to their shape, such as cocci (round) or bacilli (rod-shaped or cylinder-shaped).

bacteriuria   The presence of *bacteria* in urine.

basal cell carcinoma   A slow-growing form of skin cancer in the outer layer of skin that rarely spreads to other parts of the body. Basal cell carcinoma accounts for about 90 percent of all skin cancers.

B cell   Also called B *lymphocyte.* A type of *white blood cell* that has an important role in the *immune system,* protecting the body from infections and cancer.

benign   Not cancerous.

beta carotene   An *antioxidant* found in orange and deep-yellow fruits and vegetables that converts to *vitamin* A in the body.

bile   A greenish yellow fluid produced by the liver, stored in the gallbladder, and released into the small intestine to help break down fats and remove waste products during digestion.

bilirubin   A yellowish orange pigment in *bile* produced by the breakdown of *red blood cells.* An accumulation of bilirubin in the blood or skin is called *jaundice.*

biofeedback   A relaxation technique in which a person learns to control involuntary body functions such as *heart rate.*

biopsy   A diagnostic test in which a small sample of tissue is removed from the body and examined under a microscope. Biopsies are usually performed to determine if an abnormal growth is cancerous.

bite   See *occlusion, dental.*

bite guard   Also called a dental splint. A plastic dental appliance that fits over the biting surface of the upper or lower teeth and helps prevent a person from grinding his or her teeth.

blood clot   A clump of coagulated blood. See also *thrombus* and *embolus.*

blood poisoning   See *septicemia.*

blood pressure   A measure of the amount of force that blood exerts against the walls of the *arteries* as it is pumped through the body by the heart.

blood type   The classification of a person's blood according to the presence of different marker *proteins* on the surface of *red blood cells.*

B lymphocyte   See *B cell.*

BMI   See *body mass index.*

board certified   A term that refers to doctors who have had at least 7 years of medical training and have passed a comprehensive examination in a medical specialty (such as internal medicine, ophthalmology, or pediatrics).

body mass index   Also called BMI. A measurement used to determine if a person's body weight is in the healthy range.

bone density   A measure of the amount of *calcium* and other *minerals* in bone in relation to the width of the bone. A person's bone density is used to determine his or her risk of developing *osteoporosis.*

bone marrow   The spongy tissue inside the large bones that contains *stem cells,* which produce all the different types of blood cells.

bone marrow transplant   A procedure to replace diseased *bone marrow* with healthy bone marrow. In an autologous bone marrow *transplant,* some of a person's own bone marrow is collected, treated with powerful anticancer drugs, and frozen until needed. His or her remaining bone marrow is destroyed with *chemotherapy,* and possibly with *radiation therapy,* and he or she is given the treated, stored bone marrow (injected through a needle into a vein). In an allogeneic bone marrow transplant, all of a person's bone marrow is destroyed with chemotherapy, and possibly with radiation therapy, and then healthy bone marrow from a donor is injected into a vein.

botulism   A serious but relatively rare type of food poisoning that results from eating improperly canned or preserved foods that contain a powerful bacterial *toxin.*

brachytherapy   Also called internal *radiation therapy*. A type of radiation therapy in which a radioactive substance is inserted directly into a cancer site. Brachytherapy is performed to keep a cancer from spreading by destroying or slowing the growth of abnormal cells.

bradycardia   A *heart rate* below 60 beats per minute.

bulimia nervosa   Also called bulimia. An eating disorder characterized by binge overeating followed by self-induced vomiting or laxative abuse.

C

CA-125   A blood test in which a sample of a woman's blood is examined in a laboratory for the presence of an *antigen* called CA-125. An elevated level of CA-125 can indicate ovarian cancer or non-cancerous conditions such as fibroid tumors and pelvic infections.

calcium   A *mineral* that is essential for strong bones and teeth and that also has an important role in muscle contraction, blood clotting, and nerve function.

calculus   Also called a stone. A small, hard mass (such as a *gallstone* or a *kidney stone*), usually composed of *mineral* deposits, that forms in body tissues.

calculus, dental   Also called tartar. A hard *mineral* deposit that forms on teeth.

calorie   A measurement used in nutrition to represent the amount of energy contained in food.

capillaries   The smallest blood vessels in the body. Capillary walls are only one cell thick.

carcinogen   A substance that can cause cancer.

carcinoma   A cancerous tumor that arises from cells in the surface layer or lining membrane of an organ. Carcinomas commonly develop in the skin, lungs, breast, cervix, and prostate gland.

cardiopulmonary resuscitation   Also called CPR. A lifesaving technique in which chest compressions and *artificial ventilation* are performed on someone whose heart has stopped beating, to maintain the flow of blood to the brain.

cardiovascular system   Also called the circulatory system. The network formed by the heart and blood vessels that pumps blood and carries it to organs and tissues throughout the body.

caries, dental   Also called cavities. Tooth decay.

cartilage   A type of *connective tissue* that is an important structural component of certain parts of the skeletal system such as the *joints.*

cataract   A cloudy area in the normally clear lens of the eye that causes impaired vision.

catheter   A thin, flexible tube that is inserted into a blood vessel or body cavity to withdraw or instill fluids or to widen a passageway.

cerebrospinal fluid   The liquid that surrounds the brain and spinal cord.

cerebrovascular accident   See *stroke.*

chemotherapy   A cancer treatment that uses powerful drugs to destroy cancer cells throughout the body.

chlamydia   A *sexually transmitted disease* caused by the *bacterium* Chlamydia trachomatis.

cholesterol   A fatlike substance that is an important component of cells and is involved in the transport of fats in the blood. Types of cholesterol include *HDL cholesterol, LDL cholesterol,* and *VLDL cholesterol.*

chromosomes   Threadlike structures inside the nuclei of cells that contain *genes*. Each human cell, except egg and sperm cells, contains 46 chromosomes arranged in 23 pairs, one member of each pair contributed by each parent.

chronic   A term used to describe a disease or disorder that persists for a long time.

circulatory system   See *cardiovascular system.*

collagen   The most common structural *protein* in the body, found in *connective tissue.*

coma   A state of unconsciousness in which a person does not respond even to strong stimulation.

congenital   Present from birth.

connective tissue   A type of tissue, such as *cartilage, tendons,* or *ligaments,* that holds various body structures together.

contagious   A term used to describe diseases that can spread from one person to another by direct or indirect contact.

contracture   Irreversible shortening of a muscle or *tendon,* or shrinkage of scar tissue or *connective tissue* that produces deformity or distortion, usually in a *joint.*

contusion   A bruise.

CPR   See *cardiopulmonary resuscitation.*

crymotherapy   See *cryotherapy.*

cryosurgery   A type of surgery in which diseased or abnormal tissue is destroyed or removed by freezing.

cryotherapy   Also called crymotherapy. Any treatment technique that uses low temperatures. *Cryosurgery* is a type of cryotherapy.

curettage   A procedure using a surgical instrument called a curet to remove a thin layer of skin or tissue (such as the lining of the uterus). Curettage is used either to remove abnormal tissue or to obtain a sample of tissue for microscopic analysis.

cyanosis   Bluish coloration of the skin and *mucous membranes* caused by a lack of oxygen in the blood. Cyanosis usually results from respiratory or heart problems.

D

defibrillation   A procedure in which a brief electric shock is administered to the heart through electrodes placed on the chest to restore a rapid or irregular *heartbeat* to normal.

defibrillator   A device that restores the *heartbeat* to normal by delivering a brief electric shock to the heart muscle.

dehydration   A potentially dangerous decrease in the amount of water in the body, often as a result of persistent vomiting or diarrhea.

delusion   A false, irrational belief. Delusions are a symptom of some mental disorders such as schizophrenia.

dementia   A progressive loss of intellectual function that includes personality changes and impairment of memory, judgment, and thought processes. *Alzheimer's disease* is a common cause of dementia.

deoxyribonucleic acid   See *DNA.*

depression   A mood disorder characterized by feelings of sadness, hopelessness, and helplessness, combined with apathy, poor self-esteem, and withdrawal from social situations.

diabetes   The term commonly used to describe a disorder in which the body is unable to properly use the sugar *glucose.* The two major forms are type 1 diabetes and type 2 diabetes.

dialysis   A technique used to filter waste products from the bloodstream when kidney function is impaired.

diastolic blood pressure   The second, lower number in a *blood pressure* reading, which indicates the amount of pressure in the blood vessels when the heart rests between beats and fills with blood.

diathermy   A treatment technique that uses high-frequency electric current, microwaves, or ultrasound waves to produce heat in body tissues. Diathermy is sometimes used to increase blood flow and relieve pain in people who have rheumatoid arthritis or *osteoarthritis.*

dilate   To widen, either naturally or by using a medical instrument or a drug.

DNA   Deoxyribonucleic acid. The molecular structure inside every cell that carries genetic information. *Genes* are made of DNA.

do-not-resuscitate order (DNR)   An *advance directive* that states that no heroic measures (including *cardiopulmonary resuscitation* or mechanical life support) be used to restart a person's heart if it stops beating.

durable power of attorney for health care   An *advance directive* in which a competent person gives another person the authority to make health care decisions for him or her if the person can no longer do so.

dysplasia   Abnormal growth of cells or body structures; sometimes precedes cancerous changes in cells.

dysuria   Painful or difficult urination.

E

edema   Abnormal accumulation of fluid in body tissues.

effusion   The escape of fluid from a blood vessel or a lymphatic vessel into nearby tissues, or an abnormal accumulation of fluid.

electrolytes   Essential *minerals,* such as *sodium, potassium,* and *magnesium,* that are involved in regulating various body processes such as maintaining water balance and *blood pressure,* conducting nerve impulses, contracting muscles, and maintaining a normal *heartbeat.*

embolism   Sudden blockage of a blood vessel by an *embolus.*

embolus   A *blood clot* or other material—such as a fragment of fat or a tiny piece of tissue—that travels through the bloodstream and can block an *artery.*

endocrine system   A network of glands, organs, and tissues that produces and secretes *hormones* directly into the bloodstream to regulate many essential body processes.

endorphins   Chemicals in the brain that can improve mood and help control a person's response to pain and stress.

enzymes   *Proteins* that control chemical reactions in the body.

epinephrine   Also called adrenaline. A *hormone* produced by the *adrenal glands* that increases *heart rate* and blood flow and improves breathing.

erectile dysfunction   Also called impotence. The persistent inability to achieve and maintain an erection sufficient to complete sexual intercourse.

essential hypertension   See *primary hypertension.*

estrogen   The female sex *hormone* produced mainly in the ovaries. Estrogen stimulates the development of the female sex organs and secondary sexual characteristics such as growth of pubic hair and breast development.

F

fecal impaction   Accumulation of hardened stool in the rectum.

fiber   An indigestible nutrient (found in plant-based foods including fruits, vegetables, and whole grains) that passes through the digestive tract without being absorbed. Fiber provides bulk to help keep the digestive tract functioning properly and may reduce the risk of colon cancer.

fibrillation   Irregular, disorganized, ineffective muscle contractions, especially of the heart muscle. Fibrillation can affect either the atria (the small upper chambers of the heart) or the ventricles (the large, lower, pumping chambers of the heart).

fibrin   A stringy, insoluble *protein* that gives *blood clots* their semisolid form to enable them to plug and seal damaged blood vessel walls.

folic acid   A B *vitamin* essential for cell growth and repair and for the production of *red blood cells;* essential during pregnancy to reduce the risk of birth defects such as *neural tube defects.*

fracture   A break in a bone.

free radicals   Also called oxygen free radicals. *Molecules* produced in the body through normal cell activity or as a result of external factors such as radiation or cigarette smoke that damage or destroy cells. Free radicals are a major cause of disease and aging.

G

gallstone   A small, hardened mass composed of *cholesterol, calcium* salts, and *bile* pigments. A gallstone can form in the gallbladder or in the bile duct.

gamma globulin   The pooled *antibodies* taken from the blood of healthy donors, used to prevent or treat infections.

genes   Segments of *DNA* that are the basic functional units of *heredity.* There are about 35,000 genes in each human cell, and each gene carries instructions for making *proteins.*

genetics   The study of *heredity.*

glaucoma   Abnormally high pressure inside the eyeball that damages peripheral (side) vision, causing the visual field to become increasingly narrow, leading to total blindness.

glucose   A simple sugar that is the body's main source of energy.

glucose meter   A device used by people with *diabetes* to measure blood *glucose* levels.

graft   Healthy tissue taken from one part of the body (or from a donor) and surgically implanted in another part of the body to repair or replace damaged tissue.

granulocyte   A type of *white blood cell* that has an important role in the *immune system,* protecting the body from infections and cancer.

H

hallucination   Abnormal *sensory* perceptions not based on reality that occur without an external stimulus. Hallucinations can involve any of the senses and may be a symptom of some mental disorders.

hay fever   See *allergic rhinitis.*

HDL cholesterol   High-density lipoprotein *cholesterol.* A type of cholesterol made in the liver and transported by the blood. Also called the good cholesterol, HDL cholesterol protects against heart disease by clearing harmful *LDL cholesterol* from blood vessels.

heart attack   Also called myocardial infarction. Sudden death of a section of the heart muscle from lack of blood, usually as a result of a blockage of blood flow in one of the coronary *arteries* by a *thrombus.*

heartbeat   A contraction of the heart muscle that pumps blood from the heart into the *arteries* and throughout the body.

heart rate   The number of *heartbeats* per minute. A normal heart rate is between 60 and 100 beats per minute.

hematoma   A collection of blood in an organ or tissue caused by bleeding from an injured blood vessel.

hematuria   Blood in the urine.

hemoglobin   The oxygen-carrying *protein* in *red blood cells.*

hemolysis   The natural breakdown of *red blood cells* at the end of their life span. If hemolysis occurs prematurely, it can lead to *anemia* or *jaundice.*

hemorrhage   Excessive bleeding.

heredity   The transmission of *traits* and disorders from parents to children through *genes.*

hernia   Protrusion of a portion of an organ or tissue through a weakened area in the muscle wall that normally contains it.

high blood pressure   Also called hypertension. A condition in which *blood pressure* is persistently raised.

high-density lipoprotein cholesterol   See *HDL cholesterol.*

hip replacement   See *arthroplasty.*

histamine   A chemical released by the body during an *allergic reaction* that produces signs of inflammation, including redness, swelling, itching, heat, and pain.

HIV   Human immunodeficiency virus. A *virus* that infects specific cells of the *immune system,* causing *AIDS.*

Holter monitor   A portable device worn around the neck, at the waist, or over the shoulder that records the electrical activity of the heart during a 24-hour period or longer. A Holter monitor is used to detect *arrhythmias* and other *heartbeat* abnormalities.

hormone therapy   Use of natural or synthetic *hormones* to treat various diseases and disorders. Treatment of *diabetes* with *insulin* is one type of hormone therapy.

hormones   Chemical messengers that are produced by a network of glands called the *endocrine system* and released directly into the bloodstream, which carries them to target organs and tissues throughout the body to perform specific functions. Some examples of hormones are *estrogen, testosterone,* and *insulin.*

hospice   A concept of caring for people who are in the final phase of terminal illness that emphasizes comfort and quality of life and focuses on relieving pain and controlling other symptoms.

human immunodeficiency virus   See *HIV.*

hydrogenated fats   See *trans fats.*

hypertension   See *high blood pressure.*

I

ICU   See *intensive care unit.*

immune deficiency   See *immunodeficiency.*

immune system   A network of specialized cells and organs that produces *proteins* called *antibodies* to protect the body from infectious *microorganisms* and cancer.

immunity   Resistance to disease conferred by activities of the *immune system*. Immunity can be present at birth, can develop from having a specific disease, or can be induced through a *vaccine* that contains small doses of an infectious *microorganism* or *antibodies* to that microorganism.

immunization   Also called vaccination. The active or passive process by which resistance to specific infectious *microorganisms* is induced. In active immunization, a person is given small doses of an inactive form of a specific microorganism in a *vaccine,* providing lifelong resistance to infection by that microorganism. In passive immunization, a person is injected with *antibodies* that fight the specific microorganism, providing temporary resistance to infection by that microorganism.

immunodeficiency   Also called immune deficiency. Impaired effectiveness of the *immune system.*

immunoglobulins   See *antibodies.*

immunotherapy   Therapy to gradually build up a person's *immunity* to a substance to which he or she is allergic *(allergen)* by exposing the person to increasing doses of the substance.

implant   To insert an object or substance into the body to treat disease, deliver drugs, alter appearance, or restore or improve function. Examples of implants include breast implants, lens implants after cataract surgery, *joint replacements, pacemakers,* and radioactive implants to treat cancer.

impotence   See *erectile dysfunction.*

incubation period   The time lag (ranging from days to months) between exposure to a disease-causing *microorganism* and the appearance of symptoms. During this period, infectious microbes are multiplying but are not yet numerous enough to cause symptoms.

informed consent   Agreement to undergo a surgical or diagnostic procedure after receiving a complete explanation of the procedure and the risks involved.

in situ   Means "in place"; often used to describe cancer that has not spread from its original site.

insulin   A *hormone* produced by the pancreas that enables the body to use the sugar *glucose.*

intensive care unit   Also called the ICU. A section in most hospitals in which lifesaving surgical and medical care is given to premature babies or people who are severely injured, seriously ill, or recovering from major surgery.

intramuscular   Inside or into a muscle.

intravenous   Also called an IV. Giving medication or fluids directly through a *vein.*

intravenous drip   Also called intravenous infusion. Introducing a liquid into the body from an elevated sterile container through a needle inserted into a *vein.* The flow rate of the liquid is measured by counting the rate at which the liquid drips through a transparent chamber.

intravenous fluid   Fluid—containing essential substances such as salt, water, sugar, *protein, minerals, vitamins,* or *electrolytes*—that is infused through a *vein.*

intravenous infusion   See *intravenous drip.*

invasive   Describes a medical procedure in which body tissues are penetrated. Is also used to refer to cancer that has spread.

iron   A *mineral* that is essential for the production of many *enzymes* and for the formation of *hemoglobin,* which delivers oxygen to cells.

ischemia   Decreased blood supply to an organ or tissue.

IV   See *intravenous.*

J

jaundice   Yellow discoloration of the skin and whites of the eyes caused by an excess of the pigment *bilirubin* in the bloodstream. Jaundice may be caused by excessive destruction of *red blood cells (hemolysis)* or by a liver disorder that impairs the normal excretion of bilirubin in *bile.*

joint   A point where bone meets bone, such as the hip, knee, or elbow. Most but not all joints are capable of motion, allowing the bones to move in relation to one another.

joint replacement   See *arthroplasty.*

K

keratin   A *protein* that is the main component of the outermost layer of skin, hair, and nails.

kidney stone   A small, hard mass of *mineral* salts that can form in a kidney.

knee replacement   See *arthroplasty.*

L

laceration   A torn, jagged wound.

lactase   An *enzyme* needed to break down the milk sugar *lactose* during digestion.

lactose   One of the sugars found in milk.

lactose intolerance   The inability to digest *lactose* due to a deficiency of *lactase.*

laser   A device that produces a highly concentrated, powerful beam of light that can be used as a surgical tool.

LDL cholesterol   Low-density lipoprotein cholesterol. A harmful type of *cholesterol* made by the liver and transported in the blood. Eating foods that are high in *saturated fats* (such as red meat and whole-milk products) and *trans fats* (such as stick margarine) increases LDL.

leukocyte   A type of infection-fighting *white blood cell.*

ligament   Tough, fibrous tissue that connects bone to bone and provides stability to *joints.*

light therapy   See *phototherapy.*

lipids   Fats that are stored in the body and used for energy.

lipoproteins   Substances made of *lipids* and *protein.* Most fats, including *cholesterol,* are carried in the blood in the form of lipoproteins.

living will   An *advance directive* prepared by a competent person that indicates his or her wishes regarding life-sustaining medical treatments. A living will goes into effect only after the person is unable to speak for himself or herself and can be revised or withdrawn by the person at any time.

low-density lipoprotein cholesterol   See *LDL cholesterol.*

lymph   A milky fluid that has an important role in the *immune system* and the absorption of fats from the intestines during digestion.

lymphatic system   A network of organs, vessels, nodes, and ducts that drain *lymph* from the body's tissues back into the bloodstream. The lymphatic system is an important part of the *immune system.*

lymph nodes   Small glands throughout the body (clustered in the neck, armpits, abdomen, and groin) that are part of the *immune system.* They supply infection-fighting cells to the bloodstream and act as a barrier to the spread of infection.

lymphocyte   A type of infection-fighting *white blood cell.*

M

macula   The part of the *retina* of the eye that provides sharp sight in the center of the visual field; essential for seeing fine detail.

macular degeneration   Age-related damage to the *macula,* which leads to impaired vision.

magnesium   An essential *mineral* that has several vital roles in the body, including transmission of nerve signals.

malabsorption   Inefficient absorption of nutrients through the lining of the small intestine.

malignant   Cancerous.

malignant melanoma   See *melanoma, malignant.*

mast cell   A type of cell that plays a part in the *immune system* and in *allergic reactions.* Mast cells release inflammatory substances in response to *allergens.*

melanin   The pigment that gives skin, hair, and eyes their color.

melanoma, malignant   The most serious form of skin cancer, the first sign of which is often a change in an existing mole. Malignant melanoma spreads quickly and can be fatal. The main cause of melanoma is overexposure to sunlight.

meninges   Membranes surrounding the brain and spinal cord.

meningitis   Inflammation of the *meninges,* usually as the result of an infection.

menopause   The end of menstruation.

metabolism   The chemical processes that take place in the body.

metastasis   The spread of diseased cells or *microorganisms* from one part of the body to another part. Metastasis can occur through the *lymphatic system* or bloodstream or across a body cavity.

metastasize   To spread from one part of the body to another. Most cancerous tumors have the capacity to metastasize.

microorganism   Any microscopic life form, such as *bacteria* or *viruses.*

migraine   A severe, persistent, sometimes disabling headache that occurs on one side of the head and may spread to the other side; can be accompanied by symptoms such as nausea, vomiting, sensitivity to light and noise, fever, chills, aches, and sweating.

minerals   Chemicals in food, such as *iron, calcium,* and *phosphorus,* that are essential for good health.

ministroke   See *TIA.*

molecule   The smallest particle into which an element or compound can be divided without changing its chemical or physical properties.

monocyte   A large *white blood cell* with a single *nucleus* found in *lymph nodes,* the spleen, and *bone marrow.*

monounsaturated fat   A type of fat (found in high quantities in olive, canola, and peanut oils) that lowers harmful *LDL cholesterol* and raises beneficial *HDL cholesterol.*

mucous membrane   The thin, skinlike lining of cavities and tubes in the body, such as the digestive tract, urinary tract, and respiratory tract.

mucus   A thick, slimy fluid secreted by a *mucous membrane* to lubricate and protect the part of the body it lines.

mutation, genetic   A change in the genetic material *(DNA)* within a living cell. Mutations can be harmless, harmful, or beneficial.

myocardial infarction   See *heart attack.*

N

nebulizer   A device that disperses a drug into a fine mist that can be inhaled through a face mask. Nebulizers are usually used to treat asthma.

neonatal   Younger than 4 weeks old.

nephrons   The basic filtering units of the kidneys.

neural tube defects   Abnormalities in the development of a fetus's spinal cord or brain. The most common neural tube defect is spina bifida, a disorder in which the bones of the spine fail to develop normally, leaving part of the spinal cord exposed.

neuron   A nerve (brain) cell.

neurotransmitters   Chemical messengers that enable *neurons* to communicate with each other.

neutrophil   A type of *white blood cell.*

noninvasive   Describes a medical procedure in which the body is not penetrated. May also be used to refer to cancer that has not spread.

noradrenaline   See *norepinephrine.*

norepinephrine   Also called noradrenaline. A *hormone* that helps regulate *heart rate* and *blood pressure* by narrowing blood vessels and increasing heart rate when blood pressure drops below the normal level.

nucleus, cell   An oval or round mass inside cells that contains genetic material *(DNA)* and directs all the activities of the cell.

O

obesity   A condition in which a person's weight is 20 percent or more over the maximum desirable weight for his or her height or whose *body mass index* is 30 or greater.

occlusion   Blockage of an opening or passage in the body (such as a blood vessel) by a clot or bubble.

occlusion, dental   Also called bite. The way in which the upper and lower teeth come together when the mouth is closed.

occult blood   Blood in body fluids or in feces that is not visible to the naked eye but can be detected by tests; occult blood tests are often used to detect colon and rectal cancer.

opportunistic infections   Infections that rarely occur in healthy people but frequently occur in people who have an impaired *immune system*—such as people with *AIDS.* Examples of opportunistic infections include cytomegalovirus, Kaposi's *sarcoma* (a type of skin cancer), and pneumocystis carinii pneumonia.

osteoarthritis   Also called simply arthritis. Progressive, gradual thinning or destruction of *cartilage* in the *joints,* usually resulting from aging, injury, or overuse.

osteoma   A noncancerous bone tumor.

osteoporosis   A disorder in which bones become thin, brittle, and more susceptible to *fracture;* occurs most frequently in women.

oxidation   A damaging chemical reaction in cells caused by the actions of *free radicals;* a major factor in disease and aging.

oxygen free radicals   See *free radicals.*

P

pacemaker   An electronic device implanted in the chest to regulate the *heartbeat.*

palpitations   *Heartbeats,* usually more rapid or stronger than normal, that a person is aware of.

papillomaviruses   A group of *viruses* that can cause warts including genital warts, which can lead to cervical cancer in women.

peak flow meter   An instrument that measures how swiftly a person can expel air from the lungs; used to determine lung efficiency in people who have asthma or other respiratory diseases and to monitor their response to treatment.

perforation   A hole in the wall of an organ or tissue caused by disease or injury.

perimenopause   The transition phase that begins years before a woman's last menstrual period during which the body begins to slow its production of *estrogen.*

peristalsis   Wavelike contractions of muscles that move food and waste products through the digestive system. Occurs from the moment of swallowing to the elimination of waste from the rectum. Also transports urine from the kidneys to the bladder.

pharmacogenomics   The study of how *heredity* affects the body's response to drugs.

pheresis   See *apheresis.*

phosphorus   An essential *mineral* (found in food) that is important for strong teeth and bones and that plays a role in many processes in the body.

photophobia   An abnormal sensitivity to or intolerance of light; the sensation that light is painful to the eyes. Photophobia is a symptom of some nervous system diseases and eye disorders.

photosensitivity   An abnormal skin reaction to exposure to sunlight, usually in the form of a rash. Photosensitivity may be a symptom of some disorders or a side effect of particular medications.

phototherapy   Also called light therapy or ultraviolet light therapy. Treatment of disease by exposure to light, particularly by concentrated light rays or light of specific wavelengths. Sunlight is the most basic form of phototherapy.

placenta   Also called the afterbirth (because it is expelled after the baby is born). The organ that develops in the uterus during pregnancy and nourishes a fetus; transfers oxygen from the mother's blood to the fetus's blood and removes waste products from the fetus's blood to the mother's blood for excretion by her lungs and kidneys.

plaque, arterial   Also called atheroma. A patch of fatty tissue in an *artery* wall that can reduce blood flow or cause *thrombosis.*

plaque, dental   A sticky coating on the teeth (made up of saliva, food particles, and *bacteria*) that can cause tooth decay and gum disease if not removed.

plasma   The nutrient-filled, liquid part of the blood that remains after the blood cells have been removed.

plasma exchange   See *plasmapheresis.*

plasmapheresis   Also called plasma exchange. A procedure used to remove or reduce the amount of unwanted substances in the liquid part of blood *(plasma).* In plasmapheresis, blood is removed from a *vein* (usually in an arm) with a needle and tubing that is attached to a machine called a cell separator. The machine separates the plasma from the blood cells by spinning the blood at a high speed or by filtering the blood through a membrane; the plasma is discarded. The separated blood cells are then mixed with a plasma substitute and reinjected (usually into the other arm).

platelet   Also called a thrombocyte. A blood cell fragment needed for normal blood clotting.

polyp   A mushroomlike growth of tissue on the skin or on a *mucous membrane.*

polyunsaturated fat   A type of fat (found in corn, sunflower, safflower, sesame, flaxseed, and soybean oils) that reduces total blood *cholesterol* level but may also lower beneficial *HDL cholesterol.*

postmortem   See *autopsy.*

posttraumatic stress disorder   A persistent disturbance of emotions and behavior that develops after experiencing extreme trauma, such as being the victim of or witnessing a violent crime.

postural hypotension   Abnormally low *blood pressure* that occurs when a person sits up or stands suddenly.

potassium   An essential *mineral* that helps the body maintain water balance, conduct nerve signals, contract muscles, and maintain a normal *heartbeat.*

precancerous   Describes a condition that has the potential to become cancerous.

primary hypertension   Also called essential hypertension. *High blood pressure* with no known cause.

progesterone   A female sex *hormone* produced by the ovaries that is essential for a healthy pregnancy by promoting the growth and functioning of the *placenta.*

prolapse   Partial or complete slipping of a body organ or structure (such as the uterus, a disk between two vertebrae, or a segment of the rectum) from its normal position. Prolapse is usually caused by a weakening of surrounding supportive tissues.

prophylactic   Preventing disease.

prostaglandins   Substances similar to *hormones;* secreted in many tissues. Prostaglandins produce a variety of effects throughout the body, such as pain and inflammation in damaged tissue.

prostate-specific antigen   A *protein* produced only by the prostate gland. High levels of the protein in blood can indicate a problem with the prostate gland such as enlargement or cancer.

prosthesis   A man-made replacement (such as an artificial arm or leg, dental bridge, breast implant, or glass eye) for a diseased or missing body part.

proteins   Complex substances composed of *amino acids.* Proteins are the basis of all living matter.

PSA   See *prostate-specific antigen.*

PSA test   Prostate-specific antigen test. A test to measure the levels of *prostate-specific antigen* in the blood; an increased level of PSA may indicate prostate enlargement or prostate cancer.

psychosis   A severe mental disorder in which a person loses touch with reality.

pus   A creamy yellow or pale green liquid composed of dead *white blood cells, bacteria,* and other substances that forms at the site of an infection.

R

radiation therapy   Treatment with a stream of particles or electromagnetic waves emitted by the atoms and *molecules* of a radioactive substance; used to destroy abnormal growths such as cancer.

radiation therapy, internal   See *brachytherapy.*

red blood cells   Doughnut-shaped blood cells that carry oxygen to and remove wastes from organs and tissues.

rejection   An attack by the *immune system* on grafted tissue or a transplanted organ; may be prevented by treatment with drugs that suppress the immune system.

remission   A temporary disappearance of symptoms of a chronic disease (such as cancer or multiple sclerosis). If remission lasts more than 5 years, the disease is usually considered cured.

respirator   See *ventilator.*

retina   The light-sensitive membrane at the back of the eye on which light rays focus.

ribonucleic acid   See *RNA.*

RNA   Ribonucleic acid. A type of genetic material that carries out the instructions of a cell's *DNA.*

S

SAD   See *seasonal affective disorder.*

salt-sensitive   Describes a person whose *blood pressure* goes up or down in relation to the amount of *sodium* in his or her diet.

sarcoma   A rare, difficult-to-treat cancerous tumor of *connective tissue,* blood vessels, or fibrous tissue surrounding and supporting organs.

saturated fat   A type of fat (found in meat, dairy products, and coconut and palm oils) that is converted to harmful *LDL cholesterol* and is thought to increase the risk of heart disease and *heart attacks.*

seasonal affective disorder   Also called SAD. A

form of *depression* that tends to occur during the fall and winter, when there are fewer hours of daylight.

secondary hypertension   *High blood pressure* that has a known underlying cause.

seizure   Excessive electrical activity in the brain that causes temporary loss of consciousness or memory, or uncontrolled movements.

sensitization   The initial exposure to an *allergen,* which causes a reaction by the *immune system.* On subsequent exposure to the allergen, the reaction becomes stronger.

sensory   Of or relating to the senses; transmitting impulses from the senses to nerve centers in the brain.

septicemia   Also called blood poisoning. A life-threatening blood infection in which *bacteria* enter the bloodstream, multiply rapidly, and release *toxins.*

serotonin   A *neurotransmitter* that conveys messages between brain cells; involved in regulating mood.

sex chromosomes   The X and Y *chromosomes,* which determine sex. Females have two *X chromosomes;* males have one X chromosome and one *Y chromosome.*

sexually transmitted diseases   Also called STDs. Infections transmitted through sexual activity.

sleep apnea   See *apnea, sleep.*

sodium   An essential *mineral* that helps the body maintain water balance and *blood pressure.*

spasm   Uncontrollable contraction of one or more muscles.

splint, dental   See *bite guard.*

sprain   Tearing or stretching of a *ligament* in a *joint.*

squamous cell carcinoma   A common type of skin cancer that develops in cells on the surface of the skin. Squamous cell carcinoma is usually caused by long-term overexposure to ultraviolet radiation from the sun.

STDs   See *sexually transmitted diseases.*

stem cells   Immature cells (found mostly in *bone marrow*) that produce all the blood cells in the body.

stem cell transplant   The infusion of healthy stem cells to replace cancer cells or other diseased cells in the body. The stem cells may be the person's own stem cells (called an autologous stem cell transplant) or stem cells from a closely matched donor (called an allogeneic stem cell transplant). Before receiving the healthy stem cells, the person undergoes high-dose *chemotherapy,* possibly with *radiation therapy,* to destroy the diseased cells. The infused stem cells make healthy new cells to replace those that were destroyed.

stenosis   The narrowing of a channel in the body, especially the *arteries* or the openings of the heart valves.

stent   A tiny metal or plastic wire mesh placed inside an *artery* to keep it open.

stethoscope   An instrument for listening to sounds inside the body, especially the lungs, heart, and intestines.

stone   See *calculus.*

strain   Injury to a muscle resulting from excessive physical force.

stridor   Noisy, high-pitched breathing, usually caused by inflammation of the larynx (voice box) or trachea (windpipe).

stroke   Also called a cerebrovascular accident. Sudden damage to part of the brain caused by an interruption in blood flow to the brain. Ischemic stroke, the most common type of stroke, results from blockage of a blood vessel in the brain. Hemorrhagic stroke results from a ruptured blood vessel in the brain.

suppository   A solid cylindrical (usually cone- or bullet-shaped) pellet inserted into the rectum or vagina that melts at body temperature to release medication.

suture   A surgical stitch used to close an incision or wound. Also the name for the firmly joined interlocking joints of the skull.

systolic blood pressure   The first, higher number in a *blood pressure* reading. The systolic pressure indicates the pressure in the blood vessels when the *ventricles* of the heart contract and blood pumps through the *arteries.*

T

tachycardia   A rapid *heart rate,* especially one above 100 beats per minute.

tartar   See *calculus*, *dental*.

T cell   Also called a T *lymphocyte*. A type of *white blood cell* that protects the body from infectious *microorganisms* and cancer.

tendons   Strong, fibrous tissue that connects muscle to bone.

testosterone   The male sex *hormone* that stimulates the development of male characteristics.

thrombocyte   See *platelet*.

thrombosis   The formation of a *thrombus* inside a blood vessel or the heart.

thrombus   A *blood clot* that forms inside the heart or in an intact blood vessel, as opposed to a blood clot that forms normally in the wall of a blood vessel to seal it after injury.

TIA   Transient ischemic attack. Also called a ministroke. A brief interruption in blood flow to the brain, causing temporary symptoms such as impaired vision, sensation, movement, or speech, or memory loss.

tinnitus   A common disorder characterized by hearing persistent ringing, hissing, or other sounds in the ear when there is no external source of those sounds.

T lymphocyte   See *T cell*.

toxemia   The presence of bacterial *toxins* in the bloodstream. Toxemia of pregnancy is a disorder in which a woman has *high blood pressure*, tissue swelling, and leaking of *protein* from the kidneys into the urine.

toxic   Poisonous.

toxin   A poisonous substance produced by *bacteria* or other infectious agents and by some plants and animals.

traction   A procedure in which part of the body is placed under tension to correct alignment or to hold two adjoining structures in position. Traction is usually used as a treatment to align and immobilize *fractures* to promote healing.

trait   Any characteristic or condition (such as eye color and hair color) that is determined by *genes*.

trans fats   Also called hydrogenated fats. Fats that are made during the manufacturing of stick margarine and canned shortening and used in many processed, baked, and deep-fried foods. Trans fats can raise total blood *cholesterol* level and the level of harmful *LDL cholesterol*.

transfusion   Infusion of large amounts of blood (or the components of blood) directly into the bloodstream, usually to replace severe blood loss or to correct *anemia*. Before donor blood is used for transfusion, it is screened for infectious *microorganisms* and then matched for compatibility with the recipient's blood type.

transient ischemic attack   See *TIA*.

transplant   Transfer of an organ or tissue from one part of the body to another or from one person to another. Or an organ or tissue that has been transplanted.

trauma   Any physical or mental wound or injury.

tremor   Temporary or permanent involuntary trembling or quivering caused by rapidly alternating contraction and relaxation of the muscles; can be brought on by drugs (including alcohol) or by physical or emotional disorders.

triglycerides   One of the major fats in the blood. A high level in the blood can indicate an increased risk of heart disease, *high blood pressure,* and *diabetes*.

U

ulcer   An open sore on the skin or on a *mucous membrane*.

ultraviolet light therapy   See *phototherapy*.

unsaturated fat   A type of fat that lowers the risk of cardiovascular disease. Eating *monounsaturated fats* instead of *saturated fats* reduces harmful *LDL cholesterol* and raises beneficial *HDL cholesterol*. *Polyunsaturated fats* reduce LDL cholesterol but also lower HDL cholesterol. Monounsaturated and polyunsaturated fats tend to be soft or liquid at room temperature.

urea   A waste product from the breakdown of *protein* in the body.

uremia   Excess *urea* and other waste products in the bloodstream as a result of kidney failure.

uric acid   A waste product from the breakdown of *protein* in cells. Uric acid is eliminated from the body in urine.

V

vaccination   See *immunization*.

vaccine   A preparation containing killed or

weakened or otherwise altered versions of a specific infectious *microorganism;* given to provide *immunity* to infection with the microorganism.

valve   A structure inside a blood vessel or other passageway that allows fluid, such as blood, to flow in one direction only.

vein   A blood vessel that carries oxygen-depleted blood from the organs and tissues back to the heart and lungs for a fresh supply of oxygen.

ventilator   Also called a respirator. A machine that takes over a person's breathing by regularly pumping air into the lungs; air is expelled by the natural elasticity of the lungs and rib cage.

ventricle   A normal cavity or chamber in a body or organ, especially the right or left ventricle of the heart or any of the interconnecting ventricles of the brain.

venules   Very small *veins.*

very low-density lipoprotein cholesterol   See *VLDL cholesterol.*

viruses   Simple *microorganisms* that are responsible for most coughs, colds, and childhood fevers. Viruses are smaller than *bacteria* and can multiply only by invading a cell and using the cell's *DNA* to make copies of themselves.

vitamin   A chemical that is essential for normal functioning of the body.

VLDL cholesterol   Very low-density lipoprotein cholesterol. A type of *cholesterol* made by the liver and transported in the blood. A high VLDL cholesterol level increases the risk of heart disease.

W

weight-bearing exercise   Any exercise, such as jogging, brisk walking, or stair climbing, that works the large muscles of the lower body, stimulating bone growth and building *bone density.*

white blood cells   Colorless blood cells—including *lymphocytes, monocytes,* and *granulocytes*—that have a central role in the *immune system,* protecting the body from infections and cancer.

X

X chromosome   One of the two *sex chromosomes.* Females have two X chromosomes; males have one X chromosome and one *Y chromosome.*

Y

Y chromosome   One of the two *sex chromosomes.* Males have one *X chromosome* and one Y chromosome; females have two X chromosomes.

Drug Glossary

Most Frequently Prescribed Classes of Drugs

This glossary provides brief descriptions of the classes, or types, of drugs that are most often prescribed in the United States. The terms in italics indicate other drug categories that are also defined in this section of the glossary; the drugs that are underlined can be found in the Most Frequently Prescribed Drugs part of the glossary, which starts on page 1140. If you want to learn more about a particular drug you are taking, talk to your doctor or pharmacist.

A

abortifacients Cause muscular contractions of the uterus strong enough to expel its contents. Used to induce abortion.

ACE inhibitors See *angiotensin-converting enzyme inhibitors.*

alkylating agents *Anticancer drugs.* Interfere with cell division, which helps prevent cancer cells from multiplying. Used to treat cancer.

aminoglycosides *Antibiotics.* Kill bacteria. Used to treat serious bacterial infections.

amphetamines *Stimulants.* Increase activity in the central nervous system. Used to treat the sleep disorder narcolepsy and attention deficit disorders. In the past, often used to treat obesity because they suppress the appetite. Strictly regulated because they are highly addictive.

anabolic steroids *Hormone drugs.* Imitate the actions of the male sex hormone testosterone. Used to grow tissue, promote muscle growth, and repair and strengthen bone. Derived from male sex hormones (androgens). Abusing anabolic steroids carries significant health risks.

analgesics Relieve pain. Nonnarcotic analgesics treat mild to moderate pain, and most reduce fever; many are also *anti-inflammatories.* Narcotic analgesics treat severe pain. Can be addictive.

androgens *Hormone drugs.* Stimulate development of male sexual characteristics. Used to treat hypogonadism. Derived from male sex hormones (androgens).

anesthetics Interfere with sensory nerves and brain function. Used to relieve or prevent pain. Topical (applied directly to the skin) anesthetics relieve minor skin irritations. Injected local anesthetics eliminate pain sensation in a specific area before or during surgery, dental procedures, or labor and delivery. General anesthetics produce loss of consciousness before and during surgery.

angiotensin-converting enzyme inhibitors (ACE inhibitors) *Antihypertensives.* Relax narrowed blood vessels, reduce expanded blood volume, and decrease elevated blood pressure. Used to treat high blood pressure, to prevent or treat heart failure, and to treat kidney damage in people with diabetes.

angiotensin II receptor antagonists *Antihypertensives.* Prevent a protein called angiotensin II from narrowing the blood vessels and increasing blood pressure. Used to treat high blood pressure.

antiadrenergics Interfere with the functioning of the sympathetic nervous system by affecting the release or action of the neurotransmitter norepinephrine and the hormone epinephrine (also called adrenaline). Used to treat high blood pressure, angina, arrhythmias, and benign prostatic hyperplasia.

antiangina drugs Increase blood flow to the heart and reduce its workload. Used to relieve the chest pain called angina that occurs when part of the heart muscle does not receive enough oxygen.

antianxiety drugs *Psychotropics; sedatives; tranquilizers.* Used to relieve anxiety, induce sleep, or relax a person before surgery. Can be addictive.

antiarrhythmics Alter the electrical impulses that control the heartbeat or the way the heart responds to the impulses. Used to prevent, control, or correct an abnormal heartbeat. Include *beta blockers* and *calcium channel blockers.*

antibacterials *Antibiotics.* Used to treat bacterial infections.

antibiotics Used to prevent or treat bacterial infections. Some are used to treat specific infections; broad-spectrum antibiotics are used to treat a wide variety of infections. Have no effect on viruses. The entire course of antibiotic treatment must be completed to help prevent bacteria from developing resistance to the drug. Include *aminoglycosides, cephalosporins, macrolides, penicillins, quinolones, sulfa drugs,* and *tetracyclines.*

anticancer drugs Kill or prevent the growth of abnormal cells. Used to treat cancer. Include *alkylating agents* and *antimetabolites* (which interfere with cell division), *cytotoxics* (which kill or damage cells), and *interferons* and *interleukins* (which stimulate the immune system to attack cancer cells).

anticholinergics Block the effects of the chemical neurotransmitter acetylcholine on the nervous system. Used to dilate (widen) pupils and control muscle spasms and to treat asthma, incontinence, irritable bowel syndrome, and Parkinson's disease.

anticoagulants Interfere with blood clotting. Used to prevent and treat transient ischemic attacks, heart attack, and stroke. Include *antiplatelets* such as aspirin and clopidogrel.

anticonvulsants Control or eliminate abnormal electrical activity in the brain. Used to prevent or reduce the frequency or severity of seizures in epilepsy and other seizure disorders.

antidepressants *Psychotropics.* Used to prevent or treat depression. Include *monoamine oxidase inhibitors, selective serotonin reuptake inhibitors, heterocyclic antidepressants,* and *tricyclic antidepressants.*

antidiabetic drugs Stimulate the pancreas to release more insulin, which helps cells take in glucose to use for energy or to store, lowering the level of glucose in the blood. Used to treat type 2 diabetes.

antidiarrheals Absorb fluids and slow intestinal contractions. Used to relieve diarrhea. Include substances such as kaolin, chalk, or charcoal mixtures as well as drugs. Long-term use can lead to chronic constipation.

antiemetics Used to prevent or relieve nausea and vomiting. Usually taken orally as a tablet or liquid but may be given as a suppository or by injection, especially if a person is likely to vomit oral medication before it can take effect. Not recommended when the cause of vomiting is not known.

antifungals Used to treat fungal infections.

antihistamines Counteract the effects of histamine (one of the substances involved in allergic reactions and stomach acid production). Used to relieve the symptoms of hay fever and peptic ulcers. Include H_1 *(histamine) blockers* and H_2 *(histamine) blockers.*

antihypertensives Used to lower blood pressure. Include *angiotensin-converting enzyme inhibitors, angiotensin II receptor antagonists, beta blockers, calcium channel blockers,* and *diuretics.*

anti-inflammatories Reduce redness, swelling, heat, and pain. Used to treat osteoarthritis or rheumatoid arthritis. Include *analgesics, antirheumatics, corticosteroids, COX-2 inhibitors,* and *nonsteroidal anti-inflammatory drugs.*

antimetabolites *Anticancer drugs.* Interfere with cell division, which helps prevent cancer cells from multiplying.

antiparasitics   Kill parasites such as lice or pinworms and their eggs. Used to treat infestations.

antiplatelets   *Anticoagulants.* Help prevent blood clots by binding to platelets (cell fragments that enable blood to clot) and keeping them from clumping on blood vessel walls. Used to prevent or treat heart attack or stroke. Can cause excessive bleeding in some people. Include <u>aspirin</u> and <u>clopidogrel</u>.

antipsychotics   *Psychotropics; tranquilizers.* Block the actions of dopamine (a chemical messenger in the brain). Used to treat mental disorders such as schizophrenia and bipolar disorder or agitation or aggressive behavior in people with Alzheimer's disease or other forms of dementia.

antipyretics   Reduce fever. Include the *analgesics* <u>acetaminophen</u>, <u>aspirin</u>, and <u>ibuprofen</u>.

antiretrovirals   Inhibit the ability of retroviruses (such as HIV) to multiply.

antirheumatics   *Anti-inflammatories; immunosuppressants.* Used to relieve the symptoms of rheumatoid arthritis and other autoimmune disorders. Usually prescribed if treatment with *nonsteroidal anti-inflammatory drugs* has been ineffective.

antispasmodics   Prevent or relieve spasms in the smooth muscles of the bladder or the intestines. Used to treat irritable bladder disorders and irritable bowel syndrome.

antithyroid drugs   Reduce production of thyroid hormones in the thyroid gland and destroy excessive thyroid gland tissue. Used to treat an overactive thyroid gland.

antitussives   Suppress the area of the brain that controls coughing. Used in over-the-counter cough remedies to prevent coughing or to stop coughs caused by irritation that don't produce phlegm (called dry coughs).

antivirals   Interfere with a virus's chemical processes or prevent a virus from entering cells. Used to treat infections caused by viruses or to provide temporary immunity from viral infections such as influenza.

B

barbiturates   *Sedatives.* Depress brain activity. Used to relieve anxiety or induce sleep. Strictly regulated because they are highly addictive.

benzodiazepines   *Sedatives; muscle relaxants.* Depress some brain activities, reducing feelings of restlessness, slowing mental activity, and relaxing muscles. Used to relieve anxiety or to induce sleep.

beta₂ agonists   *Bronchodilators.* Relax the smooth muscles of the airways, making breathing easier. Used to treat asthma.

beta blockers   *Antiangina drugs; antiarrhythmics; antihypertensives.* Lower the oxygen needs of the heart by reducing the heart rate; also help maintain a regular heartbeat. Used to prevent migraine headaches and to treat palpitations, angina that results from exertion, high blood pressure, and tremors in people with anxiety.

beta-lactamase inhibitors   *Antibiotics.* Inhibit the bacterial enzymes called beta lactamases that can destroy *penicillins* before they can kill bacteria. Used in combination with penicillin to treat bacterial infections.

birth-control pills   See *oral contraceptives.*

bone-resorption inhibitors   Decrease rate of bone loss and increase bone growth. Used to prevent and treat osteoporosis and bone loss from some types of bone cancer. Include <u>alendronate</u>, <u>calcitonin</u>, and <u>risedronate</u>.

bronchodilators   Widen narrowed airways, increase air flow, and improve breathing. Used to treat chronic respiratory diseases such as asthma. Most often administered as aerosol sprays but in an emergency (such as a severe asthma attack) may be given by injection. Include *beta₂ agonists.*

C

calcium channel blockers   *Antiangina drugs; antiarrhythmics; antihypertensives.* Widen narrowed blood vessels, decrease blood pressure, and reduce the heart's workload by decreasing the movement of calcium through cell membranes. Used to treat high blood pressure, angina, and abnormal heart rhythms.

cardiac glycosides   *Antiarrhythmics.* Used to improve the efficiency of the heart in congestive heart failure and to treat heart rhythm disorders (arrhythmias).

cephalosporins   *Antibiotics.* Kill bacteria or prevent their growth. Used to treat a wide variety of bacterial infections or to prevent bacterial infections before, during, or after surgery.

combination drugs Contain two or more medications in a single dose.

contraceptives, oral See *oral contraceptives.*

corticosteroids *Anti-inflammatories; hormone drugs.* Imitate the actions of the natural corticosteroid hormones produced by the adrenal glands and suppress the immune system. Used to supplement or replace natural hormones in hormone therapy; to relieve inflammation associated with disorders such as Crohn's disease, ulcerative colitis, asthma, osteoarthritis, rheumatoid arthritis, eczema, and hay fever; and to prevent the body from rejecting transplanted organs or tissues.

COX-2 inhibitors *Nonsteroidal anti-inflammatory drugs.* Block the action of an enzyme (COX-2) that produces inflammation; cause less stomach irritation than other nonsteroidal anti-inflammatories. Used to treat osteoarthritis and rheumatoid arthritis and to relieve pain.

cytotoxics *Anticancer drugs.* Damage or kill abnormal cells.

D

decongestants Reduce swelling in the mucous membranes that line the nasal cavity. Used to relieve nasal congestion. Although most effective when taken as a nasal spray or nose drops, also can be taken orally as an ingredient in over-the-counter cold remedies. Large doses taken orally may increase heart rate and cause insomnia.

diuretics *Antihypertensives.* Remove excess fluid and sodium from the body and reduce tissue swelling by increasing the amount of urine produced by the kidneys. Used to treat high blood pressure and disorders of the heart, kidneys, and liver. Include thiazide diuretics (which cause a moderate increase in urine production and are appropriate for long-term use), loop diuretics (which are fast-acting and often used in emergency treatment of congestive heart failure), and potassium-sparing diuretics (which are used to help prevent potassium loss in urine).

dopamine-boosting drugs Help raise abnormally low levels of the chemical messenger dopamine in the brain by converting to dopamine in the brain. Used to treat Parkinson's disease.

dopamine-releasing drugs Increase the availability of the chemical messenger dopamine in the brain without increasing dopamine levels. Used to treat Parkinson's disease

E

emetics Induce vomiting by acting directly on the stomach lining or by stimulating the part of the brain that controls vomiting. Used to treat poisoning or drug overdose.

enteric-coated drugs Pills or tablets covered with a substance that prevents them from dissolving and releasing their contents until they reach the small intestine, where the contents are absorbed. Used to protect the stomach lining or prevent stomach acid from neutralizing the medication's intended effects.

estrogens *Hormone drugs.* Used to treat menstrual disorders and to relieve symptoms of menopause. In *oral contraceptives,* used to prevent pregnancy.

expectorants Help bring up mucus and other secretions. Used in over-the-counter cough remedies to treat coughs that produce phlegm (called productive coughs).

F

fertility drugs *Hormone drugs.* Used to treat female infertility.

fibrinolytics Increase blood levels of plasmin, a substance that dissolves fibrin (the insoluble protein that gives blood clots their form). Used to help dissolve blood clots.

fungicidals See *antifungals.*

G

generic drugs Drugs marketed under their official chemical names rather than under a patented brand name. For example, sildenafil is the generic name for Viagra.

H

H₁ (histamine) blockers *Antihistamines.* Prevent the release of histamine (a substance released during an allergic reaction). Used to treat allergic reactions.

H₂ (histamine) blockers *Antihistamines.* Prevent histamine (a substance that stimulates stomach acid production) from triggering production of stomach acid. Used to treat peptic ulcers.

hemostatics Enable blood to clot normally, reducing the risk of excessive bleeding. Used to stop bleeding in disorders such as hemophilia.

heterocyclic antidepressants *Antidepressants.* Balance neurotransmitters (chemical messengers in the brain), particularly serotonin and norepinephrine. Used to treat depression. Cause more side effects than antidepressants such as *selective serotonin reuptake inhibitors.*

hormone antagonists Block the actions of specific hormones. For example, the hormone antagonist tamoxifen, which is used to treat breast cancer, blocks the actions of estrogen on breast tissue.

hormone drugs Synthetic or natural hormones that replace the hormones that are produced naturally by the endocrine glands and released into the bloodstream. Used to treat disorders or conditions (such as diabetes or menopause) in which the body does not produce enough of a specific hormone.

hypnotics See *sleep medications.*

hypoglycemics See *antidiabetic drugs.*

I

immunostimulants Increase the efficiency of the immune system. Used to treat viral infections, some types of cancer, and immune system disorders such as AIDS.

immunosuppressants Reduce the activity of the immune system. Used to treat autoimmune diseases (in which the immune system mistakenly attacks the body's own tissues) and to help prevent rejection of a transplanted organ or tissues. Most are *anticancer drugs* or *corticosteroids.* Include *antirheumatics.*

interferons *Anticancer drugs.* Boost the body's immune response. Used to treat viral infections and some types of cancer. Prepared from blood proteins.

interleukins *Anticancer drugs.* Boost the body's immune response. Used to treat some types of cancer. Prepared from blood proteins.

K

keratolytics Soften and peel away the skin's tough outer layer (keratin). Used to treat skin conditions such as acne, calluses, dandruff, warts, and psoriasis.

L

laxatives Stimulate intestinal contractions (stimulant laxatives), increase the bulk of the contents of the colon (bulk laxatives), or lubricate the contents of the colon (stool softeners). Used to increase the frequency and ease of bowel movements. May be taken orally or as suppositories or enemas; bulk laxatives must be taken with lots of water. May be addictive. Overuse can lead to chronic constipation.

leukotriene inhibitors Block a group of chemicals (leukotrienes) that produce inflammation. Used to reduce inflammation of the airways in asthma.

lipid-lowering drugs Reduce cholesterol levels in the blood. Used to treat atherosclerosis (a condition in which fatty deposits called plaque clog the arteries and interfere with blood flow).

M

macrolides *Antibiotics.* Include azithromycin, clarithromycin, clindamycin, and erythromycin. Used to prevent or treat bacterial infections.

MAOIs See *monoamine oxidase inhibitors.*

mast cell stabilizers Prevent the release of histamine and other inflammatory substances in the body by mast cells, which are part of the immune system and play a role in allergic reactions. Used to prevent acute asthma.

mineral supplements Preparations containing chemical elements that must be present in the diet to maintain health. Doctors recommend a daily multivitamin/mineral supplement for most people. Supplements of a specific mineral may be used to treat a mineral deficiency caused by factors such as a poor diet, some disorders, and some medications. Include potassium.

miotics Constrict (narrow) the pupil of the eye. Used to treat glaucoma.

monoamine oxidase inhibitors (MAOIs) *Anti-*

depressants. Block the actions of a protein that breaks down specific neurotransmitters (chemical messengers in the brain) needed for feelings of well-being. Can interact adversely with many prescription and over-the-counter drugs and with red wine and some foods (such as aged cheese), causing life-threatening symptoms including dangerously high blood pressure.

mucolytics Make mucus in the lungs thinner, less sticky, and easier to cough up. Used to treat lung conditions in which abnormal amounts of mucus make breathing difficult.

muscle relaxants Relax skeletal muscles and relieve muscle spasms. Used to relieve low back pain and for anesthesia and artificial ventilation during surgery. Some *antianxiety drugs* and *sedatives* also are muscle relaxants.

mydriatics Dilate (widen) the pupil of the eye. Used before eye examinations and before and after eye surgery to enable the doctor to see into the back of the eye and to treat certain eye conditions.

N

narcotics See *analgesics.*

nitrates *Vasodilators.* Relax the blood vessels and improve blood flow and pressure, reducing the heart's workload. Used to prevent or treat angina, heart attack, and congestive heart failure.

nonsteroidal anti-inflammatory drugs (NSAIDs) *Anti-inflammatories; analgesics; antipyretics.* Block the production of prostaglandins (chemicals in the body that cause inflammation and help transmit pain signals to the brain). Used to relieve pain and reduce inflammation and stiffness in the joints and soft tissues, and to reduce fever in disorders such as osteoarthritis, rheumatoid arthritis, and gout. Include aspirin, celecoxib, ibuprofen, naproxen, and rofecoxib.

NSAIDs See *nonsteroidal anti-inflammatory drugs.*

O

opiates Any drug derived from or chemically similar to opium, which is an *analgesic.* Include codeine and morphine. Used to relieve moderate to severe pain.

oral contraceptives *Hormone drugs.* Block ovulation (the release of an egg from an ovary). Used to prevent pregnancy. Contain *estrogens* and *progestins*, either alone or in combination.

P

penicillins Broad-spectrum *antibiotics.* Used to treat a wide variety of bacterial infections, including tonsillitis, bronchitis, pneumonia, endocarditis, and many sexually transmitted diseases (STDs).

phosphodiesterase type 5 inhibitors Prevent the action of a chemical in the body called phosphodiesterase type 5. Used to treat erection problems. Include sildenafil, vardenafil, and tadalafil.

progestins *Hormone drugs.* Progesterone (a female sex hormone) or progesteronelike medications that have the same effects as natural progesterone. Used to treat bleeding of the uterus, endometriosis, and abnormalities in the menstrual cycle, and to prevent miscarriage. Protect the lining of the uterus from the effect of *estrogens* in hormone therapy.

prostaglandins Act like naturally occurring hormonelike prostaglandins (substances that have many functions in the body, including controlling blood pressure, stimulating muscle contractions, and triggering inflammation). Stimulate strong contractions of the uterus and relax the smooth muscle of blood vessels. Used to induce labor at full term and as *abortifacients.* Also used to treat glaucoma.

protease inhibitors Prevent T cells (a type of infection-fighting white blood cell) that have been infected with HIV from producing new copies of the virus. Used in combination with other drugs to block the replication of HIV in an infected person's blood.

proton pump inhibitors Inhibit the production of stomach acid. Used to treat conditions such as heartburn, peptic ulcers, and gastroesophageal reflux disease (GERD), in which the stomach produces too much acid.

psoralens Slow the growth and multiplication of skin cells and stimulate the production of skin pigment. Used to treat the skin conditions psoriasis and vitiligo.

psychotropics Affect the mind. Include *antianxiety drugs, antidepressants, antipsychotics,* and *sleep medications.* Used to induce sleep and to treat anxiety, depression, and other mental disorders.

Q

quinolones   Broad-spectrum *antibiotics*. Used to treat a wide variety of bacterial infections. Include ciprofloxacin.

S

salicylates   Relieve pain and reduce fever. Used to relieve swelling, stiffness, and joint pain. Include aspirin.

sedatives   Produce a calming, relaxing effect. Include *antianxiety drugs, barbiturates, benzodiazepines, sleep medications,* and *tranquilizers.* Some sedatives (such as *analgesics, antihistamines,* and *muscle relaxants*) cause sedation as a secondary effect.

selective serotonin reuptake inhibitors (SSRIs) *Antidepressants.* Increase the availability of serotonin (a chemical messenger in the brain). Used to treat depression. Have fewer side effects than other antidepressants.

sleep medications   *Psychotropics; sedatives.* Used to induce sleep. Include *antianxiety drugs* and *barbiturates.* Should be taken only for short periods and discontinued gradually under doctor's supervision. Restlessness and vivid dreams may persist for weeks after discontinuation.

SSRIs   See *selective serotonin reuptake inhibitors.*

statins   *Lipid-lowering drugs.* Inhibit an enzyme that controls the rate of cholesterol production, and stimulate the liver to remove bad low-density lipoprotein (LDL) cholesterol from the blood. Used to lower cholesterol in the blood.

stimulants   Increase central nervous system activity to promote wakefulness and enhance thought processes. Used to overcome attention deficit disorders and the sleep disorder narcolepsy. Include *amphetamines* and *xanthines.*

sulfa drugs   *Antibiotics.* Used to prevent or treat bacterial infections.

sulfonylureas   *Antidiabetic drugs.* Stimulate the pancreas to release more insulin into the bloodstream, effectively lowering blood glucose. Used to treat type 2 diabetes.

T

tetracyclines   Broad-spectrum *antibiotics.* Used to treat a wide variety of bacterial infections, including acne, bronchitis, and many sexually transmitted diseases (STDs).

thrombolytics   Used to help dissolve blood clots in the lungs. Often given intravenously (through a vein) during a heart attack to dissolve a clot that is blocking a coronary artery. May cause bleeding in some people. Include streptokinase and tissue plasminogen activator.

tranquilizers   Produce a calming effect. *Antianxiety drugs* are sometimes called minor tranquilizers; *antipsychotics* are sometimes called major tranquilizers.

tricyclic antidepressants   *Antidepressants.* Balance neurotransmitters (chemical messengers in the brain) such as serotonin, norepinephrine, and dopamine. Used to treat moderate to severe depression. Cause more side effects than antidepressants such as *selective serotonin reuptake inhibitors* and *heterocyclic antidepressants.*

V

vasodilators   *Antihypertensives.* Widen the blood vessels to reduce blood pressure. Used to treat high blood pressure and congestive heart failure.

vitamin supplements   Preparations containing the natural food constituents that are needed for normal body function. Doctors recommend a daily multivitamin/mineral supplement for most people. May be used to treat vitamin deficiencies (caused by factors such as poor diet, reduced nutrient absorption by the intestines, and some disorders) or to prevent deficiencies (such as during pregnancy and breastfeeding). Include folic acid.

X

xanthine oxidase inhibitors   Reduce the level of uric acid in the blood.

xanthines   *Bronchodilators; stimulants.* Relax the smooth muscles of the airways. Used to help relieve symptoms of asthma. Include caffeine and theophylline.

Most Frequently Prescribed Drugs

Here are brief descriptions of some of the drugs that are prescribed most often in the United States. Most of the entries include the generic name of the drug, its class (in italics), and a brief explanation of the drug's actions and its main uses. For a definition of the drug class, look in the front part of this glossary on pages 1133 to 1139. If you do not know the generic name of a drug you are taking, or if you need more information about a particular drug, talk to your doctor or pharmacist. Drugs that are underlined can be found in this part of the glossary.

A

acetaminophen   Nonnarcotic *analgesic; antipyretic.* Used to relieve mild to moderate pain and to reduce fever. Using acetaminophen regularly with alcohol can cause liver problems.

acetaminophen and codeine   *Combination drug.* Nonnarcotic *analgesic* and *antipyretic* (acetaminophen), and narcotic *analgesic* and *antitussive* (codeine). Used to relieve mild to moderate pain. Can be addictive.

acetaminophen and oxycodone   *Combination drug.* Nonnarcotic *analgesic* and *antipyretic* (acetaminophen), and narcotic *analgesic* (oxycodone). Used to relieve moderate to moderately severe pain. Highly addictive.

acyclovir   *Antiviral.* Used to treat herpesvirus and cytomegalovirus infections.

albuterol   *Bronchodilator; beta$_2$ agonist.* Relaxes the muscles in the bronchioles (the airways in the lungs) to ease breathing. Used to treat asthma, chronic bronchitis, and emphysema.

alendronate   *Bone-resorption inhibitor.* Builds healthy bone and helps restore lost bone. Used to prevent or treat osteoporosis.

allopurinol   *Xanthine oxidase inhibitor.* Reduces the level of uric acid in the blood. Used to prevent attacks of gout and kidney stones.

alprazolam   *Antianxiety drug.* Used to treat anxiety, panic disorders, and phobias.

amitriptyline   *Tricyclic antidepressant.* Used primarily to treat depression that is accompanied by anxiety or sleep disturbances.

amlodipine   *Antiangina drug; antihypertensive; calcium channel blocker.* Relaxes the blood vessels, decreases blood pressure, increases the supply of blood and oxygen to the heart, and reduces the heart's workload. Used to treat angina and high blood pressure.

amlodipine and benazepril   *Combination drug. Antiangina drug, antihypertensive,* and *calcium channel blocker* (amlodipine), and *angiotensin-converting enzyme inhibitor* (benazepril). Relaxes the blood vessels, decreases blood pressure, increases the supply of blood and oxygen to the heart, and reduces the heart's workload. Used to treat high blood pressure and congestive heart failure.

amoxicillin   Penicillinlike *antibiotic.* Used to treat bacterial infections of the ear, skin, respiratory tract, and urinary tract.

amoxicillin and clavulanate   *Combination drug.* Penicillinlike *antibiotic* (amoxicillin), and *beta-lactamase inhibitor* (clavulanate). Clavulanate protects the antibiotic amoxicillin from the enzyme beta lactamase, which could destroy the antibiotic before it can kill the bacteria. Used to treat bacterial infections of the ear, skin, respiratory tract, and urinary tract.

aspirin   *Nonsteroidal anti-inflammatory drug; analgesic; antipyretic; anticoagulant; antiplatelet; salicylate.* Used to relieve inflammation, reduce fever, relieve mild to moderate pain, and help prevent heart attack and stroke. Should not be used by children or adolescents because it is associated with a life-threatening disorder called Reye's syndrome.

atenolol   *Beta blocker.* Used to treat angina, high blood pressure, and some types of arrhythmias and often is used after a heart attack.

atorvastatin   *Lipid-lowering drug; statin.* Blocks the production of cholesterol in the liver, lowering the level of harmful low-density lipoprotein (LDL) cholesterol and other fatty substances in the blood. Used to prevent angina, heart disease, heart attack, and stroke.

azithromycin   *Macrolide; antibiotic.* Used to treat bacterial infections throughout the body but primarily in the respiratory tract and on the skin.

B

benazepril   *Angiotensin-converting enzyme inhibitor.* Relaxes the blood vessels, decreases blood volume, lowers blood pressure, and reduces the heart's workload. Used to treat high blood pressure and congestive heart failure.

benzonatate   *Antitussive.* Used to treat a dry cough.

bisoprolol   *Beta blocker.* Relaxes the blood vessels, reducing the heart's workload. Used to treat high blood pressure.

bupropion   *Antidepressant.* Used to treat depression and to help people stop smoking.

butalbital, acetaminophen, and caffeine   *Combination drug. Sleep medication* (butalbital), nonnarcotic *analgesic* and *antipyretic* (acetaminophen), and *stimulant* and *xanthine* (caffeine). Used to relieve tension headaches. Can be addictive.

C

calcitonin   *Hormone drug; bone-resorption inhibitor.* Reduces the rate of calcium loss from bones. Used to treat Paget's disease of the bone and hypercalcemia (too much calcium in the blood) and to help prevent bone loss in people with osteoporosis.

captopril   *Angiotensin-converting enzyme inhibitor.* Used to treat high blood pressure, congestive heart failure, and kidney disease that results from diabetes.

carisoprodol   *Muscle relaxant.* Relaxes muscles and relieves pain and discomfort caused by strains, sprains, and other muscle injuries.

cefprozil   *Antibiotic.* Used to treat bacterial infections of the ear, skin, and respiratory tract.

cefuroxime   *Antibiotic.* Used to treat bacterial infections of the ear, skin, respiratory tract, and urinary tract.

celecoxib   *Nonsteroidal anti-inflammatory drug; COX-2 inhibitor.* Used to relieve pain, tenderness, and stiffness caused by osteoarthritis.

cephalexin   *Antibiotic.* Used to treat bacterial infections of the skin, bones, respiratory tract, urinary tract, digestive system, and middle ear.

cerivastatin   *Lipid-lowering drug; statin.* Blocks the production of cholesterol in the liver, lowering the level of bad low-density lipoprotein (LDL) cholesterol and other fatty substances in the blood. Used to prevent angina, heart disease, heart attack, and stroke.

cetirizine   *Antihistamine.* Used to relieve symptoms of hay fever and other seasonal allergies and to treat the itching and hives that result from skin conditions such as eczema and dermatitis.

cimetidine   *Antihistamine; H_2 (histamine) blocker.* Decreases the amount of acid produced by the stomach. Used to treat heartburn, indigestion, and peptic ulcers.

ciprofloxacin   *Antibiotic.* Used to treat bacterial infections of the skin, bones, joints, respiratory tract, abdomen, and urinary tract.

citalopram   *Selective serotonin reuptake inhibitor.* Increases the level and activity of serotonin (a chemical messenger in the brain that is involved in regulating mood). Used to treat depression.

clarithromycin   *Macrolide; antibiotic.* Used to treat bacterial infections throughout the body; often used to treat peptic ulcers caused by the bacterium Helicobacter pylori.

clindamycin   *Antibiotic.* Used to treat serious bacterial infections that have not responded to treatment with other antibiotics or that are resistant to treatment with more commonly used antibiotics such as *penicillins*.

clomiphene   *Fertility drug.* Stimulates ovulation in women with ovulation problems. May produce multiple fetuses.

clonazepam   *Benzodiazepine; tranquilizer.* Used to treat epilepsy and panic disorders.

clonidine   *Antihypertensive.* Controls nerve impulses from the brain to the heart and blood vessels. Relaxes the blood vessels, decreases heart rate, and lowers blood pressure. Used to treat high blood pressure and withdrawal from narcotics.

clopidogrel   *Antiplatelet.* Prevents blood clot formation. Used to relieve circulation problems and reduce the risk of stroke or heart attack.

clotrimazole and betamethasone   *Combination drug. Antifungal* (clotrimazole), and *corticosteroid* (betamethasone). Kills and prevents the growth of fungi (clotrimazole) and relieves symptoms of inflammation such as redness, swelling, and itching (betamethasone). Used to treat fungal infections such as athlete's foot, jock itch, and ringworm.

conjugated estrogens and medroxyprogesterone *Combination drug. Hormone drug.* Conjugated estrogens are combined natural hormones and have properties similar to those of estradiol. Medroxyprogesterone contains the female hormone progesterone, which balances the effects of estrogen on the lining of the uterus. Conjugated estrogens are used to relieve the symptoms of menopause, while medroxyprogesterone reduces the risk of estrogen-related endometrial cancer.

cyclobenzaprine *Muscle relaxant.* Used to treat muscle spasms, stiffness, and pain that result from muscle injuries such as strains and sprains.

D

desogestrel and ethinyl estradiol *Combination drug. Oral contraceptive.* Prevents ovulation (the release of an egg from an ovary), preventing pregnancy.

diazepam *Benzodiazepine; tranquilizer.* Used to treat short-term symptoms of anxiety and anxiety disorders and seizure disorders such as epilepsy, and to relieve muscle spasms. Can be addictive.

diclofenac *Nonsteroidal anti-inflammatory drug; analgesic; antipyretic.* Used to relieve the swelling, stiffness, and joint pain caused by inflammatory disorders such as osteoarthritis and rheumatoid arthritis.

digoxin *Cardiac glycoside.* Increases the strength and efficiency of the heart and improves circulation. Used to treat congestive heart failure and irregular heart rhythms; usually prescribed with a *diuretic* to relieve swelling and an *angiotensin-converting enzyme inhibitor* to further improve circulation.

diltiazem *Calcium channel blocker.* Widens blood vessels to improve blood flow, decreases blood pressure, slows the heart rate, and reduces the heart's workload. Used to treat angina and high blood pressure.

divalproex *Anticonvulsant.* Used to treat seizure disorders such as epilepsy and the manic phase of bipolar disorder, and to help prevent migraine headaches.

doxazosin *Antiadrenergic; antihypertensive.* Relaxes the blood vessels (improving blood flow throughout the body and reducing blood pressure) and relaxes the muscles of the bladder and the prostate gland. Used to treat high blood pressure and to relieve symptoms of benign prostatic hyperplasia. The first dose can cause fainting in some people.

doxepin *Tricyclic antidepressant.* Elevates mood, relieves tension, and increases energy. Used to treat depression and anxiety.

doxycycline *Antibiotic.* Used to treat a wide variety of bacterial infections, including urinary tract infections, some tickborne and fleaborne infections, and severe acne.

E

enalapril *Angiotensin-converting enzyme inhibitor.* Used to treat high blood pressure and congestive heart failure.

erythromycin *Macrolide; antibiotic.* Used to treat a wide variety of infections—including acne, respiratory tract infections, urinary tract infections, pelvic inflammatory disease, and sexually transmitted diseases (STDs) such as gonorrhea and syphilis—and to prevent heart infections in people who are allergic to *penicillins* and who have congenital heart disease or rheumatic heart disease.

esomeprazole *Proton pump inhibitor.* Reduces the amount of acid produced by the stomach. Used to treat duodenal ulcers and gastroesophageal reflux disease (GERD) and to treat ulcers resulting from infection with the bacterium Helicobacter pylori.

estradiol *Hormone drug.* A natural *estrogen* used to relieve symptoms of menopause—including hot flashes, abnormal bleeding, and vaginal dryness and irritation—and to treat some types of breast cancer and prostate cancer.

ethinyl estradiol and norethindrone *Combination drug. Oral contraceptive. Estrogen* (ethinyl estradiol), and *progestin* (norethindrone). Prevents ovulation (the release of an egg from an ovary), preventing pregnancy.

F

famotidine   *Antihistamine; H₂ (histamine) blocker.* Reduces the amount of acid produced by the stomach. Used to treat gastroesophageal reflux disease (GERD) and peptic ulcers and to relieve heartburn and indigestion.

felodipine   *Calcium channel blocker; vasodilator.* Relaxes the blood vessels, improving blood flow and reducing blood pressure. Used to treat high blood pressure.

fenofibrate   *Lipid-lowering drug.* Lowers blood levels of cholesterol and triglycerides. Used to help prevent angina, heart disease, heart attack, and stroke.

fexofenadine   *Antihistamine; H₁ (histamine) blocker.* Used to relieve symptoms of hay fever such as sneezing and itchy, watery eyes. Causes less drowsiness than other antihistamines.

fexofenadine and pseudoephedrine   *Combination drug. Antihistamine and H₁ (histamine) blocker* (fexofenadine), and *decongestant* (pseudoephedrine). Used to relieve symptoms of hay fever (such as sneezing and itchy, watery eyes) and nasal congestion.

fluconazole   *Antifungal.* Used to treat yeast infections in the throat, the vagina, and other parts of the body.

fluoxetine   *Antidepressant; selective serotonin reuptake inhibitor.* Adjusts the balance of serotonin (a chemical messenger) in the brain. Used to treat depression, obsessive-compulsive disorder, and eating disorders such as obesity and bulimia nervosa.

fluticasone   *Corticosteroid.* Relieves inflammation of the nasal passages and eases breathing. Used to prevent or treat the symptoms of hay fever or other nasal allergies such as itchy, watery eyes and nasal congestion.

fluticasone and salmeterol   *Combination drug. Corticosteroid* (fluticasone), and long-acting *beta₂ agonist* (salmeterol). Reduces swelling in the airways (fluticasone) and relaxes and widens the airways (salmeterol). Used to treat wheezing, shortness of breath, and difficulty breathing caused by asthma and other chronic lung diseases such as chronic bronchitis and emphysema.

fluvastatin   *Lipid-lowering drug; statin.* Blocks cholesterol production in the liver, lowering the level of bad low-density lipoprotein (LDL) cholesterol and other fatty substances in the blood. Used to prevent angina, heart disease, heart attack, and stroke.

folic acid (folate)   B *vitamin supplement.* Repairs cells and helps with cell function, tissue growth, red blood cell production, and the synthesis of DNA. Found in fruits, dried beans and peas, liver, and dark green, leafy vegetables. Taking 400 micrograms of folic acid daily during the first 3 months of pregnancy prevents birth defects of the brain and spine.

fosinopril   *Angiotensin-converting enzyme inhibitor.* Relaxes the blood vessels, improving blood flow, reducing blood pressure, and enabling the heart to pump blood more efficiently. Used to treat high blood pressure and heart failure.

furosemide   Loop *diuretic.* Acts directly on the kidneys to increase the quantity of urine and eliminate excess fluid from the body. Used to treat high blood pressure and other conditions (including congestive heart failure and kidney disease) that can cause fluid to accumulate in the body.

G

gabapentin   *Anticonvulsant.* Used to help control some types of seizures that occur in epilepsy and to help relieve persistent or recurring pain associated with a herpesvirus infection (a condition called postherpetic neuralgia).

gatifloxacin   *Antibiotic.* Used to treat bacterial infections of the sinuses, respiratory tract, and urinary tract, and some sexually transmitted diseases (STDs).

gemfibrozil   *Lipid-lowering drug.* Reduces the levels of triglycerides (fatty substances in the blood). Used to prevent pancreatitis (inflammation of the pancreas) and to treat heart disease.

glimepiride   *Antidiabetic drug.* Stimulates the pancreas to release more insulin, thereby reducing the blood glucose level. Used to treat type 2 diabetes.

glipizide   *Antidiabetic drug.* Stimulates the pancreas to release more insulin, thereby reducing the blood glucose level. Used to treat type 2 diabetes.

glyburide *Antidiabetic drug.* Stimulates the pancreas to release more insulin, thereby reducing the blood glucose level. Used to treat type 2 diabetes.

glyburide and metformin *Combination drug. Antidiabetic drug.* Stimulates the pancreas to release more insulin (glyburide), and prevents the liver from producing glucose and helps the body use insulin more efficiently (metformin). Used to treat type 2 diabetes.

H

hydrochlorothiazide Thiazide *diuretic.* Stimulates the kidneys to increase urine production, eliminating excess fluid and sodium from the body and lowering blood pressure. Used to treat high blood pressure and other conditions that cause fluid to accumulate in the body, such as congestive heart failure and kidney disease.

hydrocodone and ibuprofen *Combination drug.* Narcotic *analgesic* (hydrocodone), and *nonsteroidal anti-inflammatory drug, analgesic,* and *antipyretic* (ibuprofen). Acts in the central nervous system to relieve pain (hydrocodone) and swelling and inflammation (ibuprofen). Used to treat acute pain for short periods only (because hydrocodone is highly addictive).

hydroxyzine *Antihistamine; H_1 (histamine) blocker; sedative.* Used to relieve itching caused by allergic skin reactions, to induce sleep, and to treat anxiety and nausea.

hyoscyamine *Antispasmodic.* Used to relieve painful cramps and muscle contractions caused by some disorders of the urinary tract or intestinal tract, to relieve the pain of kidney stones or gallstones, or to dry up excess secretions before anesthesia is administered.

I

ibuprofen *Nonsteroidal anti-inflammatory drug; analgesic; antipyretic.* Relieves inflammation and mild to moderate pain, and reduces fever. Used to treat osteoarthritis and rheumatoid arthritis.

indomethacin *Nonsteroidal anti-inflammatory drug; analgesic; antipyretic.* Relieves inflammation, swelling, stiffness, and pain. Used to treat osteoarthritis, rheumatoid arthritis, ankylosing

spondylitis, bursitis, tendinitis, gout, and patent ductus arteriosus.

insulin *Hormone drug.* Chemically identical to the natural insulin produced by the pancreas in the body. Used to regulate blood glucose levels in people with type 1 diabetes.

ipratropium Aerosol *bronchodilator; anticholinergic.* Relaxes and opens the airways, improving breathing. Used to prevent wheezing, shortness of breath, and difficulty breathing caused by chronic obstructive pulmonary diseases such as asthma, chronic bronchitis, and emphysema.

ipratropium and albuterol *Combination drug.* Aerosol *bronchodilator* and *anticholinergic* (ipratropium), and *bronchodilator* (albuterol). Relaxes and opens the airways, improving breathing. Used to prevent wheezing, shortness of breath, and difficulty breathing caused by chronic obstructive pulmonary diseases such as asthma, chronic bronchitis, and emphysema.

irbesartan *Angiotensin II receptor antagonist.* Widens narrowed blood vessels, improves blood flow, reduces blood volume, decreases blood pressure, and reduces the heart's workload. Used to treat high blood pressure.

isosorbide dinitrate *Nitrate.* Used to prevent or relieve angina and to treat congestive heart failure. Should not be taken with sildenafil (combining sildenafil with a nitrate drug can lower blood pressure and cause dizziness, light-headedness, fainting, and, in some cases, death).

isosorbide mononitrate *Nitrate.* Used to prevent angina but cannot relieve an angina attack. Should not be taken with sildenafil (combining sildenafil with a nitrate drug can lower blood pressure and cause dizziness, light-headedness, fainting, and, in some cases, death).

L

lansoprazole *Proton pump inhibitor.* Reduces the amount of acid produced by the stomach. Used to treat duodenal ulcers, gastroesophageal reflux disease (GERD), and ulcers resulting from infection with the bacterium Helicobacter pylori.

latanoprost *Prostaglandin.* Increases the outflow of fluid from the eye, which lowers pressure inside the eyeball. Used to treat eye disorders (including glaucoma and ocular hypertension) in which increased pressure can lead to a gradual loss of vision.

levofloxacin *Antibiotic.* Helps fight bacterial infections in many different parts of the body. Used to treat some types of sinus infections, pneumonia, chronic bronchitis, bladder infections, acute kidney infections, bacterial eye infections, and some skin infections.

levonorgestrel and ethinyl estradiol *Combination drug. Oral contraceptive.* A combination of *estrogens* and *progestins* that blocks ovulation (the release of an egg from an ovary), preventing pregnancy.

levothyroxine Thyroid *hormone drug.* Used to treat hypothyroidism, congenital hypothyroidism, and goiter.

lisinopril *Angiotensin-converting enzyme inhibitor.* Used to treat high blood pressure and congestive heart failure, and to improve a person's chances of survival when taken within 24 hours of a heart attack.

lisinopril and hydrochlorothiazide *Combination drug. Angiotensin-converting enzyme inhibitor* (lisinopril), and *diuretic* (hydrochlorothiazide). Improves blood flow, reduces blood volume, decreases blood pressure, and reduces the heart's workload. Used to treat high blood pressure and edema (swelling) caused by a variety of conditions, including heart disease.

loratadine *Antihistamine; H₁ (histamine) blocker.* Used to relieve hay fever and allergy symptoms including hives, sneezing, runny nose, and red, itchy, watery eyes. May cause less drowsiness than other antihistamines.

loratadine and pseudoephedrine *Combination drug. Antihistamine and H₁ (histamine) blocker* (loratadine), and *decongestant* (pseudoephedrine). Used to relieve symptoms of colds and hay fever such as sneezing, nasal congestion, and itchy, watery eyes.

lorazepam *Antianxiety drug; benzodiazepine.* Used for short-term relief of anxiety symptoms and to treat insomnia, seizures, and nausea. May be addictive.

losartan *Angiotensin II receptor antagonist.* Widens narrowed blood vessels, improves blood flow, reduces blood volume, decreases blood pressure, and reduces the heart's workload. Used to treat high blood pressure.

losartan and hydrochlorothiazide *Combination drug. Angiotensin II receptor antagonist* (losartan), and *diuretic* (hydrochlorothiazide). Widens narrowed blood vessels, improves blood flow, reduces blood volume, decreases blood pressure, reduces the heart's workload, and helps eliminate excess water and sodium from the body. Used to treat high blood pressure.

M

meclizine *Antihistamine; antiemetic; H₁ (histamine) blocker.* Used to treat nausea and vomiting caused by vertigo or motion sickness.

medroxyprogesterone *Hormone drug.* Used to treat menstrual disorders, some types of kidney cancer, and endometrial cancer.

medroxyprogesterone and ethinyl estradiol *Oral contraceptive.* Prevents ovulation (the release of an egg from an ovary), preventing pregnancy.

metaxalone *Muscle relaxant.* Used to relieve the pain and discomfort of strains, sprains, and other muscle injuries.

metformin *Antidiabetic drug.* Slows the absorption of glucose in the small intestine, prevents the liver from converting stored glucose into blood glucose, and helps the body use insulin more efficiently. Used to treat type 2 diabetes.

methocarbamol *Muscle relaxant.* Used to relax muscles and relieve discomfort and pain caused by strains, sprains, and other muscle injuries and, in an injection, to treat tetanus.

methylphenidate *Amphetamine;* central nervous system *stimulant.* Alters the levels of specific chemicals in the brain. Used to treat attention deficit disorders and the sleep disorder narcolepsy.

methylprednisolone *Corticosteroid; hormone drug; anti-inflammatory; immunosuppressant.* Similar to a natural hormone produced by the adrenal glands. Used to relieve inflammation and to treat asthma, some types of arthritis, severe allergies, skin disorders, kidney disorders, thyroid gland disorders, and some types of cancer. Used as hormone therapy when the body does not produce enough of the natural hormone.

metoclopramide *Antiemetic.* Stimulates emptying of the stomach into the small intestine. Used to treat nausea and vomiting associated with the use of anticancer drugs.

metoprolol *Beta blocker.* Used primarily to treat angina and high blood pressure and to prevent migraine headaches.

metronidazole *Antibacterial; antibiotic.* Used to treat a wide variety of bacterial infections, including some types of urinary tract infections in both men and women, and infections of the skin, bones, joints, abdomen, lungs, and brain.

minocycline *Tetracycline; antibiotic.* Used to treat a variety of bacterial infections, including acne, pneumonia, some infections of the urinary system, and some sexually transmitted diseases (STDs).

mirtazapine *Heterocyclic antidepressant.* Adjusts the balance of neurotransmitters (chemical messengers) in the brain, particularly serotonin and norepinephrine. Used to treat depression.

mometasone *Corticosteroid.* Used to relieve itching and inflammation caused by allergic skin reactions and a variety of skin conditions.

montelukast *Leukotriene inhibitor.* Blocks the actions of substances that cause inflammation, fluid retention, mucus secretion, and constriction (narrowing) of the lungs. Used for long-term treatment of asthma to prevent symptoms and reduce the number of acute asthma attacks; cannot be used to relieve an asthma attack.

mupirocin *Antibiotic.* Used to treat impetigo and staphylococcal infections inside the nose that have become resistant to treatment with the antibiotic methicillin.

N

nabumetone *Nonsteroidal anti-inflammatory drug; analgesic; antipyretic.* Relieves inflammation, swelling, stiffness, and joint pain. Used to treat osteoarthritis and rheumatoid arthritis.

naproxen *Nonsteroidal anti-inflammatory drug; analgesic; antipyretic.* Relieves inflammation, swelling, stiffness, and pain. Used to treat osteoarthritis, rheumatoid arthritis, juvenile rheumatoid arthritis, ankylosing spondylitis, bursitis, tendinitis, gout, and menstrual cramps.

nefazodone *Heterocyclic antidepressant.* Increases the amounts of specific chemicals in the brain. Used to treat severe depression.

nifedipine *Calcium channel blocker.* Widens narrowed blood vessels, decreases blood pressure, increases the supply of blood and oxygen to the heart muscle, and reduces the heart's workload. Used to prevent angina and to treat high blood pressure.

nitrofurantoin *Antibacterial.* Used to prevent or treat urinary tract infections.

nitroglycerin *Nitrate.* Relaxes the veins, reducing blood return to the heart and the heart's workload. Used to prevent and treat angina. Should not be taken with ergot alkaloids (which interfere with its effectiveness) or sildenafil (which can cause low blood pressure, dizziness, light-headedness, fainting, and, in some cases, death).

norgestimate and ethinyl estradiol *Combination drug. Oral contraceptive.* Prevents ovulation (the release of an egg from an ovary), preventing pregnancy.

norgestrel and ethinyl estradiol *Combination drug. Oral contraceptive.* Prevents ovulation (the release of an egg from an ovary), preventing pregnancy.

nortriptyline *Tricyclic antidepressant.* Used to relieve the symptoms of depression and to treat attention deficit disorders and bed-wetting.

nystatin *Antifungal.* Used to treat yeast infections of the skin, mouth, vagina, and intestinal tract.

O

olanzapine *Antipsychotic.* Decreases unusually high levels of some brain activities, relieving symptoms such as hallucinations, delusions, and hostility. Used to treat severe mental disorders such as schizophrenia or mania.

omeprazole *Proton pump inhibitor.* Reduces the amount of acid produced by the stomach. Used to treat duodenal ulcers, gastroesophageal reflux disease (GERD), and peptic ulcers resulting from infection with the bacterium Helicobacter pylori.

oxycodone Narcotic *analgesic.* Used to relieve moderate to severe pain. Can be addictive.

P

pantoprazole   *Proton pump inhibitor.* Reduces the amount of acid produced by the stomach. Used to treat duodenal ulcers, gastroesophageal reflux disease (GERD), and ulcers resulting from infection with the bacterium Helicobacter pylori.

paroxetine   *Selective serotonin reuptake inhibitor.* Increases the level and activity of serotonin (a chemical messenger in the brain involved in regulating mood). Used to treat depression, obsessive-compulsive disorder, panic disorder, social anxiety disorder, and posttraumatic stress disorder.

penicillin V potassium   *Antibiotic.* Used to treat pneumonia, scarlet fever, and bacterial infections of the ear, skin, and throat, and to prevent recurrent rheumatic fever and muscle spasms.

phenazopyridine   *Analgesic.* Used for short-term relief of pain, burning, and irritation in the urinary tract caused by infection, injury, catheter placement, or surgery. Also used to relieve an urgent or frequent need to urinate.

phenobarbital   *Barbiturate; sleep medication.* Used to treat anxiety and some types of epilepsy and to induce sleep.

phenytoin   *Anticonvulsant.* Used to control grand mal seizures caused by epilepsy and to prevent or control seizures that occur during or after surgery on the brain or spinal cord.

pioglitazone   *Antidiabetic drug.* Increases the body's sensitivity to insulin. Used to treat type 2 diabetes.

potassium   *Mineral supplement.* Used to maintain fluid electrolyte balance and normal heart rhythms in people who have a low potassium level because of disease or treatment with some medications (including loop and thiazide *diuretics*).

pravastatin   *Lipid-lowering drug; statin.* Blocks the production of cholesterol in the liver, lowering the level of harmful low-density lipoprotein (LDL) cholesterol and other fatty substances in the blood. Used to prevent angina, heart disease, heart attack, and stroke.

prazepam   *Antianxiety drug; benzodiazepine.* Used to relieve the symptoms of anxiety and to treat irritable bowel syndrome.

prednisone   *Anti-inflammatory; corticosteroid; hormone drug; immunosuppressant.* Used to treat inflammatory disorders such as lupus, rheumatoid arthritis, and multiple sclerosis, and flare-ups of asthma or emphysema.

promethazine   *Antihistamine; H$_1$ (histamine) blocker.* Used to relieve symptoms of hay fever or other allergies (such as sneezing, itchy skin, and itchy, watery eyes), to relieve anxiety before and after surgery, and to prevent and treat motion sickness and nausea and vomiting.

promethazine and codeine   *Combination drug. Antihistamine* (promethazine), and narcotic *analgesic* and *antitussive* (codeine). Used to relieve the symptoms of hay fever and other allergies. Can be addictive.

propoxyphene   Mild narcotic *analgesic.* Used to relieve mild to moderate pain and to treat withdrawal from narcotics. Can be addictive.

propoxyphene and acetaminophen   *Combination drug.* Mild narcotic *analgesic* (propoxyphene), and nonnarcotic *analgesic* and *antipyretic* (acetaminophen). Used to relieve mild to moderate pain and to reduce fever. Can be addictive.

propranolol   *Beta blocker.* Decreases the heart's workload, decreases blood pressure, and helps regulate heartbeat. Used to treat angina, heart attack, high blood pressure, irregular heartbeat, tremors, and some phobias. Also used to prevent migraine headaches.

Q

quinapril   *Angiotensin-converting enzyme inhibitor.* Used to treat high blood pressure and congestive heart failure.

R

rabeprazole   *Proton pump inhibitor.* Reduces the amount of acid produced by the stomach. Used to treat duodenal ulcers, gastroesophageal reflux disease (GERD), and ulcers resulting from infection with the bacterium Helicobacter pylori.

raloxifene   *Hormone drug.* Works like the female sex hormone estrogen. Stops bone loss and bone fractures and may increase bone density. Used to help prevent and treat osteoporosis (thinning of bone) in women who are past menopause.

ramipril *Angiotensin-converting enzyme inhibitor.* Used to treat high blood pressure and congestive heart failure.

ranitidine *Antihistamine; H₂ (histamine) blocker.* Reduces the amount of acid produced by the stomach. Used to treat gastroesophageal reflux disease (GERD) and peptic ulcers and to relieve heartburn and indigestion.

risedronate *Bone-resorption inhibitor.* Builds healthy bone and helps restore lost bone. Used to prevent or treat osteoporosis.

risperidone *Antipsychotic.* Decreases unusually high levels of some brain activities, relieving symptoms such as hallucinations, delusions, and hostility. Used to treat severe mental disorders such as schizophrenia.

rofecoxib *Nonsteroidal anti-inflammatory drug; COX-2 inhibitor.* Relieves symptoms such as inflammation, swelling, stiffness, and joint pain. Used to treat osteoarthritis and rheumatoid arthritis and to relieve headaches, menstrual pain, and pain after surgery.

rosiglitazone *Antidiabetic drug.* Increases the body's sensitivity to insulin. Used to treat type 2 diabetes.

S

sertraline *Selective serotonin reuptake inhibitor.* Increases the levels and activity of serotonin (a chemical messenger in the brain involved in regulating mood). Used to treat depression, panic disorder, posttraumatic stress disorder, premenstrual syndrome, and obsessive-compulsive disorder.

sildenafil *Phosphodiesterase type 5 inhibitor.* Widens the blood vessels that supply blood to the penis. Helps maintain an erection produced by sexual stimulation. Should not be used with *nitrates* (combining sildenafil with a nitrate drug can cause low blood pressure and dizziness, light-headedness, fainting, and, in some cases, death).

simvastatin *Lipid-lowering drug; statin.* Blocks the production of cholesterol in the liver, lowering the level of bad low-density lipoprotein (LDL) cholesterol and other fatty substances in the blood. Used to prevent angina, heart disease, heart attack, and stroke.

spironolactone Potassium-sparing *diuretic.* Used to treat high blood pressure and overproduction of the hormone aldosterone and to relieve fluid retention resulting from congestive heart failure, heart disease, cirrhosis of the liver, and nephrotic syndrome.

sumatriptan Hormonelike drug that acts like the chemical messenger serotonin in the brain. Relieves pain, nausea, vomiting, and sensitivity to light and sound. Used to treat symptoms of migraine headaches and cluster headaches.

T

tamoxifen *Hormone antagonist.* Blocks the action of estrogen on breast tissue. Used to treat breast cancer and to prevent breast cancer in women who are at high risk of breast cancer.

tamsulosin *Antiadrenergic.* Relaxes the muscles of the prostate and the opening of the bladder, easing the flow of urine from the bladder and through the urethra. Used to treat an enlarged prostate gland.

temazepam *Benzodiazepine; antianxiety drug.* Reduces feelings of restlessness, slows mental activity, and relaxes the muscles. Used to relieve insomnia.

terazosin *Antiadrenergic; antihypertensive.* Relaxes the blood vessels (reducing blood pressure) and relaxes the muscles of the prostate and the opening of the bladder (easing the flow of urine from the bladder and through the urethra). Used to treat high blood pressure and an enlarged prostate gland.

tetracycline Broad-spectrum *antibiotic.* Used to treat a wide variety of bacterial infections, including severe acne, conjunctivitis, tickborne diseases (such as Lyme disease), respiratory tract infections such as pneumonia, urinary tract infections, sexually transmitted diseases (STDs) such as gonorrhea, and ulcers resulting from infection with the bacterium Helicobacter pylori.

theophylline *Bronchodilator; xanthine.* Widens the airways in the lungs, increasing air flow and making breathing easier. Used to prevent or relieve the symptoms of asthma, chronic bronchitis, and emphysema, and to treat neonatal apnea.

tobramycin   *Antibacterial.* Used to treat bacterial infections of the eye and bacterial infections in people with cystic fibrosis.

tolterodine   *Antispasmodic.* Prevents contractions of the bladder. Used to treat symptoms of bladder disorders such as the frequent need to urinate or the inability to control urination.

tramadol   Nonnarcotic *analgesic.* Relieves moderate to moderately severe pain. Used to treat pain after surgery, chronic joint pain, or pain caused by cancer. May be addictive.

trazodone   *Heterocyclic antidepressant.* Used to treat anxiety and depression.

triamcinolone   *Anti-inflammatory; corticosteroid; hormone drug; immunosuppressant.* Used for long-term treatment of asthma to reduce the frequency and severity of asthma attacks, to relieve the symptoms of hay fever, and to treat nasal polyps.

triamterene   Potassium-sparing *diuretic.* Causes the kidneys to eliminate excess water and sodium from the body, reducing blood pressure and easing the heart's workload. Used to treat high blood pressure and heart disease.

triamterene and hydrochlorothiazide   *Combination drug. Diuretic.* Stimulates the kidneys to increase urine production, eliminating excess water and sodium from the body and easing the heart's workload. Used to relieve fluid retention caused by high blood pressure, congestive heart failure, or heart disease.

trimethoprim and sulfamethoxazole   *Combination drug. Antibacterial.* Used to prevent or treat severe middle ear infections, some chronic urinary tract infections, chronic or recurring bronchitis, intestinal infections (such as traveler's diarrhea), and Pneumocystis carinii pneumonia (a severe form of pneumonia that mainly affects people who have AIDS).

V

valacyclovir   *Antiviral drug.* Relieves pain and itching caused by viral infections, helps viral sores heal, and prevents new viral sores from forming. Used to treat herpes zoster (shingles) and genital herpes infections, but does not cure herpes infections.

valsartan   *Angiotensin II receptor antagonist.* Widens narrowed blood vessels, improves blood flow, reduces blood volume, decreases blood pressure, and reduces the heart's workload. Used to treat high blood pressure.

valsartan and hydrochlorothiazide   *Combination drug. Angiotensin II receptor antagonist* (valsartan), and *diuretic* (hydrochlorothiazide). Widens narrowed blood vessels, improves blood flow, reduces blood volume, decreases blood pressure, reduces the heart's workload, and helps eliminate excess water and sodium from the body. Used to treat high blood pressure.

venlafaxine   *Heterocyclic antidepressant.* Used to treat depression and generalized anxiety disorder.

verapamil   *Calcium channel blocker.* Used to treat angina, irregular heartbeat, and high blood pressure and to prevent migraine headaches.

W

warfarin   *Anticoagulant.* Prevents blood clots. Used after heart valve replacement surgery or after a heart attack to reduce the risk of clot formation and the risk of having a stroke or another heart attack.

Z

zolpidem   *Sleep medication.* Helps people fall asleep faster and sleep through the night. Used for short-term treatment of insomnia. May be addictive.

Credits

Index